Clinical Techniques

American Academy of Orthopaedic Surgeons

Athletic Training
and Sports Medicine

Chad Starkey, PhD, ATC
Glen Johnson, MD
Editors

JONES AND BARTLETT PUBLISHERS
Sudbury, Massachusetts
BOSTON   TORONTO   LONDON   SINGAPORE

Jones and Bartlett Publishers

World Headquarters
Jones and Bartlett Publishers
40 Tall Pine Drive, Sudbury, MA 01776
978-443-5000
info@jbpub.com

Jones and Bartlett Publishers Canada
2406 Nikanna Road
Mississauga, ON L5C 2W6
Canada

Jones and Bartlett Publishers International
Barb House, Barb Mews
London W6 7PA
United Kingdom

Jones and Bartlett's books and products are available through most bookstores and online booksellers. To contact Jones and Bartlett Publishers directly, call 800-832-0034, fax 978-443-8000, or visit our website www.jbpub.com.

Substantial discounts on bulk quantities of Jones and Bartlett's publications are available to corporations, professional associations, and other qualified organizations. For details and specific discount information, contact the special sales department at Jones and Bartlett via the above contact information or send an email to specialsales@jbpub.com.

American Academy of Orthopaedic Surgeons

Editorial Credits
Chief Education Officer: Mark W. Wieting
Director, Department of Publications: Marilyn L. Fox, PhD
Managing Editor: Barbara A. Scotese

Production Credits
Chief Executive Officer: Clayton Jones
Chief Operating Officer: Don W. Jones, Jr.
President, Higher Education and Professional Publishing:
    Robert W. Holland, Jr.
V.P., Design and Production: Anne Spencer
V.P., Manufacturing and Inventory Control: Therese Brauer
V.P., Sales and Marketing: William J. Kane
Acquisitions Editor: Jacqueline Mark-Geraci
Senior Production Editor: Julie Champagne Bolduc
Associate Editor: Nicole Quinn

Editorial Assistant: Erin Murphy
Senior Marketing Manager: Ed McKenna
Photo Researcher: Kimberly Potvin
Director of Interactive Technology: Adam Alboyadjian
Interactive Technology Manager: Dawn Mahon Priest
Composition: Graphic World
Text and Cover Design: Anne Spencer
Cover Image: © Photodisc
Printing and Binding: Edwards Brothers
Cover Printing: Edwards Brothers

Library of Congress Cataloging-in-Publication Data
Athletic training and sports medicine / edited by Chad Starkey, Glen Johnson, American Academy of Orthopaedic Surgeons.— 4th ed.
    p. ; cm.
  Includes bibliographical references and index.
  ISBN 0-7637-0536-5 (alk. paper)
1. Sports medicine. 2. Physical education and training.
  [DNLM: 1. Sports Medicine. 2. Athletic Injuries. 3. Physical Education and Training. QT 261 A8718 2005] I. Starkey, Chad, 1959- II. Johnson, Glen, 1952- III. American Academy of Orthopaedic Surgeons.
  RC1210.A84 2005
  617.1'027—dc22

                              2005006220

Printed in the United States of America
09 08 07 06 05 10 9 8 7 6 5 4 3 2 1

Photo Credits
p. 1, © Steve Skjold/Alamy Images; p. 2, © Jeff Greenberg/age fotostock; p. 13, © Image Source/Alamy Images; p. 31, © Photodisc; p. 47, © Photos.com; p. 62/63, © Dennis MacDonald/Alamy Images; p. 64, © Ilene McDonald/Alamy Images; p. 135, © Comstock Images/Alamy Images; p. 191, © Photos.com; p. 221, © Photodisc; p. 251, © Photos.com; p. 267, © Photodisc; p. 337, © Dynamic Graphics Group/Creatas/Alamy Images; p. 385, © Photodisc; p. 445, © Photos.com; p. 457, © Photodisc; p. 491, © PhotoLink/Photodisc/Getty Images; p. 517, © Dynamic Graphics Group/IT Stock Free/Alamy Images; p. 551, © Photodisc; p. 557, © Corbis/Creatas; p. 579, © Photodisc; p. 597, © Rubberball Productions/Alamy Images; p. 616/617, © Robert Giroux/AP Photo; p. 618, © Harry V. Reidy/Alamy Images; p. 639, © Photodisc; p. 657, © Photodisc/Creatas; p. 675, © Robert W. Ginn/Alamy Images.

CONTENTS

PREFACE

First published in 1984, *Athletic Training and Sports Medicine* is now one of the longest continually updated and durable texts dedicated to the physical medicine and rehabilitation of musculoskeletal injuries. The 20 years that *Athletic Training and Sports Medicine* has been published have seen remarkable advances in diagnosis, management, and rehabilitation of orthopaedic injuries. Conditions that were career ending when the first edition was published are now reversible thanks not only to improved surgical techniques but also to increased emphasis on injury prevention, improved diagnostic modalities, and more aggressive rehabilitation techniques.

These changes have led to a rather significant shift in the focus and tone of the fourth edition of *Athletic Training and Sports Medicine*. The fourth edition is now focused on the integrated management, diagnosis, surgical and nonsurgical management, and rehabilitation of common orthopaedic pathologies. This edition was written under the premise that the reader has a good understanding of human anatomy, clinical diagnostic skills, and is familiar with the basic principles of acute injury management, therapeutic modalities, and therapeutic exercise.

The text is divided into three sections:

- Section 1: Overview
- Section 2: Regional Pathologies
- Section 3: Specific Populations

The overview section describes the concept of integrated injury management, the basic pathological response and management of soft tissue and bony injuries, and the role of therapeutic medications in the management of these conditions. Section 2 presents a detailed integrated management plan for common conditions affecting each major body area. An overview of population-specific concerns is presented in Section 3.

Each chapter within Section 2 presents the considerations in the immediate management, surgical/medical interventions, follow-up management (such as short-term bracing or immobilization), and considerations influencing the patient's care. The medical techniques described in this text are not a "how to." Rather, they describe "how, what, when, and why" approach regarding the medical procedures that are used to return athletes and other patients to activity and describe the implication(s) of these procedures on the treatment and rehabilitation protocol.

Template (as opposed to "cookbook") rehabilitation protocol are described. The basis of the finite points of injury evaluation, therapeutic modalities, and rehabilitation addressed in other texts are detailed. This text describes how each of these areas is integrated into patient care.

The production team at Jones and Bartlett Publishers have dedicated countless hours in seeing this project from conception to completion: Jacqueline Mark, Acquisitions Editor; Nicole Quinn, Associate Editor; Erin Murphy, Editorial Assistant; Ed McKenna, Senior Marketing Manager; Julie Bolduc, Senior Production Editor; and Anne Spencer, Vice President of Production and Design. This effort would not have come to fruition without the efforts of Barbara Scotese, Managing Editor with the American Academy of Orthopaedic Surgeons and Leslie Neistadt, Developmental Editor.

A special note of thanks to the editor of the first edition, Arthur E. Ellison, MD, the second edition, Letha "Etty" Griffin, MD; and the third edition, Robert C. Schenck, MD; and their Editorial Boards. These individuals laid the framework for a remarkable and time-tested resource for athletic trainers, physical therapists, and physicians who are involved in orthopaedic medicine.

Chad Starkey, PhD, ATC

CONTRIBUTORS

Peter J. Apel, BA
Center for Orthopaedics & Biomechanics
    Research
Boise State University
Intermountain Orthopaedics
Boise, Idaho

Marc-Andre Bergeron, MD
Fellow of AAOS
Fellow of ABIME
Private Practice
Hillsdale, New York

Ned Bergert, PTA, ATC
Head Athletic Trainer
Los Angeles Angels of Anaheim
Anaheim, California

Samuel Bradbury, MAOM, ATC, CEA
President
Quality Essential Health Systems
Liberal, Kansas

L. Michael Brunt, MD
Associate Professor of Surgery
Washington University School of Medicine
Attending Surgeon
Barnes-Jewish Hospital
St. Louis, Missouri

Douglas J. Casa, PhD, ATC, FACSM
Director, Athletic Training Education
Associate Professor, Department of Kinesiology
Research Associate, Human Performance
    Laboratory
Neag School of Education
University of Connecticut
Storrs, Connecticut

Peter F. DeLuca, MD
Associate Professor of Orthopedic Surgery,
Drexel University College of Medicine
Associate Director, Hahnemann Sports
    Medicine
Head Team Physician, Philadelphia Eagles
Orthopedic Consultant, Philadelphia Flyers
    and Phantoms
Philadelphia, Pennsylvania

E. Randy Eichner, MD, FACSM
Team Internist, Oklahoma Sooners Football
Professor of Medicine, University of Oklahoma
    Medical Center
Norman, Oklahoma

Michael Ellerbush, MD
Alabama Orthopaedic and Spine Center
Northport, Alabama

Michael S. Ferrara, PhD, ATC
Professor
Department of Exercise Science
The University of Georgia
Athens, Georgia

Kevin M. Guskiewicz, PhD, ATC
Professor, Department of Exercise and Sport
    Science
Professor, Department of Orthopaedics
University of North Carolina at Chapel Hill
Chapel Hill, North Carolina

Bick Harmon, PT, ATC
Physical Therapist
Harmon Physical Therapy
West Covina, California

Christine Heilman, MS, L/ATC, CSCS
Athletic Trainer
University of Wisconsin Oshkosh
Oshkosh, Wisconsin

Dennis D. Hedge, PharmD
Professor, Department of Clinical Pharmacy
College of Pharmacy
South Dakota State University
Brookings, South Dakota

Peggy A. Houglum, PhD, ATC, PT
Assistant Professor
Rangos School of Health Sciences
Athletic Training Department
Duquesne University
Pittsburgh, Pennsylvania

Christopher D. Ingersoll, PhD, ATC, FACSM
Associate Professor
Department of Human Services
University of Virginia
Charlottesville, Virginia

Glen Johnson, MD
Parkcrest Orthopedics
St. Louis, Missouri

David M. Kahler, MD
Associate Professor
Department of Orthopaedic Surgery
University of Virginia
Charlottesville, Virginia

K. Stuart Lee, MD, FACS
Clinical Associate Professor of Neurosurgery
Brody School of Medicine of East Carolina
    University
Greenville, North Carolina

Paul A. Marchetto, MD
Associate Professor of Orthopedic Surgery,
    Drexel University College of Medicine
Director, Hahnemann Sports Medicine
Team Orthopedic Surgeon, Philadelphia Eagles
Head Team Physician, Drexel University and
    Rutgers University-Camden
Philadelphia, Pennsylvania

Allen E. Mathieu, PAC, MS, ATC
Parkcrest Orthopedics and Sports Medicine
St. Louis, Missouri

Michael McCrea, PhD, ABPP
Director, Neuropsychology Service
Waukesha Memorial Hospital
Waukesha, Wisconsin

Frank C. McCue, III, MD
Alfred R. Shands Professor of Orthopedic
    Surgery and Plastic Surgery of the Hand
Director, Division of Sports Medicine and
    Hand Surgery
University of Virginia Medical Center
Professor, Curry School of Education
Team Physician
University of Virginia
Charlottesville, Virginia

Dilaawar J. Mistry, MD, MS, ATC
Assistant Professor
Department of Physical Medicine and
    Rehabilitation
University of Virginia
Charlottesville, Virginia

Ronald P. Pfeiffer, EdD, LAT, ATC
Professor of Kinesiology/COE
Center for Orthopaedics and Biomechanics
    Research
Boise State University
Boise, Idaho

David A. Porter, MD, PhD
Methodist Sports Medicine Center
Foot and Ankle Consultant, Indianapolis Colts,
    Indiana University, Purdue University
Co-Director Research and Education Methodist
    Sports Medicine Foundation
Indianapolis, Indiana

Jeff Ryan, PT, ATC
Director of Operations
Hahnemann Sports Medicine
Hahnemann University Hospital
Philadelphia, Pennsylvania

Susan Saliba, PhD, PT, ATC
Senior Associate Athletic Trainer
Assistant Professor
Curry School of Education
Clinical Instructor in Orthopaedic Surgery
University of Virginia
Charlottesville, Virginia

John P. Salvo, MD
Assistant Professor of Surgery
UMDNJ-Robert Wood Johnson
Assistant Director, Sports Medicine
Cooper Bone & Joint Institute
Camden, New Jersey

Mitchell D. Seemann, MD
Panorama Orthopedics, P.C.
Golden, Colorado

Kevin G. Shea, MD
Center for Orthopaedics & Biomechanics
    Research
Boise State University
Intermountain Orthopaedics
Boise, Idaho

Brett A. Taylor, MD
Barnes-Jewish Hospital at Washington
    University
Department of Orthopaedic Surgery
Washington University School of Medicine
St. Louis, Missouri

Paula Sammarone Turocy, EdD, ATC
Chairperson and Associate Professor
Rangos School of Health Sciences
Athletic Training Department
Duquesne University
Pittsburgh, Pennsylvania

Katie Walsh, EdD, ATC
Director of Sports Medicine/Athletic Training
Associate Professor, Department of Health
    Education & Promotion
East Carolina University
Greenville, North Carolina

Lewis Yocum, MD
Orthopedic Surgeon
Kerlan-Jobe Clinic
Los Angeles, California

REVIEWERS OF THE FOURTH EDITION

Shari Bartz, MAEd, ATC, CSCS
Grand Valley State University
Allendale, Michigan

W. David Carr, PhD, ATC
University of Tulsa
Tulsa, Oklahoma

Marisa Colston, PhD, ATC/L
University of Tennessee at Chattanooga
Chattanooga, Tennessee

Richard G. Deivert, PhD, ATC
Ohio University
Athens, Ohio

Jennifer E. Early, PhD, L-ATC
University of Wisconsin, Milwaukee
Milwaukee, Wisconsin

Craig Elder, PhD, ATC, CSCS
Southeast Missouri State University
Cape Girardeau, Missouri

Todd A. Evans, PhD, ATC, CSCS
University of Northern Iowa
Cedar Falls, Iowa

Jay Hertel, PhD, ATC
University of Virginia
Charlottesville, Virginia

Michael Higgins, PhD, ATC/PT
University of Delaware
Newark, Delaware

Shawna Jordan, MSEd, ATC
Kansas State University
Manhattan, Kansas

Christopher J. Joyce, PhD, ATC, CSCS
University of North Florida
Jacksonville, Florida

Leamor Kahanov, EdD, ATC
San Jose State University
San Jose, California

David A. Kaiser, EdD, ATC
Brigham Young University
Provo, Utah

Larry J. Leverenz, PhD, ATC/L
Purdue University
West Lafayette, Indiana

John E. Massie, PhD, ATC/L
Southern Illinois University, Carbondale
Carbondale, Illinois

Patricia McGinn, MS, ATC/L
University of South Carolina
Columbia, South Carolina

Bill Miller, DPE, LATC
Westfield State College
Westfield, Massachusetts

Lee Ann Price, MS, ATC/L
Eastern Illinois University
Charleston, Illinois

Angela Sehgal, EdD, ATC/L
Florida State University
Tallahassee, Florida

Patrick Sexton, EdD, ATC/R, CSCS
Minnesota State University, Mankato
Mankato, Minnesota

Rene Revis Shingles, PhD, ATC
Central Michigan University
Mount Pleasant, Michigan

Christine Stopka, PhD, ATC/L, CSCS, CAPE, MTAA
University of Florida
Gainesville, Florida

Thomas G. Weidner, PhD, ATC/L
Ball State University
Muncie, Indiana

William R. Whitehill, EdD, ATC, LMT
Middle Tennessee State University
Murfreesboro, Tennessee

Gary B. Wilkerson, EdD, ATC
University of Tennessee at Chattanooga
Chattanooga, Tennessee

Richard Biff Williams, PhD, ATC/L
University of Northern Iowa
Cedar Falls, Iowa

SECTION 1 Overview

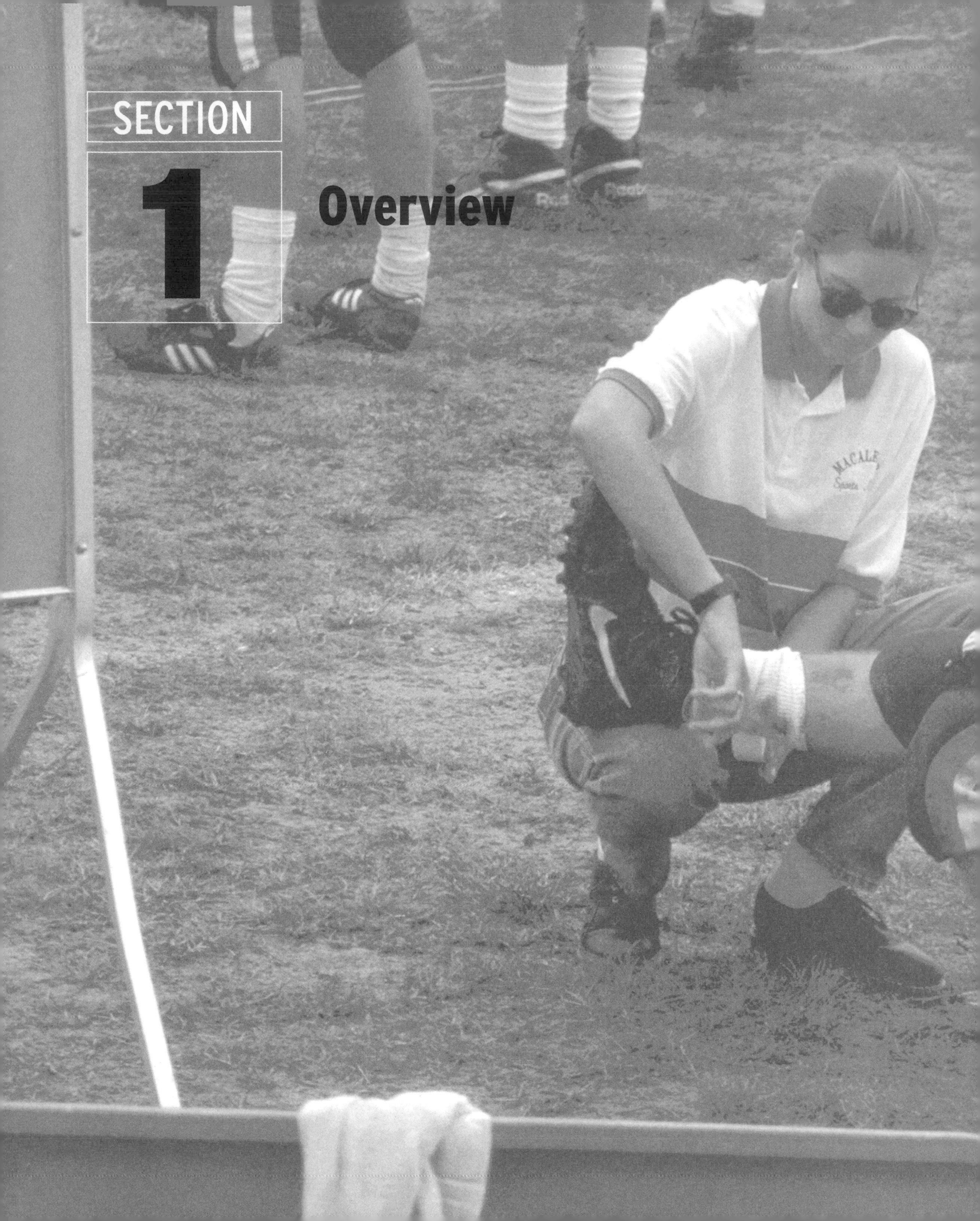

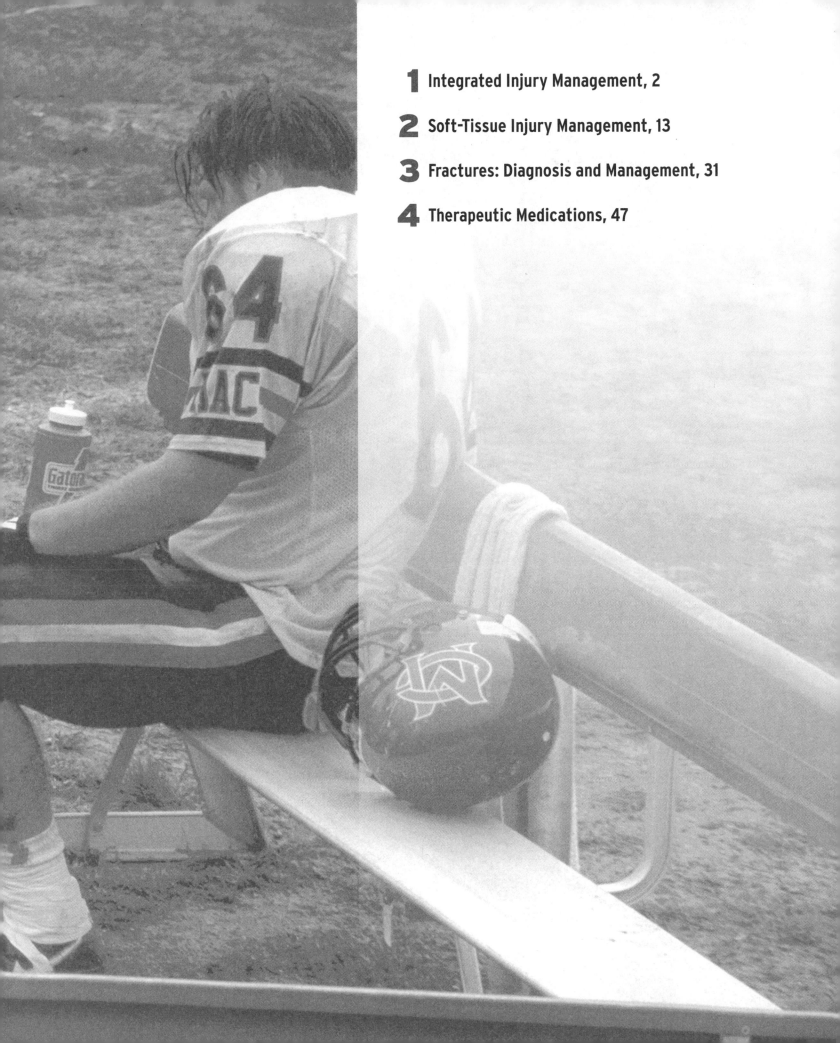

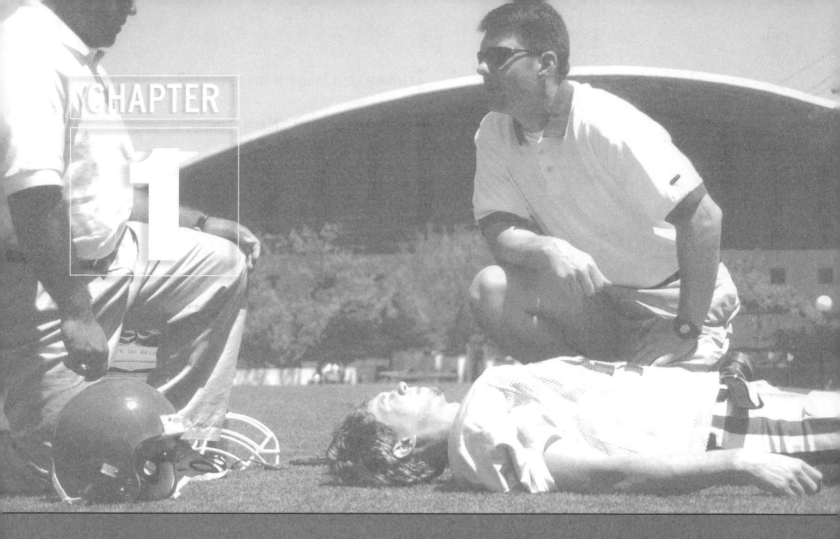

Integrated Injury Management

Introduction

Musculoskeletal trauma can be an unfortunate consequence of physical activity. When tissues are traumatized, a series of events are triggered that influence the patient's return to activity. Although the primary tissue destruction has already occurred, the initial and follow-up management affect the healing process.

The proper course of postinjury management depends on obtaining a correct diagnosis. The initial diagnosis—often determined immediately after the traumatic event—has two purposes: (1) to determine if the patient requires immediate transportation to a medical facility; and (2) to decide what procedures will be required to protect the injured body part while the patient is moved, so that a more thorough evaluation can be conducted. Furthermore, in catastrophic instances, emergency medical procedures must be performed to preserve the patient's life, limbs, and/or neurologic function.

A definitive diagnosis is based on the careful analysis of the findings of the clinical evaluation, imaging studies, and, when applicable, medical diagnostic tests. Some conditions are readily apparent on simple visual inspection, whereas further diagnostic testing may be needed to identify confounding structural defects, rule out concomitant trauma, and determine the functional integrity of the surrounding tissues. When definitive findings are present, the final diagnosis may be established by excluding other possible conditions.

Discerning a differential diagnosis is a systematic method of examining a condition that lacks unique signs or symptoms, has signs and symptoms that closely resemble multiple conditions, or has signs and symptoms that can mask another injury. Due diligence mandates that all other possible maladies be considered and ruled out before the final, definitive diagnosis is reached. Similarly, if an injury does not respond to treatment as anticipated, a complete reevaluation should be conducted and the patient referred to an appropriate specialist if applicable.

Pathomechanics and Functional Limitations After Injury

Traumatized or improperly healed tissues can lead to the alteration of a joint's normal biomechanics (pathomechanics). With time, this pathomechanical change can disrupt the normal function of other joints and muscle groups along the kinetic chain, leading to further biomechanical deficiencies.

Injury to ligaments and joint capsular structures can produce instability during movement as the joint fails to maintain its optimal position, causing weakness and inhibiting normal biomechanics. Alterations in normal range of motion (ROM) can result in compensatory postures, increasing stresses on the other joints and muscles. The ensuing biomechanical changes lead to functional shortening of some tissues and elongation of others, creating imbalances in muscle length and strength. Subsequent pathomechanical changes include muscular compensation or substitution.

Imaging Techniques

The role of diagnostic imaging in the evaluation process has significantly increased during the past decade. Diagnostic imaging was once primarily limited to the inclusion or exclusion of bony defects (including joint malalignment). Advances in radiographic imaging techniques, nuclear medicine, and computer technology have expanded the imaging modalities available to physicians, including magnetic resonance imaging (MRI) and computed tomography (CT) (Figure 1-1). Diagnostic ultrasound is a useful diagnostic tool for identifying tendinous lesions and soft-tissue masses and cysts.

The views obtained for each body area are relatively consistent for each imaging modality (Table 1-1). Limitations do exist and multiple views—or multiple imaging devices—are often required to obtain accurate images of the involved area.

Radiographs

Radiographic images are obtained by passing an x-ray beam through the tissues. The x-ray energy is collected on a film cassette or, more recently, digitally (digital or computed radiography). On a gray-scale continuum, radiographic images are white in areas of high x-ray uptake (primarily bone), filtering down to black in areas where no x-ray energy is absorbed by the tissues. Although skin, adipose tissues, some degree of soft tissue, and, in certain cases, edema or hemorrhage can be identified on radiographs, the quality and contrast resolution are often insufficient for a definitive diagnosis. For bony defects, however, radiographs are the most sensitive imaging modality, capable of detecting objects as small as 0.05 to 0.1 mm (depending on the equipment used),

---

Kinetic chain A series of body parts linked together by joints and muscles through which action/reaction forces are transmitted.

Compensation Changes in biomechanical function to overcome muscular weakness or joint dysfunction.

Substitution A secondary muscle or muscle group performing the action that would otherwise be performed by a primary muscle.

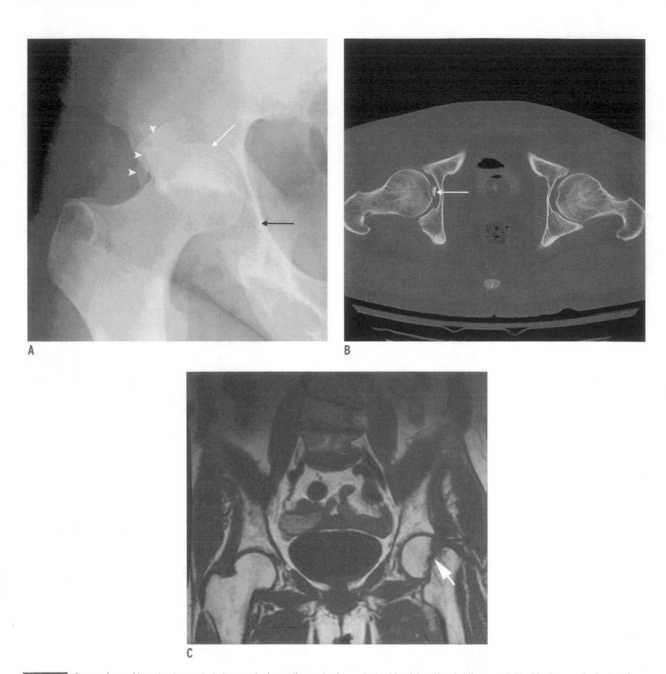

Figure 1-1 Comparison of imaging types. **A.** Anteroposterior radiograph of a posterior hip dislocation (white arrow). The black arrow indicates the acetabulum; the white arrowheads identify fracture segments. **B.** An axial CT scan of the hip shows an intra-articular fracture (white arrow) that was not visible on the radiograph in (A). This scan can be "windowed" to better illustrate soft tissue but at the expense of bony images. **C.** Coronal T1-weighted MRI of a femoral neck fracture. (Reproduced with permission from Johnson TR, Steinbach LS (eds): *Essentials of Musculoskeletal Imaging.* Rosemont, IL, American Academy of Orthopaedic Surgeons, 2004, pp 9, 435.)

compared with 0.4 to 1 mm on high-resolution CT scans.[1] Another limitation of radiographs is their two-dimensional views.

Fluoroscopy is the process of obtaining radiographic images in real time, allowing joint kinematics and guidance during surgical procedures.

◼ Magnetic Resonance Imaging

In MRI, a strong static magnetic field with intermittent radiofrequency (RF) pulses is delivered to the tissues to form an image of the internal tis-

sues. A powerful magnetic generator affects the hydrogen atoms that are found in all tissues. Similar to a compass, these atoms align with the magnetic field. When a brief (millisecond) RF pulse is introduced, the atoms deflect from their axis. When the RF pulse terminates, the atoms wobble as they align back with the magnetic field, in the process emitting weak RF signals of their own. Atoms in different types and densities of tissues realign themselves at different rates, producing a magnetic resonance signal. These signals

Table 1-1

Routine Imaging Views by Body Area

Upper Extremity

Fingers	PA, lateral, oblique (fingers should be separated)
Hand	PA, oblique, lateral
Wrist	PA, lateral (both with neutral positioning)
Forearm	AP, lateral
Elbow	AP (supinated), lateral (90° flexed); oblique views may be added for trauma patients
Humerus	AP, lateral
Glenohumeral joint	AP in internal and external rotation, true AP of the scapula, axillary; a 30° caudal tilt view is added for suspected impingement; a transscapular view is helpful in assessing glenohumeral dislocation and acromion morphology
Acromioclavicular joint	AP, 10° cephalad AP (Zanca view)

Lower Extremity

Hip	AP internal rotation, frog lateral (or cross-table lateral)
Femur	AP, lateral
Knee	AP, lateral (30° flexion)
Knee: arthritis	Add AP weight-bearing views or PA flexed weight-bearing views, lateral weight-bearing views, and occasionally Merchant axial views
Knee: intercondylar notch	Tunnel view (angulated PA or AP 45° flexed)
Patellofemoral joint	Merchant view
Lower leg	AP, lateral
Ankle	AP, lateral, mortise
Foot	AP, lateral, medial (internal) oblique (weight-bearing AP and lateral for foot alignment abnormality)
Subtalar joint	Lateral view, posterior tangential
Calcaneus	Lateral, AP, axial
Toes	AP, lateral, AP oblique

Axial Skeleton

Cervical spine	AP and lateral views; a lateral flexion-extension view can be added in patients with rheumatoid arthritis and suspected instability; a trauma spine series should include an open mouth odontoid view and a swimmer's view if C7 is not visualized
Thoracic spine	AP, lateral
Lumbar spine	AP, lateral
Sacrum	30° cephalad angulated AP, lateral
Coccyx	10° caudal angulated AP lateral
Sacroiliac joint	30° cephalad angulated AP (Ferguson view)
Pelvis	AP (Judet view and/or inlet/outlet views for pelvic ring fractures)

PA indicates posteroanterior (ie, beam of x-ray originates from the patient's posterior and travels to the anterior); AP, anteroposterior (ie, beam of x-ray originates from the patient's anterior and travels to the posterior).

Reprinted with permission from Johnson TR, Steinbach LS (eds): *Essentials of Musculoskeletal Imaging.* Rosemont, IL, American Academy of Orthopaedic Surgeons, 2004, p 6.

Table 1-2

Relative Signal Intensities of Selected Structures on Spin Echo in Musculoskeletal Magnetic Resonance Imaging

	Sequence		
Structure	T1-Weighted	Proton Density	T2-Weighted
Fat*	Bright	Bright	Intermediate
Fluid†	Dark	Intermediate	Bright
Fibrocartilage‡	Dark	Dark	Dark
Ligaments, tendon§	Dark	Dark	Dark
Muscle	Intermediate	Intermediate	Dark
Bone marrow	Bright	Intermediate	Dark
Nerve	Intermediate	Intermediate	Intermediate

*Includes bone marrow.

†Includes edema, most tears, and most cysts.

‡Includes labrum, menisci, triangular fibrocartilage.

§Signal may be increased because of artifacts.

Reprinted with permission from Johnson TR, Steinbach LS (eds): *Essentials of Musculoskeletal Imaging*. Rosemont, IL, American Academy of Orthopaedic Surgeons, 2004, p 12.

are collected by the unit and reconstructed into relatively high-resolution, high-contrast images by a computer and its software.

MRI excels in imaging soft tissue and is sensitive enough to detect stress fractures more acutely than radiographs. MRI is superior in detailing soft tissue such as ligaments, cartilage, tendons, and muscles. In some instances, a contrast medium may be injected into the tissues to improve the quality of the image. The individual RF properties (spin echo) of different tissue types can be filtered to accentuate different tissue types (**Table 1-2**). Depending on the weighting used—T1, proton density, or T2—the tissue resolution is altered for more or less prominence (**Figure 1-2**).

Most MRIs take 20 to 60 minutes, a potential complication if the patient is claustrophobic and a closed (tubelike) scanner is being used. Metal within the magnetic field is of particular concern. Most implanted metal is MRI-compatible, but other metals can be affected by–and violently pulled toward–the magnet. MRI of areas with certain tattoo inks that contain metal can cause burns.

Computed Tomography

CT scans use thin x-ray beams that are passed through the body and read by multiple detectors. Similar to radiographs, the amount of x-ray energy received by the detector is a function of the tissue density through which the beam passes, but the CT scan also detects the amount of energy scattered by the tissue. Select soft tissues such as joint spaces and vasculature can be imaged by injecting a contrast medium.

The final image is formed by computer analysis and manipulation of the energy collected by the detector. Contrast resolution is superior to that obtained on plain-film radiographs, and the gray-scale continuum can be digitally altered to display only those tissues that fall within a defined density range ("windowing"). Different views, or slices, can be extracted to create an image of the body part in various planes. Some CT scanners can construct three-dimensional images.

CT scans are primarily used to identify cortical bone, bony lesions that are not normally visible on radiographs, and (using a contrast medium) joints; however, CT lacks the contrast needed to image most soft tissues.

Diagnostic Ultrasound

Similar to therapeutic ultrasound, diagnostic ultrasound transmits high-frequency sound waves into the tissues. However, diagnostic ultrasound uses a lower frequency than therapeutic ultrasound and does not heat the tissues. Depending on the density and consistency of the underlying tissues, the sound waves are then reflected back at different speeds and amplitudes. This information is then collected by a receiver and transmitted to a computer, where it is reconstructed to form an image. Doppler ultrasound is used to detect motion, particularly in vascular studies.

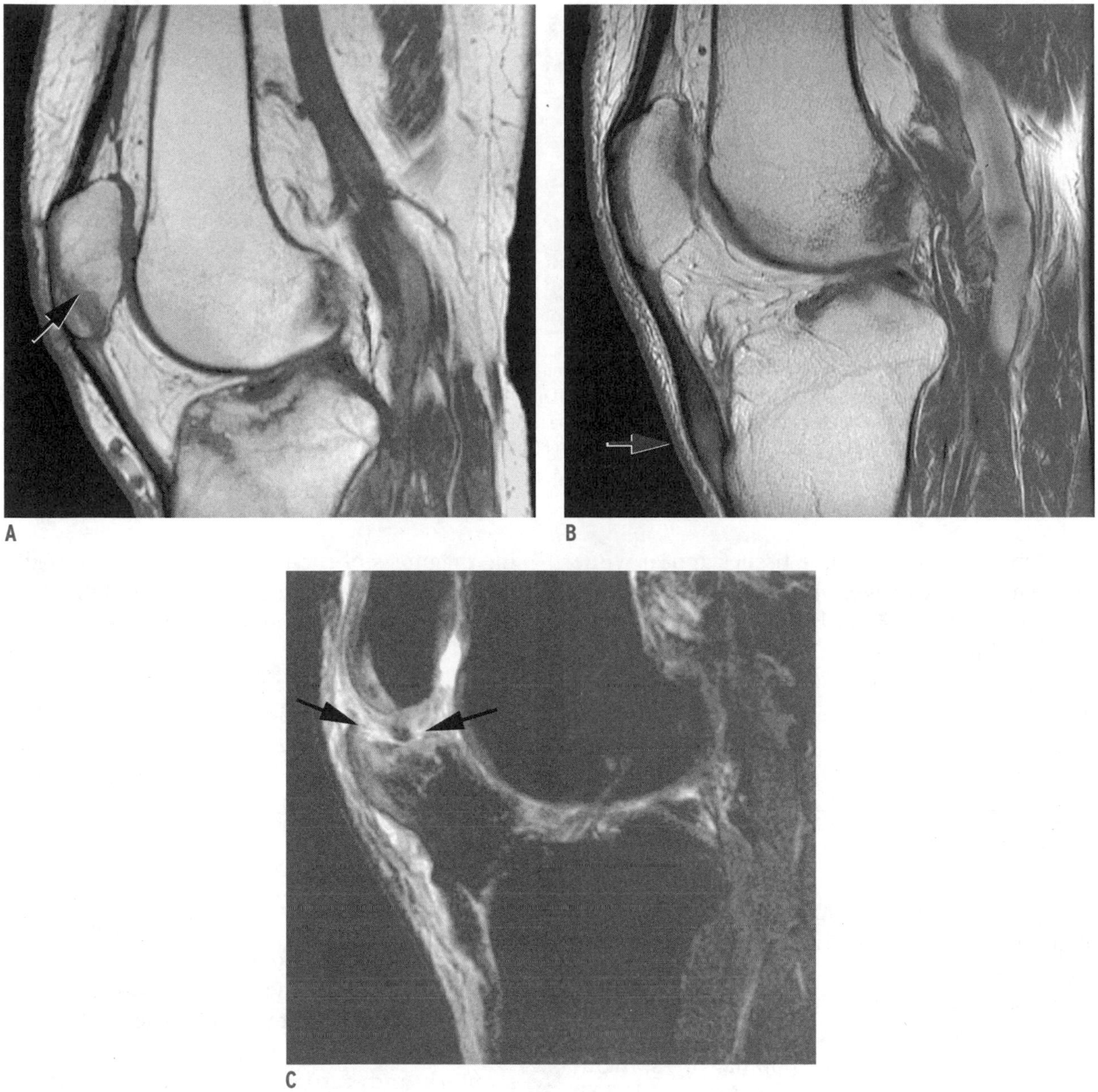

Figure 1-2 MRI tissue weighting. **A.** A sagittal T1-weighted image demonstrating bone marrow edema (arrow) consistent with a stress fracture. **B.** A sagittal proton-density-weighted image demonstrating thickening of the patellar tendon (arrow) consistent with patellar tendinitis. **C.** A sagittal T2-weighted, fat-suppressed image demonstrating a tear within the proximal patellar tendon (arrows). The altered signal intensity above the arrows indicates edema. (Reproduced with permission from Johnson TR, Steinbach LS (eds): *Essentials of Musculoskeletal Imaging.* Rosemont, IL, American Academy of Orthopaedic Surgeons, 2004, pp 488, 489, 496.)

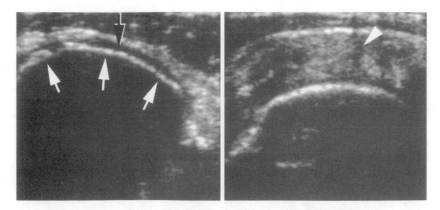

Figure 1-3   Ultrasonic image of a glenohumeral rotator cuff tear. This transverse bilateral view demonstrates a massive rotator cuff tear of the right shoulder (black arrow). The supraspinatus tendon is not visible on the left image but is visible on the right (white arrowhead). Also note that the humeral head on the left image (white arrows) is riding higher than on the right. (Reproduced with permission from Johnson TR, Steinbach LS (eds): *Essentials of Musculoskeletal Imaging.* Rosemont, IL, American Academy of Orthopaedic Surgeons, 2004, p 243.)

Dense, highly reflective tissues appear white on the ultrasonic image, whereas less reflective tissues appear darker (**Figure 1-3**). Although ultrasonic images allow better spatial resolution than CT or MRI, the interpretation of these images depends more on the skill and experience of the individual reading them.

Therapeutic Medications

Both prescription and nonprescription medications are useful during the short- and long-term care of musculoskeletal injury in modulating the injury response process, controlling pain, preventing infection, and reducing muscle spasm. Despite being somewhat maligned in the popular press, therapeutic medications that are properly prescribed by a physician and properly taken by the patient assist the healing process or help to resolve impediments to a formal rehabilitation program. However, medication should not be used as a substitute for a rehabilitation program that addresses the underlying cause of pain and inflammation.

Refer to chapter 4 for more detailed information regarding therapeutic medications.

Postinjury Management

Postinjury management encompasses the nonsurgical, preoperative, and/or prerehabilitation injury care that occurs after the immediate management of the injury and after acquiring a working diagnosis of the injury. Examples of postinjury management include suturing and the closed reduction of fractures and dislocations (see chapters 2 and 3).

Most postinjury management involves the continued use of ice, compression, and elevation. If indicated, an immobilization device is continued, splinting the extremity in a specific position and/or restricting a certain ROM.

Crutches

Crutches and, on occasion, canes are used to reduce or eliminate lower extremity weight-bearing forces. The two primary forms of crutches used in orthopaedic medicine are full-length and forearm crutches. Forearm crutches only run to the forearm, but require greater upper extremity strength and better balance than full-length crutches.

Full-length crutches are fitted by placing the tips 4″ to 6″ anterior and lateral to the foot and adjusting the length to allow 2″ to 3″ of clearance between the axilla and the top of each crutch. The hand grips are adjusted so that the elbows are flexed to approximately 30°. The body weight should be borne on the hands rather than the axillae. Improper crutch mechanics that place the body weight on the axilla can result in axillary nerve neuropathy.

Crutches can be used for either nonweight bearing (NWB) or partial weight bearing (PWB). When the patient is instructed to remain NWB, the crutch and injured extremity move in unison during normal ambulation. When ascending stairs, the patient leads with the good leg; when descending stairs, the involved leg leads (remembered by "up with the good, down with the bad").

When PWB, the involved extremity and crutches move together, but the patient bears as much weight as tolerable on the injured leg. The amount of pressure used must still allow for a proper heel-toe walking gait. If the gait is improper, the patient should be instructed to decrease the amount of pressure on the involved leg.

A cane should be held in the hand opposite the side of the injury, and the length should be adjusted so the elbow is flexed to 20° to 30° when the tip is placed 6″ in front and 6″ to the side of the foot. When walking, the cane moves forward with the involved extremity. If the patient leans or places too much weight on the cane, then two crutches should be used.

Prehabilitation

A relatively new emphasis in postinjury management is rehabilitation before surgery, or prehabilitation. The concept of prehabilitation is to maximize the strength of the surrounding muscles and increase joint ROM within tolerable limits before the patient undergoes the physical stress of surgery. Because the patient goes into the surgery with the involved extremity strong and with increased ROM, the postsurgical rehabilitation starts at an advanced point (relative to the patient with no prior conditioning) and prevents postoperative complications. Prehabilitation that addresses ROM normalization in acute anterior cruciate ligament injuries significantly decreases the incidence of arthrofibrosis after reconstruction.

Bracing

A variety of braces is commercially available and can be found for virtually every joint of the body. Braces fall into three categories: rehabilitative, functional, and prophylactic.[2] Rehabilitative braces are designed to provide protection and control motion during the healing and rehabilitative phases after injury or surgery. Functional braces allow motion and support the joint as the patient is returning to activity. These braces provide protection to the injury without hindering motion and include derotation braces, patellar stabilization braces, and ankle braces. Prophylactic braces are intended to provide protection against potentially injurious forces. Other forms of support include specific pads and orthotic devices that can help protect injured structures or shield them from injury.

Splinting and Casting

Made of plaster, moldable plastics, or fiberglass, splints cover only two or three sides of the extremity, are used for relatively short-term immobilization, and can be easily removed for treatment or evaluation. Braces and immobilizers can also be used to splint a body part. Casts completely surround the joint and are worn for extended periods.

The following general considerations are important in the application of splints and casts[3]:

1. Clothing should be removed from the area of any suspected fracture or dislocation to inspect the extremity for open wounds, deformity, swelling, and ecchymosis.
2. Any jewelry items are removed immediately if possible, including finger and toe rings.
3. The pulse, capillary refill, and neurologic status distal to the site of injury are noted and recorded. If pulses are compromised, reduction should be attempted and the patient immediately transported to an emergency care facility.
4. All wounds should be covered with a dry sterile dressing before applying a splint. The physician should be informed of all open wounds in case further evaluation is necessary.
5. The splint should immobilize the joints above and below the suspected fracture.
6. With injuries in and around the joint, the splint should immobilize the bones above and below the injured joint.
7. All rigid splints should be padded to prevent local pressure.
8. Clinicians should use their hands to minimize limb movement and support the injury site until the splint has been placed and the limb is completely immobilized.
9. A severely deformed limb should be aligned with constant, gentle manual traction so that it can be placed in a splint.
10. After the alignment, pulses and neurologic status should be checked.
11. If resistance to limb alignment is encountered when applying traction, the limb should be splinted in the position of deformity.
12. When in doubt, the clinician should splint, monitor neurovascular status, and arrange for transportation to an emergency care facility.

Surgical Intervention

Surgical intervention is indicated when an injury will leave lasting consequences of functional deficits and restoration of the anatomy will improve the prognosis and functional outcome. Although surgery is a restorative process, the scalpel's contact with the tissues creates additional trauma. The fact that this trauma is created in a controlled environment does not negate the ensuing inflammatory response and the short- and long-term functional limitations. The choice of timing of the surgical intervention, the surgical procedure used, the severity of the condition, and the surgeon's skill all influence the postoperative care, rehabilitation protocol, and long-term outcomes, as do the patient's ability and willingness to comply with the postoperative program.

Most orthopaedic surgical procedures have very specific influences on activity progression and functional limitations that must be adhered to when designing the rehabilitation program. These limitations are highly individualized and can vary even with similar procedures; they can be surgeon-specific, procedure-specific, and injury-specific. If questions exist regarding the indications and contraindications of rehabilitation techniques, clarification should be obtained from the physician to facilitate complete commitment to the postoperative protocol.

Postoperative Management

The immediate postoperative care involves protection of the repair and care of the surgical wound. Protecting the repair (including reconstructions and fixations) includes limiting the stress on the skin closure by immobilization with bracing, casting, splinting, or wrapping. After lower extremity surgery, NWB or PWB crutch ambulation is often necessary to protect the surgical site.

Basic postoperative wound care is directed at preventing contamination of the incision and optimizing the tissues' healing environment by limiting swelling and inflammation. Basic ice, compression, and elevation principles are employed. Clean wound care techniques and dressing changes help prevent contamination. The incision should be kept dry to avoid skin maceration and contamination. Sutures or staples are removed only after adequate healing has been demonstrated, usually a minimum of 7 to 14 days.

As healing progresses and it becomes safe to start mobilization, controlled passive and active ROM exercises are started. Once motion has been normalized, a comprehensive progressive resistance exercise program is begun. This is accompanied in the later phases by cardiovascular conditioning activities.

Functional evaluations determine progression to the next phase of rehabilitation and return to play.

Injury-Specific Treatment and Rehabilitation Concerns

The principles of rehabilitation are founded on an understanding of anatomy, pathophysiology, biomechanics, and tissue healing. Better incorporation of biomechanics and improvements and changes in postinjury and surgical techniques have allowed for accelerated rehabilitation programs. These changes have been made possible through sound scientific studies and constant introspection.

General rehabilitation goals are presented in **Table 1-3**. Most injuries have specific concerns that must be addressed during the rehabilitation program. Similarly, surgical procedures carry short- and long-term limitations on rehabilitation techniques.

Although rehabilitation goals are presented sequentially, in practice there is considerable overlap of goals and the specific rehabilitation protocols used to address the problems within each area (**Figure 1-4**). The physiologic ability of the patient to properly and completely perform any given exercise should be the criterion to progress through that activity. The exercises should be performed without compensation or the risk of injuring the healing tissues. Use of criterion-based progression allows patients to advance, if activity can be tolerated, yet

Table 1-3
General Rehabilitation Goals
Control inflammation, swelling, and pain.
Restore range of motion.
Restore strength.
Restore neuromuscular function.
Restore power and endurance.
Regain full function.
Return to pain-free activity.

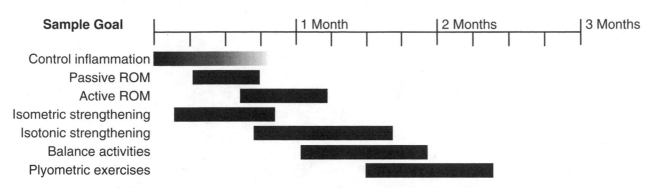

Figure 1-4   A sample rehabilitation sequence. The individual components (goals) of the rehabilitation progression often overlap. ROM indicates range of motion.

protects patients who are not physically ready to progress. **The rehabilitation timelines presented in Section II are presented as approximations of a typical rehabilitation progression, not as definitive references.** These timelines also demonstrate how particular activities overlap and interrelate with other parts of the program.

If permitted by the physician during the convalescence period, the patient should exercise the uninvolved extremities. A stationary bicycle, stair stepper, or elliptical trainer can be used if the upper extremity is involved (and for certain lower extremity injuries). If the patient is unable to bicycle or bear weight, an upper body ergometer can be used to maintain cardiovascular endurance.

Amount of Time Lost

The estimated amount of time lost is an average of the time loss for patients with similar conditions. Although the minimum amount of time required to recover from an injury is more easily predicted, the maximum recovery time is affected by numerous other variables, such as the severity of the injury, patient age, vascular integrity in the healing tissues, nutrition, medication, and steroid use. Older patients with reduced cardiac function require a longer time for recovery. Poor nutrition status or anabolic steroid use may also delay healing.

Another factor influencing the recovery time is patient compliance. With regard to the rehabilitation program, home-care instructions and activities to avoid should be carefully delineated. Noncompliant patients can increase the amount of time needed to return to activity if they do not follow through with home rehabilitation instructions,

thus delaying the anticipated progression. Failure to adhere to activity limitations, such as avoiding weight bearing can further traumatize the tissues and set back the healing process.

Return-to-Play Criteria

Before returning to sport participation or other strenuous activity, the patient should be pain free; demonstrate bilaterally equal strength, ROM, and proprioception; and be able to perform sport-specific or work-specific tasks. Muscle strength should be at least 85% to 90% of that in the uninvolved extremity.

The athlete should be able to perform all sport activities such that an observer would be unable to identify the extremity that had been injured, and the athlete should display confidence in himself or herself and the injured segment. Athletes should also be psychologically prepared to return to activity, demonstrating confidence in their ability to perform appropriately. Once all these factors are satisfied, return to activity may be allowed. Return to play should start in controlled situations with the athlete's own team and in friendly confines in a practice and scrimmage situation.

References

1. Curry TS III, Dowdey JE, Murry RC Jr: *Christensen's Physics of Diagnostic Radiology*, ed 4. Malvern, PA, Lea & Febiger, 1990.

2. France EP, Paulos LE: Knee bracing. *J Am Acad Orthop Surg* 1994;2:281-287.

3. Lucas GL (ed): General orthopaedics: Splinting principles, in Greene WB (ed): *Essentials of Musculoskeletal Care*, ed 2. Rosemont, IL, American Academy of Orthopaedic Surgeons, 2001, pp 81-87.

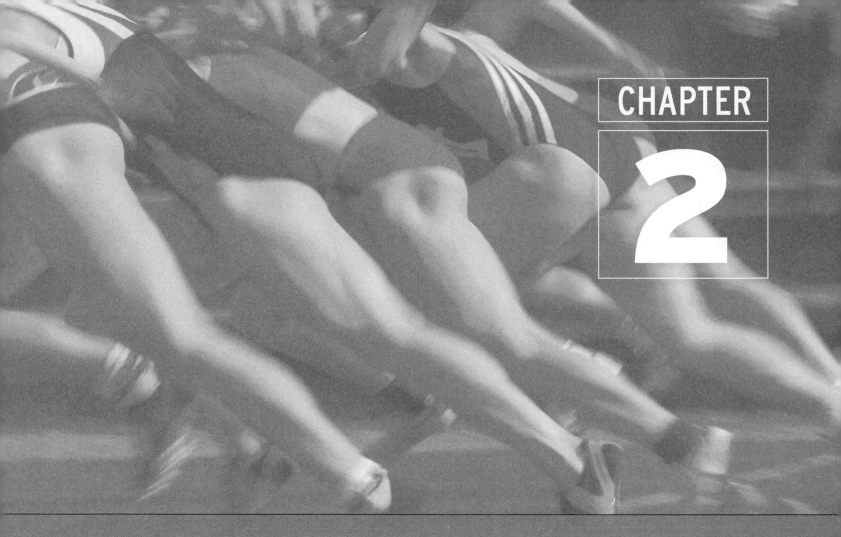

Soft-Tissue Injury Management

Christopher D. Ingersoll,
PhD, ATC, FACSM
Dilaawar J. Mistry, MD,
MS, ATC

Introduction

Soft tissue is classified into four types—epithelial, muscle, connective, and nervous—that are differentiated by **histology** and function. This chapter will address epithelial, muscle, and connective tissues, collectively referred to as "soft tissue." Topics in this chapter include the qualities of tissue; inflammation; and injuries to skin, muscle, ligaments, fascia, and synovial tissue.

Qualities of Soft Tissue

Connective tissues are composed of cells and extracellular matrix, but the amounts of each vary. In tendon, ligament, and cartilage, cells constitute 20% of the total tissue volume. The response of these tissues to injury relies on the migration of reparative cells. By contrast, muscle contains **pluripotential cells** that initiate the repair process. The extracellular matrix, which is 70% water and 30% solid, determines the form and function of connective tissue and may modulate protein synthesis by cells in response to loading or use. The two most abundant solid components of the extracellular matrix are collagen and proteoglycans.

Collagen consists of stiff, helical, insoluble protein macromolecules that provide scaffolding and tensile strength in fibrous tissues. Collagen is dif-

ferentiated into various types depending on its histologic composition. Type I collagen, the most common type, is a component of tendon, ligament, and muscle.

Proteoglycans form part of the extracellular matrix and serve to retain water within the tissues. Proteoglycans bind most of the water of tissues, making the matrix a gel-like substance rather than an amorphous solution. Proteoglycans enhance the strength of tissues by serving as cement between collagen fibers. This helps stabilize the collagenous skeleton and improves the strength of the tissue.

Response to Loading

The soft tissues that make up tendons, ligaments, and joint capsules exhibit specific types of behavior under loading. When a ligament is loaded, microtrauma occurs before the yield point is reached. When the yield point is reached, the ligament begins to plastically deform and abnormally displace (**Figure 2-1**). If load continues to be applied, plastic deformation will go on until the failure point is reached. Surrounding structures, such as the joint capsule and other ligaments, may also be damaged.

Soft tissues exhibit **viscoelastic** behavior, including stress relaxation, creep, and hysteresis. *Stress relaxation* is the decrease in force required to maintain the tissue over time when it is subject to a constant deformation. *Creep* is characterized by continued deformation in response to a maintained

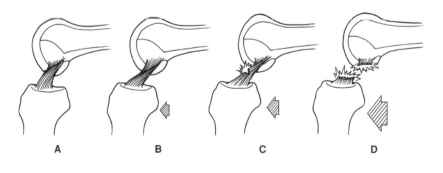

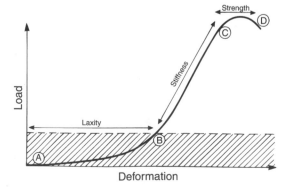

Figure 2-1 Schematic and graphic descriptions of laxity, stiffness, and strength. **Top,** Mechanisms of joint failure. A = flexion (some fiber recruitment), B = Lachman end point (100% fiber recruitment), C = sprain (microfailure), D = rupture (catastrophic failure). **Left,** Graph depicts load-deformation behaviors of a ligament with mechanisms defined. Hatched area represents range of loads during normal daily activity. (Reproduced with permission from Frank CB: Ligament healing: Current knowledge and clinical applications. *J Am Acad Orthop Surg* 1996;4:74-83.)

load (**Figure 2-2**). The *hysteresis* response is the amount of relaxation, or variation in the load-deformation relationship, that takes place within a single cycle of loading and unloading. The shape of the load-deformation curve for viscoelastic soft tissues depends on the previous loading and unloading history and the tissue's histology.

When tendons and ligaments are not being stretched, the collagen fibers display *crimp*, which is a regular undulation or wave-type pattern of cells and matrix. Crimp provides a buffer or shock absorber that protects the tissue from damage during elongation. Under loading, the tendon or ligament straightens out and the crimp disappears, similar to a rubber band. When a rubber band is "relaxed," curves can be seen throughout its length. When the band is stretched, the curves (crimps) disappear. When the tension is released from the band, the crimps reappear.

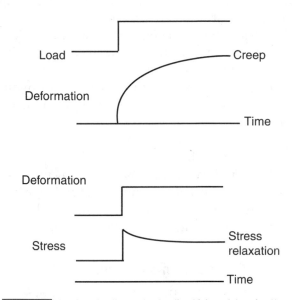

Figure 2-2 Previous loading and unloading history determine the shape of the load-deformation curve for viscoelastic soft tissues.

Inflammation

A process common to all injuries, inflammation is a localized tissue response initiated by injury to or destruction of vascularized tissues that are exposed to excessive mechanical load or antagonistic agents (**Table 2-1**). It is a time-dependent, evolving process, characterized by complex but orderly vascular, chemical, and cellular events that ultimately lead to tissue repair, regeneration, or scar formation. The inflammatory response may progress to resolution of the injury and repair of the damaged tissue or persist as chronic inflammation.

When significant tissue damage has occurred, inflammation is a necessary element of wound repair. The inflammatory process is initiated by tissue cell death, or necrosis, which results from

Table 2-1		
Inflammatory Tissue Responses		
Source	**Effect**	**Examples**
Physical and environmental agents	Tissue is directly injured as the result of physical contact	Sunburn via exposure to ultraviolet radiation
		Frostbite via excessive tissue cooling
		Burns
		Extended physical activities at high altitude
Inadequate tissue oxygenation	Inadequate cellular adenosine triphosphate (ATP) causing decreased protein synthesis and/or disordered membrane transport	Ischemia secondary to swelling
		Arterial compromise
Microbes	Microbes cause an inflammatory response by releasing toxins (bacteria), intracellular reproduction (virus), or local multiplication (fungus)	Bacterial, viral, or fungal infection
Hypersensitivity	Erroneous and disproportionate immune responsiveness can induce inflammation via various cellular or chemical mediators	Foreign substances (antigens)
		Microbes and allergens (dust, pollen, cat dander)
		Human tissue and cellular elements (autoimmune)
Chemical damage	Inflammation as the result of gross tissue damage	Acids and liquid nitrogen (used commonly to freeze warts)
		Contact dermatitis (eg, poison ivy)

damage and hypoxia at the site of injury. This non-specific response to physical trauma resembles the body's response to infection and chemical or thermal injury. Inflammation is the body's attempt to limit the extent of injury, remove devitalized tissue from the wound, and initiate tissue repair. Inflammation protects healthy tissue by three primary functions. Inflammation (1) provides the inflamed area with an exudate that contains proteins and immune cells (neutrophils, macrophages) to boost local defense mechanisms and destroy infective agents (viruses, bacteria, fungi); (2) purges the body of necrotic debris; and (3) repairs, regenerates, revitalizes, and strengthens affected tissue.

Pathophysiology

The inflammatory response is not dose related. Severe local inflammation can result from relatively minor trauma. The sudden swelling of a bursa or tendon is a good example of a disproportionate inflammatory reaction. The inability to finely regulate the inflammatory process in these situations may further damage local tissues. Various forms of anti-inflammatory and analgesic medications are administered to modulate the severity and duration of the inflammatory response (see chapter 4).

Inflammation is, however, an essential element of the injury response process. Some physicians will delay prescribing anti-inflammatory medications for 5 to 7 days following the initial injury to allow the body to initiate the acute inflammatory process.

Remodeling Gradual changes in alignment or size of a fractured bone back to normal.

Inflammatory Cells

Leukocytes, or white blood cells, are the primary buttress of the immune system that protects the body after a disruption in homeostasis. White blood cells exist in five types.

Neutrophils After tissue injury, neutrophils—the pivotal cells of the acute inflammatory response—are released from the bone marrow in response to various chemical mediators present at the site of tissue injury. Subsequently, neutrophils traverse the intravascular space and migrate through blood vessel walls (emigration) to arrive at the site of inflammation in the extravascular tissue within 12 hours of release from the bone marrow. Their main function is to ingest (phagocytose) and destroy microbes by means of various intracellular mechanisms.

Monocytes The largest of the leukocytes, monocytes mature to macrophages after their release from bone marrow into the bloodstream. Subsequently, macrophages emigrate into tissue spaces, where they may reside for several weeks or even years. At the site of inflammation, macrophages phagocytose particulate matter and process and present immune information from foreign proteins (antigens) to B and T lymphocytes, a crucial step in the future recognition of offending agents.

Lymphocytes Lymphocytes are classified into B lymphocytes and T lymphocytes. B lymphocytes have surface immunoglobulins. After antigenic stimulation, they are transformed into plasma cells that secrete antibodies. Antibody production is a vital immune mechanism that allows the human body to counteract future antigenic stimuli. Unlike B lymphocytes, T lymphocytes participate in the cell-mediated immune response, which is independent of the production of circulating antibodies.

Eosinophils Similar to the action of neutrophils and macrophages, eosinophils emigrate into extravascular tissues, where they can survive for several weeks and phagocytose particulate matter. They also exert toxic effects on microbes.

Basophils Basophils are analogous to neutrophils and eosinophils. They are motile and emigrate into extravascular tissues. After stimulation by immunoglobulins, they phagocytose microbes and particulate matter.

The Phases of Inflammation

Inflammation has three well-defined phases—inflammatory, fibroblastic, and remodeling. Inflammation has both beneficial and harmful effects on the body. The beneficial effects include stimulating the immune system, producing antibodies, diminishing the strength of toxins, and providing nutrition to the tissues. Harmful effects include destroying otherwise viable tissues and impairing tissue function. The magnitude of the inflammatory response is marked by the cardinal (clinical) signs and symptoms of inflammation (**Table 2-2**).

Inflammatory Phase

During this phase, as a result of sequential processes, leukocytes arrive at the site of injury and destroy abnormal agents, permitting healing to progress. The inflammatory phase is a chronology of events beginning with blood stasis and ending with the onset of the fibroblastic phase and may be active for a matter of hours or a month or more depending on the severity and magnitude of the injury and the tissues involved.

Blood stasis Chronologic alterations in the microcirculation adjacent to the injured area after injury are readily apparent and play a pivotal role in tissue healing. During the first 15 minutes, the small arteries known as arterioles contract, an action that perhaps has little relevance to inflammation. When

Table 2-2

The Cardinal (Clinical) Signs and Symptoms of Inflammation

Sign/Symptom	Cause
Redness (rubor)	Produced by dilation of small blood vessels
Heat (calor)	Secondary to increased blood supply (hyperemia)
Swelling (tumor)	Caused by increased fluid in the tissue space (edema)
Pain (dolor)	From stimulation of free nerve endings produced by tissue distortion and local chemical mediators of inflammation
Loss of function	Result of reflex inhibition of the inflamed area

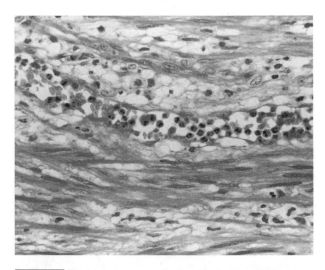

Figure 2-3 Electron micrograph showing margination of leukocytes. (Image © Biophoto Associates/Photo Researchers, Inc.)

the arterioles subsequently relax (vasodilation), however, blood flow to the injured area first increases (hyperemia) and then slows dramatically (stasis).[1] This process eventually allows leukocytes to migrate to injured tissues and promote healing.

Increased vascular permeability The walls of the smallest blood vessels are lined by a sheet of a single layer of cells (endothelium). In good health, the endothelium is intact and acts as a highly selective microfilter that prevents the escape of blood cells and excess fluid into the surrounding tissues. After injury, however, the endothelium is damaged by toxins and physical agents, and the endothelial cells contract. As a result, the endothelium becomes porous (increased vascular permeability) to the passage of protein-rich fluid (exudate) and blood cells.

Margination As a consequence of blood stasis and increased vascular permeability, leukocytes that are generally present in the central portion of blood flow begin to flow adjacent to the vascular endothelium. Subsequently, influenced by chemical substances (inflammatory mediators) released by tissues at the site of injury,[2-4] leukocytes aggregate and adhere to the endothelium in a process called margination (**Figure 2-3**).

Emigration After margination, neutrophils, eosinophils, and macrophages initially introduce extensions of cytoplasm (pseudopodia) into the breaches between constricted endothelial cells of small veins (venules) and, in some instances, arterioles. By active amoeboid movement, they move through the walls of blood vessels into the tissues surrounding blood vessels (extravascular space) in a process termed emigration. Ironically, temporary defects in vessel walls are self-limiting, and endothelial cells are not damaged during this process.

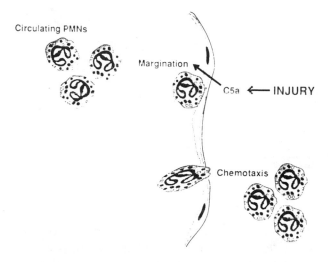

Figure 2-4 A schematic of inflammation. In chemotaxis, leukocytes migrate unidirectionally toward concentrations of mediators at the injury site. (PMN: polymorphonuclear neutrophils)

Chemotaxis After arriving in the extravascular space (**Figure 2-4**), leukocytes are directed to the site of injury by chemical mediators in a process called chemotaxis (chemo: chemical; taxis: movement). The focused movement of leukocytes follows a concentration gradient of chemical inflammatory mediators (chemotactic factors). These factors bind to receptors on the surface of leukocytes, increase calcium in the cytoplasm, and, by a complex mechanism, induce the formation of pseudopodia that are critical to amoeboid movement toward the site of injury.

Chemotactic factors that specifically attract neutrophils include components of bacteria, histamine, lymphokines, prostaglandins, leukotrienes, serotonin, and lysosomal compounds. Other physiologic mechanisms present in the plasma that also

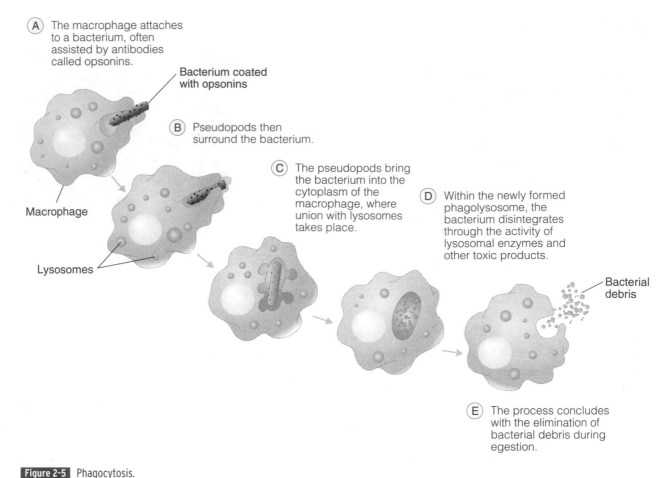

(A) The macrophage attaches to a bacterium, often assisted by antibodies called opsonins.

Bacterium coated with opsonins

(B) Pseudopods then surround the bacterium.

(C) The pseudopods bring the bacterium into the cytoplasm of the macrophage, where union with lysosomes takes place.

(D) Within the newly formed phagolysosome, the bacterium disintegrates through the activity of lysosomal enzymes and other toxic products.

Macrophage

Lysosomes

Bacterial debris

(E) The process concludes with the elimination of bacterial debris during egestion.

Figure 2-5 Phagocytosis.

serve as chemotactic factors include the complement,[5] kinin, coagulation, and fibrinolytic systems.[1]

Adhesion and phagocytosis After arriving at the site of injury, leukocytes first attach themselves to microbes and other tissue debris (adhesion) using receptors on their surface, a process that makes the microbes more suitable for ingestion (**Figure 2-5**). Adhesion is accomplished by the formation of pseudopodia that engulf microbes and debris. The pseudopodia subsequently fuse, a process that entraps microbes and debris into the cytoplasm of leukocytes.

Intracellular killing of microorganisms The entrapped microbes and debris are then exposed to several toxic chemicals and enzymes within the leukocyte cytoplasm, eventually resulting in microbial death and digestion of debris. Mechanisms responsible for this process include production of antimicrobial substances by neutrophils that combine hydrogen peroxide with myeloperoxidase, and release of potent enzymes stored in small sacs (lysosomes) in the cytoplasm of leukocytes. Release of lysosomal products then damages the injured

tissue further, a process that also activates chemotactic factors such as the coagulation system, resulting in enhanced vascular permeability, margination, and emigration of leukocytes. Thus the intracellular killing of organisms, via a feedback mechanism, serves to further the process of acute inflammation.

Fibroblastic Phase

The fibroblastic phase lasts 3 to 4 weeks and represents a continuum of several distinctive yet overlapping processes. Within 5 to 7 days of injury, the number of fibroblasts increases substantially (fibroplasia). Fibroblasts initially synthesize the protein tropocollagen. Three strands of tropocollagen linked together by chemical bonds form procollagen, which is secreted into the extracellular space between fibroblasts to form collagen. Fibroblasts also secrete heparin sulfate, hyaluronic acid, chondroitin sulfate, keratin sulfate, and proteoglycans that contribute to matrix deposition, a critical step in increasing the tensile strength of the healing tissue. Steered by growth factors, endothelial cells fi-

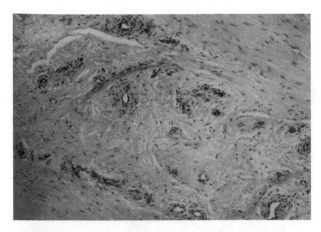

Figure 2-6 Proliferation of fibroblasts and new capillaries are often found in areas of tendon degeneration. (Reprinted with permission from Arendt EA (ed): *Orthopaedic Knowledge Update: Sports Medicine*, ed 2. Rosemont, IL, American Academy of Orthopaedic Surgeons, 1999, p 32.)

Table 2-3

Skin Layers and Function

Layer	Function
Stratum corneum	Barrier to noxious substances
Epidermis	Protects against ultraviolet damage
	Provides cutaneous immunity
Dermis	Provides the skin with elasticity and strength
Subcutaneous adipose tissue	Insulates and protects the body

---

nally migrate, divide, and mature, leading to the formation of new blood vessels (angiogenesis) (**Figure 2-6**). This process promotes the delivery of vital nutrients and oxygen to the healing tissues.

Remodeling Phase

After the third week, inflamed tissue undergoes steady modifications that can persist for several years after the initial injury. Collagen is broken down (lysis) and subsequently deposited (synthesis) in a cyclic fashion without any change in the net magnitude of collagen. Concurrently, myofibroblast proliferation produces a contraction of healing tissue and is supported by collagen alignment. Maximal tensile strength of the wound is achieved by week 12 after injury.

Skin Injuries

The skin is more than just a covering for the body; it provides structure, form, and protection, and also helps regulate temperature. The skin is composed of various layers, each serving a well-defined purpose (**Table 2-3**). Any of the skin components can be injured and produce a local inflammatory response. The most common traumatic injuries to the skin are abrasions, avulsions, contusions, lacerations and incisions, punctures, and vesiculations (blisters).

Abrasions

An abrasion is a scraping away of skin or mucous membrane as a result of a shearing force that causes partial-thickness skin loss.

Pathophysiology

The skin surrounding an abrasion undergoes normal inflammatory processes. An infection can develop from bacterial contamination, delaying healing and enhancing scar formation.

Symptoms

The dermis and epidermis are worn away, leaving blood capillaries exposed.

Immediate Management

Abrasions should be aggressively cleaned with mild soap. Debriding foreign matter prevents future discoloration of the skin ("tattooing"). An aseptic dressing is applied to prevent infection. Ice may be applied to the area to reduce the formation of a contusion secondary to the abrasive force.

Medical Management

Application of an antibiotic cream is typically sufficient. However, repeated trauma to the abrasion can prolong healing and be a precursor to infection. An abrasion surrounded by increasing redness, purulent discharge, and enlarged lymph nodes draining the affected area is likely to be infected and warrants oral or intravenous antibiotic therapy. Closed-space infection can be life threatening. A tetanus booster should be administered for all wounds, especially puncture wounds, if the previous inoculation was administered more than 5 years earlier.

Tissue Avulsions

Tissue avulsions occur as a result of a tensile load presented to the tissue. The tissue undergoes ultimate failure and separates from the body.

Symptoms

Deformity and pain are present with a skin or nail avulsion. Avulsion fractures are discussed in chapter 3 (see p 38).

Immediate Management

The avulsed area should be cleansed with a mild soap. An aseptic dressing should be applied to prevent infection.

Medical Management

Avulsed tissue may need to be sutured to attain hemostasis. Small flaps (less than 1.0 cm²), especially on the fingertips, typically do not need to be sutured. Butterfly and skin-closure tapes can be applied to flaps that do not have a dusky discoloration, which is a sign of compromised blood flow. However, larger flaps should be sutured to obtain thorough hemostasis. The gauge of suture material used and the elapsed time before suture removal are determined by the site of injury (**Table 2-4**). Because the appropriate management varies with the individual and the severity of injury, these guidelines should not be construed as the standard of care in a clinical setting.

Other common medical management guidelines include:

- Flaps adjacent to joints should be splinted after suturing to provide support and prevent flap dehiscence.
- Tetanus prophylaxis should be administered to individuals who have not received a tetanus booster for 10 years before the injury.
- Flaps that are contaminated and have been open for longer than 6 hours may not be amenable to suturing.
- Antibiotics may be needed, depending on the degree of contamination and elapsed time to suturing.

Histoacryl blue, a medicinal glue, can be substituted for suturing in specific circumstances. Considerations for appropriate use of this bonding agent include:

- The surface of the flap should be approximated and the glue applied to the surface of the flap. The glue should not touch the tissue below the surface of the flap.
- The glue generates some heat during application.
- The glue is not absorbed but separates from the surface of the flap as healing progresses.
- The agent can be used on flaps with clean edges, over areas of the body not subjected to tension forces, and on flaps and wounds less than 5 cm.
- This relatively atraumatic method for flap closure is ideal for children.

■ Contusions

A contusion, or bruise, results from compressive forces that rupture the subcutaneous vessels.

Pathophysiology

Compressive forces crush tissues, resulting in extravasated bleeding into the interstitial space.

Symptoms

Local pain, swelling, and later discoloration are present.

Immediate Management

Cryotherapy should be used to decrease secondary injury and pain. Compression should be applied and the extremity elevated, if appropriate, to control edema.

Medical Management

A hematoma—swelling caused by extravasated blood confined within a discrete body area—can form and become infected beneath a laceration or abrasion (see p 21). If the hematoma is large and organized, aspiration assists in pain control, the healing response, and prevention of infection. An infected hematoma can form an abscess that may

---

Extravasated Having escaped from the blood or lymph vessels into the tissues.

Table 2-4		
Suturing Guidelines for Skin Avulsions		
Site of Injury	Suture Gauge and Material	Suture Removal (days)
Mouth	4.0 Dexon* absorbable	Absorbed
Extremities	4.0-5.0 Monosof*	7 to 10 days
Trunk	4.0-5.0 Monosof	7 to 10 days
Scalp	5.0 Monosof	7 days
Face	6.0 Monosof	5 to 7 days
*Dexon, Davis & Geck, Danbury, CT; Monosof, US Surgical, Norwalk, CT.		

require surgical intervention. Radiographs may be needed to rule out a fracture.

Tissue Lacerations and Incisions

A laceration is an irregular wound or tear of the flesh caused by a shear force. An incision is a cut made by a sharp object, such as a knife. A shear force presented to the tissue with a sharp edge separates adjacent tissue in a straight line.

Symptoms

Local pain and bleeding are present.

Immediate Management

The incision should be cleaned thoroughly with a solution of 1 part Betadine and 10 parts water.[6] Ice can be used to diminish secondary injury and reduce pain.

Medical Management

The decision to suture can be difficult. Generally, depth, location, and length are the determining factors. Deep incisions or lacerations that allow the tissue to spread, exposing the underlying subcutaneous

or adipose tissues, should be reapproximated to prevent infection and promote healing. Facial trauma is more likely to require suturing (**Figure 2-7**). Lacerations and incisions over areas that challenge healing due to poor blood supply, bony prominences, or tension are also good candidates for suturing.

Suturing for primary closure should occur within 12 hours for an uncontaminated wound. With lacerations, the wound margins may need trimming to obtain good approximation of the skin flaps (**Figure 2-8**). Contaminated wounds should be allowed to heal via secondary intention, with regular follow-up visits to change dressings, assess healing, and check for latent infection.

Once the decision is made to suture, the type of suture must be selected (see Table 2-4). Subcutaneous sutures are usually bioabsorbable and can be monofilament or braided. If prolonged strength is needed because of tension placed on tissues, however, nonabsorbable sutures are recommended. Skin sutures can be monofilament or braided bioabsorbable. Nonabsorbable sutures can

Secondary intention
Healing that occurs secondary to the formation of a scar or other indirect union.

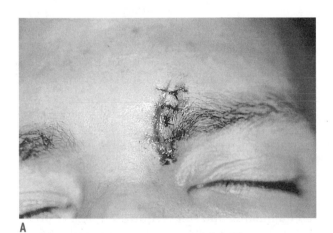

A

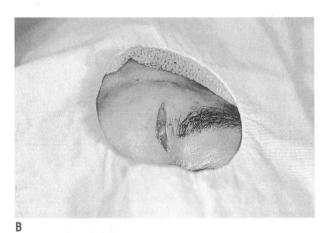

B

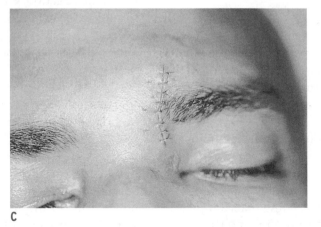

C

Figure 2-7 Monofilament sutures are used to approximate the epidermis. **A.** Hastily repaired laceration illustrating overlapping and jagged skin margins. **B.** Wound edges cleaned and sharply debrided. **C.** Precise layered repair allows for better healing and a more acceptable cosmetic outcome.

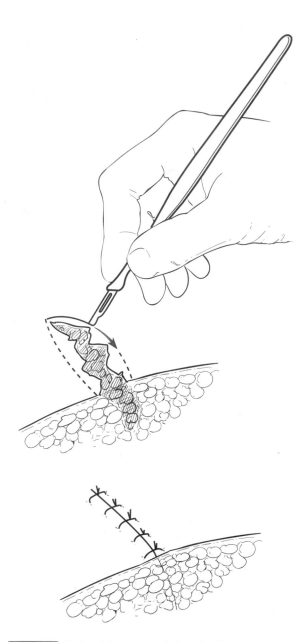

Figure 2-8 Contused, jagged wound edges should be sharply debrided to allow for better and faster healing of the laceration.

also be used but need to be removed after the healing is well underway, which varies depending upon anatomical location. Sutures are named for their constituent material and the size of the needle and suture: 0 is larger than 00 (2-0), which is larger than 000 (3-0), etc.

A variety of suture techniques can be employed by the physician. The decision is determined by the amount of tension on the closure during the healing process, the location of the wound, and the blood supply available for healing. Facial injuries are closed with very fine suture (5-0 or 6-0), using a small needle, and removed quite early (approximately 5 to 7 days later) to prevent scarring. Extensor surfaces generally are under more tension

than flexor surfaces and, therefore, require lower suture grades (stronger suture material). The type of surface may influence suture type, suture technique, and suture healing time.

■ Puncture Wounds

A puncture is a hole or wound made by a sharp, pointed instrument that disrupts tissue with compressive forces.

Pathophysiology

Puncture wounds are subject to normal inflammatory processes. Puncture wounds carry an increased risk of infection, because agents such as *Tetanus bacillus* or *Pseudomonas* can be introduced and may not be removed with routine wound care.

Symptoms

Pain and bleeding are present at the entry site of the wound.

Immediate Management

The incision should be cleaned thoroughly with a solution of 1 part Betadine and 10 parts water.[6]

Medical Management

The puncture site should be examined for any residual foreign bodies. If the puncture is caused by a sting, the sting should be scraped gently without compressing the affected area in order to prevent spreading of potential venom or toxins. The wound must be thoroughly irrigated and closely monitored for signs of infection.

Deep punctures are difficult to cleanse completely. The offending object, its environmental location, and substances it passed through on its way to the skin determine the level of concern for contamination. Puncture wounds occurring in contaminated water, grass fields, or footwear are often contaminated and may require surgical debridement and irrigation. Oral or intravenous antibiotics should be seriously considered in immediate management. Tetanus status should also be assessed and addressed if deficient.

■ Vesiculations (Blisters)

Vesiculations are blisters formed as the result of friction and are common on feet and the throwing hands of baseball pitchers. Using properly fitting footwear and "breaking in" shoes before wearing them in competition are the best ways to prevent blisters. If "hot spots" begin to form, double socks, powder, lubricant cream (petroleum gel), moleskin, donut pads, or other skin coverings can also help prevent blisters. Because of league rules, baseball pitchers cannot use foreign substances on their hands.

Pathophysiology

Blisters occur as extracellular fluid extravasates into a closed space in response to trauma (friction).

Symptoms

A burning or hot sensation is felt at the site of the blister or forming blister. A small, fluid-filled sac forms at the site of friction.

Immediate Management

If the blister is intact, it should be left alone and protected with a donut pad. If the blister is open, it should be cleaned thoroughly with a solution of 1 part Betadine and 10 parts water.[6]

Medical Management

Cooling the blistered surface can be an effective treatment. Leaving the skin in place keeps the underlying subcutaneous tissue sterile. Antibiotics are recommended for recurrent blisters, which typically become infected and thus delay the healing process. Another management approach is to drain the blister using a sterile syringe and needle, leaving the overlying skin as a protective covering. Tincture of benzoin, zinc oxide, and other home remedies have also been found useful.

Muscle

All skeletal muscles are supplied with arteries, veins, and nerves. Blood carries oxygen and nutrients to muscles and carries away the waste produced by muscle contractions. Muscle morphology depends on a fibrous connective-tissue framework in addition to the arrangement of the muscle fibers. Connective tissue surrounds whole muscle (epimysium), each fascicle or bundle of fibers (perimysium), and individual muscle fibers (endomysium). This connective-tissue framework attaches to tendon and is essential for the efficient generation of force. Disruption of any of these processes decreases the strength of the muscle and/or range of motion (ROM) of the joint. Muscles are subject to traumatic injuries and inflammatory conditions and, because of their contractile properties, are prone to hypotonic and hypertonic conditions.

Traumatic Injuries to Muscle

◼ Contusions

A contusion, or bruise, is an injury in which the skin is not broken secondary to compressive forces. A muscle contusion differs from a skin contusion in that the blood extravasates into muscle tissue, not into the skin.

Pathophysiology

A muscle contusion is created by extravasation of blood into the muscle as a result of trauma.

Symptoms

Localized tenderness, pain, swelling, and ecchymosis are present.

Immediate Management

Contusions are first treated with ice, compression, elevation, and protection.

Medical Management

Treatment with ice, compression, elevation, and protection should be continued while the inflammatory response is still active. Moist heat and massage are contraindicated early in the healing process to prevent the development of myositis ossificans (see p 25). Radiographs may be required early to rule out underlying fractures and later to rule out ossification within muscle for contusions that heal with a loss of strength and muscle contracture.

◼ Hematomas

A hematoma is a swelling or mass of blood (usually clotted) confined to an organ, tissue, or space and caused by a break in a blood vessel as the result of a compressive force.

Pathophysiology

A hematoma is caused by extravasation of blood and lymph fluid into a localized region, usually encapsulated by a connective-tissue membrane.

Symptoms

Localized tenderness, pain, swelling, and ecchymosis are present.

Immediate Management

Initial treatment for hematomas includes ice, compression, elevation, and protection.

Medical Management

Treatment with ice, compression, elevation, and protection should be continued while the inflammatory response is still active. Some anecdotal evidence suggests that early injection of hyaluronidase into the hematoma can enhance dissolution and speed the healing process. A hematoma that does not produce neurovascular compromise should not be aspirated. If neurovascular compromise is present, the patient should be referred for aspiration.

◼ Strains

A strain is trauma to the muscle or the musculotendinous unit from violent contraction or excessive forcible stretch. Strains occur as a result

Ecchymosis A bluish discoloration of the skin caused by bleeding under the skin; a bruise.

Morphology Pertaining to a tissue's structure and form without regard to function.

Hyaluronidase An enzyme that increases the permeability of connective tissue.

of tensile forces on the muscle. When stretched to failure, most muscle fails near the proximal musculotendinous junction. Failure occurs in the Z-disks when the muscle is not stimulated but external to the membrane of the myotendinous junction in stimulated muscle (**Figure 2-9**). Damaged tissue is subject to the inflammatory process.

Muscle strains are graded according to the amount of damage to the muscle fibers and the ability to palpate defects in the muscle. A grade I strain is an overstretching of the muscle fibers, with less than 10% of the muscle fibers tearing; no defect is palpable. A grade II strain is a partial tear of the muscle, usually between 10% and 50% of the muscle fibers, with a palpable defect in the muscle belly. A grade III muscle strain is an extensive tear or a complete rupture of the muscle fibers, affecting 50% to 100% of the muscle fibers. A large defect in the muscle is palpable, and normal contraction is impossible.

Symptoms

The severity of symptoms depends on the magnitude of injury. Symptoms generally include local pain, strength loss, mild swelling, ecchymosis, and local tenderness.

Clinically, grade III strains (muscle ruptures) present with muscle irregularity, a palpable defect, significant weakness, and loss of function. Patients describe the feeling during injury as a "pop"; pain and swelling occur acutely, secondary to intramuscular hemorrhage.

Differential Diagnosis

It may be necessary to differentiate a strain from a sprain, which can be done by assessing pain during ROM. Active and resisted ROM exercises may cause pain with a strain but not necessarily with a sprain.

Imaging Techniques

Muscle strains (including grade III ruptures) can be identified using axial T2-weighted magnetic resonance imaging views (**Figure 2-10**). Strains are not visible on plain radiographs.

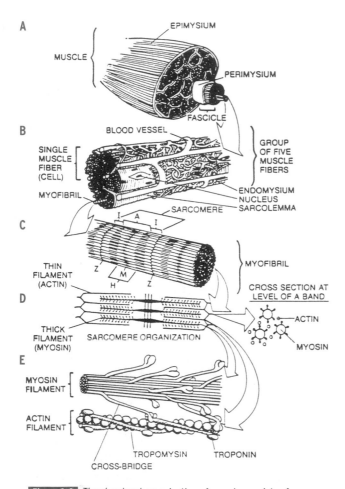

Figure 2-9 The structural organization of muscle consists of a connective-tissue framework and arranged muscle fibers. **A** and **B.** Connective tissue surrounds the epimysium, perimysium, and endomysium. **C.** Intricately arranged thick and thin filaments allow fibers to slide past each other in the sarcomere. Z-lines represent the ends of a sarcomere. **D.** Thick filaments are made up of a protein aggregate that consists of myosin, and thin filaments are made up of a protein aggregate that consists of actin, troponin, and tropomyosin. **E.** Bands and zones make up the sarcomere, enabling effective and efficient muscle contraction at the subcellular or molecular level. (Reproduced with permission from Pitman MI, Peterson L: Biomechanics of skeletal muscle, in Frankel VH, Nordin M (eds): *Basic Biomechanics of the Skeletal System*, ed 2. Philadelphia, PA, Lea & Febiger, 1989, p 90.)

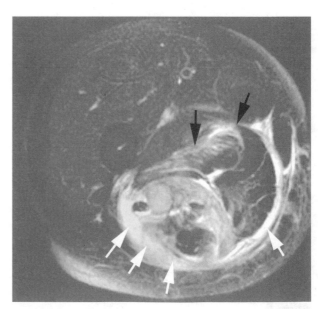

Figure 2-10 Magnetic resonance image of a hamstring strain showing increased fluids in the fascial planes (white arrows) and high signal intensity consistent with a strain of the hamstring muscles (black arrows). (Reproduced with permission from Johnson TR, Steinbach LS (eds): *Essentials of Musculoskeletal Imaging*. Rosemont, IL, American Academy of Orthopaedic Surgeons, 2004, p 556.)

Immediate Management

Strains are first treated with ice, compression, elevation, and protection.

Medical Management

A severe strain may be associated with the formation of a hematoma. Moist heat and massage are contraindicated early in the healing process to prevent the development of myositis ossificans (see next section).

Grade III strains may require surgical intervention for full recovery and optimal musculoskeletal performance. Grade III tendinous injuries are more amenable to surgical repair than intramuscular ruptures.

Inflammatory Conditions of Muscle and Tendon

Myositis/Myositis Ossificans

Myositis is an inflammation of muscle tissue as the result of infection (infectious myositis), trauma (traumatic myositis), diathetic states (polymyositis, dermatomyositis, and inclusion body myositis), or infestation by parasites (parasitic myositis). Traumatic myositis is the most common type seen in athletes. Through a metaplastic process similar to fracture callus formation, chondroid and osteoid scars form rather than the expected fibroblastic scar; this results in myositis ossificans, a myositis marked by ossification of the muscle.

Pathophysiology

Myositis is an inflammation of the connective tissue within a muscle.

Symptoms

Muscle weakness, heat, swelling, and pain are present. With myositis ossificans, a mass may be palpable. An ossified mass may be detectable radiographically after 2 to 3 weeks of persistent symptoms.

Imaging Techniques

Typically, myositis ossificans takes approximately 6 to 12 months to mature, and three-phase bone scans have been shown to be helpful in determining the maturity of the lesion. Computed tomography scans are useful for identifying subacute myositis (**Figure 2-11**). Mature (hardened) myositis eventually becomes apparent on plain radiographs.

Immediate Management

Myositis is first treated with ice, compression, elevation, and protection.

Medical Management

Surgical management of myositis ossificans is controversial. Early surgical intervention has been associated with deterioration of the condition, resulting in recurrence and lengthened disability. Some authors[7,8] have recommended surgical excision for persistent muscle atrophy, decreased ROM, and worsening pain after obtaining radiographic evidence that the lesion has matured. Delayed surgical intervention of symptomatic myositis ossificans has been associated with recurrence rates of up to 67%.

Tendinitis

Tendinitis is an inflammation of a tendon that is most commonly caused by overuse; however, trauma can also produce acute tendinitis. Pathologic changes consistent with chronic inflammation are usually observed. Tissue degeneration, characterized by cell atrophy, may also be noted. Calcium can be deposited along the course of the tendon (calcific tendinitis), with the shoulder being the most common site.

Histologically, tendon injury is characterized by mucoid degeneration, which is the loss of the normal cellularity and organized, crimped collagen fiber architecture that characterizes healthy tendon. Granulation tissue may also form, but inflammatory cells are usually absent unless the tendon is torn. The inflammation that characterizes tendinitis and paratenonitis with tendinosis may result from associated local vascular disruption.

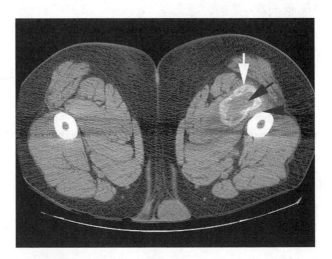

Figure 2-11 Computed tomographic scan of traumatic quadriceps myositis ossificans showing a well bounded mass with an ossified rim (white arrow) and a central unaffected area (black arrow). Note that the myositis is not in contact with the femur (black arrowhead). (Reproduced with permission from Johnson TR, Steinbach LS (eds): *Essentials of Musculoskeletal Imaging.* Rosemont, IL, American Academy of Orthopaedic Surgeons, 2004, p 49.)

The mechanism of tendon failure is believed to be inadequate production of maintenance collagen and matrix in response to increased loading. In addition, diminished vascularity also contributes by leading to decreased cellularity and consequently to decreased collagen production.

Tendinosis

Tendinosis is an intratendinous avascular degeneration that results in collagen disorientation, disorganization, and fiber separation because of an increase in mucoid ground substance, increased prominence of cells and vascular spaces with or without neovascularization, and focal necrosis or calcification. Tendinosis can refer to degeneration of a tendon from repetitive microtrauma, tendinitis without inflammation, or collagen degeneration.

Paratenonitis

Paratenonitis is inflammation of the paratenon and is synonymous with peritendinitis, tenosynovitis, and tenovaginitis. Paratenonitis occurs because the tendon sheath is susceptible to repeated pressure and friction.

Symptoms

Tendinitis causes pain over the affected tendon close to its insertion into the muscle. The pain is usually worsened by repetitive motion, but it can also be present at rest. Mild swelling may be seen over the tendon. Tendinosis is often asymptomatic or may present with a nontender, palpable nodule.

Immediate Management

Initial treatment of tendinitis is with ice, compression, elevation, and protection.

Medical Management

A severe strain may be associated with the formation of a hematoma. Extracorporeal shockwave therapy and ultrasound have shown good results with calcific tendinitis but remain under study. Extracorporeal shockwave therapy is currently approved by the US Food and Drug Administration only for treatment of plantar fasciitis and lateral epicondylitis. Use of this therapy for patellar tendinitis and fracture nonunion is awaiting approval.

Hypotonic and Hypertonic Conditions

Muscle Cramps

Muscle cramps are painful, involuntary contractions of muscles. Exercise-associated muscle cramps are the type generally encountered in sports medicine settings. Exercise-associated muscle cramps are painful, spasmodic, involuntary contractions that occur during or immediately after muscular exercise.

Muscles cannot function properly without both a continuous supply of nutrients and the continuous removal of waste. Cramps result when insufficient oxygen or nutrients are available or when waste products, such as lactic acid, accumulate. Muscle cramps can be the result of dehydration and electrolyte imbalance or an abnormal, sustained increase in α-motoneuron activity.

Symptoms

Muscle cramp symptoms include painful, sudden, involuntary contraction of the muscle, with visible or palpable localized knotting of the muscle.

Immediate Management

For mild cases, oral rehydration, stretching, ice, and gentle massage can eliminate the cramps.

Medical Management

For more severe cramps, intravenous rehydration is indicated to prevent the more serious forms of heat illness. Various intravenous solutions are used, including lactated Ringer's solution, normal saline, and various combinations of dextrose with saline. Athletes are apt to develop hyponatremia during prolonged exercise if fluid consumption exceeds fluid losses. In addition, hypotonic solutions used for intravenous rehydration of individuals with muscle cramps can exacerbate hyponatremia, leading to respiratory distress and mental status changes. Accordingly, hypotonic solutions for rehydration should be avoided.

See chapter 20, p 598 for further discussion regarding the management of heat-related muscle cramps.

Muscle Spasms

A spasm is an involuntary, sudden movement or muscular contraction that occurs as a result of an irritant, muscle injury, overuse, stress, dehydration, electrolyte imbalance, or poor posture.

Symptoms

Muscle spasms are characterized by restricted motion and painful or "tight" muscles that are tender to the touch.

Immediate Management

Oral rehydration, stretching, ice, and gentle massage can eliminate the spasms.

Medical Management

Nonsedating antispasmodics (eg, diazepam or metaxolone) are preferable for athletes. However, the use of antispasmodics should be deferred pending other modalities and nonpharmacologic therapies such as massage, acupressure, tissue mobilization, and electric muscle stimulation.

Contractures

Contractures may be caused by muscle imbalance, pain, prolonged bed rest, or immobilization that results in a fibrosis of connective tissue in skin, fascia, muscle, or a joint capsule that prevents normal mobility of the related tissue or joint.

Symptoms

Loss of joint motion is significant, resulting in immobility. Pain without any voluntary joint movement may be present in severe cases.

Immediate Management

Joint mobilization, soft-tissue stretching, continuous passive motion, or some combination of these should be instituted.

Medical Management

In severe cases, surgery or joint manipulation under general anesthesia may be necessary. These approaches are rare in sports medicine, however.

Arthrogenic Muscle Inhibition

Arthrogenic muscle inhibition is a presynaptic, ongoing reflex inhibition of the musculature surrounding a joint after distention or damage to structures of that joint.[9] Arthrogenic muscle inhibition is caused by presynaptic and postsynaptic inhibition at the motoneuron.

Symptoms

Arthrogenic muscle inhibition is characterized by diminished force output and control of the muscle.

Immediate Management

Early exercise after joint injury, particularly cryokinetics programs, and transcutaneous electric nerve stimulation may overcome the inhibitory response.

Medical Management

Medical management of arthrogenic muscle inhibition is largely undefined. Persistent arthrogenic muscle inhibition is thought to be unresolvable.

Atrophy

Atrophy is a wasting—a decrease in size of an organ or tissue as a result of disuse, aging, or disease. In orthopaedics, atrophy most commonly refers to muscular atrophy.

When atrophy occurs, cell size and function decrease in response to an environmental signal. Protein synthesis decreases, as does cell division, energy production, energy storage, and contractility. Immobilization is one cause of muscle cell atrophy. Other causes include denervation, inadequate oxygen supply or nutrition, hormonal deficiency, chronic inflammation, and aging.

Tissue degeneration implies a weaker structure. Tissues become more vulnerable to sudden dynamic overload or cyclic overloading, which may lead to fatigue and failure. Traumatic disruption can cause vascular injury and initiate a renewed inflammation repair process.

Symptoms

Atrophy is characterized by loss of muscle mass and force-producing capabilities.

Immediate Management

The first line of treatment is active exercise, possibly augmented by submotor neuromuscular electric stimulation.

Medical Management

The most commonly encountered form of atrophy following musculoskeletal trauma is disuse atrophy. Recovery of an atrophied cell requires a balance of rest and physical stimulation. Returning to activity after prolonged inactivity without substantially improved tissue integrity increases the risk of reinjury of the involved tissue. For this reason, protected activity or controlled therapeutic exercise is usually a better treatment than complete rest to maintain musculoskeletal integrity.

General principles to prevent disuse atrophy and to restore form and function include:

- Encourage early mobilization activities.
- Reduce pain (pain can cause muscle inhibition during rehabilitation).
- Restore muscle flexibility, endurance, and strength with a graded program.
- Return the patient to sport-specific training.
- Protect the area of atrophy against further injury.
- Restore cardiovascular endurance.
- Optimize nutrition with an emphasis on moderate increase in protein intake without compromising nutritional balance.

Ligament Injuries

Ligaments and joint capsules connect bone to bone and augment the mechanical stability of joints, guide joint motion, and prevent abnormal motion. Type I collagen is the major structural component of ligaments, accounting for 70% of dry weight.[10] Ligaments and tendons share a similar ultrastructure with comparable fascicular arrangements of highly oriented, highly packed collagen fibers that provide tensile strength and flexibility.[11] Ligaments also have much lower thickness-to-width ratios, and their fiber orientation varies more. In addition, ligaments contain less collagen, more glycosaminoglycans, and more elastin than tendons.

Some ligaments are composed of more than one band of fibrils or bundles. As the joint moves through its ROM, different bands of fibrils become taut to allow for greater flexibility. For example, the anteromedial bundle of the anterior cruciate ligament becomes tight as the knee flexes, and the posterolateral bundle becomes taut during knee extension.

Ligaments receive their blood supply from their insertion site on bone. They house mechanoreceptors that provide proprioceptive feedback and initiate protective reflexes.

■ Sprains

A sprain occurs when trauma from tensile or shear forces (or both) is delivered to a joint, causing pain and disability, depending on the degree of injury to the ligaments. The collagen fibers within the ligament lose their crimp and progressively fail as these forces increase. In sports medicine, a sprain is typically defined as any disruption to the integrity of a ligament.

Sprains are graded according to the magnitude of the tear and resultant joint instability. A grade I sprain is a partial tear to the ligament without instability or joint opening during a stress maneuver. A grade II sprain is a partial tear with some instability and partial opening of the joint during a stress maneuver. A grade III sprain is a complete tear of the ligament with complete opening of the joint during a stress maneuver.

Pathophysiology
Damaged ligaments are subject to inflammation.

Symptoms
Local tenderness, swelling, ecchymosis, and impaired function are present.

Differential Diagnosis
Sprains may need to be differentiated from avulsion fractures or muscle strain. Muscle strain can be identified by assessing pain during ROM; active and resisted ROM exercises may cause pain with a strain but not necessarily with a sprain.

Imaging Techniques
Plain radiographs may be ordered to rule out an avulsion fracture. Magnetic resonance imaging or computed tomography can identify complete or partial tearing of the ligament.

Immediate Management
Initial treatment includes ice, compression, elevation, and protection to avoid further injury.

Medical Management
General indications for surgical repair of sprains include:

- Persistent dysfunction despite conservative management
- Associated bony avulsion
- Most injuries with multidirectional instability
- Ankle sprains in prepubescents with Salter-Harris type III through V fractures (see p 40)
- Displaced osteochondral avulsion of the talar dome
- Most grade III sprains not amenable to medical management. However, many exceptions exist to this rule. For example, medial collateral ligament sprains in soccer players are rarely repaired surgically because of equivocal results, both from conservative management as well as surgical intervention.

Fascia

Fascia is a flat band of tissue below the skin that covers underlying tissues and separates different layers of tissue; fascia also encloses muscle. The most common injuries to the fascia are myofascial pain syndrome and fasciitis.

■ Myofascial Pain Syndrome

Specific definitions of myofascial pain syndrome vary in the literature. It is generally characterized as a painful musculoskeletal response after muscle trauma involving sensory, motor, and autonomic phenomena.[12] The key feature of myofascial pain syndrome is the presence of trigger points, which may be caused by any of the following:

- Sudden trauma to the musculoskeletal tissues
- Injury to the intervertebral disks
- Generalized fatigue
- Repetitive motion, excessive exercise, or muscle strain due to overactivity
- Inactivity
- Nutritional deficiencies

- Hormonal changes (eg, premenstrual syndrome or menopause)
- Nervous tension or stress
- Chilling of areas of the body (eg, sitting under an air-conditioning duct or sleeping in front of an air conditioner)

Symptoms

Myofascial pain syndrome is distinguished by the development of myofascial trigger points that are locally tender when active and refer pain through specific patterns to other areas of the body. A trigger point develops from any number of causes and is usually associated with a taut band, a rope-like thickening of the muscle tissue. Pressing on a trigger point typically causes referred pain.

Immediate Management

Stretch and spray (a vapocoolant is sprayed on the trigger point to lessen the pain and then the muscle is stretched), massage, and exercise are used in the early management of myofascial pain.

Medical Management

Therapeutic massage seems to be the most effective treatment. Chronic pain modulation with analgesics can be detrimental to the patient's long-term health. Trigger points can be injected with a local anesthetic. Dry needling may also be used.

Fasciitis

Fasciitis, inflammation of the fascia, results from repetitive trauma to the fascia. Often, the fascia is exposed to repetitive tensile loads that result in an inflammatory process. This repeated trauma frequently causes microscopic tearing of the fascia at or near the point of attachment of the tissue. The result of the damage and inflammation is pain.

Symptoms

Fasciitis is characterized by dull, aching pain that may improve with rest.

Immediate Management

Initial treatment is ice and rest.

Medical Management

Treatment may be augmented by ultrasound, phonophoresis, Neuroprobe (Accelerated Care Plus, Sparks, NV), contrast baths, transverse friction and deep tissue massage, or augmented soft-tissue mobilization.

Synovial Tissue

The synovium is a thin, weak layer of tissue only a few cells thick that lines the joint space. The synovium controls the environment within the joint in two ways. First, it acts as a membrane to determine what can pass into the joint space and what stays outside. Second, the synovial cells produce substances such as hyaluronan, which is a component of joint fluid. The most common injuries to the synovium are synovitis and bursitis.

Synovitis

Synovitis is inflammation of a synovial membrane (**Figure 2-12**).

Symptoms

Pain, particularly with movement, and swelling are present.

Immediate Management

Initial management of synovitis is with ice and rest.

Medical Management

Management of synovitis is based on the cause. Rheumatologic causes of synovitis must be ruled out using comprehensive blood tests. A synovial biopsy may be needed to determine the exact cause (ie, inflammatory, infectious, or posttraumatic).

Bursitis

Bursitis is an inflammation of a bursa as a result of repetitive movement or direct trauma to the bursal sac.

Pathophysiology

Inflammation of the bursal sac occurs as a result of repetitive movement or trauma.

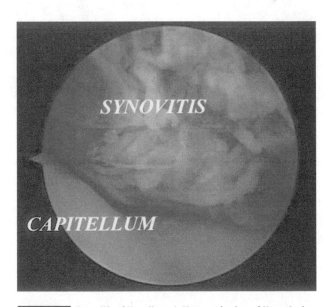

Figure 2-12 Synovitis of the elbow. Arthroscopic view of the anterior aspect of the elbow joint as seen from the anterolateral portal. Proliferative synovial tissue is visible over the capitellum. (Reproduced with permission from Horiuchi K, Momohara S, Tomatsu T, et al: Arthroscopic synovectomy of the elbow in rheumatoid arthritis. *J Bone Joint Surg Am* 2002;84:342-347.)

Symptoms

Bursitis is characterized by a dull ache or stiffness, pain worsening with movement or pressure, swelling, palpable warmth, and occasionally redness of the skin overlying the bursa.

Immediate Management

Initial treatment is with ice, compression, elevation, and protection.

Medical Management

The goal of medical management is to treat the cause of the bursitis, such as leg-length discrepancy, exaggerated Q-angle, or overuse issues.

■ References

1. Guyton AC, Hall JE: *Textbook of Medical Physiology,* ed 10. Philadelphia, PA, WB Saunders, 2001.

2. Luster AD: Chemokines: Chemotactic cytokines that mediate inflammation. *N Engl J Med* 1998;338:436-445.

3. Efron DT, Barbul A: Modulation of inflammation and immunity by arginine supplements. *Curr Opin Clin Nutr Metab Care* 1998;1:531-538.

4. Polla BS, Bachelet M, Elia G, Santoro MG: Stress proteins in inflammation. *Ann N Y Acad Sci* 1998;851:75-85.

5. Malm C, Nyberg P, Engstrom M, et al: Immunological changes in human skeletal muscle and blood after eccentric exercise and multiple biopsies. *J Physiol* 2000;529:243-262.

6. Claus EE, Fusco CF, Ingram T, Ingersoll CD, Edwards JE, Melham TJ: Comparison of the effects of selected dressings on the healing of standardized abrasions. *J Athl Train* 1998;33:145-149.

7. Jackson DW: Quadriceps contusions in young athletes. *J Bone Joint Surg Am* 1973;55:95-105.

8. Ryan JB, Wheeler JH, Hopkinson WJ, et al: Quadriceps contusions: West Point update. *Am J Sports Med* 1991;19:299-304.

9. Starkey C: *Therapeutic Modalities,* ed 3. Philadelphia, PA, FA Davis, 2004, p 24.

10. Fu FH, Harner CD, Vince KG (eds): *Knee Surgery*. Baltimore, MD, Williams & Wilkins, 1994.

11. Hopkins JT, Ingersoll CD: Arthrogenic muscle inhibition: A limiting factor in joint rehabilitation. *J Sport Rehabil* 2000;9:135-159.

12. Travell J, Simons D: *Myofascial Pain and Dysfunction: The Trigger Point Manual. The Upper Extremities*. Baltimore, MD, Williams & Wilkins, 1983.

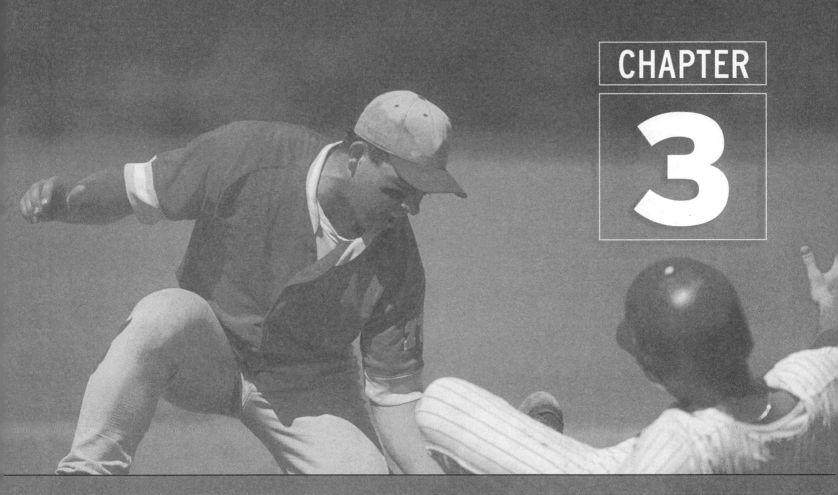

Fractures: Diagnosis and Management

Christopher D. Ingersoll,
PhD, ATC, FACSM
David M. Kahler, MD

After injury, most tissues in the human body heal by replacing the injured tissue with a dense collagen scar. This same general healing process is seen in all injured soft-tissue structures. Bone is unique as the only tissue in the body that can completely restore itself to its original form after injury via inflammatory, early reparative, late reparative, and remodeling phases. Through the process of fracture healing and remodeling, bone eventually assumes its original microscopic structure and form, ultimately regaining the same resistance to further stress as the original, uninjured structure. The goal of fracture management is to restore form and function. The rigid, biphasic composition of bone allows use of treatment options that are not available for soft tissue.

Many fractures will heal without surgical intervention. In general, surgical intervention to stabilize a fractured bone actually slows down the normal healing process. The goals of treatment for osseous injuries are to maintain anatomic length and alignment during the healing process while doing as little as possible to disturb the normal biology of fracture healing. For particular fracture patterns in certain locations, optimal preservation of form and function is provided by early surgical fixation of the fracture; this allows early motion of adjacent joints while preserving anatomic length and alignment. A fracture in a high-performance athlete may, therefore, be treated more aggressively than a fracture in a more sedentary person to expedite the athlete's return to function and participation. Athletes may also be candidates for adjunctive therapies such as low-intensity ultrasonic bone growth generators or electromagnetic bone growth stimulators that may accelerate the normal biology of fracture healing (**Figure 3-1**).

Anastomose The junction or connection between two structures such as blood vessels.

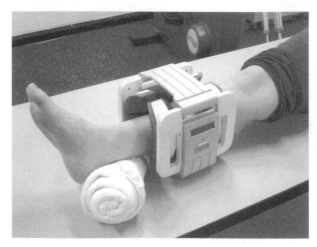

Figure 3-1 Electrical bone growth stimulator. This device, used once per day, uses electromagnetic fields to stimulate osteogenesis.

Qualities of Bone Tissue

Bone is designed to provide support and protection. It is a biphasic composite material, providing rigidity, yet also allowing flexibility.[1] Like other tissues, bone contains an organic extracellular matrix of fibers and a ground substance. However, bone is unique because of its high content of inorganic materials. Mineral salts combine with organic components to make bone both hard and rigid while allowing flexibility and resilience. The mineral portion of bone is primarily calcium and phosphate. These minerals account for 65% to 70% of the dry weight of bone.

Protein collagen, the fibrous portion of the extracellular matrix, is tough and pliable but resists stretching and has little extensibility. This collagen accounts for 95% of the extracellular matrix and 25% to 30% of the dry weight of bone.

Ground substance is a gelatinous material that surrounds the mineralized collagen fibers. It is composed primarily of protein polysaccharides called glycosaminoglycans (GAGs), which serve as a glue between the layers of the mineralized collagen fibers. The ground substance comprises approximately 5% of the extracellular matrix.

Water is also abundant in bone, accounting for up to 25% of live bone weight. Most (85%) of the water is in the organic matrix, with the remaining 15% found in various canals and cavities throughout the bone.

The osteon (also called the haversian system) is the fundamental structural unit of bone and consists of concentric layers of mineralized matrix, called lamellae, surrounding a central haversian canal (**Figure 3-2**). The outer edges of the lamellae contain small cavities called lacunae. A single osteocyte is contained within the lacunae. Small channels called canaliculi radiate out from each lacuna, connecting lacunae in adjacent lamellae. This interconnecting network of canaliculi ultimately contacts the haversian canal, allowing nutrients to reach the osteocytes.

Osteons, approximately 200 μm in diameter, usually run longitudinally but can branch and anastomose with one another. The haversian canals of individual osteons are interconnected to one another via Volkmann canals.

Osteons form two types of osseous tissue—cortical bone and cancellous bone. Cortical, or compact, bone forms the hard, outer shell of the bone. Also called the cortex, cortical bone has a dense structure similar to ivory (**Figure 3-3**). Cancellous,

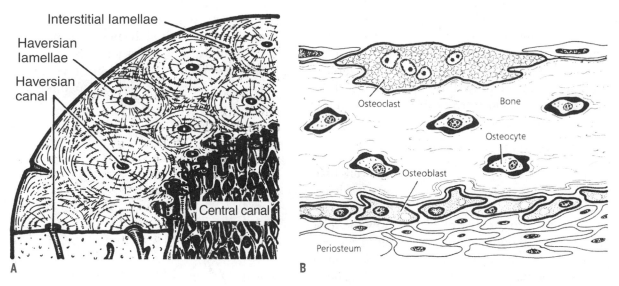

Figure 3-2 Cellular anatomy of bone. **A.** Osteon consists of concentric layers of mineralized matrix around a central canal. The haversian canal is at the center of the osteon. **B.** Bone cells are composed of osteoclasts, osteoblasts, and osteocytes.

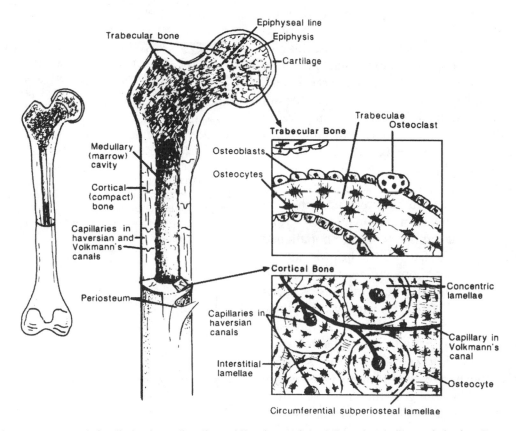

Figure 3-3 All bones are composed of cortical and cancellous tissue at the microscopic level. (Reproduced with permission from Keaveny TM, Hayes WC: Mechanical properties of cortical and trabecular bone, in Hall BK (ed): *Bone, Volume VII: A Treatise*. Boca Raton, FL, CRC Press, 1992, pp 285-344.)

or trabecular, bone is contained within the cortical shell. It is formed of thin plates called trabeculae, in a loose mesh structure. Red marrow is contained within the trabeculae. Cancellous bone is arranged in lamellae but does not contain haversian canals. Nutrients pass through the red marrow to the canali-

culi. The percentage of cortical and cancellous bone varies among individual bones, depending on the functional requirements of that bone.

Bones are classified according to their morphology into three groups—long, short, and flat. Bones are further described according to certain anatomic characteristics. Long bones, for example, have a diaphysis (shaft), metaphyses (flares at the ends), and epiphyses (rounded ends at a joint). A physis separates the epiphysis from the metaphysis and serves as the growth center for a long bone. Other areas on bones are described based on their shape, function, or both.

Biomechanical Properties

Bone is an anisotropic material,[2] which means that it exhibits different mechanical properties when loaded along different axes. A classic example of anisotropic bone is the proximal femur just below the lesser trochanter. All human bone is stronger in compression than in tension. The subtrochanteric region of the femur is placed in pure compressive load on the medial cortex and pure tensile load on the lateral cortex during normal ambulation or running. Its anatomic structure is well designed to withstand these stresses. If the pattern of stresses is reversed, or if a severe torsional load is applied to this area, the proximal femur may fail by fracturing. Because this area of bone is never subjected to expansile forces from within, insertion of an implant into the canal of the femur may result in increased barrel or hoop stresses and cause a longitudinal fracture. Anisotropy refers to the fact that the bone behaves differently when stressed in directions other than those usually encountered during physiologic loading.

Bone also has the unique ability to remodel along lines of stress. In immature bone in the very young and in new bone formation after a fracture, the bone trabeculae and osteons are not aligned along lines of stress. During the healing and remodeling process, the bony architecture is gradually remodeled into a form that best resists stresses applied to the bone. During normal growth, bone is subjected to various tensile and compressive stresses during daily activities, and the immature bone is remodeled into a structure ideally suited to withstand these stresses. If new stresses are applied—whether from growth, a new conditioning drill, or a new sport—the bone can gradually remodel to accommodate the new lines of stress. When this remodeling process is too slow to accommodate a rapid change in stress applied to the bone, a stress fracture may occur. After injury, the architecture of the bone is gradually remodeled into a form that best resists the applied stresses. For this reason, rehabilitating acute fractures and stress fractures requires that stresses be gradually applied to the bone during the healing process in order to avoid refracture.

The stress-strain curve (**Figure 3-4**) provides a key to understanding the mechanical properties of bone. The various forces and torques that may be presented to bone result in tension, compression, bending, and shear (**Figure 3-5**). Combinations of these loads can also occur.[3]

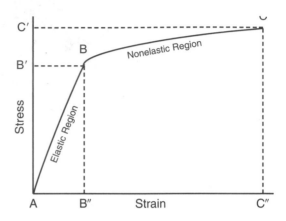

Figure 3-4 A stress-strain curve illustrates the strain that results from placing a standard specimen of tissue in a testing device and loading it to failure. Yield point B represents the point past which some permanent deformation of bone occurs, yield stress B' represents the load per unit area that the bone sample sustained before nonelastic deformation, and yield strain B" represents the total amount of deformation the sample sustained before nonelastic deformation. Ultimate failure point C is the point past which the sample failed, ultimate stress C' is the load per unit area the sample sustained before failure, and ultimate strain C" shows the amount of deformation that the sample sustained before failure. (Reproduced with permission from Frankel VH, Nordin M (eds): *Basic Biomechanics of the Skeletal System*, ed 2. Philadelphia, PA, Lea & Febiger, 1989.)

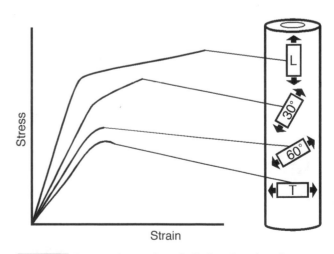

Figure 3-5 Forces and moments applied to bone in various directions produce tension, compression, bending, shear, torsion, and combined loading. (Reproduced with permission from Frankel VH, Nordin M (eds): *Basic Biomechanics of the Skeletal System*, ed 2. Philadelphia, PA, Lea & Febiger, 1989.)

Fracture Categories

Fractures are characterized according to the injured bone, the location of the fracture in that bone, the amount of fracture displacement or malalignment, and the condition of the soft-tissue envelope about the injured bone[4] (**Table 3-1**).

Fractures are generally categorized using a mechanistic classification that describes both the orientation of the fracture line and the degree of displacement. The initial clinical examination, however, separates fractures into closed fractures, with various degrees of soft-tissue injury, and open fractures, in which the bone has either protruded through the skin or a penetrating injury has caused the fracture. The descriptive terms *open* and *closed* are now preferred to the older traditional terms *compound* and *simple*. Further classification includes differentiation between nondisplaced fractures, in which a radiographic cleft can be seen but no gap exists between the fracture fragments, and displaced fractures, in which a gap or malalignment can be seen on radiographs (**Figure 3-6**).

Fracture displacement can be described as distracted, shortened, translated, or angulated. Distracted displacement (a visible gap at the fracture site) generally occurs due to the weight of an unsupported, injured limb. This condition is often seen in a midshaft humeral fracture. Oblique and spiral fractures of long bones frequently shorten due to muscular forces, and the degree

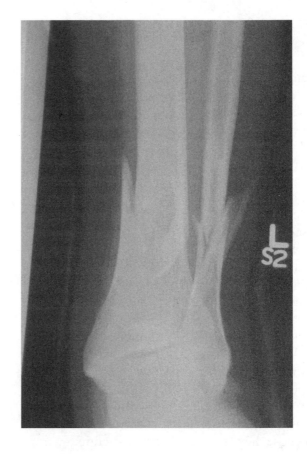

Figure 3-6 Radiograph demonstrates displaced fractures of the shaft of the tibia and fibula. The displaced fractures show translational displacement, shortening, and angulation. The spiral pattern of the fractures suggests a twisting mechanism combined with axial loading.

of shortening can often be estimated by measuring the radiographic displacement. Translational displacement occurs when traumatic or muscular forces cause malalignment, with or without angulation of the fracture fragments; in other words, a fracture may be well aligned (axes of the bone are parallel) but translationally displaced in any direction.

Angulation is described based on the apex of angulation. The apex of angulation may be described as medial, lateral, anterior, or posterior in any extremity. For example, a midshaft femoral fracture that has assumed a flexed position has the apex of angulation directed anteriorly. In the forearm, the apex of angulation is frequently described as toward the radius or ulna, or the volar or dorsal direction. Specific orthopaedic terms used to describe angulation in the coronal plane are varus (away from the midline) or valgus (toward the midline).

Table 3-1

Basic Fracture Categories

Fracture Type	Description
Nondisplaced	Bone fragments are in anatomic alignment.
Displaced	Bone fragments are no longer in their usual anatomic alignment.
	Malaligned fragments: angulated displacement
	Distal fragment longitudinally overlaps the proximal fragment: bayonetted displacement
	Distal fragment separated from the proximal fragment by a gap: distracted displacement
Closed	A fracture with no associated penetrating skin wound
Open	Fragments of bone protrude through the skin, or an external wound leads to the fracture site.

Radiologic Techniques

Plain radiographs, fluoroscopy, computed tomography (CT), and magnetic resonance imaging (MRI) described in chapter 1 are used to definitively diagnose fractures. Plain radiography is often the only radiologic technique required to confirm the presence, shape, and severity of a fracture. Fractures involving the articular surface may require the use of CT or MRI. MRI is also useful in identifying intra-articular loose bodies, skeletal malformations, and associated soft-tissue lesions.

Scintigraphy (bone scans) is a type of nuclear medicine used to image increased bone-related metabolic activity associated with stress fractures or diseases. A radioisotope such as technetium Tc 99m is injected into the patient's body. Once enough time has been allotted to allow the isotope to be absorbed, the body part is imaged. Areas of increased uptake of the isotope may be indicative of a stress fracture. Scintigraphy indicates only the area of increased metabolic activity, lacks the precise anatomic detail of other imaging techniques, and does not definitively diagnose the presence of a stress fracture.

Evaluation of a Suspected Fracture

The typical signs and symptoms of a suspected fracture are pain, swelling, tenderness, loss of function, and occasionally crepitus or deformity.[4] The diagnosis is obvious when angulation is severe. Nonetheless, with a deformity near the end of a long bone, ligament injury, joint dislocation, and growth plate injury must be included in the differential diagnosis. A deformed extremity such as a protruding bone is always a dramatic physical finding that can distract from other, potentially more serious trauma such as chest, abdominal, or brain injury.

The initial evaluation of a suspected fracture should always include a careful neurologic and vascular examination distal to the injury. The presence and symmetry of pulses and motor and sensory function for all major nerves crossing the injury site must be documented. The initial examination is extremely important because a worsening neurologic presentation usually warrants aggressive intervention.

Radiographic evaluation of a suspected fracture should include two views taken 90° from each other and encompassing both adjacent joints. If a fracture is suspected but not seen on initial radiographs, additional special views may be taken, or CT or MRI studies may be considered.

Fracture Types

Greenstick Fracture

A greenstick fracture occurs in response to a bending force (**Figure 3-7**). The side that experiences tension will fracture. The cortex on the side experiencing compression remains intact but undergoes plastic deformation; bone fails on the weaker tension side, and the stronger compression side maintains integrity, despite bending through plastic deformation. The resultant fracture appears as a transverse fracture into the midsubstance of the bone, intersecting with a longitudinal fracture. Bones in children tend

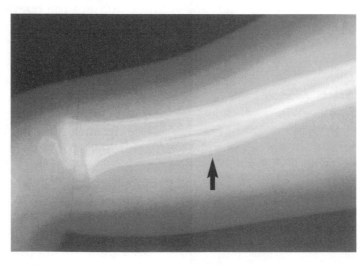

Figure 3-7 Greenstick fracture. This type of fracture is prevalent in children because of their pliable bones.

to have a relatively low content of inorganic material and higher extracellular matrix content compared with adults. Therefore, the child's bone is more pliable and more likely to bend without breaking.

Because greenstick fractures occur exclusively in children, the differential diagnosis for any deformity near the end of a long bone must include injury to the growth plate or ligaments. However, greenstick fractures usually occur in the diaphysis or metadiaphysis and typically remain significantly angulated after injury, leaving little doubt as to the diagnosis.

Prognosis

The prognosis for a greenstick fracture depends on the degree of initial displacement. In nearly every greenstick fracture involving a long bone in a growing patient, 10° of angulation may be acceptable. In certain patients (varus angulation of the tibia, for example), more precise restoration is required. Angulation of up to 10° in the diaphysis of a long bone is usually readily remodeled to normal alignment during the healing process. A greenstick fracture near the end of the long bone, however, may sometimes develop progressive angulation, particularly in the proximal tibia, requiring long-term follow-up. Although a greenstick fracture can often be partially reduced by applying external forces and a cast, it is sometimes nec-

essary to anesthetize the patient and complete the fracture on the compression side to adequately reduce the malalignment. This reduction of the malalignment without a skin incision is termed a closed reduction. Greenstick fractures are almost always treated with closed reduction rather than open surgical reduction, and reduction is maintained by external means such as a cast or splint rather than internal fixation.

Remodeling is generally far more rapid in children than in adults. Remodeling of angular deformities is particularly rapid when the deformity is in the same plane of motion as the nearest joint or when the deformity is near a rapidly growing physis. Remodeling of rotational deformities is less reliable and should not be expected to provide an acceptable result. Closed reduction for rotational deformities is recommended.

■ Transverse Fracture

Transverse fractures result from a direct blow or pure bending forces, producing a fracture line that is perpendicular to the long axis of the bone (**Figure 3-8**). The weaker tension side of the bone fails before the compression side. If an axial load is applied to the bone at the time of the bending force, the bone typically fails with a "butterfly" fragment on the concave side of the bending forces.

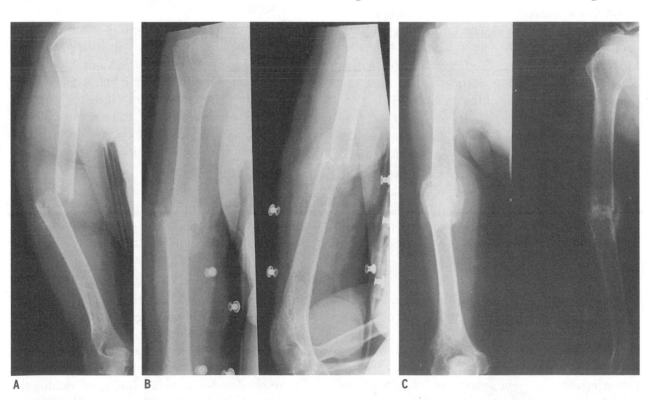

A   B   C

Figure 3-8 This transverse fracture of the humeral shaft was treated with application of an external fracture brace. **A.** Initial radiograph. **B.** Radiographs at 4 weeks demonstrate the formation of early peripheral callus. **C.** Radiographs at 4 months. The fracture healed with minimal varus angulation. (Reproduced with permission from Sarmiento A, Latta LL: Functional fracture bracing. *J Am Acad Orthop Surg* 1999;7:66-75.)

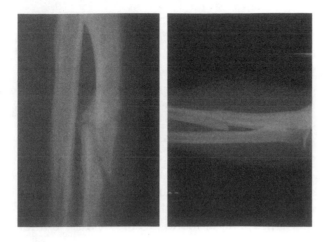

Figure 3-9 Radiographs showing nightstick, or tapping, fractures of the ulna.

An example of a typical transverse fracture is a "nightstick" fracture of the ulna, which is caused by a direct blow to the subcutaneous surface of the ulna. This is sometimes called a "tapping" fracture and is often seen in lacrosse players (**Figure 3-9**).

Prognosis

These low-energy injuries can often be treated nonsurgically. The prognosis is generally good if there is no displacement and the fracture is closed.

■ Oblique Fracture

Oblique fractures occur in response to compressive (axial) loads, and the bone fails through shear forces, producing a fracture line approximately 45° to the long axis (**Figure 3-10**). The failure mechanism is usually oblique breaking of the osteons, and these fractures tend to occur in the metaphysis.

Differential Diagnosis

Oblique fractures typically demonstrate some shortening due to the mechanism of injury (longitudinal or axial loading) and angulation at the fracture site. Oblique fractures may be differentiated from spiral fractures by their radiographic appearance. Oblique fractures appear to have blunt ends, whereas spiral fractures usually have sharp ends like the nib of a fountain pen.

Prognosis

The prognosis for an oblique fracture depends on the amount of initial displacement. Minimally displaced fractures are frequently treated nonsurgically. Fractures that have significantly shortened the bones disrupt the blood supply to the bone ends and often require surgery. The amount of initial displacement has also been correlated with the time required for bone healing. Severely displaced oblique fractures may require bone grafting to obtain bony union.

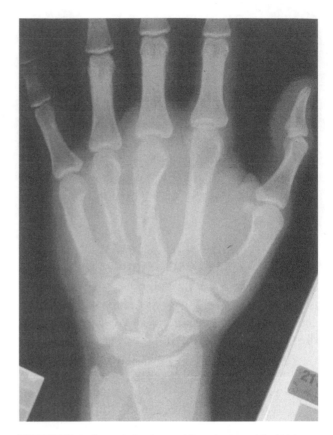

Figure 3-10 Radiograph showing an oblique fracture of the third metacarpal of the thumb.

■ Spiral Fracture

Spiral fractures occur as a result of torsion, a twisting about the long axis of the bone that produces a helical fracture line (**Figure 3-11**). A spiral fracture is characterized by a fracture line that twists around the bone and is connected by a longitudinal fracture line. Shear, compressive, and tension loads occur during torsion. The fracture occurs due to failure in shear followed by failure in tension.

Prognosis

Internal fixation, either with an intramedullary rod for a midshaft fracture or a plate and screws near the end of a bone, is often the treatment of choice for severely displaced spiral fractures.

■ Avulsion Fracture

Avulsion fractures occur from tensile loading at the site of ligament or tendon insertion (**Figure 3-12**). A sudden traction load applied to the ligament or tendon pulls, or avulses, a fragment of bone away from the epiphysis or metaphysis. Common sites for avulsion fractures include the greater tuberosity of the humerus, the various apophyses about the pelvis, the tibial tubercle, and the tip of the fibula.

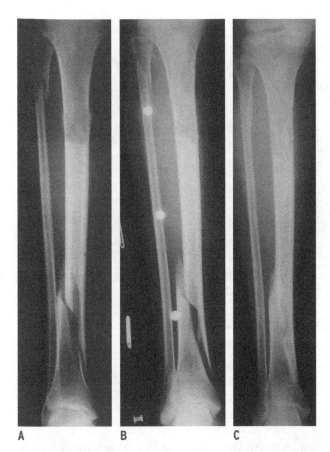

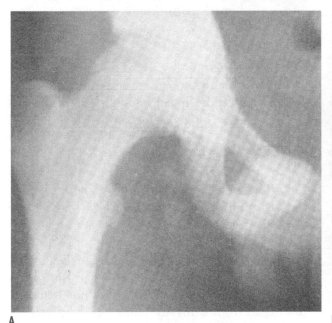

A   B   C

Figure 3-11 A spiral fracture of the distal tibia and proximal fibula.
A. Initial radiograph. **B.** Radiograph 10 days later (taken through a brace).
C. Radiograph at 1 year. (Reproduced with permission from Sarmiento A,
Latta LL: Functional fracture bracing. *J Am Acad Orthop Surg* 1999;7:66-75.)

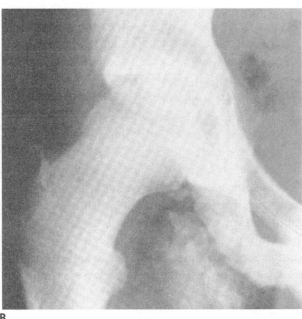

A   B

Figure 3-12 Radiographs of an avulsion fracture of the ischial tuberosity. **A.** Anterior view. **B.** Posterior view.

Prognosis

The prognosis for an avulsion fracture depends on the location and amount of displacement. As little as 5 mm of displacement in a greater tuberosity fracture may warrant surgical reduction and fixation in order to restore normal rotator cuff function. Conversely, avulsions of the ischial apophysis or anterior-superior iliac spine of the pelvis are often widely displaced but rarely require surgical management. In general, avulsion fractures are treated surgically if they are very close to a joint or if the degree of displacement suggests they may not heal in a position allowing restoration of normal function.

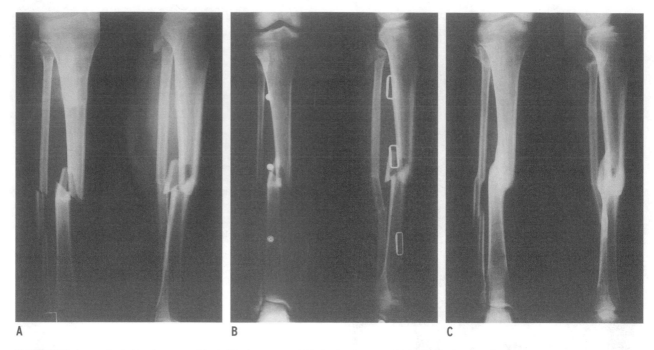

Figure 3-13 A comminuted fracture associated with a two-segment fibular fracture. **A.** Initial radiographs. **B.** Radiographs at 2 weeks (taken through a brace). **C.** Radiographs at 11 months. (Reproduced with permission from Sarmiento A, Latta LL: Functional fracture bracing. *J Am Acad Orthop Surg* 1999;7:66-75.)

Comminuted Fracture

A comminuted fracture involves failure of the bone at two or more sites (**Figure 3-13**). This fracture is the result of compression, tensile, or shearing forces or some combination of these forces. Comminution at a fracture site indicates that the bone has absorbed a large quantity of energy before fracture and significant soft-tissue injury may have occurred to the nerves, muscles, and blood vessels around the fracture site. The term *segmental fracture* is used to describe a fracture of the bony diaphysis in two separate places, a pattern seen exclusively in high-energy injuries such as violent collisions. Another common type of comminuted fracture is a shattering injury to either the tibial plateau or tibial plafond or the distal radius, in which the joint surfaces are broken into multiple pieces by a sudden, violent axial load.

Prognosis

The goals of treatment for comminuted fractures are generally the same as for other fracture patterns. However, because these are high-energy injuries, it is usually more difficult to maintain anatomic length and alignment with closed methods, and surgery is often indicated. Fractures involving the articular surface usually require open reduction to restore normal alignment of the joint surface, followed by internal fixation using screws and buttress plates or, occasionally, an external fixator. Even if the frac-

ture heals in anatomic position, joint stiffness, pain, and posttraumatic arthritis are common outcomes.

Epiphyseal Fracture

Epiphyseal fractures involve the separation of the epiphysis from the bone between the shaft and its growing end. Epiphyseal fractures can occur as a result of shearing, avulsion, splitting, or crush mechanisms.

The Salter-Harris classification describes damage to the epiphyseal plate, with or without a fracture (**Figure 3-14**). A type I injury has no bony fracture, but the epiphysis separates at the level of the entire physeal plate. Type II injuries, the most common pediatric fractures, involve separation of part of the epiphysis from the metaphysis through the physeal plate, plus a metaphyseal fracture. Type III injuries rarely occur. The fracture line extends from the joint space to the physeal plate and then laterally to the edge of the plate, separating the fractured epiphysis from the metaphysis. Type IV fractures extend from the joint space through the growth plate and across the metaphysis. Type V is a severe crush injury of the physeal plate itself. Displacement is unusual, and the injury may be unnoticed.

Prognosis

If adequately reduced by closed reduction, type I and II Salter-Harris epiphyseal fractures usually have a good prognosis, even if less than perfectly reduced.

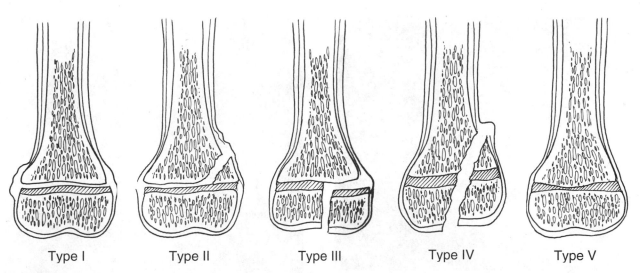

Figure 3-14   Salter-Harris classification of fractures. Type I is characterized by physeal separation; type II by a fracture line that extends transversely through the physis and exits through the metaphysis; type III by a fracture that traverses the physis and exits through the epiphysis; and type IV by a fracture line that passes through the epiphysis, across the physis, and out the metaphysis. Type V is a crush injury to the physis. (Reproduced with permission from Kay RM, Matthys GA: Pediatric ankle fractures: Evaluation and treatment. *J Am Acad Orthop Surg* 2001;9:268-278.)

Type II injuries, however, lead to growth disturbances in 5% of children. Type III fractures must be reduced perfectly and may require an open technique and wire fixation; even so, the prognosis is usually poor. Type IV fractures almost always necessitate open reduction and smooth wire fixation. The prognosis is poor for type IV and V fractures. Interruption of growth of the epiphyseal growth plate often accompanies type V fractures.

The significance of a fracture involving the epiphysis or physis is that a subsequent disturbance in growth may occur. Early fusion of the epiphysis may lead to a growth disturbance, and asymmetric fusion through a fracture line may result in progressive angulatory deformity as the uninjured portion of the physis grows while the injured portion does not. Physeal and epiphyseal injuries should generally be followed by a pediatric orthopaedic surgeon for assessment of potential growth disturbance until the patient is skeletally mature.

Impacted Fracture

A result of compressive forces, impacted fractures have one side of the fracture wedged into the interior of the other end of the bone (**Figure 3-15**). Impacted fractures generally occur in the metaphyseal regions because of axial loading: the more rigid cortical diaphysis is typically forced into the cancellous metaphysis. These fractures occur most frequently in aging individuals with osteoporosis. Many impacted fractures can be treated nonsurgically, provided there is no worrisome angulation through the fracture site or significant (> 5 mm) intra-articular depression.

Prognosis

The prognosis for impacted fractures is generally good unless the fracture extends into the joint and causes articular irregularities. Severe impaction leading to angulation of the metaphysis or articular surface may also require open reduction to restore normal joint range of motion. In general, the cancellous bone surfaces in impacted fractures heal very rapidly and therapeutic motion may be started immediately because these fractures are usually stable.

Intra-articular Fracture

Articular fractures involve a portion of the articular surface of the joint and are frequently caused by severe axial loads or combined axial loading and angular deviation (**Figure 3-16**). The articular cartilage and underlying bone are typically fractured. Intra-articular fractures involve the joint surfaces at the ends of the bone and often require surgical management to restore articular congruity.

Differential Diagnosis

Pain, swelling, significant joint effusion, and severe restriction of joint motion occur. A **lipohemarthrosis** is essentially always present in articular fractures because of leakage of the bone marrow contents into the articular space. Lipohemarthrosis is sometimes visible on plain radiographs as the fat layers above the blood in the joint. Occasionally, the fracture line is not visible, but lipohemarthrosis confirms the diagnosis, either radiographically or with aspiration of the affected joint. Intra-articular fractures commonly affect the tibial plateau of the knee, the

Lipohemarthrosis
Fatty cells within the synovial membrane.

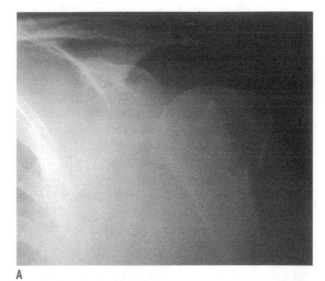

A

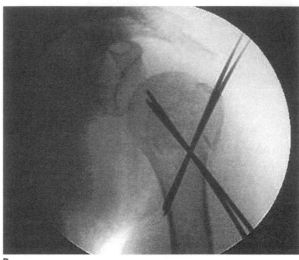

B

Figure 3-15 Impacted fracture of the humerus. **A.** Anteroposterior view demonstrating a nondisplaced 4-part fracture of the humeral shaft. **B.** Radiograph obtained after open reduction and fixation using Kirschner wires and transosseous sutures. (Reproduced with permission from Naranja RJ Jr, Iannotti JP: Displaced three- and four-part proximal humerus fractures: Evaluation and management. *J Am Acad Orthop Surg* 2000;8:373-382.)

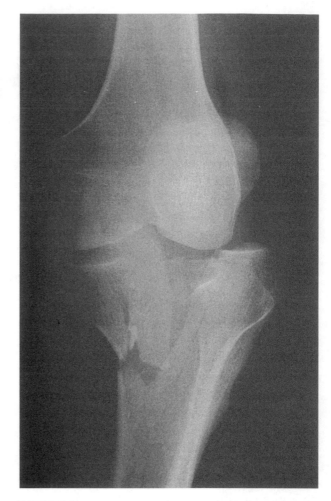

Figure 3-16 A displaced intra-articular fracture of the tibial plateau.

articular surface of the ankle, and the radial head in the elbow joint.

Prognosis

Articular fractures can occasionally be treated nonsurgically if displacement is minimal. In general, fractures with less than 1 mm of articular displacement can be managed nonsurgically, but any step displacement greater than this usually mandates open reduction to restore a smooth joint surface. Fractures of the tibial plateau may have a smooth depression in the center of the articular surface; in these cases, up to 5 mm of depression can be managed nonsurgically. Occasionally, external

fixation with pins and a frame can be used to stabilize the fracture. Provided stable fixation can be achieved, early motion of articular injuries can result in excellent function, although the risk of post-traumatic arthritis is increased.

Stress Fracture

Stress fractures occur in bone that is actively remodeling because of the application of new or unfamiliar stresses to the bone (**Figure 3-17**). When a runner suddenly increases mileage or an athlete adds a conditioning technique such as plyometric squats, new stresses are applied to normal bone. The bone responds by reabsorbing some of the existing bone and laying down new osteons along the lines of the new stress. During this period of remodeling, the bone temporarily becomes weaker and may be unable to withstand the new stresses. This weakening often occurs about 3 weeks after a new activity is initiated and manifests itself as a stress reaction or stress fracture. Stress fractures are often not visible on initial radiographs, as the in-

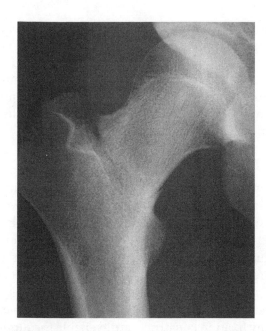

Figure 3-17 Anteroposterior radiograph of the proximal femur of a 19-year-old Marine recruit reveals a fatigue fracture on the superior portion of the femoral neck. (Reproduced with permission from Shin AY, Gillingham BL: Fatigue fractures of the femoral neck in athletes. *J Am Acad Orthop Surg* 1997;5:293-302.)

jury is generally at the microscopic level. Confirmation of the diagnosis often occurs only after subsequent radiographs reveal a healing response.

Insufficiency fractures, a subset of stress fractures, occur in abnormal bone that is unable to withstand the normal stresses of daily activity. These fractures are common in elderly osteoporotic women and frequently occur about the hip or knee.

The signs and symptoms of a stress fracture are pain and tenderness without deformity. Tibial shaft stress fractures typically present with little pain at rest, but pain is experienced when arising and taking the first few steps in the morning. This pain generally subsides with modest activity such as walking, and the patient may even be able to run a short distance before progressively acute pain limits activity. In severe or neglected stress fractures, the symptoms may progress to the point that weight bearing is not possible and pain is experienced even at rest.

Most stress fractures are treated nonsurgically, with restriction of painful activity and a gradual return to weight-bearing exercise within the limits of pain. Radiographs are usually obtained at intervals during healing to ensure that a fracture line has not developed and that the injury is healing. Surgical management is generally reserved for fractures that persist for a long period or develop a nonhealing fracture line. Stress fractures that are usually treated surgically include the Jones fracture of the proximal fifth metatarsal and the tibial fracture that devel-

ops the "dreaded black line," indicating a fracture with poor potential for healing.

A stress fracture of the femoral neck is a special case. The consequences of undertreating a stress fracture of the femoral neck are potentially more dire than in other anatomic locations; developing a complete fracture of the femoral neck may result in loss of the blood supply to the femoral head and subsequent need for hip replacement. Athletes with stress fractures of the femoral neck are typically runners who present with groin pain about 3 weeks after adding mileage or changing their running surface or shoe type. A change in activity almost always precedes the development of a stress fracture; the only exception is the distance runner with osteoporosis who develops an insufficiency fracture without a change in activity. Pain is generally relieved by modest activity but builds up during the course of a run and eventually necessitates a cessation of activity. Initial radiographs of the hip are usually normal. Any patient with a suspected femoral neck stress fracture should be immediately placed on restricted weight bearing with crutches until a confirmatory test such as a bone scan or MRI can be obtained.

Stress fractures of the femoral neck are classified into two types that differ radiologically and in clinical outcome. The first is the tension stress fracture, which originates at the superior surface of the femoral neck and results in a transverse fracture directed perpendicular to the line of force transmitted in the femoral neck. These injuries carry the risk of further advancement of the fracture line superiorly and eventual displacement, leading to **nonunion** and **osteonecrosis**. Hence, early diagnosis and treatment are essential.

The second type is a femoral neck compression stress fracture, which shows internal callus formation in radiographs. The fracture is usually located at the inferior margin of the femoral neck without cortical discontinuity and is thought to be mechanically stable. The compression fracture occurs mostly in younger patients, and continued stress typically does not cause displacement. The earliest radiographic evidence of a compression stress fracture is a haze of internal callus in the inferior cortex of the femoral neck. Eventually, a small fracture line appears in this area and gradually scleroses.

Differential Diagnosis

Initial radiographs are generally negative in the evaluation of the suspected stress fracture; consequently, other potential differential diagnoses must be ruled out. With tibial pain, these include medial tibial stress syndrome and compartment syndrome.

Nonunion Failure of a bone to heal within 9 months following the initial fracture.

Osteonecrosis Bone death secondary to a decreased blood supply; avascular necrosis.

For suspected stress fractures of the femoral neck, differential diagnoses include iliopsoas bursitis and referred pain from the low back. Additional imaging, such as a bone scan or MRI, is often required to confirm the diagnosis of a stress fracture.

Prognosis

Stress fractures from tension may advance, leading to possible displacement, nonunion, and osteonecrosis. Early diagnosis and treatment are essential to prevent these sequelae. Stress fractures due to compression are generally thought to be mechanically stable. After the internal callus develops, a small fracture line appears and gradually scleroses.

> **Sequelae** A condition resulting from an injury or disease.

Fracture Management

Fracture management can be considered in seven steps (**Table 3-2**). In general, fractures in athletes are treated more aggressively than in the general population to allow early motion of the adjacent joints, preserve muscle tone and mass, and expedite return to activity. Although internal fixation of a fracture does not speed healing, it may allow accelerated rehabilitation. Considerations differ depending on the nature of the fracture. Unique requirements of nondisplaced, displaced, and angulated closed and open fractures should be addressed.

■ Nondisplaced Fracture

Nondisplaced fractures often require little treatment beyond initial rest, analgesics, and time to heal. If the fracture is stable and nondisplaced, all

---

Table 3-2

Basic Steps in Fracture Management

Step 1 – History

Step 2 – Physical examination

Step 3 – Laboratory and radiographic investigations

Step 4 – Obtain reduction if the fracture is not in an acceptable position (closed reduction by manipulation or surgical open reduction)

Step 5 – Maintain reduction (application of external immobilization using an external splint, cast, or brace, or surgical internal fixation using a plate and screws, intramedullary rod, or external fixator)

Step 6 – Systemic therapeutic exercise such as cardiovascular exercise to maintain conditioning level; therapeutic exercise can also be performed on the uninvolved extremities

Step 7 – Rehabilitation of the involved body part once healing has occurred

---

that may be required is protection (cast or splint) along with measures to decrease swelling and pain (ice; elevation; and analgesics, NSAIDs, or both) for 24 to 48 hours, followed by progressive mobilization with weight bearing as comfort permits. An appropriate rehabilitation program should be carried out as the fracture heals.

■ Displaced and Angulated Fracture

Angulated and displaced fractures may not be in acceptable positions. Angulation can often be corrected by manipulation under anesthesia. Displaced fractures can occasionally be treated with closed reduction under anesthesia followed by a cast, but more often they require surgery. Unstable fractures are at risk of shifting during healing and usually need surgery for stabilization and realignment. Many fixation constructs are available for surgical intervention. They can be used individually or in combination and include screws, a variety of fracture-specific plates, intramedullary nails, wires, and external fixators. The device selection depends on the type of fracture and the surgeon's preference.

In general, fracture treatment attempts to preserve the biology of fracture healing while restoring the anatomy. Although open application of plates and screws provides excellent and immediate stability, stripping the periosteum and removing the normal fracture hematoma often slow the healing process. Contemporary techniques of percutaneous fixation and intramedullary nailing help to preserve the normal fracture biology and speed healing.

■ Closed Fracture

Closed fractures are managed based on their angulation and displacement (as described above).

■ Open Fracture

Open fractures are a surgical emergency requiring emergent evaluation and treatment. Appropriate management includes early surgical debridement and irrigation of the fracture site. These fractures are usually stabilized acutely with internal or external fixation in order to splint the soft tissues and allow wound management. Although excellent results can be expected with lower-grade open fractures, fractures involving extensive stripping of the periosteum, contamination, or vascular injury often require multiple surgical procedures in order to prevent infection and obtain bony union. Even in the best of settings, open fractures with compromised blood supplies have an ominous prognosis. Fractures associated with vascular injuries

Table 3-3

Fracture Complications

Life Threatening	Limb Threatening	Local Effects
Fat-embolism syndrome	Compartment syndrome	Delayed union
Shock	Joint contracture	**Malunion**
Sepsis (cellulitis, gas gangrene, necrotizing fasciitis)	Chronic osteomyelitis	Nonunion
Pulmonary embolism	Chronic vascular insufficiency	Chronic nerve damage
Acute compartment syndrome	Reflex sympathetic dystrophy (complex regional pain syndrome)	Avascular necrosis
Vascular damage		

Malunion Healing of a bone in a faulty position, creating an imperfect union.

Sepsis The spread of an infection into the bloodstream, creating a systemic condition.

that compromise the perfusion of the distal limb result in a 50% amputation rate.

Complications

Complications with fractures can be grouped into three categories—life-threatening complications, limb-threatening complications, and complications having local effects (**Table 3-3**).

Rehabilitation Implications

The goal of surgical management of any fracture is to provide an anatomic reduction and enough stability to allow accelerated rehabilitation. A limb that needs to be immobilized after surgical treatment of a fracture is generally considered a failure of surgical management. The exceptions are segmental fractures, significantly comminuted fractures, and fractures involving vascular injuries.

Stable fracture patterns (transverse, short oblique, and minimally displaced) can generally be treated with aggressive mobilization of adjacent joints and partial weight bearing. Full weight bearing is allowed as soon as fracture healing is apparent on follow-up radiographs. Unstable fracture patterns (comminuted, long oblique, and most spiral fractures) are generally treated surgically and then with protected weight bearing, whereas adjacent joints are mobilized. Weight bearing is restricted until fracture healing is documented.

Therapeutic modalities have also been used as adjuncts to therapy. Low-intensity ultrasound has been approved by the US Food and Drug Administration to accelerate healing in new fractures and to treat nonunions. Electric bone stimulation has been used for traumatic fractures of long bones, failed joint fusion, infantile pseudarthrosis, and pseud-

arthrosis of the spine (see Figure 3-1). Some practitioners have begun using low-power lasers to promote healing in stress fractures.

Other interventions claimed to promote bone healing include growth hormone, thyroid hormones, calcitonin, insulin, vitamin A, vitamin D, anabolic steroids, chondroitin sulfate, hyaluronidase, hyperbaric oxygen, growth factors, demineralized bone matrix, and bone marrow cells.

Healing times vary greatly, but bone is generally stable in 6 to 8 weeks. Age, nutrition, smoking, type of bone, and location of fracture all influence fracture healing time.

Communication forms the foundation of developing a rehabilitation plan. The perceived compliance of the patient and the fracture pattern dictate the amount of activity allowed. Most surgeons approve an accelerated rehabilitation protocol performed under the strict supervision of an athletic trainer or physical therapist. Such a protocol is also predicated on stable internal fixation and a compliant patient. A prescription for prolonged immobilization should be questioned because the long-term deleterious consequences of immobility have been well documented.

References

1. Bassett CAL: Electrical effects in bone. *Sci Am* 1965;213: 18-25.
2. Frankel VH, Burstein AH: *Orthopaedic Biomechanics.* Philadelphia, PA, Lea & Febiger, 1970.
3. Frankel VH, Nordin M (eds): *Basic Biomechanics of the Musculoskeletal System*, ed 2. Philadelphia, PA, Lea & Febiger, 1989.
4. Harkness JW, Ramsey WC, Harkness JW: Principles of fractures and dislocations, in Rockwood CA, Green DP, Buchholz RW (eds): *Rockwood and Green's Fractures in Adults*, ed 3. Philadelphia, PA, JB Lippincott, 1991.

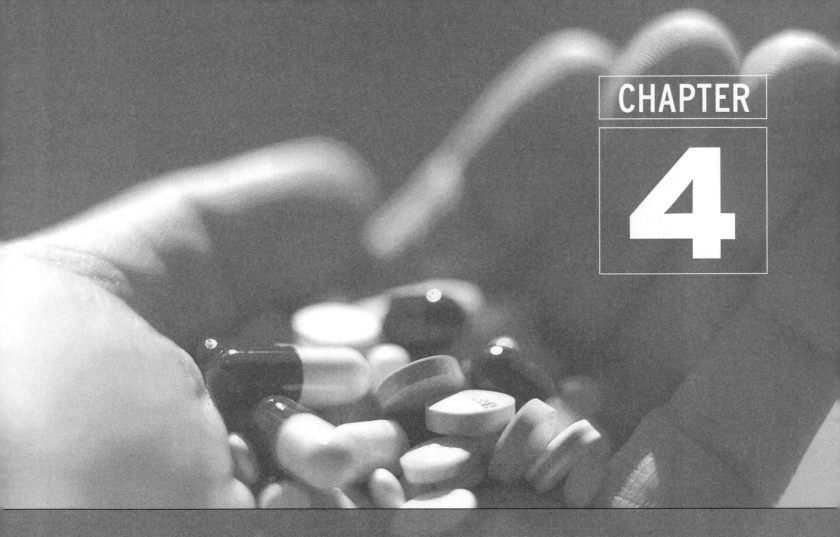

Therapeutic Medications

Dennis D. Hedge, PharmD

Medications are routinely prescribed for the treatment of various ailments and conditions. Anti-inflammatory agents, analgesics, anesthetics, antibiotics, and antiseptics are among the most common medications used in orthopaedics and sports medicine. Considering the frequency with which these agents are used and the potential harm that can occur if they are used inappropriately, an understanding of their mechanisms of action, common adverse effects, and potential drug interactions is essential. This chapter will provide a discussion of these issues as they pertain to common pharmacologic agents used in sports medicine.

Medications discussed in this chapter include both prescription and over-the-counter (OTC) products. Prescription medications are also called "legend drugs" because they carry the following federal warning (or legend) on the package:

CAUTION: Federal Law prohibits dispensing without a prescription.

A prescription for a medication is a legal document admissible in a court of law and written specifically for use by an individual. Sharing a prescription medication or using it for a person other than the individual for whom the prescription was written is a violation of the law. OTC medications may be purchased without a prescription. However, it is important that the instructions for use on the product's label be followed to avoid potential harm.

Given the complex nature of modern medications and their administration, it is impossible to cover all aspects of medication use in this textbook. Accordingly, a comprehensive resource on commonly used medications should also be available. Among the more commonly used drug references are *The Physicians' Desk Reference* (PDR), *American Hospital Formulary Service Drug Information*, and *Drug Facts and Comparisons*. Such a reference should be consulted whenever questions arise involving drug interactions, contraindications for use, adverse effects, and instructions for administration. In addition, all sports medicine personnel should have the most current lists of banned medications maintained by the various sport-regulating bodies, such as the National Collegiate Athletic Association, the US Olympic Committee, and the International Olympic Committee. These lists can be accessed via the Internet and should be reviewed frequently so updates are not missed.

Medication Storage and Dispensing

Medication dispensing is the preparing, packaging, and labeling of a prescription drug for use by an individual.[1] Athletic trainers cannot be delegated authority for dispensing prescription medications; this is not authorized by current drug laws. Most states have strict regulations for drug labeling, record maintenance, patient counseling, and drug storage for both prescription and OTC medications. Failure to adhere to these drug laws and regulations can put the sports medicine staff at risk for legal disciplinary action.

In addition to ensuring compliance of all personnel with state and federal drug laws and regulations, all prescription and OTC medications should be stored in a designated and secure location and under proper environmental conditions (as indicated on the package labeling). On a regular basis, the entire medication inventory should be examined for outdated, recalled, and damaged or deteriorated drugs; these agents should be properly destroyed.

Whenever a medication is dispensed, the individual receiving the drug should be informed about its function, adverse effects, and how to take it. Before receiving a medication, the individual should also be screened for the possibility of drug-related problems by reviewing the drug-allergy history, medication history, and medical condition list. Therefore, maintenance of up-to-date records for the patient is vital. Follow-up should be undertaken to ensure compliance with the therapy and ascertain that the therapy has been effective and free of harmful adverse effects.

Routes of Drug Administration

Drug administration is regarded as giving or applying a single dose of a medication.[1] Primary routes for delivering drugs to the body include enteral, parenteral, and topical administration. The enteral route of drug administration includes giving medications sublingually, rectally, and orally, with the latter generally regarded as the most convenient method. Parenteral methods of medication administration include subcutaneous, intramuscular, and intravenous injections. With subcutaneous administration, drugs are injected into the subcutaneous tissue under the skin that overlies muscle. The medication is absorbed slowly via this delivery method, thus delaying the onset of drug action. Drugs are injected directly into muscle tissue with intramuscular administration. Intravenously administered medications have a rapid onset of action and can be given in the form of an intravenous bolus or a slower intravenous infusion. Although the rapid onset of action with intravenous administration is often desirable, medications administered intravenously have the greatest potential for causing adverse reactions. Topical drug administration offers several advantages. It eliminates the inconvenience of parenteral administration, reduces the risk for systemic side effects, focuses the agent's effects at the site of inflammation, and allows for easy termination of therapy if needed.

Drug delivery through the skin can be enhanced by application of low-level electric current (iontophoresis) or ultrasound (phonophoresis). Although these are common clinical techniques, their efficacy has not been substantiated.

Iontophoresis uses a low-amperage direct current to drive ions from drug solution into tissue (**Figure 4-1**).[2] Iontophoresis has been used to treat musculoskeletal inflammatory disorders with nonsteroidal anti-inflammatory drugs (NSAIDs) and corticosteroids. Iontophoresis treatment regimens (measured in milliampere seconds of current) vary depending on the medication used and the medical condition being treated.

Phonophoresis is the application of therapeutic ultrasound to increase drug delivery through the skin.[3] In phonophoresis, ultrasonic energy is transferred through a compound capable of transmission. The ultrasonic waves create two primary physical consequences within the skin—heating

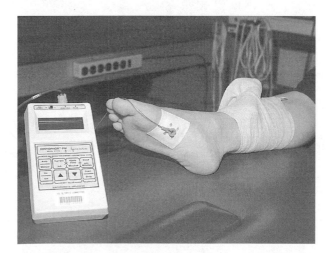

Figure 4-1 Iontophoresis uses direct current to introduce NSAIDs or corticosteroids into the subcutaneous tissues.

and cavitation. The overall result is thought to be increased skin permeability, which enhances drug diffusion through the skin. Although a variety of medicinal agents have been administered via phonophoresis, hydrocortisone and dexamethasone are the agents most frequently used for treating musculoskeletal injuries.

Anti-inflammatory and Analgesic Medications

Musculoskeletal pain is a common result of athletic-related injury. Musculoskeletal pain usually occurs as a result of trauma that arises secondary to the physical forces placed on the body. In general, acute pain continues until the injury heals. Effective pain management is often needed to improve the patient's quality of life, allow earlier incorporation of therapeutic exercise into the treatment protocol, and expedite return to activity.

Medication options for acute pain management include acetaminophen, NSAIDs, steroidal anti-inflammatory agents, and opioid analgesics. Acetaminophen is used for its analgesic effects in mild pain situations. In addition to the analgesic effect of acetaminophen, the medication also has **antipyretic** properties. The NSAIDs include salicylates, such as acetylsalicylic acid (aspirin), and nonsalicylates, such as ibuprofen. These agents exhibit anti-inflammatory, analgesic, and antipyretic properties. Because of these actions, NSAIDs are routinely used for relieving mild to moderate pain associated with acute or chronic inflammatory conditions and fever control (**Table 4-1**). Opioid analgesics are employed to treat moderate to severe acute or chronic pain. Opiates are used for severe acute pain if a nonopioid agent fails to offer relief and may be combined with a nonopioid medication when the nonopioid is not completely effective on its own.

Corticosteroids, or steroidal anti-inflammatory agents, have a number of medicinal uses. Corticosteroids can be administered in various ways depending on the condition and indications for treatment. Certain corticosteroids are used in the immediate care of spinal cord trauma to reduce edema and subsequent secondary cell death.

Nonsteroidal Anti-inflammatory Drugs

NSAIDs act primarily by inhibiting the cyclooxygenase (COX) enzymes COX-1 and COX-2. The anti-inflammatory, analgesic, and antipyretic effects of the NSAIDs are mediated through the COX-2 isoenzyme,

Antipyretic Having fever-reducing properties.

Table 4-1

Pharmacologic Property Comparison

	Analgesic Effects	Anti-inflammatory Effects	Antipyretic Effects
Acetylsalicylic acid (aspirin)	YES	YES	YES
Other NSAIDs	YES	YES	YES
Acetaminophen	YES	NO	YES

which, when inhibited, results in a blockade of prostaglandin production.[4-7] The prostaglandins sensitize nerves to painful stimuli and are produced from arachidonic acid, which is released when an injury occurs.

Both COX-1 and COX-2 inhibitors interfere with the process by which arachidonic acid converts to prostaglandin. COX-1 is found in most tissues and is responsible for helping to maintain homeostatic functions such as gastric, renal, and platelet function. Theoretically, the COX-2 inhibitors act directly on the inflammatory sites without increasing risk for gastrointestinal ulceration. The COX-2 inhibitors are being scrutinized, however, for possibly increasing the risk for development of thrombotic cardiovascular events, such as heart attacks and strokes[8] (**Figure 4-2**).

Salicylates

The salicylate NSAID aspirin is used for mild pain and is available in both oral and topical forms. When given orally, the usual adult dose of aspirin for pain management is 325 to 650 mg every 4 to 6 hours. Among the concerns associated with aspirin use are gastrointestinal (GI) disturbances and bleeding (**Table 4-2**). Because of the potential adverse effects on the GI system, aspirin is available in buffered and enteric-coated formulations and should be taken with food or a large glass of water to minimize irritation. Other adverse reactions associated with aspirin therapy are tinnitus and hypersensitivity reactions.

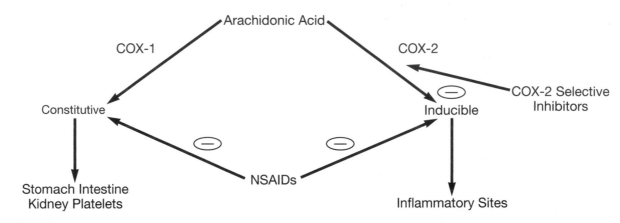

Figure 4-2   NSAIDs inhibit the production of prostaglandins to limit the inflammatory response to injury.

Table 4-2

Salicylates

Generic Compound	Generic or Brand Name	Common Adult Dose
Acetylsalicylic acid	Aspirin	325–650 mg every 4 h
Choline salicylate	Arthropan	435–870 mg every 4 h
Magnesium salicylate	Doan's Pills	325–650 mg every 4 h
Salsalate	Disalcid	1,000 mg every 12 h
Sodium salicylate	Various generic names	325–650 mg every 4 h
Choline magnesium trisalicylate	Trilisate	1,000 mg every 12 h

Instructions

Take with food. Do not chew tablets or crush enteric-coated products. Do not combine with other NSAIDs.

Cautions

Acetylated salicylates may worsen ulcers and cause internal bleeding. Caution should be used in individuals who consume alcohol or use blood thinners and those with aspirin sensitivity.

In asthma patients, aspirin sensitivity often results in bronchospasm.[6] Aspirin-associated bronchospasm is most likely to occur in individuals with severe asthma and those with perennial rhinitis and nasal polyps. Other aspirin sensitivity reactions include urticaria, angioedema, hypotension, and syncope. The similarities between aspirin and other NSAIDs can create cross-sensitivity to these medications.

Aspirin inhibits blood-platelet aggregation, prolonging bleeding for as long as 1 week after a single aspirin dose.[4-7] Considering the potential for bleeding complications, aspirin should not be used after injuries such as concussions or in any other situation in which bleeding and bruising may lead to complications. In addition, persons with known aspirin hypersensitivity should avoid aspirin and other products containing aspirin. Aspirin should be used with extreme caution in individuals with a history of GI disease and those with an increased risk of bleeding, including persons on anticoagulation medications such as Coumadin (generic name warfarin). In addition, aspirin is contraindicated in children younger than 12 years with a viral illness because of an increased risk for the development of Reye syndrome.[4-6]

Nonsalicylate NSAIDs

The nonsalicylate NSAIDs are available in both prescription and nonprescription forms and provide analgesia that is equal to or better than aspirin (**Table 4-3**). Individuals may have different responses to various NSAIDs; therefore, if an NSAID is being administered at the optimal dose and a response is lacking, another medication within the class should be tried. One prescription agent, ketorolac tromethamine (Toradol), is available in injectable and oral formulations.

Like aspirin, nonsalicylate NSAIDs can cause adverse GI and hematologic effects and hypersensitivity reactions.[9-11] When administered orally, these medications should be taken with food and at the lowest possible dose that provides adequate analgesia. Each of these medications inhibits the activity of prostaglandin synthetase, leading to inhibition of platelet aggregation and subsequent increased bleeding time. Because these agents have also been shown to induce renal insufficiency, persons with diminished renal function should consult a physician or, when in doubt, not use them.

Inhibition of COX-1 is primarily responsible for the GI and bleeding effects associated with NSAID use. To decrease these unwanted effects, selective inhibitors of COX-2 have been developed (**Table 4-4**). These agents, originally thought to have an improved

Urticaria Hives, characterized by the development of a wheal that itches.

Angioedema Edema of the skin, mucous membranes, or viscera.

Reye syndrome Condition usually affecting children younger than 15 years, commonly the result of taking aspirin and characterized by liver, spleen, kidney, and lymph node dysfunction.

Table 4-3

Traditional Nonsalicylate Nonsteroidal Anti-Inflammatory Agents

Generic Name	Brand Name	Common Adult Dose
Diclofenac potassium	Cataflam	50 mg every 8 h
Diclofenac sodium	Voltaren	50 mg every 8 h
Diclofenac/ Misoprostol	Arthrotec	50 mg/200 μg 2-4 times/day 75 mg/200 μg twice daily
Diflunisal	Dolobid	500 mg every 12 h
Etodolac	Lodine	200-400 mg every 6-8 h XL formulation 400-1,000 mg daily
Fenoprofen	Nalfon	200-300 mg every 4-6 h
Flurbiprofen	Ansaid	200-300 mg/d in 2-4 divided doses
Ibuprofen	Motrin	800-3,200 mg per day in 4 divided doses
Indomethacin	Indocin	25 mg 2-3 times per day
Ketoprofen	Orudis	25-50 mg every 6-8 h
Ketorolac	Toradol	10 mg every 4-6 h
Meloxicam	Mobic	7.5-15 mg daily
Nabumetone	Relafen	500 mg every 12 h
Naproxen	Naprosyn	250 mg every 6-8 h
Naproxen sodium	Anaprox	275 mg every 6-8 h
Naproxen sodium (controlled release)	Naprelan	550-1,100 mg daily
Oxaprozin	Daypro	600-1200 mg daily
Piroxicam	Feldene	20 mg daily
Sulindac	Clinoril	150 mg every 12 h
Tolmetin sodium	Tolectin	200-400 mg every 8 h

Instructions

NSAIDs should not be taken with other prescription or OTC NSAIDs. Take with food, or a glass of milk or water. Do not take for more than 10 days for pain or more than 3 days for fever unless directed to do so by a physician.

Cautions

Caution should be exercised in individuals who regularly consume alcohol or use blood thinners, and those with sensitivity to aspirin and similar medications, asthma, or ulcers.

---

adverse effects profile, are under scrutiny for possibly increasing the risk of thrombotic cardiovascular events.[9,12,13]

Inhibition of the COX-2 isoenzyme with NSAIDs impedes the growth of new bone, potentially delaying fracture healing or stabilization of

Table 4-4

COX-2 Inhibitors

Generic Name	Brand Name	Common Adult Dose
Celecoxib	Celebrex	200 mg/d in 1 or 2 doses or 400 mg/d in 2 doses.
Valdecoxib	Bextra	10 mg/d in a single dose

Instructions

NSAIDs should not be taken with other prescription or OTC NSAIDs. Take with food, or a glass of milk or water. Do not take for more than 10 days for pain or more than 3 days for fever unless directed to do so by a physician.

Cautions

Caution should be taken in individuals who regularly consume alcohol or use blood thinners and in those with sensitivity to aspirin and similar medications, asthma, or ulcers.

an implanted joint.[14] This finding suggests that individuals with a bone fracture or those with cementless joint replacement surgery should not receive NSAIDs, and an alternative agent such as acetaminophen or a codeine product should be considered for pain management. Currently, no specific recommendations exist with regard to a specific period for avoiding NSAIDs after a fracture or joint replacement.

The injectable agent ketorolac tromethamine provides analgesia comparable to 6 to 12 mg of intramuscular morphine.[15] After therapy initiation with intramuscular or intravenous ketorolac, a switch to the oral formulation should be made as soon as possible. To prevent the emergence of adverse effects, the total duration of injectable and oral ketorolac therapy should not exceed 5 days.[4,5,7] Accordingly, a switch to an alternative analgesic agent should be made before the sixth day of therapy. Caution must be exercised when ketorolac is used postoperatively because severe bleeding complications have been documented.[4,5,7]

The patient must not exceed the recommended daily dose of the NSAID or use more than one NSAID at a time. Using multiple NSAIDs or exceeding the prescribed dose can result in adverse effects. These agents should be used cautiously in individuals taking anticoagulant medications or angiotensin-converting enzyme (ACE) inhibitors, and they can increase the risk of GI bleeding in individuals who drink three or more alcoholic beverages each day.[4-7]

■ Acetaminophen

Acetaminophen is similar to aspirin in its analgesic and antipyretic effects but has little or no effect on inflammation. The advantages of acetaminophen over aspirin include its absence of effect on blood platelets and gentler effects on the GI tract. However, acetaminophen is generally regarded as a less effective analgesic than prescription NSAIDs and is, therefore, used primarily for mild pain situations and fever relief.

Acetaminophen is well tolerated in doses up to 4,000 mg/d, with a usual dosage range of 325 mg to 1,000 mg every 4 to 6 hours. Overdoses of acetaminophen can result in hepatic injury and failure. Acetaminophen is contraindicated in patients with liver disease and chronic alcohol users.[16] In addition to an increased risk of acetaminophen liver toxicity associated with alcohol consumption, concomitant use of acetaminophen with other potentially hepatotoxic medications, such as isoniazid, may increase the risk of liver injury. Also, acetaminophen elevates the level of anticoagulation in patients receiving warfarin therapy.[4-6] Therefore, patients receiving oral anticoagulation therapy should have their international normalized ratio or prothrombin time values checked by the physician more frequently when concomitant acetaminophen therapy is used, with subsequent dosage adjustments being made as necessary.

■ Opioid Analgesics

The opioid analgesic agents are used for managing acute severe pain or pain that does not respond to the nonopioid pain relievers.[6] These medications interact with central nervous system receptors and alter pain perception, although the precise mechanism is unknown. Opioid medications are available either as single-entity drugs or in combination with nonopioids such as acetaminophen, ibuprofen, or aspirin (**Table 4-5**). Opioid analgesics can be administered via several different routes. For acute pain, the opioids are generally administered orally or by intramuscular or intravenous injection.

The opioid analgesics should be used for the shortest duration possible and only under the supervision of a physician. A switch to a nonopioid analgesic should be made as soon as the patient's pain decreases to a level at which opioid medications are no longer needed because the opioid medications have the potential to become addicting; they also can cause adverse effects in athletes.[4-6,9] Sedation and mental confusion are adverse effects of the

Table 4-5

Opioid Analgesics

Generic Content	Brand Name	Common Adult Dose
Morphine	MS Contin (SR)	15-30 mg orally every 8-12 h
	MS IR	10-30 mg orally every 4 h
Hydromorphone	Dilaudid	2-4 mg orally every 4-6 h
Oxycodone	OxyContin (SR)	10 mg orally every 12 h
	OxyIR	5 mg orally every 6 h
Oxycodone 5 mg Acetaminophen 500 mg	Tylox	1 tablet orally every 6 h
Oxycodone 2.5 mg Acetaminophen 325 mg	Percocet 2.5/325	1 tablet orally every 6 h
Oxycodone 5 mg Acetaminophen 325 mg	Percocet 5/325	1 tablet orally every 6 h
Oxycodone 7.5 mg Acetaminophen 500 mg	Percocet 7.5/500	1 tablet orally every 6 h
Oxycodone 10 mg Acetaminophen 650 mg	Percocet 10/650	1 tablet orally every 6 h
Oxycodone HCL 4.5 mg Oxycodone terephthalate 0.38 mg Aspirin 325 mg	Percodan	1 tablet orally every 6 h
Meperidine	Demerol	50-150 mg orally, subcutaneously, or intramuscularly every 3-4 h
Codeine	Codeine	15-60 mg orally or intramuscularly every 4-6 h
Acetaminophen 300 mg Codeine 15 mg	Tylenol No. 2	1-2 tablets orally every 4 h
Acetaminophen 300 mg Codeine 30 mg	Tylenol No. 3	1-2 tablets orally every 4 h
Acetaminophen 300 mg Codeine 60 mg	Tylenol No. 4	1-2 tablets orally every 4 h
Codeine 30 mg Acetaminophen 325 mg Caffeine 40 mg Butalbital 50 mg	Fioricet with codeine	1-2 capsules orally every 4 h
Codeine 30 mg Aspirin 325 mg Caffeine 40 mg Butalbital 50 mg	Fiorinal with codeine	1-2 tablets orally every 4 h
Hydrocodone 2.5 mg Acetaminophen 500 mg	Lortab 2.5/500	1-2 tablets orally every 4-6 h
Hydrocodone 5 mg Acetaminophen 500 mg	Lortab 5/500	1-2 tablets orally every 4-6 h
Hydrocodone 7.5 mg Acetaminophen 500 mg	Lortab 7.5/500	1-2 tablets orally every 4-6 h
Propoxyphene	Darvon 65 mg (HCL)	65 mg orally every 4 h
	Darvon-N 100 mg (napsylate)	100 mg orally every 4 h
	Darvon-N 50 mg/5mL (napsylate)	
Acetaminophen 650 mg Propoxyphene napsylate 100 mg	Darvocet N-100	1-2 tablets orally every 4-6 h
Tramadol	Ultram	50-100 mg orally every 4-6 h

Instructions

Do not crush or chew extended-release products. Do not exceed prescribed dosage.

Cautions

May cause dizziness, drowsiness, mental clouding, nausea, vomiting, constipation, and respiratory depression.

opiate medications that can impair an athlete's ability to perform and potentially increase the risk of injury. The opioids can also cause respiratory depression, nausea, vomiting, and constipation.

Codeine is a popular oral opioid that is used for analgesia by itself or in combination with nonopioid analgesics. As with all opioid analgesics, codeine should be given in the smallest effective dose. When given as a single agent, the dosage range of codeine is 15 to 60 mg every 4 to 6 hours. When codeine is combined with a nonopioid such as acetaminophen or aspirin, the nonopioid component is the agent that limits the dose given. Thus, an analgesic combination of codeine and acetaminophen should be dosed in a manner that does not exceed 4,000 mg/d of the acetaminophen component.

Other commonly used opioid agents are hydrocodone, oxycodone, hydromorphone, morphine, propoxyphene, and meperidine. Hydrocodone, similar to codeine in its analgesic effect, is available as an analgesic agent in combination with nonopioid medications. The usual adult dose of hydrocodone is 2.5 to 10 mg every 4 to 6 hours; the amount of the nonopioid agent must not exceed the daily maximum dosage in these combination products. Oxycodone is available orally as an oxycodone-only medication and in combination with a nonopioid analgesic. The usual adult dose of oxycodone is 20 mg/d, given in divided doses.

Morphine is used for severe pain management and is generally regarded as the gold standard of opiate agents. As a result, morphine is not routinely used for athletic injuries. If morphine is required for managing pain, the smallest effective dose should be prescribed and administered as infrequently as possible, as with other opiates, to minimize the development of tolerance and physical dependence. A typical dose of morphine is in the range of 5 to 15 mg every 4 hours when given parenterally and 10 to 30 mg every 4 hours when administered orally. Hydromorphone is closely related to morphine and has a strong analgesic effect but may produce less nausea, vomiting, and constipation than morphine. The usual dose of hydromorphone is 2 mg every 4 to 6 hours as necessary when given orally or parenterally.

Propoxyphene is available orally and used for mild to moderate pain, but it is not sufficiently potent for treating severe pain. Most commonly, propoxyphene is given with acetaminophen or aspirin, 65 mg every 4 hours for the hydrochloride salt and 100 mg every 4 hours for the napsylate form. With repetitive dosing, propoxyphene and its metabolite, norpropoxyphene, can accumulate, increasing the potential for adverse effects. Adverse effects seen with propoxyphene are similar to those of other opioid analgesics; however, the incidence of seizures in an overdose situation is higher with propoxyphene.

Meperidine is a synthetically derived opiate agonist that has historically been used for the management of severe pain. Meperidine is available in both oral and injectable forms, but the oral form is generally not recommended. The primary concern with meperidine is that it is metabolized to normeperidine, a central nervous system stimulant. As normeperidine accumulates in the central nervous system, agitation, tremors, myoclonus, and seizures can occur. Orally administered meperidine is of particular concern in this regard; it has only about one fourth of the analgesic effectiveness of similar parenteral doses, yet produces an equal quantity of the toxic metabolite. The elimination half-life of normeperidine is extended in patients with renal dysfunction, increasing the risk of toxic effects. Considering the potential for these adverse effects, meperidine should only be used for acute pain situations of 48 hours or less in patients who do not have a history of renal insufficiency or neurologic disease. Also, meperidine should not be used by any person taking a monoamine oxidase inhibitor; the resulting interaction could trigger a life-threatening situation. In addition, meperidine has a relatively short duration of analgesic effect, necessitating frequent dosing.

Tramadol is an oral medication with weak opioid-receptor agonist activity and inhibits the reuptake of norepinephrine and serotonin, which appears to add to its analgesic effect. The usual dose of tramadol is 50 mg every 4 to 6 hours. Adverse effects are similar to those seen with other opioid medications and include dizziness, somnolence, constipation, nausea, and vomiting. Tramadol can also increase the risk of seizures, particularly when the dosage exceeds the recommended range.

◼ Topical Anti-inflammatory Agents

Trolamine salicylate is a commercially available, topical anti-inflammatory medication used for the treatment of muscle or joint pain in adults. The topical salicylates are not intended for self-medication beyond 10 days. Physician referral is indicated if the pain increases or continues beyond 10 days because pain of such intensity and duration could indicate a medical condition that requires supervised medical therapy. Topical salicylates should be liberally applied and rubbed into the affected area two to four times per day. If the medication is used regularly, moderate peeling of the skin can occur. The patient should not apply the medication to acutely inflamed or raw skin, and should avoid topical salicylate contact with mucous membranes or eyes. If excessive skin irritation develops during therapy, treatment should be halted.

■ Corticosteroids

The corticosteroid agents can be classified into two groups—glucocorticoids and mineralocorticoids—based on their main pharmacologic activity. The agents with primarily glucocorticoid activity have anti-inflammatory properties and are used for musculoskeletal conditions (**Table 4-6**). Glucocorticoids can be administered via several routes (oral, parenteral, topical), but systemic therapy is not routinely recommended for anti-inflammatory effects in sports medicine because of their adverse-effects profile. When taken systemically for an extended period, corticosteroids can increase an individual's susceptibility to infection; lead to osteoporosis; cause GI disturbances, including peptic ulcer disease; cause hypokalemia and sodium retention, which may lead to edema; increase the risk for cataract development; and precipitate **iatrogenic Cushing syndrome**.[4,5]

Mineralocorticoids affect the balance of water and electrolytes and are not commonly prescribed for musculoskeletal injuries.

Glucocorticoid medications can relieve local symptoms when injected into or near an area of inflammation (**Table 4-7**). However, glucocorticoid injections into a joint should be infrequent, not exceeding three or four injections per year (even less frequently in weight-bearing joints), because of the possibility of cartilage damage.[6] This damage is believed to be the result of either inhibition of protein synthesis in articular cartilage by the steroid or increased use of diseased joints once symptoms are relieved. After the injection, the patient should minimize activity and stress to the joint for several days. When corticosteroids are injected into or near inflamed tissue, care should be taken to avoid injecting weight-bearing tendons such as the Achilles tendon, and the injection site should be rested for 1 to 2 weeks. These injections should not be repeated more frequently than three or four times over 6 months.

Iontophoresis and phonophoresis are alternative methods of administering corticosteroids to areas of inflammation. Refer to page 49 for more information regarding these drug-delivery methods.

Table 4-6

Traditional Corticosteroid Anti-Inflammatory Agents

Product Name	Relative Glucocorticoid Potency	Relative Mineralocorticoid Potency
Short-Acting Products		
Cortisone	0.8	2
Hydrocortisone	1	2
Intermediate-Acting Products		
Prednisone	4	1
Prednisolone	4	1
Methylprednisolone	5	0
Triamcinolone	5	0
Long-Acting Products		
Betamethasone	25	0
Dexamethasone	30	0

Table 4-7

Common Injectable Corticosteroids

Medication	Relative Potency	Onset	Duration
Hydrocortisone	1	Fast	Short
Prednisolone terbutate	4	Fast	Intermediate
Methylprednisolone acetate	4	Slow	Intermediate
Triamcinolone acetonide	5	Moderate	Intermediate
Triamcinolone hexacetonide	5	Moderate	Intermediate
Betamethasone	25	Fast	Long

Adapted with permission from Greene WB (ed): *Essentials of Musculoskeletal Care*, ed 2. Rosemont, IL, American Academy of Orthopaedic Surgeons, 2001, p 20.

Iatrogenic Condition inadvertently caused by medical treatment.

Cushing syndrome The hypersecretion of the adrenal cortex, resulting in the overproduction of glucocorticoids.

Corticosteroids for Acute Spinal Cord Trauma

The anti-inflammatory corticosteroid methylprednisolone has been used to minimize disability associated with acute spinal cord injury. In the second National Acute Spinal Cord Injury Study (NASCIS 2), a subset of patients treated within 8 hours of injury with methylprednisolone demonstrated improvement in motor and sensory function at 6 weeks and 6 months when compared with other groups in the trial.[17,18] The 24-hour dosing protocol of methylprednisolone 30 mg/kg intravenously over 15 minutes followed by a 5.4 mg/kg/hr infusion for 23 hours, when administered within the 8-hour window, has become the standard treatment for acute spinal cord injury (see chapter 16). A follow-up study, the National Acute Spinal Cord Injury Study III (NASCIS 3), confirmed the findings of NASCIS 2 and suggested that individuals receiving therapy between 3 and 8 hours after suffering the acute spinal cord injury have improved outcomes when the infusion of methylprednisolone is for 48 hours instead of 24 hours.[17,18] One concern raised in NASCIS 3, however, is that patients receiving the longer duration of therapy had an increased risk of severe sepsis and pneumonia when compared with those receiving the 24-hour treatment regimen. For more information on the role of corticosteroids and other medications in the management of acute spinal cord trauma, see page 532.

Local Anesthetics

Local anesthetics reversibly block nerve impulse conduction and produce temporary loss of sensation in the area of application or injection. These agents are valuable for pain relief from oral lesions and abrasions when applied topically (eg, viscous lidocaine) and for pain prevention during medical procedures when injected. In sports medicine, injectable local anesthetics are used for infiltration anesthesia—the injection of a local anesthetic solution intradermally, subcutaneously, or submucosally in the area needing to be anesthetized. This technique is commonly employed during minor medical procedures such as laceration repair.

Lidocaine is one of the most commonly used local anesthetic agents; it has an onset of action of less than 2 minutes and a duration of approximately 2 hours.[5] Lidocaine is available in various strengths (0.5%, 1%, 1.5%, 2%) and in combination with epinephrine. The epinephrine-containing lidocaine products prolong the duration of anesthetic effect by slowing vascular absorption. Because of the vasoconstricting effects of epinephrine, the combination lidocaine and epinephrine products can also reduce bleeding, which may be helpful when repairing lacerations. As a general rule, the smallest dose and concentration of lidocaine needed to produce the desired anesthetic effect should be administered. If a longer duration of anesthesia is required, alternative anesthetics such as bupivacaine (4-hour duration) may be used.

Local anesthetics can have potentially dangerous and life-threatening effects if high plasma concentrations occur as the result of systemic absorption. These risks include excitation and then depression of the central nervous system and adverse cardiovascular effects. In addition, a burning sensation at the site of injection can occur, and the potential for hypersensitivity reactions ranges from a benign rash to anaphylaxis. The cross-reactivity among related local anesthetics must also be noted.

Antibiotics

Antibiotics can be used to treat a variety of infections, including upper and lower respiratory tract infections, cellulitis, and infected wounds. When using antibiotics, several key principles need to be understood. Antibiotics should not be used for the treatment of viral illness, only for bacterial infections. In addition, the patient must complete the entire course of therapy prescribed by a physician. Failure to completely eradicate the bacterial organisms causing an infection can result in a relapse of the infection and development of resistance to the antibiotic. In the modern era, bacteria that are resistant to the effects of antibiotics have become a major concern. Consequently, the microorganism causing the infection should be cultured whenever possible. If an organism is isolated, antibiotic-susceptibility tests should be conducted and, if necessary, the results of these tests should then be used to modify the original empiric therapy.

Several methods of categorizing antibiotics exist. This chapter will group commonly prescribed antibiotics by separating them into classes based on molecular structure (**Table 4-8**).

Penicillins

In addition to penicillin itself, several derivatives of penicillin are available as treatment options for infection. The penicillin medications are also called beta-lactam agents because of their chemical structure. These agents disrupt the cell wall of bacteria, resulting in a **bacteriocidal** effect. Penicillin has generally been viewed as the drug of choice for the treatment of streptococcal infections. Over the past few years, however, bacteria have become increasingly resistant to the effects of penicillin and its derivatives.[6] Among the more commonly prescribed penicillins are dicloxacillin, ampicillin, amoxicillin, and amoxicillin/clavulanate. Dicloxacillin is active against the microorganism *Staphylococcus aureus* and is often used for the treatment of skin infections resulting from these bacteria. Ampicillin and amoxicillin have a broader spectrum of antimicrobial activity and can be used to treat several commonly occurring infec-

Bacteriocidal An agent that kills bacteria.

Table 4-8

Commonly Used Antibiotics

Antibiotic Class	Agents Within the Class	Adverse Effects
Penicillins	Penicillin, ampicillin, amoxicillin, amoxicillin/clavulanate, dicloxacillin	Diarrhea, nausea, vomiting, rash
Cephalosporins	Cefadroxil, cephalexin, cefuroxime, cefprozil, cefdinir, cefpodoxime, cefixime, cefaclor	Diarrhea, nausea, vomiting, rash
Macrolides	Erythromycin, azithromycin, clarithromycin	Nausea, vomiting, diarrhea, rash, hearing loss
Quinolones	Ciprofloxacin, levofloxacin, gatifloxacin, moxifloxacin	Nausea, vomiting, diarrhea, dizziness, lightheadedness, vertigo, rash, arthralgias, tendinitis
Tetracyclines	Doxycycline, minocycline, tetracycline	Nausea, vomiting, diarrhea, rash, photosensitivity
Lincosamides	Clindamycin, lincomycin	Nausea, vomiting, diarrhea, rash
Oxazoladinone	Linezolid	Thrombocytopenia, nausea, vomiting, rash
Sulfonamides/sulfonamide combinations	Sulfisoxazole, sulfamethoxazole, trimethoprim/sulfamethoxazole	Rash, methemoglobinemia, leukopenia, thrombocytopenia, nausea, vomiting, headache

tions, such as those involving the upper and lower respiratory tracts. Amoxicillin/clavulanate thwarts the effects of beta-lactamase produced by bacteria as a mechanism of resistance.

For the most part, penicillin and its derivatives are fairly well tolerated. Among the more common adverse effects of the penicillins are rash, nausea, and diarrhea. Anaphylactic hypersensitivity reactions associated with the penicillins are rare but can occur.

■ Cephalosporins

The cephalosporin antibiotics are popular beta-lactam medications that can be divided into generational groupings based upon their antimicrobial coverage spectrum. Four generations of cephalosporin antibiotics are currently available. In general, the first-generation cephalosporin agents are used for treating gram-positive bacterial infections (*Streptococcus, Staphylococcus*). Gram-negative bacterial activity (*Escherichia coli, Klebsiella, Haemophilus influenzae*) is greater in the later generations. Cephalosporins are very well tolerated and are used for several different types of infection, including cellulitis, respiratory tract infections, urinary tract infections, and bone infections. Adverse effects are similar to those of the penicillin medications but occur less frequently. Hypersensitivity reactions can result, and patients with a penicillin allergy are at increased risk of an allergic reaction to cephalosporins.

■ Macrolides

The macrolide medications have long been popular treatment selections for individuals with penicillin and cephalosporin allergies. The macrolide agents have a **bacteriostatic** effect. Commonly prescribed macrolides include erythromycin, azithromycin, and clarithromycin, which are used for skin and respiratory tract infections. The adverse effects of erythromycin include nausea and diarrhea. Although taking oral erythromycin with food may improve tolerability, in some individuals these side effects are severe enough to warrant discontinuation of the medication. The latest generation of macrolides (azithromycin, clarithromycin) has similar adverse effects to erythromycin but generally to a lesser degree. These newer medications also have a broader coverage spectrum than erythromycin.

Bacteriostatic
Inhibits the replication of bacteria.

■ Quinolones

The quinolone antibiotics are bacteriocidal agents that have become increasingly popular since the emergence of bacterial resistance to penicillins, cephalosporins, and macrolides. The quinolone medications are now often classified into generational groupings. The earliest quinolone medications had primarily a gram-negative coverage spectrum, but the latest quinolones to reach the market have enhanced gram-positive activity. The wide spectrum of coverage makes quinolones appropriate for treating many types of infection.

However, in order to ensure safe and effective quinolone use, several important clinical findings must be understood. Quinolones are contraindicated in children because of concerns over skeletal growth and development. In addition, when quinolone antibiotics are orally administered, they should not be given concurrently with antacids or calcium or iron supplements. The quinolone antibiotics are usually well tolerated; adverse effects include dermatologic reactions, GI upset, dizziness and confusion, the potential to induce arrhythmias in susceptible individuals, and tendon disorders.[19] The tendon disorders associated with fluoroquinolone administration have been estimated to occur at a rate of 15 to 20 per 100,000 patients and manifest as both tendinitis and tendon rupture. Although any tendon can be affected, the Achilles tendon is frequently involved. The tendon problems associated with quinolone therapy are primarily seen in individuals older than 60 years and in patients receiving corticosteroid therapy. Although tendon effects are typically seen after quinolone therapy within 2 weeks of administration, these effects have also been seen weeks and months after therapy.

It is extremely difficult to prove clear cause-and-effect relationships between medications and adverse effects such as tendon rupture. Thus, the actual risk for development of such problems is unknown, and the data should be used simply as a guide for making more informed medication decisions.

Miscellaneous Antibiotics

Clindamycin, tetracyclines, trimethoprim/sulfamethoxazole, and linezolid are among the other antibiotics that may be used to treat infection. In general, these agents are used less commonly than the antibiotics described previously because of bacterial resistance, adverse effects, and cost considerations. For example, clindamycin is active against aerobic gram-positive organisms such as streptococcal, staphylococcal, and anaerobic bacteria, but it can cause diarrhea and other GI effects.

The tetracycline antibiotics are used for a variety of infections. Adverse effects include GI upset and photosensitivity and hypersensitivity reactions. The tetracyclines should not be used in children 8 years of age or younger because they can cause enamel hypoplasia and tooth discoloration in developing teeth. Medication interactions can also be a problem. Antacids containing aluminum, calcium, or magnesium, and laxatives containing magne-

sium given concurrently with tetracyclines interfere with tetracycline absorption. Iron products should also not be given concurrently with tetracycline antibiotics.

Trimethoprim/sulfamethoxazole has a broad application of use as an antibiotic agent. The most frequent adverse reactions associated with trimethoprim-sulfamethoxazole therapy are nausea and dermatologic reactions, such as rash and itching. Trimethoprim/sulfamethoxazole has also been shown to prolong the prothrombin time of persons receiving warfarin therapy; accordingly, the dosage of warfarin and prothrombin time must be carefully monitored if the medications are given concurrently.

Linezolid is a newer antibiotic agent with activity against gram-positive bacteria. Because of cost, linezolid is generally reserved for treating infections that are resistant to other antibiotics. A unique adverse effect associated with linezolid therapy is an increased risk of thrombocytopenia, especially when therapy lasts longer than 14 days.[4,5] Thus, blood platelet levels should be monitored in patients receiving prolonged linezolid therapy.

Natural Products

Over the past few years, natural therapeutic products have steadily increased in popularity. Natural products are routinely used for a variety of medicinal purposes. Reasons for using the natural products include enhancement of overall health and performance, and treatment and prevention of disease.

A few considerations are in order when selecting a natural product. The term natural product does not necessarily mean safe product. Natural products with medicinal properties should be treated with the same respect accorded any other medication with potential adverse effects and medication interactions. Therefore, anyone taking these products should inform his or her physician and pharmacist. Also, only standardized products from reputable manufacturers should be used, and the dosage recommendations on the product's label should be within the appropriate therapeutic range for the product. Patients who are pregnant or breastfeeding should only use these products under the supervision of a physician. Finally, it is extremely important to recognize that many natural products have more than one name and are often marketed in combinations. Failure to rec-

Thrombocytopenia
An abnormal decrease in the number of blood platelets.

ognize either of these facts could have dangerous consequences.

Ephedra (Ma huang)/Ephedrine

Ephedrine is derived from the plant *Ephedra sinica* and has been used therapeutically as a decongestant and central nervous system stimulant for thousands of years.[20,21] Recently, however, ephedra and ephedra-containing products have come under considerable scrutiny regarding safety. Manufacturers of ephedra products make claims that their products improve athletic performance, improve concentration, and facilitate weight loss. Sales of ephedrine and ephedrine-containing substances have been banned in the United States.

Ephedra is a sympathomimetic agent that causes vasoconstriction, cardiac stimulation, and bronchial muscle relaxation. It also inhibits perspiration. Potential adverse effects associated with ephedra usage are heart arrhythmias, elevated blood pressure, heart attack, stroke, headache, dizziness, seizures, and psychosis. Ephedra use has been linked to several deaths as well.[22] An additional concern is that caffeine potentiates the effects of ephedrine, and the combination can result in added danger.

Caffeine

Caffeine has long been used to enhance endurance and stay alert. Caffeine is found in many readily available products.[20,21] Benefit claims made by manufacturers of caffeine products include improved athletic performance, increased energy, delayed fatigue, and glycogen-sparing effects. When caffeine is used, blood epinephrine levels rise, resulting in an increased heart rate, higher blood pressure, and central nervous system stimulation. An additional pharmacologic effect of caffeine is diuresis, so the potential for dehydration exists when caffeine products are used. Other adverse events that can occur with caffeine use include heart palpitations, headache, nausea, and tremor.

Creatine

Creatine is a supplement used to enhance athletic performance by promoting protein synthesis for muscle building and providing a readily available source of energy for muscle contraction.[20,21] This is believed to occur via an increase in the amount of phosphocreatine available for conversion of adenosine diphosphate to adenosine triphosphate, an energy source for muscle contraction. Adverse effects associated with creatine supplementation include weight gain resulting from water retention, increased water requirements, and the potential for muscle cramps and heat-related illness secondary to electrolyte abnormalities. Creatine should be used cautiously in patients with renal or liver abnormalities.

Glucosamine

Glucosamine is an amino-sugar substrate used in the synthesis of the major structural components of cartilage.[20,21] In addition to a cartilage-synthesis function, glucosamine also appears to have anti-inflammatory effects. Because of these pharmacologic functions, glucosamine products are marketed as antiarthritic agents. Although more research studies need to be conducted to analyze long-term safety and efficacy, available data indicate that glucosamine is more beneficial in the treatment of mild arthritis than in severe forms of the disease. Glucosamine is not known to have any major toxicities, and the adverse events seen with glucosamine have been primarily limited to mild GI upset.

Chondroitin

Chondroitin sulfate is a natural substance that is a critical component of connective tissue and joint cartilage.[20,21] When used as a supplement, chondroitin sulfate is claimed to support the maintenance of healthy cartilage and joints. Chondroitin sulfate absorbs water, leading to increased cartilage thickness. This increased thickness results in greater absorption and distribution of compression forces on joints. Chondroitin sulfate is often given in combination with glucosamine and has not been associated with any significant adverse effects to date.

Methyl Sulfonyl Methane (MSM)

Methyl sulfonyl methane (MSM) is a derivative of dimethyl sulfoxide (DMSO) with anti-inflammatory and analgesic properties.[20,21] The advantage of MSM over DMSO is that it causes less odor and produces sustained concentrations in the body. Many theoretic mechanisms exist regarding the pain relief seen with MSM therapy, including inhibiting pain transmission along type c nerve fibers, enhancing blood flow, and reducing muscle spasm. The anti-inflammatory properties of MSM are thought to possibly occur via inhibited release of inflammatory mediators. MSM is a well-tolerated agent; no serious adverse effects or toxicity have been routinely seen.

References

1. The National Collegiate Athletic Association: *NCAA Sports Medicine Handbook 2003-04*. Indianapolis, IN, The National Collegiate Athletic Association, 2003.

2. Kanikkannan N: Iontophoresis-based transdermal delivery systems. *Biodrugs* 2002;16:339-347.

3. Machet L, Boucaud A: Phonophoresis: Efficiency, mechanisms and skin tolerance. *Intl J Pharm* 2002;243:1-15.

4. *American Hospital Formulary Science Drug Information*, ed 2003. Bethesda, MD, American Society of Health-System Pharmacists, 2003.

5. *Drug Facts and Comparisons*, ed 56. St. Louis, MO, Facts & Comparisons, 2001.

6. Dipiro JT, Talbert RL, Yee GC, Matzke GR, Well BG, Posey LM (eds): *Pharmacotherapy: A Pathophysiologic Approach*, ed 5. New York, NY, McGraw-Hill Medical Publishing Division, 2002.

7. *Physicians' Desk Reference 2003*, ed 57. Montvale, NJ: Medical Economics, 2002.

8. Mukherjee D, Nisson SE, Topol EJ: Risk of cardiovascular events associated with selective COX-2 inhibitors. *JAMA* 2001;286:954-959.

9. Barkin RL, Barkin D: Pharmacologic management of acute and chronic pain: Focus on drug interactions and patient-specific pharmacotherapeutic selection. *South Med J* 2001;94:756-770.

10. McCarthy DM: Comparative toxicity of nonsteroidal anti-inflammatory drugs. *Am J Med* 1999;107:37S-47S.

11. Rainsford KD: Profile and mechanisms of gastrointestinal and other side effects of nonsteroidal anti-inflammatory drugs (NSAIDs). *Am J Med* 1999;107:27S-36S.

12. Jackson LM and Hawkey CJ: COX-2 selective nonsteroidal anti-inflammatory drugs: Do they really offer any advantages? *Drugs* 2000;59:1207-1216.

13. Urban MK: COX-2 specific inhibitors offer improved advantages over traditional NSAIDs. *Orthopedics* 2000;23 (suppl):761S-764S.

14. Goodman S, Ma T, Trindade M, et al: COX-2 selective NSAID decreases bone ingrowth in vivo. *J Orthop Res* 2002;20:1164-1169.

15. Brown C, Mazzula JP, Mok MS, Nussdorf RT, Rubin PD, Schwesinger WH: Comparison of repeat doses of intramuscular ketorolac tromethamine and morphine sulfate for analgesia after major surgery. *Pharmacotherapy* 1990;10(6 Pt 2):45S-50S.

16. Zimmerman HJ, Maddrey WC: Acetaminophen (paracetamol) hepatotoxicity with regular intake of alcohol: Analysis of instances of therapeutic misadventure. *Hepatology* 1995;22:767-773.

17. Nesathurai S: Steroids and spinal cord injury: Revisiting the NASCIS 2 and NASCIS 3 trials. *J Trauma* 1998;45:1088-1093.

18. Walker J, Criddle LM: Methylprednisolone in acute spinal cord injury: Fact or fantasy? *J Emerg Nurs* 2001; 27:401-403.

19. Casparian JM, Luchi M, Moffat RE, Hinthorn D: Quinolones and tendon ruptures. *South Med J* 2000;93: 488-491.

20. *Natural Products Pocket Guide, 2000-2001.* Hudson, OH, Lexi-Comp, Inc, and Cincinnati, OH, Natural Health Resources, 2000.

21. *Physicians' Desk Reference for Herbal Medicines*, ed 2. Montvale, NJ, Medical Economics, 2000.

22. Haller CD, Benowitz NL: Adverse cardiovascular and central nervous system events associated with dietary supplements containing ephedra alkaloids. *New Engl J Med* 2000;343:1833-1838.

4

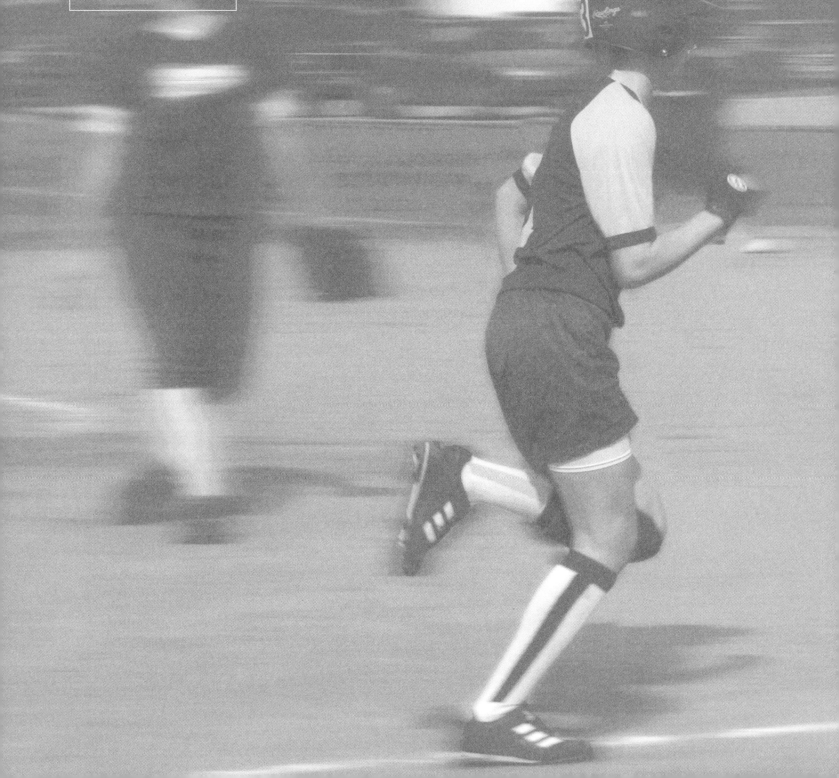

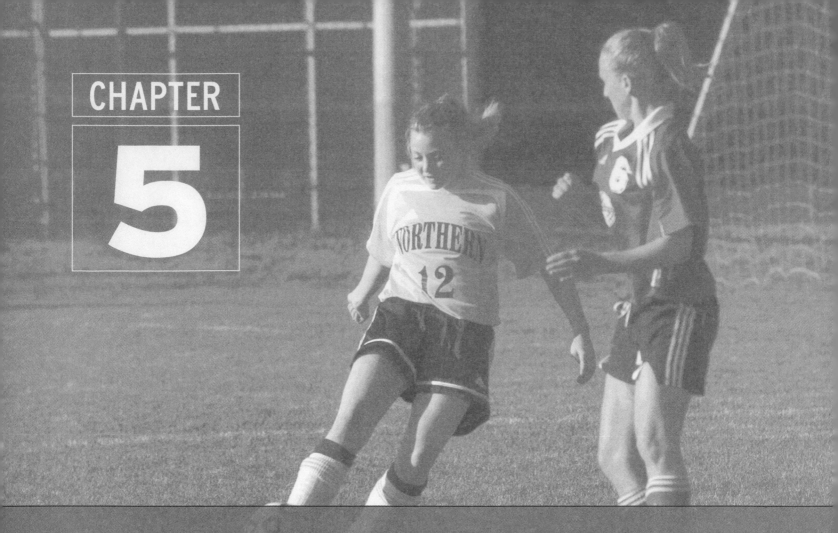

CHAPTER 5

Foot, Ankle, and Leg Injuries

Peggy A. Houglum, PhD, ATC, PT
David A. Porter, MD, PhD

TOE

First Metatarsophalangeal Joint Sprain (Turf Toe)

Hyperextension, hyperflexion, varus stress, and valgus stress of the first metatarsophalangeal (MTP) joint can sprain the capsuloligamentous structures, causing "turf toe." Turf toe is a nondescript term used to describe a wide range of injuries, including dorsal capsule sprains, capsule inflammation, and plantar plate injuries.

The most frequent cause of injury is joint hyperextension.[1] Turf toe is common in football players and is thought to occur more on artificial turf, especially older turf that has lost its resiliency and absorbs less shock than newer surfaces. A softer, more flexible shoe that is less resistant to toe extension may further contribute to the onset of turf toe, as may a stiff MTP joint, reduced ankle motion, history of prior injury, player position, player weight, age, and years of participation.[2]

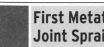

CLINICAL PRESENTATION

History

First MTP joint hyperextension, especially when the ankle is dorsiflexed[2]
First MTP joint pain

Observation

Swelling and possible discoloration of the first MTP joint

Functional Status

Antalgic gait with toe-off occurring laterally

Physical Evaluation Findings

Reduced or painful range of motion (ROM)
First MTP joint valgus stress or hyperextension may cause pain

Differential Diagnosis

First metatarsal fracture, proximal first phalanx fracture, sesamoid fracture, MTP joint dislocation (grade III turf toe), sesamoiditis, plantar fascia rupture, hallux rigidus, hallux valgus, degenerative joint disease

Imaging Techniques

Radiographs should be obtained during the initial diagnostic workup. Anteroposterior (AP) and lateral radiographs may be ordered to rule out bony injury and evaluate joint alignment. Degenerative changes may be noted in chronic conditions. Magnetic resonance imaging (MRI), computed tomography (CT), or supplementary radiographs should be obtained to rule out other possible injuries when symptoms do not subside with treatment. In addition, MRI can be useful in determining plantar plate integrity.

Definitive Diagnosis

The definitive diagnosis is made based on the patient's history, clinical findings, and the absence of evidence of acute trauma on radiographs.

Pathomechanics and Functional Limitations

Normal foot mechanics place a significant amount of stress on the first MTP joint. When walking, 30% to 50% of the body weight is transferred to the joint. During activities such as running and jumping, the forces applied to the first MTP joint are magnified to three to eight times body weight. Stresses applied to an injured MTP joint must be limited until healing is sufficient to tolerate even the relatively low-level forces experienced during walking. Prolonged injury can result in hallux rigidus, hallux valgus, or both.

■ Immediate Management

Immediate treatment includes the usual course of rest, ice, compression, and elevation. Cold application remains the initial modality of choice; an ice bag or ice bucket may be used.

■ Medications

Nonsteroidal anti-inflammatory drugs (NSAIDs) may be prescribed in the early postinjury phase of rehabilitation. In higher-level athletes, the physician may inject the joint directly with a combination of anti-inflammatory and analgesic medications.

■ Surgical Intervention

Surgery is indicated if an MTP joint dislocation cannot be reduced. However, surgery is unnecessary for routine turf toe conditions unless the plantar plate is ruptured.

■ Postinjury/Postoperative Management

Rest, including partial or non–weight-bearing crutch ambulation, and limiting the amount of toe extension decrease the symptoms.[1] Full weight bearing is permitted when the patient can ambulate normally without assistive devices. It may be necessary to progress from non–weight bearing to partial weight bearing with crutches before normal weight bearing is possible.

A firm-soled shoe is helpful in relieving weight-bearing pain. A steel foot plate beneath the innersole of the shoe or taping the toe can splint the first MTP joint during functional activities.

■ Injury-Specific Treatment and Rehabilitation Concerns

Specific Concerns

Limit first MTP joint extension.
Encourage early, pain-free ROM.
Control inflammation.
Restore joint motion.

Once pain and swelling have decreased, joint mobilization and active and passive stretching exercises can be started to regain MTP joint ROM. If ankle motion is deficient, the treatment program should include a regimen of activities to restore normal motion.

Strengthening of the extrinsic and intrinsic muscles of the foot, ankle, and leg is included in the rehabilitation program. Once strength has improved, stress levels applied to the joint are gradually increased. Activities begin with bilateral heel raises, progressing to single-leg heel raises and then to resisted heel raises. Resisted heel raises begin in slow, controlled motion and progress to faster motions with rapid changes in direction as the patient's tolerance for these activities improves. Weight-bearing activities during treatment should be performed with a stiff shoe insert to protect the MTP joint, and the patient should be allowed time to adjust to the device.

■ Estimated Amount of Time Lost

If normal ambulation and running are possible with a grade I sprain, the patient may continue sport participation with shoe modifications and toe taping. A grade II sprain can restrict participation for 2 to 4 weeks, whereas a grade III sprain can result in 6 to 8 weeks lost.[1] Although a properly treated turf toe can heal in 2 to 8 weeks, disability may be prolonged because of the secondary effects of injury and the MTP joint stress applied during normal activity. If the condition is chronic or has not been treated appropriately, disability may be even more prolonged.

Chronic turf toe delays the return to normal participation. Older patients with compromised distal lower extremity circulation require a longer recovery period.

■ Return-to-Play Criteria

Full ROM (70° to 90° of extension) and strength of the intrinsic foot muscles, especially the first digit flexors and abductors, must be restored to preinjury levels. The patient should be able to push off from each foot, jump and land, cut and stop suddenly, sprint forward and laterally, and run posteriorly on the involved foot without difficulty.

Functional Bracing

A stiff-soled shoe or a stiff insert such as a steel foot plate placed in the shoe reduces pain during ambulation. Such a modification should be continued once the athlete has returned to activity to further protect the toe and reduce stresses applied to it. Graphite or Rolled Steel innersoles can be manufactured and inserted in any shoe. Toe-spica taping to restrict extension can also allow the patient to return to function more comfortably (**CT** 5-1).

Sesamoiditis

CLINICAL PRESENTATION

History

Overuse or direct trauma to the plantar aspect of the first MTP joint may be reported.
Abnormal foot posture may be noted.
Generalized pain around the great toe may be reported.
A sudden "snap" or "pop" during running may be described.
Pain occurs with great toe hyperextension during terminal stance and preswing.

Observation

Swelling may be localized under the first MTP joint.
The foot may be supinated.
Reduced great-toe active flexion and extension may be present.
Pes cavus or a plantar-flexed first ray may be noted.

Functional Status

Antalgic gait secondary to pain when bearing weight on the first ray
Decreased first MTP joint extension

Physical Evaluation Findings

The sesamoids are point tender.

The sesamoids are attached to each other by a strong intersesamoid ligament and plantar plate and to the plantar surface of the head of the first metatarsal. Lined with hyaline cartilage, the sesamoids are embedded within the flexor hallucis brevis tendon and are stabilized by intrinsic ligaments (**Figure 5-1**). During MTP joint flexion, they move proximally into the metatarsal's head-neck region and distally to the end of the metatarsal during extension. The sesamoids elevate the tendon away from the axis of joint motion, thereby increasing the tendon's mechanical advantage. They also help to absorb weight-bearing forces, protect the tendon, and reduce friction.[3]

CT Clinical Technique 5-1

Turf Toe Taping

Application

1. Cut a 2-in-wide piece of moleskin as indicated in **(A)**.
2. Position the great toe in neutral. Place anchors around the distal phalanx of the great toe and one around the midfoot **(B)**.
3. Using the moleskin, apply a checkrein that spans the plantar surface of the foot and toe between the anchors **(C)**.
4. Use 1-in tape to connect the anchors, taping from the toe to the foot. Apply strips on the plantar surface to prevent hyperextension, on the dorsal surface to restrict hyperflexion, or on both surfaces to keep the toe immobile **(D)**.
5. Spica wraps may be applied to further support the joint **(E)**.
6. Complete the taping by repeating the anchor strips around the distal toe and midfoot **(F)**.

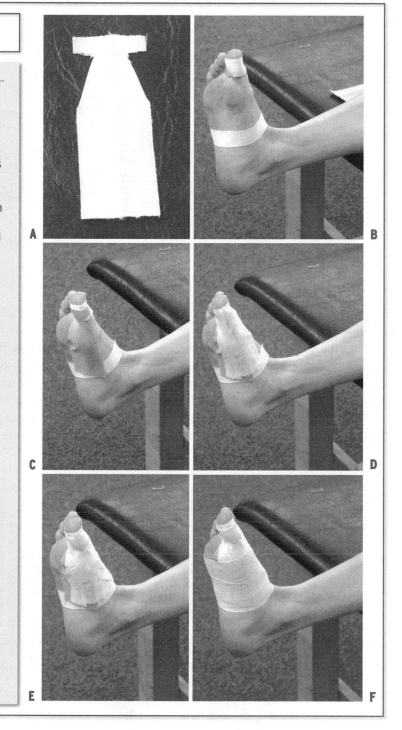

Repetitive tensile forces applied to the sesamoids during activity, especially while the great toe is extended, and combined with compressive weight-bearing loads can easily irritate the sesamoids. The larger medial sesamoid bears more weight than the lateral sesamoid and, therefore, receives more stress, but sesamoiditis can affect either bone.[4] Individuals with a cavus or pronated foot, plantar-flexed first ray, or tight plantar fascia are more susceptible to sesamoid injuries. Sesamoiditis is sometimes referred to as "dancer's toe" because of its prevalence in this population.

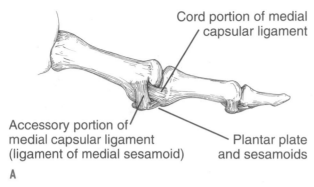

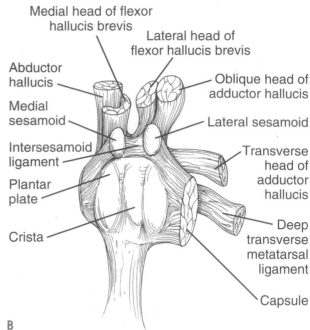

Figure 5-1 Anatomy of the hallux. **A.** Components of the medial capsular ligament. **B.** Intrinsic muscles and ligaments surrounding the sesamoids. The intrinsic muscles have been dissected and moved distally to show the plantar aspect of the first metatarsophalangeal joint. (Adapted with permission from Richardson EG: Injuries to the hallucal sesamoids in the athlete. *Foot Ankle* 1987;7: 228-244.)

Differential Diagnosis

Acute sesamoid fracture, sesamoid stress fracture, first MTP joint sprain, hallux rigidus, hallux valgus, avascular necrosis, osteochondritis, arthritis, bursitis, medial plantar nerve neuropathy

Bipartite A congenital or traumatic splitting of a structure into two parts.

Imaging Techniques

Sesamoid views are helpful in conjunction with AP views to rule out a sesamoid fracture or **bipartite** sesamoids (**Figure 5-2**). A bone scan can reveal increased uptake, consistent with periosteal inflammation or disruption of the capsuloligamentous structures.

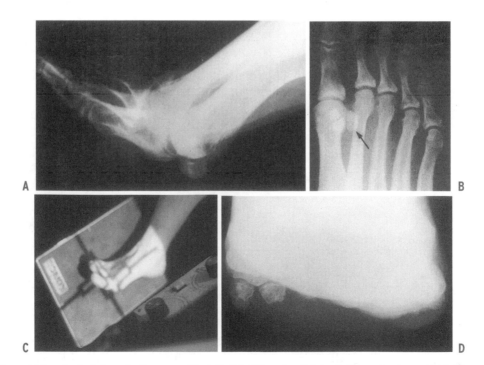

Figure 5-2 Radiographic imaging techniques for the sesamoids. **A.** Medial oblique view. **B.** Lateral oblique view (arrow highlights sesamoids). **C.** Technique for posteroanterior axial view. **D.** Axial view demonstrating medial sesamoid degeneration. (Reproduced with permission from Richardson EG: Hallucal sesamoid pain: Causes and surgical treatment. *J Am Acad Orthop Surg* 1999;7:270-278.)

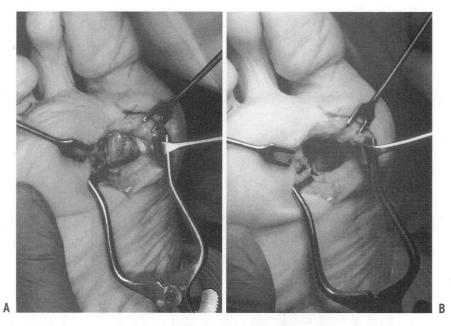

Figure 5-3 Surgical excision of the lateral sesamoid. **A.** The incision is made from the plantar aspect of the foot. The flexor hallucis longus tendon and neurovascular bundle must be identified and protected. **B.** View after sesamoid removal. (Reproduced with permission from Richardson EG: Hallucal sesamoid pain: Causes and surgical treatment. *J Am Acad Orthop Surg* 1999;7:270-278.)

Definitive Diagnosis

Diagnosis is confirmed through a thorough physical examination, radiographic findings, and elimination of other possible diagnoses.

Pathomechanics and Functional Limitations

Pain is the primary factor limiting activity. If weight-bearing stresses under the first metatarsal head are not reduced, the inflammatory process continues, further limiting function. With time, pain, muscular compensation, and deterioration of the joint surfaces alter first MTP joint biomechanics and lead to other conditions such as hallux rigidus or hallux valgus.

■ Immediate Management

Ice and protected weight bearing should be implemented. The extent of protected weight bearing is dictated by the severity of symptoms. Padding and other pressure-relief techniques may allow normal activities to continue, but MTP joint hyperextension should be avoided.

■ Medications

An NSAID in conjunction with the immediate management can help to control pain and inflammation. Corticosteroids can also aid in treating this problem; an injection resolves pain more quickly than oral medication.

■ Surgical Intervention

Open excision of a sesamoid may be required if the problem fails to improve with conservative measures. Two thirds of the sesamoid can be removed without altering the joint's ligamentous structure.[3]

The lateral sesamoid is approached through a plantar incision (**Figure 5-3**). The medial sesamoid is approached via a medial incision (**Figure 5-4**). The sesamoid is excised with a scalpel, taking care not to damage the tendon or ligaments. If the patient has been diagnosed with plantar fascia tightness, that condition may be addressed during this surgical procedure (see plantar fasciitis, p 78).

After surgery, the patient is restricted from first MTP joint extension, which stresses the joint capsule and associated muscles until healing is complete. Rehabilitation focuses on strengthening the flexor hallucis longus and brevis muscles and maintaining joint ROM.

■ Postinjury/Postoperative Management

Postoperatively, the tendon and incision are protected by limiting weight bearing and MTP joint hyperextension. Instruct patients to avoid wearing high-heeled shoes, which extend the great toe and focus weight-bearing forces on the sesamoids. Taping and padding may assist the athlete in returning to sport sooner but should not be used after surgery to shorten the recovery process (**Figure 5-5**).

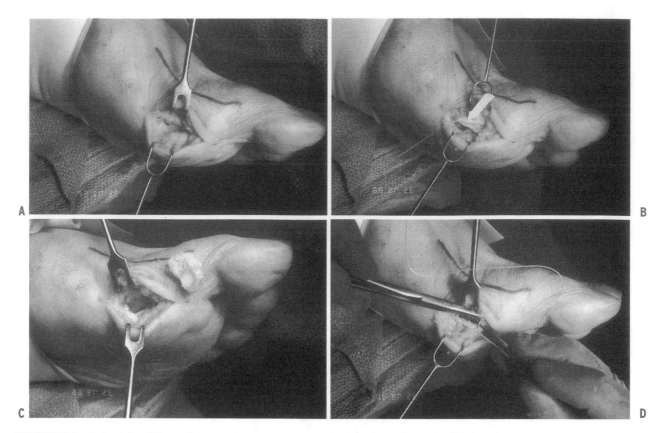

Figure 5-4 Surgical excision of the medial sesamoid. **A.** This incision is made along the medial joint line. **B.** the plantar medial hallucal nerve is identified and avoided. **C.** The medial sesamoid is excised. **D.** The joint capsule is stitched closed, and the flexor hallucis brevis tendon is repaired. (Reproduced with permission from Richardson EG: Hallucal sesamoid pain: Causes and surgical treatment. *J Am Acad Orthop Surg* 1999;7:270-278.)

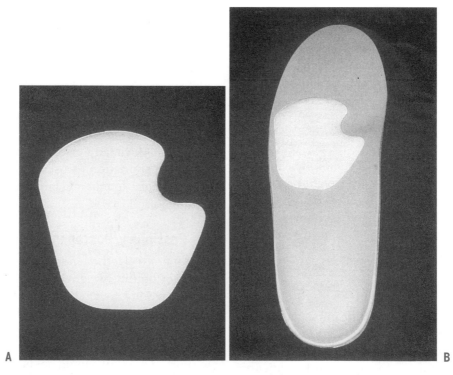

Figure 5-5 Padding to reduce weight-bearing forces on the sesamoids. **A.** Pad cut from felt or similar material with a cutout for the sesamoids (upper right). **B.** The pad is then affixed to the patient's orthosis or shoe insert. Note the added dimple under the weight-bearing area of the sesamoids. (Reproduced with permission from Richardson EG: Hallucal sesamoid pain: Causes and surgical treatment. *J Am Acad Orthop Surg* 1999;7:270-278.)

Injury-Specific Treatment and Rehabilitation Concerns

Specific Concerns

Reduce weight-bearing forces on the sesamoids.

Limit great toe extension, especially during weight bearing, in the early stages of treatment.

Progress to flexion-extension ROM exercises.

Strengthen the toe flexors.

Accommodative changes in footwear can help to relieve symptoms[4,5](**Table 5-1**). If footwear alterations do not sufficiently reduce pain, crutches, a short leg cast, or a brace may be necessary.[5]

If palpation reveals scar tissue adhesions, soft-tissue mobilization techniques may improve the mobility of the sesamoids and permit their movement during toe flexion and extension. If the MTP and interphalangeal joints have lost their normal accessory movement, grade III and IV AP, posteroanterior, and lateral glides and rotational joint mobilization can aid in restoring mobility once inflammation has subsided.

If these techniques are not successful, a below-knee, non–weight-bearing brace or cast for 4 to 8 weeks may be necessary to accomplish the desired goals. If symptoms persist despite this conservative approach, surgical excision may be necessary.

Estimated Amount of Time Lost

If adequate stress reduction can be accomplished with footwear modifications, no time may be lost. If pain is severe, the patient may need to restrict the pressure applied to the area by reducing or halting the offending activity until inflammation subsides. If surgical excision is the treatment, an extended recovery time is necessary, perhaps 3 to 4 months.

Return-to-Play Criteria

Before returning to competition, the patient should have no pain during sesamoid palpation or during activity, and the first MTP joint should have at least 60° to 75° of extension and be pain free.

Functional Bracing

A stiff shoe insert reduces the shear forces applied to the sesamoids. An orthotic or taping may also help in returning the athlete to play (see **Figure 5-5**). Taping reduces great toe MTP joint hyperextension (see **CT** 5-1).

Hallux Valgus

Hallux valgus is deviation of the first toe at the MTP joint, which leads to the formation of a bunion. The proximal phalanx angulates laterally, and the medial aspect of the first metatarsal head is prominent and painful (**Figure 5-6**). With time, **exostosis** begins to form on the medial side of the joint, leading to characteristic bunion development. The deformity is more prevalent in women than in men and can

> **Exostosis** A bone spur or bony overgrowth.

Table 5-1

Footwear Modifications to Relieve Sesamoiditis

Lower heels of the shoes.

Use a shoe with a thick, medium to firm outer sole.

Use a stiff-soled shoe to decrease first MTP joint extension.

Insert a pad with a soft innersole.

Insert a pad that extends just proximal to the head of the first metatarsal to decrease weight-bearing loads on the sesamoids.

Carve a depression in the innersole of the shoe to accommodate the sesamoids.

Use a custom-made orthotic.

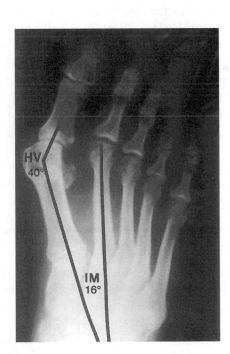

Figure 5-6 The hallux valgus (HV) angle is formed by the intersection of lines bisecting the first metatarsal and the first phalanx of the great toe. The normal angle is approximately 15°. (The radiograph demonstrates a 40° angle.) The angle between the first and second metatarsals (intermetatarsal [IM] angle) should be less than 9°. (Reproduced with permission from Mann RA: Disorders of the first metatarsophalangeal joint. *J Am Acad Orthop Surg* 1995;3:34-43.)

History

This deformity occurs over time.

Observation

Obvious first MTP joint deformity, with valgus angulation and prominence medially

The medial joint may be red and swollen secondary to pressure and irritation from footwear.

A bunion may be present.

Pes planus is often noted.

Functional Status

Full weight bearing is possible, but the patient is more comfortable without shoes.

The first toe is abducted and may override or underride the second toe.

The lower extremity may remain in external rotation during gait.

Physical Evaluation Findings

The medial MTP joint is tender to the touch.

ROM is commonly within normal limits.

be seen in young athletes, especially gymnasts and dancers. In adults, the onset occurs during the third decade of life.

The first MTP joint contributes to the windlass mechanism, raising the arch when the toe is dorsiflexed (see Plantar Fasciitis, p 78) and acting as a cam to control balance during ambulation.[6] During gait, the valgus stress applied to the first MTP joint from terminal stance to preswing increases joint forces and eventually affects the joint's medial collateral ligament.

Hallux valgus conditions range in deformity and pain from a mild medial eminence to a lateral first MTP joint subluxation of significant magnitude, causing problems in the second toe. Often pain is caused by more than one source and can be associated with pes planus.

Stretching of the medial joint capsule with repetitive stress applied during ambulation ultimately causes capsule inflammation and can contribute to pain.[7] The shoe rubbing against the soft tissues can also cause pain. A compressive force on the lateral joint and the increased stress applied to the second MTP joint can add to hallux valgus pain and exacerbate bunion development. Occasionally, the second MTP joint can develop secondary laxity in compensation for first MTP joint rigidity; both conditions can cause pain in more advanced cases.

Differential Diagnosis

Hallux rigidus, gout, rheumatoid arthritis, sesamoiditis

Imaging Techniques

Weight-bearing radiographs help to determine the extent of the condition and associated malalignment that may affect the MTP joint (**Figure 5-7**). The angle between the first and second metatarsals should be determined to help predict the rate of deterioration: the greater the divergence, the greater the chance of progression and continued symptoms.

Definitive Diagnosis

An angle greater than 15° between the proximal phalanx and first metatarsal; positive physical findings, and confirmatory radiographic findings are diagnostic.

Pathomechanics and Functional Limitations

When the joint is altered, normal function is impaired, and during terminal stance to preswing, the foot passively rolls over the lateral metatarsal heads rather than over the first MTP joint. A hallux valgus deformity commonly develops in a hypomobile foot as the forefoot remains pronated during the last half of stance, when it should be supinating. As the heel is raised from the ground in terminal stance and the foot remains pronated, the forces are directed to the medial aspect of the great toe, with little force distribution to the lateral aspect of the foot. Over time, repetitive great toe stress first causes a callus build-up over the medial aspect of the toe, and then the MTP joint and the sesamoid bones subluxate, resulting in medial capsule stretching and stress to the great toe tendons and the second toe.

■ Immediate Management

Ice, immobilization, and protective weight bearing in symptomatic patients

■ Medications

One of the NSAIDs may be prescribed to control the acute local inflammatory process. Although not commonly used, a corticosteroid injection may be considered with severe pain and associated MTP joint degeneration.

■ Surgical Intervention

Several different surgical techniques can be used to correct a hallux valgus deformity. The nature and cause of the deformity, the patient's complaints, the radiographic findings, and the sur-

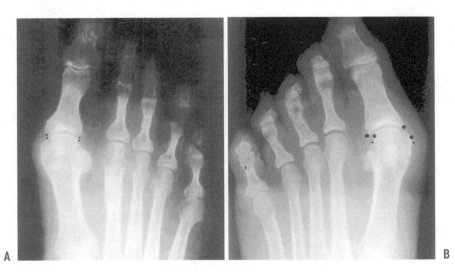

Figure 5-7 Congruency of joint surfaces in the presence of hallux valgus. **A.** Congruent joint surfaces. The surfaces are parallel, and there is no lateral subluxation of the metatarsal head. **B.** Subluxation associated with hallux valgus. The joint surfaces are not parallel, and the proximal phalanx is subluxated laterally relative to the metatarsal head. (Reproduced with permission from Mann RA: Disorders of the first metatarsophalangeal joint. *J Am Acad Orthop Surg* 1995;3:34-43.)

geon's preference factor into the decision-making process.[7] In competitive athletes, hallux valgus surgery is indicated only after the career is completed or when shoe modifications, inserts, and NSAIDs have failed, *and* the patient is unable to compete because of pain.

A distal osteotomy with a soft-tissue procedure and occasionally a proximal phalanx osteotomy is most often performed on competitive athletes[8] (ST 5-1). If hallux rigidus is concurrent, the dorsal 25% to 35% of the first metatarsal head

and spurs is removed. Some surgeons include a dorsal closing-wedge osteotomy of the proximal phalanx. The goal is to obtain 90% of MTP joint extension at surgery.

■ Postinjury/Postoperative Management

The patient is instructed to wear shoes that have adequate forefoot width and a low heel. Avoid high-heeled and pointed-toe shoes because of the compressive forces they place on the first MTP joint.

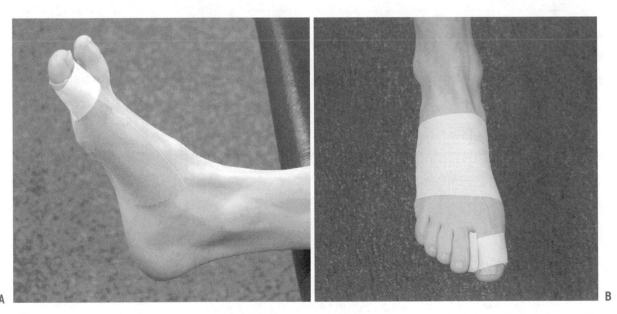

Figure 5-8 Taping for hallux valgus. **A.** Moleskin is used to apply a mild varus force to the great toe. **B.** Padding between the first and second toes assists in discouraging the valgus alignment.

S|T Surgical Technique 5-1

Correction of Hallux Valgus (Chevron Procedure)

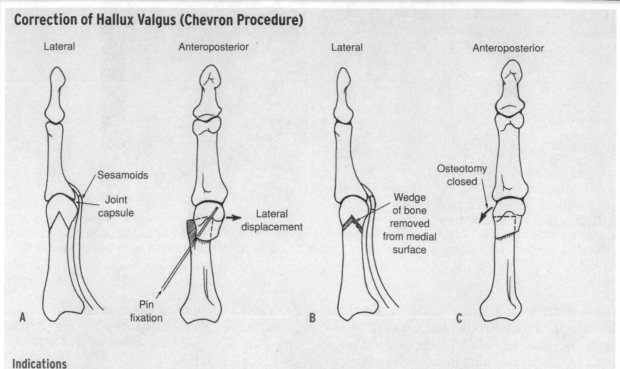

Indications

Hallux valgus angle less than 30° and an intermetatarsal angle of less than 13° that fail to respond to conservative treatment

Overview

1. The incision is made over the medial aspect of the joint.
2. A chevron (V-shaped) wedge is cut into the distal metatarsal (**A**).
3. The head is translated laterally 4 to 5 mm. Occasionally a 1- to 3-mm wedge of bone is removed to correct the distal metatarsal articular angle (**B**).
4. The osteotomy is closed and fixated with a pin (**C**).

Functional Limitations

Great toe extension is often limited. Appropriate early great toe passive and active-assisted exercise can maximize extension. First ray shortening often results from this procedure.

Implications for Rehabilitation

High-impact activity must be avoided after osteotomy until radiographically proven healing occurs. MTP joint extension is emphasized, and tight-fitting shoes should be avoided.

Potential Complications

If the valgus deformity is too great, correction may be incomplete. Loss of internal fixation and avascular necrosis are also possible.

Figure reproduced with permission from Mann RA: Disorders of the first metatarsophalangeal joint. *J Am Acad Orthop Surg* 1995;3:34-43.

Orthotics to correct pes planus do not correct the hallux valgus but may reduce the rate of deformity progression.

The toe can be taped with a medial checkrein to reduce the valgus deformity. A felt or soft rubber insert can be placed between the first and second toes to further reduce the angulation (**Figure 5-8**). A doughnut pad reduces pain caused by a bunion.

■ Injury-Specific Treatment and Rehabilitation Concerns

Specific Concerns

Proper footwear to decrease external forces on the deformity
If a bunion is present, protect it with a donut pad.
Correct foot biomechanics with an orthotic if indicated.

The most important issues when treating hallux valgus nonsurgically are identifying possible causes and reducing pain. Individuals with this condition commonly have pes planus and may benefit from orthotics. Although the orthotics do not resolve the hallux valgus, they may stop the degenerative progression. Pain relief is primarily accomplished by altering footwear. Shoes with rigid or leather uppers are more irritating to hallux valgus than shoes with soft uppers made of cloth or nylon mesh. MTP joint padding to reduce pressure on the tender area may also reduce pain. Shoes should have a toe box of adequate width into which the forefoot fits comfortably.

After surgical correction, active ROM activities, joint mobilization, and gradual return to activities as pain allows are sufficient for the patient to resume a normal level of function. Strengthening the intrinsic foot muscles is necessary. Gait training may be necessary if the patient reverts to the previous gait style.

◼ Estimated Amount of Time Lost

This condition is self-limiting. If the patient can wear a shoe that does not irritate the bunion, normal activities may be possible. If surgery is required, 3 to 6 months may be needed before full return to participation is possible, primarily because of the time required to relieve pain, wear shoes, and run without pain after surgery.

◼ Return-to-Play Criteria

The patient must be able to wear the appropriate athletic shoe and run, cut, and jump without pain. The MTP joint must have near full ROM (at least 60° of dorsiflexion), full intrinsic muscle strength of the great toe muscles, and restored joint proprioception, balance, and agility.

Functional Bracing

Taping and protective inserts may help to support the first MTP joint; a donut pad under the medial aspect of the great toe can relieve pressure. Realigning the toe with anchor tapes (as in taping for turf toe) may be helpful: the tape strips between the two anchors are applied to the medial side of the toe from the interphalangeal joint anchor to the midarch anchor while the toe is passively positioned in normal alignment. Once the toe tape strips maintain the toe in proper alignment, closing anchors are applied.

◼ Hallux Rigidus

Hallux rigidus, restricted first MTP joint dorsiflexion, is usually seen in 1 in 40 adults older than 50 years as the result of degenerative arthritis.[9] A long first metatarsal may predispose younger individuals to hallux rigidus.[10] Arthritis may be the result of previous injuries, such as an intra-articular fracture, turf toe, or osteochondral injury of the first metatarsal head,[2] although it may also occur insidiously without a history of trauma.[7] A dorsal or lateral osteophyte near the metatarsal head may become irritated from friction caused by the shoe's toe box (**Figure 5-9**).

CLINICAL PRESENTATION

History

Pain when climbing stairs
Pain when going up hills
Pain during preswing
Pain while wearing shoes

Observation

Gross deformity is often not present.
A dorsal or medial presence may represent an osteophyte.
Triceps surae atrophy may be noted in chronic conditions.
A relatively long first metatarsal may be present.

Functional Status

Decreased first MTP joint extension
Flexion ROM is within normal limits.
Premature or absent preswing phase in weight bearing

Physical Evaluation Findings

Pain during palpation of the dorsal and medial aspect of the first MTP joint
Pain with forced joint extension
Inability to stand on the toes

Differential Diagnosis

Hallux valgus, first MTP joint sprain, gout, sesamoiditis, degenerative arthritis

Imaging Techniques

The presence of a dorsal osteophyte on the first metatarsal head is not necessarily diagnostic but suggests hallux rigidus (**Figure 5-10**).

Definitive Diagnosis

Physical examination demonstrating limited ROM in dorsiflexion and positive radiographic studies

Pathomechanics and Functional Limitations

Normal gait requires 60° to 75° of first MTP joint extension. When dorsiflexion is limited, the patient may ambulate with the foot supinated, vault over the toe during the terminal stance and preswing phases of gait,[2] or walk on the lateral foot border. Because the patient does not extend the first MTP or have a normal heel-off to toe-off gait, atrophy may be present in the involved calf.[11] Compensatory conditions at the knee or hip may be secondary to gait alteration.

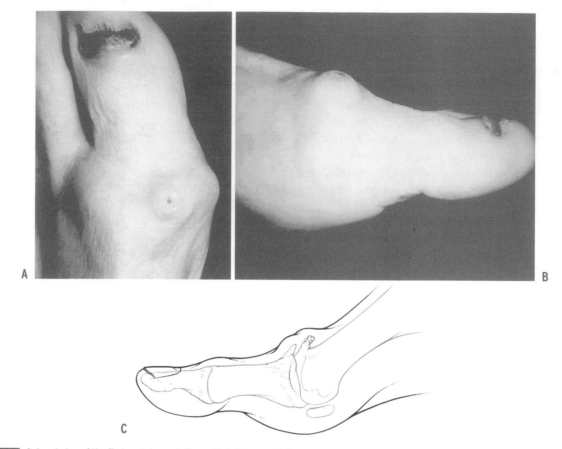

Figure 5-9 Osteophytes of the first metatarsophalangeal joint. **A.** Dorsal view. **B.** Lateral view. **C.** Illustration of osteophyte. (Parts A and B reproduced with permission from Greene WB (ed): *Essentials of Musculoskeletal Care*, ed 2. Rosemont, IL, American Academy of Orthopaedic Surgeons, 2000, pp 463-464. Part C reproduced with permission from Mann RA: Hallux rigidus, in Greene WB (ed): *Instructional Course Lectures XXXIX*. Park Ridge, IL, American Academy of Orthopaedic Surgeons, 1990, pp 15-21.)

■ Immediate Management

Ice and immobilization are initiated for pain relief. Firm-soled shoes or rigid inserts to prevent excessive MTP joint motion are recommended.

■ Medications

Although NSAIDs are helpful in decreasing inflammation, they do little for the overall problem. In severe cases, a corticosteroid injection may be helpful to control pain.

■ Surgical Intervention

Hallux rigidus is common, but the optimal surgical treatment is unclear.[9,10,12,13] Hallux rigidus surgery is indicated in competitive athletes for debilitating pain or when shoe modifications, taping, inserts, and NSAIDs have failed and the athlete cannot compete because of the pain.

Surgical techniques include cheilectomy, proximal phalanx osteotomy, and arthroplasty and may include excision of the phalanx or metatarsal or a prosthetic replacement.[10] A cheilectomy is the surgical technique recommended for athletes.[2] Proximal os-

Cheilectomy Surgical removal of bone spurs.
Arthroplasty Joint replacement surgery.

teotomies, in which the base of the proximal phalanx is resected, are not used on athletes because they would disrupt the plantar plate and flexor hallucis attachments, resulting in decreased push-off strength.[2] Distal osteotomies with soft-tissue procedures are most often used for competitive athletes (see ⓢⓣ 5-1). Hallux rigidus surgery involves removing the dorsal 25% to 35% of the first metatarsal head and spurs. The goal is to achieve 90% of great toe MTP joint extension at surgery.

Great toe extension is often limited after surgery. Appropriate early great toe passive and active-assisted exercises can minimize this limitation. High-impact activity must be avoided after osteotomy surgery until radiographically proven healing occurs. Extension of the MTP joint should be emphasized. After hallux valgus surgery, tight-fitting shoes should be avoided, and the use of orthotics to limit or protect extension can be helpful.

■ Postinjury/Postoperative Management

Postinjury management is directed at preventing reinjury, which is accomplished with rigid inserts to limit MTP joint motion and irritation and a wide

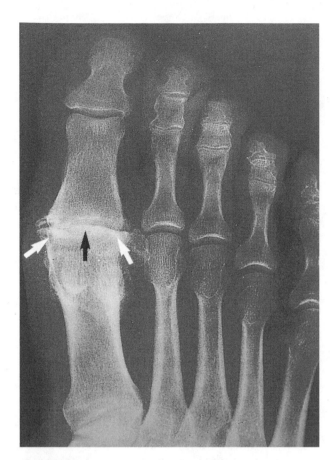

Figure 5-10 Anteroposterior view of hallux rigidus. Weight-bearing view demonstrates narrowing of the joint space (black arrow) and medial and lateral osteophytes (white arrows). (Reproduced with permission from Johnson TR, Steinbach LS (eds): *Essentials of Musculoskeletal Imaging.* Rosemont, IL, American Academy of Orthopaedic Surgeons, 2004, p 631.)

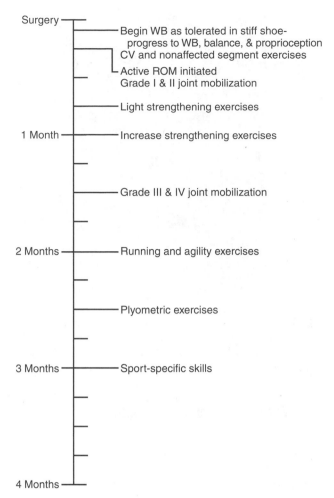

Note: Time frames are approximate. Function is the guide.

toebox to prevent metatarsal head compression. High-heeled shoes are avoided. After surgery, routine incision care is provided to the surgical site; weight bearing is protected, and impact activities are avoided. Activities can be advanced after 6 to 8 weeks.

■ Injury-Specific Treatment and Rehabilitation Concerns

> **Specific Concerns**
>
> Remove compressive MTP joint forces with footwear.
> Limit forced extension.
> Restore pain-free ROM into extension.

Primary nonsurgical management includes reducing first MTP joint stress. This can be accomplished with shoe modifications, such as a rocker-soled shoe, stiff insert, or custom orthosis

(**Figure 5-11**). If an osteophyte is present, it may be necessary to use a shoe that has an extra-deep or extra-wide toe box. Donut pads may also assist in reducing pressure on the osteophyte. Rest and an NSAID reduce any inflammation.

Weight bearing is permitted in a wooden-soled or other stiff-soled shoe for 6 weeks postoperatively. At 1 to 2 weeks, when type I collagen begins to form in earnest at the operative site, MTP joint dorsiflexion exercises are initiated to encourage the newly forming collagen to align for optimal strength. As the athlete continues to heal and achieves adequate flexibility, strength gains are followed by the normal progression of therapeutic exercises for balance, coordination, and agility.

Grade II joint mobilization may be used for initial pain relief, advancing to grade III and IV mobilizations after the surgical site is healed.

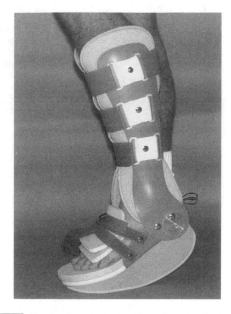

Figure 5-11 The "Rock Boot" (Röck Orthopädie, Schopfloch, Germany) has an interchangeable elevated heel rocker and an open posterior aspect. (Reproduced with permission from Saltzman CL, Tearse DS: Achilles tendon injuries. *J Am Acad Orthop Surg* 1998;6:316-325.)

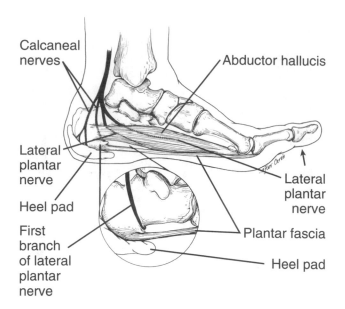

Figure 5-12 Location of nerves in proximity to the heel. Arrow indicates dorsiflexion. Insert: Windlass mechanism involving fascial attachment at the base of the proximal phalanges. (Reproduced with permission from Gill LH: Plantar fasciitis: Diagnosis and conservative management. *J Am Acad Orthop Surg* 1997;5:109-117.)

■ Estimated Amount of Time Lost

Patients treated nonsurgically are self-restricted by pain. Those who undergo surgical correction have recovery times varying from 2 to 12 months, although the average time is less than 6 months.[12]

■ Return-to-Play Criteria

The patient must be able to wear the appropriate athletic shoe; run, cut, and jump without pain; and have full MTP joint ROM (at least 60° of dorsiflexion), full intrinsic muscle strength of the great toe muscles, and restored joint proprioception, balance, and agility.

Functional Bracing

Rigid inserts can protect against excessive MTP joint motion and prevent recurrence. Footwear modifications may be necessary, depending on whether osteophytes are present.

FOOT

Plantar Fasciitis

The cause of plantar fasciitis is probably multifactorial.[14] Typically, the plantar fascia thickens, with reduced vascularity and elasticity near its insertion on the medial plantar calcaneus. The area becomes inflamed, resulting in nociceptor changes that may trigger persistent pain.[15]

The plantar fascia is composed of collagen and elastin fibers. When at a relaxed length, the elastin fibers are wavy and unstressed. When tension is applied, the fibers straighten, increasing the amount of load the structure can receive and still return to

---

CLINICAL PRESENTATION

History

Insidious onset of pain that originates in the plantar heel and progresses distally
Increased pain when standing after a prolonged period of non-weight bearing, such as arising from bed in the morning
Pain decreases with activity.
Patients tend not to seek medical attention until the condition becomes chronic.

Observation

Swelling may be noted over the plantar medial aspect of the heel.

Functional Status

Antalgic gait
Decreased ankle dorsiflexion

Physical Evaluation Findings

Pain with palpation over the medial calcaneal tubercle

its normal resting condition. The plantar fascia distributes the stress applied to the foot and lower extremity during weight bearing. As repetitive loads caused by these activities are applied to the fascia and tissue breakdown occurs, the fascia may become stiff.[15] The development of plantar fasciitis may be related to the amount of stress applied to the plantar fascia.[16]

The foot's windlass mechanism provides stability for propulsion. In terminal stance, the arch is shortened by the winding of the windlass mechanism.[16] As the body's weight is propelled over the first ray, tension increases in the medial plantar fascia and can entrap the first branch of the lateral plantar nerve[16] (**Figure 5-12**). Repetitive stress to the fascia from this mechanism is exaggerated by the Achilles tendon as it pulls with an upward force on the calcaneus.

Individuals with pes planus or pes cavus seem susceptible to plantar fasciitis. Both foot postures place additional stress on the plantar fascia.

Plantar Fascia Rupture

Patients who have a plantar fascia rupture experience effects similar to those who opt for surgical release to relieve the pain. However, the long-term effects include a variety of possible injuries and deformities, such as longitudinal arch sprain, midfoot sprain, lateral plantar nerve dysfunction, stress fracture, hammer toe deformity, swelling, lateral column pain, and antalgic gait.[15]

Many patients who experience a plantar fascia rupture have received corticosteroid injections. For this reason, corticosteroid injections and surgery as treatment options should be carefully considered.

Differential Diagnosis
Tarsal tunnel syndrome, contusion, calcaneal stress fracture, sciatica, seronegative spondyloarthropathy, calcaneal or plantar tumor

Medical Diagnostic Tests
This diagnosis is frequently one of exclusion: negative imaging studies, negative electromyography and nerve conduction testing for tarsal tunnel syndrome, and negative bone scan for calcaneal stress fracture.

Imaging Techniques
The presence or absence of a calcaneal plantar spur on lateral radiographs is *not* diagnostic and represents only long-standing inflammation and/or calcific deposits within the flexor brevis muscle (**Figure 5-13**). Radiographs may also be taken to determine the foot posture and identify the calcaneal

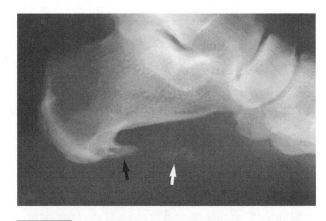

Figure 5-13   Lateral view of a heel spur. The black arrow highlights a large spur emanating from the distal calcaneal tubercle. Calcification is also seen distal to the spur (white arrow), representing calcification within the plantar fascia or a fracture of a preexisting spur. (Reproduced with permission from Johnson TR, Steinbach LS (eds): *Essentials of Musculoskeletal Imaging.* Rosemont, IL, American Academy of Orthopaedic Surgeons, 2004, p 567.)

pitch angle, used to indicate the presence of pes planus or pes cavus.

Definitive Diagnosis
The diagnosis is based on the classic history and area of tenderness. Radiographs may reveal a bone spur, but this is not necessarily the cause of the plantar fasciitis. In 10% of patients, another diagnosis, such as tarsal tunnel syndrome, is also present.[15]

Pathomechanics and Functional Limitations
Loss of normal foot flexibility and decreased dorsiflexion ROM redistribute the weight-bearing loads across the foot. Altered foot and ankle biomechanics can affect lower extremity biomechanics and predispose the patient to other repetitive stress injuries. Excessive plantar fascia load can be induced by barefoot walking, excessive or prolonged pronation, and being overweight.

Immediate Management

Ice and stretching with plantar fascia support are the foundations of treatment. See Postinjury/Postoperative Management (p 80) and Functional Bracing (p 82).

Medications

Initially, a course of an NSAID in conjunction with aggressive Achilles tendon stretching is indicated. If NSAIDs are ineffective, phonophoresis or iontophoresis is tried. Corticosteroid injections may provide immediate relief. However, they should be used cautiously because they predispose the patient to plantar fascia rupture and fat pad atrophy.[17]

Seronegative spondyloarthropathy
An inflammatory condition of the spine that progresses to affect tendinous insertions throughout the body.

■ Surgical Intervention

Surgical intervention is necessary if conservative management fails. Various surgical approaches are available. Orthotripsy, or extracorporeal ultrasonic shock-wave therapy, is a noninvasive technique used to interrupt the inflammatory cycle. This procedure can be effective for patients with recalcitrant plantar fasciitis. Arthroscopic or open techniques are used to surgically release the inflamed medial band of the plantar fascia (**S T** 5-2). When tarsal tunnel syndrome has also been documented, a simultaneous tarsal tunnel release is performed.

■ Postinjury/Postoperative Management

A dorsiflexion night splint can be an adjunctive treatment in plantar fasciitis. Worn only at night, the splint provides a low-grade, prolonged stretch to the foot and ankle to lessen early morning pain.[18] For daytime activities, a heel cup or pad is inserted into the shoe to raise the heel and may relieve plantar fascia stress, reducing pain. The heel cup or pad may also provide a shock-absorbing cushion against weight-bearing forces. An orthosis is often used to support the arch during the healing phase as a part of conservative treatment or after surgical release or extracorporeal shock-wave therapy (see p 82). Arch taping can decrease pain during athletic participation (**CT** 5-2).

Patients with significant inflammation should be treated before being allowed to return to activity because inflammation can weaken soft tissue and result in plantar fascia rupture during a sudden sprint or explosive motion. This possibility is especially likely if the plantar fascia has been previously injected with corticosteroid.

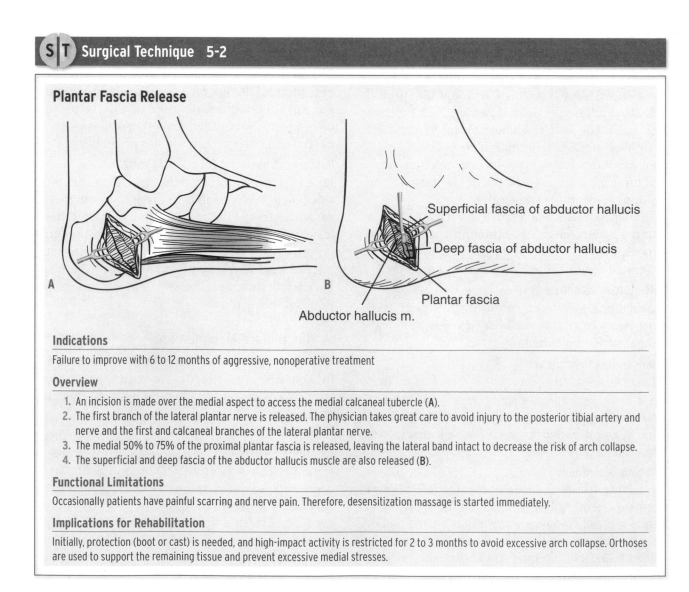

S|T   Surgical Technique   5-2

Plantar Fascia Release

Indications

Failure to improve with 6 to 12 months of aggressive, nonoperative treatment

Overview

1. An incision is made over the medial aspect to access the medial calcaneal tubercle (**A**).
2. The first branch of the lateral plantar nerve is released. The physician takes great care to avoid injury to the posterior tibial artery and nerve and the first and calcaneal branches of the lateral plantar nerve.
3. The medial 50% to 75% of the proximal plantar fascia is released, leaving the lateral band intact to decrease the risk of arch collapse.
4. The superficial and deep fascia of the abductor hallucis muscle are also released (**B**).

Functional Limitations

Occasionally patients have painful scarring and nerve pain. Therefore, desensitization massage is started immediately.

Implications for Rehabilitation

Initially, protection (boot or cast) is needed, and high-impact activity is restricted for 2 to 3 months to avoid excessive arch collapse. Orthoses are used to support the remaining tissue and prevent excessive medial stresses.

CT Clinical Technique 5-2

Taping for Plantar Fasciitis

Application

1. Apply anchor strips over the plantar surface of the metatarsal heads, spanning from the lateral aspect of the fifth MTP joint to the medial aspect of the first MTP joint (do not cross the dorsal aspect of the foot). Another anchor runs from the lateral aspect of the fifth MTP joint to the medial aspect of the first MTP joint, crossing the midportion of the posterior calcaneus.
2. Pulling snugly, apply a 2- or 3-in-wide piece of moleskin from the posterior anchor on the calcaneus to the metatarsal anchor (**A**).
3. Using 1-in adhesive tape, apply "X" strips from lateral to medial, circling behind the calcaneus, starting with the fifth MTP joint. Repeat this process, moving the starting point medially with each strip (**B**).
4. To ensure calcaneal inversion and support the bone with a thicker fat pad beneath it, starting distally on the foot, apply stirrups from the lateral to medial anchors, overlapping one half of the tape's width each time (1- or 1½-in tape may be used) (**C**).
5. End the procedure using 1½-in stretch tape (**D**).

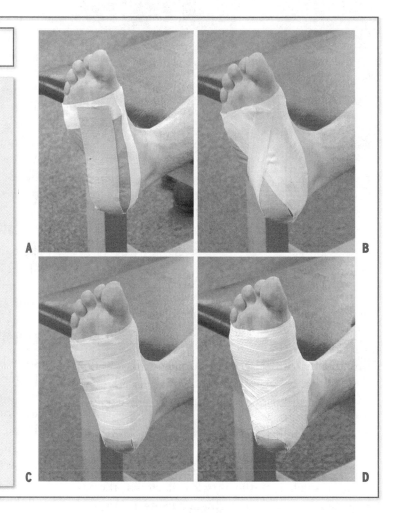

Injury-Specific Treatment and Rehabilitation Concerns

Specific Concerns

Stretch the Achilles tendon complex.
Elongate the plantar fascia.
Strengthen the supporting musculature.
Control inflammation.
Correct the biomechanical causes contributing to the condition.

Plantar fasciitis is a chronic condition that frequently goes unattended for several months after onset, and 10% to 20% of patients may not experience complete pain relief.[15,19] If pain levels can be controlled with conservative treatment, patients may be willing to endure occasional bouts of pain rather than undergo surgery. Avoiding unsupported weight bearing (bare feet, stocking feet, "flip-flops") prevents further aggravation of the inflammatory condition.

The patient should be instructed in performing regular flexibility exercises for the Achilles tendon complex and gently stretching the plantar fascia.[17] Because of the amount of collagen in both the plantar fascia and the Achilles tendon, prolonged stretches that affect the plastic qualities of these structures provide the most benefit. Heating modalities should be applied before the stretches to optimize the tissues' viscoelastic properties.

Standing on an incline board with the heel down and the knee straight for 10 to 15 minutes can provide sufficient Achilles complex stretching. The patient can stretch the plantar fascia by passively extending the toes or, if pain and strength permit, standing on the toes. Each of these mechanisms relies on the windlass effect to stretch the fascia. The patient may also roll the arch over a rolling pin, bottle, or ball to stretch the fascia. To prevent discomfort, do not roll the heel over the object (**Figure 5-14**).

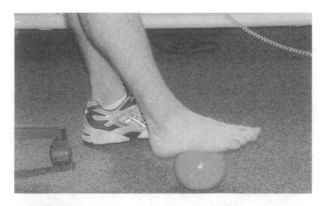

Figure 5-14 A ball, glass bottle, or roller can be used to stretch the plantar fascia. The patient presses down against the object and rolls it back and forth along the fascia, increasing pressure as tolerated. To prevent discomfort, instruct the patient to avoid placing pressure on the heel.

In addition to a night splint and orthosis, taping the heel and plantar surface to stabilize and centralize the calcaneal fat pad under the calcaneus may provide more cushion for ambulation (see p 81). A soft or rigid orthosis to reduce overpronation or an accommodative orthosis for a rigid foot decreases torque or impact forces placed on the plantar fascia. A cast is sometimes used for 2 weeks in an attempt to reduce heel pain.

If the patient has a foot deformity contributing to the problem, orthoses may provide symptomatic control of the inflammatory process. If lower extremity strength is deficient, the muscles affected by the antalgic gait should be strengthened using a variety of exercises. Although any lower extremity muscle group can be affected by an antalgic gait, the hip abductors, hip extensors, and knee extensors are most often involved. If the patient has developed a habitual antalgic gait, gait correction is included in the treatment program. An antalgic gait also results in muscle imbalances and weakness, so once an assessment of the entire lower extremity has been made, strengthening exercises for the affected muscles are included.

Once the proper orthoses are provided, if needed, running mechanics should be assessed to ensure proper execution. The primary site of concern is rearfoot mechanics. Heel movement from inversion or an erect position just before initial contact, moving rapidly into eversion in the first half of weight bearing, with the heel moving into inversion or an erect position in the last half of weight bearing in preparation for preswing, should be examined.

Extracorporeal Shock-Wave Therapy

Extracorporeal shock-wave therapy has been used to treat plantar fasciitis in Europe for several years. In 2000, the US Food and Drug Administration approved the use of extracorporeal shock-wave ther-

apy devices for the treatment of plantar fasciitis in the United States.

Some controversy exists concerning the efficacy of extracorporeal shock-wave treatments. They have been reported to be of no benefit[3] and a successful treatment modality.[20] Although the therapy was not recommended as the first procedure for recalcitrant heel pain, significant improvements were noted.[21] However, the researchers caution that pain is difficult to measure, their subjects had other procedures that might have contributed to the overall effects, and patients with heel pain often experience resolution without treatment.

■ Estimated Amount of Time Lost

The pain is self-limiting in this chronic condition. If pain is severe, the patient may be unable to perform sport activities until pain is reduced. This extreme situation, however, is not common.

■ Return-to-Play Criteria

If foot biomechanics are abnormal (eg, a very mobile foot with excessive pronation or a rigid foot with no pronation), an orthosis or taping may relieve the excessive stresses otherwise placed on the plantar fascia (see **CT** 5-2).

Only patients with severe pain need to modify or restrict activities. Pain reduction may occur with the use of orthoses, but some pain may still be present; however, this level is not sufficient to decrease the ability to perform.

Functional Bracing

Support for the fascia starts with not walking barefoot or in stocking feet or slippers and using tape, heel cups, orthoses, or cross-trainer footwear. An accommodative orthosis may benefit patients with rigid arches. In contrast, the individual with a flexible foot benefits from a rigid or semirigid orthosis, which supports the arch and corrects excessive or early pronation.

Interdigital Neuroma (Morton Neuroma)

Morton neuroma is also referred to as an interdigital neuroma, perineural fibroma, and plantar interdigital neuroma. More accurate nomenclature may be interdigital nerve compression syndrome or interdigital neuritis.[22] Although the condition can occur in any of the intermetatarsal head spaces, it is most common between the third and fourth metatarsal heads or between the second and third metatarsal heads; the interdigital nerve makes its

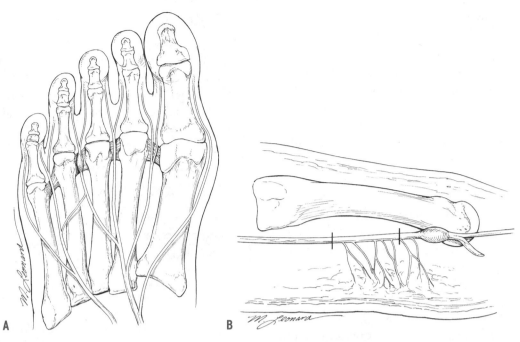

A   B

Figure 5-15   Anatomy of the interdigital nerves. **A.** Normal anatomy of the plantar aspect of the foot. **B.** Lateral view of the plantar branches of the digital nerve. (Reproduced with permission from Weinfled SB: Interdigital neuritis: Diagnosis and treatment. *J Am Acad Orthop Surg* 1996;4:328-335.)

most acute direction changes at those sites as it travels toward the distal digits (**Figure 5-15**) and is most susceptible to stress at those locations. Repetitive nerve irritation can result in a buildup of protective scar tissue (fibrosis) around the nerve, producing a neuroma.

CLINICAL PRESENTATION

History

Pain originating from the plantar foot and radiating into the toes
An advanced Morton neuroma produces pain that migrates proximally.
Some degree of pain relief is obtained when the patient is barefoot.

Observation

No deformity is noted.
An antalgic gait may be evident.

Functional Status

Weight bearing is limited.

Physical Evaluation Findings

Intense pain when the neuroma is palpated
Pain increases when the foot is squeezed while pressure is applied to the area of the neuroma (Mulder sign).[23]

Although interdigital neuroma was initially thought to be the result of digital nerve compression, the condition is now believed to be po-

tentially more complex. Increased fibrotic connective tissue, arteriosclerosis, and other changes in the arterial wall leading to ischemia, inflammation of nearby bursae that leads to secondary fibrosis, tethering of the nerve by restricted soft tissue, and digital nerve compression during weight bearing have all been identified as factors that may lead to Morton neuroma.[18] Interdigital nerve compression can also occur from wearing tight shoes, using inappropriate shoes for athletic workouts, and wearing high heels.[2] Women experience Morton neuroma five times more frequently than men. Although the condition can occur at any age, most patients are between 20 and 50 years old.

Differential Diagnosis

Metatarsalgia, MTP synovitis, stress fracture, arthritis

Medical Diagnostic Tests

The diagnosis is based on the history and physical examination. Resolution of symptoms with a lidocaine injection in the distal web space can help confirm the diagnosis.

Imaging Techniques

Although the diagnosis of interdigital neuroma is primarily based on the clinical symptoms, MRI with gadolinium can identify the lesion. Ultrasonic imaging has also been successfully used to identify the presence and location of an interdigital neuroma.

Plain radiographs may be ordered to rule out MTP joint changes, arthritis, and fracture.

Definitive Diagnosis

Interdigital neuroma pain arises from between the metatarsal heads rather than from the metatarsal or the MTP joint. Burning and numbness are classic symptoms of nerve irritation that are not reported with other possible diagnoses. A positive Mulder sign is diagnostic.

Pathomechanics and Functional Limitations

Repetitive digital nerve compression or irritation is the cause. Weight bearing is painful, and the increased stresses of impact can exacerbate pain, numbness, and eventual paralysis in the nerve distribution. The interdigital nerve injury affects two toes because of the branching of the common interdigital nerve. Altered biomechanics in an attempt to reduce pain can lead to stress-related lower extremity injury from muscular compensation and the redistribution of weight-bearing forces.

■ Immediate Management

Remove the patient from activity and treat the area with ice. If normal weight-bearing activities produce pain, fit the patient for crutches.

■ Medications

Inflammation can be relieved with NSAIDs. Persistent symptoms may respond to a corticosteroid injection. No more than one or two injections, however, should be given because they may cause fat pad atrophy, worsening the problem.

■ Postinjury Management

Continue with crutch walking as indicated. A metatarsal pad, orthotic inserts, and shoe modifications help relieve the offending weight-bearing stresses. Proper footwear (wide toe box with cushioned forefoot and a low heel) is instituted, and impact activities are limited.

■ Surgical Intervention

Surgery is a last resort, performed only if the patient's symptoms fail to respond to conservative treatment and pain continues for up to 1 year or significantly affects activity. The interdigital nerve is excised and, therefore, after surgery, numbness occurs in the area of skin innervated by the excised nerve (ST 5-3). The ensuing numbness is not typically a major complaint if only the interdigital nerve is excised.

■ Postoperative Management

With a dorsal incision, immediate weight bearing is usually permitted. Postoperative side effects such as swelling and pain are treated with ice, elevation, and active ROM. Complete recovery is usually possible within 4 to 8 weeks, with full return to participation after the normal healing process.

■ Injury-Specific Treatment and Rehabilitation Concerns

Specific Concerns

Relieve pressure on and irritation to the nerve.
Prevent pressure on the nerve during activities with a pad, orthotic inserts, and/or shoe modifications.

The initial treatment is designed to relieve inflammation and reduce stress on the neuroma. Shoes with a thicker outer sole for added shock absorption, a wide toe box to relieve lateral compression, and a low heel relieve downward pressure on the neuroma. A neuroma pad inserted in the shoe can spread the metatarsal heads and relieve nerve pressure (**Figure 5-16**). Modalities to relieve inflammation may be indicated, depending on the source of irritation. If the nerve tethering

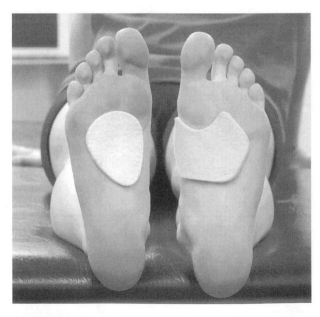

Figure 5-16 Metatarsal pads: Left: "Teardrop" pad used to support the transverse metatarsal arch. Right: "Moon pad" used to support and/or protect the first metatarsophalangeal joint.

Surgical Technique 5-3

Excision of an Interdigital Neuroma

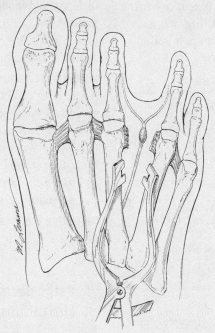

Indications

Recalcitrant pain despite properly sized shoes

Overview

1. A dorsal incision is made to expose the nerve.
2. The nerve is resected distally at least 1 cm distal to its bifurcation.
3. The plantar-directed branch is **cauterized**.
4. The nerve is resected proximally in the foot to allow the stump to be clear of the weight-bearing surface of the plantar foot.
5. Typically the transverse metatarsal ligament is cut to expose the nerve. In some elite athletes, the ligament is only partially cut to reduce postoperative spreading of the metatarsals and reduce pain.

Functional Limitations

The patient has permanent numbness between the adjacent toes (eg, between the third and fourth toes with intermetatarsal resection between toes three and four).

Implications for Rehabilitation

Early desensitization massage assists in recovery from nerve pain. After the wound is well healed (2 to 4 weeks), rehabilitation can be aggressive.

Figure reproduced with permission from Weinfled SB: Interdigital neuritis: Diagnosis and treatment. *J Am Acad Orthop Surg* 1996;4:328-335.

Cauterized Sealed off by using heat.

is caused by scar tissue or soft-tissue adhesions, deep tissue mobilization is needed.

■ Estimated Amount of Time Lost

Because the injury is self-limiting, time lost depends on the pain level, specific sport activity (how much stress is applied to the foot), and whether sufficient pain relief can be achieved with treatment.

■ Return-to-Play Criteria

Return to full sport participation is permitted when the patient can don athletic shoes and perform sport activities without pain. The cause of irritation (eg, soft-tissue restriction, narrow shoes, plantar-flexed ray) should be relieved or removed before return to participation.

Functional Bracing

Proper shoe wear with a wide toe box is more important than bracing. However, padding properly placed behind the metatarsal heads can help relieve interdigital nerve pressure (see Figure 5-16).

Navicular Stress Fracture and Accessory Navicular

CLINICAL PRESENTATION

History

Insidious onset of vague pain over the foot's dorsum or medial longitudinal arch
Pain may radiate into the first or second ray or the cuboid.
Pain increases with activity and decreases with rest.

Observation

Deformity is seldom observed.
A prominent medial navicular may be noted with a pronated foot.

Functional Status

Antalgic gait favors the affected extremity.
Ankle strength and ROM are usually within normal limits.
Hopping on the involved extremity produces pain.

Physical Evaluation Findings

Pain may be elicited during palpation of the stress fracture site.

The vague symptoms associated with navicular stress fractures may result in the underdiagnosis of this condition.[24] The navicular is the keystone for the medial longitudinal arch; significant stresses are applied to the bone, even during simple ambulation. The stress is magnified as dynamic weight-bearing loads increase during activities such as sprinting, running, and jumping. Contractile forces applied by muscles during forceful activities combined with the compressive forces are thought to contribute to over-stressing the navicular.[24] Morton toe, hallux valgus, limited dorsiflexion, and restricted subtalar motion may also contribute to navicular stress fractures.[25]

An accessory navicular is a genetic deviation that may become apparent during adolescence, especially in girls. The medial aspect of the navicular bone forms a secondary ossification protuberance (**Figure 5-17**). Reports of tenderness and some edema over the medial aspect of the navicular are often accompanied by tenderness to resisted inversion and a flexible pes planus foot. The diagnosis is confirmed by radiographs. Although the problem is

not usually debilitating, pain can be relieved with shoe modifications to ease pressure over the area. The pain may resolve once bone growth is completed but can persist in active individuals.

Differential Diagnosis

Tarsal tunnel syndrome, neuroma, periostitis, synovitis, tendinitis, gout, traumatic metatarsal fracture, anterior ankle impingement

Imaging Techniques

Acute stress fractures are not visible on plain radiographs. A bone scan shows increased periosteal uptake in the area of the stress fracture, but increased uptake does not always indicate a stress fracture. An immature stress fracture may be imaged with CT scan or MRI. Acute navicular fractures are frequently visible on plain radiographs (**Figure 5-18**).

Definitive Diagnosis

A positive bone scan with CT scan or MRI confirming a stress fracture

■ Pathomechanics and Functional Limitations

As the fracture matures, pain occurs earlier in the workout and persists longer after the activity. Unstable muscular and ligamentous attachment sites for the medial longitudinal arch decrease the arch's stability and alter the biomechanics during foot pronation and supination. If stress continues, the fracture may become a nonunion or displace and require surgical fixation.

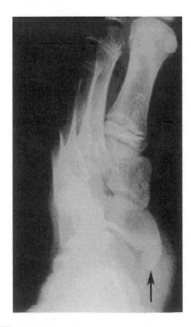

Figure 5-17 Oblique radiograph of an accessory navicular (arrow). (Reproduced with permission from Greene WB (ed): *Essentials of Musculoskeletal Care*, ed 2. Rosemont, IL, American Academy of Orthopaedic Surgeons, 2000, p 602.)

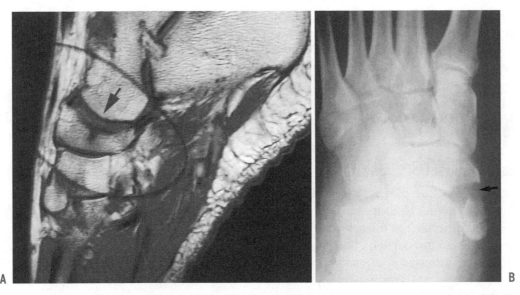

Figure 5-18   Radiographic views of the navicular. **A.** Magnetic resonance imaging indicating a stress fracture of the navicular midsection (arrow). **B.** Anteroposterior radiograph demonstrating an avulsion fracture of the accessory navicular. Contraction of the tibialis posterior muscle has caused proximal migration of the fragment. (Reproduced with permission from Johnson TR, Steinbach LS (eds): *Essentials of Musculoskeletal Imaging.* Rosemont, IL, American Academy of Orthopaedic Surgeons, 2004, pp 595-596.)

Immediate Management

Protected weight bearing based on symptoms displayed during the workup helps limit the pain and inflammatory response. Ice and NSAIDs also are helpful in the immediate management. Immobilization may be indicated in certain situations, such as acute trauma or intense pain.

Medications

An NSAID is helpful for pain relief. With extreme trauma or pain, oral narcotics are indicated.

Surgical Intervention

Surgery is indicated for fractures that fail to heal with 6 weeks of non–weight bearing or for a patient who is unwilling to accept nonoperative treatment, such as a professional athlete. The most common surgical technique involves the fixation of the fractured segment using one or two screws and may involve a bone graft.

Most patients require 6 weeks of non–weight bearing after surgery. The most common complications include recurrent stress fracture, nonunion, and degenerative arthritis. Motion can be initiated early as long as the wound is healing well and the patient remains non–weight bearing.

Postinjury/Postoperative Management

Navicular stress fractures are often resistant to conservative treatment. To allow healing and prevent a nonunion, the patient should remain non–weight bearing for 6 to 8 weeks. Because the bone is a keystone for the arch, excessive stresses are applied to the navicular during ambulation, which should, therefore, be limited. A controlled ankle motion (CAM) boot can also be used to decrease weight-bearing forces on the navicular. Recovery is slow, so the foot may require protection from stress, including weight-bearing exercises and return to sport participation, for an extended time, possibly 4 to 6 months. Most athletes benefit from orthosis use during their sports careers.

Injury-Specific Treatment and Rehabilitation Concerns

> **Specific Concerns**
> Prevent excessive stress application to the navicular.
> Restore function as healing progresses.

Weight bearing is restricted for 6 to 8 weeks, with or without a cast. The patient is reexamined at 3 weeks and again at 6 weeks. If tenderness persists at 6 weeks, the cast (if used) and non–weight-bearing status are continued for another 2 weeks. Once the cast is removed, the patient may experience generalized foot discomfort with weight bearing and paresthesia, but these complaints vary from the initial complaints. Because non–weight bearing and immobilization may be prolonged, soft-tissue and joint-mobilization techniques may be required to restore the athlete's motion and function. These techniques may be performed during the non–weight-bearing period if the foot is not in a cast. If a cast was applied, these techniques are used once the cast is removed. When weight bearing is permitted, progressive rehabilitation for strength, balance, coordination, agility, and functional activities is instituted, using the patient's pain as a guide for advancement.

■ Estimated Amount of Time Lost

In nonsurgical cases, the patient is restricted to non–weight bearing for 6 to 8 weeks. This may be followed by an additional 2 to 6 weeks of rehabilitation before return to full participation is feasible. After surgery, 4 to 6 months of activity may be lost.

■ Return-to-Play Criteria

Once the fracture demonstrates radiographic healing and no point tenderness to palpation or pain during activities, the patient may return to full participation. In addition, the patient's gait should be normal, in both walking and running, and he or she should be able to perform all required sport activities pain free on return to full participation.

Functional Bracing

Because a navicular stress fracture may be secondary to a shortened first metatarsal, a firm, full-length insert that extends under the first ray may reduce the stress on the bone. If the predisposing factor was reduced navicular or subtalar motion, a flexible orthotic insert may limit forces applied to the navicular. A heel insert relieves stresses by reducing dorsiflexion.

Metatarsal Fracture

The fifth metatarsal is unique in its predisposition to different types of fractures. Avulsion fractures tend to occur at the attachment site of the peroneus brevis, abductor digiti quinti, and/or lateral band of the plantar fascia. Stress fractures are usually observed at the most proximal portion of the bone along the shaft, and Jones fractures affect the transition between the shaft and the base (**Figure 5-19**). A Jones fracture can occur with an ankle sprain and be overlooked during the initial examination and postinjury care. If localized pain persists, follow-up radiographs may reveal a fracture. Jones fractures may require surgical repair because healing is often delayed.

Although stress fractures can develop in any of the metatarsals, the second metatarsal is most fre-

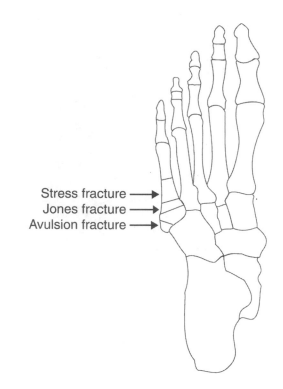

Stress fracture →
Jones fracture →
Avulsion fracture →

Figure 5-19 Common fracture locations of the fifth metatarsal.

quently involved, and the first and fourth metatarsals are the least frequent locations. Second, third, and fourth metatarsal stress fractures constitute 90% of metatarsal injuries.[26] Athletes participating in running or racquet sports, aerobics, ballet, gymnastics, and basketball experience the most metatarsal stress fractures, even though those in other sports, such as football, hockey, and soccer, are not immune.[2,27,28]

Similar to other stress fractures, metatarsal stress fractures occur most often from a rapidly increased activity level or a dramatic change in sport with repetitive bone overloading and insufficient recovery time. Metatarsal stress fractures can be oblique, longitudinal, or transverse. Transverse stress fractures are common in the fifth metatarsal, whereas compression stress fractures are more likely in the first metatarsal.[27]

A cavus or planus foot may be a predisposition to metatarsal stress fractures, but people with a planus foot have more stress fractures than those with a cavus foot. Pes cavus, genu varum, and chronic ankle instability may increase the risk of fifth metatarsal stress fractures. This is thought to be the result of increased adduction forces placed on the fifth metatarsal by proximal instability or medially directed forces from foot or knee malalignment. A cavus foot tends to absorb stress in the metatarsal rather than transferring it to the tibia and fibula.[27]

Pes planus feet have more first and second metatarsal stress fractures.[27] Hyperpronation associated with pes planus increases forces on the medial aspect of the foot. A short first metatarsal and a long second metatarsal have also been implicated as contributing factors to second metatarsal stress fractures. With such a configuration, an increased load is applied more laterally to the foot, increasing second metatarsal stress. This is particularly problematic if the hallux is rigid or abducted.

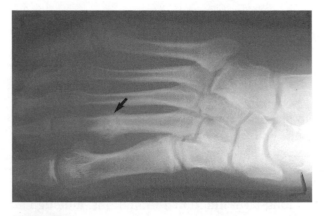

Figure 5-20 Late-stage stress fracture of the second metatarsal. Arrow depicts callus formation. (Reproduced with permission from Johnson TR, Steinbach LS (eds): *Essentials of Musculoskeletal Imaging.* Rosemont, IL, American Academy of Orthopaedic Surgeons, 2004, p 623.)

CLINICAL PRESENTATION

History

A sudden change in the distance, duration, or type of exercise
Pain over the forefoot that may radiate into the toes
No discrete onset of pain but a gradual, progressive onset of symptoms related to activity
As the fracture matures, pain persists after activity has stopped.
Acute fractures have a sudden onset of symptoms.
Mild swelling may be noted.

Observation

Findings are often unremarkable.
Redness may be noted over the dorsal foot.
As the fracture progresses, swelling may be noted and the foot may feel warm.
Acute fractures may present with obvious deformity.

Functional Status

An antalgic gait favoring the affected extremity may be noted.
A first or second metatarsal stress fracture may cause the patient to walk on the lateral aspect of the foot.
Active and resisted ROM may cause pain.

Physical Evaluation Findings

Pain with palpation of the site; a first metatarsal stress fracture may result in tenderness and swelling over the metatarsal base.[29]
With a mature stress fracture, a palpable mass may represent the formation of a bony callus.
Long-bone compression test may give positive result.
Squeeze test may give positive result.
A tuning fork placed along the involved metatarsal may elicit pain.

Differential Diagnosis

Synovitis, Jones fracture, metatarsalgia, avulsion fracture, neuroma

Imaging Techniques

Plain radiographs may show a healing stress fracture, but rarely do they demonstrate an acute stress fracture. Serial radiographs may document the healing progression. Bone scan, CT scan, or MRI may be diagnostic if the radiographs are negative (**Figure 5-20**).

Definitive Diagnosis

Positive radiographs, bone scan, CT scan, or MRI; fifth metatarsal stress fractures tend to remain relatively asymptomatic until a complete fracture suddenly occurs

Pathomechanics and Functional Limitations

The loss of bony integrity or pain redistributes the weight-bearing surfaces of the foot, altering foot and, therefore, gait biomechanics, thereby increasing the possibility of new stress fractures or lower extremity overuse conditions. The athlete's ability to perform sport-specific activities, such as explosive starts, cutting, jumping, and landing, may also be impaired. Metatarsal stress fractures are the result of overuse stress. Adequate healing time before returning to activities helps avoid recurrence.

■ Immediate Management

A high suspicion of stress fracture initiates the workup. Symptomatic treatment is indicated: ice, elevation, and protective weight bearing with crutches limits the symptoms.

■ Medications

The use of NSAIDs for pain relief is helpful.

■ Surgical Intervention

Surgical intervention is common in failed union or nonunion of a fifth metatarsal Jones fracture. Intervention during the competitive season may allow the athlete to return before the season ends.

Because the fifth metatarsal is at increased risk of a nonunion in response to conservative treatment, many physicians elect to surgically repair the fracture once diagnosed. The two predominant surgical techniques are a bone graft and an intermedullary screw. Although internal screw fixation allows a more rapid return to participation, it can also cause soft-tissue irritation.[30] To decrease the likelihood of refracture, the screw is normally left in place during the athlete's competitive life. With bone grafting, complications are usually fewer, but recovery is slower.[30]

After surgery, hardware failure and/or nonunion may still occur. Successful surgeries do not result in long-term functional limitations, although an orthosis may be prescribed before return to activity to minimize the refracture risk.

◼ Postinjury/Postoperative Management

The most common treatments of metatarsal stress fractures are a short leg walking cast, CAM boot, or other functional cast-brace for 5 to 6 weeks (see Figure 5-11). Sometimes a wooden shoe or other stiff-soled shoe is used to minimize metatarsal stress.

Activity limitations focus on eliminating the stress that caused or aggravated the existing problem. Identifying the fracture cause is important so that when the athlete returns to activities, the same mistakes can be avoided. Often training errors or changes in shoe wear or running surfaces are contributors to, if not the root of, the problem.

◼ Injury-Specific Treatment and Rehabilitation Concerns

> **Specific Concerns**
> Relieve stress on the metatarsal.
> Stabilize and protect the fracture site.

Second, third, and fourth metatarsal stress fractures should heal with rest and conservative care. First metatarsal stress fractures are managed with reduced activity and shoe modifications and result in the least amount of time lost.[29] Fifth metatarsal fractures do not respond as well to conservative treatment as other metatarsal stress fractures.

◼ Estimated Amount of Time Lost

On average, the athlete is restricted from normal activity for 4 to 8 weeks, which does not include the time necessary for rehabilitation and a gradual return to full participation. Depending on the indi-

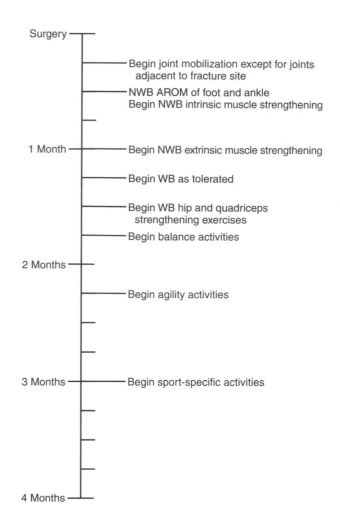

Surgery —

— Begin joint mobilization except for joints
adjacent to fracture site

— NWB AROM of foot and ankle
Begin NWB intrinsic muscle strengthening

1 Month —— Begin NWB extrinsic muscle strengthening

— Begin WB as tolerated

— Begin WB hip and quadriceps
strengthening exercises
— Begin balance activities

2 Months —

— Begin agility activities

3 Months —— Begin sport-specific activities

4 Months —

Note: Time frames are approximate. Function is the guide.

vidual's response to treatment and rehabilitation, full recovery may take 6 to 12 weeks.

◼ Return-to-Play Criteria

As with a navicular fracture, the patient should be able to perform all activities without pain before returning to play. The athlete is tested on sport-specific activities and drills and must demonstrate normal performance without favoring or hesitating to use the foot. The foot should be in a stable, supportive shoe, and the causative factors that initially led to a stress fracture should be resolved.

Functional Bracing

A shoe with a stiff sole or rigid insert reduces metatarsal stress. A rocker-bottom shoe also decreases metatarsal stress during the last half of the stance phase. A stiff foot plate insert with a viscoelastic insole covering the stiff foot plate may also be used; the former splints the metatarsal, and the latter attenuates impact force.

ANKLE

Tarsal Tunnel Syndrome

Pressure on the posterior tibial nerve posterior to the medial malleolus can occur from trauma, a space-occupying lesion, or foot deformity[31] (**Table 5-2**). Trauma and space-occupying lesions place direct pressure on the nerve. Rear-foot varus shortens the abductor hallucis to reduce the tarsal tunnel size. Rear-foot valgus stretches the nerve during pronation. Attempts to correct pronation with a medial wedge have also been suspected of narrowing the tarsal tunnel to impinge the nerve.[31]

A high-arched foot or rear-foot varus shortens the abductor hallucis; these conditions increase stress on the posterior tibial nerve. A flaccid foot or valgus foot deformity that stretches the nerve as the foot rotates laterally increases medial nerve tension. Swelling from trauma or another space-occupying condition creates pressure on the larger branch of the posterior tibial nerve, the medial plantar nerve.

Tension, stress, and pressure on a nerve result in initial pain that can be sharp, shooting, aching, or cramping and radiating into the plantar foot. Pain can also be nonspecific and described as all over the foot and radiating proximally to the an-

kle. As the irritation continues, paresthesia, numbness, and burning are reported, with weakness in later stages. Symptoms are relieved with rest and aggravated with activity.

The effects of tarsal tunnel syndrome can occur distal or proximal to the tarsal tunnel. Proximal symptoms result from entrapment of the entire posterior tibial nerve; distal symptoms occur with entrapment of the medial or lateral plantar nerves, branches of the posterior tibial nerve[32] (**Figure 5-21**). Although the lateral plantar nerve becomes entrapped at the tarsal tunnel, the medial plantar nerve is believed to become entrapped in the fibromuscular tunnel between the abductor hallucis and navicular tuberosity.[32] The latter entrapment is called "jogger foot" and is commonly related to excessive pronation secondary to a valgus deformity.[32]

If the ankle is placed in extreme dorsiflexion, whether during squatting, uphill running, or landing from a jump, the posterior tibial nerve is stretched. If the nerve is already weakened by tarsal tunnel impingement, such activity worsens the condition.

Differential Diagnosis
Lumbar disk herniation, diabetic or alcohol-related neuropathy, vascular insufficiency, plantar fasciitis, flexor hallucis longus tendinitis, flexor digitorum longus tendinitis, posterior tibial tendinitis

Medical Diagnostic Tests
Positive electromyography and nerve conduction velocity tests indicate nerve dysfunction; a diagnostic injection of bupivacaine (Marcaine) and/or a corticosteroid preparation that temporarily relieves the pain confirms the condition.

Table 5-2

Causes of Tarsal Tunnel Syndrome

Trauma	Space-occupying Lesions	Foot Deformities
Fracture of the distal tibia	Varicosities	Rear-foot valgus
Fracture of the calcaneus	Lipoma	Pes planus
Medial ankle sprain	Edema	Rear-foot varus
Posterior tibial injury	Exostosis	Pes cavus
Flexor digitorum longus trauma	Weight gain	
Flexor hallucis longus trauma	Ganglion cyst	
Secondary soft-tissue scarring		
Medial capsular adhesions		

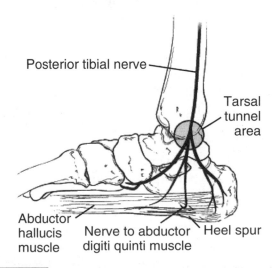

Figure 5-21 Anatomy of the tarsal tunnel. (Reproduced with permission from Greene WB (ed): *Essentials of Musculoskeletal Care*, ed 2. Rosemont, IL, American Academy of Orthopaedic Surgeons, 2000, p 511.)

Posterior tibial nerve

Tarsal tunnel area

Abductor hallucis muscle

Nerve to abductor digiti quinti muscle

Heel spur

CLINICAL PRESENTATION

History

Foot or ankle trauma may have triggered tarsal tunnel syndrome.

Abnormal foot posture may be noted.

Intermittent pain, burning, tingling, or numbness may occur along the medial aspect of the foot and ankle.

Symptoms may interfere with sleep.

Those with advanced symptoms may demonstrate intrinsic muscle weakness.

Symptoms may migrate proximally up the lower leg.

Symptoms may increase when wearing high-cut shoes or high heels.[33]

Symptoms are reduced with rest, elevation, and loose-fitting shoes.[34]

Observation

Rear-foot varus or valgus may be noted.

Possible hypertrophy of the abductor hallucis muscle

Possible swelling posterior to the medial malleolus

Functional Status

Running may be difficult to continue once symptoms occur during the workout.

Physical Evaluation Findings

End-range dorsiflexion may reproduce pain.

Positive Tinel sign along the posterior tibial nerve

Placing tension on the nerve by dorsiflexing and everting the foot and ankle may cause pain.

Imaging Techniques

Radiographs may be ordered to rule out a bony condition that impinges on the tarsal tunnel. MRI or a CT scan may be used to identify nerve entrapment or the presence of a ganglion cyst.

Definitive Diagnosis

Positive electromyography and nerve conduction velocity test results for tarsal tunnel or pain relief with bupivacaine injection (or both).

Pathomechanics and Functional Limitations

A valgus foot deformity is a common predisposing element of tarsal tunnel syndrome. The posterior tibial nerve becomes tensioned, a condition that increases during ambulation. Lesions occupying the space in the tarsal tunnel, such as a nodule or swelling from an injury, reduce the space within the tunnel, applying pressure to the nerve. Abductor hallucis hypertrophy may also be a source of the problem by pushing the lateral plantar nerve against the navicular tuberosity.

The patient's function is self-limited by pain. In severe cases, the patient may be unable to run for the time or intensity required for sport because of pain. Identifying the cause of the lesion and correcting the problem or eliminating the nerve pressure allows resumption of pain-free activity.

▇ Immediate Management

Relieving nerve pressure eliminates the patient's pain. Most patients report reduced symptoms with rest. Modalities such as ice, electric stimulation, heat, and ultrasound may be used to reduce symptoms. For permanent relief, the underlying cause must be identified and resolved (eg, foot deformity, space-occupying lesion, intrinsic muscle hypertrophy, tight retinaculum).

▇ Medications

Initially, NSAIDs are used to decrease the inflammatory process. However, the cause of the problem may limit NSAID effectiveness. Corticosteroid injections or nerve-desensitizing medications such as gabapentin (Neurontin) can also be tried for patients with recalcitrant symptoms.

▇ Surgical Intervention

Surgical decompression of the tarsal tunnel is indicated for recalcitrant pain that is unresponsive to custom orthotic inserts, NSAIDs, and therapeutic injections. The release must include the medial flexor retinaculum (lanciate ligament) and medial plantar nerve distal to the navicular. The nerve is just posterior to the posterior tibial tendon and flexor digitorum longus tendon.

Continued pain after surgery is not rare, but complete, pain-free, full return of motion should be the goal. Early ROM of the toes and subtalar and ankle joints is encouraged. Excessive dorsiflexion with eversion during the first 3 weeks can aggravate pain and inhibit wound healing.

▇ Postinjury/Postoperative Management

Postoperatively, the patient is non–weight bearing for 7 to 10 days. At about 5 days, active ROM of the toes, ankle, and subtalar joint can begin. A CAM boot may be used once partial weight bearing is permitted (see Figure 5-11).

▇ Injury-Specific Treatment and Rehabilitation Concerns

Specific Concerns

Avoid dorsiflexion and eversion early in the rehabilitation program.
Prevent denervation atrophy.

Modalities such as ice, electric stimulation, heat, and ultrasound may be used to relieve inflammation. Orthotic appliances can reduce the nerve stresses caused by some foot deformities. Once pain and inflammation are under control, stretching and strengthening exercises can be beneficial in preparing the athlete to return to sport participation.

After 7 to 10 days, weight bearing to tolerance is permitted and exercises for stretching and strengthening are initiated. Once the patient is bearing full weight, swelling has subsided, and muscle strength and function are restored, the patient should be measured for orthotic appliances. Closed kinetic chain exercises should be performed in the orthotic appliances. A progression of strengthening exercises for the intrinsic and extrinsic foot muscles is introduced, with steady advancement to agility, plyometric, functional, and sport-specific activities before the athlete returns to full participation.

After 2 weeks, mild isometric exercises of the ankle and subtalar joint can start. By the end of the third week, resistive toe exercises such as marble pick-ups can begin along with isotonic ankle and subtalar exercises. Once the patient is bearing full weight, balance activities to restore proprioception are initiated, followed by a progression of activities leading to coordination and then agility skills. Because the athlete will be out of normal activity for a time, exercises for the uninvolved extremities and cardiovascular conditioning activities that do not stress the injured foot are necessary. A progressive return to full activity can begin once the athlete's agility skills reflect appropriate performance.

Estimated Amount of Time Lost

In nonsurgical cases, the patient may be restricted to no or limited activity for up to 4 weeks. If surgery is the treatment of choice, up to 3 months may be required before return to activity is possible.[35]

Return-to-Play Criteria

Because pain is the primary limiting factor, activities must be pain free. If surgery has been performed, the soft tissue surrounding the scar and adjacent tissue must be mobile. The cause of the problem must be identified and resolved. Balance, coordination, agility, motion, and strength must be restored if the athlete has been unable to participate for a time. The athlete must demonstrate the ability to perform sport-specific activities without hesitation or favoring the affected side.

Functional Bracing

Orthotic appliances to relieve nerve pressure by correcting a valgus or varus foot deformity may be required. Care should be taken in shoe selection to prevent rubbing the medial aspect of the heel, especially if surgery has been part of the treatment. Shoe modifications may be needed if pressure on the surgical site is uncomfortable.

Ankle Sprains: Lateral, Medial, and Syndesmosis

Ankle ligaments provide proprioceptive information to allow the joint to function normally, contribute to joint stability to prevent excessive joint motion, and act as guides to direct joint motion[36] (**Figure 5-22**). When these ligaments are damaged in an ankle sprain, their ability to serve these functions is compromised.

Lateral Ligaments

The ankle is the most frequently injured joint. Lateral ankle sprains represent 85% of all athletic-related ankle injuries, and the anterior talofibular

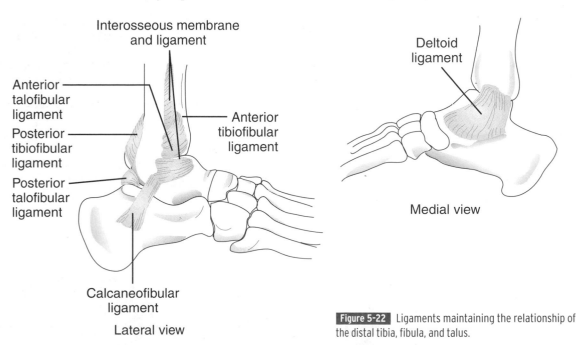

Interosseous membrane and ligament

Anterior talofibular ligament

Posterior tibiofibular ligament

Posterior talofibular ligament

Anterior tibiofibular ligament

Calcaneofibular ligament

Lateral view

Deltoid ligament

Medial view

Figure 5-22 Ligaments maintaining the relationship of the distal tibia, fibula, and talus.

ligament is the most frequently injured.[33,37-40] The lateral aspect of the ankle is more frequently sprained than the medial aspect because of the joint's anatomy and biomechanics. A lateral ankle sprain results from an inversion stress and plantar flexion and frequently involves multiple lateral ligaments. The injury extent depends on the amount of stress applied and the position of the talus within the ankle mortise.

The anterior talofibular ligament is sprained when the athlete lands on the foot in a plantar-flexed and inverted position; once the foot makes contact with the ground, the foot continues to roll from plantar flexion toward dorsiflexion as more of the body's weight is placed on the extremity. If the ankle remains inverted while the ankle moves from plantar flexion toward dorsiflexion, the calcaneofibular ligament is also injured. Less often, the posterior portion of the lateral ligament complex is injured. When the posterior talofibular ligament is injured, the foot is in extreme inversion and dorsiflexion, as when the athlete inverts the foot and continues forward motion, either by propulsion from another player or by the momentum of running.

Medial Ligaments

The deltoid (medial) ligament is sprained less frequently than the lateral ligaments. The injury mechanism involves extreme subtalar joint eversion, and the extent of injury is directly proportional to the amount of stress applied to the ligament. With the subtalar joint in an everted position, the ankle may be in plantar flexion, a neutral position, or dorsiflexion at the time of stress application. Because of the deltoid ligament strength, when a sprain occurs, a distal tibial avulsion fracture should be suspected until ruled out with radiographs.

Distal Tibiofibular Syndesmosis

A sprain of the distal tibiofibular syndesmosis joint is a sprain of the anterior tibiofibular ligament, posterior tibiofibular ligament, and/or distal portion of the interosseous membrane. The lay term for this in-

CLINICAL PRESENTATION

	Lateral Sprain	Medial Sprain	Syndesmosis Sprain
History	Subtalar inversion and/or plantar flexion or dorsiflexion Pain arises from the lateral aspect of the ankle	Subtalar eversion and/or talocrural rotation Pain arises from the medial malleolus.	Weight bearing on the leg with a sudden pivoting motion (external rotation) Pain arises from just proximal to the malleoli.
Observation	Initial swelling is localized to the lateral aspect of the ankle. With time, the entire foot and ankle may become swollen. Grade II and III sprains may present with ecchymosis 3 or 4 days postinjury.	Immediately postinjury, swelling is localized to the medial malleolus. Acute injuries may be associated with swelling and ecchymosis throughout the foot.	Generalized postinjury swelling is localized above and medial to the lateral malleolus. The patient is unable to bear weight or walks with an antalgic gait.
Functional Status	Dysfunction is proportional to the injury severity. Antalgic gait may be noted. ROM is decreased secondary to pain, edema, and muscle spasm.	Pain and dysfunction are usually proportional to the trauma severity. The patient is unable to bear weight, or an antalgic gait may be noted.	Pain and dysfunction are usually proportional to the trauma severity. The patient is unable to bear weight, or an antalgic gait may be noted.
Physical Evaluation Findings	Pain with palpation of the involved ligament(s)	Pain with palpation of the deltoid ligament; pain at a bony insertion site may indicate a fracture To complete the physical evaluation, palpation over the proximal fibula is necessary to fully evaluate syndesmosis integrity. Decreased ROM in all planes of motion	The region between the distal tibia and fibula is tender. Painful ROM in extremes of dorsiflexion and plantar flexion
Positive Special Tests	Inversion stress test (calcaneofibular ligament) Anterior drawer test (anterior talofibular ligament)	Eversion stress test External rotation test (Kleigler test)	Dorsiflexion stress test Lateral rotation test (Kleigler test) Squeeze test

jury is a "high ankle sprain." A sprain of this structure must be recognized immediately, so that proper management, which is different from that for other ankle sprains, can be instituted. When lateral rotation of the leg or dorsiflexion occurs in weight bearing, a lateral force from the talus is exerted on the fibula. A sufficient force can stretch or tear the tibiofibular ligament as the malleoli are pushed away from each other. This mechanism is commonly seen during planting and pivoting maneuvers. In severe cases, the distal interosseous membrane is also affected. Because of the mechanism, a medial ankle sprain (deltoid ligament rupture) is often associated with syndesmosis injury. See Imaging Techniques in the Fibular Fractures section (p 123).

Injury to this ligament is unique. The lateral and medial ankle ligaments are stressed with medial and lateral movements, but the tibiofibular ligament is stressed whenever weight is borne on the extremity, and this stress is increased with external rotation. One purpose of the ligament is to hold the distal tibia to the distal fibula, forming the ankle mortise joint, so the injured ligament is stretched each time weight is transmitted from the calcaneus to the talus within the talus joint.

Differential Diagnosis

Avulsion fracture, lateral malleolar fracture, fifth metatarsal fracture, osteochondral talar dome fracture, syndesmosis sprain, subtalar ligament lesion, peroneal strain, subluxating peroneal tendons; additional differential diagnoses for syndesmosis sprains include extensor digitorum longus strain, extensor hallucis longus strain, and Maisonneuve fracture

Imaging Techniques

If pain occurs over the bony structures, radiographs are necessary to rule out a fracture. The Ottawa Ankle Rules were designed to enable emergency room physicians to reduce the number of ankle radiographs performed for ankle injuries, minimizing patient waiting and costs without inadvertently missing a fracture.[41,42] Radiographs should be taken within 10 days of injury if the patient has bony tenderness over the lower 6 cm of the tibia or fibula and is unable to bear weight on the limb.[36,37] In addition, foot radiographs are indicated if the patient has bony tenderness over the navicular or fifth metatarsal and is unable to bear weight, both immediately after the injury and at the time of examination (**Figure 5-23**).[43]

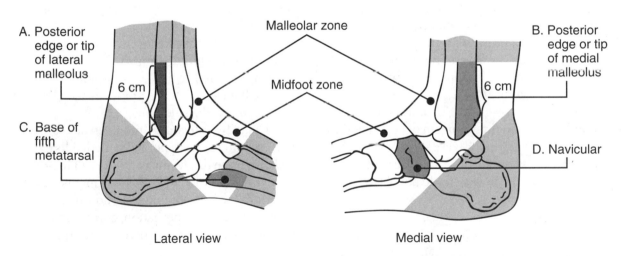

An ankle radiographic series is only required if there is any pain in the maleolar zone and any of these findings is present:
(1) bone tenderness at A
(2) bone tenderness at B
(3) inability to bear weight both immediately and in the ED

A foot radiographic series is only required if there is any pain in midfoot zone and any of these findings is present:
(1) bone tenderness at C
(2) bone tenderness at D
(3) inability to bear weight both immediately and in the ED

Figure 5-23 The Ottawa Ankle Rules. An ankle radiographic series is required only if there is pain in the malleolar zone and if there is bone tenderness in zones A or B or if the patient is unable to bear weight immediately or in the emergency department. A foot radiographic series is needed if there is pain in the midfoot zone or there is bone tenderness in zones C or D or if the patient is unable to bear weight immediately or in the emergency department. (Reproduced with permission from Stiell IG, Greenberg GH, McKnight RD, Wells GA: The "real" Ottawa Ankle Rules. *Ann Emerg Med* 1996;27:103-104.)

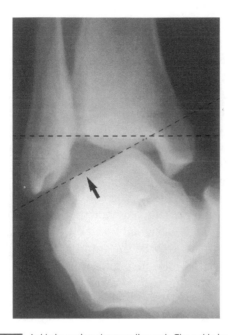

Figure 5-24 Ankle inversion stress radiograph. The ankle is manually inververted (ie, talar tilt test) during the radiograph. The angle formed between the superior border of the ankle mortise and the talus demonstrate the amount of laxity (arrow). (Reproduced with permission from Johnson TR, Steinbach LS (eds): *Essentials of Musculoskeletal Imaging.* Rosemont, IL, American Academy of Orthopaedic Surgeons, 2004, p 645.)

<table>
<tr><td>Table 5-3</td></tr>
</table>

Possible Factors Contributing to Recurring Ankle Sprains

The ligaments heal in a lengthened and stretched position, so support becomes deficient.

Scar tissue replacing the ligament is never as strong as the original ligament and lacks sufficient strength to restrict motion.

Peroneal muscles are not properly rehabilitated after a sprain and may, therefore, be too weak to provide active protection.

Instability of the distal tibiofibular joint

Genetic ligamentous laxity

Loss of proprioception after the original injury to the ligaments

Impingement of the distal fascicle of the anterior talofibular ligament

The damaged capsule's scar tissue is impinged in the talofibular joint.

Tight Achilles tendon

Tarsal coalition

Adapted with permission from Safran MR, Zachazewski JE, Benedetti RS, Bartolozzi AR III, Mandelbaum R: Lateral ankle sprains: A comprehensive review: Part 2. Treatment and rehabilitation with an emphasis on the athlete. *Med Sci Sports Exerc* 1999;31(suppl 7):S438-S447.

If pain occurs during palpation of the malleoli, base of the fifth metatarsal, or navicular, radiographs are taken. If no pain is present, the patient is asked to ambulate. Ambulating four steps without assistance, two on each foot, is considered weight bearing, even if the gait is antalgic.[41,42]

If a moderate to severe ankle sprain is suspected, lateral ankle stress radiographs may be ordered to compare laxity bilaterally (**Figure 5-24**). However, this procedure is painful when performed on an acute injury, so many physicians do not obtain stress radiographs of acute sprains.

Definitive Diagnosis

The history of an inversion injury and positive physical examination provide the basis for a definitive diagnosis. Concomitant injuries, such as malleolar avulsion fracture, medial ankle injury, syndesmosis sprain, peroneal tendon subluxation, and peroneal avulsion fracture, often go unnoticed, especially with moderate and severe ankle sprains, so all areas of pain must be investigated.

Pathomechanics and Functional Limitations

Several factors contribute to the high rate of ankle ligament reinjury (**Table 5-3**). Functional ankle instability is a frequent by-product of lateral ankle sprains, occurring in 29% to 42% of sprains;[40] however, mechanical ankle instability is much less frequent. Functional ankle instability is a perceived

instability by the patient and includes a sensation of the ankle giving way.

Recurrent or severe inversion ankle sprains can result in osteochondral injury to the talus or distal tibia. The patient complains of pain arising from the medial aspect of the ankle, especially during inversion and dorsiflexion.

The deltoid ligament provides medial subtalar joint stability and supports the medial longitudinal arch. Injury to this ligament may result in prolonged disability because of these requirements and stress. If the athlete has a preinjury condition such as pes planus or excessive pronation, chronic instability of the medial aspect of the ankle can result.

■ Immediate Management

Rest or immediate immobilization with tape, wrap, or splint; ice; compression; and elevation are included in the initial treatment of ankle sprains. Focal compression with a horseshoe or circular pad can further reduce edema (**Figure 5-25**).[44,45]

■ Medications

The early use of NSAIDs can help limit the inflammatory response and speed recovery. However, whether to use NSAIDs during the first 24 to 48 hours after injury or withhold them for the anticoagulation effect (which may increase swelling) is unresolved.

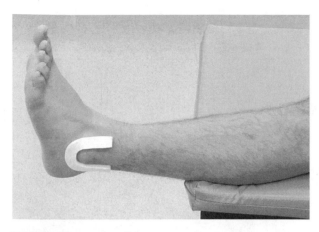

Figure 5-25   A U-shaped focal compression pad. This pad prevents excess fluid accumulation within the ankle joint capsule by forcing it to move over the fibula and proximally on the lower leg.

During the immediate care of severe ankle sprains, narcotic analgesics may be necessary to help control pain.

■ Postinjury Management

Electric stimulation may also be used to relax muscle spasm, relieve pain, and reduce edema. If the athlete is unable to ambulate normally, crutches for partial or non–weight bearing are recommended.

Early treatment should include open basket-weave taping to control edema.

Because of the tibiofibular ligament's unique responsibilities, the injured athlete needs to use crutches with weight bearing only to tolerance (no pain) or non–weight bearing to avoid stressing the injured ligament. Failure to do so delays the healing process and return to participation and could create a chronic condition. Radiographs should always be considered for this injury because an accompanying fibular (Maisonneuve) fracture is common.

■ Surgical Intervention

Most surgery is conducted using an open procedure. Anatomic reconstruction is preferred for young competitive athletes. Reattachment of the ligament to the fibula with augmentation from the inferior extensor retinaculum is often the preferred approach (**s t** **5-4**). Several other procedures, including tenodesis with peroneus brevis, plantaris, or hamstring have also been used to rebuild the lateral ligaments (**Figure 5-26**).

Deltoid ligament repair often requires concurrent repair of the distal syndesmosis (**s t** **5-5**). If a

Tenodesis The surgical relocation and fixation of a tendon.

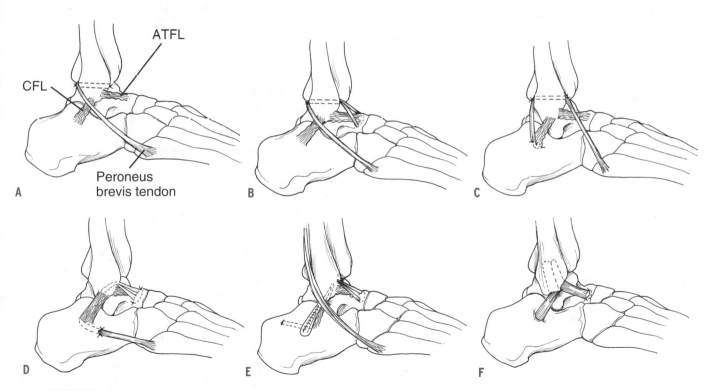

Figure 5-26   Augmented reconstructions. **A.** The Evans reconstruction uses a tenodesis of the peroneus brevis tendon to the fibula. **B.** The Watson-Jones procedure reconstructs the anterior talofibular ligament in addition to tenodesis of the peroneus brevis tendon. **C.** The Chrisman-Snook procedure uses a split peroneus brevis tendon to reconstruct the anterior talofibular and calcaneofibular ligaments. **D.** The Colville procedure also uses a split peroneus brevis tendon to reconstruct the anterior talofibular and calcaneofibular ligaments in an anatomic manner without limiting subtalar motion. **E.** The Anderson procedure uses the plantaris tendon to anatomically reconstruct both lateral ligaments without limiting subtalar motion. **F.** The Sjølin technique uses periosteal flaps to augment an anatomic repair. (Reproduced with permission from Colville MR: Surgical treatment of the unstable ankle. *J Am Acad Orthop Surg* 1998;6:368-377.)

S|T Surgical Technique 5-4

Nonaugmented Lateral Ankle Reconstruction

Indications

Chronic instability of the lateral aspect of the ankle requires surgery when rehabilitation or ankle bracing fails or when instability with daily activity and/or with use of a brace and/or limits activity level.

Overview

Nonaugmented lateral reconstruction (Bröstrom and modified Bröstrom, pictured above)
1. A curvilinear incision is made to expose the distal fibula, lateral ligaments, and calcaneus.
2. The repair is completed with the torn ligaments and inferior extensor retinaculum being reflected and sutured in place.
3. If a tenodesis is performed, the tendon is harvested and routed through drill holes or held in position with suture anchors to reproduce the lateral ligamentous structures.

Augmented lateral reconstructions (Evans, Watson-Jones, Elmslie-Trillat, Chrisman-Snook; see Figure 5-26).
1. The tendon (often the peroneal brevis) is identified and harvested, retaining as much length of the tendon as possible.
2. Often the tendon is left attached distally.
3. The tendon is then rerouted with various combinations of soft-tissue tunnels, bone tunnels, and suture anchors.
4. Retinacula are repaired, and tissues are closed.

In all techniques, the ankle is immobilized postoperatively to protect the repair or reconstruction.

Functional Limitations

Tenodesis (augmented) surgery has relatively poor long-term results, with degenerative changes and restricted subtalar motion. Tenodesis techniques cross the subtalar joint and thereby limit that joint's motion, and subsequent pathomechanics can occur. Anatomic reconstruction (nonaugmented) can provide full ROM after surgery because the procedure does not cross the subtalar joint, but degenerative ankle changes can still result. The ligament repair and extensor retinaculum reflection (nonaugmented) are more anatomic and less restrictive.

Implications for Rehabilitation

The repair is protected with immobilization during the early healing phase. After 3 to 4 weeks, the ankle can be moved through a gentle ROM exercise program and bear partial weight. Generally, the athlete must avoid plantar flexion and inversion for 4 weeks after surgery (some surgeons allow dorsiflexion and eversion after 1 week). After 6 weeks, the patient can bear weight as tolerated with brace support for the repair. Early progressive resistance exercises with plantar flexion and dorsiflexion can begin. Gradual progression occurs through the next 8 weeks. The lateral repair continues to be protected during this period with a lace-up or lateral stabilizer brace.

Comments

Return to sport is allowed after 3 months. Many physicians require the use of an ankle brace for the first full season after return. Nonaugmented repairs are preferred by most specialists.

Figure reproduced with permission from Colville MR: Surgical treatment of the unstable ankle. *J Am Acad Orthop Surg* 1998;6:368-377.

S|T Surgical Technique 5-5

Repair of Deltoid (Medial) Disruption and Syndesmosis Disruption

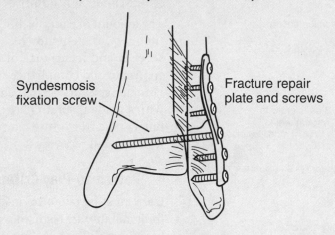

Syndesmosis fixation screw

Fracture repair plate and screws

Indications

A deltoid ligament (medial) sprain is often associated with syndesmosis injury and may require surgical intervention. If any mortise widening is seen on radiographs, surgery is required to repair the deltoid ligament and syndesmosis.

Overview

1. A curvilinear incision is made medially over the medial malleolus, and the injury is identified and repaired with sutures. Caution is needed to protect the distal tendons and posterior tibial artery that pass inferior to the medial malleolus.
2. Laterally, the fibula is approached just above the tibial plafond. If a concurrent fracture is present, it is fixated using a plate and screws. A syndesmosis screw is placed across from the fibula into the tibia with the ankle dorsiflexed.
3. Reduction of the syndesmosis is visualized under fluoroscopy.

Functional Limitations

The patient is maintained non-weight bearing while the syndesmosis screw is in place.

Implications for Rehabilitation

The placement of a syndesmosis screw necessitates non-weight bearing to prevent screw breakage. Once the screw is removed as an outpatient procedure after 6 to 12 weeks, ambulation can begin. ROM exercises and light resistance exercises can be introduced after the immobilization period.

syndesmosis screw has been placed, some surgeons restrict weight bearing until the screw is removed at 6 to 12 weeks. Strength and ROM exercises with partial weight bearing are then initiated. Full weight bearing is allowed after 8 weeks, and impact activities are permitted after 12 weeks.

■ Postoperative Management

Protecting the injured ligaments during the healing process is necessary to optimize healing. Postoperative management begins with immobilization and non–weight bearing. Partial weight bearing and ROM exercises are started after the initial healing response. Refer to the Functional Limitations and the Implications for Rehabilitation (in **S T** 5-5) for the specific surgery that was performed.

Pain and edema control are important. The most effective methods for these goals are compression, elevation, and minimizing stress to the damaged structures. Weight bearing is to tolerance; a general rule of thumb is if the athlete is unable to ambulate normally, crutches or other assistive devices to allow normal gait are necessary.

■ Injury-Specific Treatment and Rehabilitation Concerns

Specific Concerns

Prevent unwanted stresses on the healing ligament.
Control edema formation.
Maintain weight-bearing and ROM within limits of pain.

For both surgically repaired and conservatively treated ankle sprains, timing of the healing process and the patient's response are the primary factors pacing the rehabilitation progression. Active ROM is

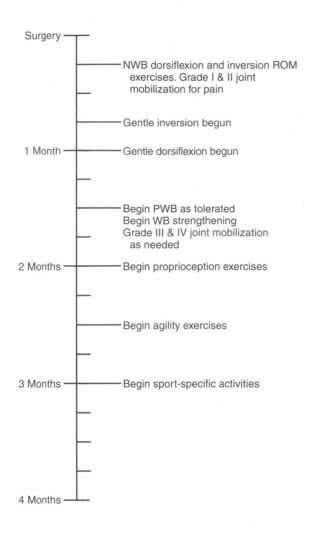

Surgery —

— NWB dorsiflexion and inversion ROM exercises. Grade I & II joint mobilization for pain

— Gentle inversion begun

1 Month —   — Gentle dorsiflexion begun

— Begin PWB as tolerated
Begin WB strengthening
Grade III & IV joint mobilization as needed

2 Months —   — Begin proprioception exercises

— Begin agility exercises

3 Months —   — Begin sport-specific activities

4 Months —

Note: Time frames are approximate. Function is the guide.

started when the injury is in the proliferation phase of healing. For surgical repairs, active ROM may begin after the first postoperative week. The initiation of active ROM exercises for conservatively treated ankles depends on injury severity: anywhere from day 2 for very minor injuries to days 3 to 5 for moderate injuries. If the ankle is immobilized, soft-tissue adhesions and joint restrictions have likely developed secondary to edema, tissue damage, and immobilization. These problems must be treated with soft-tissue and joint mobilization before full ankle and foot motion are restored. These mobilization techniques and active and passive motion exercises together restore normal mobility of the segment.

When the patient is in the mid to late proliferation phase of healing, more aggressive strengthening exercises can be started. Once the athlete is bearing full weight on the involved extremity, strength is increased with closed kinetic chain activities. Proprioceptive exercises begin with bal-ance activities, progressing to coordination and then agility activities in preparation for plyometric and finally functional and sport-specific activities.

▉ Estimated Amount of Time Lost

The amount of pain, swelling, and disability and the time requirements for recovery are related to the severity and recurrence of injury, the patient's response to and compliance with treatment, and the clinician's ability to manage the injury. A patient with a grade II sprain may recover in 2 to 6 weeks, but a grade III rupture may require 6 to 8 weeks or more for full recovery.

▉ Return-to-Play Criteria

Care must be taken to ensure that soft-tissue and joint mobility are restored, especially if the ankle has been immobilized. An antalgic gait can cause muscle imbalances to develop between the left and right lower extremities, so examination should reveal full strength restoration throughout the involved extremity. Return of proprioceptive function is evaluated by comparing balance, coordination, and agility between the extremities.

Functional Bracing

A stirrup-type brace can also be applied to provide stability to the injured ligament. Once the athlete begins activities, taping or an ankle brace may provide some sense of stability and improve proprioception during activities. Moleskin stirrups can provide additional stability when taping the ankle.

Controversy exists regarding the ability of high-top shoes to reduce the incidence of ankle sprains, but many people advocate their use.[46,47] Taping and bracing after an ankle sprain is also debated. Backers indicate that additional support is useful,[48] whereas others have found little or no difference in preventing additional injury.[49] Recent evidence suggests that although taping and bracing do not help athletes without injury, they do increase joint awareness in subjects who have had a prior injury.[50] If an athlete feels more confident in his or her ability and more secure if the ankle is taped or braced, providing the support may be advantageous physically or psychologically, or both.

Ankle Fractures and Dislocations

Talocrural dislocations often occur with accompanying fracture to the medial or lateral malleolus (or both). An isolated talocrural dislocation without concomitant fracture of the malleoli or posterior

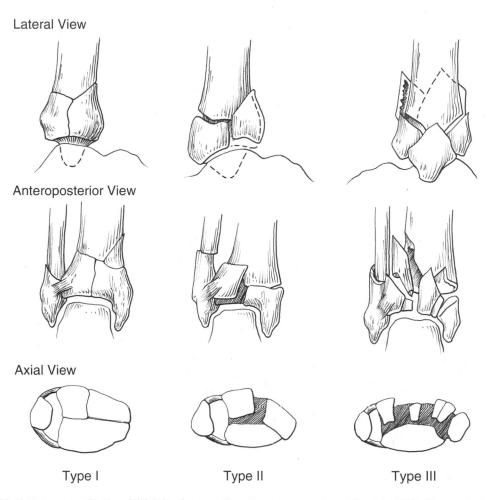

Lateral View

Anteroposterior View

Axial View

Type I   Type II   Type III

Figure 5-27   Rüedi-Allgöwer classification of tibial pilon fractures. Type I is a cleavage fracture of the distal tibia, with a nondisplaced articular surface. Type II is characterized by mild to moderate displacement of the articular surface but minimal to no comminution of the joint surface or adjacent metaphysis. Type III shows comminution of the articular surface and metaphysis with significant impaction of the metaphysis. (Adapted with permission from Mueller ME, Allgower M, Schneider R, Willenegger H (eds): *Manual of Internal Fixation: Techniques Recommended by the AO-ASIF Group,* ed 3. New York, Springer-Verlag, 1991, p 279.)

tibia is rare.[51] Ankle fractures can involve the lateral malleolus, medial malleolus, collateral ligament structures, posterior tibia (posterior malleolus), and talar dome. Among the most serious ankle fractures are those that involve the tibial weight-bearing articular surface or the adjacent tibial metaphysis, or both (**Figure 5-27**).[52]

Fractures involving one side of the ankle are stable and can be successfully treated symptomatically. A bimalleolar fracture includes the tibial and fibular malleoli or a distal fibular fracture with deltoid ligament disruption. A trimalleolar fracture involves the posterior tibia and a bimalleolar fracture. Because both of these fractures occur on the medial and lateral aspects of the ankle, they are considered unstable, and surgical repair has the best results. In addition, a fracture of the posterior tibia or talus (talotibial osteochondral defect) can also occur with a dislocation. Because of the proximity to the bones, the skin covering the malleoli can be disrupted, causing an open fracture-dislocation.

Combined ankle plantar flexion and forced subtalar inversion or eversion can result in the fractures described in the preceding paragraphs and a posterior talar dislocation. If inversion occurs, the displacement is posteromedial; an eversion force produces a posterolateral displacement. Posteromedial dislocations occur more frequently because the ankle tends to be in an inverted and plantar-flexed position when an athlete lands from a jump. Ankle dislocations also occur from a severe rotation or twisting mechanism while the foot is planted.

Predisposing factors for ankle dislocations include ligamentous laxity, medial malleolus hypoplasia, a history of ankle sprains, and peroneal muscle weakness.[51] Support for the ankle region is primarily medial-lateral and not anterior-posterior, the direction of ankle dislocations. If the angle of force application causes a dislocation, osteochondral defects of the posterior tibia and talus can also occur but are frequently overlooked because of the more obvious dislocation.

CLINICAL PRESENTATION

History

High-force impact to the ankle, often involving inversion and
    plantar flexion
Exquisite pain

Observation

In most cases, gross joint deformity and malalignment are noted.
    However, some talar dislocations may present more subtly.

Functional Status

ROM cannot occur secondary to disrupted joint alignment.
Inability to bear weight on the extremity

Physical Evaluation Findings

Obvious joint disruption
Fracture of the lateral and/or medial malleolus

Differential Diagnosis

Syndesmosis sprain, talar dome fracture

Imaging Techniques

Radiographs confirm the presence of the fracture-
dislocation suggested by the deformity. A CT scan
or an MRI may be required to define the fracture
configuration and possible presence of soft-tissue
injury or bone bruises (**Figure 5-28**).

Definitive Diagnosis

Positive radiographic findings

Pathomechanics and Functional Limitations

A pure dislocation without fracture, although rare,
can result in a good outcome when treated by closed
reduction, followed by immobilization and a progressive rehabilitation program.[51] Some motion may
be lost, but the ankle will be functional.

In an ankle with a fracture-dislocation, the
effects are more profound. If the medial malleolus fracture occurs proximal to the deltoid ligament, the ankle is unstable and requires surgical
fixation. Displaced fractures of any bone also
need open reduction and internal fixation. Talar
fractures are more complex and demand removal
of osteochondral fragments and prolonged
non–weight bearing.

An open fracture requires surgical debridement to reduce the risk of osteomyelitis. This injury causes extensive damage to soft tissue, bone,
and joints. Recovery occurs with proper treatment
and rehabilitation, but eventual posttraumatic
arthritis is common.

■ Immediate Management

Immobilization in the position of dislocation, application of ice and elevation, and transport to
an emergency department are necessary, especially with an accompanying open fracture or
suspected bimalleolar, trimalleolar, or talar dome
fracture. Neurovascular examination should always be performed before immediate treatment.
Continued periodic examinations should take
place until emergency department treatment is
provided.

■ Medications

Oral or injectable narcotic analgesics are used because of the traumatic nature of the injury. Massive
damage occurs to the ankle and subtalar soft tissues from this high-energy injury.

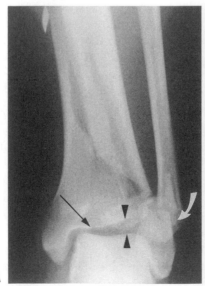 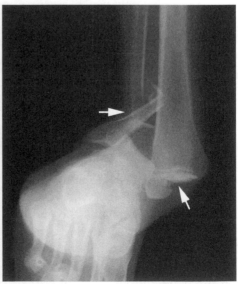

Figure 5-28   **A.** Radiograph of an ankle mortise fracture. The black arrow highlights an intra-articular pilon fracture and the white arrow highlights a distal fibular fracture. The mortise is unstable and marked by widening of the lateral joint line (arrowheads). **B.** Bimalleolar fracture-dislocation of the ankle mortise. The arrows demonstrate the fractures of the malleoli. (Reproduced with permission from Johnson TR, Steinbach LS (eds): *Essentials of Musculoskeletal Imaging*. Rosemont, IL, American Academy of Orthopaedic Surgeons, 2004, p 650.)

■ Surgical Intervention

All dislocations require immediate closed or open reduction and documentation of congruent joint alignment. Surgery might be required to obtain acceptable anatomic joint and bony alignment. **Table 5-4** lists other conditions warranting surgery after ankle mortise fracture. The surgical technique depends on the fracture type and requires rigid fixation, anatomic alignment, and restoration of joint surfaces.

Rigid internal fixation allows near-immediate ROM (**Figure 5-29**). Weight bearing is limited or delayed in articular surface injuries. Arthritis, stiffness, and pain are common after these injuries.

Table 5-4

Indications for Surgery After a Talocrural Fracture or Dislocation

Bimalleolar fracture

Trimalleolar fracture

Lateral malleolar fracture with concomitant medial (deltoid) ligament rupture

Displaced or angulated tibial fracture

Unstable syndesmosis injury

Fracture of the weight-bearing articular surface 1 mm or larger

Dislocation that cannot be reduced by closed means

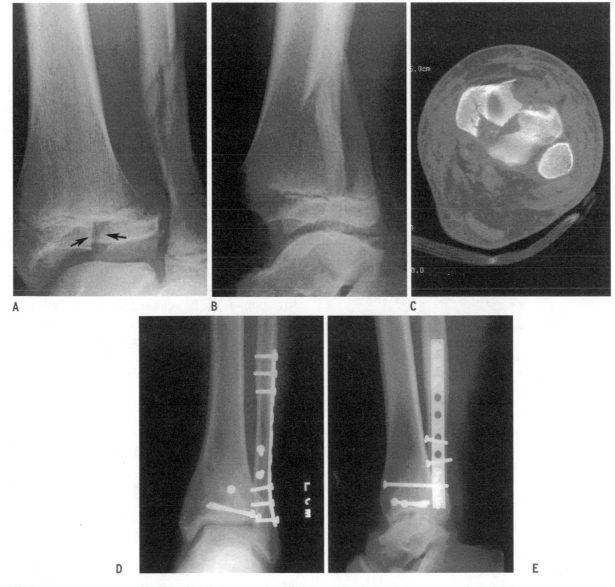

Figure 5-29 **A.** Anteroposterior radiograph of a two-part lateral triplane fracture (arrows) and a comminuted fracture of the distal fibula. **B.** Lateral radiograph of A. **C.** Computed tomography scan demonstrating marked external rotation of the lateral portion of the distal fibula, fracture displacement, and comminution of the distal tibia. **D.** Anteroposterior view of subsequent repair. **E.** Lateral view of repair. (Reproduced with permission from Kay RM, Matthys GA. Pediatric ankle fractures: Evaluation and treatment. *J Am Acad Orthop Surg* 2001;9:268-278.)

■ Postinjury/Postoperative Management

Immobilization after surgical reconstruction is necessary to allow soft-tissue and bone healing. Allowances for motion depend on the presence of associated fractures and degree of soft-tissue injury.

■ Injury-Specific Treatment and Rehabilitation Concerns

> **Specific Concerns**
>
> Protect the bones from unwanted stresses.
> Delay the onset of atrophy.
> If applicable, protect the traumatized ligaments and/or surgical
>   repair.
> Restore soft-tissue mobility.
> Restore joint ROM.
> Restore muscular strength.

After surgery, the ankle is usually placed in a CAM boot with a brief period of no or partial weight bearing to tolerance at the outset (see Figure 5-11). The an-

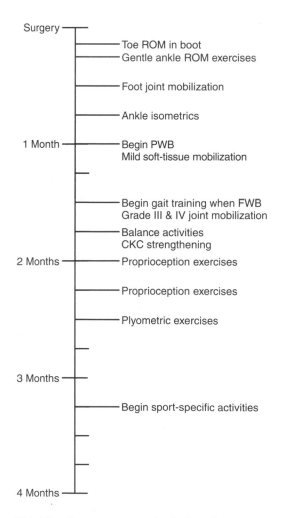

Surgery	
	Toe ROM in boot
	Gentle ankle ROM exercises
	Foot joint mobilization
	Ankle isometrics
1 Month	Begin PWB
	Mild soft-tissue mobilization
	Begin gait training when FWB
	Grade III & IV joint mobilization
	Balance activities
	CKC strengthening
2 Months	Proprioception exercises
	Proprioception exercises
	Plyometric exercises
3 Months	
	Begin sport-specific activities
4 Months	

Note: Time frames are approximate. Function is the guide.

kle may be removed from the boot after about 7 days for mild passive or active ROM. After 2 to 3 weeks, isometrics within the pain-free range may be initiated.

Once the surgical site is well healed, soft tissue around the site and the scar itself should be examined for adhesions. If the tissue is restricted, soft-tissue mobility techniques are used to restore movement. Care should be taken, however, because the tissue is new and very easy to tear. Mobilization of the involved joints should be avoided for the first 6 to 8 weeks. After that time, if examination reveals tightness in any of the joints of the unaffected foot, mobility should be increased.

While the patient is restricted in activities, maintain cardiovascular fitness and maintain or develop muscle strength in the uninvolved extremities. Open kinetic chain exercises for the hip, knee, and foot of the involved extremity can also be included during the non–weight-bearing phase.

■ Estimated Amount of Time Lost

Time lost can range from 3 months in uncomplicated cases to 12 months or more in severe cases. Complicating factors such as neurovascular compromise and talar dome or tibial osteochondral defects can also prolong recovery.

■ Return-to-Play Criteria

Patients with this type of injury participate in rehabilitation programs for extended periods. Thus, a thorough examination of the athlete's abilities must be made before return to athletic participation. With immobilization and swelling, soft tissue in the area commonly becomes restricted; these restrictions must be released to restore full motion and function. Joint mobility and ROM should be fully regained. Muscle strength of the entire lower extremity can be significantly affected by prolonged inactivity and needs to be normal before the athlete returns to play.

Functional Bracing

The athlete may feel more confident if the ankle is taped or an ankle brace applied. Neither may offer protection against a repeated injury, but proprioception may benefit from such a technique or device.

Peroneal Tendon Subluxations and Dislocations

Most peroneal tendon subluxations and dislocations primarily involve the peroneus brevis tendon (PBT). The least severe injury occurs when the PBT

CLINICAL PRESENTATION

History

Mechanism of sudden, strong peroneal contractions, especially when the ankle is dorsiflexed
Pain arising from the posterior aspect of the lateral malleolus
A "snap" or "pop" may be described as the tendon dislocated from the groove.

Observation

Swelling posterior to the lateral malleolus

Functional Status

If the tendon remains dislocated, ambulation is difficult or impossible.
Complaints of the ankle "giving way" as the tendon dislocates are common in chronic conditions.

Physical Evaluation Findings

Motion into plantar flexion and inversion is normal.
An avulsed segment of the superior peroneal retinaculum may be palpated.
Resisted eversion causes pain and may reproduce the symptoms.
Crepitus may be palpated over the tendons as they pass behind the lateral malleolus.

displaces anterior to the lateral malleolus but remains within the peroneal retinaculum. In more severe cases, the retinaculum tears and a bony segment avulses from its posterior attachment, so the retinaculum lies posterior to the PBT.

The mechanism of injury is a sudden, severe contraction of the peroneals while the ankle is dorsiflexed. Snow skiers are susceptible to this mechanism when the ski tips dig into the snow and the skier falls forward or digs the inner ski borders into the snow during a turn. These injuries are also seen in skating, water skiing, gymnastics, basketball, football, tennis, and dancing.

Peroneal dislocations can be acute or chronic. Acute injuries may be misdiagnosed as lateral ankle sprains. The dislocated tendons often relocate spontaneously, so the actual injury remains undiagnosed. Patients with a history of recurrent ankle sprains should be evaluated for peroneal tendon subluxation or dislocation.

Predisposing anatomic conditions that may contribute to this injury include the following: (1) a shallow fibular groove for the peroneal tendons, (2) a prominent calcaneofibular ligament, (3) congenital absence of the peroneal retinaculum, (4) acquired or congenital laxity of the peroneal retinaculum, and (5) a low peroneus brevis muscle belly that crowds the fibular malleolar groove.[53]

Differential Diagnosis

Lateral ankle sprain, chronic ankle instability, anterolateral impingement syndrome, nerve injury, osteochondral lesions, arthritis

Imaging Techniques

A CT scan or an MRI with axial views may assist in diagnosing peroneal inflammation, tendon disruption, or dislocation. A superior peroneal retinaculum avulsion can result in a bony fragment being laterally displaced, the "fleck sign"[54] (**Figure 5-30**).

Definitive Diagnosis

The definitive diagnosis is based on a positive history of complaints indicating that the tendon is slipping out of its groove, such as snapping and popping, and confirmed by visualization or palpation of the dislocating tendon.

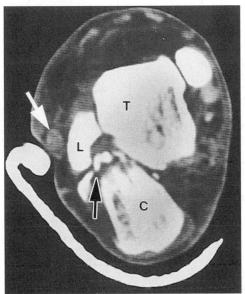

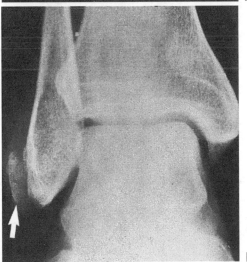

Figure 5-30 Radiographic images of peroneal tendon dislocations. **A.** Computed tomography scan showing lateral displacement of the peroneal tendon (white arrow). There is also an associated subluxation of the subtalar joint (black arrow). **B.** The "fleck sign" associated with a rupture of the superior peroneal retinaculum. As the retinaculum avulses from the anterior fibula, a piece (fleck) of bone may be displaced (white arrow). (Reproduced with permission from Johnson TR, Steinbach LS (eds): *Essentials of Musculoskeletal Imaging.* Rosemont, IL, American Academy of Orthopaedic Surgeons, 2004, p 650.)

Pathomechanics and Functional Limitations

In addition to pain and swelling affecting normal function, repeated PBT subluxation against the fibula can cause a longitudinal tear or shredding of the tendon. Chronic ankle instability is also a complication of chronic PBT subluxation. If left untreated, adaptive tendon shortening occurs, resulting in reduced power and function during ambulation.

Gait is also mechanically altered when the tendon dislocates from the peroneal groove. When the tendons displace anteriorly, their mechanical angle of pull changes from that of a plantar flexor to a dorsiflexor with a strong eversion component.

Immediate Management

Acute injuries are managed using ice, compression, and elevation.

Medications

Pain and the inflammatory process that can accompany a dislocating or subluxating tendon can be limited by the use of NSAIDs.

Postinjury Management

Successful conservative treatment can occur but is rare. Conservative attempts to maintain the tendon in place can include adhesive strapping with a pad to restrict subluxation, J-shaped pads that anchor in front of the fibula and wrap around laterally and posteriorly to hold the tendon in place, and non–weight bearing for 3 weeks (**Figure 5-31**). If the foot is kept relatively stable and the tape restricts the tendon's movement, scar-tissue formation may allow the tendon to be managed without surgery.

If an acute injury is treated conservatively with a short leg, non–weight-bearing cast for 6 weeks and results are successful, the time lost may be an additional 3 to 6 weeks, depending on the individual's response to treatment. Although most reports of conservative management indicate poor success rates,[55-57] some physicians attempt conservative treatment in acute cases.

Surgical Intervention

Chronic injuries are more universally treated with surgical repair.[55,58,59] The surgery typically involves deepening the posterior fibular groove and reconstructing the superior retinaculum. After surgery, concomitant dorsiflexion and eversion are avoided to remove stress from the retinacular reconstruction, but plantar flexion and inversion actively create smooth tendon excursion. Return to athletic competition is expected after 3 to 4 months of rehabilitation.

Postoperative Management

After surgery, the ankle is maintained for 4 weeks in a non–weight-bearing cast, followed by 2 weeks in a weight-bearing cast. Active and resisted dorsiflexion and eversion are prevented during the early rehabilitation phase (approximately 6 to 8 weeks). This is followed by progressive resistance and ROM exercises within 2 weeks.

Injury-Specific Treatment and Rehabilitation Concerns

> **Primary Goals**
> _____
> Avoid eversion and dorsiflexion motions to reduce stress on the superior retinaculum.
> Restrict motion, especially dorsiflexion with eversion, for the first 6 to 8 weeks.

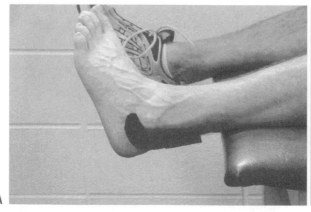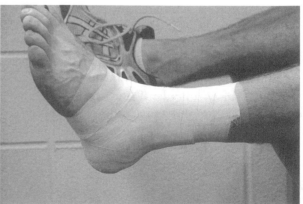

Figure 5-31   Use of a J-pad to control peroneal subluxations. **A.** A foam or felt pad is cut to conform to the path of the peroneal tendons as they pass around the lateral malleolus. **B.** The pad is secured using athletic or elastic tape.

Early in the rehabilitation process, superior peroneal retinaculum stresses are reduced by avoiding dorsiflexion and eversion. Once the patient begins partial weight bearing in a CAM boot, active plantar flexion and inversion can begin, but the return to the starting position (the motion of dorsiflexion and eversion) must be passive. Talar mobilization exercises and active dorsiflexion and eversion begin when the patient can bear weight without pain.

The progression of resisted strengthening, proprioception, and agility exercises is initiated when the patient can bear weight without pain when not wearing a brace. As strength and proprioception improve, the patient can progress through plyometric and functional activities that lead to a return to competition.

■ Estimated Amount of Time Lost

Conservative approaches to management may result in 6 to 12 weeks of time lost. After surgical repair, the patient may be withheld from competition for 2 to 4 months.

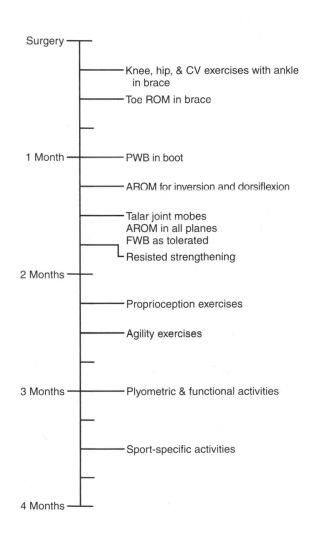

Surgery
— Knee, hip, & CV exercises with ankle
  in brace
— Toe ROM in brace

1 Month — PWB in boot

— AROM for inversion and dorsiflexion

— Talar joint mobes
  AROM in all planes
  FWB as tolerated
  └ Resisted strengthening

2 Months —

— Proprioception exercises

— Agility exercises

3 Months — Plyometric & functional activities

— Sport-specific activities

4 Months —

Note: Time frames are approximate. Function is the guide.

■ Return-to-Play Criteria

Before returning to full participation, the patient must have full motion without pain or tendon subluxation during functional activities.

Functional Bracing

A J-pad may be used in an attempt to decrease the forces on the superior peroneal retinaculum (see Figure 5-31).

ACHILLES TENDON

Retrocalcaneal Bursitis

Retrocalcaneal bursa inflammation is also known as Haglund disease, "pump bump," and tendo Achilles bursitis. Mechanical disorders such as repetitive retrocalcaneal compression or friction can lead to the condition.[34]

The bursa's anterior wall lies against the calcaneus, and its posterior wall merges with the epitenon of the Achilles tendon[60] (**Figure 5-32**). Its fluid is highly viscous, and when the bursa becomes inflamed, the walls become thickened and edematous. During normal ambulation, the enlarged bursa is compressed between the calcaneus and the Achilles, a condition that intensifies when shoes are worn.

Foot pathomechanics resulting from excessive pronation contribute to this condition. Wearing negative-heeled shoes can increase the bursal compression by stretching the Achilles tendon during initial contact and midstance. A shortened Achilles also increases the compression force on the bursa.

Epitenon A glistening, synovial-like membrane that envelops the tendon surface.

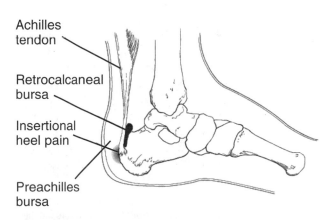

Achilles tendon

Retrocalcaneal bursa

Insertional heel pain

Preachilles bursa

Figure 5-32 Sites of posterior heel pain. (Reproduced with permission from Greene WB (ed): *Essentials of Musculoskeletal Care*, ed 2. Rosemont, IL, American Academy of Orthopaedic Surgeons, 2000, p 493.)

CLINICAL PRESENTATION

History

Pain arising from the posterior calcaneus

Observation

Retrocalcaneal exostosis (pump bump)
Swelling

Functional Status

Plantar flexion compresses the soft tissues, resulting in pain.
Pain may be decreased when walking barefoot.
Walking on the toes or in high heels may increase pain.

Physical Evaluation Findings

Pain occurs when pressure is applied to the soft tissue anterior
   to the Achilles tendon. The tendon itself is not painful.
Increased tissue temperature and swelling may be noted lateral
   to the Achilles tendon.

Differential Diagnosis

Achilles tendinitis, plantar fasciitis, calcaneal stress
fracture

Imaging Techniques

Bursography differentiates between retrocalcaneal
bursitis and insertional Achilles tendinitis.[60] An enlarged Haglund process can be noted on lateral radiographs. Sagittal MRI can demonstrate an enlarged
retrocalcaneal bursa (**Figure 5-33**).

Definitive Diagnosis

Positive physical examination and exclusion of
other conditions

Pathomechanics and Functional Limitations

Alteration of the patient's gait secondary to Achilles
tendon tightening or foot overpronation can redistribute forces along the foot and lower extremity.
Retrocalcaneal bursitis can, therefore, lead to
Achilles tendinitis, metatarsal stress fractures, and
lower extremity inflammatory conditions.

■ Immediate Management

Ice and immobilization may help to decrease the
inflammatory process. Relief of external pressure
from shoes or heel straps is also helpful.

■ Medications

Pain and inflammation can be controlled by the use
of NSAIDs. With recalcitrant symptoms, corticosteroid injections can be used in an attempt to decrease the inflammatory reaction.

■ Postinjury Management

The three primary concerns are to (1) identify and correct the cause of retrocalcaneal bursitis, (2) reduce
the inflammation, and (3) restore all deficiencies to
allow the individual to return to full participation.

A donut pad can be placed over the bursa to reduce friction. During peak inflammation, however,
the patient will likely prefer to wear a slipper or san-
dal without a back or back strap. A heel lift may reduce the biomechanical forces on the Achilles tendon.

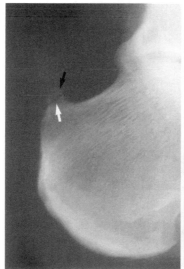
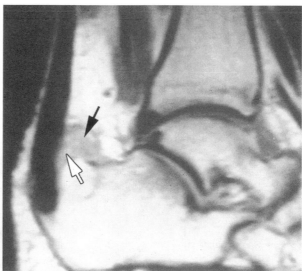

Figure 5-33   Imaging of retrocalcaneal bursitis. **A.** Lateral radiograph of the calcaneus demonstrating an enlarged Haglund process (white arrow). The exostosis has fragmented (black arrow). The clouding around the structure indicates soft-tissue inflammation. **B.** Sagittal magnetic resonance image demonstrating enlargement of the retrocalcaneal bursa (black arrow) and inflammation of the Achilles tendon insertion on Haglund process (white arrow). (Reproduced with permission from Johnson TR, Steinbach LS (eds): *Essentials of Musculoskeletal Imaging.* Rosemont, IL, American Academy of Orthopaedic Surgeons, 2004, p 572.)

■ Surgical Intervention

Surgery for retrocalcaneal bursitis is rarely indicated. Surgery involves excision of the exostosis and the superior border of the calcaneal tuberosity. If the Achilles tendon is calcified, the involved portion may be removed through a longitudinal incision. After surgery, a padded short leg cast or brace is applied with the ankle maintained in approximately 20° of plantar flexion for 3 weeks.

■ Postoperative Management

The patient is non–weight bearing for approximately 3 weeks after surgery and then uses a walker boot. Active plantar-flexion and dorsiflexion exercises can be initiated once the patient transitions to the boot.

■ Injury-Specific Treatment and Rehabilitation Concerns

> **Specific Concerns**
>
> Decrease compressive forces on the calcaneus and Achilles tendon caused by footwear.
> If present, protect the exostosis with a donut pad.
> Correct improper foot mechanics.
> Increase Achilles tendon flexibility.

Resolving this condition is rooted in correcting the underlying cause and reducing inflammation. Two common factors contributing to retrocalcaneal bursitis are a tight Achilles tendon and a flaccid foot that promotes excessive pronation. When the foot is pronated during the gait phase as it should be supinating, a medial torque is applied to the Achilles tendon; this torque increases pressure on the bursa. Placing a lift in the shoe heel reduces the stretching stress on the Achilles and compression on the bursa. (Both shoes should have the same-size lift to prevent lumbosacral injury.) Custom orthotic appliances may correct foot alignment to place less pressure on the bursa and can also lift the heel. Ice, whirlpool, and ultrasound can reduce the inflammation.

■ Estimated Amount of Time Lost

At least 4 to 6 weeks may be required for the condition to resolve.

■ Return-to-Play Criteria

Return to full sport participation is permitted once inflammation has subsided and the causes of the condition have been resolved. At this point, the patient should be able to wear an athletic shoe without discomfort.

Functional Bracing

If the patient has a flaccid, excessively flexible, or planus foot, orthotic appliances should be provided and used for all activities.

Achilles Tendinitis (Tendinopathy)

"Tendinitis," or "tendonitis," is actually a misnomer. Very rarely is the tendon itself inflamed. More often, this problem involves the synovial sheath (tenosynovitis) or the paratenon sheath (paratendinitis) that surrounds a tendon. In some cases, the tendon actually has microscopic tears from repeated trauma (tendinosis). The proper term is "tendinopathy" or "tendon stress syndrome." Because tendinitis is not an accurate term, "tendinopathy" will be used here.

Achilles injuries result from external influences and inherent factors or a combination of both. Acute Achilles injuries are most often the result of external influences. Tendinopathy usually involves a number of factors that combine to put more stress on the tendon than it can tolerate. This segment deals with tendinopathy injuries, whereas the following section presents acute Achilles injuries.

Inflammation occurs when repetitive stresses applied to the structures do not allow full recovery before the stress is reapplied. The site of inflammation in the Achilles, about 2 to 6 cm proximal to the tendon's distal insertion on the calcaneus, is poorly vascularized (**Figure 5-34**).

> **CLINICAL PRESENTATION**
>
> **History**
> Insidious onset of pain
> Repetitive stress to the ankle and leg
>
> **Observation**
> Swelling may be noted over the Achilles tendon in the area 2 to 6 cm proximal to the calcaneal insertion.
> Achilles tendon nodules may be palpable in advanced cases.
>
> **Functional Status**
> Hamstrings and triceps surae ROM may be decreased.
> In severe cases, walking may be difficult, and pronounced gait changes may be observed.
>
> **Physical Evaluation Findings**
> A nodule may be felt on the medial tendon about 2 to 6 cm proximal to the tendon's calcaneus insertion.
> The nodule is tender to palpation.
> Pain may be elicited during passive Achilles tendon stretching.
> Decreased plantar-flexion strength may be noted.
> Hyperpronation and decreased dorsiflexion ROM may be present.

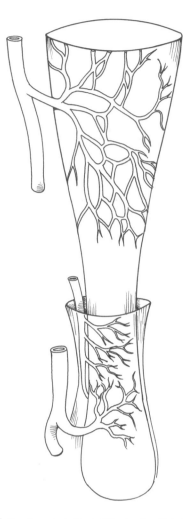

Figure 5-34 Blood supply to the Achilles tendon. Note that longitudinal vessels supply the tendon proximally and distally, whereas transverse vessels supply the middle portion. (Reproduced with permission from Jones DC: Tendon disorders of the foot and ankle. *J Am Acad Orthop Surg* 1993;1:87-94.)

Achilles tendinosis presents with gradual, progressive pain, usually with an insidious onset. The athlete generally does not report the injury until it begins to interfere with performance or the pain occurs during rest or simple ambulation. At this time, the patient can usually point to the pain location in the Achilles tendon midsubstance.

Factors contributing to tendinopathy include training errors such as running too far, increasing distance or intensity too quickly, too much hill work, running on hard surfaces, inappropriate or worn shoes, specialized workouts without variety, poor technique, and fatigue.[61] Restricted dorsiflexion, restricted subtalar joint mobility, decreased hamstring mobility, leg-length discrepancy, and muscle imbalances are also thought to contribute to Achilles tendinopathy.[62] The largest contributors to Achilles disorders are believed to be malalignments and biomechanical faults.[62] Of these, foot

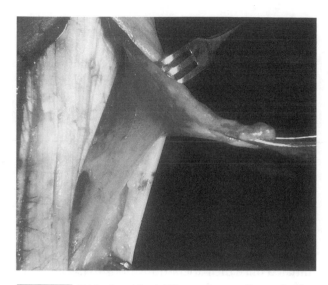

Figure 5-35 Thickening of the Achilles paratenon as the result of inflammation. (Reproduced with permission from Jones DC: Tendon disorders of the foot and ankle. *J Am Acad Orthop Surg* 1993;1:87-94.)

hyperpronation is believed to be the most prevalent cause. Hyperpronation can become exaggerated if the Achilles is tight, and the combination applies even greater stress to the Achilles than either problem alone. During midstance, the foot normally begins to move toward supination, but a hyperpronated foot does not, so the Achilles contracting to propel the body forward is simultaneously stretched. This stress is especially predominant along the medial tendon at the site of reduced vascular supply, where palpation tenderness is usually greater. Individuals involved in middle-distance and long-distance running, soccer, volleyball, tennis, and badminton have the highest incidence of Achilles tendinopathy.[62]

The cause of Achilles tendon overuse disorders has been disputed. Tendon inflammation was thought to be the degeneration source, but this theory has not been substantiated by the presence of inflammatory agents.[62] One of the current predominant theories is the mechanical theory initially stated by Leadbetter:[63] when a tendon is repeatedly brought to 4% to 8% beyond its normal length, fatigue occurs in the tendon tissues. This fatigue restricts the tendon tissue's ability to repair itself, and the microtraumatic process takes over. Collagen becomes denatured, and crosslinks break, progressively weakening the collagen and negatively affecting the matrix and vascular supply (**Figure 5-35**). Eventually, tendinosis results.

Differential Diagnosis

Retrocalcaneal bursitis, calcaneal stress fracture, tibial stress fracture, posterior tibial tendinitis, tarsal tunnel syndrome, ossicle formation posterior to the talus (os trigonum)

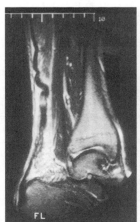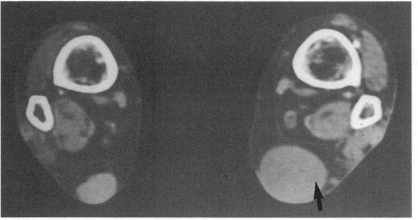

Figure 5-36 Imaging of the Achilles tendon. **A.** Magnetic resonance imaging demonstrating a partial longitudinal tear of the Achilles tendon associated with tendinopathy. (Reproduced with permission from Jones DC: Tendon disorders of the foot and ankle. *J Am Acad Orthop Surg* 1993;1:87-94.) **B.** Axial computed tomography scan of both legs. The Achilles tendon of the right leg is notably thicker than the left. (Reproduced with permission from Johnson TR, Steinbach LS (eds): *Essentials of Musculoskeletal Imaging.* Rosemont, IL, American Academy of Orthopaedic Surgeons, 2004, p 641.)

Imaging Techniques

Radiographs are obtained to rule out the presence of an os trigonum or Haglund process inflammation (see Figure 5-18). MRI can be used to identify Achilles tendon tears. Axial CT scans can identify paratenon thickening (**Figure 5-36**).

Definitive Diagnosis

Clinical symptoms are often sufficient to make the diagnosis of Achilles tendinopathy, once other possible diagnoses have been ruled out. The diagnosis is further confirmed through radiographic findings. In some cases, an Achilles tendon nodule is palpated as the patient plantar flexes and dorsiflexes the ankle (**Figure 5-37**).

Pathomechanics and Functional Limitations

Pain can decrease triceps surae strength, leading to a weak toe-off phase of gait and reducing the ability to perform functional activities such as jumping. If the condition is advanced, the athlete is unable to perform normal workouts or has pain during workouts. The athlete may also report sleep disturbances. Over time, a longitudinal tendon tear may develop.

■ Immediate Management

The causative factors must be identified and corrected for any lasting improvement in Achilles tendinopathy to occur. Inflammation and pain relief can be achieved with a variety of options, including medications prescribed by the physician, modalities such as ultrasound and ice, and cross-friction massage (to reduce adhesions secondary to the inflammation).

■ Medications

The treatment of Achilles tendinopathy routinely includes NSAIDs. Recalcitrant symptoms may respond to phonophoresis or iontophoresis. Corticosteroid injections into the tendon sheath are contraindicated because of the increased risk of

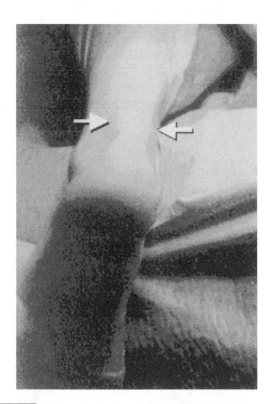

Figure 5-37 Photograph of chronic Achilles tendinopathy. A tender, nodular swelling (arrows) can be seen moving as the ankle is plantar flexed and dorsiflexed. (Reproduced with permission from Paavola MP, et al: Current concepts review: Achilles tendinopathy. *J Bone Joint Surg Am* 2002;84:2062-2076.)

Achilles tendon rupture. Injection into the retro-calcaneal bursae can be done safely.

Postinjury/Postoperative Management

A heel lift may reduce Achilles tendon forces sufficiently to allow for pain-free gait. Patients with advanced cases need to walk with crutches for a pain-free gait. Footwear should not compress the Achilles tendon and calcaneus.

Surgical Intervention

Surgical intervention is indicated when pain and dysfunction persist despite 3 to 6 months of aggressive Achilles tendon stretching and eccentric strengthening and/or a 1- to 2-month trial of immobilization. Via a medial incision, the tendon sheath is dissected and a tenosynovectomy is performed, removing the nonviable degenerative tissue and bone spurs (**Figure 5-38**). If the inflammation involves the tendon insertion, the superior calcaneus prominence may also be removed.

After surgery, return to activity is anticipated in 3 to 4 months, but the surgical results are highly variable. If the calcaneus was debrided, 6 weeks of immobilization are warranted.

Postoperative Management

After paratenonitis surgery, the patient is non–weight bearing for 7 to 10 days, progressing to full weight bearing as tolerated. With tendinosis, the patient can bear full weight, protecting the tissues using a rocker boot with an adjustable heel for 2 to 4 weeks

(see Figure 5-11). During this time, ROM exercises can be performed.

Injury-Specific Treatment and Rehabilitation Concerns

> **Specific Concerns**
> _____
> Decrease Achilles tendon stress.
> Improve Achilles tendon, ankle, and hamstring ROM.
> Restore Achilles tendon soft-tissue mobility.

The primary goal is to identify and correct (as much as possible) the causative factors. Changes in the athlete's workout may be required. The athlete who is restricted in activities can maintain cardiovascular fitness and preserve or develop muscle strength in the uninvolved extremities. Pool running may be possible if it does not irritate the Achilles tendon. Open kinetic chain exercises for the involved extremity's hip, knee, and foot can also be included during the non–weight-bearing phase. Once inflammation is alleviated, a gradual progression of eccentric exercises effectively treats tendinitis.[64]

Heel lifts can be inserted in the shoes to relieve Achilles tendon stress; arch supports or orthotic appliances should be used to correct biomechanical or structural deviations. Stretching exercises improve Achilles, ankle, and hamstring flexibility. Ice, ultrasound, cross-friction massage, and NSAIDs may all assist in relieving inflammation. A progressive program of eccentric exercises is initiated

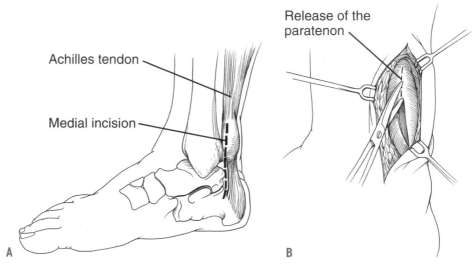

Figure 5-38 Surgical intervention of Achilles tendon inflammation. **A.** A medial longitudinal incision minimizes cutting of the sural nerve and short saphenous venous system. **B.** After full-thickness flaps are created, the paratenon is released and any thickened areas are excised. (Reproduced with permission from Saltzman CL, Tearse DS: Achilles tendon injuries. *J Am Acad Orthop Surg* 1998;6:316-325.)

once the inflammation is manageable: when the athlete performs 3 sets of 10 heel raises at a moderate eccentric pace without pain.

Estimated Amount of Time Lost

Activity is limited primarily by pain. The time lost varies greatly; the condition is self-limiting, and return is also governed by the degree of inflammation, the individual's tolerance, and the success of efforts to reduce inflammation. Reduced activity is recommended until the inflammation can be controlled and causative factors resolved.

Return-to-Play Criteria

The causative factors involved in the athlete's tendinopathy must be identified and corrected or diminished. To avoid pain during activity, inflammation should be resolved before the athlete is allowed to fully resume sport participation.

Functional Bracing

Orthoses may be necessary to correct biomechanical or structural deviations contributing to Achilles tendinopathy. If calf flexibility remains a problem, inserting heel lifts into the shoes may reduce some of the Achilles stress.

Achilles Tendon Rupture

Interruption of the Achilles tendon occurs 5 to 7 cm above the tendon insertion on the posterior calcaneus. At this location, the tendon rotates, so the lateral fibers become medially situated as the tendon travels to the triceps surae. This is also the site of reduced tendon vascularity (see Figure 5-34). The injury is most often seen in male athletes 30 to 40 years of age who participate in sudden stop-and-go, quick-change-of-position activities such as basketball and racquet sports. The injury can also occur in athletes who are moving forward when the foot suddenly becomes anchored, as when a falling player lands on the foot.

Although the exact cause is unclear, repetitive microtrauma to the tendon is thought to predispose the athlete to Achilles rupture when the tendon is suddenly and aggressively stretched while simultaneously contracting eccentrically. The athlete reports a sudden "pop" and immediate, intense pain in the calf. It is typically described as a sensation of being "shot," kicked, or hit by a racquet.

Differential Diagnosis

Achilles tendinitis, triceps surae strain, plantaris strain, deep venous thrombosis

Imaging Techniques

Radiographs are not required in frank Achilles tendon ruptures. Partial tendon ruptures can be visualized on MRI or CT scan (**Figure 5-39**; see Figure 5-34).

frank clearly or visibly evident.

Definitive Diagnosis

A clinical diagnosis of a complete Achilles tendon rupture can be made based on a positive Thompson test result, in which squeezing of the triceps surae group fails to produce plantar flexion. Partial tendon tears are diagnosed based on the findings of MRI studies.

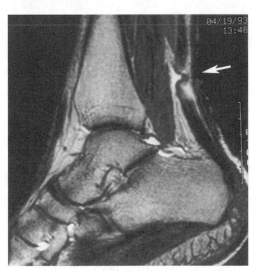

Figure 5-39 Sagittal magnetic resonance imaging demonstrating an acute, incomplete tear of the Achilles tendon. (Reproduced with permission from Saltzman CL, Tearse DS: Achilles tendon injuries. *J Am Acad Orthop Surg* 1998;6:316-325.)

Pathomechanics and Functional Limitations

The athlete is unable to ambulate or does so with difficulty and cannot stand on the toes of the involved leg.

■ Immediate Management

Rest, ice, compression, and elevation; non–weight bearing with crutches; referral to an orthopaedic physician is indicated

■ Medications

Narcotic pain medication may be used to control severe pain. However, pain is often not an overriding problem.

■ Postinjury Management

The ankle is immobilized in a position that approximates the Achilles tendon, approximately 20° or less of plantar flexion (if this position does not appropriately realign the tendon, surgical repair should be performed). Immobilization and non–weight bearing are maintained for at least 2 weeks. The patient progresses to a short leg cast or boot for an additional 6 to 8 weeks and then is gradually weaned from it. When normal footwear is introduced, a ½- to ¾-in heel lift is used for 1 month, followed by 1 month of a 1-cm lift. Progressive resistance exercises can be started at 8 to 10 weeks.

■ Surgical Intervention

Athletes benefit from surgical repair because of the prolonged recovery required and greater risk of recurrence with conservative treatment. For Achilles tendon rupture, surgical treatment is favored for the competitive athlete but optional for the noncompetitive athlete, although nonsurgical treatment can be successful. For Achilles tendinitis, surgical treatment is considered when pain persists after 3 to 6 months of aggressive Achilles stretching and/or eccentric strengthening and a trial of immobilization (1 to 2 months). Surgical reapproximation of the tendon ends reestablishes "normal" gastrocnemius-soleus tendon length (ST 5-6).

■ Postinjury/Postoperative Management

The initial postoperative boot positions the ankle in approximately 15° to 30° of plantar flexion to limit stress on the surgical repair. Weight bearing is not permitted for the first 1 to 3 weeks to avoid pushing off with the Achilles. Pain and edema are controlled with modalities of choice. A walking boot can be used for 6 weeks. A heel lift, as described in postinjury management, should be used when normal footwear is introduced.

Passive plantar flexion and active dorsiflexion to 20° can begin at 3 to 7 days after surgery. Conditioning for the cardiovascular system and unaffected segments can be performed during this time.

■ Injury-Specific Treatment and Rehabilitation Concerns

Specific Concerns

Avoid forceful motion for the first 8 to 12 weeks.
Restore Achilles tendon length.
Restore triceps surae strength.

With conservative management, the athlete begins in a cast or CAM boot in plantar flexion; the cast is changed or the CAM boot is adjusted monthly to gradually increase dorsiflexion to reach the neutral position by 3 months. A foot orthotic appliance that restricts dorsiflexion to neutral is then worn for an additional 4 to 8 weeks.

Because surgical repair of a ruptured Achilles tendon offers quicker recovery and a lower rerupture rate than nonsurgical management, athletes usually undergo surgical repair. Different surgical techniques are available; the athlete's recovery depends on the surgical technique and the postoperative protocol. A more liberal protocol uses a postoperative posterior splint that is removed on the third day to allow early passive ROM within a pain-free range throughout the day.[65] Early weight bearing is permitted after the sutures are removed during the second or third week. A CAM boot that allows full plantar flexion but limits dorsiflexion to −10° is used for the next 2 weeks. At week 4, neutral dorsiflexion is permitted.

A more conservative postoperative protocol uses a below-knee cast with progressive decreases in ankle plantar flexion every 3 weeks for 6 weeks.[66] At 6 weeks, the cast is removed, and active ankle exercises, including strengthening, and full weight bearing, are allowed. Jogging can begin in a pool and is permitted on land at 3 months. Provided the athlete has fully recovered in all areas, unrestricted activity is allowed at 6 months.

Two extremes of care exist, and most surgeons opt for a postoperative protocol that lies in between. The foot is placed in a boot with the ankle positioned in 15° to 30° of plantar flexion, and no weight bearing is permitted for 1 to 3 weeks. During this time, the athlete can perform toe exercises and ac-

| S|T | Surgical Technique 5-6 |

Achilles Tendon Repair

After Alvarado

Indications

Ruptured Achilles tendon

Overview

1. A medial incision is made over the Achilles tendon to expose the stumps.
2. The stumps are approximated using two to four sutures. If the rupture occurred at the bony attachment, suture anchors are required.
3. Some surgeons also advocate repair of the paratenon.
4. If Achilles tendinitis is present, the nonviable degenerative tissue is debrided, and the bone spurs and prominence of the posterior superior calcaneus are removed.
5. The ankle is immobilized in 20° of plantar flexion.

Functional Limitations

Calf size is smaller; the involved extremity must be isolated to regain full strength and size. The tendon is thicker after surgery.

Implications for Rehabilitation

Achilles stretching is avoided for 3 to 6 months after surgery to protect the tendon from "stretching out." Plantar-flexion mobility and strengthening can begin early (2 to 4 weeks).

Comments

After Achilles repair, return to sport requires 6 to 12 months.

Figure reproduced with permission from Saltzman CL, Tearse DS: Achilles tendon injuries. *J Am Acad Orthop Surg* 1998;6:316-325.

tive ankle and foot ROM within the boot. Knee and hip exercises can also be performed as long as the boot is worn. After the third week, toe-touch weight bearing is started, and by week 6, the athlete begins progressing to full weight bearing as tolerated. During the toe-touch weight-bearing period, slow isometric exercises can be initiated with the foot in the boot. Starting in the third week, the plantar-flexion angle of the boot is decreased 5° each week until the patient can wear a shoe with a heel lift by week 8. Gentle active ROM moving into dorsiflexion can also begin in the third week. At 6 weeks, slow, progressive, passive Achilles stretching can start, along with intrinsic muscle strengthening and stationary bicycling, with push-off only from the heel, not the toes. Aggressive rehabilitation has the patient stationary bicycling while wearing a boot at 2 weeks and full weight bearing at 3 weeks.

When full weight bearing is permitted, gait training is required. After week 8, a gradual progression of resistive exercises is started, beginning with light resistance and limited excursion, which gradually increase to tolerance. Running activities are delayed until about 6 months.

■ Estimated Amount of Time Lost

Time lost depends on the treatment technique selected, ranging from 6 to 12 months for surgical repair to more than a year for conservative care.

■ Return-to-Play Criteria

If the Achilles remains tight, a heel lift in the shoes may relieve some tendon stress. Rehabilitation after an Achilles repair is prolonged, and significant deficiencies occur in motion, strength, proprioception, and sport performance for several months, so these factors must be restored before the athlete can safely return to full sport participation.

Functional Bracing

A heel lift may be required if full ROM into dorsiflexion is not present.

LEG

Acute Compartment Syndrome

Acute compartment syndrome most commonly arises from a traumatic event that results in increased pressure within the compartment, which is surrounded by restrictive fascia that prevents expansion. Pressure compromises the vascular structures, leading to limb-threatening ischemia and, if left untreated, eventual death of the tissues enclosed in the compartment.

Sudden, severe injuries cause significant swelling. These injuries may range from contusions and strains to crush fractures. Swelling places ever-increasing pressure on blood vessels, nerves, and muscles within the compartment (**Figure 5-40**). With inadequate blood supply to tissues within the compartment, tissue necrosis ensues as swelling remains unchecked.

Pain may be elicited by attempts to passively stretch the muscles, but if the nerve has been damaged by the swelling, pain may not occur with a stretch (**Table 5-5**). Paralysis results if the nerve is damaged or the pressure within the compartment inhibits the nerve; by this time, damage can be severe and irreversible.[67] Paresthesia was thought to be the most reliable finding,[68] but it has more recently been demonstrated that the five Ps of vascular insufficiency (pallor, pain, paralysis, pulselessness, and paresthesia) are not reliable.[67] Each compartment has its own

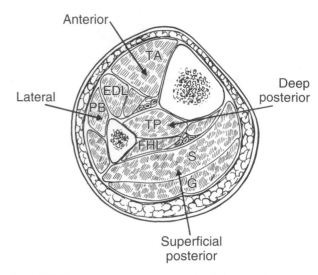

Figure 5-40   Cross-section of the proximal half of the leg shows the direction of needle insertion for testing each compartment. EDL, extensor digitorum longus; FHL, flexor hallucis longus; G, gastrocnemius; PB, peroneus brevis; S, soleus; TA, tibialis anterior; TP, tibialis posterior. (Reproduced with permission from Whitesides TE, Heckman MM: Acute compartment syndrome: Update on diagnosis and treatment. *J Am Acad Orthop Surg* 1996;4:209-218.)

unique characteristics of sensory deficit. If the anterior or lateral compartment is affected, numbness occurs on the dorsum of the foot. If the deep posterior compartment is affected, numbness is reported on the plantar surface of the foot.

It is important to note that if the five Ps are present, surgical compartment release will be too delayed to produce optimal results.[67] In addition, by the time sensory deficits are apparent, ischemia has been present for an hour or more, and complete recovery even after release is unlikely.[67] The most reliable symptoms are disproportionate pain in the area and increased pain with passive stretching of the muscles within the compartment.[67]

Differential Diagnosis

Tibial stress fracture, tibial stress reaction, periostitis, tibial fracture, popliteal artery claudication, peripheral nerve entrapment, medial tibial syndrome, muscle strain

Table 5-5

Pain Produced During Passive Muscle Stretching Correlated With the Compartment Involved

Pain With Muscle(s) Stretching	Compartment Involved
Extensor hallucis longus	Anterior compartment
Peroneals	Lateral compartment
Triceps surae	Superficial posterior compartment
Flexor hallucis longus	Deep posterior compartment

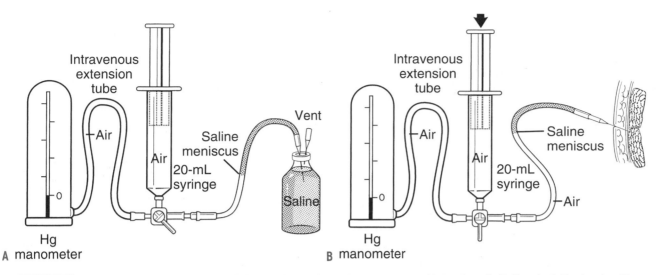

Figure 5-41 Whitesides infusion technique to identify increased compartmental pressure. **A.** Assembled equipment with the valve in the closed position. **B.** Testing configuration. The needle is inserted into the involved compartment, and the intracompartmental pressure is determined. (Reproduced with permission from Whitesides TE, Heckman MM: Acute compartment syndrome: Update on diagnosis and treatment. *J Am Acad Orthop Surg* 1996;4:209-218.)

Medical Diagnostic Tests

Intracompartmental pressure can be monitored using the infusion technique or the Howmedica Slit catheter or Stryker STIC devices (**Figure 5-41**). In certain cases, such as concurrent tibial fractures, time-series pressure measurements may be ordered.[67]

CLINICAL PRESENTATION

History
A direct blow to the lower leg
Pain reported may be disproportionate to apparent injury severity.

Observation
The skin overlying the compartment is distended.
Vascular disruption can cause the skin to appear pale or discolored.

Functional Status
Pain and weakness limit the patient's ability to walk.

Physical Evaluation Findings
Pain may be elicited during passive elongation of the muscles in the involved compartment.
Sensation over the dorsal or plantar foot may be decreased.
In severe cases, distal pulses may be absent.

Imaging Techniques

Swelling and distension within the compartment are shown by MRI studies. Muscle edema may also be noted after direct trauma.

Definitive Diagnosis

A clinical diagnosis of acute compartment syndrome can be based on the injury history and the patient's signs and symptoms. If intracompartmental pressure measurements are taken, the diagnosis is confirmed if the diastolic pressure minus the intracompartmental pressure is less than or equal to 30 mm Hg.

Pathomechanics and Functional Limitations

The patient is unable to bear weight on the involved limb. As pressure increases within the compartment, the neurovascular structures become compressed, increasing pain and decreasing the distal blood supply and innervation. The distal extremity may swell secondary to impaired venous return. In the worst-case scenario, vascular and neurologic compromise can lead to permanent disability of the distal extremity.

◼ Immediate Management

This is a limb-threatening orthopaedic emergency. The limb is managed using ice and elevation, but a compression wrap is not applied because external compression further increases the compartment pressure and exacerbates the condition. The athlete must be immediately referred for a possible emergency fasciotomy.

◼ Medications

Intravenous, intramuscular, or oral narcotic medications may be administered for short-term pain relief, but it is inappropriate to use them to delay the need for surgical intervention. The failure to control pain with narcotics should be a warning of potential acute compartment syndrome.

◼ Postinjury Management

The extremity should be elevated to decrease interstitial pressures and to encourage venous and lymphatic return. Ice packs placed on the extremity can minimize swelling and limit secondary hypoxic injury. A compression wrap should not be applied until permitted by the attending physician. Crutch use is often indicated.

Surgical Intervention

Most patients with acute compartment syndromes, especially those with one or more clinical signs or symptoms, require surgical intervention. All four compartments must be released. An anterior incision is made from the proximal tibia to the distal tibia to identify the intermuscular septum that separates the anterior and lateral compartments, taking care to avoid the superficial peroneal nerve. These two compartments can be released through this single incision. The deep posterior and posterior compartments are released through a medial incision, avoiding the saphenous vein and nerve. The deep posterior compartment is approached through a medial tibial periosteal approach. The skin incisions are not sutured, and the incisions must be packed open.

Postoperative Management

The incisions are left open and packed with gauze. Repeated wash-out procedures and secondary closures are required. Tissue jacks have become popular to close the wounds after repetitive wash-out procedures once tissue viability is assured. These tissue jacks can speed the healing process because they avoid the necessity for split-thickness skin grafts.

After healing progresses, a compression dressing is applied, and immediate weight bearing is permitted as tolerated. Knee and ankle ROM exercises can also begin once the incisions are healed. Stretching and strengthening exercises are added as tolerated, and the rehabilitation program is progressed accordingly. Dressing checks and changes for infection prevention are necessary for the fasciotomy release sites.

Fasciotomy Surgical incision of the fascia.

Injury-Specific Treatment and Rehabilitation Concerns

> ### Specific Concerns
> Monitor and change dressings to prevent infection.
> Prevent unwanted pressure increases within the compartment.
> Stretch compartmental muscles as tolerated.

Once healing of the surgical incisions has been deemed appropriate by the physician, ankle ROM and strengthening can begin. The rehabilitation program progresses as described for ankle sprains.

Estimated Amount of Time Lost

Approximately 12 weeks are required after surgery for complete recovery.[69] Posterior compartment release requires more time for recovery than anterior or lateral compartment release because of the more extensive dissection and healing of a larger muscle mass.

Return-to-Play Criteria

Even after the surgical sites are healed, the tissue remains relatively fragile for several months, so if the patient participates in contact or collision sports, protective padding over the wounds may be necessary to prevent skin breakdown. If the surgical release was performed in a timely manner, the patient may have no deleterious effect on motor or sensory innervation. If permanent sensory deficit has occurred, return to sport participation may still be possible, but this depends on the extent of the deficit and the sport.

Functional Bracing

Protective covering of the healed surgical sites may be indicated if there is a risk of damaging the cutaneous scar tissue. Once healing is complete, approximately 12 weeks, protective padding is not needed.

Chronic Exertional Compartment Syndrome

Although chronic compartment syndrome can occur in any of the four leg compartments, it most often affects the anterior compartment. Chronic compartment syndrome, often referred to as chronic exertional compartment syndrome, is an exertional condition brought on with exercise and relieved with rest. Pain results from eccentric muscle contractions, which increase intracompartmental pressure and likely impair venous blood egress.

Vascular flow to the muscles is diminished and leads to ischemia.[70] Osmotic pressure in the interstitial fluid of the compartment increases with the release of proteins during eccentric muscle activity. Increased pressure reduces blood flow, resulting in tissue ischemia. Pain from ischemia and compartment pressure is the primary limiting factor in functional performance.

Athletes most commonly affected include distance runners, those involved in running sports such as soccer and lacrosse, and skaters. Once the symptoms develop, they continue throughout the activity, remaining at the same intensity or increasing as the activity continues. In the early stages, pain is reduced or ceases soon after the activity is stopped.[71] Because symptoms persist with activity, pain may intensify after a workout.[22]

History

Anterior lower leg pain that increases with activity and decreases with rest

Muscle cramping, burning, and tightness may be described.

Symptoms may radiate into the ankle and dorsum of the foot.

A "slop-foot" gait may be noted with significant anterior compartment involvement.

Observation

Usually no outward signs of recurrent anterior compartment syndrome are present.

Functional Status

No remarkable changes in strength and ROM during periods of nonstrenuous activity

Muscle weakness and pain that develop during activity may alter gait.

Physical Evaluation Findings

Anterior compartment palpation may reveal tenderness and a hard feel.

The area may be painful to the touch.

Differential Diagnosis

Periostitis, fibular stress fracture, tibial stress fracture, tibial stress reaction, medial tibial syndrome, tenosynovitis, tarsal tunnel syndrome, muscle disorders, infection, popliteal artery claudication, peripheral nerve entrapment, tumor

Medical Diagnostic Tests

Diagnostic studies are undertaken when there is a clinical suspicion of chronic exertional compartment syndrome. This involves compartment pressure measurements pre- and postactivity after onset of symptoms, using the commercially available Slit catheters as described earlier. Elevated pressures preactivity (>15 mm Hg) and/or postactivity (>30 mm Hg) aid in the diagnosis.

Imaging Techniques

Radiographs are unremarkable. Bone scan and MRI are occasionally used to rule out stress reactions.

Definitive Diagnosis

Elevated compartment pressures and symptoms during activity

Pathomechanics and Functional Limitations

Pain and increased compartmental pressure limit functional performance.

■ Immediate Management

Ice and stretching for pain relief

■ Medications

Pain can be reduced and the patient can safely return to activity with the assistance of NSAIDs.

■ Postinjury Management

Taping, orthotic appliances, and shoe modifications can help by allowing the athlete to continue participation. However, relief with immediate management is variable and not often long term.[22]

■ Surgical Intervention

Elevated compartmental pressures and symptoms during exercise, although not a medical emergency, may require surgical release of the fascia. Most symptoms arise from elevated anterior and lateral compartment pressures. Rarely do pressures elevate to a degree to cause symptoms in the posterior compartments. Surgical release for the anterior and lateral compartments can be accomplished with a single incision.

If the involved fascia has herniated, a small (3 to 5 cm) incision is made directly over the defect, otherwise the incision is made midway between the tibial crest and fibular shaft (**Figure 5-42**). The intermuscular septum and nearby superficial peroneal nerve are identified. A **fasciotome** is passed superiorly and inferiorly, 1 cm medial and 1 cm lateral to the intermuscular septum, to release the anterior and lateral compartments, respectively. If necessary, the posterior compartments are easily released through a second incision along the medial border, mid one-third of the tibia. Following the procedure, the skin incisions are closed and a pressure dressing is applied.

Fasciotome A device used to split subcutaneous or intramuscular fascia.

■ Postinjury/Postoperative Management

After surgical release, the patient usually bears weight to tolerance, but activities causing swelling must be avoided. Crutch weight bearing as tolerated, stretching, and stationary bicycling with progressive walking are advanced for the first 2 weeks. Active ROM and stretching exercises can be started immediately postoperatively. Monitoring the dressings and preventing wound infections are important during the first week. As the skin heals, active motion and mild massage may assist in maintaining good soft tissue mobility. Care must be taken to avoid excessive friction on new scar formation that will tear or shear the immature tissue; massage should not be performed until at least week 6, and then emphasis should be more on the adjacent tissue than directly over the new scar tissue. The patient normally has only mild postoperative pain and experiences a rapid recovery, with resumption of full sport participation within 3 to 6 weeks.

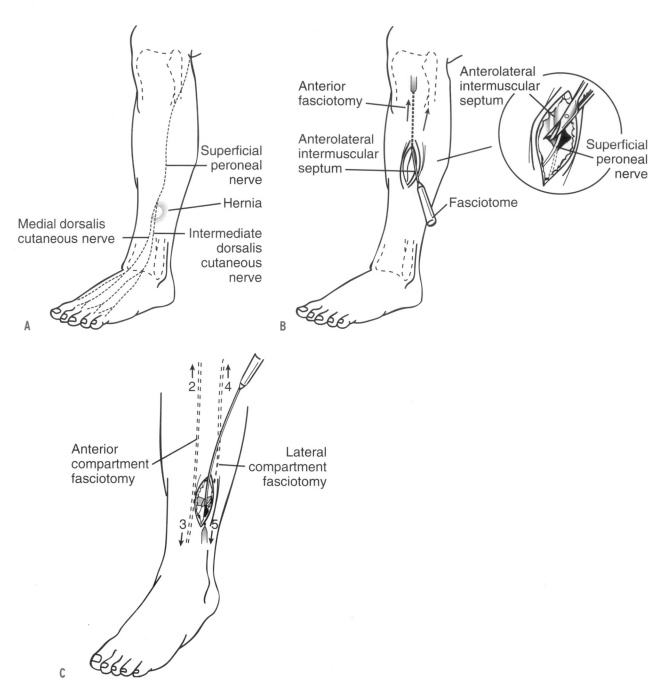

Figure 5-42 Single-incision release of the anterior compartment. **A.** The compartment's neurovascular structures are identified and avoided during the procedure. The incision is made directly over the defect if present. Otherwise the incision is made between the tibial crest and fibular shaft. **B.** The fasciotome is first passed superiorly. **C.** A second pass is made to release the fascia.

■ Injury-Specific Treatment and Rehabilitation Concerns

Specific Concerns

Prevent infection of fasciotomy wounds.
Promote active ROM immediately postoperatively.
Prevent recurrence by accelerating rehabilitation.

Postoperative care usually includes ice for the first 48 hours and immediate ROM and stretching exercises. Full weight bearing is possible within a day or two. Once the incisions are healed, cycling and swimming can be initiated. Strength loss is usually minimal, and the athlete responds quickly to treatment. Recovery is usually complete within 3 to 6 weeks but can extend for 12 or more weeks.

Estimated Amount of Time Lost

Recovery time is usually 3 to 6 weeks but can extend to 12 weeks. The type of surgery, the size of the fasciotomy required, the athlete's pain tolerance, and healing complications all influence recovery time.

Return-to-Play Criteria

All surgical sites must be completely healed before the athlete returns to full participation. If the sport involves collision or contact, protective padding is advised over the area for several weeks or months until the scar tissue is stable and under no threat of breakdown.

Functional Bracing

Shoe orthoses are sometimes used to reduce compartment stress. Protective padding may be initially applied to surgical scars to maintain scar integrity against abuse during activity.

Tibial Stress Fractures

One of the most common sites for stress fractures is the tibia in its middle or distal one third. A stress fracture occurs with the application of a nonviolent, repetitive stress that does not allow sufficient recovery between stress applications for the bone to adapt. Microfractures develop and advance to a stress fracture. The bone fails biomechanically when bone resorption occurs at a faster rate than bone formation.[72]

Changes in training factors such as intensity, terrain, and shoes can be causative factors leading to tibial stress fractures. Athletes beginning a season with little or no preseason preparation are more susceptible to stress injuries. Sudden changes in terrain, such as running downhill or on soft surfaces such as sand or mud, increase impact and muscle stresses. Tibial stress is greatest during the push-off and landing phases of running.[73] Shoes without appropriate support or cushion may increase leg stresses. Women with menstrual dysfunction who have reduced bone mineral density are also susceptible to stress fractures.

Athletes in endurance and jumping sports (eg, distance running, dance, aerobics, soccer, and basketball) are most commonly affected by tibial stress fractures. Typically, weight-bearing activities cause the insidious onset of pain, which is eased with rest. The athlete often does not report the pain until it interferes with workouts or performances or occurs even at rest or with simple ambulation.

CLINICAL PRESENTATION

History

A sudden increase in the duration, frequency, and/or intensity of training

The patient may describe a change in activity surface, such as grass to concrete.

The patient may report changes in shoes or use of excessively worn shoes.

Observation

The lower leg may have no remarkable abnormalities.

Functional Status

Initially, only mild pain may be described during activity.

As the fracture matures, pain begins earlier in the workout, creates more discomfort, and persists longer after the activity.

Active and passive ROM is usually within normal limits.

Physical Evaluation Findings

Tenderness and a bony prominence may be palpated over the fracture site.

Pain may be elicited when low-intensity therapeutic ultrasound is applied over the fracture site.[48]

Pain may be experienced during resisted ROM.

Differential Diagnosis

Fibular stress fracture, tibial periostitis, anterior tibial tendinitis, posterior tibial tendinitis, popliteal artery entrapment,[74] chronic exertional compartment syndrome, medial tibial stress syndrome, nerve entrapment

Imaging Techniques

Most early radiographs are negative for immature stress fractures. Bone scans can be used to identify areas of increased periosteal activity, but this in and of itself does not always indicate a stress fracture (**Figure 5-43**). MRI is as sensitive as a bone scan but is more specific in diagnosing stress fractures. MRI is becoming the imaging method of choice.[75]

Definitive Diagnosis

A clinical diagnosis may be made based on the patient's symptoms, especially increased pain during exertional activity such as running, even in the absence of positive radiographic studies.

Pathomechanics and Functional Limitations

Minimizing stresses during the preswing and initial contact phases of gait by wearing stress-reducing shoes or running on a firm yet giving surface such as a composite may allow the athlete to continue workouts relatively pain free. If these modifications are not possible, alternative workouts may be required until the pain is resolved. If the pain becomes too intense, the athlete may have to stop activity until the pain becomes manageable or resolves.

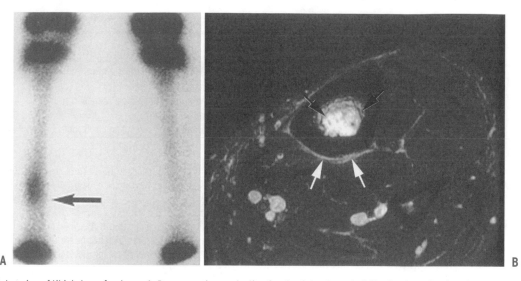

Figure 5-43 Imaging of tibial stress fractures. **A.** Bone scan demonstrating focal uptake characteristic of a stress fracture (arrow). (Reproduced with permission from Greene WB (ed): *Essentials of Musculoskeletal Care*, ed 2. Rosemont, IL, American Academy of Orthopaedic Surgeons, 2000, p 375.) **B.** Magnetic resonance image indicating bone marrow edema (black arrows) and periosteal edema (white arrows) indicative of a stress fracture. (Part A reproduced with permission from Sullivan JA, Anderson SJ (eds): *Care of the Young Athlete*. Rosemont, IL, American Academy of Orthopaedic Surgeons and American Academy of Pediatrics, 1999, p 308. Part B reproduced with permission from Johnson TR, Steinbach LS (eds): *Essentials of Musculoskeletal Imaging*. Rosemont, IL, American Academy of Orthopaedic Surgeons, 2004, p 519.)

■ Medications

Inflammation and the associated pain can be reduced by using NSAIDs. Some physicians avoid prescribing NSAIDs if a stress fracture is suspected because of the potential interruption of bone healing.

■ Postinjury Management

The patient is restricted from activities that cause pain, and alternative forms of exercise such as stationary bicycling or swimming are used. Identifying and correcting the probable causes of the tibial stress fracture may assist in reducing the athlete's pain. If the pain is restrictive, the athlete may use a CAM boot, or if the pain is severe, limiting ambulation to non–weight bearing may be necessary.

■ Surgical Intervention

When surgery is indicated, the procedures for a traumatic tibial fracture are followed (see p 124).

■ Postoperative Management

Initially, the patient can bear weight to tolerance with crutches, advancing to full weight bearing as pain allows.

■ Injury-Specific Treatment and Rehabilitation Concerns

Ice, whirlpool, and conditioning activities for the uninvolved segments should be a part of the initial treatment program. Pool running and non–weight-

bearing exercises can keep the athlete in good condition during this time.

Specific Concerns

Remove the insulting forces to the lower leg.
Emphasize knee-extension activities.

Obtaining full knee extension is an early goal of rehabilitation, using a protocol similar to that for anterior cruciate ligament rehabilitation (see p 141). At 1 week postoperatively, the patient can begin exercise on a bicycle, stair stepper, or elliptical trainer. When the patient can exercise on an elliptical trainer for 30 to 45 minutes, a running progression can be instituted.

■ Estimated Amount of Time Lost

Depending on the amount of pain, the patient may or may not lose any time from activity. In some cases, the patient may need to refrain from sport participation and weight bearing for 6 to 8 weeks.[72] In severe cases, postinjury rehabilitation may take 8 to 9 months before full return to activity is possible.

■ Return-to-Play Criteria

The patient must report no pain during any sport-specific activities and should demonstrate proper performance of such activities at the preinjury level.

Functional Bracing

Correct footwear is important in reducing tibial stresses. If the patient has prolonged or exaggerated pronation during running, orthotic appliances may be necessary to limit tibial stresses.

Fibular Fractures

A Dupuytren fracture involves the lower fibular shaft just proximal to the tibiofibular syndesmosis. A fracture in the midshaft is a Hugier or high Dupuytren fracture. A fracture of the proximal fibular neck with disruption of the interosseous ligament is a Maisonneuve fracture.[76] With a fracture of the fibular shaft, the distal tibiofibular syndesmosis and interosseous ligament up to the fracture site can also be injured.[77]

CLINICAL PRESENTATION

History

An abduction and/or lateral rotation force of the leg

Observation

Displaced fractures produce obvious deformity; however, no deformity may be noted.
Swelling over the fracture site

Functional Status

Weight bearing may still be possible.
Pain is elicited during cutting activities.

Physical Evaluation Findings

Palpation of the fracture site produces pain.
Fibular compression test produces pain.

Differential Diagnosis

Lateral ankle sprain, bimalleolar fracture, talar dome fracture, syndesmotic ankle sprain, Achilles tendon rupture

Imaging Techniques

Bone tenderness and severe swelling with ecchymosis or bruising require radiographic evaluation using AP and lateral views (**Figure 5-44**). When possible, weight-bearing radiographs produce a physiologic stress on the ankle that allows better assessment of the ankle ligaments, in particular the syndesmosis and deltoid ligament.

Definitive Diagnosis

The definitive diagnosis is based on positive radiographic findings.

Pathomechanics and Functional Limitations

If the fracture is isolated to the fibula, weight bearing may be possible because only about 6% of the body weight is distributed over the fibula during the stance phase of gait. The fibula bears essentially

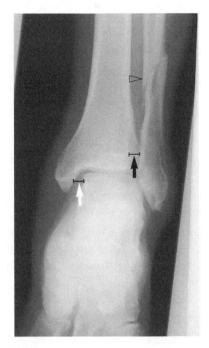

Figure 5-44 Fibular fracture. Non-weight-bearing anteroposterior view shows a fibular fracture caused by pronation and eversion. Note the increased space between the medial malleolus and talus and the medial clear space (white arrow), indicating a deltoid ligament rupture. The space between the distal tibia and fibula (the tibiofibular clear space) is widened (black arrow). For this to occur, the anterior tibiofibular ligament and the syndesmosis must be ruptured. An oblique fracture of the fibula (arrowhead) is seen above the level of the syndesmosis. (Reproduced with permission from Johnson TR, Steinbach LS (eds): *Essentials of Musculoskeletal Imaging.* Rosemont, IL, American Academy of Orthopaedic Surgeons, 2004, p 647.)

no weight, so aggravation during weight bearing is unlikely. Laypersons commonly think fractures do not exist if weight bearing is possible, but walking is feasible when the fibula is fractured. With an isolated fibular fracture, a CAM boot or walking cast can be used. If the injury involves ligament or bony structures, initial weight bearing may be limited.

■ Immediate Management

Suspected fractures should be immobilized in the position found, with ice and compression applied, and the athlete transported for further medical assessment and radiographs.

■ Medications

Pain relief can be obtained using NSAIDs or narcotics. Avoid NSAIDs if surgery is contemplated.

■ Surgical Intervention

If a syndesmotic disruption is present, a syndesmotic screw is used to repair the injury once the fracture is reduced. It is common for fibular fractures to require open reduction and internal fixation, usually using a syndesmotic screw, regardless of the fracture location. Displaced distal fractures are repaired with open reduction and internal fixation using plates and screws. Fibular shaft (midshaft and above) fractures are generally left to heal without fixation.

■ Postinjury/Postoperative Management

Although there is some dispute, many physicians remove the syndesmotic screw before the patient is allowed full weight bearing on the extremity without a boot or splint.[76] This relatively minor procedure should not delay the rehabilitation process because it does not require any specific postoperative concerns except for observation and management of the new wound.

■ Injury-Specific Treatment and Rehabilitation Concerns

Specific Concerns

Reduce stiffness and fibrosis by reestablishing ROM.
Strengthen the foot, ankle, and lower leg.
Retrain gait.

While restricted in activities, the athlete can maintain cardiovascular fitness and preserve or develop muscle strength in the uninvolved extremities. Open kinetic chain exercises for the hip, knee, and foot of the involved extremity can also be included during the non–weight-bearing phase.

Once weight bearing is permitted, the patient can perform balance activities and closed kinetic chain strength exercises. Rehabilitation from this point follows a normal process with advances in mobility, strength, coordination, agility, and functional activities.

■ Estimated Amount of Time Lost

Surgically repaired fractures may require up to 6 weeks of non–weight bearing after surgery. An additional 2 to 4 months are necessary for rehabilitation. Complications after surgery, such as nonunion and infection, can prolong recovery. Nonsurgical management requires 2 to 3 months for healing.

■ Return-to-Play Criteria

Whether the injury was treated conservatively or surgically, test results for strength and agility should be normal compared with the uninvolved leg. If surgery was performed, the site should be well

healed and full motion regained in the foot and ankle before the athlete returns to participation. The sport-specific activities pursued during rehabilitation can be used to test the athlete's readiness for return to full participation. The athlete should perform equally with the left and right lower extremities and display confidence in his or her own performance. The surgical hardware for syndesmosis injuries is likely to have been removed by this time, and the physician has indicated that the fracture site is healed satisfactorily and cleared the athlete for return to participation.

Functional Bracing

Ankle taping or a brace may be used for return to participation, but this is optional. If the athlete is involved in a collision or contact sport, a pad or wrap may offer the healed surgical site some protection.

Traumatic Tibial Fractures

Fractures of the tibia are common in athletes involved in collision sports and skiing. Most tibial fractures are closed and involve the middle and lower one third.

CLINICAL PRESENTATION

History

Significant force delivered to the tibia

Observation

A displaced fracture produces obvious deformity.
Swelling and muscle spasm develop soon after the injury.

Functional Status

The patient is unable and unwilling to bear weight on the involved leg.

Physical Evaluation Findings

If visible deformity is present, no other additional information is needed before making the decision to refer the patient.
Deformity indicates tibial and associated fibular fractures.
With a nondisplaced fracture, tenderness and crepitus are present over the fracture site.
Point tenderness is palpable over the fracture site.

A significant impact or torsional force is required to fracture the tibia. Although improved ski equipment has reduced the incidence of tibial fractures, if the ski becomes embedded within the snow while the athlete is moving, the top of the boot can provide sufficient leverage against the tibia to cause a horizontal fracture. Collision and contact sports such as football, wrestling, soccer, and lacrosse can produce impact forces, either between two athletes or between the athlete and the ground, causing tibial fractures. Torque or twisting forces imparted during rotation while weight bearing cause an oblique or spiral fracture.

Differential Diagnosis

Fibular fracture, talocrural dislocation, tibiofemoral dislocation, severe contusion, stress fracture

Imaging Techniques

Lateral and AP radiographs confirm the fracture (**Figure 5-45**). An intra-articular fracture is best imaged with a CT scan to define the fracture configuration and assist in the surgical decision-making process.

Definitive Diagnosis

Positive radiographic findings

Pathomechanics and Functional Limitations

A tibial fracture disrupts normal weight bearing, so ambulation is not possible. The patient is reluctant to move the extremity because of the associated pain. The rapid onset of muscle spasm also makes movement painful and limits the patient's desire to move the leg.

Delayed union of an isolated tibial fracture is a risk. More success with fewer complications has been found with internal fixation of tibial fractures.[48]

Functional limitations are often related to the fracture configuration. More unstable fractures require increased attentiveness and patient compliance to remain non–weight bearing. Nonsurgical management can involve long leg or short leg casting and non–weight bearing. Surgical fixation of the fracture may avoid the necessity of casting and weight-bearing restrictions, but limitations depend on the construct stability and the fracture configuration.

◼ Immediate Management

Immobilization of the fracture in the position found, monitoring for neurovascular integrity throughout the extremity, applying ice to the site, and immediate transport to the emergency room for radiographs and care are important. If the fracture is open, applying a loose dressing to protect the wound during immediate care and transport to a medical facility is needed for this medical emergency.

◼ Medications

Oral and injectable narcotic analgesics decrease the pain produced by the injury.

◼ Surgical Intervention

Management of a tibial fracture depends on the location of the fracture, displacement, and associated injuries (see chapter 3). Surgical repair is indicated

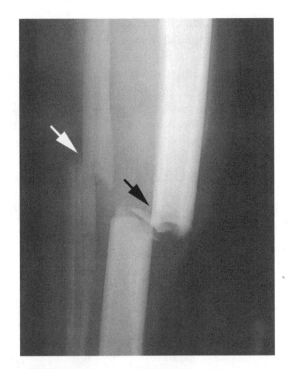

Figure 5-45 Tibial shaft fracture. Anteroposterior view of the tibia and fibula demonstrates a transverse fracture through the middiaphysis of the tibia (black arrow). Note also the transverse fracture through the midshaft of the fibula (white arrow) with lateral displacement of the distal fragments. (Reproduced with permission from Johnson TR, Steinbach LS (eds): *Essentials of Musculoskeletal Imaging.* Rosemont, IL, American Academy of Orthopaedic Surgeons, 2004, p 504.)

when the fracture involves 1 mm or more of the articular surface, the syndesmosis is unstable, or the fracture is displaced or angulated. Almost all bimalleolar and trimalleolar fractures require surgery, as do lateral malleolar fractures with concomitant medial (deltoid) ligament rupture.

◼ Postinjury/Postoperative Management

Postinjury and postoperative management is determined by the stability of the fracture and the surgical construct. Less complex fractures permit faster return of function. If the fracture is stable and does not involve multiple sites or the joint, it is likely to heal without complications and allow the athlete a more rapid recovery.

◼ Injury-Specific Treatment and Rehabilitation Concerns

Specific Concerns

Obtain anatomic fracture union.
Ensure stabilization of the fracture site.
Avoid infection of the surgical site (if applicable).

Rehabilitation concerns are multifactorial and often conflicting. Early motion is desired, but if the fracture is unstable, this may not be possible. Generally speaking, intra-articular fractures need adequate stabilization so the construct tolerates early motion, but weight bearing must be avoided to prevent loss of reduction. Intramedullary nailing is the most stable construct, allowing the earliest weight bearing and fastest functional progression. Open fractures carry a much higher risk of nonunion and infection and may be very slow to heal. Muscle strengthening of the entire closed kinetic chain is important during the rehabilitation process.

Estimated Amount of Time Lost

Without postinjury complications, recovery from a tibial fracture requires 3 to 6 weeks of non–weight bearing, followed by a period of partial weight bearing before full weight bearing on the extremity is permitted. Disability can last 3 to 12 months.

Complications such as delayed healing, nonunion, osteoporosis, compartment syndrome, and ankle pain extend the time of disability.

Return-to-Play Criteria

The fracture site must be adequately healed before return to participation can be considered. Because of the long-term disability, many of the standard elements of conditioning (eg, motion, strength, and proprioception) are deficient and require sustained rehabilitation before return to participation. All aspects must be restored to normal limits before return to play is permitted.

Functional Bracing

A protective shin guard or pad may be necessary once the athlete returns to play. An ankle brace may aid a distal fracture, whereas a knee brace may help protect a proximal fracture.

Rehabilitation

While non–weight bearing, the patient should maintain cardiovascular conditioning and strength of the upper extremities, contralateral lower extremity, and other involved extremity segments. A number of activities can be used to maintain these conditioning levels. For example, an upper body ergometer, single-leg stationary bicycling, running on crutches, or wheelchair activities maintain cardiovascular conditioning. If the cast is waterproof, aquatic exercises can be used for both cardiovascular and lower extremity fitness. Upper and lower body resistance exercises preserve strength and muscle endurance levels.

Gait training may require progressive advancement from non–weight bearing to full weight bearing: moving from two crutches without weight on the involved extremity to two crutches with partial weight, then one crutch with partial weight before the athlete discards the crutches and walks unassisted.

Therapeutic modalities initially may consist of a whirlpool to warm the foot and prepare the skin for treatment. Grade I and II joint mobilizations to relieve pain during the first week may be necessary, followed by grades III and IV to increase joint mobility if the patient has acquired a capsular pattern or joint restriction with immobilization. Massage to reduce postcast edema and open lymph vessels may be needed for the first few days. After the first week or two, passive modalities such as whirlpool and electric stimulation for pain or edema should not be necessary, because the pain and edema should be resolved. Once the athlete performs active flexibility and strengthening exercises, ice may be necessary to calm any irritation that may have occurred because of the stress of the exercises.

Flexibility Exercises

Each stretch is held for at least 15 to 20 seconds and repeated three or four times unless otherwise noted.

Dorsiflexion Stretch for the Gastrocnemius
Leaning against the table or wall, the patient stands in a lunge position with the stretch leg behind and the support leg forward. With the back heel remaining on the ground and the knee straight, the patient leans forward to put weight on the front leg and arms (**Figure 5-46**).

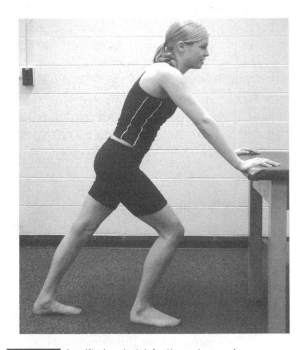

Figure 5-46 Dorsiflexion stretch for the gastrocnemius.

Dorsiflexion Stretch for the Soleus
Leaning against the table or wall, the patient stands in a lunge position with the stretch leg behind and the support leg forward. With the back heel remaining on the ground and the knee flexed, the patient leans forward to put weight on the front leg and arms (**Figure 5-47**).

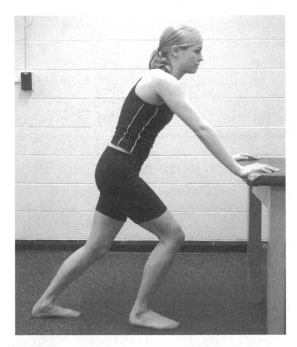

Figure 5-47 Dorsiflexion stretch for the soleus.

Prolonged Dorsiflexion Stretch

This exercise addresses tightness in the Achilles tendon or rigid scar tissue in the posterior calf. The patient stands with the back to the wall, a rolled-up towel behind the knees to prevent knee hyperextension, and the feet on an incline board with the heels on the floor and no more than 1 in from the wall. This position is maintained for 5 to 15 minutes as tolerated.

Plantar Flexion Stretch

The patient sits on the heels with the knees fully flexed and feet in plantar flexion and attempts to push the dorsum of the feet to lie flat on floor.

Strengthening Exercises

■ Isometrics

Plantar Flexion

Sitting with the involved distal foot on top of the dorsum of the uninvolved foot, the patient points the involved foot downward as the movement is resisted by the opposite foot dorsiflexing. Hold for 10 seconds, and repeat 10 times.

Dorsiflexion

Sitting with the uninvolved heel on top of the dorsum of the involved foot, the patient pushes the involved foot up as the movement is resisted by the opposite foot plantar flexing. Hold for 10 seconds, and repeat 10 times.

Inversion

Sitting with the inside of the involved ankle against a doorway or table leg, the patient pushes the foot into the stable object, holding for 10 seconds. Repeat 10 times.

Eversion

Sitting with the outside of the involved ankle against a doorway or table leg, the patient pushes the foot into the stable object, holding for 10 seconds. Repeat 10 times.

■ Rubber-Tubing Exercises

Early isotonic foot and ankle exercises can be performed using rubber tubing, starting with light resistance and increasing as strength is developed (**Figure 5-48**).

■ Intrinsic Foot Exercises

Towel Roll

A towel is placed on the floor in front of the seated patient. The heel of the involved foot is placed on the floor near the towel and the forefoot on the towel.

Keeping the heel in place, the patient rolls the towel toward the foot, curling the toes to move the towel. A weight can be added at the distal end of the towel to make the exercise more difficult (**Figure 5-49**).

Marble Pick-up

Marbles are placed on the floor, and the patient uses the toes to pick them up, one at a time. The marbles can be placed beside the opposite foot or lifted to the hand.

■ Body Resistance Exercises

Heel Raises

Standing on the floor and keeping knees extended, the patient raises up on the toes, lifting the heels off the floor. Progression for this exercise includes beginning with both feet, advancing to one foot, moving from the floor to an incline, and adding weights.

Toe Raises

Standing on the floor, the patient lifts the toes and forefoot off the floor, keeping weight on the heels. This can be progressed to standing on a decline, with the heels higher than the toes.

Ankle Weights

With a cuff weight wrapped around the forefoot, the patient is placed in an antigravity position for the motion being resisted. For inversion, the patient lies on the involved side; for eversion, the patient lies on the opposite side; and for dorsiflexion, the patient sits with the leg hanging off the table. These exercises can also be performed against manual resistance or progressively increased weights.

Orthotic Corrections

During gait, the foot initially contacts the ground in supination and immediately moves into pronation. At midstance, the rear foot moves from pronation to a neutral position and continues to move into supination, so at preswing, the foot has converted from a force absorber in the first half of weight bearing to a force deliverer during the propulsion phase at the end of weight bearing. The foot serves three functions during the weight-bearing phase of gait: it adapts and dissipates stresses at initial contact, provides balance and stability as it serves as the contact between the moving body and the ground, and acts as a rigid lever to provide propulsion just before the non–weight-bearing phase.[78]

Although the description in the previous paragraph sounds fairly simple, the mechanics occurring because of these changes in the foot are anything

5

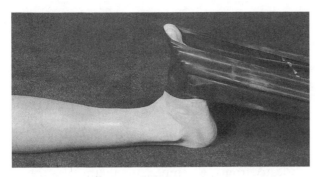

Dorsiflexion (A): With the tubing anchored in a door jamb, the patient faces the door jamb and wraps the tubing around the forefoot of the involved ankle, so the resistance occurs when the foot is dorsiflexed.

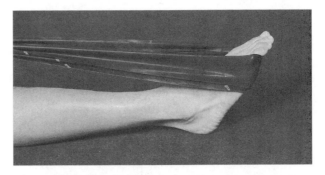

Plantar flexion (C): The patient grasps the tubing in both hands and loops the tubing around the plantar foot with the knee in extension. Taking slack out of the tubing, the foot is moved into plantar flexion against the tubing resistance. The exercise can be repeated with the knee flexed to emphasize the soleus muscle.

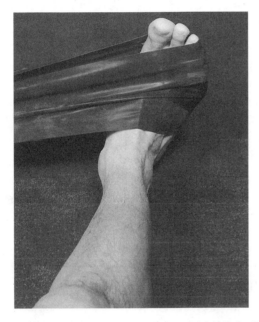

Eversion (B): With the tubing anchored in a door jamb, the patient wraps the tubing around the forefoot of the involved ankle, so the resistance occurs when the foot is everted.

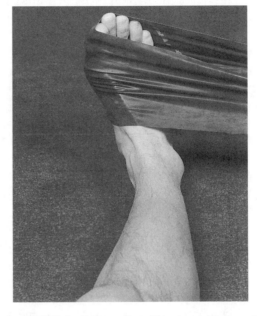

Inversion (D): With the tubing anchored in a door jamb, the patient wraps the tubing around the medial aspect of the involved ankle, so the resistance occurs when the patient inverts the foot.

Figure 5-48 Rubber-tubing exercises.

but simple. When pronation occurs in weight bearing, calcaneal eversion, talar medial rotation, tibial medial rotation, forefoot abduction on the rear foot, and depression of the medial longitudinal arch also occur. These changes cause the body's center of gravity to move medial to the foot, resulting in knee valgus with an increased Q angle and greater lateral quadriceps pull.

If joint tightness or muscle inflexibility is present, abnormal mechanics can result. Over time and with repetitive or exaggerated stress application, tissue breakdown can occur. Orthotic corrections can be the logical "fix" to alter these abnormal mechanics.

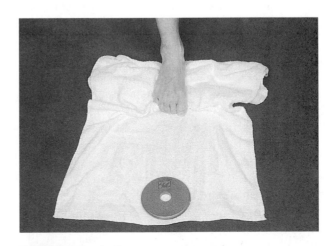

Figure 5-49 Towel roll.

■ Purposes of Orthotic Corrections

Orthotics are used to accommodate a foot deformity or compensate for abnormal function and biomechanics during gait. These abnormalities increase forces on the foot and other segments up the chain, risking injury or creating cumulative stress to weaken and break down normal tissue. The ultimate purposes of orthotic appliances, then, are to accommodate or correct alignment to relieve pain, reduce stress and injury risk, and allow optimal function.

■ Foot Orthotic Corrections

Foot orthoses can be applied to or inserted in the shoe. Some athletic shoes have external adaptations to accommodate the patient or reduce stresses applied by the athlete's sport. For example, heel flares on running shoes increase heel stability at initial contact and may reduce valgus stresses experienced during running. An elevated heel placed in a running shoe reduces Achilles tendon stress during running. The outer sole of a tennis shoe has a squared edge rather than a rounded edge to provide more stability and prevent ankle rollover during sudden lateral direction changes. An anterior-posterior rocker bottom on an outer sole reduces ankle forces at initial impact and to the toes and forefoot during preparation to toe-off.

Orthotic inserts for shoes can be made of different substances. Felt or foam pads can be used to correct alignment or absorb forces. More rigid substances help to improve alignment.

If more support is needed, various prefabricated orthotic appliances are available. They come in different styles and compositions and are designed for different functions. Some are composed of stiff materials and offer corrective assistance; others are composed of softer materials and provide accommodation rather than correction.

Custom orthoses are more expensive than over-the-counter models, but they may be necessary to relieve pain or correct the deformity sufficiently to allow normal athletic performance. Custom orthoses can also be accommodative or correctional (sometimes called functional). The purpose is determined by the constituent substance. Semirigid materials such as cork, rubber, and light-density foam provide accommodative orthoses. Those made of rigid or semirigid substances that do not easily give or lose their shape when weight is applied are correctional or functional orthoses. To determine whether an orthotic appliance is accommodative or functional, apply pressure to the mold or attempt to twist the device. If it easily gives to stress appli-

cation, it is accommodative. The more rigid the orthotic appliance, the less room for error in device construction. The individual taking measurements of the patient's feet must be as precise as possible when rigid and semirigid orthoses are to be made.

Custom orthoses are designed for a specific individual. They are made after an impression of the patient's feet is taken, and the orthosis is then formed around that impression. Custom orthoses are also fabricated from low-temperature thermoplastic materials molded through direct contact with the foot. Typically, an impression of the patient's feet is made using plaster-of-Paris casts or having the patient step into a box of foam similar to the green foam used by florists. The foam gives to the pressure of the foot in it and retains the shape when the foot is removed. The orthotist builds an orthosis based on the impressions and the information provided by the clinician on factors that may alter the orthotic requirements. For example, if the patient has limited dorsiflexion, the orthotist may build heel lifts into the orthoses to reduce Achilles tendon stress.

■ Types of Orthotic Correction

Valgus Pad

A valgus pad can be placed along the medial aspect of the shoe to reduce pronation stress by decreasing the amount of pronation and compensated forefoot varus, or it can be accommodative by supporting a supinated foot (**Figure 5-50**).

Metatarsal Pad

A metatarsal pad can be used if pressure over the distal metatarsals is painful. Modifications of this pad can be made to relieve weight bearing around the first ray by cutting out that portion or improve weight bearing by cutting out the pad from the other metatarsal areas (**Figure 5-51**).

Calcaneal Pads

A variety of calcaneal pads can relieve pressure over a calcaneal spur or reduce pronation with a medial wedge (**Figure 5-52**).

■ Footwear

Shoes have an important role in foot mechanics. Their primary purpose is to protect the foot's soft tissue from the insults it would otherwise encounter without protection. They also help to distribute force, absorb stress, provide traction, and support foot structures. They come in many styles, models, and colors. Ultimately, the shoe's function, not its color or style, should be the most important determinant in selection.

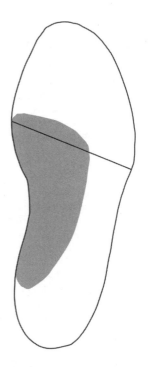

Figure 5-50 Valgus pad.

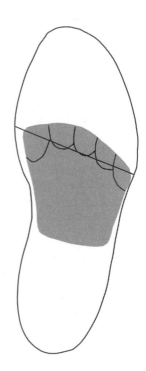

Figure 5-51 Metatarsal pad.

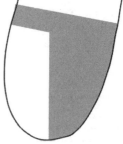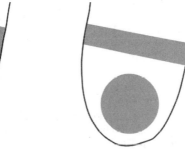

Figure 5-52 Calcaneal pads.

Athletic shoe selection should be a marriage of the shoe's function with the patient's sport demands and the foot's biomechanical and structural deviations. The clinician should inspect the patient's worn shoes and the patient's feet to obtain an idea of the abnormal biomechanical stresses created. A collapsed medial heel counter reflects pronation. Blood under the toenail indicates the toe box is too short. An unequal wear pattern of the shoes may be a sign of a leg-length discrepancy. A patient who has excessive or prolonged pronation should use a shoe with increased medial rear-foot midsole density or a medial wedge, a strong or reinforced heel counter, and a board last. A patient with a painful or rigid first ray should wear a rigid-soled shoe with a rocker bottom, especially in the forefoot, and the midsole should be thicker than normal to absorb more stress.

■ References

1. Clanton TO, Ford JJ: Turf toe injury. *Clin Sports Med* 1994;13:731-741.

2. Hockenbury RT: Forefoot problems in athletes. *Med Sci Sports Exerc* 1999;31(suppl 7):S448-S458.

3. Richardson EG: Hallucal sesamoid pain: Causes and surgical treatment. *J Am Acad Orthop Surg* 1999;7:270-278.

4. Jahss MH: The sesamoids of the hallux. *Clin Orthop* 1981;157:88-97.

5. Dietzen CJ: Great toe sesamoid injuries in the athlete. *Orthop Rev* 1990;19:966-972.

6. Nevin C: Kinematics of the first metatarsophalangeal joint in intact and surgically altered cadavers. *Foot Ankle Int* 1997;18:132-137.

7. Mann RA: Disorders of the first metatarsophalangeal joint. *J Am Acad Orthop Surg* 1995;3:34-43.

8. Moberg E: A simple operation for hallux rigidus. *Clin Orthop* 1979;142:55-56.

9. Hamilton WG, O'Malley MJ, Thompson FM, Kovatis PE: Capsular interposition arthroplasty for severe hallux rigidus. *Foot Ankle Int* 1997;18:68-70.

5

10. Grady JF, Axe TM, Zager EJ, Sheldon LA: A retrospective analysis of 772 patients with hallux limitus. *J Am Podiatr Med Assoc* 2002;92:102-108.

11. Anderson RJ: Hallux rigidus and atrophy of calf muscles. *N Engl J Med* 1999;340:1123.

12. Thomas PJ, Smith RW: Proximal phalanx osteotomy for the surgical treatment of hallux rigidus. *Foot Ankle Int* 1999;20:3-12.

13. Lau JTC, Daniels TR: Outcomes following cheilectomy and interpositional arthroplasty in hallux rigidus. *Foot Ankle Int* 2001;22:462-470.

14. Buchbinder R, Ptasznik R, Gordon J, Buchanan J, Prabaharan V, Forbes A: Ultrasound-guided extracorporeal shock wave therapy for plantar fasciitis: a randomized controlled trial. *JAMA* 2002;288:1364-1372.

15. Ogden JA, Alvarez R, Levitt R, Cross GL, Marlow M: Shock wave therapy for chronic proximal plantar fasciitis. *Clin Orthop* 2001;387:47-59.

16. Fuller EA: The windlass mechanism of the foot: A mechanical model to explain pathology. *J Am Podiatr Med Assoc* 2000;90:35-46.

17. Gill LH: Plantar fasciitis: Diagnosis and conservative management. *J Am Acad Orthop Surg* 1997;5:109-117.

18. Evans A: Podiatric medical applications of posterior night stretch splinting. *J Am Podiatr Med Assoc* 2001;91:356-360.

19. Acevedo JI, Beskin JL: Complications of plantar fascia rupture associated with corticosteroid injection. *Foot Ankle Int* 1998;19:91-97.

20. Helbig K, Herbert C, Schostok T, Brown M, Thiele R: Correlations between the duration of pain and the success of shock wave therapy. *Clin Orthop* 2001;387:68-71.

21. Rompe JD, Schoellner C, Nafe B: Evaluation of low-energy extracorporeal shock-wave application for treatment of chronic plantar fasciitis. *J Bone Joint Surg Am* 2002;84:335-341.

22. Weinfeld SB, Myerson MS: Interdigital neuritis: Diagnosis and treatment. *J Am Acad Orthop Surg* 1996;4:328-335.

23. van Wyngarden TM: The painful foot: Part I. Common forefoot deformities. *Am Fam Physician* 1997;55:1866-1876.

24. Khan KM, Brukner PD, Kearney C, Fuller PJ, Bradshaw CJ, Kiss ZS: Tarsal navicular stress fracture in athletes. *Sports Med* 1994;17:65-76.

25. Omey ML, Micheli LJ: Foot and ankle problems in the young athlete. *Med Sci Sports Exerc* 1999;31(suppl 7):S470-S486.

26. Devas M: Stress fractures, in Helal B, Rowley DI, Cracchiolo AR, Myerson MS (eds): *Surgery of Disorders of the Foot and Ankle.* Philadelphia, PA, Lippincott Williams & Wilkins, 1996, pp 761-773.

27. Weinfeld SB, Haddad SL, Myerson MS: Metatarsal stress fractures. *Clin Sports Med* 1997;16:319-338.

28. O'Malley MJ, Hamilton WG, Munyak J, DeFranco MJ: Stress fractures at the base of the second metatarsal in ballet dancers. *Foot Ankle Int* 1996;17:89-94.

29. Lucas MJ, Baxter DE: Stress fracture of the first metatarsal. *Foot Ankle Int* 1997;18:373-374.

30. Lawrence SJ, Botte MJ: Jones' fractures and related fractures of the proximal fifth metatarsal. *Foot Ankle* 1993;14:358-365.

31. Lau JTC, Daniels TR: Tarsal tunnel syndrome: A review of the literature. *Foot Ankle Int* 1999;20:201-209.

32. Beskin JL: Nerve entrapment syndromes of the foot and ankle. *J Am Acad Orthop Surg* 1997;5:261-269.

33. Swain RA, Holt WS Jr: Ankle injuries: Tips from sports medicine physicians. *Postgrad Med* 1993;93:91-100.

34. Watson AD, Anderson RB, Davis WH: Comparison of results of retrocalcaneal decompression for retrocalcaneal bursitis and insertional Achilles tendinosis with calcific spur. *Foot Ankle Int* 2000;21:638-642.

35. Kuper BC: Tarsal tunnel syndrome. *Orthop Nurs* 1998;17:9-17.

36. Safran MR, Benedetti RS, Bartolozzi AR III, Mandelbaum BR: Lateral ankle sprains: A comprehensive review. Part 1: Etiology, pathoanatomy, histopathogenesis, and diagnosis. *Med Sci Sports Exerc* 1999;31(suppl 7):S429-S437.

37. Leddy JJ, Kesari A, Smolinski RJ: Implementation of the Ottawa Ankle Rules in a university sports medicine center. *Med Sci Sports Exerc* 2002;343:57-62.

38. Hertel J, Denegar CR, Monroe MM, Stokes WL: Talocrural and subtalar joint instability after lateral ankle sprain. *Med Sci Sports Exerc* 1999;31:1501-1508.

39. Safran MR, Zachazewski JE, Benedetti RS, Bartolozzi AR III, Mandelbaum R: Lateral ankle sprains: A comprehensive review. Part 2: Treatment and rehabilitation with an emphasis on the athlete. *Med Sci Sports Exerc* 1999;31(suppl 7):S438-S447.

40. Gerber JP, Williams GN, Scoville CR, Arciero RA, Taylor DC: Persistent disability associated with ankle sprains: A prospective examination of an athletic population. *Foot Ankle Int* 1998;19:653-660.

41. Stiell IG, Greenberg GH, McKnight RD, et al: Decision rules for the use of radiography in acute ankle injuries: Refinement and prospective validation. *JAMA* 1993;269:1127-1132.

42. Stiell IG, McKnight RD, Greenberg GH, et al: Implementation of the Ottawa Ankle Rules. *JAMA* 1994;271:827-832.

43. Stiell IG, Greenberg GH, McKnight RD, Wells GA: The "real" Ottawa Ankle Rules. *Ann Emerg Med* 1996;27:103-104.

44. Garrick JG, Schelkun PH: Managing ankle sprains: Keys to preserving motion and strength. *Physician Sportsmed* 1997;25:56-58,63-64,67-68.

45. Wilkerson GB, Horn-Kingery HM: Treatment of the inversion ankle sprain: Comparison of different modes of compression and cryotherapy. *J Orthop Sports Phys Ther* 1993;17:240-246.

46. Verhagen EALM, van der Beek AJ, van Mechelen W: The effect of tape, braces and shoes on ankle range of motion. *Sports Med* 2001;31:667-677.

47. Barrett JR, Tanji JL, Drake C, Fuller D, Kawasaki RI, Fenton RM: High- versus low-top shoes for the prevention of ankle sprains in basketball players: A prospective randomized study. *Am J Sports Med* 1993;21:582-585.

48. Wilkerson GB: Biomechanical and neuromuscular effects of ankle taping and bracing. *J Athl Train* 2002;37:436-445.

49. Cordova ML, Ingersoll CD, Palmieri RM: Efficacy of prophylactic ankle support: An experimental perspective. *J Athl Train* 2002;37:446-457.

50. Callaghan MJ, Selfe J, Bagley PJ, Oldham JA: The effects of patellar taping on knee joint proprioception. *J Athl Train* 2002;37:19-24.

51. Rivera F, Bertone C, De Martino M, Pietrobono D, Ghisellini F: Pure dislocation of the ankle: Three case reports and literature review. *Clin Orthop* 2001;382:179-184.

52. Thordarson DB: Complications after treatment of tibial pilon fractures: Prevention and management strategies. *J Am Acad Orthop Surg* 2000:8:253-265.

53. Diaz GC, van Holsbeeck M, Jacobson JA: Longitudinal split of the peroneus longus and peroneus brevis tendons with disruption of the superior peroneal retinaculum. *J Ultrasound Med* 1998;17:525-529.

54. Frey C: Foot and ankle, in Johnson TR, Steinbach LS (eds): *Essentials of Musculoskeletal Imaging.* Rosemont, IL, American Academy of Orthopaedic Surgeons, 2004, p 650.

55. Brage ME, Hansen ST Jr: Traumatic subluxation/dislocation of the peroneal tendons. *Foot Ankle* 1992;13:423-431.

56. Forman ES, Micheli LJ, Backe LM: Chronic recurrent subluxation of the peroneal tendons in a pediatric patient: Surgical recommendations. *Foot Ankle Int* 2000;21:51-53.

57. Niemi WJ, Savidakis J Jr, DeJesus JM: Peroneal subluxation: A comprehensive review of the literature with case presentations. *J Foot Ankle Surg* 1997;36:141-145.

58. Krause JO, Brodsky JW: Peroneus brevis tendon tears: pathophysiology, surgical reconstruction, and clinical results. *Foot Ankle Int* 1998;19:271-279.

59. Mendicino RW, Orsini RC, Whitman SE, Catanzariti AR: Fibular groove deepening for recurrent peroneal subluxation. *J Foot Ankle Surg* 2001;40:252-263.

60. Frey C, Rosenberg Z, Shereff MJ, Kim H: The retrocalcaneal bursa: Anatomy and bursography. *Foot Ankle* 1992;13:203-207.

61. Clanton TO, Solcher BW: Chronic leg pain in the athlete. *Clin Sports Med* 1994;13:743-759.

62. Paavola M, Kannus P, Jarvinen TAH, Khan K, Józsa L, Järvinen M: Achilles tendinopathy. *J Bone Joint Surg Am* 2002;84:2062-2076.

63. Leadbetter WB: Cell-matrix response in tendon injury. *Clin Sports Med* 1992;11:533-578.

64. Stanish WD, Curwin S, Mandel S: *Tendinitis: Its Etiology and Treatment.* New York, NY, Oxford University Press, 2000.

65. Myerson MS: Injuries in the athlete, in Helal B, Rowley DI, Cracchiolo AR, Myerson MS (eds): *Surgery of Disorders of the Foot and Ankle.* Philadelphia, PA, Lippincott-Raven, 1996, pp 793 809.

66. Leppilahti J, Forsman K, Puranen J, Orava S: Outcome and prognostic factors of Achilles rupture repair using a new scoring method. *Clin Orthop* 1998;346:152-161.

67. Whitesides TE, Heckman MM: Acute compartment syndrome: Update on diagnosis and treatment. *J Am Acad Orthop Surg* 1996;4:209-218.

68. Hutchinson MR, Ireland ML: Common compartment syndromes in athletes: Treatment and rehabilitation. *Sports Med* 1994;17:200-208.

69. Schepsis AA, Lynch G: Exertional compartment syndromes of the lower extremity. *Curr Opin Rheumatol* 1996;8:143-147.

70. Garcia-Mata S, Hidalgo-Ovejero A, Martinez-Grande M: Chronic exertional compartment syndrome of the legs in adolescents. *J Pediatr Orthop* 2001;21:328-334.

71. Blackman PG: A review of chronic exertional compartment syndrome in the lower leg. *Med Sci Sports Exerc* 2000;32(suppl 3):S4-S10.

72. Touliopolous S, Hershman EB: Lower leg pain: Diagnosis and treatment of compartment syndromes and other pain syndromes of the leg. *Sports Med* 1999;27:193-204.

73. Ekenman I, Tsai-Fellander L, Westblad PPT, Turan I, Rolf C: A study of intrinsic factors in patients with stress fractures of the tibia. *Foot Ankle Int* 1996;17:477-482.

74. Batt ME, Ugalade V, Anderson MW, Shelton DK: A prospective controlled study of diagnostic imaging for acute shin splints. *Med Sci Sports Exerc* 1998;30:1564-1571.

75. Haims A, Jokl P: Knee and lower leg, in Johnson TR, Steinbach LS (eds): *Essentials of Musculoskeletal Imaging.* Rosemont, IL, American Academy of Orthopaedic Surgeons, 2004, p 517.

76. Yablon I, Forman ES: Ankle fractures, in Helal B, Rowley DI, Cracchiolo AR, Myerson MS (eds): *Surgery of Disorders of the Foot and Ankle.* Philadelphia, PA, Lippincott-Raven, 1996.

77. Ebraheim NA, Mekhail AO, Gargasz SS: Ankle fractures involving the fibula proximal to the distal tibiofibular syndesmosis. *Foot Ankle Int* 1997;18:513-521.

78. Subotnick SI: Conservative treatment for the foot in sport, in Helal B, Rowley DI, Cracchiolo AR, Myerson MS (eds): *Surgery of Disorders of the Foot and Ankle.* Philadelphia, PA, Lippincott-Raven, 1996, pp 867-869.

5

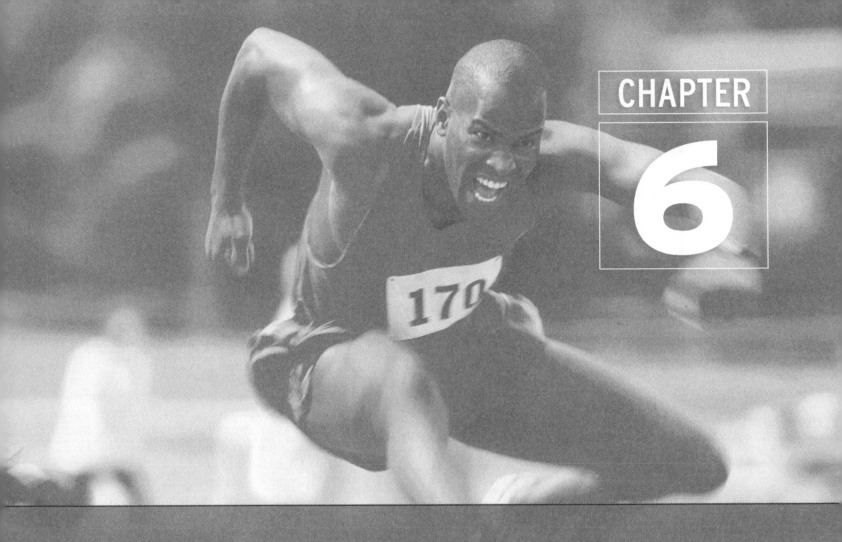

Knee Injuries

Jeff Ryan, PT, ATC
Peter DeLuca, MD

Anterior Cruciate Ligament Sprain

CLINICAL PRESENTATION

History

Mechanism of injury:
- Acute tensile load from knee rotation with the foot planted
- Knee hyperextension
- Contact injury

A "pop" may be associated with the injury.

Initial pain that may subside

Swelling occurs within hours of the injury.

Observation

Joint effusion

Patient postures the knee in slight flexion due to effusion or to reduce ACL stress.

Functional Status

Weight bearing may be limited by pain and instability.

Active and passive range of motion (ROM) is decreased by joint effusion and inflammation.

The quadriceps musculature may be inhibited by pain and joint effusion.

The patient avoids complete knee extension.

Physical Evaluation Findings

The following special tests may be positive:
- Lachman
- Anterior drawer
- Alternate Lachman
- Pivot shift

Anterior cruciate ligament (ACL) sprains frequently occur secondary to noncontact forces associated with "cutting" on a planted foot and externally rotating the lower leg. This position, combined with a valgus force during the cutting motion, can place a tensile force on the ACL (**Figure 6-1**) that exceeds the tissue strength. ACL injury can also occur when landing or planting the foot with the knee extended, a mechanism common in sports such as basketball, gymnastics, and volleyball.

A contact-related ACL sprain commonly occurs with contact to the posterolateral knee. This load causes anterior tibial shear and creates the possibility of a medial collateral ligament (MCL) sprain and medial meniscal injury from a valgus load. Lateral knee compression might cause a lateral meniscal injury.

Specific types of meniscal injuries are associated with ACL injuries. The lateral meniscus is more commonly torn in acute ACL injuries. The medial meniscus is more commonly injured in the chronically ACL-deficient knee.[1]

Articular surface changes and osteochondral defects (see p 174) can also occur after ACL injury.[1] The incidence of chondral surface changes with chronic ACL tears is at least twice that associated with acute injuries.

Differential Diagnosis

Patellar dislocation, posterior cruciate ligament (PCL) injury, tibiofemoral dislocation, osteochondral defect, meniscal tear

Medical Diagnostic Tests

Aspiration of a hemarthrosis limits the differential diagnosis to structures with a vascular supply. This procedure also relieves pain caused by joint distention. The lateral knee is cleansed with alcohol, and the skin is numbed with a topical or local anesthetic. The physician inserts the needle below the patella at the lateral joint line or, if knee flexion is limited, a suprapatellar approach is used. One hand applies pressure to the medial aspect of the knee, pushing on the joint effusion, and the plunger is then slowly withdrawn in the syringe, siphoning out the fluid.

Imaging Techniques

Standard anteroposterior (AP) and lateral radiographs are helpful to rule out an avulsion fracture. Magnetic resonance imaging (MRI) may demonstrate several signs indicating a tear—poor or nonvisualization of the ligament with sagittal images, irregular contour of fibers, interrupted fibers, and/or a focally increased signal reflecting edema within

Hemarthrosis A collection of blood within a joint.

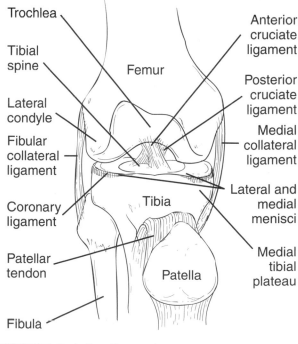

Trochlea

Tibial spine

Femur

Lateral condyle

Fibular collateral ligament

Coronary ligament

Tibia

Patellar tendon

Patella

Fibula

Anterior cruciate ligament

Posterior cruciate ligament

Medial collateral ligament

Lateral and medial menisci

Medial tibial plateau

Figure 6-1   Illustration of knee anatomy.

the ligament (**Figure 6-2**). Bone bruises, which may lead to long-term lateral knee pain and be clinically significant as osteochondritis dissecans, are more common in the lateral compartment. Bone bruises are often visualized in the mid lateral femoral condyle and the posterior lateral tibial plateau after an acute ACL injury. The long-term clinical significance of these bone bruises has not been determined (**Figure 6-3**).

Definitive Diagnosis

Positive Lachman test, positive findings on MRI, KT-2000 manual maximum test with more than 3 mm of laxity compared with the uninjured side

Pathomechanics and Functional Limitations

Most patients are unable to continue activity secondary to pain and instability. Joint effusion causes loss of full knee extension and flexion. Ambulation is impaired by pain, quadriceps inhibition due to the joint effusion, and the lack of full extension.

Patients with a chronic ACL-deficient knee may not experience dysfunction with normal activities of daily living (ADLs) and sports activities that do not involve cutting, pivoting, or sudden starting and stopping. With repeated giving-way episodes, however, these patients may have increased instability, even with low-level function. Most are unable to participate in activities that require pivoting on the planted foot. Joint instability is common, creating actual giving way during these activities or a sensation that the knee will give way or shift. Often patients demonstrate the sensation of the shift phenomenon by wringing their hands.

◼ Immediate Management

The patient is removed from activity, and ice is applied to the knee. The patient is placed in an immobilizer in slight flexion for comfort and fitted with crutches until further clinical workup is completed and the extent of injury determined.

◼ Medications

Nonsteroidal anti-inflammatory drugs (NSAIDs) are useful in the lower-grade injuries. However, in grade II and III injuries, acute pain management with narcotic analgesics may be used to allow patients to participate in the rehabilitation program and sleep more comfortably.

◼ Postinjury Management

Most patients benefit from using crutches until full ROM and quadriceps activity have been restored. Patients with a concurrent collateral ligament sprain may benefit from a hinged knee brace (**Figure 6-4**). Aspirating the joint effusion decreases pressure within the joint, reducing pain, promoting restoration of ROM, preventing arthrogenic muscle inhibition, and allowing muscle activity through exercise.

In some patients, a conservative approach to treating the ACL injury may be chosen. These patients are less active, especially in sports requiring cutting and pivoting. Some in-season athletes attempt to conservatively rehabilitate the ACL injury

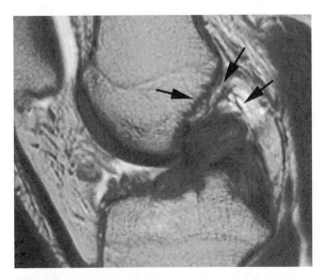

Figure 6-2 MRI sagittal view of an ACL tear. Arrows show tears in the proximal fibers from the femoral attachment, and the ligament stump is seen doubled over onto itself. (Reproduced with permission from Johnson TR, Steinbach LS (eds): *Essentials of Musculoskeletal Imaging.* Rosemont, IL, American Academy of Orthopaedic Surgeons, 2004, p 548.)

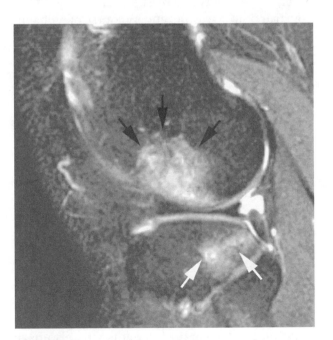

Figure 6-3 Femoral and tibial bone bruises. The black arrows indicate marrow edema in the anterolateral femur. The white arrows indicate tibial marrow edema. (Reproduced with permission from Johnson TR, Steinbach LS (eds): *Essentials of Musculoskeletal Imaging.* Rosemont, IL, American Academy of Orthopaedic Surgeons, 2004, p 485.)

Endoscope (endoscopic) A flexible instrument equipped with a lens and light that allows the inspection of a cavity.

Autogenic graft Graft tissue transplanted from one part of the patient's body to another part.

Allogenic graft Graft tissue obtained from the same species but not from the patient (eg, from a cadaver).

Harvest morbidity The death, failure, or rejection of the implanted tissue.

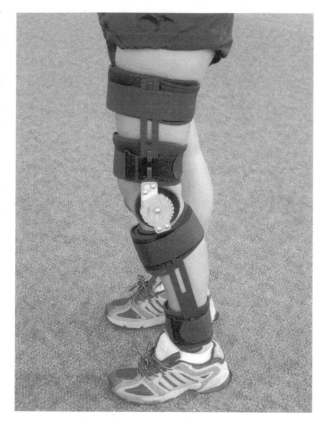

Figure 6-4   Hinged knee brace. This type of controlled-range of motion brace maybe be used for most types of knee sprains. The available range of motion can be adjusted by the clinician.

to return to activity that season, and then opt for reconstruction at season's end. A course of prehabilitation can decrease joint inflammation and restore ROM and muscle activity in the lower extremity before reconstruction.[2] Thorough knee evaluation should be performed for associated injuries (eg, meniscal or other ligamentous injury) that would eliminate the possibility of a quick return to activity. MRI findings must rule out other injuries including mensical abnormality.

■ Surgical Intervention

Proper timing of ACL reconstruction is important in order to minimize the risk of postsurgical arthrofibrosis.[3] The initial inflammatory reaction should subside, full extension and near full flexion should be obtained, and quadriceps tone should be restored before surgery (approximately 21 days) for an isolated ACL injury and 4 to 6 weeks with an associated MCL sprain.[3] Patients who also have sustained a locked bucket-handle meniscal tear (see p 159) causing a fixed flexion contracture—usually a chronic condition—need to undergo a staged sur-

Arthrofibrosis Abnormal formation of fibrous tissue within a joint.

gical procedure to prevent the development of arthrofibrosis. In this case, the meniscus is repaired first, followed by later ACL reconstruction.

An endoscopic procedure is preferred (ST 6-1). The surgical goal is to place the graft in a position that replicates the original anatomic position of the ACL and recreate a functionally stable knee. Several autogenic graft and allogenic graft options are available.[4] Autograft options include bone-patellar tendon-bone, quadrupled semitendinosus/gracilis tendons, and quadriceps tendon. Allograft choices include the Achilles tendon with attached calcaneal bone, bone-patellar tendon-bone, anterior tibial tendon, and posterior tibial tendon.

Surgeon experience and preference, graft availability, and tolerance to harvest morbidity determine which graft will be used (ST 6-2). The patient's graft choice can also factor into the decision-making process. Some patients may choose an allograft to potentially decrease postoperative pain because there is no donor site. Other patients may choose not to have an allograft because they do not want cadaveric tissue implanted into their body for an elective procedure such as ACL reconstruction.

Certain conditions may favor the use of one graft over another. An autogenous bone-patellar tendon-bone graft may be excluded in patients with a history of patellofemoral disease or a significant history of Osgood-Schlatter disease because of the possibility of a weakened tibial tuberosity bone plug. In general, however, the autogenous bone-patellar tendon-bone graft offers a strong graft with bone-to-bone fixation points that make fixation stronger early in rehabilitation.

Autogenous soft-tissue grafts may be ruled out for larger males because the available graft may not offer a large enough construct. Although hamstring grafts tend to be more lax after reconstruction, this finding has not proven to be clinically significant, and hamstring muscle function is not disrupted. A double-looped tendon of gracilis and semitendinosus offers a good graft construct. Newer techniques with soft-tissue screws provide effective fixation that is closer to the joint surfaces, decreasing graft movement within the bone tunnels.

With stringent testing and preoperative care, allografts have minimal potential for disease transmission, making them a safe choice. Tissue rejection is typically not the problem seen during vital organ transplantation. Allografts can be larger than autografts, significantly increasing tensile strength. Without donor site morbidity, allografts tend to produce less postoperative pain, and exercise may begin more quickly and more vigorously in the early stages of rehabilitation. The allograft is also the graft of choice for revision ACL surgery so that a second donor site is not created around the knee.

■ Postoperative Management

After surgery, the wounds are covered with a sterile dressing; a compressive bandage is applied from the toes to the proximal thigh; and the leg is placed in a postoperative, long leg, hinged knee brace. Dressings are changed several days later, and any bulky, compressive cotton dressings are removed. The elastic bandage is continued.

Continuous cold therapy can be applied over the dressings. Although patients subjectively favor continuous cold application, evidence is limited that the use of continuous cold is advantageous immediately postoperatively.[5] Similarly, patients may subjectively report increased comfort with the use of continuous passive motion (CPM), but long-term efficacy has not been substantiated.[6-8]

Patients are instructed to bear weight as tolerated with the brace locked in full extension. The brace can be unlocked for ambulation once extension is full, flexion is greater than 120°, and adequate leg control is demonstrated by a straight-leg raise without a lag and a normal gait pattern.

Quadriceps setting with the knee in full extension and straight-leg raises with the brace locked in extension begin on the second postoperative day. Patients start formal rehabilitation at 5 to 7 days postoperatively.

■ Injury-Specific Treatment and Rehabilitation Concerns

Specific Concerns

Protect the graft.
Restore full patellar motion and knee ROM.
Prevent early rotation forces on the knee.
Avoid early weight-bearing flexion (with associated meniscal tears).

Patients should begin weight bearing as tolerated with the knee fully extended in a locked knee brace as soon as possible. The goal is to bear full weight without assistance 1 week after surgery. Patients should sleep with the knee locked in extension until full, active extension can be maintained. The brace can be removed for rehabilitation. When good muscular control of the leg and full extension

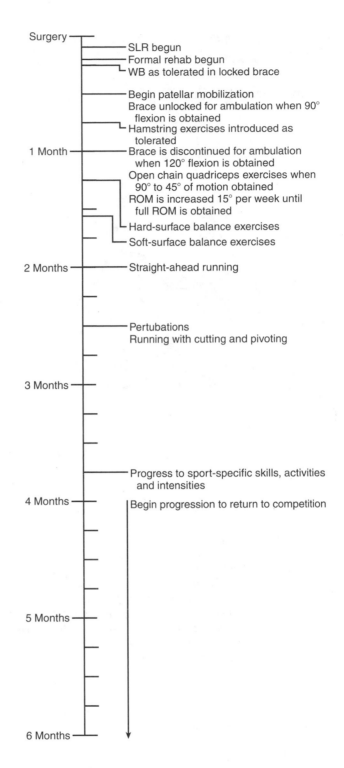

Surgery — SLR begun
— Formal rehab begun
— WB as tolerated in locked brace

— Begin patellar mobilization
Brace unlocked for ambulation when 90° flexion is obtained
— Hamstring exercises introduced as tolerated

1 Month — Brace is discontinued for ambulation when 120° flexion is obtained
Open chain quadriceps exercises when 90° to 45° of motion obtained
ROM is increased 15° per week until full ROM is obtained
— Hard-surface balance exercises
— Soft-surface balance exercises

2 Months — Straight-ahead running

— Pertubations
Running with cutting and pivoting

3 Months —

— Progress to sport-specific skills, activities and intensities

4 Months — Begin progression to return to competition

5 Months —

6 Months —

Note: Time frames are approximate. Function is the guide.

to flexion past 90° are achieved, the brace can be unlocked for ambulation. The brace can be discontinued when flexion is 120°.

To restore tibiofemoral motion, the patella is mobilized until it is moving normally compared with

S|T Surgical Technique 6-1

ACL Reconstruction

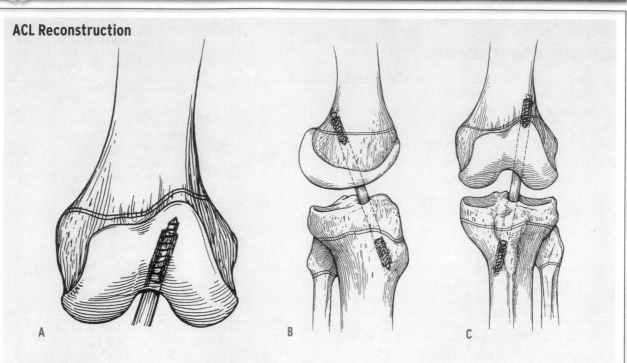

Indications

Failure to control giving way by limiting twisting activities or continual giving way with ADLs; individuals involved in high-risk activities that lead to giving-way episodes

Overview

1. The knee is visually inspected and physically examined to assess the injury.
2. Routine arthroscopy portals are developed (see Knee Arthroscopy). If autogenous grafts are chosen, a medial parapatellar tendon incision is made and the patellar tendon is identified. If a hamstring graft is used, a short medial incision is made over the insertion extending along the medial hamstrings.
3. If an autograft is chosen, it is harvested from the knee (see Surgical Technique 6-2).
4. Any additional procedures such as meniscal repair or resection (see Meniscal Repair, p 162) are performed.
5. The knee is prepared to accept the graft with a notchplasty, and tunnels are drilled through the femur (**A**) and tibia (**B**) to reproduce the anatomy. An attempt is made to place the graft through the tunnels in the original ACL footprint.
6. The graft is passed into position and then fixated into the tunnels (**C**). Various fixation options exist, depending on the specific graft choice and the surgeon's preference.
7. Full motion and negative Lachman and pivot-shift tests should be demonstrated as part of the final phase of surgery.

Functional Limitations

Dictated by the surgical procedure, graft source, and associated concomitant surgeries or comorbid conditions. Partial weight bearing (until quadriceps control is sufficient), avoidance of weight bearing and weight-loaded deep flexion (with meniscal repair), and restricted lateral movements are usually implemented postoperatively.

Implications for Rehabilitation

Accelerated rehabilitation focuses on regaining motion and full weight bearing in the early postoperative phase. Strengthening exercises are then instituted to regain function.

Potential Complications

The most feared complication is the development of arthrofibrosis, which limits the patient's functional ability. Other potential complications include graft failure, meniscal repair failure, donor site injury (with autogenous graft harvest), infection, deep vein thrombosis, and tibial or femoral fracture.

Figure reproduced with permission from Staniski CL: Anterior cruciate ligament injury in the skeletally immature patient: Diagnosis and treatment. *J Am Acad Orthop Surg*, 1995;3:146-158.

Notchplasty A surgical enlargement of the intercondylar notch to increase the space available to the ACL.

S|T Surgical Technique 6-2

Harvesting an Autograft

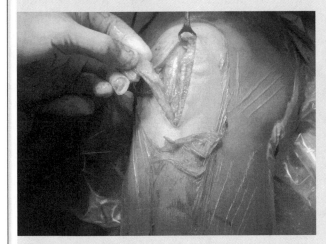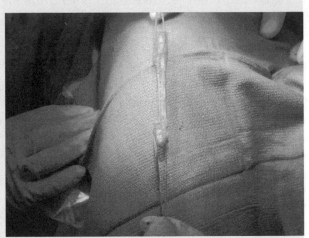

Bone-Patellar Tendon-Bone (shown above)

Through an anterior incision, the central one third (9 to 10 mm) of the patellar tendon is harvested with a scalpel; associated bone plugs from the superior aspects of the patella and tibial tubercle are obtained with a saw.

Semitendinosus and Gracilis

Through an anteromedial incision, a long harvesting instrument slides along the tendon and separates it from its muscular attachment and the semimembranosus tendon/muscle unit. Once the semitendinosus and gracilis tendons are identified, the harvesting instrument is placed around the tendons and run up the medial hamstring group, amputating at the proximal extent. Most physicians leave the distal attachment to the pes anserine and deliver the graft into the tibial and femoral tunnels after appropriate preparation.

the contralateral knee. Patients who have had a bone-patellar tendon-bone graft are closely monitored for patellar mobility, especially a superior glide.

ROM exercises are started immediately using various active-assisted and passive ROM techniques. To restore full extension, prone hanging or sitting with the knee in an extended position while the ankle is supported is used. The patient should have at least 90° of flexion by 2 weeks and 120° of motion by 4 weeks postoperatively. If these goals are not met, passive motion should be performed more aggressively. Bicycles are not recommended to regain ROM, as they tend to place high-load, low-duration stretches on the knee, which will be compensated for by the hip and ankle.

Early quadriceps muscle reeducation is also emphasized. In addition to active quadriceps setting and exercises, motor-level electrical stimulation is applied to the quadriceps with the knee fully extended. In full extension, the vector forces of the contracting quadriceps tendon should be more compressive than translatory. Counterweights can be applied to the proximal tibia to reduce or eliminate any unwanted translatory forces (**Figure 6-5**).

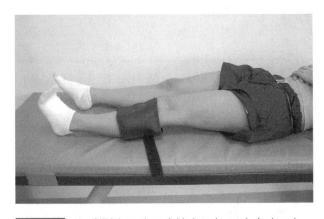

Figure 6-5 Use of tibial counterweights to reduce anterior translation of the knee during electrical stimulation. (Note: the electrodes have not yet been applied.)

Good quadriceps firing is emphasized during all exercises. Biofeedback may be helpful in reinforcing quadriceps muscle recruitment. The patient begins a partial or minisquat program as soon as weight bearing is full and joint effusion is controlled. Weights can be held in the hands and increased as tolerated. One-leg minisquats or step-up exercises begin when the patient's control is adequate to perform the exercise smoothly and maintain the knee in a straight plane.

Open chain quadriceps exercises are initiated from 90° to 45° of motion 4 weeks after surgery, increasing extension 15° every 2 weeks until extension is full. This protocol is followed not only to protect the graft but, more important, to protect the patellofemoral joint. Early on, when an effusion is present, the vastus medialis oblique (VMO) may be inhibited. Quadriceps exercises are performed in a range in which patellar control is not as dependent on the VMO.

Hamstring exercises can begin as soon as tolerated. In patients who underwent a hamstring tendon graft, the donor site may be sore for several weeks. Active or very light resistance exercises are performed when the soreness diminishes. Hamstring activity is increased as tolerated. Open and closed chain exercises for the hip and ankle also begin early in the rehabilitative process.

Bicycling activity is initiated when the patient has adequate ROM to cycle without any compensation in the hip, knee, or ankle. Stair-stepper machines can be introduced when the patient begins unilateral minisquats, emphasizing shorter arcs of motion with a great deal of quadriceps activity. Use of an elliptical glider or ski machine and treadmill walking begin when the patient can ambulate unbraced with a normal gait pattern. However, none of these repetitive exercises should be started in the presence of active inflammation.

Balance and proprioception exercises are essential to a functionally stable knee. Weight-shifting exercises are begun early in the process to prepare the knee to accept full weight-bearing stresses. Simple exercises with a straight leg on a hard, stationary surface can start as soon as the patient is walking without a brace. These are done in a controlled, protected environment. More challenging situations, such as soft or moving surfaces, can be introduced about 6 to 8 weeks after surgery if leg control is good. More challenging dynamic activities with perturbations or simultaneous upper extremity and trunk activities are started at about 12 weeks postoperatively.

A straight-ahead running program can begin at about 8 weeks if strength and endurance are adequate to permit running without any deviations. At about 12 weeks, gentle cutting and pivoting activities can be initiated, progressing to more acute angles of cutting, shuttle drills, and pivoting. Plyometrics are added for further challenge. Additional agility drills should be designed to challenge the patient in manners similar to the activities he or she will encounter in returning to sport.

Estimated Amount of Time Lost

Some patients may try to rehabilitate and complete the sport season. Attempts to cope with the injury through rehabilitation and bracing may require at least 4 to 6 weeks. Surgical reconstruction typically sidelines the patient from full sport or strenuous work activities for 4 to 9 months.[9,10] Good results with return to activity as soon as 8 weeks postoperatively have been reported,[11] but some experts have recommended that the return to full activity should not occur until 1 year postoperatively.[12]

An accelerated rehabilitation program focusing on early restoration of motion, quadriceps muscle activity, and full weight bearing may have the greatest influence on decreasing time lost after reconstruction.[11] Fewer complications after surgery, including patellofemoral pain, have also been demonstrated.[13]

Return-to-Play Criteria

The patient may return to competition when there is no pain, full ROM, restored strength of the quadriceps and hamstrings, and successful completion of functional tests for the lower extremity and an agility program with activities similar to the sport activities.

Functional Bracing

The patient may be fitted with a functional knee brace designed for ACL injuries or use an off-the-shelf brace. Those who need a streamlined brace for an activity such as gymnastics may prefer a custom brace (**Figure 6-6**). Some physicians choose not to brace because of the paucity of scientific evidence that bracing is effective in preventing future knee injury or improving functional performance.

Medial Collateral Ligament Sprain

CLINICAL PRESENTATION

History

Valgus stress to the knee on a loaded extremity
External rotation may also be reported.
Pain is described along the MCL.
Pain may extend distally to the medial tibial flare and proximally to the medial epicondyle.

Observation

Initial observation may not reveal significant findings.
With time, swelling may develop over the medial knee.

Functional Status

Functional status depends on injury severity:
* Grade I: little to no loss of ROM or ability to bear weight
* Grade II: difficulty bearing weight due to pain and loss of ROM, especially at the end ranges
* Grade III: severe functional limitations

If the MCL is torn proximal to the joint line, motion loss is greater.[18]

Physical Evaluation Findings

The following special tests are positive:
* Valgus stress at 25° to 30°: MCL injury
* Valgus stress at 0°: damage to the MCL, medial joint capsule, and possibly the cruciate ligaments
* Slocum drawer

Tests for cruciate ligament stability may be positive if the valgus stress test at 0° is positive.

Tests for meniscal tears are less reliable in the presence of an acute MCL injury.

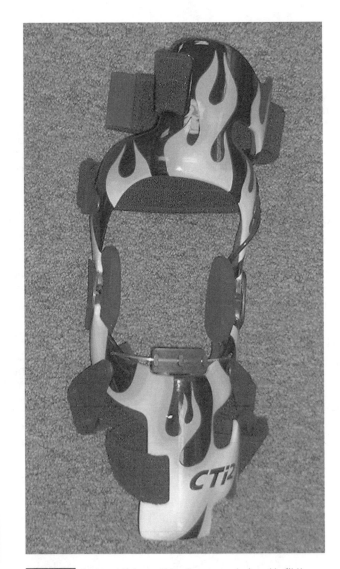

Figure 6-6 Custom ACL brace. These braces are designed to fit the contour of the patient's femur and tibia and allow for precise alignment of the knee joint. As the patient grows, or muscle mass increases, the brace should be rechecked for fit and replaced if necessary.

MCL sprains frequently occur from a direct valgus force across the knee while the foot remains planted or, less frequently, by an indirect force as the knee is forced into valgus during an activity such as skiing. Indirect injuries are also seen in soccer when two players simultaneously contact the ball from opposite sides (a "50-50 ball").

After an indirect injury mechanism, a purely valgus force must be differentiated from a torsional force. Noncontact torsional injuries may result in a combined MCL-ACL injury and have a higher incidence of meniscal damage.[14,15] Although less frequent, a valgus force to the knee while the tibia is externally rotated may result in trauma to the MCL and PCL.[16] In this mechanism, the unloaded foot contacts the ground. Contact to the leg (but not necessarily the knee) forces the knee into valgus and external rotation.

The medial-side structures form three distinct layers[17] (**Figure 6-7**). The first layer, the superficial layer, is the deep fascia encompassing the patellar tendon anteriorly and the popliteal fossa, including the medial hamstrings, posteriorly. The second layer, the MCL, blends with the third layer, the posteromedial capsule, forming the posterior oblique ligament.

The tissues involved and the extent of injury depend on the knee position and the applied stresses. When the knee is extended, valgus forces are absorbed by the entire complex. If the knee is flexed

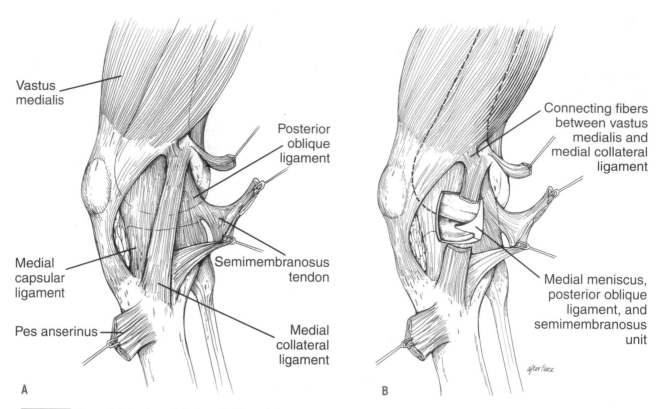

Vastus medialis

Posterior oblique ligament

Medial capsular ligament

Semimembranosus tendon

Pes anserinus

Medial collateral ligament

A

Connecting fibers between vastus medialis and medial collateral ligament

Medial meniscus, posterior oblique ligament, and semimembranosus unit

after Pearce

B

Figure 6-7 The medial structures of the knee. **A.** The medial capsuloligamentous complex. **B.** The MCL is dynamized by the connecting fibers of the vastus medialis, and the posterior oblique ligament is dynamized by the semimembranosus. (Reproduced with permission from Indelicato PA: Isolated medial collateral ligament injuries in the knee. *J Am Acad Orthop Surg* 1995;3:9-14.)

beyond 20°, the superficial tissues are most responsible for dissipating forces.

The MCL deep layers communicate with the medial joint capsule and medial meniscus. Damage to these structures should be suspected if the deep layer of the MCL is injured by the valgus force. A bone bruise or osteochondral trauma may occur in the lateral joint secondary to compressive forces.

Differential Diagnosis
Meniscal tear, ACL sprain, patellar retinaculum sprain, patellar dislocation, epiphyseal fracture (pediatric patients), medial hamstring strain, pes anserinus strain

Imaging Techniques
Radiographs are obtained to rule out avulsion fracture, intra-articular fracture, and patellar injury. MRI is used to identify MCL trauma and rule out damage to other ligaments and the menisci (**Figure 6-8**).

Definitive Diagnosis
Pain elicited on valgus stress with or without the presence of laxity in the acute setting; a positive MRI finding for MCL injury. If the examination is

delayed by a few days, extension may be limited secondary to edema, making it difficult to perform a clinical examination.

Pathomechanics and Functional Limitations
MCL disruption results in pain and possible joint instability. Grade I injuries are marked by pain with activity, no instability, and minimal loss of ROM. Patients typically have minimal limitations in normal ADLs. Grade II MCL sprains produce increased pain, swelling, loss of ROM, and the inability to perform low-intensity activities without pain. Although knee laxity is increased and an end point can still be identified, valgus instability often results. Grade III sprains are painful and produce significant limitations in ROM, especially toward the end ranges. Complete ligament disruption causes significant instability during activity.

■ Immediate Management
An acute MCL injury should be protected until the full extent of injury is appreciated. Initially, the knee may be more comfortable immobilized in slight flexion, especially with more severe injuries. The patient should use crutches to decrease stress through

the knee. Ice, compression, and elevation control early inflammation and limit edema formation.

Medications

NSAIDs are useful in the lower-grade injuries. However, in grade II and III injuries, acute pain management with narcotic analgesics may be used to allow the patient to participate in the rehabilitation program and sleep more comfortably.

Surgical Intervention

Primary repair of an isolated MCL injury is typically not needed but may be considered in a combined MCL-ACL injury; the decision to repair the MCL is made during the ACL surgery.[19,20] The ACL is reconstructed first, and then the knee is re-examined in full extension. If the knee is still unstable while in or near full extension, the MCL is repaired (**ST** 6-3). If valgus laxity is restored to grade I after ACL reconstruction alone, primary MCL repair is not performed.

Surgical treatment of the MCL is prone to high complication rates, including stiffness and patellofemoral dysfunction.[21] These issues must be addressed early in the rehabilitation program.

Postinjury/Postoperative Management

Isolated MCL injuries are usually successfully treated with a conservative program of rest from aggravating activities, NSAIDs, and functional rehabilita-tion. However, such injuries must be protected against recurrent valgus stress. A hinged knee brace can protect against injurious forces while allowing the patient to perform ROM exercises. Some grade III injuries may require a brief period of immobilization until pain subsides. A hinged brace can be initially locked in a comfortable position and then unlocked as the ligament heals. The brace is continued until the patient has at least 100° of motion, demonstrates good muscular control of the leg, and walks without a limp.

Patients with grade II or III MCL injuries should ambulate with crutches. In general, weight bearing is encouraged, and weight can be placed on the injured extremity as tolerated. Patients should begin a formal rehabilitation program to restore ROM, strength, and function as soon as tolerable.

Injury-Specific Treatment and Rehabilitation Concerns

Specific Concerns

Maintain patellar mobility.
Encourage early strengthening.
Emphasize early, pain-free ROM.

All patients with isolated MCL injuries undergo a similar course of rehabilitation, but they progress at different rates depending on the extent

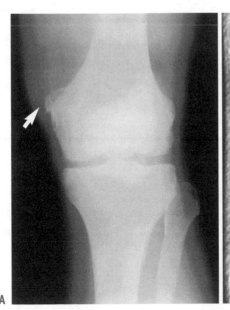 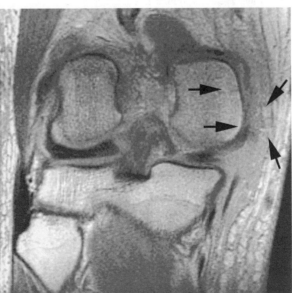

Figure 6-8 Imaging techniques for MCL sprains. **A.** AP radiograph demonstrates a Pellegrini-Stieda lesion (arrow), indicating a chronic MCL injury. (Reproduced with permission from Cosgarea AJ, Jay PR: Posterior cruciate ligament injuries: Evaluation and management. *J Am Acad Orthop Surg* 2001;9:297-307.) **B.** Coronal MRI scan of an MCL tear. The arrows indicate a complete tear of the MCL. (Reproduced with permission from Johnson TR, Steinbach LS (eds): *Essentials of Musculoskeletal Imaging.* Rosemont, IL, American Academy of Orthopaedic Surgeons, 2004, p 550.)

S|T Surgical Technique 6-3

MCL Repair

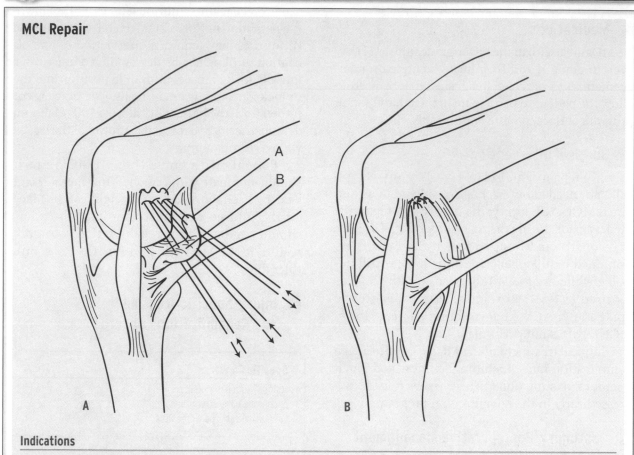

Indications

Persistent laxity with symptoms of valgus laxity and failure of conservative management

Overview

Acute Combined MCL-ACL Injuries

1. ACL reconstruction is performed (see Surgical Technique 6-1), and valgus laxity is reassessed. If the knee remains unstable in near or full extension, primary repair is performed.
2. The incision site is the same one used for the ACL reconstruction and autogenous graft harvest. With an allograft, a limited medial incision can be used.
3. The MCL and posterior oblique ligament are exposed.
4. Sutures are inserted into the stump of the posterior oblique ligament (POL) on the adductor tubercle (**A**).
5. With the knee in 60° of flexion, the POL is tied to the adductor tubercle (**B**).
6. The MCL is repaired, and the tibial end of the POL is attached to the tibia (**C**).
7. The anterior border of the POL is sutured over the posterior portion of the MCL (**D**).

of injury. The progression of rehabilitation exercises and activities is based on ability rather than set time periods.

Patients with grade I and II injuries can begin ROM exercises within a pain-free range as soon as tolerated. Simple quadriceps-setting exercises and leg raises may start immediately if tolerated. Other strengthening exercises can begin once pain and swelling begin to subside. The knee must not incur

any valgus forces at any point during the early rehabilitation period. A valgus brace should be worn during adduction leg-raising exercises.

When full, pain-free ROM is obtained and no pain is elicited on clinical examination, proprioceptive exercises are instituted. These exercises should stress the knee in full extension as well as some flexion. Activities that place limited, controlled stress on the medial knee should be added

S|T Surgical Technique 6-3, cont'd

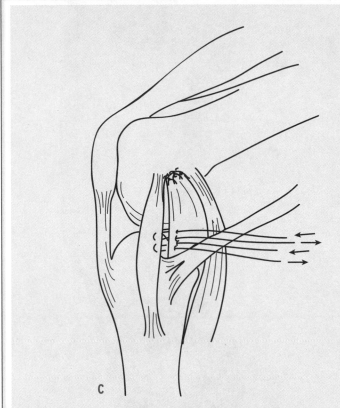
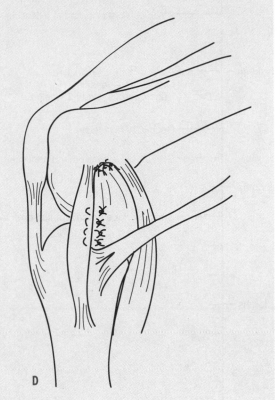

Chronic Instability of the MCL Despite an Adequate Healing Period
1. The MCL and posterior oblique ligament are exposed.
2. The medial capsular is **reefed** or advanced to restore medial stability.

Functional Limitations

MCL repairs may result in some postoperative stiffness. Care should be taken to mobilize the joint without injuring the repair.

Implications for Rehabilitation

ROM and strengthening exercises are implemented early to prevent arthrofibrosis. The repair is protected with a brace, and valgus stress is limited to prevent injury to the repair.

Potential Complications

Arthrofibrosis, repair failure, and other surgical complications such as deep vein thrombosis and infection are possible.

Figures are reproduced with permission from Hughston JC, Eilers AF: The role of the posterior oblique ligament in repairs of acute medial (collateral) ligament tears of the knee. *J Bone Joint Surg Am* 1973;55:923-940.

> **Reef (reefing)** A folding or tucking of tissues.

to the program. These include cup pick-ups and standard proprioceptive exercises with multiplanar activities and functions such as ball catching while balancing (see chapter 9).

Once the clinical examination is pain free, ROM is full, and strength is adequate, straight-ahead activities such as jogging and straight up-and-down jumping may begin, followed by nonlinear agility activities as tolerated. Patients with grade II or III injuries should be braced during agility activities.

■ Estimated Amount of Time Lost

Time lost to MCL injury varies with the grade of the sprain. Grade I MCL sprains may result in loss of 1 to 2 weeks. Grade II sprains may lose 2 to 4 weeks, whereas grade III sprains may require 2 to 3 months until full return to activity is possible.

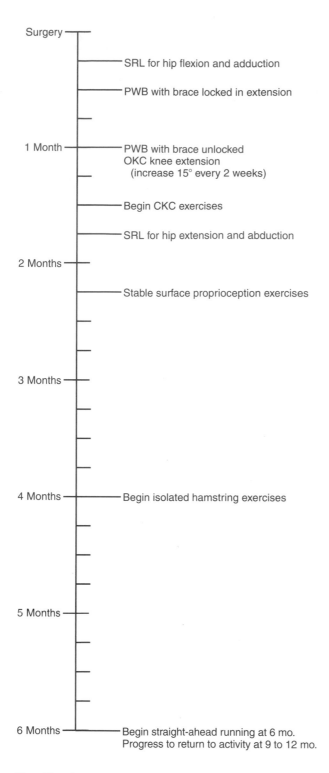

Surgery

— SRL for hip flexion and adduction

— PWB with brace locked in extension

1 Month — PWB with brace unlocked
OKC knee extension
(increase 15° every 2 weeks)

— Begin CKC exercises

— SRL for hip extension and abduction

2 Months

— Stable surface proprioception exercises

3 Months

4 Months — Begin isolated hamstring exercises

5 Months

6 Months — Begin straight-ahead running at 6 mo.
Progress to return to activity at 9 to 12 mo.

Note: Time frames are approximate. Function is the guide.

■ Return-to-Play Criteria

The patient may return to competition when there is no pain, full ROM, restored strength to the quadriceps and hamstrings, normal balance, and successful completion of an agility program with activities similar to the sport activities.

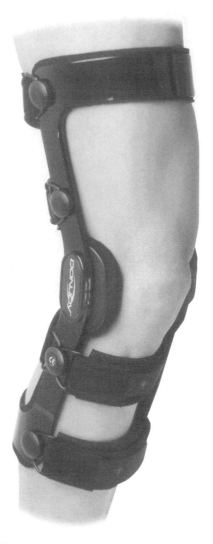

Figure 6-9 Collateral ligament brace. These off-the-shelf braces are used to protect and provide stability to the medial and lateral collateral ligaments.

Functional Bracing

A hinged knee brace with medial and lateral stays designed for MCL injuries is used with grade II and III sprains. It may be used in a grade I injury if the risk of reinjury is increased, as in a football lineman, or if the patient feels more confident returning to activity with the knee braced. An off-the-shelf brace designed for ACL instability is most suitable for grade III injuries and patients with grade II sprains requiring added protection (**Figure 6-9**). The brace is used only until the season is completed and is not required in subsequent seasons.

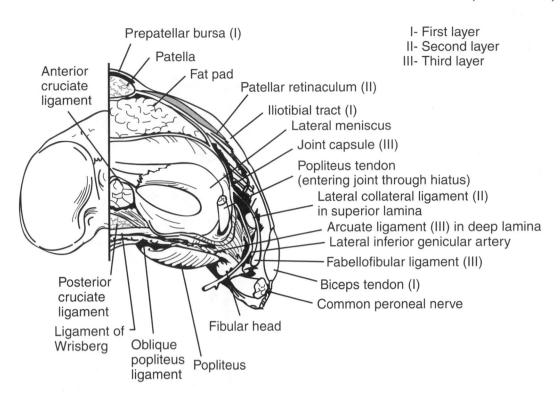

I- First layer
II- Second layer
III- Third layer

Figure 6-10 The structures of the lateral complex. (Reproduced with permission from Seebacher JR, Inglis AE, Marshall JL, Warren RF: The structure of the posterolateral aspect of the knee. *J Bone Joint Surg Am* 1982;64:536-541.)

Lateral Complex Injuries

The lateral complex, also known as the posterolateral complex, is divided into three anatomic areas. The first layer consists of the prepatellar bursa, iliotibial tract, and biceps tendon; the second layer consists of the patellar retinaculum and the lateral collateral ligament; and the third layer includes the joint capsule and arcuate and fabellafibular ligaments (**Figure 6-10**). Isolated lateral collateral ligament (LCL) sprains are rare. Forces that would otherwise be applied to the medial knee are usually deflected as the contralateral extremity is contacted first.

Most injuries involving the LCL also affect other tissues that form the lateral complex of the knee. Injuries to these tissues can be debilitating to the patient, even during regular gait, creating a varus thrust.[22] Lateral complex injuries may also include the cruciate ligaments.[23]

Differential Diagnosis

Fibular head avulsion fracture, lateral meniscal injury, ACL sprain, PCL sprain, tibiofemoral dislocation, physeal fracture in the pediatric patient

Imaging Techniques

AP radiographs are helpful to rule out a fibular head avulsion fracture (**Figure 6-11**). An AP view while varus thrust is applied may be useful in determin-

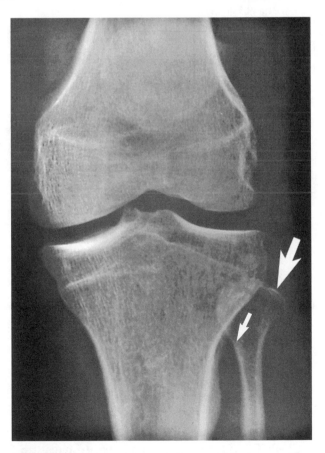

Figure 6-11 AP radiograph demonstrating an avulsion fracture of the fibular head (arrow) in a patient with combined PCL, posterolateral corner, and LCL injuries. (Reproduced with permission from Cosgarea AJ, Jay PR: Posterior cruciate ligament injuries: Evaluation and management. *J Am Acad Orthop Surg* 2001;9:297-307.)

CLINICAL PRESENTATION

History

Traumatic contact to the anteromedial knee, hyperextension, or a noncontact varus force to the knee[22]

Lateral knee pain with instability[24]

Patients with a concomitant peroneal nerve injury may describe paresthesia along the lateral foot.

Observation

Swelling, especially along the lateral knee

Possible lateral thrust during ambulation

Functional Status

Weight bearing limited by pain and sensation of instability

ROM decreased both actively and passively by pain

Physical Evaluation Findings

Manual muscle test of ankle dorsiflexors or great toe extension to document peroneal nerve function. Peroneal nerve injury has been reported in 15% to 56% of grade III LCL injuries.[24,25]

The following special tests may be positive:
- Varus stress at 30°: isolated LCL injury
- Varus stress at 0°: concomitant tear of ACL or ACL and PCL
- External-rotation recurvatum
- Posterolateral rotation
- Lachman
- Anterior drawer
- Alternate Lachman
- Pivot shift
- Posterior drawer

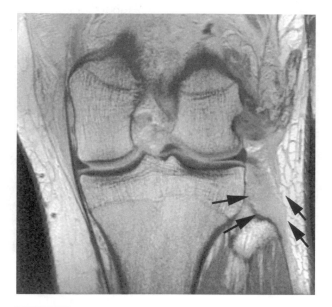

Figure 6-12 Coronal MRI view of the lateral complex. Arrows point to an avulsion of the LCL and biceps femoris tendon from the fibular head. (Reproduced with permission from Johnson TR, Steinbach LS (eds): *Essentials of Musculoskeletal Imaging.* Rosemont, IL, American Academy of Orthopaedic Surgeons, 2004, p 550.)

ing the extent of lateral compartment joint-line opening.[26] With chronic instability, the amount of medial compartment arthritis must be assessed. A bilateral standing posteroanterior view with the knee flexed at 45° assesses tibiofemoral joint-space narrowing.[27]

MRI is used to confirm the extent of injury to the lateral complex, cruciates, and menisci. Standard coronal, sagittal, and axial cuts are obtained. If a lateral injury is suspected, thin-sliced (2-mm), proton-density, coronal oblique images including the entire fibular head and styloid are useful[28] (**Figure 6-12**). An **arteriogram** is obtained to assess vascular injury if clinically indicated or if a tibiofemoral dislocation is suspected.

Arteriogram A radiograph of a blood vessel after the injection of a radiopaque dye into the bloodstream.

Definitive Diagnosis

The definitive diagnosis is based on positive findings of the varus stress test at 30° (isolated LCL), varus stress test at 0° (concomitant tear of ACL or ACL-PCL), external-rotation recurvatum test, and posterolateral rotation test. Passive knee extension results in hyperextension and external rotation of the involved leg. In chronic cases, a varus-thrust gait may be demonstrated. A posterior dynamic pivot shift may also be present.

MRI findings are used to confirm the clinical findings. Peroneal nerve damage is confirmed by electromyographic studies and nerve conduction tests, but it may take 3 to 4 weeks for these tests to become diagnostic.

Pathomechanics and Functional Limitations

Isolated lateral complex injuries result in varus laxity. Combined LCL and cruciate ligament injuries create a complex pattern of laxity leading to instability. Patients with isolated grade I LCL injuries present with ADL limitations secondary to pain. Patients with grade II and III injuries and combined cruciate ligament tears are limited in all weight-bearing activities due to instability.

■ Immediate Management

Acute lateral complex injuries should initially be protected until the injury extent is determined. The patient may be more comfortable with the knee immobilized in slight flexion, especially with a severe LCL injury. Crutches decrease stress through the knee.

Ice, compression, and elevation are used to control early inflammation and limit edema formation.

■ Medications

NSAIDs are useful in the lower-grade injuries. In grade II and III injuries, acute pain management with narcotic analgesics may be used to allow the patient to participate in the rehabilitation program and sleep more comfortably.

◼ Postinjury Management

Early recognition of the structures involved and injury severity forms the basis for successful treatment.[23,24,29] Isolated grade I and II injuries to the LCL or lateral complex can be treated conservatively. Patients with grade II injuries must be followed closely with a period of rehabilitation. Those with continued complaints of pain and instability may require surgical repair. Because of the high success rate with acute repair, some physicians elect to surgically repair all grade II lateral complex injuries to more adequately restore normal anatomy and function.

Patients with lateral complex and cruciate ligaments injuries should have angiographic studies to rule out vascular injury.[30] Vascular injury should be assessed by a vascular surgeon for immediate repair of the injured vessel.

◼ Surgical Intervention

Symptomatic grade II and III injuries require surgical anatomic repair of the tissues within 10 to 14 days.[23,29,31] After this time, retraction of the injured tissues may prevent an adequate anatomic restoration via primary repair. Failing to recognize the injury or the degree of laxity in the early postinjury period (2 weeks) dictates a late reconstruction with a graft or tissue advancement rather than primary repair of the injured structures. Late reconstruction yields results inferior to primary repair. Patients with chronic insufficiency require late reconstruction and/or high tibial osteotomy, which should be considered salvage procedures.

Primary tissue repair is favored over late reconstruction because of better restoration of normal knee biomechanics. Optimal techniques for repairing lateral complex injuries include direct repair back to bone and side-to-side suturing of soft tissues (ST 6-4). Restoring normal anatomic position with secure fixation allows ROM to be pursued early and safely postoperatively.[26] Any concurrent reconstructions of the ACL and/or PCL are performed at the time of the primary repair of the lateral complex.

◼ Postoperative Management

If secure repair of the lateral complex tissues is performed to restore anatomic position, the patient can commence ROM immediately after surgery. The physician determines the limits of early ROM in a safe zone during surgery. With complex injuries, a brief 1- to 2-week immobilization period may be warranted.

Delayed signs of neuropathy should be followed with serial electromyographic and nerve conduction tests.

◼ Injury-Specific Treatment and Rehabilitation Concerns

> **Specific Concerns**
>
> Encourage pain-free ROM within limits set by physician.
> Avoid knee hyperextension, external rotation, and varus forces.
> Maintain patellar mobility.

Nonsurgical Treatment of Grade I and II Injuries

Patients are initially protected in a knee immobilizer in full extension for 3 to 4 weeks with no weight bearing. Patellar mobilizations may be conducted. Quadriceps setting and straight-leg raising into hip flexion are performed in the immobilizer.

After the initial immobilization period, the patient is placed in a hinged brace while ROM, strength, and weight bearing progress as tolerated. The brace can be discontinued when ROM is full and control of the leg is adequate, as demonstrated by a normal gait pattern and straight-leg raising without a lag. No specific limitations are placed on restoring ROM, which is advanced as tolerated. Hip muscle strengthening with flexion and abduction exercises is progressed. Adduction and hip-extension exercises are introduced after 6 weeks, when tissue healing is more advanced. Quadriceps strengthening can begin with both open and closed chain activity. Hamstring activity starts at 6 weeks, as adequate tissue healing is achieved.

Primary Repair to the Lateral Complex

Lateral complex injuries are associated with greater morbidity than PCL injuries. With a concurrent LCL-PCL reconstruction, ROM restrictions for the lateral complex override the PCL guidelines presented below and in the PCL section (see p 158).

The patient bears no weight for 2 weeks. Partial weight bearing with the knee locked in extension for 2 weeks is then initiated. If sufficient leg control is established, the patient may bear weight as tolerated in an open-hinged brace for 2 more weeks. As long as adequate anatomic repair has been accomplished, the patient can immediately begin passive ROM, avoiding knee hyperextension. Any motion restrictions because of tension placed on the primary repair noted during surgery must be strictly followed. Active hamstring motion must be limited.

Straight-leg raises for hip flexion and adduction can begin after 1 week. Abduction and extension exercises start after adequate healing of the

S|T Surgical Technique 6-4

Repair of the Lateral Complex

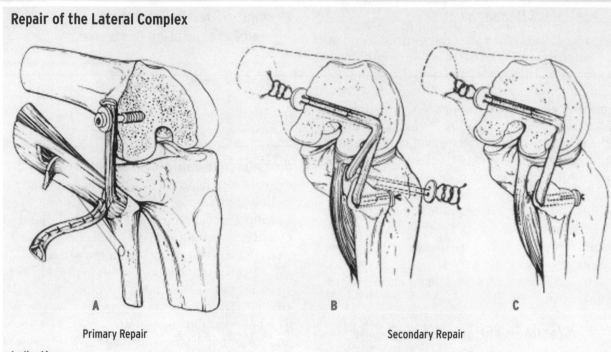

A — Primary Repair

B   C

Secondary Repair

Indications

Injury to the lateral structures with lateral instability

Overview

Primary Repair

1. A curvilinear incision is made midway between the Gerdy tubercle and fibular head and extending up to the lateral femoral epicondyle in the midportion of the iliotibial band.
2. Dissection is carried through the iliotibial band, and the injury is identified.
3. If the injury involves the fibular head or peroneal nerve, the peroneal nerve is identified and moved out of the surgical field.
4. The tissue is repaired back to bone.
5. Sutures are placed through the tissue. If the tissue has been torn off the fibular head, a suture anchor may be passed to fixate it back to the fibular head.
6. A **curette** is used to produce a fresh bony bed to accept the tissue.
7. The tissue is advanced to the prepared bony bed and fixated (**A**).

Secondary Repair

1. The incision is similar to that used for a primary repair.
2. The graft tissue (such as the patellar tendon) is harvested.
3. A tunnel is bored through the lateral femoral condyle.
4. A **bifurcated** graft is fixated distally via tunnels bored through the proximal tibia and fibular head and fixated using anchors (**B**).
5. An isolated reconstruction involves fixation through a tunnel bored through the fibular head (**C**).

Functional Limitations

Postoperative motion limitations are determined by the surgical procedure, structures repaired, and fixation strength. Other limitations may be dictated by associated neurovascular injuries.

Implications for Rehabilitation

Avoidance of varus stress through weight bearing is required in order to prevent excessive stresses to the repair. Motion limitations may also be necessary, especially with secondary reconstructions.

Potential Complications

Repair failure and continued varus instability can limit the patient's functional outcome.

Figures reproduced with permission from Covey DC: Injuries of the posterolateral corner of the knee. *J Bone Joint Surg Am* 2001;83:106-118.

Curette A scoop-shaped surgical instrument used to remove tissue.

Bifurcated Made up of, or divided into, two parts.

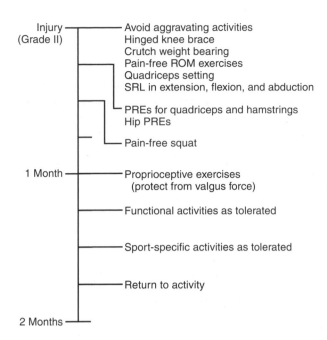

Injury (Grade II)
- Avoid aggravating activities
- Hinged knee brace
- Crutch weight bearing
- Pain-free ROM exercises
- Quadriceps setting
- SRL in extension, flexion, and abduction

- PREs for quadriceps and hamstrings
- Hip PREs

- Pain-free squat

1 Month
- Proprioceptive exercises (protect from valgus force)

- Functional activities as tolerated

- Sport-specific activities as tolerated

- Return to activity

2 Months

Note: Time frames are approximate. Function is the guide.

primary repair at about 6 to 8 weeks. Quadriceps activity may begin with leg-extension exercises at 4 weeks. Initially, these are performed from 90° to 30° and extension is increased 15° every 2 weeks until full ROM is obtained. Closed chain activities can begin at approximately 4 to 6 weeks postoperatively. Isolated hamstring activity is delayed until 4 months postoperatively.

The patient can begin proprioception exercises on a stable surface as soon as weight bearing is full. At approximately 12 weeks, less stable and more challenging exercises may be introduced.

Walking, swimming, and cycling may start 8 to 12 weeks after surgery. Running straight ahead on level surfaces can begin at 6 months, followed by agility and sport-specific drills if the patient demonstrates adequate strength and balance. Full return to activity may take 9 to 12 months.

■ Estimated Amount of Time Lost

Isolated grade I injuries require 2 to 4 weeks of rehabilitation. Grade II and III injuries and those involving the cruciate ligaments require surgical intervention and 6 to 9 months of rehabilitation, similar to isolated cruciate reconstruction. Surgical intervention and acute versus chronic surgical treatment of the lateral complex increase the time lost, possibly up to 1 year.

■ Return-to-Play Criteria

The patient must have grade I or less laxity of the lateral knee; full restoration of ROM, strength, and proprioception; and the ability to compete in sport-specific activities without instability.

Functional Bracing

Patients use a hinged knee brace for isolated lateral-side injuries. Patients with concomitant cruciate injuries use a functional knee brace designed to stabilize anterior and/or posterior laxity, as dictated by the involved structures.

Posterior Cruciate Ligament Sprain

CLINICAL PRESENTATION

History

Knee hyperflexion
A fall onto a flexed knee
A posteriorly directed force to the anterior tibia with a flexed knee
Mechanisms involving cutting, pivoting, or hyperextension could lead to multiple-ligament injury.
Patients may report minimal or no pain in acute injuries.
Over time, patients may complain of vague symptoms related to the patellofemoral joint.

Observation

Swelling is slight to moderate.
Ecchymosis may be present in the popliteal space.
A posterior sag may be noted.

Functional Status

Isolated grade I or II tears may initially be overlooked by the patient.
Gait may be normal or antalgic.
ROM may be normal.
Terminal flexion may be limited secondary to pain, especially with a partially torn PCL.
Concomitant injuries to other ligaments cause greater motion loss.

Physical Evaluation Findings

Any or all of the following special tests may be positive:
- Posterior drawer
- Godfrey
- External rotation

PCL tears, although less common than ACL and MCL tears, are more prevalent than previously thought. A literature review demonstrated PCL tears in as many as 44% of all acute knee injuries.[32] The underrecognition of PCL tears is due, in part, to the asymptomatic nature of most of these injuries.

The PCL is the primary restraint to posterior translation of the tibia on the femur (**Figure 6-13**). The MCL, LCL, and posterolateral corner of the knee all form secondary restraints to this motion.[31] In knees with an intact PCL, these secondary restraints play a minimal role in preventing posterior translation. However, in the PCL-injured knee, the secondary restraints play a vital role in maintaining stability.[31]

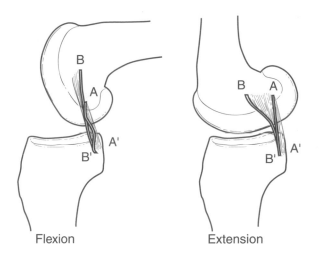

Flexion   Extension

Figure 6-13 The insertion of the PCL extends 2 cm below the surface of the posterior aspect of the tibial plateau. With flexion, the bulk of the ligament (B-B′) becomes taut. The posterior band (A-A′) becomes taut in extension.

An isolated PCL tear increases posterior translation of the tibia on the femur. Concomitant tearing of the MCL, LCL, or posterolateral corner can further and significantly increase posterior translation. The PCL also acts as a secondary restraint to external rotation, with the posterolateral corner of the knee providing the primary restraint. When the posterolateral corner is injured but the PCL remains intact, forces on the PCL increase.[31]

Differential Diagnosis
Posterior capsular sprain; meniscal tear; ACL sprain; symptomatic or ruptured Baker cyst; hamstring, gastrocnemius, popliteus, or plantaris muscle strain

Imaging Techniques
Radiographic evaluation should consist of AP, lateral, tunnel, and patellofemoral views. MRI is highly accurate for diagnosing the location of PCL tears and aids in assessing possible posterolateral corner injury[31] (**Figure 6-14**). This information may influence the treatment approach; femoral attachment injuries may be more amenable to surgical repair.[31]

Definitive Diagnosis
Positive orthopaedic tests demonstrating posterior laxity, conclusive findings on MRI

Pathomechanics and Functional Limitations
Patients with an isolated PCL tear may have few functional limitations. The types and descriptions of these limitations differ depending on the injury.

Acutely, patients may be unable to perform activities due to pain and swelling; however, because instability is not always present, they may not seek immediate treatment. In chronic PCL tears, functional limitations tend to be similar to those of patellofemoral disease, including generalized discomfort, pain on descending stairs, and the sensation of giving way during activity. Particular difficulty may occur when slowing down while running, as the hamstrings contract more forcefully and displace the tibia.

Anterior shear forces of the femur on the tibia produce pain and instability. When the foot is fixed on the ground and the femur decelerates, such as in a basketball jump-stop or a gymnastics dismount, the femur displaces anteriorly relative to the tibia.

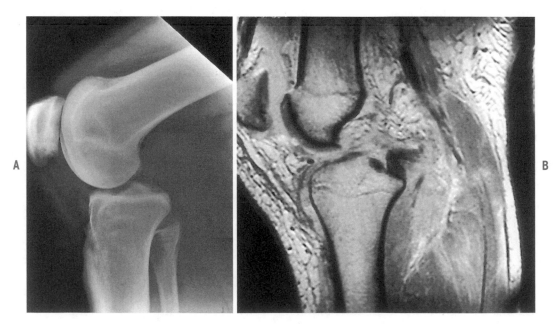

Figure 6-14 Imaging of PCL tears. **A.** Posterior subluxation of the tibia seen on a lateral view of a posterior stress radiograph of a patient with combined grade III PCL-MCL injury. **B.** MRI demonstrating an acute complete tear of the PCL. (Reproduced with permission from Cosgarea AJ, Jay PR: Posterior cruciate ligament injuries: Evaluation and management. *J Am Acad Orthop Surg* 2001;9:297-307.)

Immediate Management

The patient should be placed in a hinged, controlled-motion brace as close to full extension as pain allows until a thorough assessment is conducted to rule out concomitant posterolateral corner injury. Keeping the leg near full extension removes stress from the injured structures by properly aligning the tibia. Ice, compression, and elevation control the early inflammatory process and limit edema formation.

Medications

NSAIDs are helpful in the lower grade injuries. However, in grade II and III injuries, acute pain management with narcotic analgesics may be used to enable the patient to participate in the rehabilitation program and sleep more comfortably.

Postinjury Management

Patients with isolated grade I and II PCL injuries are treated with protected weight bearing until pain and swelling are eliminated. Rehabilitation can begin immediately. Conservatively treated, isolated grade III injuries are immobilized for 2 to 4 weeks in a hinged-motion brace as close to full extension as pain allows. Partial weight bearing to tolerance is permitted. Quadriceps setting and straight-leg raises should be performed.

Surgical Intervention

Immediate PCL reconstruction for an isolated grade III injury is indicated with a "peel-off" injury that can be replaced in its bony attachment and in young, active patients. Failure to improve with conservative treatment of grade III sprains may also warrant PCL reconstruction. In addition, surgical intervention may be appropriate if symptoms occur in the medial compartment of the knee and the patellofemoral joint or if the PCL is injured along with other ligaments or the posterolateral corner. If the posterolateral corner must be repaired, surgery should be performed within 2 weeks of injury.

Techniques to reconstruct the ligament are controversial. PCL reconstruction may be attempted arthroscopically or performed with an open technique. Arthroscopically, fluid may extravasate into the lower leg. If this occurs, the arthroscopy must be abandoned and the surgery completed through an open technique.

Surgical techniques have focused on reconstructing just the larger anterolateral bundle of the PCL (one-bundle technique) or both bundles (two- or double-bundle technique) (**Figure 6-15**). The one-bundle technique reduces but does not eliminate the laxity. Recent cadaveric studies of the double-bundle technique demonstrate better restoration of joint biomechanics,[33] but long-term, in vivo studies of stability and function with this technique have not been performed.

The other controversy in PCL reconstruction involves tibial graft placement. The traditional technique places the graft through a tibial tunnel; the major disadvantage is that the graft exits the tibial tunnel just below the posterior tibial plateau and bends around ("killer turn") toward its eventual insertion into the femur (ST 6-5). This procedure is technically challenging and may place unwanted forces on the graft, resulting in eventual failure.

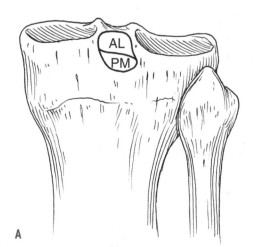
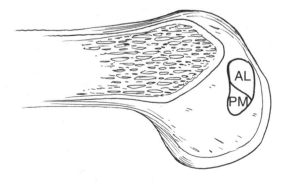

A   B

Figure 6-15 Anatomy of the PCL insertion. **A.** Outline of the anterolateral bundle (AL) and posteromedial bundle (PM) of the tibial insertion. **B.** Femoral origin. (Adapted with permission from Harner CD, Hoher J: Evaluation and treatment of posterior cruciate ligament injuries. *Am J Sports Med* 1998;26:471-482.)

S|T Surgical Technique 6-5

Tibial Tunnel ("Killer-Turn") Technique for PCL Reconstruction

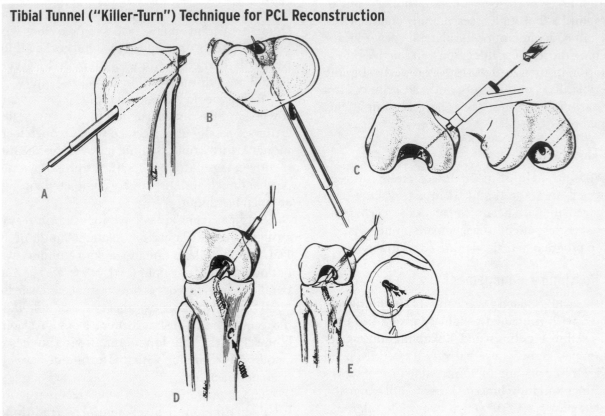

Indications

Patients with grade III PCL injuries who remain symptomatic after a course of formal rehabilitation

Overview

1. The knee is examined; PCL remnants are identified and debrided.
2. The course of the tibial tunnel is identified, a guide wire is placed, and correct placement is confirmed with a radiograph before the tunnel is drilled.
3. A tibial tunnel from the anteromedial tibia to the tibial attachment footprint is created (**A** and **B**).
4. The femoral tunnel(s) are then identified and drilled (**C**).
5. If a single bundle is used, it is placed, tensioned, and fixated.
6. With a double bundle, a semitendinosus autograft is harvested and prepared with an Achilles tendon allograft.
7. The graft is placed through the tibial tunnel and into the femoral tunnel. In double bundles, the allograft is typically used for the anterolateral bundle and the autograft for the posteromedial bundle (**D**).
8. The bundles are fixated at the femoral side (**E**).
9. The knee is cycled, and the graft is tensioned and fixated at the tibia. (If a single bundle is used, the graft is fixated at 90°. If a double bundle is used, the anterolateral bundle graft is fixated at 90°, whereas the posteromedial graft is fixated at 30°.)

Functional Limitations

Repaired isolated PCL tears rarely create functional limitations. However, when combined with other ligament injuries, multidirectional instability of the knee may result.

Implications for Rehabilitation

The graft sustains the greatest tension at 90° of flexion. This position should be avoided until healing is adequate.

Potential Complications

Complications include graft loosening and typical surgical complications such as deep vein thrombosis, infection, etc. The tibial tunnel approach may create excess stress along the graft as it makes the "killer turn" around the posterior tibia, but no conclusive evidence demonstrates that this technique significantly affects the surgical outcome.

Figures reproduced with permission from Miller MD, Harner CD, Koshiwaguchi S: Acute posterior cruciate ligament injuries, in Fu FH, Harner CD, Vince KG (eds): *Knee Surgery*. Philadelphia, PA, Williams & Wilkins, 1994, pp 749-767.

S|T Surgical Technique 6-6

Tibial Inlay Method of PCL Reconstruction

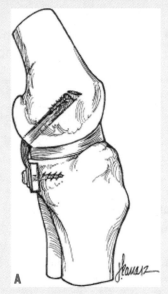 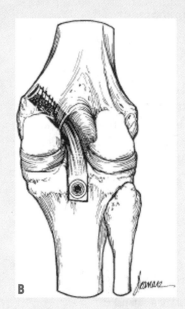

Indications

Patients with Grade III PCL injuries who remain symptomatic after a course of formal rehabilitation

Overview

1. The patient is placed prone or in the lateral decubitus position with the operative leg up.
2. A single- or double-bundle technique can be used. If a single bundle is chosen, it is placed in a position to replicate the anterolateral bundle of the original PCL.
3. The PCL remnants are identified and debrided.
4. The femoral tunnels are drilled to simulate the double bundle's footprints of the PCL in the anteromedial notch (**A**).
5. The leg is extended, and an oblique incision is made at the medial gastrocnemius head, exposing the area between the medial head and the semimembranosus tendon.
6. The neurovascular structures are retracted.
7. The posterior capsule is incised, and the PCL attachment is visualized.
8. An inlay window is prepared in the tibia to accept the bone block of the allograft tissue.
9. The graft is placed and fixated in the tibial inlay with one or two screws (**B**).
10. The graft is placed, tensioned, and fixated in the femoral tunnel.

Implications for Rehabilitation

The graft sustains the greatest tension at 90° of flexion. This position should be avoided until healing is adequate.

Potential Complications

Graft loosening and typical surgical complications, such as deep vein thrombosis and infection

Comments

The tibial inlay technique is technically demanding. The lateral decubitus or prone position is necessary for this procedure; other surgical procedures for multiple-ligament injuries require the supine position. The position change extends surgical time and can be burdensome to the surgeon and operative team.

Figures reproduced with permission from Bergfeld J, McAllister DR, Parker RD, Valdevit ADC, Kambic HE: A biomechanical comparison of posterior cruciate ligament reconstruction techniques. *Am J Sports Med* 2001;29:129-136.

More recently, a tibial inlay technique has been described (**S|T** 6-6).[34] A bone trough is created at the PCL footprint. Bone attached to the graft is then inlaid in the trough and fixated, creating a more natural graft attachment and eliminating the bend that occurs with the tibial tunnel technique.

Many graft options are available, including patellar tendon autograft, quadriceps tendon autograft, hamstring autograft, patellar tendon allograft, and Achilles tendon allograft. If the tibial inlay technique is used, the graft must have a bone block attached.

Postoperative Management

The knee is immobilized in full extension for 4 weeks. The patient is carefully followed for signs and symptoms of arthrofibrosis, including increasing stiffness or pain and decreasing function. If any of these are detected, knee mobility becomes more aggressive. The patient is allowed to weight bear as tolerated with the knee extended. Quadriceps setting and straight-leg raises are performed during

this period. The brace is unlocked at 4 weeks for ambulation and discontinued at 8 weeks if the patient has good leg muscle control and at least 100° of flexion.

■ Injury-Specific Treatment and Rehabilitation Concerns

> **Specific Concerns**
>
> Protect the injury/graft from unwanted stresses.
> Avoid hamstring contractions.
> Emphasize quadriceps reeducation.
> Encourage weight bearing and ROM as tolerated.

Conservative Rehabilitation

Rehabilitation of isolated grade I and II PCL injuries focuses on quadriceps muscle strengthening initiated with leg raises, open chain knee extension from 60° to 0°, and minisquats. As tolerated, the patient can begin proprioceptive training, progressing to straight-ahead running, agility skills, and sport-specific activities and then to full activity. Typically, patients return to full activity in 2 to 4 weeks.

Four weeks after injury, patients with grade III PCL injuries progress to full weight-bearing and ROM exercises. Strengthening of the quadriceps musculature is initiated with open knee extension from 60° to 0° and minisquats. At 8 weeks, strengthening exercises can advance to 90° of motion and hamstring exercises can begin. The patient can begin proprioceptive training as tolerated, progressing to straight-ahead running, agility skills, and sport-specific activities and then to full activity. Typically, patients return to full activity in about 3 months.

Postoperative Rehabilitation

Two weeks after PCL reconstruction, patients can begin formal rehabilitation. Patellar mobilization is important because of the prolonged period of immobility. ROM exercises are commenced with the clinician or patient applying an anterior translatory force to the posterior tibia while the knee is flexed. The anterior translation force decreases or eliminates tensile stress that may be placed upon the PCL graft with flexion and is used until about 8 weeks after surgery. Initially, ROM is progressed to 60°. Full extension should be obtained as soon as possible. At 6 weeks, ROM can advance as tolerated.

Strengthening focuses on the quadriceps and initially includes high-intensity electrical stimula-

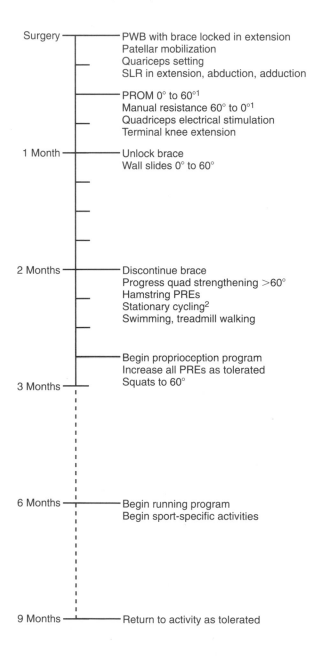

Surgery — PWB with brace locked in extension
Patellar mobilization
Quariceps setting
SLR in extension, abduction, adduction

PROM 0° to 60°[1]
Manual resistance 60° to 0°[1]
Quadriceps electrical stimulation
Terminal knee extension

1 Month — Unlock brace
Wall slides 0° to 60°

2 Months — Discontinue brace
Progress quad strengthening >60°
Hamstring PREs
Stationary cycling[2]
Swimming, treadmill walking

Begin proprioception program
Increase all PREs as tolerated
3 Months — Squats to 60°

6 Months — Begin running program
Begin sport-specific activities

9 Months — Return to activity as tolerated

[1]Apply a proximal anterior counterforce when the knee is flexed
[2]Seat high, resistance low, no toe clips
Note: Time frames are approximate. Function is the guide.

tion, straight-leg raising, and manual resistance from 60° to 0° while a manual anterior translatory force is applied to the posterior tibia. Closed chain exercises such as wall slides in a 0° to 60° range can begin at 4 weeks. Hip flexion should be minimized during closed chain exercises to decrease activity in the hamstring musculature. No active hamstring contractions are allowed until at least 8 weeks after surgery, at which time hamstring exercises begin with simple cuff weights. The patient can progress ROM during quadriceps strengthening exercises to 90° to 0° and increase exercise intensity as tolerated.

Proprioceptive and balance exercises are begun at 8 weeks, when the graft can start to accept posterior translation forces from hamstring contractions. These are progressed as tolerated.

Stationary bicycling, swimming, and treadmill walking can be initiated 8 weeks after surgery. Running is allowed at 6 months, and agility and sport-specific drills start as tolerated. The patient must be able to perform these activities without any compensation before advancing to more challenging levels. Sports activities can begin at 9 months, but it may take as long as 12 months before the patient can participate successfully.

Estimated Amount of Time Lost

Time lost to injury is 2 to 4 weeks after an isolated grade I or II injury. Grade III injuries are less predictable; conservative treatment may include prolonged rehabilitation of about 3 months, with PCL reconstruction taking 9 to 12 months before return to full activity.

The greatest influences on time lost are whether the PCL tear is isolated or part of a multiple-ligament injury and tear severity. Isolated injuries can often be treated nonsurgically, whereas patients with grade III isolated injuries and PCL tears with concomitant ligamentous injuries are good candidates for surgical repair.

Return-to-Play Criteria

The patient may return to competition when there is no pain, full ROM, restored quadriceps and hamstrings strength, and successful completion of lower extremity functional tests and an agility program with activities similar to the sport activities.

Functional Bracing

The patient may be fitted with a functional knee brace designed for PCL injuries (**Figure 6-16**).

Meniscal Tears

The menisci are integral to the normal function and long-term health of the knee joint. The fibrocartilaginous structures provide stability, shock absorption, and joint lubrication. The blood supply to each meniscal portion determines whether a tear will heal spontaneously or require surgical repair. The peripheral 20% to 30% of the medial meniscus and 10% to 25% of the lateral meniscus—the "red zones"—are relatively well vascularized, making these areas more conducive to healing and repair.[35,36] The avascular, or white, zone is the inner third and not conducive to healing. The red-white zone, which may have some blood supply, has limited healing potential (**Figure 6-17**).

The type of meniscal injury is affected by age. Younger patients tend to tear the meniscus and injure the ACL. The tear is likely to occur in the red and red-white zones, making those injuries more conducive to surgical repair. Older patients who have degenerated menisci may be more prone to acute, isolated tears in the white zone and through degenerative intrameniscal tissue. The type of tear

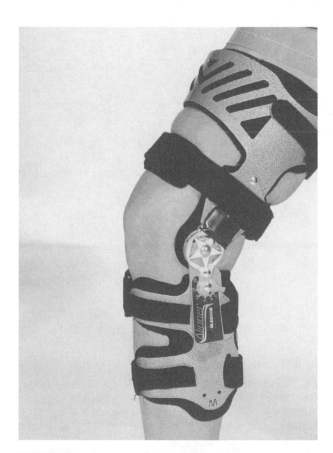

Figure 6-16 PCL brace. Note the suprapatellar strap used to stabilize the femur and prevent posterior displacement on the tibia.

CLINICAL PRESENTATION

History

Shearing or torsional forces through the knee
Pain along the joint line
The patient may describe giving way or locking of the joint.
Meniscal tears should be suspected with an acute ACL injury.

Observation

A joint effusion is common with a medial meniscal tear but less common with a lateral meniscal tear.
The patient with a locked knee lies on the examination table with the knee flexed.

Functional Status

Weight bearing may be limited by pain and the sensation of instability.
ROM may not be limited unless the knee is locked.
Full flexion is usually painful as the meniscus is compressed between the articular surfaces.

Physical Evaluation Findings

The joint line is painful to palpation. Typically, posterior joint-line pain on the medial side reflects a medial meniscal tear, and middle joint-line pain on the lateral side indicates a lateral meniscal tear. Pain along the anterior joint line may be related to patellofemoral injury.[37,40]
Positive McMurray test; however, test reliability is low
Positive Apley compression/distraction test

sustained by the meniscus is the major determinant of the surgical procedure used (**Figure 6-18**). The tear configuration also dictates the physician's repair choice. Complex tears, or tears that occur in multiple planes, are not generally conducive to repair.

Medial meniscal injuries tend to cause more symptoms than those of the lateral meniscus.[37] Most medial meniscal tears occur in the posterior portion, causing pain with weight bearing. Medial meniscal tears are more common in chronic ACL-deficient knees and more amenable to repair.[37,38] Lateral meniscal tears are more common in acute ACL injuries.[38] The lateral meniscus is more mobile than the medial meniscus, leading to an increased number of insidious-onset tears.

Because of the important role of the meniscus, tissue preservation is attempted whenever possible. Loss of meniscal tissue decreases the contact surface area and increases the peak local contact stress on the joint surfaces.[39] Over time, loss of meniscal tissue can lead to an earlier onset of arthritis.

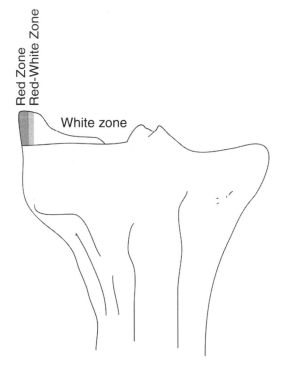

Figure 6-17 Vascular zones of the meniscus. The red zone formed by the outer 10% to 30% of the meniscus has sufficient blood supply to permit healing. The large white zone is avascular, and healing is not possible. The red-white zone is partially vascularized and has limited healing potential.

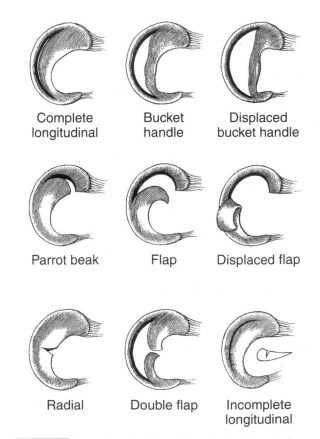

Figure 6-18 Types of meniscal tears. (Reproduced with permission from Tria AJ, Klein KS: *An Illustrated Guide to the Knee.* New York, NY, Churchill Livingstone, 1992.)

Differential Diagnosis

Patellofemoral syndrome, symptomatic synovial plica, osteochondritis dissecans, loose body, chondral fracture, ligamentous injury

Medical Diagnostic Tests

Positive MRI findings

Imaging Techniques

Standard radiographs should be obtained to rule out osteochondral fracture or osteochondritis dissecans. Narrowed joint space, the Fairbank sign, may be associated with osteophyte formation.[41] MRI is more than 90% accurate in detecting acute meniscal tears but less reliable in detecting degenerative tears.[42,43] MRI is not accurate in determining repair potential.[39] False-negative findings are most common in smaller peripheral tears that are conducive to repair.[39] MRI can also detect asymptomatic tears that do not require surgery (**Figure 6-19**).

Definitive Diagnosis

The definitive diagnosis is based on the history and mechanism considered with other signs, such as joint-line pain with palpation, pain with flexion, and a positive McMurray test with associated clinical findings. MRI is helpful in the conclusive diagnosis of meniscal injury.

A sensation of giving way may be related to quadriceps inhibition or weakness from a variety of knee ailments. A meniscal tear should be suspected when true giving way or buckling of the knee is described. Although many patients may describe locking, true locking is the inability to completely extend the knee. This may be transient and related to a bucket-handle tear of the meniscus that wedges between the articular surfaces.

Pathomechanics and Functional Limitations

Patients complain of pain with weight-bearing and squatting activities. Acute meniscal tears may be more functionally limiting due to pain and joint effusion. Pain occurs with deep flexion and/or twisting activities.

▨ Immediate Management

The patient should be removed from activity, and ice applied to the knee. If the patient cannot tolerate weight bearing, crutches are needed until further clinical workup is completed and the extent of the injury is ascertained.

▨ Medications

NSAIDs are useful.

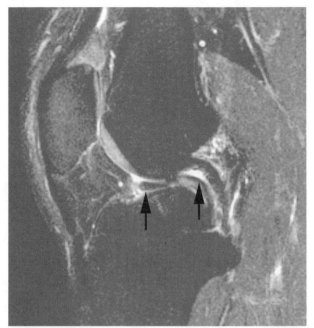
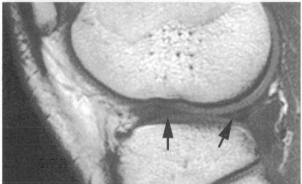
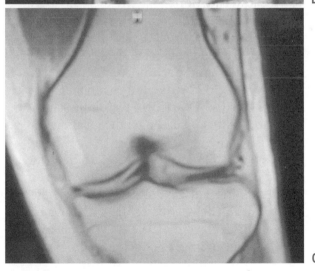

Figure 6-19 MRI of meniscal tears. **A.** The darkened areas of the meniscus (arrows) are consistent with a displaced bucket-handle tear on a sagittal MRI. **B.** Sagittal view demonstrating tears of the anterior and posterior horns of the lateral meniscus. **C.** Coronal view of bucket handle tear. (**A** and **B** are reproduced with permission from Johnson TR, Steinbach LS (eds): *Essentials of Musculoskeletal Imaging*. Rosemont, IL, American Academy of Orthopaedic Surgeons, 2004, p 553.)

Postinjury Management

If the knee is locked or unstable, the patient needs the protection afforded by using crutches. A locked knee requires immediate surgery so that no further damage is sustained. If a meniscal tear is suspected but the knee is not locked, the patient should be allowed pain-free function with normal ADLs. If pain or a sensation of giving way is experienced, crutches are helpful until the knee becomes asymptomatic.

Conservative treatment is usually indicated in the patient with an intact ACL and a stable meniscal tear. Treatment includes rehabilitation to strengthen the entire lower extremity, followed by a progressive return to more stressful weight-bearing activities. Patients who begin or continue to experience mechanical symptoms are candidates for surgery.

Surgical Intervention

Partial meniscectomy involves arthroscopic removal of unstable or symptomatic torn tissues (**ST** 6-7). Tears within the avascular zone that are more complex, involve numerous cleavages within the tear, change the contour of the meniscal body, or are degenerative may not be repairable.[39] These tears are removed so that a smooth surface is left for femoral condyle contact. The surgeon preserves as much tissue as possible to decrease the risk of joint degeneration.

Tears in the outer third and some tears in the middle third of the meniscus may be non-repairable, especially a complex tear that extends into the avascular zone in patients younger than 20 years.[44] Partial meniscectomy would necessitate removal of a large portion of the meniscus, resulting in loss of meniscal function and a greater risk of arthritis. A variety of techniques are available for the surgeon based on the location and extent of the repair (**ST** 6-8).

In an unstable knee, the rate of successful meniscal repair along with ACL reconstruction is higher than that of isolated meniscal repair.[45,46] The stability provided by the reconstruction and the hemarthrosis created by the ACL reconstruction may produce a more conducive healing environment for the meniscal repair.[47,48]

Meniscal transplantations are being used on a limited basis, and the surgical techniques are still being refined. They are technically demanding and not routinely offered as surgical options. However, in patients who have had a subtotal to total meniscectomy, this option is attractive in preventing degenerative changes. Cadaver menisci must be matched in size to ensure appropriate function. The meniscal allograft is harvested and implanted with bone plugs attaching to the anterior and posterior meniscal horns. The allograft is then firmly sutured along its periphery to ensure stability.

Postoperative Management

The meniscal repair must be protected in the early healing phases. The patient is placed in a hinged brace, non–weight bearing, for 1 week and then progressed to full weight bearing with the brace locked in extension. The brace is discontinued when the patient has full ROM and demonstrates normal leg control by being able to straight-leg raise without a lag, walk normally, and perform stair climbing in a normal step-over-step manner.

Injury-Specific Treatment and Rehabilitation Concerns

> **Specific Concerns**
>
> Avoid early weight-bearing flexion.
> Emphasize early low-impact activities.

Conservative Rehabilitation

Initial treatment focuses on controlling inflammation with ice and therapeutic exercise. Active or active-assisted ROM exercises such as heel slides are used. When adequate ROM is obtained, low-impact activity such as bicycling, elliptical gliding, and aquatic exercise can be initiated. The hip, quadriceps, and hamstrings are strengthened. At first, these exercises are performed in an open chain, progressing to weight-bearing strengthening exercises when pain abates. Weight-bearing activities such as the stair stepper and treadmill can be added gradually.

When strength is within normal limits, the patient can complete agility drills, beginning with controlled tasks such as forward and backward running and side shuffling. More complex activities such as figure-of-8 and jumping and cutting drills are introduced as tolerated.

Partial Meniscectomy

Using crutches, the patient bears partial weight until pain and inflammation are controlled, typically in 3 to 4 days. Subsequent treatment is similar to the conservative treatment for meniscal tears. Flexion is not forced early in rehabilitation so that residual soreness does not worsen.

Meniscal Repair

The knee is immobilized, non–weight bearing. Passive ROM begins immediately with a limit of 90° of flexion until approximately 4 weeks after surgery to avoid compressing the meniscal repair and then progresses to full flexion. Full, immediate mo-

Partial Menisectomy

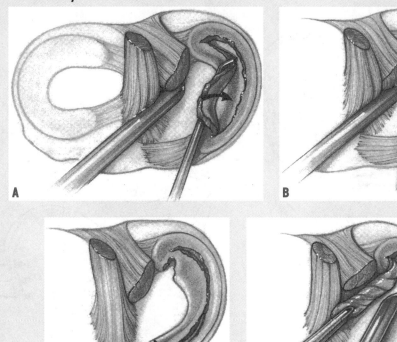

Indications

A meniscal tear location and configuration not conducive to repair; therefore, the unattached segment must be removed

Overview

1. Arthroscopic portals are made anteromedial and anterolateral to the patellar tendon at joint line. Inflow portal is superomedial or superolateral to the patella.
2. The meniscus is visualized, and a nonrepairable tear (a tear within the white zone or a radial tear communicating with the free edge of the meniscus) is identified (**A**).
3. The tear is debrided to a smooth margin using various biters and shavers (**B**).
4. A smooth, stable rim margin is made, sculpting the borders of the tear to form a smooth transition between the remaining portion of the meniscus (**C**).
5. The excised portion of the meniscus is removed (**D**).

Functional Limitations

Early motion limitations are secondary to the trauma of the arthroscopy and swelling. Early strength deficits are secondary to VMO inhibition from the joint distention and arthroscopic trauma.

Implications for Rehabilitation

The more tissue removed, the more compromised the shock absorption, and the greater the stresses that will be transferred to the articular surfaces. Early motion and progressive resistance exercises allow the patient to regain function quickly.

Figures reproduced with permission from Canale ST (ed): *Campbell's Operative Orthopaeics*, ed 9. St. Louis, MO, Mosby-Year Book, 1998.

tion and weight bearing have also demonstrated good results.[49-51]

Motor-level electrical stimulation along with concurrent voluntary exercise is used for reeducating the quadriceps. Straight-leg raises are performed in all planes except extension. Quadriceps exercises are started when the patient can fully recruit the muscle and perform straight-leg raises without a lag. Light hamstring exercises with cuff weights are not begun until 4 weeks after surgery.

S|T Surgical Technique 6-8

Meniscal Repair

Indications

Mechanical symptoms of a meniscal tear, positive clinical examination, and positive findings on MRI

Overview

Several methods are available for meniscal repair. In all methods, the rim of the tear should be abraded to create bleeding and an environment more conducive to healing.

Inside-Out Meniscal Repair
1. A small posteromedial or posterolateral incision is made.
2. Sutures are placed through the inner rim of the tear and out through the outer tear rim and the joint capsule.
3. The sutures are tensioned, and the tear is probed. If stably reduced, the sutures are tied over the joint capsule.

Outside-In Meniscal Repair (shown)
1. A small posteromedial or posterolateral incision is made.
2. A spinal needle is placed through the joint capsule and across the tear (**A** and **B**).
3. Sutures are passed through the needle and tied down to secure the tear (**C** and **D**).
4. The outside-in technique may be preferred when the surgeon wants better control passing needles and sutures near the neurovascular bundles. These structures can be retracted and the needles and sutures passed.

All-Inside Repair
1. The all-inside technique is specifically for posterior horn tears.
2. A special 70° arthroscope is advanced into the posterior compartment.
3. Sutures are placed and tied without piercing the posterior capsule, protecting the posterior neurovascular structures.

Functional Limitations

Limitations in weight bearing and deep flexion are often prescribed postoperatively to protect the repair. No impact activities should be permitted during the healing of the meniscal repair.

Implications for Rehabilitation

Protected motion and weight bearing naturally slow the rehabilitation process.

Comments

Biodegradable surgical "darts" and "arrows" have been used in place of sutures to repair the meniscus. However, these materials can dislodge and float in the joint, causing pain and dysfunction.

Figure reproduced with permission from Hanks GA, Kalenek A: Alternative arthroscopic techniques for meniscal repair: A review. *Orthop Rev* 1990;19:541-548.

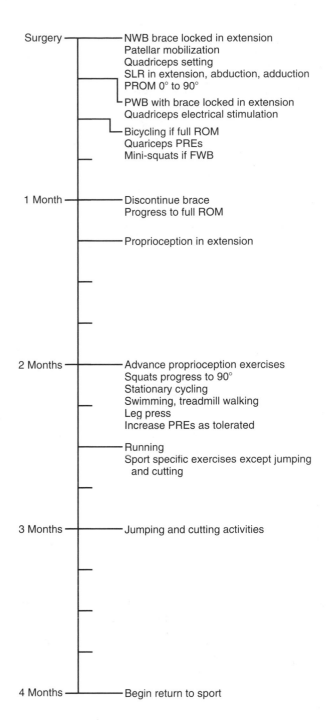

Surgery — NWB brace locked in extension
Patellar mobilization
Quadriceps setting
SLR in extension, abduction, adduction
PROM 0° to 90°

— PWB with brace locked in extension
Quadriceps electrical stimulation

— Bicycling if full ROM
Quariceps PREs
Mini-squats if FWB

1 Month — Discontinue brace
Progress to full ROM

— Proprioception in extension

2 Months — Advance proprioception exercises
Squats progress to 90°
Stationary cycling
Swimming, treadmill walking
Leg press
Increase PREs as tolerated

— Running
Sport specific exercises except jumping
and cutting

3 Months — Jumping and cutting activities

4 Months — Begin return to sport

Note: Time frames are approximate. Function is the guide.

The patient can transition to heavier weights with machines at 6 weeks as the repair heals further. Light closed chain activities such as minisquats and wall slides start when weight bearing is full. More stressful activities such as the leg press and deeper squatting to 60° can be introduced at 8 weeks.

Bicycling exercises may commence when ROM is adequate. Other activities that include weight bearing start at 8 weeks, with running and a progression of functional activities instituted at 10 weeks. Activities involving jumping and cutting are allowed at 12 weeks and are advanced carefully.

■ Estimated Amount of Time Lost

Conservative treatment of smaller peripheral tears may require 2 to 6 weeks before activity can be resumed. A patient with a partial meniscectomy may miss 4 to 6 weeks of activity. Time lost after meniscal repair ranges from 10 weeks[50] to 6 months.[52]

With conservative treatment, smaller peripheral tears on the medial side quickly become asymptomatic relative to the lateral side. The aggressiveness of the rehabilitation program for a repaired meniscus is the determining factor regarding the time lost after surgery.[50]

■ Return-to-Play Criteria

The patient can return to play when sport-specific drills can be completed and the knee is relatively asymptomatic. Both good function and confident use of the knee should be demonstrated before the athlete returns to full competition. A knee sleeve may be helpful in the management of meniscal injuries to enhance joint warmth.

Distal Femur and Proximal Tibia Fractures

CLINICAL PRESENTATION

History

The mechanism is usually a high-energy force.
Distal femur and tibial plateau fractures are usually the result of axial compression with varus or valgus force.
Medial tibial plateau fractures usually involve a varus force, whereas lateral tibial plateau fractures usually involve a valgus force.
Immediate pain

Observation

Joint effusion in intra-articular fractures
More generalized swelling from extra-articular fractures
Deformity may be noted in severe fractures.
Skin integrity should be checked to rule out an open fracture.

Functional Status

Immediate inability to bear weight due to pain
Depending on fracture severity and displacement, partial ROM may be possible.

Physical Evaluation Findings

Although ligaments may be concurrently injured, a thorough examination may be contraindicated by the presence of the fracture.
Distal pulses and nerve function should be thoroughly assessed.

Fractures of the distal femur or proximal tibia rarely occur in sports because high-velocity forces are required to cause these injuries in young, healthy individuals. These fractures can be extra- or intra-articular. In skeletally immature patients, lower-velocity forces can fracture the growth plate.

Distal femur fractures are classified as supracondylar, intercondylar, or a combination (**Figure 6-20**). Proximal tibia fractures are commonly described as fractures of the medial or lateral tibial plateau with a fracture through the bone or a depressed fracture in the tibial plateau. Tibial plateau fractures are described using the Schatzker classification. Types I through III are associated with low-velocity forces, whereas types IV through VI are associated with high-energy forces (**Figure 6-21**).

Intra-articular fractures must be treated to minimize the long-term effects on the articular surfaces. Restoring a normal articular surface is essential for proper joint function and minimizing early post-traumatic arthritic changes.

Soft-tissue injuries should be suspected in fractures about the knee. Ligamentous injuries occur in approximately 20% of tibial plateau fractures, with the ACL and lateral meniscus most often involved.[53,54]

Differential Diagnosis

Ligament disruption, extensor-mechanism disruption, tibiofemoral dislocation

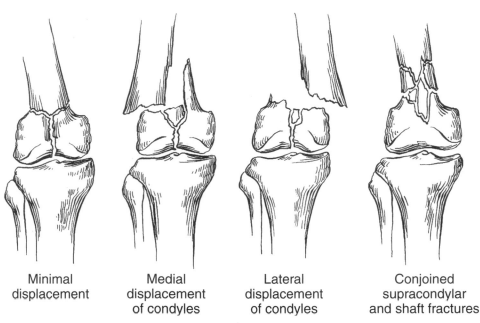

Minimal displacement   Medial displacement of condyles   Lateral displacement of condyles   Conjoined supracondylar and shaft fractures

Figure 6-20 Classification of femoral condyle fractures. (Reproduced with permission from Greene WB (ed): *Essentials of Musculoskeletal Care*, ed 2. Rosemont, IL, American Academy of Orthopaedic Surgeons, 2000, pp 376.)

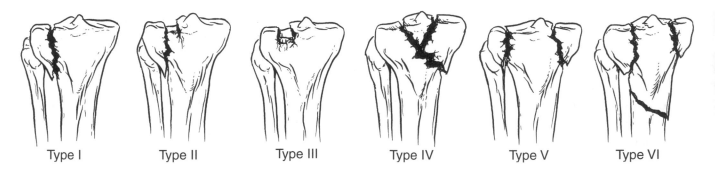

Type I   Type II   Type III   Type IV   Type V   Type VI

Figure 6-21 The Schatzker classification of tibial plateau fractures. Type I, wedge (split) fracture of the lateral tibial plateau; Type II, split depression fracture of the lateral plateau; Type III, pure central-depression fracture of the lateral plateau without an associated split; Type IV, fracture of the medial tibial plateau, usually involving the entire condyle; Type V, bicondylar fracture, consisting of split fractures of both the medial and lateral plateaus without articular depression; and Type VI, tibial plateau fracture with an associated proximal shaft fracture. (Reproduced with permission from Koval KJ, Helfet DL: Tibial plateau fractures: Evaluation and treatment. *J Am Acad Orthop Surg* 1995;3:86-94.)

Medical Diagnostic Tests

Fat droplets within the hemarthrosis confirm the breach of the bony cortex (see p 116 for a description of the aspiration technique).

Imaging Techniques

Standard AP and lateral radiographs are obtained to determine the presence and extent of the fracture configuration. Radiographs taken at internal and external oblique angles of 40° are used to profile the condyles[55] (**Figure 6-22**).

Computed tomography is used to assess the extent of articular depression and/or fracture lines and for surgical planning. MRI is helpful in imaging suspected soft-tissue injury.

Definitive Diagnosis

Radiologic findings confirm the diagnosis of distal femur and proximal tibia fractures.

Pathomechanics and Functional Limitations

Most patients experience an immediate inability to ambulate secondary to pain and instability. With the accumulation of the joint effusion, extension and flexion are lost.

■ Immediate Management

The extremity should be splinted in the position in which it is found and the patient immediately transported to the emergency room. Distal pulses are checked and serially monitored. Motor and sensory function of the tibial and peroneal branches of the sciatic nerve should be assessed. The patient is evaluated for the presence or threat of an acute compartment syndrome (see p 116). Other trauma should be ruled out.

■ Medications

These injuries require acute pain management with narcotic analgesics and NSAIDs. Deep vein thrombosis prophylaxis may need to be considered, especially in patients requiring extended periods of immobilization and activity restrictions.

■ Postinjury Management

Nondisplaced or minimally displaced and stable tibial plateau fractures can be treated nonsurgically in a controlled-motion brace, strictly non–weight bearing. The fracture should be radiographically assessed weekly for the first 3 weeks to ensure that it has remained reduced and stable.

■ Surgical Intervention

Displaced fractures may require open reduction and internal fixation to restore joint alignment and congruity.[55,56] The amount of articular depression that requires surgical intervention is controversial; surgical intervention for depressions greater than 3 mm has been recommended in athletes.[57]

Arthroscopically assisted reduction of depressed tibial plateau fractures is an effective treatment method in athletes.[54,58,59] The fracture and concomitant soft-tissue damage can be better visualized intra-articularly without a large incision and dissection of soft tissues around the knee. Depressed fractures are reduced through a small incision over the tibia. Using guides placed arthroscopically, the surgeon can then elevate the depressed fracture with bone tamps placed through the small distal incision. Once elevated, the defect is packed with **corticocancellous** bone chips.

Corticocancellous
The cortex of spongy bone.

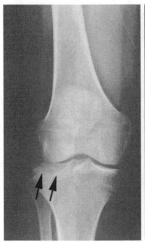
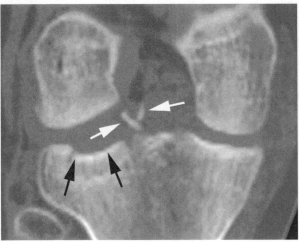
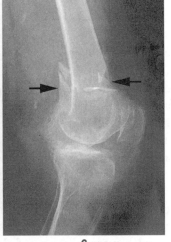

A   **B**   **C**

Figure 6-22   Imaging of fractures about the knee. **A.** Radiograph of a depressed fracture of the lateral tibial plateau. **B.** Computed tomographic scan of a depressed fracture of the lateral tibial plateau and associated tibial spine avulsion (white arrows) suggesting an associated cruciate ligament injury. **C.** Lateral radiograph of a supracondylar fracture of the femur. (Reproduced with permission from Johnson TR, Steinbach LS (eds): *Essentials of Musculoskeletal Imaging*. Rosemont, IL, American Academy of Orthopaedic Surgeons, 2004, p 501.)

Distal femur fractures require open reduction with internal fixation. The fractures are usually angulated, and joint congruity is disrupted. The fracture is fixated with intermedullary nails or a supracondylar plate with interfragmentary screws.

■ Postoperative Management

Patients with nondisplaced and minimally displaced tibial plateau fractures or arthroscopically assisted reductions of depressed tibial plateau fractures can initially be placed in a locked, hinged knee brace. After 3 to 4 weeks, the brace can be unlocked for ROM exercises. The patient remains non–weight bearing for 4 to 6 weeks.

The patient with stable internal fixation may begin CPM immediately. Active quadriceps and hamstrings exercises can start about 2 days after surgery. Minimal weight bearing can commence at 3 to 5 days, depending on fixation stability. Toe-touch weight bearing continues for about 2 to 3 months, until radiographs demonstrate adequate healing. Weight bearing is progressively increased until solid union is achieved.

External support is not required unless there is concomitant ligamentous injury or a question of fixation stability.

■ Injury-Specific Treatment and Rehabilitation Concerns

Specific Concerns

Achieve adequate fracture healing in anatomic position with maintenance of articular congruity.
Protect the healing bone.
Restore full patellar motion and knee ROM.

Although fractures about the knee must be protected, the benefits of early joint motion are considered in the rehabilitation process. Fracture management needs to provide stabilization so that passive motion can be introduced as soon as possible. Patellar mobilization is performed to restore normal joint biomechanics. Scar massage and mobilization are used after distal femur fracture surgery, because many times soft-tissue trauma and/or surgical scars cause soft-tissue contractures. Quadriceps and hamstrings stretching is important. Prone quadriceps stretching enhances normal knee flexion with internally fixated distal femur fractures; the quadriceps may have been disrupted by the fracture trauma, the surgical procedure, or the fixation plate lying underneath the quadriceps. If the quadriceps was disrupted during the surgical fixation, it must be allowed to heal adequately before tissue stretching begins.

Active lower extremity exercises are begun as early as possible, 3 to 4 weeks after injury for non-surgically treated tibial plateau fractures. The ability to begin active exercises is actually aided with stable internal fixation. Heavy progressive resistance exercises are not introduced until adequate clinical and radiographic healing is demonstrated.

As the patient advances to full weight bearing, proprioception exercises are instituted.

■ Estimated Amount of Time Lost

Patients with tibial plateau fractures may be able to return to activity approximately 3 months after the injury if the fracture was minimally displaced. Tibial plateau fractures that required open reduction and internal fixation will require longer recovery because of prolonged weight-bearing restrictions. Distal femur fractures typically take 6 to 12 months before patients can return to full participation in sports.[57]

Surgical fixation of some fractures may speed injury recovery time. Once stabilized, these fractures can be more aggressively rehabilitated with protected weight bearing.

■ Return-to-Play Criteria

Complete fracture healing must be demonstrated radiographically. The knee must be pain free with functional ROM and adequate return of strength. The patient should be able to successfully perform lower extremity functional tests.

Tibiofemoral Dislocation

The tibiofemoral, or knee, dislocation is arguably the most serious knee injury in athletics, posing significant risk of injury to the popliteal artery and peroneal nerve that could lead to the loss of the lower leg. Fortunately, this is rare in athletes. Knee dislocations also present challenges to rehabilitation. They can occur from either high- or low-velocity forces. Low-velocity injuries are more common in sports; high-velocity injuries are typical in motor vehicle, industrial, and water-skiing accidents.

Knee dislocations can occur in any direction, but most occur posteriorly. In some cases, the knee may spontaneously relocate, making timely recognition of the injury more difficult. Any injury to three or more of the knee's major ligaments (ACL, PCL, MCL, LCL) should be regarded as a knee dis-

CLINICAL PRESENTATION

History

A common sport mechanism involves a posteriorly directed force through the tibia, similar to that of a PCL injury.

Extreme pain is experienced, with immediate inability to move the leg.

A cold sensation in the foot is reported if lower leg blood flow is compromised.

Paresthesia in the associated nerve distribution may be noted with a peroneal or tibial nerve injury.

Observation

Gross malalignment of, and swelling in, the dislocated knee

Large amount of swelling in the spontaneously relocated knee

Functional Status

Immediate inability to move the leg secondary to the dislocation and pain

Inability to bear weight

Physical Evaluation Findings

Positive ligamentous tests in the spontaneously reduced knee

Absence of dorsalis pedus and/or posterior tibial pulse with vascular injury; initially present pulses need to be serially checked for changes.

Diminished function of the peroneal (toe extension) and/or tibial (toe flexion) branches of the sciatic nerve. Nerve function should be serially examined for several days after the injury.

location, even if the joint surfaces are aligned at the initial evaluation.[60,61] Different combinations of ligamentous injury occur, but the ACL and PCL are always torn when the knee dislocates.[61] Knee dislocations often produce concurrent damage to the joint capsule, menisci, articular surfaces, and muscles and tendons surrounding the knee and threaten the neurovascular structures that cross the joint.

Vascular injury has been estimated to occur in 32% of all knee dislocations; the rate is slightly higher (40%) for anterior or posterior dislocations.[62] The popliteal artery is vulnerable to injury from knee dislocation because of its close proximity to the posterior tibia and its limited mobility.[60] The artery is subject to a tension mechanism with an anterior dislocation or direct trauma from the tibial plateau during a posterior dislocation. Arterial injury can range from an intimal flap tear to total disruption. Careful assessment of the vascular supply is essential, because distal extremity circulation must be restored within 6 to 8 hours. Amputation rates as high as 85% have been reported when vascular damage has not been treated within this time frame.[62]

The peroneal nerve is also at risk of injury. The incidence has been estimated to be about 25%.[60] The nerve may be more at risk with lateral or posterolateral injuries. The tibial nerve may also be injured.

Acute compartment syndrome must be considered. Prolonged dislocation or transection of the popliteal artery further complicates this medical emergency.

Differential Diagnosis

Displaced femur or tibia fracture, dislocated patella, isolated ligament injury

Medical Diagnostic Tests

Doppler pressure measurements are more accurate in assessing vascular status than the physical examination and correlate well with arteriographic findings.[60] However, false-negative results may occur in cases of intimal tears.

Imaging Techniques

Standard radiographic views confirm the dislocation and document intra-articular or periarticular fractures (**Figure 6-23**). Arteriograms must be performed in all suspected and known knee dislocations (**Figure 6-24**). MRI should be obtained to assess the associated soft-tissue structures after the patient's vascular status has been adequately evaluated and immediately treated.

Definitive Diagnosis

Obvious visible signs of dislocation, positive radiographic findings, three or more positive major ligamentous tests on clinical examination

Pathomechanics and Functional Limitations

Patients are immediately limited in function due to gross ligamentous instability.

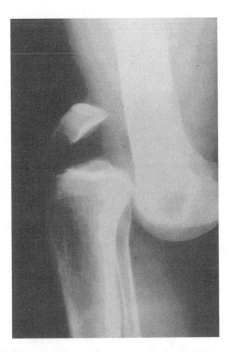

Figure 6-23 Lateral view of a typical anterior dislocation of the knee. (Reproduced with permission from Good L, Johnson RJ: The dislocated knee. *J Am Acad Orthop Surg* 1995;3:284-292.)

Intimal Relating to the innermost membrane of the vessel.

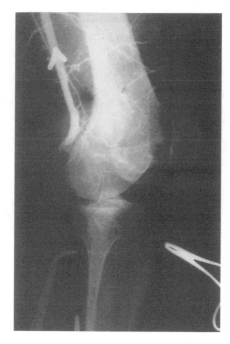

Figure 6-24 Intraoperative arteriogram demonstrates disruption of the popliteal artery just above the knee after a posterior dislocation. (Reproduced with permission from Good L, Johnson RJ: The dislocated knee. *J Am Acad Orthop Surg* 1995;3:284-292.)

Immediate Management

The leg should be splinted before the patient is moved, and the patient should be transported to the hospital as quickly as possible. While awaiting transport to the hospital, a physician can attempt a single, immediate reduction unless there is a suspected posterolateral dislocation.[63,64] These dislocations have a high incidence of medial joint-capsule interposition and should be reduced surgically to minimize the risk of skin necrosis.[63,64] If the reduction attempt fails on the first try, the leg should be splinted and the patient immediately transported. The patient is monitored for the onset of shock.

Medications

These injuries are painful and require the use of narcotic analgesics such as morphine or meperidine via intramuscular injection or intravenously. Later, NSAIDs may be indicated. Muscle relaxants may be employed with significant muscle disruption.

Surgical Intervention

Arterial injury, a dislocation that will not reduce, an open dislocation, or acute compartment syndrome are indications for immediate surgery. Addressing vascular disruption or a compartment syndrome takes precedence over the surgical re-

construction of other aspects of the knee. The additional trauma from the ligament surgery could increase compartment swelling, and the fasciotomy could pose a higher risk of infection. The risk of infection with open dislocation is too high to warrant inserting foreign material into the knee at an early stage.

After vascular repair, the repair should not be moved or stretched. With an intact vascular status and no open dislocation or risk of acute compartment syndrome, thorough evaluation of the ligaments and nerves is mandated. Rehabilitation aggressiveness is determined on a case-by-case basis by the vascular and orthopaedic surgeons.

If immediate surgical intervention is not needed, many experts believe that a delayed surgical approach to restore knee stability is preferable to conservative treatment of a knee dislocation.[61,65,66] However, the exact surgical procedure to perform and the timing of surgery are subjects of considerable controversy.

Some authors have proposed not reconstructing the ACL, whereas others recommend reconstructing the cruciates as essential to a functional, stable knee.[61,66] Although the concern over developing arthrofibrosis is real and favors delaying surgery at least 3 weeks, the ability to adequately repair the medial, lateral, and posterolateral structures becomes increasingly difficult after 2 weeks. Reestablishing posterolateral corner continuity has the highest priority and must be undertaken in a timely manner.

In the absence of overwhelming evidence to support increased symptoms related to arthrofibrosis when concomitant repairs and reconstructions are performed, surgical repair or reconstruction should be considered for all torn ligaments.[60] To minimize additional knee trauma, allografts should be considered. Because the lateral and posterolateral structures must be repaired to establish a stable joint, the surgical procedure should be performed after 2 weeks but no more than 3 weeks from the time of the initial injury.

The treatment of nerve injuries in dislocated knees remains controversial. If possible, a surgeon with expertise in nerve grafting should be available. A macroscopically intact nerve should not be treated except by careful serial assessments of function. If needed, nerve grafting using the sural nerve may be attempted, or the nerve may be tagged for later exploration if appropriate.

The patient should be prepared for a staged procedure, in which a series of surgeries is performed to address the neurologic, vascular, and musculoskeletal trauma. If the lateral corner is being addressed with nerve grafting, further surgery may be conducted after the lateral structures heal.

Postinjury/Postoperative Management

Postoperative management depends on secure fixation of repaired or reconstructed tissues. Mild instability is often preferred to an overly stiff knee; therefore, early motion is encouraged even if some instability might occur. In the presence of stable surgical treatment, bracing and mobilization should be as aggressive as possible to decrease the likelihood of stiffness. A hinged knee brace and CPM are advocated. The patient keeps the brace locked for ambulation until adequate quadriceps strength has returned and ROM is restored. However, vascular and/or nerve grafting may require prolonged motion protection with a locked brace to ensure healing and prevent traction on the repairs.

If fixation security is in question, the brace may be locked in extension and ROM advanced after healing progresses. Arthrofibrosis is the primary postsurgical complication, and measures to decrease stiffness should be made as soon as it is recognized.

Injury-Specific Treatment and Rehabilitation Concerns

Specific Concerns

Protect vascular and nerve graft repairs.
Minimize arthrofibrosis.
Reestablish joint stability.
Restore patellar mobility.
Regain ROM.
Restore motor function.

After a knee dislocation, the return to sports activities, while still possible, is secondary to less aggressive goals such as the return to normal ADLs. The patient with a knee dislocation is at great risk for arthrofibrosis, leading to significant loss of ROM.

Edema about the knee also affects ROM. Intermittent compression devices should only be used if the possibility of compartment syndrome has been ruled out. Elevation and active exercise through muscle pumping and edema-reduction massage are helpful. A compression stocking or elastic wrap helps to control edema between treatment sessions.

Early motion is advocated to minimize arthrofibrosis. Patellar mobilizations in all directions and passive and active-assisted ROM are beneficial. The surgeon should establish the safe ROM for the early rehabilitation stages. Less aggressive motion in certain ranges may be preferred, depending on tissue strength at the time of surgical repair or reconstruction.

Significant loss of quadriceps function should be anticipated. Motor-level electrical stimulation can be used to stimulate the quadriceps muscles until volitional contractions produce sufficient tension.

The surgical procedure dictates the manner in which rehabilitation proceeds. If the ACL was reconstructed, a timeline similar to that for isolated ACL reconstruction can be instituted for strengthening exercises. If the PCL was also reconstructed, isolated PCL reconstruction guidelines should take precedence.

Proprioceptive exercises are essential for the patient with a knee dislocation. Simple proprioceptive exercises, such as single-leg stance on a hard stationary surface, can begin as soon as the patient is bearing full weight and has adequate leg control. The patient may initially benefit from a functional knee brace while performing these exercises. More dynamic proprioceptive exercises can be introduced as the patient demonstrates adequate muscular control to safely perform the exercise with minimal risk to the surgical repair.

Estimated Amount of Time Lost

Substantial time is lost from sports activity. The rehabilitation process takes 6 to 12 months or more, depending on injury severity, vascular involvement, and neurologic status.

Vascular injury, compartment syndrome, and impaired neurologic status increase the time lost. Return to competition may not be practical for many patients.

Return-to-Play Criteria

A full return to playing sports at preparticipation levels is difficult secondary to loss of ROM, possible instability, and dysfunction from nerve injury. Patients must demonstrate sufficient ROM, strength, and proprioception to perform at adequate levels without placing themselves at risk for further injury. A custom functional knee brace designed to accommodate the patient's specific injury pattern is typically used.

Iliotibial Band Friction Syndrome

Iliotibial band (ITB) friction syndrome is a localized inflammation of the ITB fascia or the knee joint capsule synovium. The inflammation is created by friction as the ITB passes over the lateral femoral condyle during repetitive activities (**Figure 6-25**). This syndrome is most commonly seen in runners and cyclists.[67-69] Pain is localized over the lateral femoral condyle and may present at a specific distance or duration of the causative activity (see Trochanteric Bursitis, p 230).

Differential Diagnosis

Symptomatic synovial plica, lateral meniscal tear, patellofemoral syndrome, popliteal tendinitis

Imaging Techniques

None are usually required.

Definitive Diagnosis

Pain at or near the lateral femoral epicondyle during foot strike relieved with activity cessation; positive Noble compression test

Pathomechanics and Functional Limitations

Pain usually begins predictably after a specific time or distance into running and is localized over the lateral femoral condyle. Pain significantly improves when the patient stops activity but returns quickly if activity is resumed.

▦ Immediate Management

The patient should cease all activity and apply ice over the ITB.

CLINICAL PRESENTATION

History

Insidious onset
Repetitive activity causing the ITB to rub over the lateral femoral condyle between 20° and 30° of knee flexion as the foot strikes the ground[70]
Downhill running exacerbates the syndrome.

Observation

Genu varum and hyperpronation may be predisposing lower extremity postures.

Functional Status

A stiff knee gait may be assumed to avoid rubbing the ITB over the condyle.
Active and passive ROM is normal.
Resisted knee extension may elicit pain at 20° to 30°.

Physical Evaluation Findings

Positive Noble compression test
Positive Ober test
True leg-length discrepancy may be present.

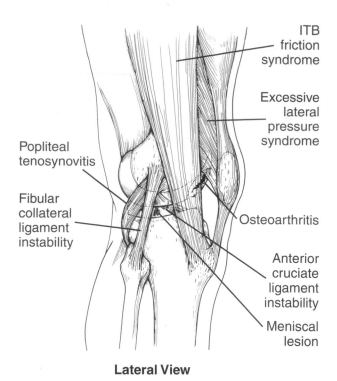

Lateral View

Figure 6-25 Inflammation of the ITB where it passes over the lateral femoral condyle can cause ITB friction syndrome. Other causes of lateral knee pain are also indicated. (Reproduced with permission from James SL: Running injuries to the knee. *J Am Acad Orthop Surg* 1995;3:309-318.)

▦ Medications

Oral NSAIDs are useful. Patients with symptoms that are initially resistant to NSAIDs, therapeutic modalities, and exercise may require a corticosteroid injection. Iontophoresis with dexamethasone (4 mg in 1-cm² suspension) and lidocaine (4% in 2-cm² suspension) can also be helpful in the early management of ITB friction syndrome.

▦ Surgical Intervention

Surgical intervention, which is rarely necessary, consists of surgical resection of only the portion of the ITB that impinges on the femoral condyle—typically the posterior 2 cm of the ITB at the condyle level.[67,68,71]

▦ Postinjury/Postoperative Management

Conservative management consists of oral NSAIDs, rehabilitation, and avoidance of aggravating activities. Ice and ITB and hamstring stretching are indicated. Patients with genu varum, true leg-length discrepancy, and hyperpronation may benefit from orthotics. Strengthening exercises for the trunk, pelvis, and extremity ensure proper biomechanics during activity.[72]

Immediate postsurgical concerns revolve around initiating knee ROM and ITB stretching to minimize scar tissue formation. The patient should perform early passive knee ROM and may resume an aggressive stretching program once wound healing is adequate.

Injury-Specific Treatment and Rehabilitation Concerns

> **Primary Goals**
>
> Eliminate localized inflammatory process.
> Correct abnormal biomechanics.
> Encourage ITB stretching.

Initial rehabilitation focuses on decreasing inflammation. Iontophoresis, ice, and pain-free flexibility exercises may be used.

As the inflammatory process diminishes, rehabilitation addresses restoration of normal length to the tensor fascia latae/ITB complex. Deep friction massage and stretching of the complex are required. Preheating the area enhances the viscoelastic properties of the tissues. Localized adhesions (approximately 10 to 15 cm^2) can be heated using 3-MHz ultrasound at continuous output and sufficient output intensity. Because of the relatively subcutaneous location of the ITB, larger areas can be adequately heated using a moist heat pack.

The ITB partially inserts on the lateral patellar soft tissues. Combining medial patellar mobilization with ITB stretching or electrically induced ITB contractions may be helpful in decreasing tension throughout this area.

Nonaggravating aerobic activities such as bicycling, upper body ergometry, or swimming may be used to maintain cardiovascular conditioning.

A complete lower extremity strengthening program to address the pelvis and thigh musculature is instituted. Functional activities such as step-ups, lunges, and side lunges are essential. Activities focus on proper neuromuscular control of the lower extremity, eliminating postures that may cause the ITB to rub over the lateral femoral condyle. These activities include proper pelvic stabilization, eliminating any contralateral drop of the pelvis as the weight is borne on the affected leg, and effectively stretching the ITB over the condyle.

Control of internal tibial rotation to prevent recurrence may be aided by limiting compensatory pronation with orthotics.

Postsurgical therapeutic interventions can begin in a similar fashion to conservative treatment once wound healing is adequate.

Estimated Amount of Time Lost

Initially, the patient must cease aggravating activities for 1 to 2 weeks while rehabilitating. Symptoms resistant to rehabilitation may require extended periods of time lost, but this is preferable to surgery. The patient may continue other nonaggravating activities such as bicycling or swimming to maintain cardiovascular conditioning. Activities such as tennis and basketball that involve more starting and stopping may be tolerated and can continue as long as the patient is symptom free.

Failure to improve with conservative measures may require surgical release of the ITB, extending the rehabilitation period. After surgery, patients can usually resume running after 4 weeks.[71]

Return-to-Play Criteria

The patient can begin return-to-play activities when symptoms are completely resolved on physical examination, beginning with low mileage and progressing to desired distances as tolerated. Orthotics should continue to be used even after return to full activity.

Popliteal Tendinitis

CLINICAL PRESENTATION

History

Insidious onset
Mechanism of repetitive stress, such as running
Pain in the posterolateral knee

Observation

Foot hyperpronation may be present.
An antalgic gait may occur during the aggravating activity.

Functional Status

Active and passive ROM is normal.
Resisted leg flexion, especially as flexion is initiated from the fully extended position and the tibia is "unscrewed," may cause pain.

Physical Evaluation Findings

Pain during palpation of the popliteus tendon, posterior to the LCL

The popliteal tendon often becomes inflamed concurrently with other knee injuries.[73,74] Because it produces pain over the posterolateral knee, popliteal tendinitis must be differentiated from ITB friction syndrome and lateral meniscal injury. Isolated popliteal tendinitis can occur from repetitive stress, such as running, and may worsen when running downhill.

Differential Diagnosis

ITB friction syndrome, lateral meniscal tear, symptomatic Baker cyst, lateral hamstring tendinitis

Imaging Techniques

MRI is helpful in differentiating between popliteal tendinitis and lateral meniscal derangement if the clinical history and examination are nonspecific.

Definitive Diagnosis

Pain over the popliteus tendon, posterior to the LCL with palpation

Pathomechanics and Functional Limitations

Pain may limit repetitive activity such as running, particularly running downhill.

■ Medications

Oral NSAIDs are useful. Phonophoresis or iontophoresis may be used for recalcitrant symptoms.

■ Postinjury Management

Conservative management consists of oral NSAIDs, rehabilitation, and avoidance of aggravating activities. Compensatory pronation may be controlled with foot orthotics. A heel lift may be used to relieve the acute symptoms and allow inflammation to resolve. Ice and hamstring stretching are also indicated. Strengthening exercises for the trunk, pelvis, and extremities ensure proper biomechanics during activity.

■ Injury-Specific Treatment and Rehabilitation Concerns

> **Specific Concerns**
>
> Eliminate localized inflammatory process.
> Correct abnormal biomechanics.

Initial rehabilitation focuses on decreasing inflammation. Iontophoresis with an anti-inflammatory agent, ice applications, and pain-free flexibility exercises may be used. Normal flexibility and strength of the lower extremities should be restored before the patient begins activities such as running, which place repetitive stresses on the tendon.

Patients should continue with nonaggravating aerobic activities such as the upper body ergometer to maintain cardiovascular conditioning. A heel lift or orthotics may also relieve pain.

■ Estimated Amount of Time Lost

Initially, the patient may need to cease the aggravating activities for 1 to 2 weeks while rehabilitating. Failure to improve with conservative treatment may increase the amount of time lost.

■ Return-to-Play Criteria

The patient can begin return-to-play activities when symptoms are completely resolved. Return to activity begins with low intensity and short time periods of activity and progresses to desired distances and durations as tolerated.

Osteochondral Defect

Chondral and osteochondral injuries can range from a simple contusion to the chondral surface and underlying bone to fractures of these structures.[75] Although other joints can sustain osteochondral injury, the knee is most commonly

---

CLINICAL PRESENTATION

History

Traumatic Mechanism

Shearing forces caused by knee translation or rotation
A compressive force is translated through the joint during landing or falling.
A combination of these forces may be reported.
Repetitive microtraumatic forces placed across the knee might also create an osteochondral lesion:[76] osteochondritis dissecans.
The patient may describe sudden pain. Instability may be reported, especially if the osteochondral injury occurred with an ACL rupture.

Nontraumatic Onset

A history of repetitive activities
Diffuse knee soreness
Increasing pain over time
Intermittent swelling may be reported.
Usually the patient notes that rest greatly improves symptoms. Pain and swelling return with resumption of activities.

Observation

Possible joint effusion
In chronic nontraumatic cases, quadriceps atrophy may be noted.

Functional Status

Depending on the injury location, an antalgic gait may be exhibited.

Physical Evaluation Findings

Positive Wilson sign
Positive ligamentous tests if ligamentous injury is also present
Area of lesion may be tender to palpation.

affected.[76] The mechanism is usually related to trauma, but the trauma may be so minor that it is not recognized at the time of injury. In more severe traumatic incidents of osteochondral injury, an acute hemarthrosis may develop. The osteochondral injury often occurs concomitantly with meniscal or ligamentous injury.

Differential Diagnosis

Meniscal injury, patellofemoral joint dysfunction, ligament sprain, tibial plateau fracture, soft-tissue overuse syndrome, degenerative joint disease

Imaging Techniques

Standard AP and lateral knee radiographs and axial views of the patellofemoral joint can be sensitive enough to diagnose osteochondral injuries. A notch view has been advocated to visualize the lateral aspect of the medial femoral condyle, the typical lesion location[77,78] (**Figure 6-26**).

Tomograms have been recommended as the best method for diagnosis and follow-up management of osteochondral defects.[78] They assess the bony contour and amount of cortical bone present on the osteochondral lesion. The amount of bone on the fragment predicts the healing response. Follow-up tomograms aid in determining the healing response to treatment.

MRI can also be used to diagnose osteochondral defects. An added benefit is the ability of MRI to detect concomitant meniscal and ligamentous injuries. Although MRI may be sensitive enough to determine the size and degree of displacement of the lesion, it may not be sensitive enough to determine the prognosis for healing.

Bone scintigraphy may be helpful in diagnosing and following up osteochondral injuries. It predicts the prognosis of nonsurgical treatment in patients with open physes but is less reliable in those with closed physes.[79]

Definitive Diagnosis

Clinical symptoms may be vague, and the defect should be confirmed with radiographs or MRI.

Pathomechanics and Functional Limitations

The osteochondral lesion creates pain with activity that is relieved with rest. ROM may be limited by pain and inflammation. A defect that becomes a loose body can create a mechanical block to motion. The patient may experience a sensation of giving way due to pain inhibition during activity or quadriceps weakness.

▓ Immediate Management

Immediate management usually consists solely of ice, because the injury is not recognized as anything more than a contusion. In the instances where a large defect is created acutely, the patient may be more comfortable in an immobilizer with crutches to unload the knee.

▓ Medications

NSAIDs are used.

> **Bone scintigraphy** A nuclear bone scan in which a radioactive substance is injected into the patient's body and the amount of absorption is identified. Increased absorption may indicate a stress fracture or periosteal inflammation.

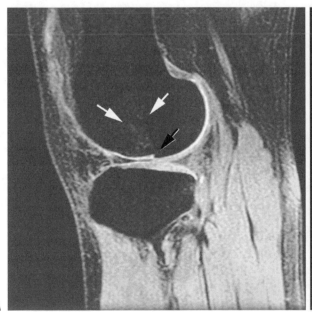 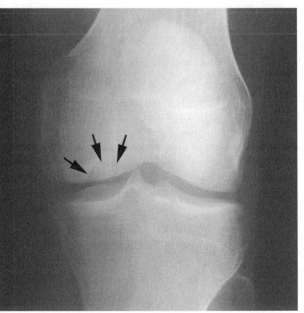

Figure 6-26 Knee osteochondral defects. **A.** Sagittal MRI demonstrating injury to the articular cartilage (black arrow) and marrow edema (white arrow). The patient has an associated ACL lesion (not shown). **B.** AP radiograph demonstrating the crescent-shaped area (black arrows) in the medial femoral condyle characteristic of osteochondritis dissecans. (Reproduced with permission from Johnson TR, Steinbach LS (eds): *Essentials of Musculoskeletal Imaging*. Rosemont, IL, American Academy of Orthopaedic Surgeons, 2004, p 511-513.)

■ Postinjury Management

In a youngster with an osteochondral lesion, conservative treatment is recommended unless a fragment is detached or the patient is within 8 months of physis closure.[80] Conservative treatment may be attempted for small lesions in patients with closed physes but is not normally recommended for adults.

During conservative treatment of an osteochondral defect, the patient must cease all stressful activities but may bear weight as tolerated without pain. Crutches decrease the load through the joint. If ROM is painful, a knee immobilizer is used, and the patient can perform ROM exercises. This initial treatment period lasts 6 to 8 weeks and is followed by repeat imaging to assess lesion status. Strengthening exercises and sport-specific activities progress as the patient's condition improves.

■ Surgical Intervention

Several surgical interventions can be used for osteochondral defects, including arthroscopic drilling with fixation. The drilling causes bleeding in the tissue, which creates a healing environment for the fragment. Mechanically fixating the fragment should improve the likelihood of holding the fragment in place during healing so that joint congruity is restored.[78] The fragment can be fixated with K-wires, compressive screws, cannulated screws, bone pegs, or absorbable pins.[78]

Abrasion chondroplasty and microfracture techniques penetrate the subchondral bone, causing bleeding and fibrin clot and primitive stem-cell formation.[81,82] These primitive stem cells then differentiate into chondrocytes, which repair the defect. The defect is filled with a mix of fibrocartilage and hyaline cartilage. The mechanical properties are not those of normal hyaline cartilage but are a better alternative than exposed bone.

Autologous chondrocyte transplantation uses chondrocyte cells that are harvested from the knee arthroscopically and then grown in a laboratory setting. These cells are transplanted into the chondral defect during a second procedure approximately 4 weeks later. The cells are held in place by a periosteal flap until they mature. This procedure may be beneficial in pure chondral defects but not when bone loss is significant.

Osteochondral autograft transplantation may be useful in focal osteochondral lesions. The size of the defect that can be treated is partially determined by the amount of hyaline cartilage that can be harvested. In this procedure, harvest "plugs" are taken from non–weight-bearing areas of the knee and placed into

> **Fibrocartilage** A mesh of collagen fibers, proteoglycans, and glycoproteins, interspersed with fibrochondrocytes.

the defect to form a mosaicplasty.[83] The mosaicplasty consists of a mosaic of hyaline cartilage plugs; interplug spaces are filled in with fibrocartilage "grout."

Most management methods require protected weight bearing for an extended period to allow healing to proceed without aggravation. ROM is encouraged, but not axial loading.

■ Postoperative Management

Postoperative care revolves around protection of the surgical site. Initially, the patient is placed on crutches, non–weight bearing, for 6 to 8 weeks unless the lesion is located in a non–weight-bearing portion, such as the trochlear groove. In this case, the patient can bear weight as tolerated in a locked, hinged knee brace. The brace also protects the knee from unwanted torsional or shearing forces on the leg. Passive ROM, either with a CPM machine or therapeutic exercises, is performed to aid in cartilage healing.

■ Injury-Specific Treatment and Rehabilitation Concerns

Primary Goals
Avoid painful weight-bearing exercise.
Avoid axial loads on the knee.
Maintain ROM.

After the initial 6- to 8-week healing period, the conservative or postsurgical management of osteochondral defects progresses to restoration of full ROM, strength, and function. Low-load aerobic exercises are beneficial. In addition to the cardiovascular benefits, the exercise physiologically warms the surrounding soft tissues before the knee is moved through ROM. The low loads, providing intermittent compression to the healing cartilage, aid in bringing nutrition to the area.

Active, active-assisted, and passive ROM exercises can be incorporated. Strengthening exercises are advanced for the entire extremity. Initially, open chain exercises are beneficial within a pain-free ROM. Closed chain exercises can progress if the knee remains asymptomatic. The physician determines the ROM that will place the greatest stress across the defect, and this position is avoided until the defect is healed. Weight-bearing exercises are added carefully.

The patient benefits from proprioceptive exercises. Initial attempts at balance and proprioception should minimize the risk of producing shearing or torsional forces across the area of the defect. The patient can begin these once weight bearing is full. Exercises that create a higher risk of shearing or torsional forces should not be initiated until 12 weeks after treatment has commenced. The patient can then progress as tolerated.

■ Estimated Amount of Time Lost

Conservative treatment of young patients with osteochondritis dissecans can last 9 to 12 months, and surgical repair requires 6 to 9 months. Children who have demonstrable healing with imaging and an asymptomatic knee may return sooner with close follow-up. Some patients undergoing surgery may return at 4 to 5 months if the knee is asymptomatic; these are usually more competitive athletes.

Adults with osteochondral lesions may attempt a period of 2 to 3 months of conservative rehabilitation and return to activities. Many times, the patient selectively modifies these activities based on symptoms. Surgical treatment options in the adult all require 6 to 9 months of rehabilitation to ensure healing of the donor graft into the osteochondral defect.

■ Return-to-Play Criteria

The patient can return to full activity when the clinical examination is normal, especially for pain and swelling. Healing should also be demonstrated on imaging studies. The patient must have adequate ROM, strength, and balance and must successfully complete a program of agility and function similar to the required sport activities.

Functional Bracing

Bracing is not needed unless the patient has a concomitant ACL or PCL reconstruction. A knee sleeve may benefit by warming the joint during activities.

Osteoarthritis

Arthritis of the knee may be caused by osteoarthritis or rheumatoid arthritis. It can involve degeneration of the articular cartilage in the medial and/or lateral compartment, patellofemoral joint, or a combination of these areas. The medial compartment is most often affected.

Arthritis may occur from progressive articular cartilage degeneration or trauma from fractures, meniscal damage, and/or ligamentous insufficiencies. Decreased meniscal load-bearing ability after subtotal or total meniscectomy correlates with arthritis development.[27] Various rheumatologic conditions can cause cartilage destruction and are usually associated with systemic symptoms as well.

CLINICAL PRESENTATION

History

Primary Arthritis

Insidious onset

Cartilage degeneration is more prevalent after 50 years of age.[27]

Increased body weight may increase the likelihood of primary osteoarthritis.

Localized joint pain becomes more diffuse as the disease progresses.

Pain initially is described with activity but may become more constant.

Chronic joint swelling

Pain leads to a decreased activity level.

Complaints of mechanical symptoms such as catching or locking may indicate an unstable meniscal injury, loose body, or gross articular-surface changes such as osteophyte formation.

Instability complaints should be further defined as a sensation of giving way, which may result from muscle weakness and pain inhibition, or true instability from ligamentous insufficiency.

Secondary Arthritis

Previous knee trauma

Because this type of arthritis is secondary to an established injury, it is more prevalent than primary osteoarthritis in younger populations. The patient may have a history of intra-articular fracture, meniscal injury, or ligamentous instability.[84]

Complaints are similar to those of patients with primary osteoarthritis.

Observation

Joint effusion is usually present.

The joint may be warm to the touch.

Medial compartment degeneration may create a varus, or bow-legged, deformity.

Lateral compartment degeneration may create a valgus, or knock-kneed, deformity.

Functional Status

Gait may be antalgic.

Patients with medial compartment arthritis and varus deformity may stretch the soft tissues on the lateral aspect of the knee, causing a lateral thrust of the knee when ambulating.

ROM is decreased both actively and passively by the joint effusion and inflammation in the early stages.

Osteophytes and irregular joint surfaces may create a mechanical block to motion.

Physical Evaluation Findings

Findings may suggest an unstable meniscal tear.

Ligamentous tests may be positive from previous injuries.

Varus instability may occur with medial compartment degeneration.

Valgus instability may occur with lateral compartment degeneration.

Osteoarthritis, the focus of this section, involves a loss of articular-cartilage integrity and biochemical and histologic changes. If the arthritis progresses, the underlying bone is eventually affected.

Differential Diagnosis

Meniscal tear, patellofemoral pain syndrome, gout, rheumatologic disorders, neoplastic synovitis, osteonecrosis, osteochondral defects, loose bodies

Medical Diagnostic Tests

Aspiration of the effusion may reveal inflammatory synovitis. Laboratory analysis of this fluid may also reveal a diagnosis of rheumatic arthritis, which may alter the treatment course. Because other joints may also be affected, medications specific to rheumatic disease may be used, and the patient may require follow-up with a rheumatologist to coordinate the total medical care of the disease, including systemic effects.

Imaging Techniques

AP, lateral, and Merchant views of both knees are required. Additionally, 45° posteroanterior, standing bilateral radiographs with the body weight evenly distributed over both legs demonstrate joint-space narrowing (**Figure 6-27**).

Because the earliest cartilage loss usually occurs between 30° and 60° of flexion, routine weight-bearing AP radiographs may not be sensitive to early arthritic changes.[27] A weight-bearing, 45°-flexed, posteroanterior radiograph may demonstrate subtle joint-space loss[85] (**Figure 6-28**).

In patients with an angular deformity, especially those who will undergo surgical intervention, weight-bearing AP radiographs from the hips to the ankles should be obtained to most accurately identify the angular deformity of the limb.

MRI is most often indicated in the patient with minimal radiographic changes, localized pain, and complaints more consistent with meniscal injury.

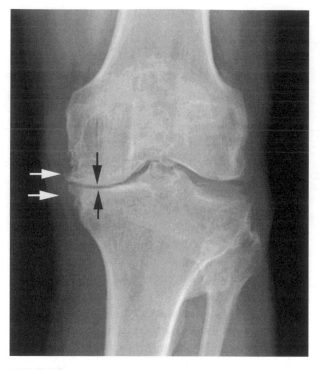

Figure 6-27 AP radiograph of osteoarthritis of the knee. Note the narrowing of the medial joint line (black arrows) and osteophytes along the medial joint line (white arrows). (Reproduced with permission from Johnson TR, Steinbach LS (eds): *Essentials of Musculoskeletal Imaging.* Rosemont, IL, American Academy of Orthopaedic Surgeons, 2004, p 531.)

It is also useful in assessing osteochondral fracture, osteonecrosis, or an isolated osteochondral defect.[27]

In patients with suspected arthritis, two radiographic views should be taken, an AP view and a posteroanterior 45°-flexed view. Radiographic sensitivity can vary dramatically with these views.

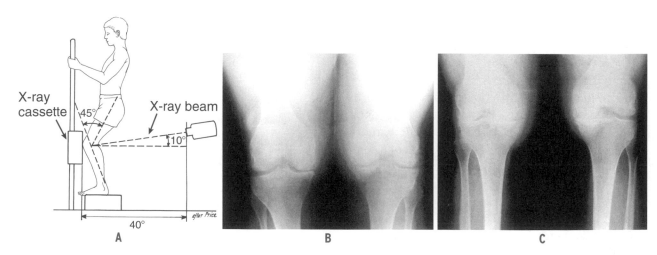

Figure 6-28 Radiographic imaging for knee arthritis. **A.** Patient positioning. **B.** Joint spacing appears normal with the knee extended. **C.** When the same patient is positioned as in **A**, decreased joint space is apparent. (**A** is adapted with permission from Rosenberg TD, Paulos LE, Parker RD, Coward DB, Scott SM: The forty-five degree posteroanterior flexion weight bearing radiograph of the knee. *J Bone Joint Surg Am* 1988;70:1479-1483. **B** and **C** are reproduced with permission from Cole BJ, Harner CD: Degenerative arthritis of the knee in active patients: Evaluation and management. *J Am Acad Orthop Surg* 1999;7:389-402.)

Definitive Diagnosis

Symptomatic knee with degenerative changes noted on radiographs

Pathomechanics and Functional Limitations

In the early stages, patients may have transient symptoms that only minimally limit function. Symptoms are usually reversible with minimal interventions such as over-the-counter NSAIDs, rest, and ice, with resultant return to activity. As the disease progresses, symptoms recur more often and more intensely and are more resistant to previous treatments. Functional activities are increasingly affected. Sports and occupational activities that place large weight-bearing stresses across the knee joint become limited, followed by progressive limitation of ADLs such as walking and normal stair climbing. This functional loss is often correlated with loss of motion and strength and increased frequency of inflammatory exacerbations.

◼ Medications

Because patients most often complain of pain, especially in the early stages of arthritis, acetaminophen may be indicated, especially when swelling is minimal to absent. Although renal and hepatic toxicity can occur when recommended dosages are exceeded, acetaminophen offers efficient pain relief with minimal side effects when taken as recommended.[86] These dosages are 650 mg every 4 to 6 hours as needed, with a maximal daily dosage of 4,000 mg. Because of the potential renal and hepatic toxicity, acetaminophen must be taken with caution when using alcoholic beverages.

NSAIDs offer both inflammatory control and analgesia. Over-the-counter or prescription NSAIDs are the pharmacologic options of choice when swelling is a persistent problem. Inhibiting the cyclooxygenase and lipooxygenase portions of arachidonic acid metabolism, NSAIDs block inflammatory mediators such as prostaglandins and leukotrienes.

Prostaglandins also have many beneficial effects in the body. Their protective effects on the gastric mucosal lining, renal blood flow, and sodium balance can all be affected by prostaglandin inhibition. The most common side effect is dyspepsia. A history of gastrointestinal disorders or renal or liver disease and ongoing anticoagulation therapy are all contraindications to the use of NSAIDs.[87]

Glucosamine and chondroitin sulfate have become popular supplements in the treatment of arthritis (see chapter 4). Glucosamine is thought to stimulate chondrocyte and synoviocyte metab-olism, whereas chondroitin sulfate is proposed to inhibit the enzymes that cause cartilage degradation and prevent the formation of fibrin thrombi in periarticular tissues.[88,89] Recommended dosages are a minimum of 1 g of glucosamine and 1,200 mg of chondroitin sulfate per day.[90]

Other pharmacologic agents that can be used for osteoarthritis include corticosteroid injections and viscosupplementation agents such as hyaluronate therapy. Corticosteroid injections may be useful in patients who fail to obtain relief from oral medications and those with contraindications to the use of NSAIDs. The corticosteroid injection is a strong anti-inflammatory medication that offers the benefit of direct delivery to the involved tissues without systemic effects. Only 3 to 4 injections per year are typically recommended and then only as needed.

Patients with osteoarthritis have reduced concentrations of hyaluronate and, thus, reduced viscoelasticity of their synovial fluid. Hyaluronate therapies should improve the viscoelastic properties of synovial fluid, making it more effective in absorbing joint loads and lubricating joint surfaces. Viscosupplements are injected weekly for 3 to 5 weeks.

◼ Postinjury Management

Nonsurgical treatment for osteoarthritis focuses on rest, pharmacologic agents, therapeutic exercise, and avoiding high-impact activities (see p 180).

◼ Surgical Intervention

Arthroscopic lavage and debridement may be suitable for some patients. Indications include a history of mechanical symptoms, symptoms for 6 or fewer months, normal knee alignment, and mild to moderate radiographic changes.[91-93] Pain relief is reported in 50% to 70% of these patients and ranges from several months to several years in duration. To be most efficacious in this population, arthroscopy should be used to treat unstable meniscal tears, significant motion-limiting osteophyte formations, and loose or unstable chondral flaps.[27,94]

High tibial osteotomy may be prudent in patients with valgus or varus alignment and subsequent medial or lateral unicompartmental arthrosis. If the contribution of arthritic disease in the other compartment or the patellofemoral joint is in question, an offset (medially for a valgus deformity and laterally for a varus deformity), short leg walking cast may be used for 3 days to assess the level of pain reduction. Patients whose pain is not reduced

Lavage The washing or cleansing of a hollow tissue space with water.

may be having symptoms from several compartments of the knee, for which an osteotomy would not be useful.[95]

In the high tibial osteotomy, a wedge of bone is removed (closed wedge) or a wedge is created (open wedge) and filled in with iliac crest bone graft to correct knee alignment and unload the diseased compartment. The surgeon determines the proper amount of wedge that must be created to correct the alignment preoperatively, through the use of ankle to hip radiographs. Once the alignment is corrected, the bone must be fixated until it heals. Staples, plates, and external fixators can be used.

An alternative for medial or lateral compartment disease without malalignment is a unicompartmental arthroplasty. In this procedure, only the diseased compartment is addressed. Surgical benefits are a smaller incision, less bone loss, good function, and ease in revising to a total knee arthroplasty if needed. Both the high tibial osteotomy and unicompartmental surgical procedures require an intact ACL.

Total knee arthroplasty remains an excellent option for active patients provided they are willing to modify joint-loading activities. The arthroplasty replaces the tibiofemoral joint surfaces and may include the patellofemoral joint if it is involved. Although arthroplasty has always been a good alternative for patients older than 60 years of age, improved materials and surgical techniques have now made it an option for younger patients. Good results without a high risk of failure have been achieved in patients younger than 55 years.[96-98]

Postinjury/Postoperative Management

Patients undergoing an arthroscopic procedure begin rehabilitation with ROM and strengthening exercises immediately. They may use crutches for several days to increase comfort.

Postoperative management of a patient with a high tibial osteotomy varies depending on the fixation used. A plate allows for immediate ROM and weight bearing.

A patient with a total knee arthroplasty spends 3 to 5 days in the hospital. During this time, the focus is on wound healing, ROM, early weight bearing, and basic strengthening exercises. CPM is used in the hospital. The patient can typically bear weight as tolerated with either crutches or a walker. Quadriceps setting and straight-leg raises are performed for strengthening. The patient then undergoes formal rehabilitation at least 3 days per week in conjunction with an extensive home program.

Injury-Specific Treatment and Rehabilitation Concerns

Specific Concerns
Control pain and inflammation.
Maintain ROM.
Correct biomechanics and other predisposing factors.
Minimize weight-bearing forces through the joint during activity.

The conservative or postoperative rehabilitation of the arthritic patient focuses on maximizing function while decreasing the load-bearing forces through the joint. Stiffness and loss of motion increase stress on the joint and pain. Patellar mobilization is especially important for restoring motion after total knee arthroplasty. Active-assisted and passive ROM exercises can be used to improve ROM. The end feel experienced while performing ROM exercises, especially in the conservative treatment of arthritis, can indicate the functional status of the knee. Patients with arthritic changes, including osteophyte formation, may experience a hard end feel of bone hitting bone. This motion should not be forced. In addition, the flexion limitations of particular total joint replacement systems must be recognized. Exceeding the flexion limits may cause prosthesis loosening and result in premature failure.

Strengthening exercises focus on the lower extremity gravity-resisting muscles. Strengthening the gluteals, quadriceps, and gastrocnemius-soleus complex helps reduce fatigue that leads to abnormal biomechanics during activity. Proper, efficient function of these muscle groups also assists in dampening forces through the lower extremity joints. Heavy weight-bearing exercises are not recommended. Pain-free open chain and low-load, high-endurance closed chain exercises are instituted.

Pain, loss of motion, aging, and ligamentous insufficiency may all affect balance in this patient population. Proprioceptive exercises are vital to improve function and decrease the incidence of falls. The patient's goals regarding the type and intensity of desired activity should be considered when designing a proprioceptive program.

Aerobic exercise is important for its cardiovascular benefits and to control the patient's body weight. Controlling body weight decreases the load-bearing forces through the joint or joint replacement. Exercises such as swimming, bicycling, elliptical gliding, ski machine, and walking are recommended.

Estimated Amount of Time Lost

Arthritis is a progressive, degenerative disease. Time lost depends on the level of symptoms and the treatment interventions used. Patients with minimal symptoms may not miss any time from activity. Others may need several weeks of rehabilitation before returning to activity. Still others may be advised not to return to their previous activities or naturally tend to alter their activity to decrease joint stress by adopting different activities and activity levels.

The amount of articular cartilage destruction, the patient's symptoms and willingness to adapt lifestyle, and treatment course chosen all influence the amount of time lost.

Return-to-Play Criteria

In the conservatively treated, active osteoarthritic population and patients undergoing arthroscopic or osteotomy procedures, pain is the most significant return-to-play criterion. The patient's inflammatory process should not be active, and pain should be minimal and controllable with medications, rest, and exercise. The patient must have adequate ROM and strength to perform activities without risk of acute injury. A knee sleeve may provide warmth to the joint, making activity more comfortable. Braces ("unloader" braces) designed to unload one of the knee compartments can be used, but tend to be bulky; active patients may find them too restrictive for certain sports activities (**Figure 6-29**).

The patient should consider activities that minimize joint loads. Some weight-bearing stresses cannot be avoided, such as those associated with tennis

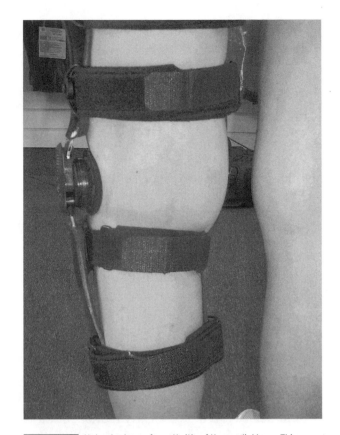

Figure 6-29 Unloader brace for arthritis of the medial knee. This brace uses adjustable tension to create a valgus force on the knee, thereby reducing weight-bearing pressures on the medial joint surfaces.

or basketball. Whenever possible, less stressful activities should be pursued for fitness. The patient may choose swimming or bicycling over running for cardiovascular exercise.

Patients who have undergone a total knee arthroplasty must make activity changes to limit joint loading. Unrestricted golfing is allowed, and some surgeons may permit a return to limited amounts of doubles tennis. Walking, swimming, and bicycling are encouraged as fitness activities. No brace is needed after arthroplasty.

Rehabilitation

A knee rehabilitation program must address trunk, pelvis, and lower extremity stability. Although isolated exercises are beneficial early in rehabilitation, functional therapeutic exercises must be included in the late stages. Synergistic kinetic chain activity should be encouraged as soon as allowed.

Proprioceptive and functional progression exercises for the knee and lower extremity are described in chapter 9.

Range of Motion

Other relevant patellar mobilization activities and range of motion activities can be found in chapters 7 and 9.

Continuous Passive Motion

A CPM device can increase early motion, but it is often better to involve the patient in active rehabilitation as soon as possible. CPM should not be used as a substitute for active or active-assisted ROM unless the specific diagnosis requires this or postsurgical restrictions are imposed by the surgeon. Although a CPM device may promote early motion, it typically does not maintain full extension or achieve full flexion.

CPM is indicated when its use will decrease postinjury or postsurgery morbidity. The CPM device can increase motion and decrease pain and swelling and may aid in healing by promoting fibrocartilage or hyaline-cartilage growth.

CPM is contraindicated in unstable fractures. It does not adequately stress full extension and is usually less effective once knee flexion has increased past 90°.

Heel Slide

The patient lies supine or sits on a table with the back supported and the involved lower extremity straight. For the passive technique, the patient uses a towel to slide the heel toward the hip, moving the knee into flexion until a pulling or restriction in motion is experienced (**Figure 6-30**). The active technique relies on hamstring contractions to move the foot. The position is held for 20 seconds. The patient then performs a slow, controlled return to the starting position. The patient may use a stretching strap, belt, or towel to assist the motion.

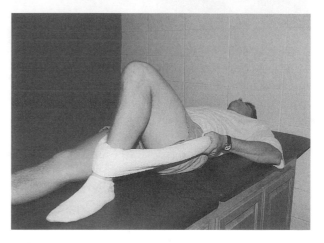

Figure 6-30   Heel slide.

Wall Slide

The patient lies supine on a table placed perpendicular to the wall, with the involved lower extremity supported by the wall. The patient allows gravity to slowly pull the foot down the wall until a pulling or restriction in motion is experienced (**Figure 6-31**). The terminal position is held for 20 seconds. The foot is then returned to the starting position.

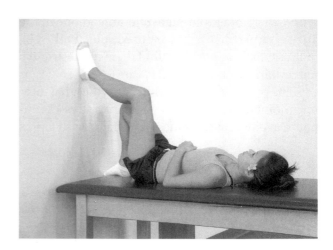

Figure 6-31   Wall slide.

Prone Hangs

The patient lies prone on a table with the thighs supported just proximal to the patella. Gravity pulls the tibia into extension as the patient relaxes (**Figure 6-32**). Light cuff weights can be added to in-

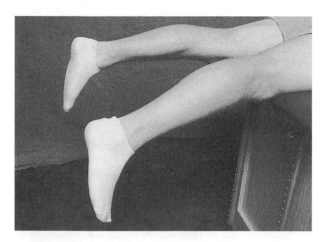

Figure 6-32 Prone hangs.

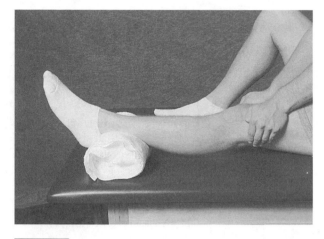

Figure 6-34 Towel propping.

crease the stretch. Higher loads should be avoided because patient guarding may occur. The patient can start at 5 minutes and work up to 10 minutes of continuous stretching or intermittently stretch for 1 minute and relax for 1 minute.

Prone Flexion

If a flexion restriction is determined to be caused by the extensor mechanism alone or in combination with the joint capsule, a prone stretch may be indicated. Lying prone on the table, the patient loops a strap around the ankle and pulls the knee into flexion (**Figure 6-33**). The stretch is held for 20 seconds. The leg is then returned to extension.

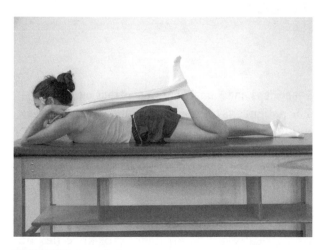

Figure 6-33 Prone flexion.

Towel Propping

The patient sits on the table with a towel roll under the ankle of the involved extremity. Gravity pulls the unsupported knee into extension. The patient can manually assist the extension by gently pressing the thigh toward the table (**Figure 6-34**). An

active quadriceps set can also be performed in this position. For a prolonged stretch, weights may be placed proximal to the patella. For a flexion contracture, heat placed behind the knee may promote further relaxation and stretch.

Strengthening Techniques

Specific knee ROM has advantages and disadvantages, based on the injury being treated. For example, closed kinetic chain exercises develop high tibiofemoral joint contact forces but low shearing forces because of compression and the cocontractions of the quadriceps and hamstring muscles. In contrast, open kinetic chain exercises result in lower tibiofemoral compression, higher anterior shearing forces with quadriceps activity, and higher posterior shearing forces with hamstring activity. **Table 6-1** provides the results of analyses of joint forces in various positions and ranges.[99,100]

See chapter 9 for more lower extremity strengthening exercises.

Isometric Exercises

Quadriceps Sets

The patient lies supine, sits, or stands with the involved knee in full extension. The quadriceps are then maximally contracted, "setting" the muscle, and held for 10 seconds. Motor-level electrical stimulation can aid the patient in recruiting motor units and holding the contraction. Biofeedback can be used to recruit motor units and aid the patient in developing and sustaining an enhanced contraction. The patient should be monitored for proper muscle activation patterns, to prevent the

Table 6-1

Analysis of Joint Forces

Knee Position	Forces
0° (Full extension)	Minimal stress on the ACL and PCL
	Minimal PFJ contact forces and stability
	Marked quadriceps activity with isometrics and moderate activity with single-leg raising
0° to 30° (Terminal knee extension)	High anterior shear forces with quadriceps activity in both OKC and CKC
	Increased PFJ stability at 20°
	Greatest quadriceps EMG activity with OKC (all groups)
	Minimal PCL stress as a result of posterior shear forces with quadriceps activity in both OKC and CKC
0° to 60°	Low ACL stress as a result of anterior shear forces with hamstring activity in OKC
	Low PCL stress as a result of posterior shear forces with hamstring activity
60° to 90°	No ACL stress as a result of anterior shear forces from quadriceps or hamstring activity in OKC or CKC
	Good PFJ stability
	High PFJ contact forces
	High PCL stress as a result of posterior shearing forces with hamstring activity in OKC or CKC
90° to 105°	Highest posterior shearing forces in both OKC and CKC
	Highest tibiofemoral compressive forces
	Greatest quadriceps EMG activity in CKC

PFJ = patellofemoral joint; OKC = open kinetic chain; CKC = closed kinetic chain; EMG = electromyography

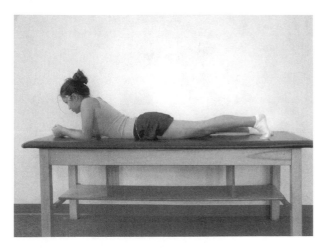

Figure 6-35   Reverse quadriceps sets.

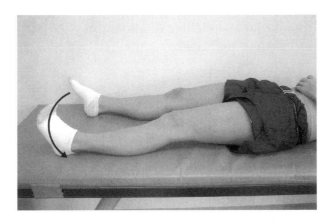

Figure 6-36   Hamstring sets.

gluteals and hamstrings from substituting for quadriceps activity.

Reverse Quadriceps Sets

The patient lies prone with the toes of the involved leg on the table. The patient then straightens the leg to lift the femur off the table (**Figure 6-35**).

Hamstring Sets

The patient sits or lies supine and presses the heel of the involved extremity into the supporting surface using the hamstring muscles. The patient should be monitored so that gluteal substitution patterns are avoided (**Figure 6-36**).

Quadriceps and Hamstrings Cocontraction

The patient sits or lies supine with the involved extremity in full extension. The patient contracts or sets the quadriceps and simultaneously uses the hamstrings to press the involved heel into the supporting surface.

Multiangle Isometrics

The quadriceps and hamstrings can be exercised isometrically at various degrees of knee flexion. These angles are determined by the patient's diagnosis, postsurgical precautions, and tolerance. The level of shearing forces on the ACL and PCL, the patellofemoral joint reaction forces, and the levels of patellar stability vary with different positions.

■ Isotonic Exercises

Straight-leg Raises

Initially, these exercises are performed using only the extremity weight. As the patient's strength improves, cuff weights can be added to the thigh, knee, or ankle. The patient should perform a quadriceps set during all planes of these motions to develop synergistic activity between the hip and thigh muscles (**Figure 6-37**).

Closed Chain Terminal Knee Extension

The patient stands with the involved knee in approximately 30° of flexion. The resistance is placed behind the knee proximal to the popliteal fossa, and the patient straightens the knee by setting the quadriceps (**Figure 6-38**). The patient should be monitored to prevent gluteal substitution.

Leg curl The patient lies prone, and resistance is placed proximal to the ankle posteriorly. Limited arcs of motion can be used (**Figure 6-39**).

Leg extension The patient is seated, and resistance is placed proximal to the ankle anteriorly. Limited arcs of motion can be used (**Figure 6-40**). If attempting a full arc, the quadriceps should be volitionally set as forcefully as possible at terminal extension to enhance recruitment.

■ Isokinetics

Isokinetics provide a useful strengthening and testing modality for speed-specific training. However, isokinetics involve a computerized, electro-

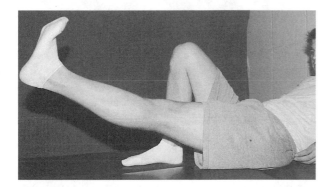

Flexion: The patient lies supine, with the uninvolved extremity flexed and the involved extremity fully extended. The patient first sets the involved quadriceps and then lifts the heel from the table. The leg is only lifted so the heel is about 1 to 1.5 feet off the table. It is slowly lowered, attempting to touch the calf before the heel. The quadriceps is then relaxed.

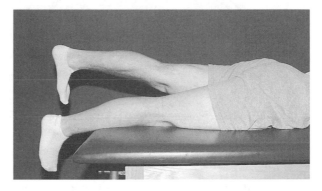

Extension: The patient lies prone with the knees fully extended. The patient first sets the involved quadriceps and then lifts the involved extremity away from the table.

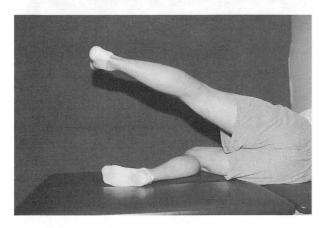

Abduction: The patient lies on the uninvolved side, with the uninvolved knee flexed and the involved extremity fully extended. The patient first sets the quadriceps and then lifts the involved extremity away from the table.

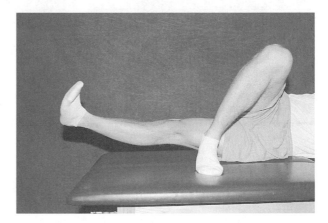

Adduction: The patient lies on the involved side, with the involved knee fully extended and the uninvolved extremity crossed over the involved extremity. The patient first sets the involved quadriceps, and then lifts the involved extremity away from the table.

Figure 6-37 Straight-leg raises.

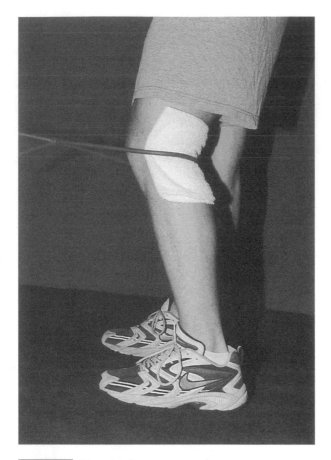

Figure 6-38   Knee extension.

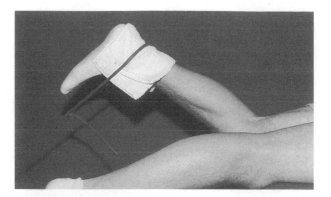

Figure 6-39   Leg curl.

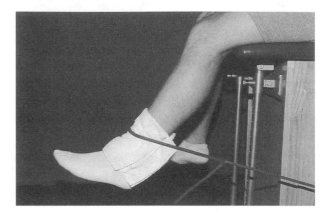

Figure 6-40   Leg extension.

mechanical device that is not readily available because of prohibitive costs. Exercise velocity and volume, contraction type (concentric, eccentric, isometric, and isotonic), and ROM can be varied according to the needs of the patient. Although isokinetic exercise is versatile, it is not a panacea or replacement for a comprehensive rehabilitation progression.

■ References

1. Fithian DC, Paxton LW, Goltz DH: Fate of the anterior cruciate ligament-injured knee. *Orthop Clin North Am* 2002;33:621-636.

2. Shelbourne KD, Trumper RV: Preventing anterior knee pain after anterior cruciate ligament reconstruction. *Am J Sports Med* 1997;25:41-47.

3. Shelbourne KD, Wilckens JH, Mollabashy A, DeCarlo M: Arthrofibrosis in acute anterior cruciate ligament reconstruction: The effect of timing of reconstruction and rehabilitation. *Am J Sports Med* 1991;19:332-336.

4. Miller SL, Gladstone JN: Graft selection in anterior cruciate ligament reconstruction. *Orthop Clin North Am* 2002;33:675-683.

5. Barber FA, McGuire DA, Click S: Continuous-flow cold therapy for outpatient anterior cruciate ligament reconstruction. *Arthroscopy* 1998;14:130-135.

6. Richmond JC, Gladstone J, MacGillivray J: Continuous passive motion after arthroscopically assisted anterior cruciate ligament reconstruction: Comparison of short- versus long-term use. *Arthroscopy* 1991;7:39-44.

7. Noyes FR, Mangine RE, Barber SD: The early treatment of motion complications after reconstruction of the anterior cruciate ligament. *Clin Orthop* 1992;277:217-228.

8. Rosen MA, Jackson DW, Atwell EA: The efficacy of continuous passive motion in the rehabilitation of anterior cruciate ligament reconstructions. *Am J Sports Med* 1992;20:122-127.

9. Howell SM, Taylor MA: Brace-free rehabilitation, with early return to activity, for knees reconstructed with a double-looped semitendinosus and gracilis graft. *J Bone Joint Surg Am* 1996;78:814-825.

10. Glasgow SG, Gabriel JP, Sapega AA, Glasgow MT, Torg JS: The effect of early versus late return to vigorous activities on the outcome of anterior cruciate reconstruction. *Am J Sports Med* 1993;21:243-248.

11. Shelbourne KD, Nitz P: Accelerated rehabilitation after anterior cruciate ligament reconstruction. *Am J Sports Med* 1990;18:292-299.

12. Bynum EB, Barrack RL, Alexander AH: Open versus closed chain kinetic exercises after anterior cruciate ligament reconstruction: a prospective randomized study. *Am J Sports Med* 1995;23;401-406.

13. Tyler TF, McHugh MP, Gleim GW, Nicholas SJ: The effect of immediate weightbearing after anterior cruciate ligament reconstruction. *Clin Orthop* 1998;357:141-148.

14. Indelicato PA: Non-operative treatment of complete tears of the medial collateral ligament of the knee. *J Bone Joint Surg Am* 1983;65:323-329.

15. Shelbourne KD, Patel DV: Management of combined injuries of the anterior cruciate and medial collateral ligaments. *Instr Course Lect* 1996;45:275-280.

16. Shelbourne KD, Mesko JW, McCarroll JR, et al: Combined medial collateral ligament-posterior cruciate rupture: Mechanism of injury. *Am J Knee Surg* 1990;3:41-44.

17. Warren LF, Marshall JL: The supporting structures and layers on the medial side of the knee: An anatomical analysis. *J Bone Joint Surg Am* 1979;61:56-62.

18. Robins AJ, Newman AP, Burks RT: Postoperative return of motion in anterior cruciate ligament and medial collateral ligament injuries: The effects of medial collateral ligament rupture location. *Am J Sports Med* 1993;21:20-25.

19. Ellsasser JC, Reynolds FC, Omohundro JR: The non-operative treatment of collateral ligament injuries of the knee in professional football players: An analysis of seventy-four injuries treated non-operatively and twenty-four injuries treated surgically. *J Bone Joint Surg Am* 1974;56:1185-1190.

20. Indelicato PA: Isolated medial collateral ligament injuries in the knee. *J Am Acad Orthop Surg* 1995;3:9-14.

21. Noyes FR, Barber-Westin SD: The treatment of acute combined ruptures of the anterior cruciate and medial ligaments of the knee. *Am J Sports Med* 1995;23:380-389.

22. LaPrade RF, Wentorf F: Diagnosis and treatment of posterolateral knee injuries. *Clin Orthop* 2002;402:110-121.

23. Krukhaug Y, Molster A, Rodt A, Strand T: Lateral ligament injuries of the knee. *Knee Surg Sports Traumatol Arthrosc* 1998;6:21-25.

24. DeLee JC, Riley MB, Rockwood CA Jr: Acute straight lateral instability of the knee. *Am J Sports Med* 1983;11:404-411.

25. LaPrade RF, Terry GC: Injuries to the posterolateral aspect of the knee: Association of injuries with clinical instability. *Am J Sports Med* 1997;25:433-438.

26. LaPrade RF: The medial collateral ligament complex and the posterolateral aspect of the knee, in Arendt EA (ed): *Orthopaedic Knowledge Update: Sports Medicine 2*. Rosemont, IL, American Academy of Sports Medicine, 1999, pp 327-340.

27. Cole BJ, Harner CD: Degenerative arthritis of the knee in active patients: Evaluation and management. *J Am Acad Orthop Surg* 1999;7:389-402.

28. LaPrade RF, Gilbert TJ, Bollom TS, Wentorf F, Chaljub G: The MRI appearance of individual structures of the posterolateral knee: A prospective study of normal and knees with surgically verified grade III injuries. *Am J Sports Med* 2000;28:191-199.

29. Rettig AC, Rubinstein RA: Medial and lateral ligament injuries of the knee, in Scott WN (ed): *The Knee*. St Louis, MO, Mosby-Year Book, 1994, pp 803-822.

30. Harner CD, Hoher J: Evaluation and treatment of posterior cruciate ligament injuries. *Am J Sports Med* 1998;26:471-482.

31. Kannus P: Nonoperative treatment of grade II and III sprains of the lateral ligament compartment of the knee. *Am J Sports Med* 1989;17:83-88.

32. Shelbourne KD, Davis TJ, Patel DV: The natural history of acute, isolated, nonoperatively treated posterior cruciate ligament injuries: A prospective study. *Am J Sports Med* 1999;27:276-283.

33. Harner CD, Janaushek MA, Kanamori A, Yagi AKM, Vogrin TM, Woo SL: Biomechanical analysis of a double-bundle posterior cruciate ligament reconstruction. *Am J Sports Med* 2000;28:144-151.

34. Berg EE: Posterior cruciate ligament tibial inlay reconstruction. *Arthroscopy* 1995;11:69-76.

35. Arnoczky SP, Warren RF: Microvasculature of the human meniscus. *Am J Sports Med* 1982;10:90-95.

36. Arnoczky SP, Warren RF: The microvasculature of the meniscus and its response to injury: An experimental study in the dog. *Am J Sports Med* 1983;11:131-141.

37. Fitzgibbons RE, Shelbourne KD: "Aggressive" nontreatment of lateral meniscus tears seen during anterior cruciate ligament reconstruction. *Am J Sports Med* 1995;23:156-159.

38. Bellabarba C, Bush-Joseph CA, Bach BR Jr: Patterns of meniscal injury in the anterior cruciate-deficient knee: a review of the literature. *Am J Orthop* 1997;26:18-23.

39. McCarty EC, Marx RG, DeHaven KE: Meniscus repair: Considerations in treatment and update of clinical results. *Clin Orthop* 2002;402:122-134.

40. Steiner ME, Grana WA: The young athlete's knee: Recent advances. *Clin Sports Med* 1988;7:527-546.

41. Brindle T, Nyland J, Johnson DL: The meniscus: Review of basic principles with application to surgery and rehabilitation. *J Athl Train* 2001;36:160-169.

42. Reicher MA, Hartzman S, Duckweiler GR, Bassett LW, Anderson LJ, Gold RH: Meniscal injuries: Detection using MR imaging. *Radiology* 1986;159:753-757.

43. Mink JH, Levy T, Crues JV III: Tears of the anterior cruciate ligament and menisci on MR imaging evaluation. *Radiology* 1988;167:769-774.

44. Noyes FR, Barber-Westin SD: Arthroscopic repair of meniscal tears extending into the avascular zone in patients younger than twenty years of age. *Am J Sports Med* 2002;30:589-600.

45. Greis PE, Holmstrom MC, Bardanna DD, Burks RT: Meniscal injury: II. Management. *J Am Acad Orthop Surg* 2002;10:177-187.

46. DeHaven KE: Decision-making factors in the treatment of meniscal lesions. *Clin Orthop* 1990;252:49-54.

47. Cannon WJ Jr, Vittori JM: The incidence of healing in arthroscopic meniscal repairs in anterior cruciate ligament–reconstructed knees versus stable knees. *Am J Sports Med* 1992;20:176-181.

48. Morgan CD, Wojtys EM, Casscells CD, Casscells SW: Arthroscopic meniscal repair evaluated by second-look arthroscopy. *Am J Sports Med* 1991;19:632-638.

49. Barber FA: Accelerated rehabilitation for meniscus repairs. *Arthroscopy* 1994;10:206-210.

50. Shelbourne KD, Patel DV, Adsit WS, Porter DA: Rehabilitation after meniscal repair. *Clin Sports Med* 1996;15:595-612.

51. Barber FA, Click SD: Meniscus repair rehabilitation with concurrent anterior cruciate reconstruction. *Arthroscopy* 1997;13:433-437.

52. DeHaven KE, Lohrer WA, Lovelock JE: Long-term results of open meniscal repair. *Am J Sports Med* 1995;23:524-530.

53. Delamarter RB, Hohl M, Hopp E Jr: Ligament injuries associated with tibial plateau fractures. *Clin Orthop* 1990;250:226-233.

54. Gill TJ, Moezzi DM, Oates KM, Sterett WI: Arthroscopic reduction and internal fixation of tibial plateau fractures in skiing. *Clin Orthop* 2001;383:243-249.

55. Bharam S, Vrahas MS, Fu FH: Knee fractures in the athlete. *Orthop Clin North Am* 2002;33:565-574.

56. Hohl M, Johnson EE, Wiss DA: Fractures of the knee, in Rockwood CA, Green DP, Bucholz RW (eds): *Fractures in Adults*, ed 3. Philadelphia, PA, JB Lippincott, 1991, pp 1725-1797.

57. Cohn SL, Sotta RP, Bergfeld JA: Fractures about the knee in sports. *Clin Sports Med* 1990;9:121-139.

58. Buchko GM, Johnson DH: Arthroscopy assisted operative management of tibial plateau fractures. *Clin Orthop* 1996;332:29-36.

59. Mazoue CG, Guanche CA, Vrahas MS: Arthroscopic management of tibial plateau fractures: an unselected series. *Am J Orthop* 1999;28:508-515.

60. Good L, Johnson RJ: The dislocated knee. *J Am Acad Orthop Surg* 1995;3:284-292.

61. Shelbourne KD, Porter DA, Clingman JA, McCarroll JR, Rettig AC: Low-velocity knee dislocation. *Orthop Rev* 1991;20:995-1004.

62. Green NE, Allen BL: Vascular injuries associated with dislocation of the knee. *J Bone Joint Surg Am* 1977;59:236-239.

63. Quinlan AG, Sharrad WJW: Posterolateral dislocation of the knee with capsular interposition. *J Bone Joint Surg Br* 1958;40:660-663.

64. Hill JA, Rana NA: Complications of posterolateral dislocation of the knee: Case report and literature review. *Clin Orthop* 1981;154:212-215.

65. Dedmond BT, Almekinders LC: Operative versus nonoperative treatment of knee dislocations: A meta-analysis. *Am J Knee Surg* 2001;14:33-38.

66. Richter M, Bosch U, Wippermann B, Hofmann A, Krettek C: Comparison of surgical repair or reconstruction of the cruciate ligaments versus nonsurgical treatment in patients with traumatic knee dislocations. *Am J Sports Med* 2002;30:718-727.

67. Noble CA: Iliotibial band friction syndrome in runners. *Am J Sports Med* 1980;8:232-234.

68. Kirk KL, Kuklo T, Klemme W: Iliotibial band friction syndrome in runners. *Orthopedics* 2000;23:1209-1214.

69. Taunton JE, Ryan MB, Clement DB, McKenzie DC, Lloyd-Smith DR, Zumbo BD: A retrospective case-control analysis of 2002 running injuries. *Br J Sports Med* 2002;36:95-101.

70. Orchard JW, Fricker PA, Abud AT, Mason BR: Biomechanics of iliotibial band friction syndrome in runners. *Am J Sports Med* 1996;24:375-379.

71. James SL: Running injuries to the knee. *J Am Acad Orthop Surg* 1995;3:309-318.

72. Kirk KL, Kuklo T, Klemme W: Iliotibial band friction syndrome. *Orthopedics* 2000;23:1209-1214.

73. Forbes JR, Helms CA, Janzen DL: Acute pes anserine bursitis: MR imaging. *Radiology* 1995;194:525-527.

74. Brown TR, Quinn SF, Wensel JP, Ki JH, Demlow T: Diagnosis of popliteus injuries with MR imaging. *Skeletal Radiol* 1995;24:511-514.

75. Farmer JM, Martin DF, Boles CA, et al: Chondral and osteochondral injuries: Diagnosis and management. *Clin Sports Med* 2001;20:299-319.

76. Birk GT, DeLee JC: Osteochondral lesions: Clinical findings. *Clin Sports Med* 2001;20:279-286.

77. Minas T, Peterson L: Advanced techniques in autologous chondrocyte transplantation. *Clin Sports Med* 1999;18:13-44.

78. Cain EL, Clancy WG: Treatment algorithm for osteochondral injuries of the knee. *Clin Sports Med* 2001;20:321-342.

79. Paletta GA Jr, Bednarz PA, Stanitski CL, Sandman GA, Stanitski DF, Kottamasu S: The prognostic value of quantitative bone scan in knee osteochondritis dissecans: A preliminary experience. *Am J Sports Med* 1998;26:7-14.

80. Cahill BR: Osteochondritis dessicans of the knee: Treatment of juvenile and adult forms. *J Am Acad Orthop Surg* 1995;3:237-247.

81. Johnson LL: Arthroscopic abrasion arthroplasty: A review. *Clin Orthop* 2001;391(suppl):S306-S317.

82. Steadman JR, Rodkey WG, Rodrigo JJ: Microfracture: Surgical technique and rehabilitation to treat chondral defects. *Clin Orthop* 2001;391(suppl):S362-S369.

83. Hangody L, Feczko P, Bartha L, Bodo G, Kish G: Mosaicplasty for the treatment of articular defects of the knee and ankle. *Clin Orthop* 2001;391(suppl):S328-S336.

84. Daniel DM, Stone ML, Dobson BE, Fithian DC, Rossman DJ, Kaufman KR: Fate of the ACL-injured patient: A prospective outcome study. *Am J Sports Med* 1994;22:632-644.

85. Rosenberg TD, Paulos LE, Parker RD, Coward DB, Scott SM: The forty-five-degree posteroanterior flexion weight-bearing radiograph of the knee. *J Bone Joint Surg Am* 1988;70:1479-1483.

86. Bradley JD, Brandt KD, Katz BP, Kalasinski LA, Ryan SI: Comparison of an antiinflammatory dose of ibuprofen, an analgesic dose of ibuprofen, and acetaminophen in the treatment of patients with osteoarthritis of the knee. *N Engl J Med* 1991;325:1716-1725.

87. Berger RG: Nonsteroidal anti-inflammatory drugs: Making the right choices. *J Am Acad Orthop Surg* 1994; 2:255-260.

88. Ghosh P, Smith M, Wells C: Second-line agents in osteoarthritis, in Dixon JS, Furst DE (eds): *Second Line Agents in the Treatment of Rheumatic Diseases.* New York, NY, Marcel Dekker, 1992, pp 363-427.

89. Muller-Fassbender H, Bach GL, Haase W, Rovati LC, Setnikar I: Glucosamine sulfate compared to ibuprofen in osteoarthritis of the knee. *Osteoarthritis Cartilage* 1994;2:61-69.

90. Bougeois P, Chales G, DeHais J, Delcambre B, Kuntz JL, Rosenberg S: Efficacy and tolerability of chondroitin sulfate 1200 mg/day vs chondroitin sulfate 3 × 400 mg/day vs placebo. *Osteoarthritis Cartilage* 1998;6(suppl A):S25-530.

91. Merchan ECR, Galindo E: Arthroscope-guided surgery versus nonoperative treatment for limited degenerative osteoarthritis of the femorotibial joint in patients over 50 years of age: A prospective comparative study. *Arthroscopy* 1993;9:663-667.

92. Wouters E, Bassett FH III, Hardaker WT Jr, Garrett WE Jr: An algorithm for arthroscopy in the over-50 age group. *Am J Sports Med* 1992;20:141-145.

93. Yang SS, Nisonson B: Arthroscopic surgery of the knee in the geriatric patient. *Clin Orthop* 1995;316:50-58.

94. Dervin GF, Stiell IG, Rody K, Grabowski J: Effect of arthroscopic debridement for osteoarthritis of the knee on health-related quality of life. *J Bone Joint Surg Am* 2003;85:10-19.

95. Krackow KA, Galloway EJ: A preoperative technique for predicting success after varus or valgus osteotomy at the knee. *Am J Knee Surg* 1989;2:164-170.

96. Gill GS, Chan KC, Mills DM: 5- to 18-year follow-up study of cemented total knee arthroplasty for patients 55 years old or younger. *J Arthroplasty* 1997;12:49-54.

97. Stern SH, Bowen MK, Insall JN, Scuderi GR: Cemented total knee arthroplasty for gonarthrosis in patients 55 years old or younger. *Clin Orthop* 1990;260:124-129.

98. Diduch DR, Insall JN, Scott WN, Scuderi GR, Font-Rodriguez D: Total knee replacement in young, active patients: Long-term follow-up and functional outcome. *J Bone Joint Surg Am* 1997;79:575-582.

99. Fox E, Bowers R, Foss M (eds): *The Physiological Basis for Exercise and Sport,* ed 5. Madison, WI, Brown and Benchmark, 1993.

100. Henning CE, Lynch MA, Click KR: An in vivo strain gauge study of elongation of the anterior cruciate ligament. *Am J Sport Med* 1985;13:22.

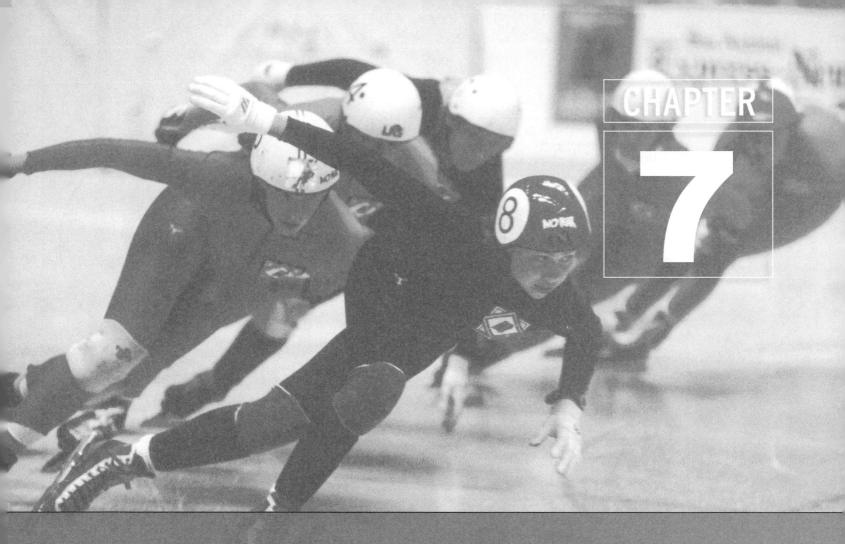

Patellofemoral Injuries

Jeff Ryan, PT, ATC
Paul Marchetto, MD

Patellofemoral Pain Syndrome

CLINICAL PRESENTATION

History

Chronic or overuse mechanism
Increased activity may be reported.
Achy, diffuse pain in the anterior knee
Pain in the medial or lateral popliteal space

Observation

Gross observation is often unremarkable.
Patellar malposition (eg, baja, alta, or squinting positions) may
    be noted
Bilateral or unilateral pronation of the foot

Functional Status

Activities that increase patellofemoral joint reaction forces,
    such as running, squatting, jumping, and stair climbing, may
    be impaired.
Prolonged flexion of the knee may increase pain (movie or the-
    ater sign).

Physical Evaluation Findings

Crepitation may be present.
No definitive, reliable special or ligamentous tests exist.

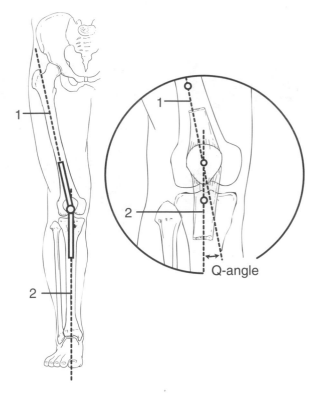

Figure 7-1   Measuring the Q angle. Three points (the anterior superior iliac spine, center of the patella, and the center of the tibial tubercle) form the Q angle. The line of pull of the quadriceps (1) is approximated by a line extending from the anterior superior iliac spine through the center of the patella and (2) from the tibial tubercle to the center of the patella.

Patellofemoral pain syndrome (PFPS) describes a range of problems characterized by diffuse, achy pain in the anterior knee. For this reason, PFPS is sometimes referred to as anterior knee pain. Symptoms increase with activities such as squatting, stair climbing, and running, which load the patellofemoral joint.

"Chondromalacia patella," a term that literally means softening of the cartilage and indicates an articular defect in the patellar articular surface, is sometimes used to describe PFPS. Many patients with PFPS do not have an articular cartilage defect, and patients with articular cartilage defects may not have anterior knee pain syndromes. Thus, this term is not preferred because it may not accurately describe the patient or the symptoms.

Pathomechanics at the foot, ankle, and hip can influence patellar biomechanics. The complete kinetic chain should be analyzed, including static and dynamic postures of the entire leg. Particular attention should be paid to the position of the subtalar joint, because hyperpronation may be evident. A leg-length difference may exist if one foot is pronated and the other foot is supinated (with the pronated foot representing the longer leg), and the Q angle may be increased (**Figure 7-1**).

Increased Q angles cause the patella to track laterally, increase the compressive forces on the patella's lateral facet, and place tension on the medial patellar restraints. Although less common than increased Q angles, small Q angles cause the patella to track medially, place compressive forces on the odd and medial facets, and increase tension on the lateral patellar restraints.

Failure to adequately stabilize the trunk through core strength can affect the biomechanics of patellar tracking and, thus, contribute to PFPS. Throughout the evaluation of a patient with suspected PFPS, the entire closed kinetic chain should be systematically and thoroughly evaluated.

Muscle tightness or weakness of the foot, ankle, and hip should be identified. Tightness of the gastrocnemius-soleus complex may produce compensatory hyperpronation. Tightness of the hip muscles can alter the biomechanical relationship between the femur and the patella. Tight hamstrings and/or a tight iliotibial band can also affect patellofemoral pressure during normal movements. Weak hip muscles, especially the hip abductors, may allow the femur to drift into adduction during weight bearing, effectively increasing the Q angle. Pelvic instability, particularly an anterior position of the pelvis, has also been implicated in patellar pain syndrome. The anterior tilt of the pelvis can internally rotate the femur, increasing lateral compression of the patella with loading of the knee in the flexed position. The position of the pelvis and the biomechanical causes of improper positioning, such as weak trunk stabilizers and pelvic muscle inflexibility, should be evaluated.

Differential Diagnosis

Patellar malalignment, patellar or quadriceps tendinitis, patellar osteoarthritis, meniscal tear, plica syndrome

Imaging Techniques

Anteroposterior (AP), lateral, and bilateral axial radiographs are obtained to rule out a fracture or bipartite patella and to assess malalignment (**Figure 7-2**). Magnetic resonance imaging (MRI) may be helpful if other soft-tissue injury in the knee is suspected. However, positive findings may be present on MRI in the absence of clinically significant symptoms. For example, a torn meniscus may be visible on the MRI, even though the patient does not have meniscal symptoms.

If patellar malalignment needs to be further assessed, an axial computed tomography (CT) scan should be obtained (see p 196, Figure 7-5).

Definitive Diagnosis

Findings on the clinical evaluation (anterior patellar pain) and the exclusion of other possible pathologic findings

Pathomechanics and Functional Limitations

Decreased extensor-mechanism efficiency and pain with patellar tendon function can produce significant changes in lower extremity biomechanics. As the condition deteriorates, running, squatting, and jumping are impaired. Eventually, pain interferes with normal activities of daily living, such as stair climbing and walking.

■ Immediate Management

Typically, PFPS does not occur acutely. If the pain affects the patient's ability to function normally during an activity, stopping the activity and applying ice are warranted.

■ Medications

A nonsteroidal anti-inflammatory drug (NSAID) to control the inflammatory response is often recommended. Rarely, an intra-articular injection of hydrocortisone is used.

■ Surgical Intervention

Surgery is not usually recommended for this condition. Persistent symptoms despite 6 to 8 months of conservative management may necessitate arthroscopic evaluation, at which time surgery may be indicated for concomitant conditions. Surgical options may then include debridement of diseased articular cartilage or abrasion chondroplasty, and microfracture techniques can be used to penetrate the subchondral bone, causing bleeding and the formation of a fibrin clot and primitive stem cells.[1,2] These primitive stem cells differentiate into chondrocytes to repair the defect, which then heals with fibrocartilage or a mix of fibrocartilage and hyaline cartilage. The mechanical properties are not those of normal hyaline cartilage but are a better alternative than exposed nonarticular bone.

■ Postinjury/Postoperative Management

If the patient has an antalgic gait, crutches or a cane should be used. The patient should avoid activities that produce pain. If surgical microfracture techniques were performed, the patient may be maintained non–weight bearing, allowing passive range of motion (ROM) for 6 to 8 weeks to allow the maturation of the chondrocytes.

■ Injury-Specific Treatment and Rehabilitation Concerns

Specific Concerns

Control pain and inflammation.
Restore normal patellar biomechanics.

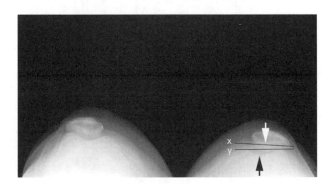

Figure 7-2 Axial view of patellar malalignment. The median ridge of the patella (white arrow) is located lateral to the most concave portion of the femoral trochlea (black arrow), indicating a patellar subluxation. The angle formed by the lateral patellar facet (x) and line drawn across the femoral condyles (y) indicates an abnormal patellar tilt. (Reproduced with permission from Johnson TR, Steinbach LS (eds): *Essentials of Musculoskeletal Imaging*. Rosemont, IL, American Academy of Orthopaedic Surgeons, 2004, p 483.)

The initial treatment of PFPS focuses on controlling pain and inflammation with cryotherapy and therapeutic exercise. A thorough evaluation of trunk, pelvis, and lower extremity posture, flexibility, and muscle activation should be performed. Hyperpronation of the feet can increase the lateral forces on the patella; if this condition is thought to contribute to PFPS, the patient should be fitted for a corrective foot orthotic device. Flexibility exercises for the hip, quadriceps, hamstrings, and gastrocnemius-soleus muscle groups are instituted as needed.

In addition to therapeutic exercises, a functional rehabilitation brace such as the Protonics bracing system to enhance proper positioning of the pelvis and lower extremity can also be considered (**Figure 7-3**). Through resistance applied by the brace, these muscles are theoretically activated while other muscles are inhibited, thereby training and reinforcing the desired pelvic and lower extremity positioning. Further benefits may be obtained through patellar taping techniques.

Synergistic activity between the quadriceps and other lower extremity muscles must also be developed. The quadriceps muscles are responsible for dynamic patellar stability but work synergistically with the hip and calf muscles. Initial quadriceps strengthening can begin in isolation with motor-level electrical stimulation. Strengthening exercises for the lower extremity should focus on restoring synergistic control of the patella during extremity movement. Cocontraction of the quadriceps (controlling the patella) and the other leg muscles moving the extremity at the hip, knee, or ankle should be emphasized.

Leg-raising activities are begun in all directions. The quadriceps and vastus medialis obliquus (VMO) are simultaneously contracted with the hip muscles during hip exercises. The patient progresses through open and closed kinetic chain strengthening, which is performed through the pain-free ROM only. As strength of the musculature and control of the patella are restored, the patient advances through proprioception exercises and agility and sport-specific drills.

Estimated Amount of Time Lost

The patient may not lose any time; in general, if pain is tolerable, no swelling is present, and the knee and lower extremity muscles function normally, activity may continue. If continued activity is impossible, however, a period of formal rehabilitation lasting 1 to 4 weeks is warranted. The patient must continue the exercise routine after returning to full activity.

Patients who do not respond to 1 to 4 weeks of conservative rehabilitation require further evaluation to rule out other injuries. In the absence of additional findings, continued formal rehabilitation or an independent exercise program is continued.

Return-to-Play Criteria

The patient may return to competition when pain is resolved, normal flexibility and strength are restored, and the ability to successfully complete

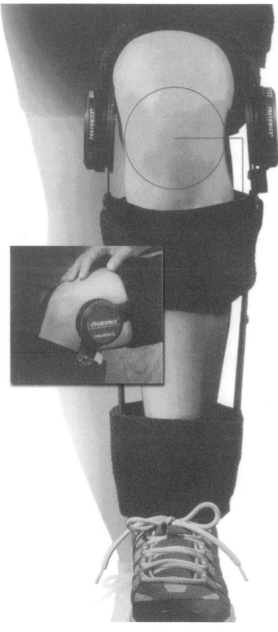

Figure 7-3 Protonics knee brace. Using variable resistance, this orthosis is used for lower extremity and pelvic neuromuscular reeducation by encouraging coactivation of the muscles.

lower extremity functional tests, agility tests, and sport-specific activities is demonstrated.

Functional Bracing

A knee sleeve with a patellar cutout may be used to increase warmth to the area. A Drytex or elastic material is preferred to neoprene to avoid skin breakdown.

Patellar Malalignment and Subluxation

CLINICAL PRESENTATION

History

Insidious onset
Pain, possibly diffuse, along the medial and/or anterior aspect of the joint
Patient may describe a "clunk" as the patella subluxates and relocates.

Observation

Swelling may be present, especially after activity
Hyperpronation of the feet may be noted.
Excessive femoral anteversion (hip internal rotation exceeds hip external rotation by 30°) may be evident.

Functional Status

Decreased ROM, especially flexion, if the patella subluxates during the motion
Weight bearing is decreased with greater degrees of subluxation
Inhibition of the quadriceps mechanism is noted as an inability to produce force.

Physical Evaluation Findings

Positive patellar apprehension test result
Hypermobile lateral glide of the patella

Patellar maltracking or subluxation is the instability of the patellofemoral joint in the absence of dislocation. Patients may have a history of trauma, but typically the onset is insidious. Malalignment is characterized by the improper tracking of the patella within the femoral trochlear groove, whereas subluxation involves greater instability. Normal patellar tracking requires proper balance in the strength and contraction timing of the medial and lateral anterior muscles of the knee. The soft-tissue restraints must be pliable enough to allow the patella to track through the femoral trochlea without drifting too far laterally (**Figure 7-4**).

A full spectrum of findings usually combine to cause malalignment or subluxation, including pathomechanics at the foot and hip, tightness of surrounding soft tissues, and weaknesses in the lower extremity.

Differential Diagnosis

Meniscal tear, symptomatic plica, hip injury

Imaging Techniques

Lateral, AP, tunnel, and axial radiographs are obtained to determine the relationship of the patella to the trochlear groove and to identify any osteochondral defects or fractures from previous episodes (see Figure 7-2).

To better determine the relationship of the patella to the trochlear groove, especially if surgical treatment is being considered, an axial CT scan is obtained, providing a more sensitive imaging technique for identifying patellar malalignment.[3] The CT scan allows imaging of the patella within the trochlear groove from 20° of flexion to full extension, when the joint relies more on soft-tissue structures for stability (**Figure 7-5**). An axial CT scan can also demonstrate a laterally positioned tibial tubercle.[4] The surrounding soft tissues are well visualized on MRI. Dynamic axial MRI images have been proposed to characterize the influence of the soft tissues on the patella.[5] These images can demonstrate the degree of knee flexion at which patellar malalignment is greatest and whether the patella reduces.

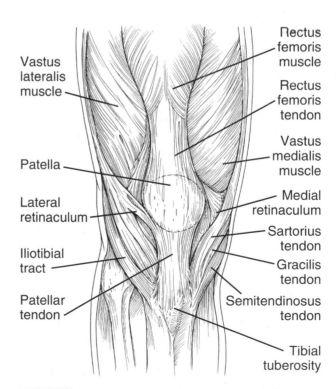

Figure 7-4 Normal anatomy of the knee's extensor mechanism. (Reproduced with permission from Matava MJ: Patellar tendon ruptures. *J Am Acad Orthop Surg* 1996;4:287-296.)

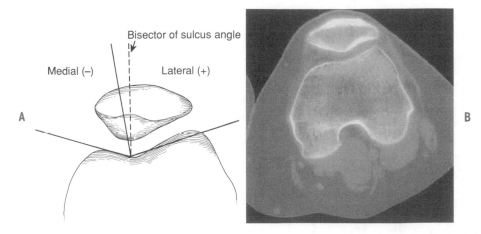

Figure 7-5 Imaging techniques for patellar maltracking and subluxation. **A.** Congruence angle obtained from a standard Merchant view should demonstrate that the patellar apex is medial to the bisected femoral trochlea. **B.** Computed tomography scans are useful for determining patellofemoral alignment. (Reproduced with permission from Fulkerson JP: Patellofemoral pain disorders: Evaluation and management. *J Am Acad Orthop Surg* 1994;2:124-132.)

Definitive Diagnosis

Patellar instability causes apprehension. Medial retinacular tearing seen on MRI is helpful in identifying subluxation. Malalignment problems are more subtle, and the diagnosis is often one of exclusion.

Pathomechanics and Functional Limitations

Tearing of the medial retinacular tissues can lead to chronic instability of the patellofemoral joint and decreased mechanical efficiency of the knee extensor mechanism (**Figure 7-6**). Patients may have recurrent subluxations, and altered biomechanics will, with time, degrade the patellar and femoral articular surfaces. Patients with patellar instability may also experience quadriceps inhibition described as the leg "giving way."

■ Immediate Management

The patient is removed from activity, and ice is applied. An immobilizer and crutches are warranted for an antalgic gait, significant swelling, or instability with weight bearing.

■ Medications

An NSAID may be recommended for pain control and anti-inflammatory effects or acetaminophen for pain control.

■ Postinjury Management

After an acute episode of subluxation, the patient applies ice intermittently to reduce pain and control inflammation. If the patella is thought to be unstable, an immobilizer can be applied. While using the immobilizer, the patient begins pain-free quadriceps-setting exercises. Ambulation is with crutches, bearing weight as tolerated.

If the subluxation caused an effusion, aspiration may be needed. Fat droplets in the aspirate may indicate an osteochondral lesion. The initial treatment is to immobilize the knee in full extension with a compressive dressing along the lateral aspect of the patella. Approximating the torn medial patellar structures may aid in healing in a satisfactory position. The patient is evaluated every 2 weeks and can begin formal rehabilitation when the tenderness over the medial patellar structures is decreased.[6,7]

■ Surgical Intervention

If conservative treatment fails to restore a normally functioning patellofemoral joint and recurrent subluxations persist, surgical treatment similar to that for patellar dislocation can be considered (see Patellar Dislocation, p 197). Surgical treatment for pain alone is not appropriate. Typically the motivation

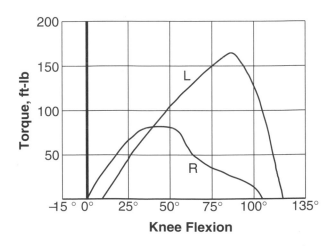

Figure 7-6 Isokinetic torque curves of the quadriceps muscle. Note the sharp decline in extensor strength of the affected leg (R) at 50° of knee flexion compared with the normal left leg (L). (Reproduced with permission from Boden BP, Pearsall AW, Garrett WE, Feagin JA Jr: Patellofemoral instability: Evaluation and management. *J Am Acad Orthop Surg* 1997;5:47-57.)

to exhaust all conservative measures is greater when considering surgery for patellar subluxation.

Postoperative Management

Postsurgical treatment is the same as for the surgical procedures described in the treatment of patellar dislocation (see Patellar Dislocation).

Injury-Specific Treatment and Rehabilitation Concerns

> **Specific Concerns**
>
> Minimize early stresses on the medial patellar restraints.
> Control inflammation.
> Encourage proper realignment of healing tissues.
> Tighten lax tissues.
> Lengthen shortened tissues.
> Restore normal patellar mobility.

The initial conservative treatment of patellar maltracking or subluxation focuses on controlling inflammation with modalities and therapeutic exercise. As the peripatellar soft tissues heal, patellar mobilization is used to restore normal medial patellar glide and patellar tilt. Knee ROM can be progressed as tolerated with active-assisted or passive ROM. A thorough evaluation of lower extremity flexibility is warranted, and exercises for the hip, quadriceps, hamstrings, and gastrocnemius-soleus muscle groups are introduced as needed.

Except for quadriceps-setting exercises, all other strengthening exercises for the lower extremity should focus on restoring synergistic control of the patella during extremity movement. The patient should contract the quadriceps mechanism to stabilize the patella while performing all other lower extremity exercises.

Leg-raising activities in all directions are begun early. The quadriceps and VMO are contracted simultaneously with the hip musculature during hip exercises. If the patient demonstrates adequate control of the trunk, pelvis, and patellofemoral articulation, exercises are progressed through open and closed kinetic chain strengthening. As muscular strength increases and control of the patella is restored, the patient advances through proprioception exercises and agility and sport-specific drills.

See Patellar Dislocation for a description of postsurgical rehabilitation.

Estimated Amount of Time Lost

Time lost to the injury varies; 3 to 6 weeks of rehabilitation are often needed for a patient who cannot perform because of symptoms. The degree of tear-

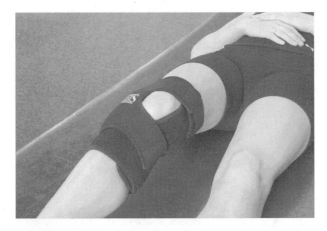

Figure 7-7   Knee sleeve used for patellar subluxations and dislocations. The lateral block is intended to improve patellar stability.

ing of the medial patellar-stabilizing structures has the greatest influence on the amount of time lost. If the patella becomes chronically unstable and the lateral retinacular tissues are tight, surgical intervention and 3 to 4 months of recovery may be necessary.

Return-to-Play Criteria

The patient may return to competition when pain is resolved, ROM is full, quadriceps strength has been restored, and functional tests for the lower extremity are successfully completed. Agility programs with activities similar to sport activities should also be pain-free.

Functional Bracing

Patellar taping may be helpful (see p 218). Knee sleeves developed specifically to place a medially directed force on the patella may be used for the return to activity (**Figure 7-7**).

Patellar Dislocation

Patellar dislocation is the most extreme outcome of patellar instability. The patient may have a history of previous malalignment or subluxation, but dislocation (which is almost always lateral) may be the result of acute trauma (**Figure 7-8**). Medial dislocation is rare and usually secondary to a contact injury while large forces are being exerted on the patella or, more commonly, to surgical error made during a realignment procedure.

When the patella dislocates laterally, the medial retinaculum and medial patellofemoral ligament tear (**Figure 7-9**). An osteochondral defect or fracture of the medial patella may also be associated with the dislocation. As the quadriceps muscles contract to relocate the patella, the medial facet

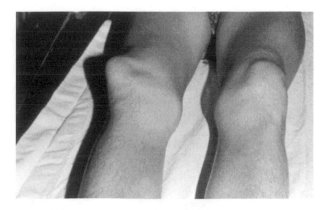

Figure 7-8 Acute lateral patellar dislocation. (Reproduced with permission from Crosby LA, Lewallen DG (eds): *Emergency Care and Transportation of the Sick and Injured*, ed 6. Rosemont, IL, American Academy of Orthopaedic Surgeons, 1995, p 555.).

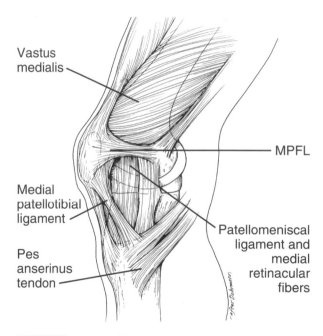

Figure 7-9 Anatomy of the medial aspect of the knee. The medial patellofemoral ligament provides 53% of the restraining force in preventing lateral displacement of the patella: the patellomeniscal ligament and medial retinacular fibers, on average, 22%. (Reproduced with permission from Boden BP, Pearsall AW, Garrett WE, Feagin JA Jr: Patellofemoral instability: Evaluation and management. *J Am Acad Orthop Surg* 1997;5:47-57.)

forcefully contacts and shears across the lateral femoral condyle, causing the bone injury.

Anatomic deviations may predispose an individual to patellar dislocations. Patella alta, shallow trochlea, increased Q angle, tight lateral retinaculum, genu valgum, femoral anteversion, pronated feet, and general ligamentous laxity have all been implicated in a high rate of patellar dislocations.[6] The injury may result from contact but more often occurs from the combination of malalignment of the extensor mechanism and laterally directed forces

on the patella from the contraction of the quadriceps muscles. The knee is usually in some degree of valgus, such as planting or cutting on the planted foot, when the quadriceps forcefully contract.

CLINICAL PRESENTATION

History

Strong quadriceps contraction
A valgus force to the knee may be described.
Pain radiates from the knee and the surrounding restraints.
A "pop" may be reported.
The patient may describe the patella dislocating and, possibly, relocating.
The patient may have a history of patella alta, genu valgum, femoral anteversion, pronated feet, and/or a large Q angle.

Observation

If the patella remains dislocated, obvious deformity is noted, including the presence of the medial femoral condyle.
The knee is usually positioned in slight flexion.
Medial effusion may be present.

Functional Status

Motion and weight bearing are not possible while the patella is dislocated.
After spontaneous reduction, knee motion may be inhibited by pain and swelling.
If the patient can flex and extend the knee, the end ROMs (especially flexion) are painful.

Physical Evaluation Findings

The physical evaluation should not be performed while the patella is still dislocated.
Positive patellar apprehension test result
Hypermobile lateral patellar glide

Differential Diagnosis

Medial collateral ligament sprain, anterior cruciate ligament sprain, patellar fracture, chondral fracture

Imaging Techniques

If the patella remains dislocated, AP and lateral radiographs of the knee are obtained. If the patella has been relocated, AP, lateral, tunnel, and axial radiographs are taken to determine the relationship of the patella to the trochlear groove and whether any osteochondral defects or fractures occurred during the dislocation.

The surrounding soft tissues are well visualized on MRI, especially when the medial retinaculum is torn (**Figure 7-10**). Dynamic axial MRI images may characterize the influence of the soft tissues on the patella,[5] displaying the degree of knee flexion at which patellar malalignment is greatest and whether the patella reduces.

An axial CT scan is obtained to better determine the relationship of the patella to the trochlear groove, particularly if surgical treatment is being

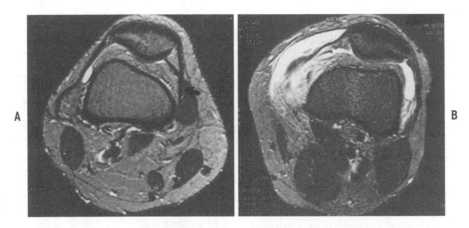

Figure 7-10   Axial magnetic resonance images of the patellofemoral joint. **A.** Normal medial patellofemoral ligament. **B.** Avulsion of the ligament off the medial femoral epicondyle. (Reproduced with permission from Boden BP, Pearsall AW, Garrett WE, Feagin JA Jr: Patellofemoral instability: Evaluation and management. *J Am Acad Orthop Surg* 1997;5:47-57.)

considered. Patellar malalignment can be more sensitively detected with a CT scan.[3] A CT scan allows imaging of the relationship of the patella to the trochlear groove from 20° of flexion to full extension, when the joint relies more on the soft-tissue structures. The axial CT scan can also be used to demonstrate a laterally positioned tibial tubercle.[4]

Definitive Diagnosis

The definitive diagnosis is based on a history of the patella subluxating and subsequently being reduced, direct visualization of the dislocated patella, radiographic findings, and/or the finding of patellar instability causing apprehension. Medial retinacular tearing evident on MRI is helpful in diagnosing dislocation if the patella spontaneously reduced.

Pathomechanics and Functional Limitations

Tearing of the medial retinacular tissues can lead to chronic instability of the patellofemoral joint, potentially causing recurrent subluxations or dislocations. Patients with patellar instability may also experience quadriceps inhibition as a feeling that the leg is giving way. Knee effusion may inhibit contraction of the VMO, thereby increasing patellar instability.

■ Immediate Management

Immediate treatment is to attempt to relocate the patella, either actively or passively. Active reduction is performed by having the patient try to extend the knee by contracting the quadriceps while a slight lateral to medial pressure is exerted on the patella. For a passive reduction, the patient should be as relaxed as possible, lying supine. The distal thigh is stabilized with one hand, while the other hand passively extends the knee. The patella relocation is recognized by the clunk as it goes back into the trochlear groove.

If the initial attempt is unsuccessful, the leg should be immobilized in the current position and the patient transported to the hospital. Further attempts to relocate the patella can then be attempted after oral or injectable pain medication has been administered. In the interim, ice and compression are applied to minimize muscle spasm and pain.

■ Medications

Narcotic analgesics may be prescribed to control the initial pain. A rapid-onset, short-acting intravenous muscle relaxant is used if the first attempt at reducing the dislocation is unsuccessful. The patient may then be prescribed a course of NSAIDs to control inflammation and relieve pain.

■ Postinjury Management

Joint aspiration may be needed to alleviate a tense effusion created by tearing of the medial structures. Fat droplets in the aspirate may indicate an osteochondral lesion. The initial treatment is to immobilize the knee in full extension with a compressive dressing along the lateral aspect of the patella. Approximating the torn medial patellar structures may aid in healing in a satisfactory position. The patient is evaluated every 2 weeks and can begin formal rehabilitation when the tenderness over the medial patellar structures has decreased. A patient with minimal effusion, no signs of malalignment, and a negative J sign is advanced with a course of conservative care.[6,7]

■ Surgical Intervention

Surgical treatment should be considered if conservative management fails to restore patellofemoral joint function; surgical treatment for pain alone is not commonly recommended. If the soft tissues around the joint are thought to be affecting joint alignment clinically, a soft-tissue realignment is an option. This may consist of a lateral release for tight lateral structures, repair or reconstruction of medial stabilizing tissues for a relaxed or torn medial retinaculum, or a combination of these procedures.

Arthroscopy is indicated if an osteochondral lesion has created a loose body within the joint. The physician can visualize the site of the lesion to determine the course of treatment. A small loose body may be removed, whereas a larger lesion may be conducive to surgical fixation to restore the joint surfaces. During arthroscopy, patellar tracking and patellar tilt can also be observed.[8]

Lateral release is most effective in patients with a documented patellar tilt but is seldom performed as an isolated procedure (ST 7-1).[9] The surgery entails sectioning the lateral retinaculum from the vastus lateralis tendon distally, including the lateral patellofemoral and patellotibial ligaments from the superior pole of the patella to the tibial tubercle. Although the lateral release is thought to allow the patella to move medially, the surgery is actually more effective in reducing the posterolateral forces on the patella. Results of the lateral release for patellar instability deteriorate over time.[10-12]

Repair of the medial stabilizing structures should be reserved for younger active athletes who have sustained a patellar dislocation through an indirect mechanism.[13] Surgical repair or reconstruction can also be performed after traumatic injury with incomplete healing of the medial stabilizing structures and recurrent instability.[10] Most often, the medial structures are tightened with a medial-reefing procedure (ST 7-2). The medial patellofemoral ligament is identified through a medial incision and repaired. Many times, the ligamentous injury involves an avulsion from the femoral attachment, which can be repaired with suture anchors.

The VMO can also be advanced distally in an attempt to stabilize the patella. This procedure continues to lose favor with some, as it is not thought to change the vector of pull on the patella.[10] The success of the surgery may result from tightening of the medial ligaments, and it is better to protect the VMO.

Lateral-release and medial-reefing procedures are commonly performed together. If the lateral tissues are tight and create abnormal mechanics and patellar tilt, release or lengthening of these tissues should be considered. In the absence of tight lateral structures, medial reefing should be considered as an isolated procedure.

A medialization procedure of the tibial tubercle should be considered for the skeletally mature patient with a lateral quadriceps mechanism angle and recurrent subluxations or dislocations.[14] In the past, medialization or medialization combined with moving the tibial tubercle distally (Hauser procedure) has also been performed for recurrent patellar instability.[15] The Roux-Elmslie-Trillat procedure combines tibial tubercle transfer with lateral release and medial reefing.[16] Anteriorization procedures (eg, Macquet procedure) have also been advocated to decompress the patellofemoral joint in chronic PFPS (ST 7-3).

More recently, the Fulkerson procedure has been used to correct patellar instability. A modification of earlier medialization procedures, this technique involves an oblique osteotomy of the tibial tubercle. The tubercle is moved medially and anteriorly, effectively decreasing the Q-angle and decompressing the joint. This procedure can be combined with soft-tissue surgeries as indicated. However, an increased incidence of proximal tibial fractures has been identified after Fulkerson procedures.[17]

■ Postinjury/Postoperative Management

Cold packs are administered to reduce pain and control inflammation. Quadriceps-setting exercises are begun within the limits of pain while the patient is wearing the immobilizer. Crutch walking with the patient bearing as much weight on the leg as tolerated begins immediately. If a tense effusion is present, aspirating the joint may help control pain and prevent VMO inhibition.

After arthroscopic debridement of a loose body or a lateral release without a realignment procedure, the patient is treated with a compressive dressing, a lateral buttress, and an elastic bandage (**Figure 7-11**). Formal rehabilitation for strengthening and restoring function begins after 5 to 7 days.

After repair of the medial patellofemoral ligament, the knee is immobilized for 1 to 2 weeks. A compressive dressing with a lateral buttress is applied to push the patella medially and take stress off the repaired tissues. The patient is initially non–weight bearing. After 2 weeks, formal rehabilitation can begin.

After a tibial tubercle transfer procedure, the patient's knee is locked in full extension. Wound healing over the tibial tubercle is a concern, especially with the Macquet procedure, and the immobilization period is required to ensure better wound healing. After 10 to 14 days of adequate healing, the patient can usually begin rehabilitation. The

Lateral Release

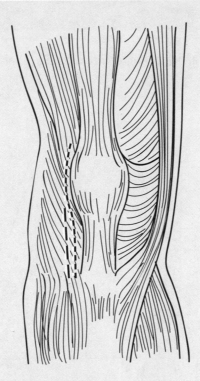

------ Retinacular release
— — — Skin incision (open procedure)

Indications

Patellar tilt and failure of conservative management to decrease patellar dislocations

Overview

Two methods are available for lateral retinacular release.

Arthroscopic

1. Anteromedial and anterolateral peripatellar tendon arthroscopic portals and a superolateral arthroscopic portal are created.
2. The retinaculum is bisected using electrocautery.
3. A needle is placed and visualized to mark the superior pole of the patella.
4. The retinaculum is released from the superior pole of the patella to the inferior aspect of the joint capsule with electrocautery.

Open Procedure

Arthroscopy is performed to visualize the patella and trochlear groove. Thorough inspection of the joint is conducted to look for loose osteochondral or chondral fragments knocked off at the time of the dislocation.

1. A small lateral incision is made over the lateral retinaculum.
2. The lateral retinaculum is incised using electrocautery, without encroaching into the joint capsule.
3. The proximal extent of the release is from the superior patellar pole, but now the release can safely be extended to the level of the tibial tubercle if necessary.

After both procedures, a compressive dressing is applied to control swelling and apply medially directed pressure on the patella, keeping the edges of the newly released tissues unopposed.

Functional Limitations

Early return to functional activity is encouraged. Functional limitations are few.

Implications for Rehabilitation

Patellar mobilization to avoid scar retraction of the release is necessary. Also, aggressive VMO strengthening encourages medialization and correction of the patellar tilt.

Potential Complications

If the lateral release is extended proximally, the vastus lateralis tendon can be separated from the extensor mechanism to the extent that medial dislocation of the patella can occur. Bleeding from the lateral geniculate artery can cause a postoperative hematoma, excessive swelling, and VMO shutdown.

Comments

Usually this procedure is combined with a distal realignment procedure and/or a proximal reefing of the VMO or medial retinaculum.

S|T Surgical Technique 7-2

Medial-Reefing Procedure, Medial Imbrication, or Proximal Patellar Realignment

Indications

Acute injury with documented tear of the medial retinacular structures; in a patient with chronic symptomatic patellar instability in whom conservative management has failed, a medial-reefing procedure can be performed in conjunction with a distal realignment procedure and/or a lateral retinacular release.

Overview

Acute Injury

1. An incision is made around the medial patella.
2. The injury is identified, which is usually easy in the acute setting because visible evidence of palpable defects helps direct the surgeon in the repair.
3. The torn borders of the defect are sutured with an absorbable material.
4. If the medial patellofemoral ligament has been torn from the femoral attachment, suture anchors may be used to repair the damage.

Chronic Injury

1. Dynamic tracking is visualized to observe the maltracking of the patella.
2. A lateral retinacular release (**A**, arrow).
3. The tissue borders are freshened with a sharp incision (**B**).
4. Depending on the quality of tissue present for repair, the surgeon must decide whether to excise a wedge of tissue or overlap the tissues and suture one over the other. Recently, these repairs have been augmented with porcine graft to provide collagen scaffolding for tissue ingrowth, which strengthens the repair (**C, D**).

Functional Limitations

The extremity is immobilized while the repair heals. Gradually advancing flexion is allowed over time.

Implications for Rehabilitation

The knee is immobilized near extension for 2 weeks. The motion allowed depends on the repair and quality of the tissue the surgeon encountered during the procedure. The porcine scaffolding graft is absorbed in 6 weeks. Open kinetic chain straight-leg raises and short-arc quadriceps exercises are initiated at week 2 and advanced to closed kinetic chain exercises by week 6.

Potential Complications

Failure of the repair can occur with time, resulting in increased patellar instability symptoms. Overcorrection can cause the patella to subluxate or dislocate medially, which results in significant extensor-mechanism dysfunction.

Comments

For a patient with chronic symptoms, an aggressive rehabilitation program precedes any surgical intervention.

hinged knee brace remains locked for ambulation until the patient has more than 90° of motion and adequate quadriceps control. After the initial period of non–weight bearing, the patient can progress weight bearing as tolerated.

■ Injury-Specific Treatment and Rehabilitation Concerns

Specific Concerns

Minimize early stresses on the medial patellar restraints.
Control inflammation.
Encourage proper realignment of healing tissues.
Tighten lax tissues.
Lengthen shortened tissues.
Restore normal patellar mobility.

Conservative Management

The initial conservative treatment of patellar dislocation involves controlling inflammation with modalities and therapeutic exercise. As the peripatellar soft tissues heal, patellar mobilization is used to restore normal medial patellar glide and patellar tilt. The patient can progress knee ROM as tolerated with active-assisted or passive exercises. A thorough evaluation of lower extremity flexibility is warranted. Flexibility exercises for the hip, quadriceps, hamstrings, and gastrocnemius-soleus muscle groups are usually instituted.

The strength and proper activation patterns of the pelvis and the entire lower extremity must be restored. The trunk and pelvic muscles are vital to providing a stable base for the lower extremity musculature and should be incorporated into the rehabilitation program. The quadriceps muscles provide dynamic stability of the patella but work in synergy with the hip and calf muscles. Except for quadriceps-setting exercises, other strengthening exercises for the lower extremity should focus on

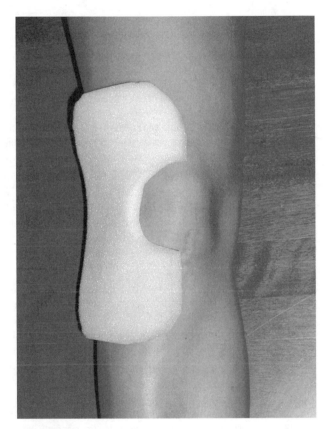

Figure 7-11 Lateral buttress. Applied postoperatively, this felt or foam pad prevents the patella from moving laterally, thereby reducing stress on the healing surgical tissues.

restoring synergistic control of the patella during extremity movement. The patient should simultaneously contract the quadriceps mechanism to stabilize the patella while performing all other lower extremity exercises.

Early on, trunk- and pelvic-stabilization exercises and leg-raising activities are begun in all directions. The quadriceps and VMO are contracted simultaneously with the hip musculature during hip exercises. The patient progresses through open and closed kinetic chain strengthening. As muscle strength and patellar control are restored, the

Fulkerson, Roux-Elmslie-Trillat, and Macquet Distal-realignment Procedures

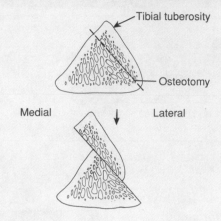

Indications

Failure of conservative management in chronic PFPS and chronic patellar dislocation

Overview

1. Before the distal-realignment procedure, arthroscopy is performed to evaluate the position of the patella, the extent of the articular surface damage, and the presence of loose bodies.
2. Lateral retinacular release and proximal reefing may accompany the distal-realignment procedure and are performed first.
3. A lateral peripatellar tendon incision is made, and the tibial tubercle attachment of the patellar tendon is identified. The proximal lateral tibia is cleaned off the periosteum, and an osteotomy is made with a saw or an osteotome.
4. Individual differences in procedures from this point follow:

Macquet Procedure

1. A long, horizontally oriented osteotomy extending at least one third the length of the tibia is made.
2. The fragment of bone is mobilized and elevated with bone graft from the iliac crest or allograft bone stock. The elevation unloads the patella to decrease the joint reaction forces.
3. The fragment and bone graft are held in position with one or two screws through the fragment into the proximal tibia.

Roux-Elmslie-Trillat Procedure

1. A shorter horizontal osteotomy is performed and medialized with a horizontal slide of 5 to 10 mm.
2. The extent of the medialization depends on the degree of correction anticipated by the preoperative planning and the visualization of patellar tracking intraoperatively.
3. One or two screws are placed through the fragment into the underlying tibia to hold the medialized position.

Fulkerson Procedure

1. An oblique osteotomy is performed through the tibial tubercle and directed from posterolateral to anteromedial.
2. The osteotomy is slid medially in an oblique manner, following the contour of the osteotomy. This oblique slide causes the tubercle to be medialized and elevated. Elevation of the extensor mechanism unloads the joint reaction forces as in the Macquet procedure, and the medial slide corrects the maltracking as in the Roux-Elmslie-Trillat procedure.
3. One or two screws are placed through the fragment into the underlying tibia to hold the elevated, medialized position.

Functional Limitations

Weight bearing is restricted and motion is protected during the early healing phases.

Implications for Rehabilitation

After surgery, the patient wears an immobilizer locked in extension, and weight bearing is limited for the first 2 weeks. Allowed motion and weight bearing progress during the next 4 weeks. At 6 weeks, the patient is out of the brace, performing rehabilitation and bearing weight as tolerated.

After a Macquet procedure, the osteotomy requires an extended time of healing to prevent complications and fracture. The healing time, as determined by radiographic examination, may delay the progression of ROM and weight bearing.

Potential Complications

Macquet: This procedure has a higher rate of nonunion because of the elevated anterior cortex. The very prominent anterior tibial cortex is cosmetically unappealing to some.

Fulkerson: A higher incidence of proximal tibia fractures *may* be related to the use of this procedure, causing some to reconsider the procedure.

Comments

The purpose of this family of procedures is to realign the force vectors pulling on the patella or decrease the joint reaction forces on the patella.

Figure reproduced with permission from Fulkerson JP: Patellofemoral pain disorders: Evaluation and management. *J Am Acad Orthop Surg* 1994;2:124-132.

patient advances through proprioception exercises and agility and sport-specific drills.

Postsurgical Rehabilitation

Lateral Release After a lateral release, medial patellar mobilization should be started as soon as possible to maintain the length of the lateral structures and decrease any contracted scar formation within the tissues. A side-lying position is often helpful for the mobilization, stretching the lateral thigh musculature. Trunk, pelvis, quadriceps, and lower extremity strengthening are begun immediately.

Medial-Reefing Procedure Following a medial-reefing procedure, medial patellar mobilization and ROM exercises can begin after 2 weeks of healing. The ROM and aggressiveness of the progression should be discussed with the surgeon and determined by the degree of flexion tension placed across the repair.

As healing occurs, strengthening progresses. Submaximal quadriceps setting and electrical stimulation can begin at 3 to 4 weeks postoperatively. Active exercises can be advanced at 6 to 8 weeks. Maximal quadriceps contractions should not begin until about 10 to 12 weeks after surgery. The patient then proceeds through proprioception exercises and agility and sport-specific drills.

Distal Realignment Procedure With a distal realignment procedure, after the initial period of immobilization for wound healing, the patient with a stable fixation of the tibial tubercle can progress knee ROM. Passive motion is used at first; flexion past 120° is not pursued until adequate bone healing is demonstrated on radiographs.

Strengthening is advanced once the osteotomy is adequately healed. Submaximal quadriceps exercises can commence at 3 to 4 weeks, with more active exercises beginning at 4 to 6 weeks. Maximal contractions are not progressed until adequate bone healing is demonstrated radiographically, usually by 8 to 10 weeks. The patient then proceeds through proprioception exercises and agility and sport-specific drills.

■ Estimated Amount of Time Lost

Time lost to the injury varies. At minimum, a first-time patellar dislocation requires approximately 3 weeks of immobilization, followed by 3 to 6 weeks of rehabilitation before the athlete begins to return to activity.

The degree of tearing of the medial patellar-stabilizing structures has the greatest influence on

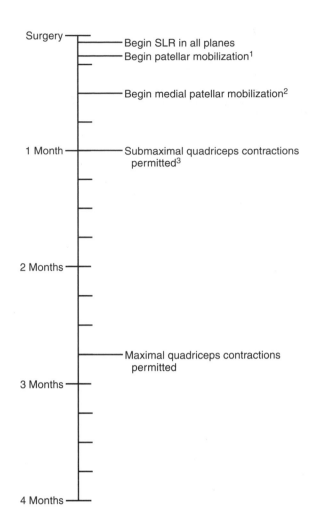

Surgery —— Begin SLR in all planes
—— Begin patellar mobilization[1]

—— Begin medial patellar mobilization[2]

1 Month —— Submaximal quadriceps contractions permitted[3]

2 Months ——

—— Maximal quadriceps contractions permitted

3 Months ——

4 Months ——

Note: Time frames are approximate. Function is the guide.

[1]Lateral release
[2]Medial reefing procedure
[3]Osteotomy

the amount of time lost. If the patella is grossly unstable and requires surgical repair, the time lost can be 4 to 6 months. The surgical procedure ultimately influences the amount of time lost.

■ Return-to-Play Criteria

The patient may return to competition when pain is absent, ROM is full, quadriceps strength has been restored, and functional tests and agility programs with sport-specific activities for the lower extremity are successfully completed.

Functional Bracing

Patellar taping may be helpful in the patient who had a dislocation but now has symptoms more typical of patellar malalignment. A knee sleeve designed to place a medially directed force on the patella may be used for the return to activity.

Patellar Tendinitis

CLINICAL PRESENTATION

History

Repetitive running, jumping, or other activities that produce large concentric and eccentric forces from the extensor mechanism

Pain at the inferior pole of the patella

Pain begins after exercising for a period and then subsides with rest.

Pain may become constant and involve sitting and ascending and descending stairs.

Observation

Swelling and redness may be present at the inferior pole of the patellar tendon.

Functional Status

Gait may be antalgic.

Usually, ROM is full but may be painful with active and resisted extension and/or passive flexion.

Physical Evaluation Findings

Pain with resisted extension

Pain with passive stretch of the extensor mechanism

Pain with palpation of the inferior pole of the patella

Patellar tendinitis is an overuse injury of the knee's extensor mechanism. The condition is characterized by pain in the anterior aspect of the knee; close inspection usually pinpoints the inflammatory process at the inferior patellar pole. Often termed "jumper's knee," the injury is more common in basketball, volleyball, and soccer players and in dancers. The forceful extension exerted during jumping and eccentric forces during landing create microtrauma and inflammation in the patellar tendon.[18] Patellar tendinitis can be classified using a 6-stage scale modified from the work of Blazina[19,20] (**Table 7-1**).

Osgood-Schlatter disease is a traction apophysitis that causes tibial osteochondrosis from the pull of the patellar tendon. It occurs in people with active growth plates, usually going through growth spurts, and is typified by pain at the tibial tubercle. Sinding-Larsen-Johansson syndrome is a traction injury that causes a patellar osteochondrosis at the insertion of the patellar tendon into the inferior pole of the patella.

Differential Diagnosis

Partial patellar tendon rupture, patellar bursitis, Osgood-Schlatter disease, Sinding-Larsen-Johansson syndrome

Table 7-1

Classification of Patellar Tendinitis According to Symptoms

Stage	Symptoms
0	No pain
1	Pain only after intense sport activity; no undue functional impairment
2	Pain at the beginning and after sport activity; still able to perform at a satisfactory level
3	Pain during sport activity; increasing difficulty performing at a satisfactory level
4	Pain during sport activity; unable to participate in sport at a satisfactory level
5	Pain during daily activity; unable to participate in sport at any level

Adapted with permission from Ferretti A, Conteduca F, Camerucci E, Morelli F: Patellar tendinosis: A follow-up study of surgical treatment. *J Bone Joint Surg Am* 2002;84:2179-2185.

Imaging Techniques

Lateral and AP radiographs are obtained to assess osteophyte formation at the inferior pole of the patella and calcification within the tendon. MRI is reserved for patients with recalcitrant symptoms and those in whom surgical intervention is being considered (**Figure 7-12**).

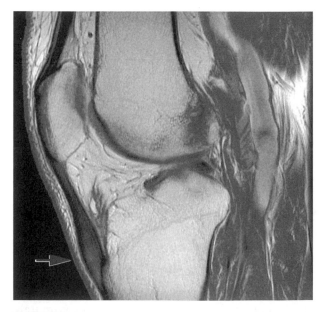

Figure 7-12   Magnetic resonance imaging demonstrating patellar tendinosis. The arrow illustrates a thickening of the patellar tendon, indicative of patellar tendinosis. (Reproduced with permission from Johnson TR, Steinbach LS (eds): *Essentials of Musculoskeletal Imaging.* Rosemont, IL, American Academy of Orthopaedic Surgeons, 2004, p 488.)

Definitive Diagnosis

Pain in the extensor mechanism during activity, resisted knee extension, and passive stretch of the extensor mechanism; pain with palpation of the tendon at and just below the inferior pole of the patella

Pathomechanics and Functional Limitations

Physical activity is limited by pain from the inflammatory process. Jumping activities are among the first to be limited, followed by running, ascending and descending stairs, and walking. Weakness of the knee extensor mechanism or patellar maltracking can alter lower extremity biomechanics and cause overuse injuries anywhere along the kinetic chain.

■ Immediate Management

Patellar tendinitis typically does not occur acutely. If the pain affects the patient's ability to function normally during an activity, ceasing activity and applying ice are warranted.

■ Medications

Initially, NSAIDs are used. Phonophoresis or iontophoresis may be attempted for recalcitrant symptoms, but the efficacy of these techniques is not substantiated. Corticosteroid injection is contraindicated because of the increased risk of tendon rupture.

■ Postinjury Management

Rest from aggravating activities is essential to reduce the inflammatory response. Patients with pain during ROM may benefit from several days of rest in an immobilizer. If gait is painful, an assistive device such as crutches, a cane, or an immobilizer should be used. After an initial period to decrease the inflammatory process, rehabilitation is started to restore normal function in a manner similar to that described in the patellofemoral pain syndrome section.

■ Surgical Intervention

Surgical intervention is rarely needed. In advanced cases, the surgeon may debride the patella near the insertion of the patellar tendon to reinitiate the healing process (ST 7-4).

■ Postoperative Management

The patient's knee is placed in a hinged knee brace locked in full extension, and the patient may bear weight as tolerated for the first 2 weeks. The patient may begin ROM exercises immediately, but extremes of flexion are avoided until the skin has healed adequately.

The patient can discontinue the brace after 4 weeks if knee flexion is at least 120°, adequate leg control is demonstrated by a normal leg raise, and the gait pattern is normal.

■ Injury-Specific Treatment and Rehabilitation Concerns

> **Specific Concerns**
>
> Control inflammation.
> Restore normal muscle firing pattern.
> Restore strength of the quadriceps and hamstrings.
> Emphasize proper biomechanics.

Initial rehabilitation focuses on controlling the inflammatory process. Iontophoresis using dexamethasone with or without lidocaine may be prescribed. Because of the superficial nature of the tissue, ice is used judiciously.

Gentle stretching exercises are begun as soon as possible; the sensation of stretch within the muscle group should be elicited. Pain at the inflamed tendon warrants modifying stretch positioning (prone with assistance from a strap vs standing) or passive stretching. Cross-friction massage may be administered before the stretch to decrease pain and improve blood flow. Beginning with light but deep massage perpendicular to the tendon, greater pressure can be applied as the area becomes less sensitive to the applied force.

The quadriceps mechanism and the hip flexor groups are the focus. A generalized stretching program for both lower extremities should also be performed. A progressive strengthening program is instituted to the patient's tolerance. In severe, longstanding patellar tendinitis, moderate to severe atrophy may be present.

Although the focus is on open and closed kinetic chain exercises for the quadriceps mechanism, a complete trunk, pelvic, and lower extremity program should be included. Proximal stabilization is essential, and eccentric control of the quadriceps musculature needs to be emphasized. Isokinetics may also be helpful to strengthen the quadriceps under conditions that better replicate the higher-speed contractions needed during jumping and landing from a jump.

When the patient is pain free and has adequate flexibility and strength, plyometric training is beneficial in preparing for the return to competitive activities. Initially, the focus must be on proper technique, progressing to endurance training for

S|T   Surgical Technique   7-4

Debridement of the Patellar Tendon

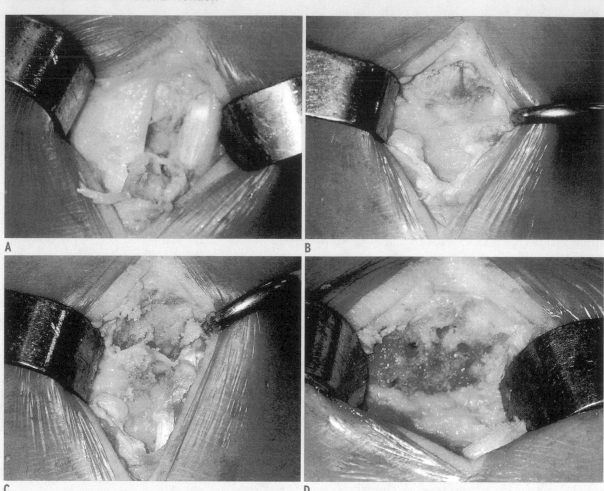

A

B

C

D

Indications

Failure of conservative management

Overview

1. An incision is made over the anterior tendon (**A**).
2. The paratenon and proximal portion of the tendon are split longitudinally (**B**).
3. The diseased areas of the tendon are identified; however, gross inspection often reveals an outwardly normal appearance.[19]
4. The inferior pole of the patella is exposed, and a small cortical bone block is removed along with the proximal central portion of the tendon (**C**).
5. The inferior pole of the patella is drilled to create a bleeding tissue bed conducive to healing (**D**).
6. Only the paratenon is closed.

Functional Limitations

The patient is restricted from weight bearing and motion is protected during the early healing phases.

Implications for Rehabilitation

After the initial non-weight bearing period, the patient is permitted to ambulate in a locked brace with limited weight bearing as tolerated.

Potential Complications

Inadequate wound healing; rarely, the patellar tendon may avulse or rupture after return to activity.

Comments

This procedure is reserved for patients whose symptoms do not respond to adequate conservative management.

Figures reproduced with permission from Ferretti A, Conteduca F, Camerucci E, Morelli F: Patellar tendinosis: A follow-up study of surgical treatment. *J Bone Joint Surg Am* 2002;84:2179-2185.

the athlete who must jump repetitively. On successful completion of a plyometric program, sport-specific drills can begin.

Estimated Amount of Time Lost

Decreased or restricted activity for 1 to 4 weeks is required for conservative treatment, which should be tried for at least 3 months before surgery is considered. For minor symptoms, activity modification is favored over surgical treatment.

Patients whose symptoms interfere with normal sports and daily activities and fail to respond to conservative measures may require surgery.[21] Time lost after surgery can vary from 3 to 6 months, depending on the patient's ability to reverse the effects of previous inactivity and postsurgical morbidity.

Return-to-Play Criteria

The patient may return to competition when pain is absent, ROM is full, lower extremity and particularly quadriceps strength has been restored, and functional, agility, and sport-specific tests are successfully completed.

Functional Bracing

A patellar strap may be worn, but the success and tolerance of this device varies widely. A simple knee sleeve with a patellar cutout may be useful in increasing warmth within the tendon (see Figure 7-7).

Patellar Tendon Rupture

The patellar tendon is placed under high tensile forces during athletic activities, especially when the quadriceps femoris muscles are contracting eccentrically. This force is magnified if a fall is sustained on the patella while the quadriceps muscles are contracting eccentrically. The resulting force can overwhelm the tendon and lead to a patellar fracture (see p 213).

Tendon ruptures are classified as suprapatellar or infrapatellar, but complete tendon ruptures are rare (**Figure 7-13**). Suprapatellar tendon ruptures are also known as quadriceps tendon ruptures. Both types of ruptures tend to occur in athletic patients who are younger than 40 years and are often the

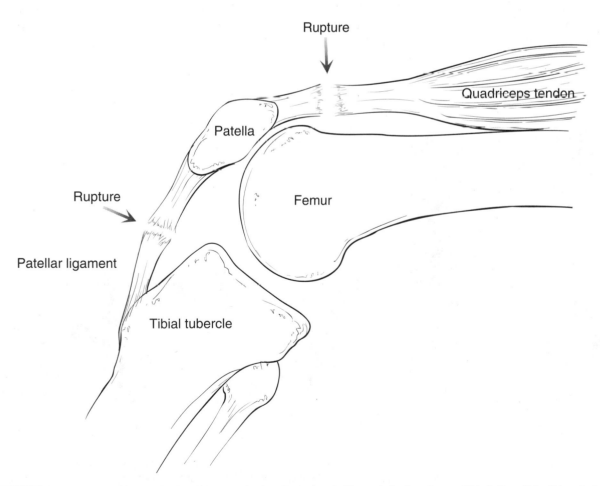

Rupture

Quadriceps tendon

Patella

Rupture

Femur

Patellar ligament

Tibial tubercle

Figure 7-13 Common areas of ruptures in the extensor mechanism. (Reproduced with permission from Greene WB (ed): *Essentials of Musculoskeletal Care*, ed 2. Rosemont, IL, American Academy of Orthopaedic Surgeons, 2000, p 404.)

CLINICAL PRESENTATION

History

Forceful contraction of the quadriceps, especially when the knee is flexed

Immediate pain and disability

Observation

Obvious defect at the rupture site

Swelling from hemarthrosis

Functional Status

Inability to straighten the leg

Inability to bear weight

Some knee extension may be possible if the patellar retinaculum is intact.

Physical Evaluation Findings

Passive flexion is limited by pain and swelling.

Inability to maintain a passively extended knee against gravity

A palpable defect is present in a complete rupture

Differential Diagnosis

Patellar fracture, patellar dislocation

Imaging Techniques

Lateral and AP views are obtained to rule out bone injury. Patella alta is easily identified using lateral radiographs. MRI is helpful if there is any question about the extent of the injury or if a concomitant injury to surrounding tissues is suspected (**Figure 7-14**). Diagnostic ultrasound can also be used to visualize a tendon rupture.

Definitive Diagnosis

A partial tear is characterized by pain and extensor-mechanism weakness. The partial defect may be palpable, and the patient can hold the knee in a passively extended position. With a complete tear, the patient is unable to actively maintain the passively extended knee against gravity; if the retinaculum is also torn, the patient cannot extend the knee against gravity. A defect may be palpable at the rupture site. The extent of the rupture can be confirmed by MRI.

Pathomechanics and Functional Limitations

Acutely, the patient with a partial tear is unable to bear weight without pain and the sensation of giving way. With a complete rupture, the patient is immediately unable to generate forces in the quadriceps mechanism and cannot maintain body weight against gravity.

end result of long-term tendinitis. The course of treatment for a partial tendon tear depends on the severity of the injury. The tear may be treated conservatively with rehabilitation, or, if most of the tendon is ruptured, the tear may need to be treated surgically. Patellar tendon rupture is a potential complication after anterior cruciate ligament reconstruction when the middle third of the patellar tendon is harvested as donor tissue.

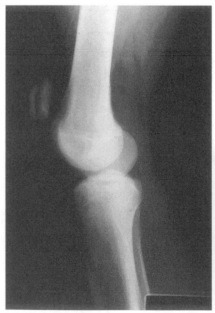
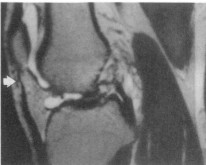
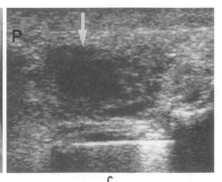

A   B   C

Figure 7-14   Imaging modalities for patellar tendon ruptures. **A**. Lateral radiograph of the knee indicates a high-riding patella (patella alta). The entire patella is superior to the Blumensaat line (a line drawn parallel to the intercondylar notch). **B**. Sagittal magnetic resonance image of the patellar tendon demonstrating a rupture near the infrapatellar pole (arrow). **C**. Sagittal ultrasonic image of an acute tear of the midsubstance of the tendon (arrow) (P, patella). (Reproduced with permission from Matava MJ: Patellar tendon ruptures. *J Am Acad Orthop Surg* 1996;4:287-296.)

■ Immediate Management

The knee should be placed in a straight-leg immobilizer and the patient given crutches. Ice can be applied. The foot should be placed on the ground with minimal weight bearing, so the patient is more stable.

■ Medications

Analgesic medications are helpful in controlling pain.

■ Postinjury Management

The knee is placed in a hinged knee brace locked in extension until surgery. Aspiration of the hemarthrosis can make the patient more comfortable.

■ Surgical Intervention

Patellar tendon rupture is best treated with surgical repair performed within 7 to 10 days. Simple end-to-end suturing of the patellar defect alone or in conjunction with a cerclage suture is most commonly performed (**S T** 7-5).[22] Suture anchors are being used more frequently, and the use of porcine scaffolding graft is also gaining acceptance to augment the surgical repair.

■ Postoperative Management

A compressive dressing is applied to the knee, which is placed in extension in a locked hinged knee brace. The patient can bear weight by toe-touch during crutch-assisted walking. Active quadriceps setting should be performed on the first postoperative day. At 2 weeks, the skin sutures are removed, and formal rehabilitation begins.

■ Injury-Specific Treatment and Rehabilitation Concerns

Specific Concerns

Control loads placed on the extensor mechanism
Delay the onset of atrophy.
Prevent arthrofibrosis secondary to decreased ROM during the immobilization period.

The patient continues to wear the locked brace for ambulation. Weight bearing is progressed at 4 weeks, with the goal of full weight bearing in the locked brace by 6 weeks. During this time, the patient can perform gait training with the brace unlocked. The brace can be discontinued when flexion is at least 120°, control of the extensor mechanism

without an extensor lag on straight-leg raise is adequate, and normal gait is possible.

Passive ROM exercises are initiated from full extension to 45°. Increasing flexion by approximately 30° per week is appropriate; flexion is not forced. At about 6 weeks, the patient can begin prone stretching for the quadriceps mechanism. Patellar mobilization can be performed, but superior glides should be performed only out of necessity and with caution. Superior glides are not recommended until at least 4 to 6 weeks postoperatively.

At approximately 2 weeks, the patient begins leg raising in all planes, performed with active quadriceps setting during the exercise; leg raises can be performed with the brace on until adequate leg control is attained. Active knee extension begins at 3 weeks through the available ROM. If an extensor lag is present, the leg can be passively extended, and the patient can first work on eccentric contractions of the muscle group. Heavy loads are

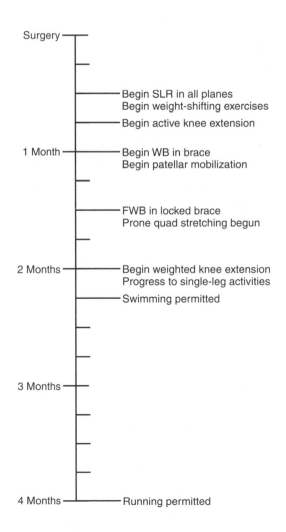

Surgery

Begin SLR in all planes
Begin weight-shifting exercises
Begin active knee extension

1 Month — Begin WB in brace
Begin patellar mobilization

FWB in locked brace
Prone quad stretching begun

2 Months — Begin weighted knee extension
Progress to single-leg activities
Swimming permitted

3 Months

4 Months — Running permitted

Note: Time frames are approximate. Function is the guide.

S|T Surgical Technique 7-5

Repair of a Patellar Tendon Rupture

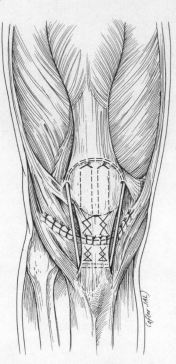

Indications

Definitive diagnosis of a patellar tendon rupture

Overview

1. The tendon is exposed through a vertical midline incision.
2. The frayed tendon ends are debrided to a bed of a viable tissue.
3. Three holes are drilled through the longitudinal length of the patella.
4. Sutures are woven through the distal tendon across the defect into the proximal portion of the tendon and then passed through the transpatellar holes. Suture anchors can replace these two steps and provide excellent fixation during the healing phase.
5. If a cerclage suture or tape is to be used, a hole is drilled transversely though the tibial tubercle posterior to the tendon insertion. Suture or surgical tape is placed through this hole, taken up over the patella, and passed posterior to the quadriceps tendon.
6. The sutures are clamped but not tied.
7. A lateral radiograph is obtained to determine whether the height of the patella is similar to that of the patella in the contralateral leg. The sutures can then be tightened or loosened until adequate tension is obtained to restore normal tendon length. The sutures are then tied over the superior pole of the patella, and the cerclage suture or tape is also tied off.
8. If the patellar tendon is avulsed from the inferior pole of the patella, suture anchors can be used with the suture woven through the tendon stump distally and tied as the tendon is reduced onto the patella.

Functional Limitations

Limitations are related to the severity of the injury and the speed of surgical repair.

Implications for Rehabilitation

Protect the extensor mechanism with a hinged knee brace to limit ROM

Potential Complications

Failure of the fixation; difficulty regaining flexion may necessitate manipulation under anesthesia to break up fibrosis once the extensor mechanism has adequate healing

Comments

A fine line exists between healing the extensor mechanism and regaining functional ROM. More problems develop in quadriceps tendon repairs than in patellar tendon repairs.

Figure reproduced with permission from Matava MJ: Patellar tendon ruptures. *J Am Acad Orthop Surg* 1996;4:287-296.

Chapter 7 Patellofemoral Injuries 213

not added until at least 8 weeks postoperatively. Closed kinetic chain strengthening exercises can begin as soon as the patient is bearing at least 50% weight on the injured leg. Single-leg closed kinetic chain activities can progress when the patient is bearing full weight.

The patient may begin stationary bicycle riding as soon as sufficient ROM is available without any compensatory movements at other joints. Walking on a treadmill or elliptical glider or exercising on a ski machine can begin when bearing full weight. However, these exercises must be performed without compensation or deviation. As the patient tires, especially early in rehabilitation, the exercise should be halted for that session. Aquatic therapy can be an excellent choice for this patient population. Exercises for ROM and strengthening can begin as the wound is healed, and actual swimming can begin at about 6 to 8 weeks. The patient can return to running at 4 months if no gait deviations are noted.

■ Estimated Amount of Time Lost

Estimated rehabilitation time is 4 to 6 months after surgical repair. Postoperative complications, including arthrofibrosis or patella baja or patella alta, that affect the ability of the quadriceps mechanism to produce force can delay the rehabilitation process.

■ Return-to-Play Criteria

The patient may return to competition when pain is absent, ROM is full, quadriceps strength is restored, and functional tests for the lower extremity are completed successfully. Typically this occurs 4 to 6 months after the repair.

Functional Bracing

A neoprene knee sleeve may be used for comfort.

Patellar Fracture

Patellar fractures are not common in the young population, but they pose great concern when they occur. The primary mechanism of injury is similar to that of a patellar tendon rupture, falling on the patella when the quadriceps is contracting eccentrically (see p 209). A patellar fracture associated only with quadriceps muscle contraction is rare and usually the result of a preexisting patellar stress fracture.[23]

Patellar fractures are classified as shown in **Figure 7-15**. After injury, articular surface congruency must be restored to prevent decreased torque pro-

CLINICAL PRESENTATION

History

A fall or direct blow to the patella
Pain arising from the patella

Observation

Swelling over and around the patella is present.
Acute hemarthrosis
Deformity of the patella may be noted, although it may be masked by edema.

Functional Status

The patient is unable to bear weight on the involved leg.
During flexion and extension, ROM is decreased; extension lags at least 10° to 30°.[23]
Inhibition of the quadriceps mechanism is noted as an inability to produce force.

Physical Evaluation Findings

Inability to generate force across the extensor mechanism to perform a straight-leg raise

duction from the extensor mechanism and to limit abnormal joint reaction force patterns at the patellofemoral articulation.

Differential Diagnosis

Patellar tendon rupture, quadriceps tendon rupture, patellar dislocation

Imaging Techniques

Lateral and AP radiographs are taken to determine the status of the fracture, including how many fragments are present and their positions (**Figure 7-16**). If axial views are attainable, they can be helpful in determining the congruity of the articular surface of the patella.

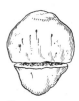

Transverse   Vertical   Marginal

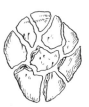 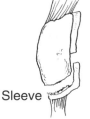

Comminuted   Osteochondral   Sleeve

Figure 7-15 Classification of patellar fractures based on the configuration of the fracture lines. (Reproduced with permission from Cramer KE, Moed BR: Patellar fractures: Contemporary approach to treatment. *J Am Acad Orthop Surg* 1997;5:323-331.)

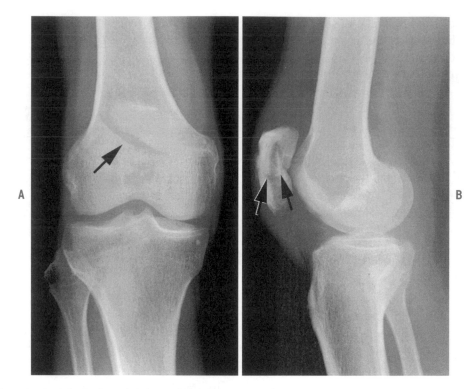

Figure 7-16 Radiographs of patellar fractures. **A.** Anteroposterior view demonstrating an oblique fracture through the superior patella (arrow). **B.** Lateral view demonstrating fracture of the body of the patella (left arrow) and a step-off of the articular surface (right arrow). (Reproduced with permission from Johnson TR, Steinbach LS (eds): *Essentials of Musculoskeletal Imaging*. Rosemont, IL, American Academy of Orthopaedic Surgeons, 2004, p 495.)

Definitive Diagnosis

Radiographic findings demonstrating the fracture

Pathomechanics and Functional Limitations

Fracturing the patella disrupts the ability of the extensor mechanism to generate forces across the knee. Normal daily living and sport activities are severely limited. Occasionally, if the fracture is nondisplaced or vertical, enough integrity may remain in the extensor mechanism to allow a weak straight-leg raise. However, with displacement, the extensor-mechanism disruption limits the ability to perform a straight-leg raise.

■ Immediate Management

The knee is immobilized in a position of comfort; full extension is preferred if possible. Ice can be applied, and crutches are used for non–weight-bearing ambulation.

■ Medications

Narcotic analgesics can be used to control the initial pain. The patient may then be prescribed a course of NSAIDs to control inflammation.

■ Postinjury Management

A tense effusion can be aspirated to provide pain relief. Lacerations and abrasions must be actively managed with a wound-care program of cleaning

and proper dressings. Adequate healing of any wounds is essential to minimize a surgical delay because of wound problems. The presence of surface wounds may constitute an open fracture and should be managed accordingly.[24,25] The knee is placed in an immobilizer in full extension to minimize stress across the extensor mechanism. Ice can continue to be used before surgery.

■ Surgical Intervention

Except when the patellar fracture is a small avulsion, the injury almost always requires fixation using various techniques, including screw fixation or Kirschner wires and tension-band loops (**ST** 7-6). Soft-tissue repairs to the retinaculum and quadriceps muscle can be performed as well.

The arthroscopically assisted surgical approach as a means of avoiding skin problems, allowing early rehabilitation, and achieving better cosmesis has been advocated.[26] With this technique, the surgical fixation is similar to that obtained from an open technique but is guided by an arthroscope and fluoroscopy.

■ Postinjury/Postoperative Management

The leg is placed in a compressive dressing and locked in extension in a hinged knee brace. Special attention must be directed at wound care and

S|T Surgical Technique 7-6

Open Reduction and Internal Fixation of Patellar Fractures

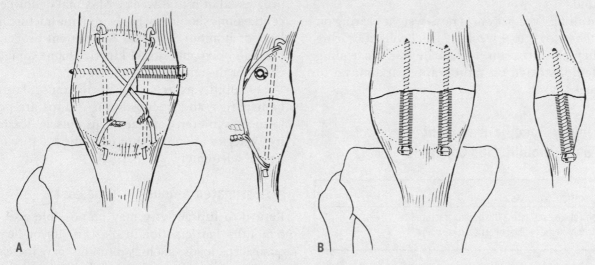

A   B

Indications

Fracture of the patella; fixation technique varies according to the type and orientation of the fracture line

Overview

1. A vertical incision is made, and the fracture is identified.
2. The joint is inspected through the defect to visualize the femoral condyles and trochlear groove for defects and damage.
3. The patellar articular surface is palpated.
4. Thorough irrigation and probing to extract any fragments are necessary.
5. The fracture configuration is determined by direct visualization. The fragment borders are cleaned to aid in the fracture reduction.
6. Fragments are drilled and Kirschner wires placed to hold the fragments in place for fixation.
7. Cannulated-screw systems have become popular because the fixation screw is placed directly over the temporary wire fixation. The fracture configuration dictates the fixation techniques.
8. Figure-of-eight cerclage wiring can augment the fixation, or if comminution is severe, it may be the only option.
9. Often, capsular defects medially and laterally accompany a transverse patellar fracture and must be sutured and repaired.

Functional Limitations

Healing must occur before aggressive ROM and strengthening exercises can be initiated.

Implications for Rehabilitation

After surgery, the knee is placed in a controlled-motion brace and the patient is limited in weight bearing. Early open kinetic chain exercises are initiated when pain allows. As healing is documented, ROM and progressive resistance exercises are advanced. Complete healing takes place in 6 to 8 weeks.

Potential Complications

Failure or loss of fixation and posttraumatic arthritis are the most common complications. Also retained hardware can become painful postoperatively.

Comments

Patellar fractures should be managed acutely. Skin defects should be thoroughly probed to determine whether the defect extends into the fracture. Reestablishing the articular surface to limit posttraumatic arthritis is preferred, but the fracture configuration dictates fixation options. High degrees of comminution (which usually occurs in the distal pole of the patella) may require excision of some of the fragments.

Figures reproduced with permission from Boden, BP, Pearsall, AW, Garrett, WE, Feagin, JA: Patellofemoral instability: Evaluation and management. *J Am Acad Orthop Surg* 1997;5:47-57.

adequate wound healing. After 3 to 4 days, the bulky dressing is removed and the wound assessed. At 1 week, the patient begins submaximal quadriceps setting and passive ROM that does not stress the wound.

Initially the patient is non–weight bearing on crutches for 3 to 4 weeks. Partial weight bearing is then permitted until adequate fracture healing is demonstrated on radiographs, at about 6 to 8 weeks.

Injury-Specific Treatment and Rehabilitation Concerns

Specific Concerns

Control stresses across the healing fracture site.
Encourage the healing of articular cartilage.

As the fracture heals, the patient can progress knee ROM, limiting the stress placed on the wound. Initially, this is performed with passive ROM and then advanced to active-assisted ROM. Flexion past 90° is not pursued until adequate bone healing has occurred, usually in 6 to 8 weeks after fixation. However, tension-band wiring may allow for mobilization at 4 to 6 weeks. Patellar mobilization is not performed until adequate fracture healing is demonstrated.

Submaximal quadriceps setting and electrical stimulation can begin at 2 to 3 weeks. Early on, leg-raising activities are begun in all directions. The quadriceps and VMO are contracted simultaneously with the hip musculature during hip exercises. Active exercises for strengthening the quadriceps are progressed at 6 to 8 weeks. Maximal quadriceps contractions should not begin until the fracture has healed, at about 8 weeks. The patient proceeds through open and closed kinetic chain strengthening for the entire lower extremity.

Flexibility exercises for the hip musculature, hamstrings, and triceps surae groups are performed as tolerated. Quadriceps muscle flexibility exercises are not begun until the fracture has healed adequately.

Estimated Amount of Time Lost

Return to full activity may be possible at 4 to 6 months. Participation in sports requiring heavy quadriceps loads, such as jumping, may increase the time required to return to full activity.

Return-to-Play Criteria

The patient may return to competition when pain is resolved, ROM is full, quadriceps strength is restored, and functional, agility, and sport-specific tests are successfully completed.

Functional Bracing

A knee sleeve with a patellar cutout may be used to increase warmth to the area. A Drytex or elastic material is preferred over neoprene to avoid skin breakdown.

Rehabilitation

This section presents treatment techniques that are unique to the patellofemoral articulation. Refer to the knee rehabilitation section (p 182) and chapter 9 for therapeutic exercises for the patellofemoral joint, knee, and lower extremity.

Patellar Mobilization

Patellar mobilization may be indicated for conditions of the interrelated patellofemoral joint and knee. An injury to one joint can adversely affect the other joint.

To perform patellar mobilization, the patient should be supine or sitting off the edge of the table. In the supine position, an adjustable bolster can be placed under the knee to modify the amount of ex-

tension. Having the patient sitting off the edge of the table assists in performing mobilizations with the knee in varying degrees of flexion. The patient's leg can then be placed over the clinician's leg to alter the amount of flexion.

Performing mobilization routines is easier if an interface between the clinician's hand and the patient's skin is used to better grasp the patella. Gauze pads, a damp towel, or a rubber material such as a jar opener can be used for this purpose. The patella is moved inferiorly, superiorly, medially, or laterally until resistance is felt, and the position is held for at least 30 seconds to attain a low-load, prolonged stretch (**Figure 7-17**). When performing medial mobilizations, position the patient side lying on the side opposite the treatment and place a pillow or towels between the legs to enhance relaxation.

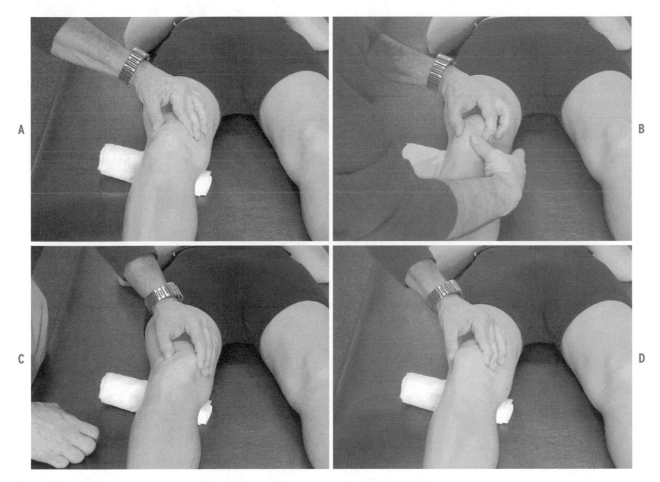

Figure 7-17 Patellar mobilization techniques. **A.** *Inferior mobilization.* Grasp the superior pole of the patella and move it distally until resistance is felt. **B.** *Superior mobilization.* Grasp the inferior patellar pole and move the patella proximally until resistance is felt. **C.** *Medial mobilization.* Grasp the patella with the thumbs on the lateral side and the forefingers on the medial side. Glide the patella medially until resistance is felt. **D.** *Lateral mobilization.* Grasp the patella firmly between the thumbs on the lateral side and the forefingers on the medial side.

Extra caution is required when performing medial patellar mobilization. This technique is similar to the apprehension test and may result in patient anxiety.

At minimum, a set of 5 repetitions should be performed, although whether more mobilization is needed can be determined for each patient. As with any stretching of soft tissues, two to three sets of the mobilization should be performed throughout the day.

Patellar Tendon Cross-Friction Massage

The patient is supine with the knee on a bolster or sitting over the edge of the table. The forefinger and middle finger deliver massage strokes perpendicularly to the patellar tendon. As the tendon becomes less sensitive, increase the pressure being applied.

Iliotibial Band Trigger-Point Massage

Numerous trigger points may form within the length of the iliotibial band as the result of patellofemoral dysfunction. Trigger-point massage is performed with the patient side lying on the side opposite the injury. Positioning a pillow or towels between the patient's legs enhances the relaxation.

With the thumb or a commercially available device, start with light but deep pressure to the trigger point. The pressure is then increased to the patient's tolerance, and the massage is performed for about 30 to 60 seconds. The iliotibial band should be stretched immediately after the massage.

Patellar Taping

Patellar taping as developed by McConnell has become a popular adjunct to the treatment of patellofemoral conditions.[27] McConnell based the taping on creating a more appropriate alignment of the patella as it tracks within the femoral groove, thus decreasing pain and improving function (**Figure 7-18**).

After a thorough evaluation, patellar taping can be used as an adjunct to rehabilitation. The specific applications of the McConnell taping techniques are beyond the scope of this text, but in general, the techniques attempt to correct patellar glide, tilt, and rotation (**Table 7-2**).

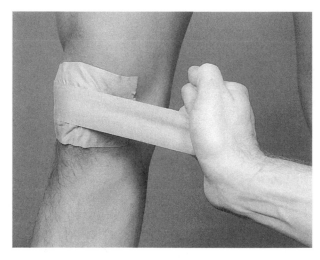

Figure 7-18   The McConnell taping technique. This figure shows the patella being moved medially.

Table 7-2

Patellar Taping

Position	Findings	Technique
Glide: the medial or lateral displacement of the patella	The critical test: The clinician manually blocks the patella into a medial glide as the patient performs isometric quadriceps contractions throughout the ROM. Decreased pain indicates a laterally gliding patella.	Tape is secured at the lateral border of the patella. The clinician applies a medial manual glide, takes up soft tissue along the medial aspect of the thigh, and secures the tape along the medial femoral condyle.
Tilt: (1) the anterior-posterior orientation with respect to the medial and lateral facet orientation to the femur. (2) the superior-inferior orientation with respect to the superior and inferior pole orientation to the femur	The clinician places the thumb and index finger along the medial and lateral borders of the patella with the knee extended and the quadriceps relaxed. The orientation of the patellar borders is assessed. (Tight lateral structures are presumed to cause the lateral border to rest lower than the medial border.) Repeated with the superior and inferior poles of the patella.	To correct a tilt, tape is placed opposite the tilt and secured to correct the alignment. For example, to correct a lateral tilt, the tape is placed along the medial aspect of the patella. The clinician applies a medial manual tilt, takes up soft tissue along the medial aspect of the thigh, and secures the tape along the medial femoral condyle.
Rotation: a comparison of the longitudinal axis of the patella with the longitudinal axis of the femur	The clinician determines the longitudinal axis of the patella by palpating the midpoint of the superior and inferior poles of the patella. The line formed by these two points is considered the axis of the patella and is compared with the axis of the femur. With an externally rotated patella, the inferior patellar pole sits laterally compared with the femur's longitudinal axis. With an internally rotated patella, the inferior patellar pole sits medially compared with the femur's longitudinal axis.	Correction of an externally rotated patella: Tape is secured laterally along the inferior border of the patella. The inferior pole of the patella is manually rotated into a neutral position, and the tape is secured superiorly along the medial aspect of the femoral condyle. Correction of an internally rotated patella: The tape is secured superiorly along the lateral border of the patella. The patella is manually corrected, and the tape is secured inferiorly along the medial aspect of the femoral condyle.

7

References

1. Johnson LL: Arthroscopic abrasion arthroplasty: A review. *Clin Orthop* 2001;391(suppl):S306-S317.

2. Steadman JR, Rodkey WG, Rodrigo JJ: Microfracture: Surgical technique and rehabilitation to treat chondral defects. *Clin Orthop* 2001;391(suppl):S362-S369.

3. Inoue M, Shino K, Hirose H, Horibe S, Ono K: Subluxation of the patella: Computed tomography analysis of patellofemoral congruence. *J Bone Joint Surg Am* 1988;70:1331-1337.

4. Jones RB, Barlett EC, Vainright JR, Carroll RG: CT determination of tibial tubercle lateralization in patients presenting with anterior knee pain. *Skeletal Radiol* 1995;24:505-509.

5. Witonski D: Dynamic magnetic resonance imaging. *Clin Sports Med* 2002;21:403-415.

6. Micheli LJ: Patellofemoral disorders in children, in Fox JM, Del Pizzo W (eds): *The Patellofemoral Joint*, New York, NY, McGraw-Hill, 1993, pp 105-121.

7. Cash JD, Hughston JC: Treatment of acute patellar dislocation. *Am J Sports Med* 1988;16:244-249.

8. Schreiber SN: Proximal superomedial portal in arthroscopy of the knee. *Arthroscopy* 1991;7:246-251.

9. Kolowich PA, Paulos LE, Rosenberg TD, Farnsworth S: Lateral release of the patella: Indications and contraindications. *Am J Sports Med* 1990;18:359-365.

10. Post WR, Teitge R, Amis A: Patellofemoral malalignment: Looking beyond the viewbox. *Clin Sports Med* 2002;21:521-546.

11. Metcalf RW: An arthroscopic method for lateral release of subluxating or dislocating patella. *Clin Orthop* 1982;167:9-18.

12. Betz RR, Magill JT III, Lonergan RP: The percutaneous lateral retinacular release. *Am J Sports Med* 1987;15:477-482.

13. Boden BP, Pearsall AW, Garrett WE, Feagin JA Jr: Patellofemoral instability: Evaluation and management. *J Am Acad Orthop Surg* 1997;5:47-57.

14. Fulkerson JP: Patellofemoral pain disorders: Evaluation and management: *J Am Acad Orthop Surg* 1994;2:124-132.

15. Hauser EW: Total tendon transplant for slipping patella. *Surg Gynecol Obstet* 1938;66:199-214.

16. Cox JS: Evaluation of the Roux-Elmslie-Trillat procedure for knee extensor realignment. *Am J Sports Med* 1982;10:303-310.

17. Fulkerson JP: Fracture of the proximal tibia after Fulkerson anteromedial tibial tubercle transfer: A report of four cases. *Am J Sports Med* 1999;27:265.

18. Richards DP, Ajemian SV, Wiley JP, Zernicke RF: Knee joint dynamics predict patellar tendonitis in elite volleyball players. *Am J Sports Med* 1996;24:676-683.

19. Ferretti A, Conteduca F, Camerucci E, Morelli F: Patellar tendinosis: A follow-up study of surgical treatment. *J Bone Joint Surg Am* 2002;84:2179-2185.

20. Blazina ME, Kerlan RK, Jobe FW, Carter VS, Carlson GJ: Jumper's knee. *Orthop Clin North Am* 1973;4:665-678.

21. Popp JE, Yu JS, Kaeding CC: Recalcitrant patellar tendinitis: Magnetic resonance imaging, histologic evaluation, and surgical treatment. *Am J Sports Med* 1997;25:218-222.

22. Matava M: Patellar tendon ruptures. *J Am Acad Orthop Surg* 1996;4:287-296.

23. Hohl M, Johnson EE, Wiss DA: Fractures of the knee, in Rockwood CA, Green DP, Buchholz RW (eds): *Rockwood and Green's Fractures in Adults*, ed 3. Philadelphia, PA, JB Lippincott, 1991, pp 1725-1797.

24. Johnson EE: Fractures of the patella, in Rockwood CA Jr, Green DP, Heckman JD (eds): *Rockwood and Green's Fractures in Adults*, ed 4. Philadelphia, PA, Lippincott-Raven, 1996, pp 1956-1972.

25. Whittle AP: Fractures of the lower extremity, in Canale ST (ed): *Campbell's Operative Orthopedics*, St. Louis, MO, Mosby, 1998, pp 2042-2179.

26. Turgut A, Gunal I, Acar S, Seber S, Gokturk E: Arthroscopic-assisted percutaneous stabilization of patellar fractures. *Clin Orthop* 2001;389:57-61.

27. McConnell J: The management of chondromalacia patellae: A long-term solution. *Aust J Physiother* 1986;32:215-223.

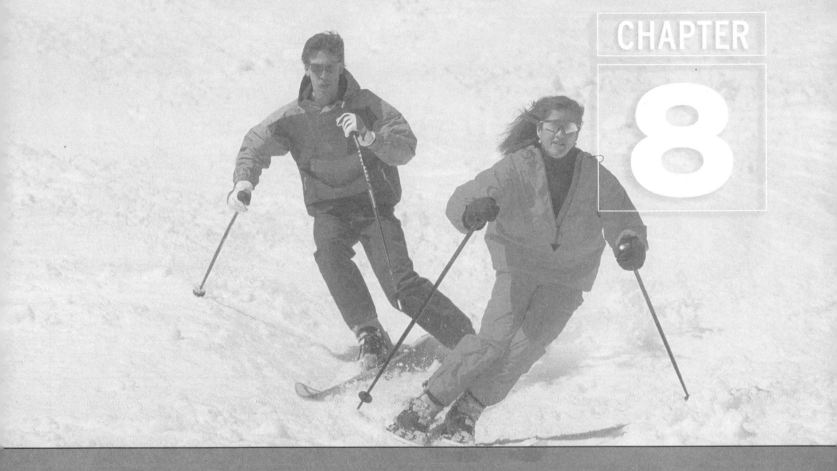

Femur, Hip, and Pelvis Injuries

Peggy A. Houglum,
PhD, ATC, PT
Glen Johnson, MD

Strains

Adductor Strains

Adductor strains ("groin strains") occur in sports that require strong eccentric muscle action of the adductors, such as hockey, fencing, handball, hurdling, high jumping, cross-country skiing, and especially soccer.[1,2] The adductor longus is the most frequently injured, possibly because of its relatively poor mechanical advantage.[1] The muscle tends to be injured at the musculotendinous junction. The mechanism of injury is usually a sudden, passive lengthening with a simultaneous active muscle contraction. The risk of adductor strains increases if the strength ratio between the adductors and abductors is less than 80%.[3] A history of previous adductor strains is also predictive of future episodes.[3]

Hamstring Strains

Hamstring muscle (semimembranosus, semitendinosus, and biceps femoris) strains are common in athletes who rely on the hamstring muscle group to decelerate the quadriceps during explosive activities, such as sprinting, jumping, and kicking. Hamstring strains are frequent injuries in athletes participating in sprinting sports such as soccer, baseball, track sprinting, football, bas-

CLINICAL PRESENTATION

Adductor Strains	Hamstring Strains	Quadriceps Strains
History		
Sudden eccentric contraction of the adductor muscles	Sudden, powerful eccentric contraction of the hamstring muscles	Sudden contraction of the quadriceps muscle
Sudden pain and tenderness at the site of injury	Risk increases when the hamstring muscles are fatigued or weak.	A sudden sprint or change of direction, a fall down steps, or a clean-and-jerk maneuver when lifting weights
Observation		
Secondary muscle spasm	Secondary spasm develops quickly.	A defect in the distal quadriceps may be apparent.
Gradual onset of swelling and discoloration	Ecchymosis may occur within 2 days.	Significant swelling
	A defect in the muscle contour may be palpated in a grade II or III injury.	Muscle spasm
		Ecchymosis
Functional Status		
		Grade I and II Strains
The patient may walk with an antalgic gait.	The patient may walk with an antalgic gait.	Decreased strength in the affected leg
Adduction against resistance is painful.	Knee extension with hip flexion against resistance is painful, as are straight-leg raises.	Antalgic gait
Abduction terminal range of motion (ROM) may be deficient secondary to pain and spasm.		**Grade III Strain**
	Full hip extension with concomitant knee-flexion ROM may be less than on the uninjured side secondary to pain and spasm.	The patient is likely unable to stand or bear weight on the extremity.
		Inability to lift leg
		A stiff-legged gait is possible, in which the knee is locked by the hamstring.
Physical Evaluation Findings		
		Grade I and II Strains
A palpable defect may be noted.		Limited flexion ROM
Moving the leg into full abduction to stretch the injured muscle results in pain.	Muscle palpation and resistance testing produce pain.	Manual muscle tests demonstrate weakness in the involved leg for knee extension and, possibly, hip flexion (if the rectus femoris is involved).
	Muscle stretching produces pain.	
	During resisted ROM, the foot rotates away from the involved portion of the muscle.	**Grade III Strain**
		Lack of active knee extension, especially against gravity, makes the diagnosis obvious.

ketball, and rugby.[4] Avulsion injuries occur during activities such as ice skating, weight lifting, and water skiing, when sudden stress loads are placed on the isometrically contracting muscle group.[5] Because the hamstring group comprises two-joint muscles that act concentrically at the hip and eccentrically at the knee during activity, it has a greater risk of injury. In addition, the biceps femoris has two heads originating from two different locations—one on the ischium and the other on the femoral shaft. Muscles with this type of compound origin and different innervations for the two heads are termed "hybrid muscles." The sudden change in function from concentric to eccentric motion during activity makes the hamstring group susceptible to injury. Hamstring strains tend to occur between the musculotendinous junction, either proximally near the tendon insertion onto the ischial tuberosity or more toward the midbelly of the muscle, where tendon slips extend (**Figure 8-1**).[5]

The rate of reinjury is high when the quadriceps-to-hamstring strength ratio, left-to-right strength comparisons, and flexibility are not restored before returning to participation. The strength of the left and right hamstring groups should not differ by more than 10%. Ratios between the quadriceps and hamstring can be determined using isokinetic equipment. Although expected ratios vary by sport, a normal isokinetic range for the hamstring is 50% to 60% of quadriceps strength.

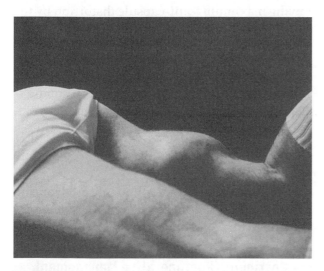

Figure 8-1 Third degree strain (rupture) of the hamstring muscle group. (Reproduced with permission from: Clanton TO, Coupe KJ: Hamstring strains in athletes: Diagnosis and treatment. *J Am Acad Orthop Surg* 1998;6:237-248.)

Quadriceps Strains

One of the quadriceps group's muscles, the rectus femoris, has a two-joint configuration, predisposing it to injury. The rectus femoris frequently works simultaneously at the hip and knee, one end performing a concentric activity and the other end performing an eccentric contraction. A severe rectus femoris strain can result in an avulsion fracture at the proximal insertion on the anterior inferior iliac spine. The large amount of torque produced by the quadriceps muscle group and the dynamic forces placed on the lower extremity predispose the muscles to rupture (grade III strain). A rupture between the patella and distal insertion is a patellar tendon rupture (see p 209). A rupture that occurs between the origin of the individual muscles of the quadriceps group and the patella is a quadriceps tendon rupture. Both injuries disrupt the knee extensor mechanism. Individuals sustaining these injuries are usually older, between 30 and 60 years, with no history of quadriceps muscle or tendon injury. Long-term use of anabolic steroids may increase the risk of rupture.[6]

In grade II and III strains, the patient should be evaluated for concurrent trauma of the cruciate ligaments, collateral ligaments, and menisci of the knee.

Differential Diagnosis

Adductors: Intra-abdominal trauma, genitourinary abnormalities, osteitis pubis, referred lumbosacral disorders, and hip injuries.[2] The possibility of hamstring or iliopsoas strain, avulsion fracture, or femoral tumor should also be considered if the injury does not respond to treatment. Adductor muscle strains may be part of a triad seen with abdominal sports hernia (see chapter 15).

Hamstring: Adductor strains, avulsion fracture, hip injury, femoral stress fracture, lumbosacral referred pain syndrome, piriformis syndrome, sacroiliac dysfunction, sciatica, ischial bursitis, hamstring tendinitis

Quadriceps: Patellar fracture, patellar tendon rupture, meniscal involvement

Imaging Techniques

Plain radiographs are helpful in visualizing avulsion fractures of the attachment (**Figure 8-2**). In suspected adductor strains, radiographs may show evidence of osteitis pubis. In quadriceps injuries, radiographs can reveal patellar fractures, and patellar retraction can also be seen with a patellar tendon rupture as the patella rides in a baja position on lateral radiograph. Magnetic resonance imaging (MRI) is the most sensitive technique to identify midsubstance defects in a muscle or tendon.

Osteitis pubis Inflammation of the pubic symphysis.

Sports hernia The combination of an adductor strain, abdominal strain, and osteitis pubis.

Baja An unexpectedly low position.

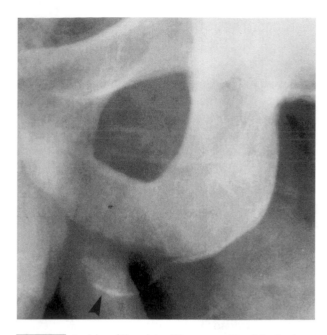

Figure 8-2   Avulsion of the origin of the common hamstring tendon from the ischial tuberosity (note arrowhead in lower left). (Reproduced with permission from Clanton TO, Coupe KJ: Hamstring strains in athletes: Diagnosis and treatment. *J Am Acad Orthop Surg* 1998;6: 237-248.)

Definitive Diagnosis

Physical evaluation findings noted in "Clinical Presentation," positive finding on MRI, or the exclusion of other conditions confirms the diagnosis. An adductor strain presents with pain along the muscle group that intensifies with passive stretching into abduction and with resistive muscle action into adduction. Pain to palpation may be difficult to elicit in minor strains, especially with high adductor strains. In a quadriceps strain with extensor mechanism disruption, the patient has difficulty performing or may be unable to perform a straight-leg raise. A palpable defect accompanies the disruption and indicates retraction.

Pathomechanics and Functional Limitations

Premorbid weakness or muscle imbalance, rather than reduced flexibility, is the best predictor and largest predisposing factor for muscle strains.[7,8] A history of previous strains also plays a large role in predicting future strains.[9] The strain produces an antalgic gait, weakness, and inability to function at a normal level of sport participation.

Adductors   When a muscle imbalance and decreased flexibility develop concurrently, the probability of injury (or reinjury) significantly increases. Initial functional limitations of adduc-

tor strains include a pathologic gait, weakness, and inability to function at a normal level of sport participation. Because the adductors stabilize the hip during hip and trunk activities, loss of adductor strength can create an imbalance between these muscles and the hip abductors. Left uncorrected, this imbalance can lead to other hip and knee injuries.

Hamstring   Functional limitations include a pathologic gait with the knee held in slight flexion, reduced hip motion in both flexion (stretching the hamstring) and extension (activating the hamstring), and reduced stride length. Weakness and a reduced ability to use the hamstring in both concentric and eccentric activities are also common functional limitations.

Quadriceps   Significant extensor mechanism disruption results in the loss of knee control. The knee's insufficient contribution to gait is compensated for by changes in the body's center of gravity relative to the knee joint and the use of other muscles to maintain knee extension during weight bearing. The knee is kept posterior to the body's center of gravity to maintain it locked in extension. The normal medial, or external, rotation of the tibia during knee flexion and extension is diminished and affects foot pronation and supination.

The knee is unstable, and the patient reports an inability to bear weight, actively move the knee, or control it. In essence, the knee is nonfunctional. Swelling is usually profound and limits the possible knee ROM. The knee is maintained at approximately 30° of flexion, a position allowing maximum joint-capsule distortion by the fluid.

■ Immediate Management

Immediate management consists of ice, compression, elevation, and mild stretching to minimize inflammation and spasm.

■ Medications

Analgesic medications are commonly used for pain and nonsteroidal anti-inflammatory drugs (NSAIDs) prescribed for acute injuries.

■ Postinjury/Postoperative Management

If the patient cannot walk normally, crutch walking with weight bearing to tolerance is necessary.

Premorbid Before the onset of the condition.

Primary Repair of a Proximal Hamstring Avulsion

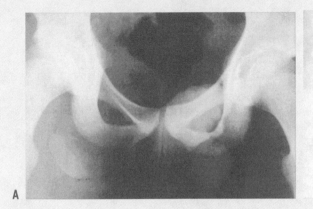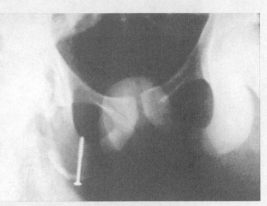

Indications

MRI demonstrating bony or tendinous avulsion from the ischial origin with > 2 cm of retraction

Overview

1. The patient is positioned prone for a posterior approach to the ischium.
2. A curvilinear (hockey stick) incision is made along the gluteal fold and extended down the medial leg.
3. The inferior border of the gluteus maximus is identified and retracted superiorly.
4. The hamstring group is identified and followed back to the avulsed ischium (**A**).
5. Care is taken not to damage the sciatic nerve, which is found under the biceps femoris and laterally as the nerve tracks proximally.
6. The avulsed tendon is fixed back to the ischium with the surgeon's choice of suture anchors or hardware (**B**).

Functional Limitations

The patient may experience pain and stiffness with hamstring stretching or contraction. The location of the scar is such that it can be tender or a neuroma may develop from sitting on hard surfaces. Some residual weakness may exist.

Implications for Rehabilitation

The repair should be protected by preventing simultaneous knee extension and hip flexion during the healing process. A knee immobilizer to restrict extension is used early in the recovery process. As healing progresses, the knee is allowed more extension with hip flexion.

Comments

Because of the muscle strength and the limited surface for reattachment of the avulsed tendon, an extended period of healing and rehabilitation is required. The patient may never return to the preinjury functional status.

■ Surgical Intervention

Adductor and Hamstring Strains

Surgery is indicated in proximal hamstring tendinous avulsion injuries with significant retraction but not for intrasubstance tears.[5] The surgery requires deep, tedious dissection into the tissues. To prevent scar tissue from hindering the repair, surgery should be performed as soon as possible once the retraction has been identified (**ST** 8-1).

Quadriceps Strains

Complete extensor mechanism disruption requires reapproximation to reestablish function. The surgical approach is a direct midline incision and direct visualization of the injury. Primary repair yields superior results over late reconstruction. Various repair techniques are available, and the appropriate procedure is determined by the tear location (**ST** 8-2). Also see **ST** 7-5.

S|T Surgical Technique   8-2

Extensor Mechanism Repair

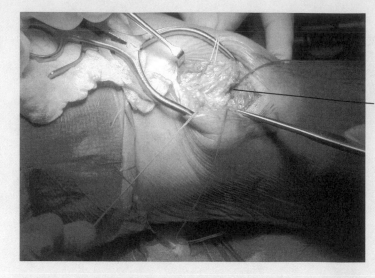

Quad tendon tear

Indications

Extensor mechanism disruption demonstrated by functional evaluation and MRI

Overview

1. The patient is placed in the supine position.
2. A midline incision is made, and dissection to the fascial plane overlying the extensor mechanism is performed, followed by peri-incisional blunt dissection.
3. The defect is identified, and the tear borders are trimmed and cleaned in preparation for the primary repair.
4. Using the surgeon's choice of suture anchors and/or locking tendon suture techniques, the ends are reapproximated and reinforced with extensor-retinaculum repair.

Functional Limitations

With healthy tissue for repair, few functional limitations are expected.

Implications for Rehabilitation

Protected flexion and weight bearing are necessary in the early postoperative period. Gradual weight bearing, flexion, and active quadriceps contractions are allowed as healing progresses.

Comments

Tears in close approximation to bony attachments can be firmly fixed to the patella or tibial tubercle with suture anchors. Some partial tears are amenable to surgical repair with similar techniques. MRI demonstrating a partial disruption and defect may reflect an injury that will respond faster to surgical reapproximation of the torn tissues.

■ Injury-Specific Treatment and Rehabilitation Concerns

Specific Concerns

Control inflammation.
Avoid early eccentric contractions of the healing muscle.
Promote tissue elongation.
Prevent contracture formation.

With a grade I or II thigh muscle strain, the patient should be examined for possible underlying causes of the injury. Biomechanical abnormalities such as leg malalignment, muscle-strength imbalances, or leg-length discrepancy should be assessed.[2] If the patient reports prior strains, the amount of old scar tissue and subsequent restrictions should be assessed.

While limited in activities, the patient can maintain cardiovascular fitness and maintain or develop muscle strength in the uninvolved extremities. Open kinetic chain exercises for the hip, knee, and foot can be included if weight-bearing exercises cause pain. Abdominal exercises should be incorporated early in the program. Hip exercises for the other motions and knee-extension exercises can be performed against resistance if pain free.

Adductors

The adductors are also hip rotators, so rotator and adductor strengthening is necessary once pain and spasm are under control. After the inflammation phase has passed, ROM should be restored. Exercises to strengthen the weakened adductors are also included. Scar-tissue management is incorporated into the program after the tissue has reached its remodeling phase and can tolerate tissue-mobilization techniques. Abdominal exercises are incorporated early in the program and focus on stabilization activities for the core muscles.

Hamstring

If an avulsed tendon has been surgically repaired, the rehabilitation process will be prolonged, with slow progression to weight bearing and muscle activity. A fine balance must be attained between sufficient stress to allow optimal healing and excessive stress that hinders healing.

Postoperative bracing with a motion-controlled knee brace may assist in protecting a proximal repair from excessive tension. The knee is placed in flexion; with time and healing, progressive extension is allowed.

Quadriceps

After a severe or surgically repaired strain, the leg is immobilized, non–weight bearing, for 3 to 6 weeks. Knee exercises are initially limited to quadriceps isometrics, active or active-assisted flexion ROM, and hamstring resistance in a limited range. Tibiofemoral joint mobilization can be used to reduce pain and maintain joint mobility. Patellofemoral joint mobilization may start with grades I and II for pain control at 10 days to 2 weeks; after week 3 or 4, depending on the surgeon's recommendation, grade III techniques may be used.

One of the concerns after a repair is wound contracture and scarring, causing patella baja or patella alta. Another issue is incomplete active knee extension, which results from dehiscing when stress is applied too early. Caution, common sense, knowledge of healing, and careful observation of treatment results must be used to gauge the appropriate amount and progression of stresses applied to the healing structures.

If an extensor lag exists with active knee extension, the lag must be identified as secondary to tightness, weakness, or overstretching of the repaired tendon. Joint mobilization, especially in the last few degrees of knee extension with rotation (ie, screw-home mechanism), and scar-tissue mobilization may be necessary if the extensor lag is caused by tightness. A lag caused by weakness can be reduced by emphasizing terminal knee strength with electrical stimulation, biofeedback, and end-range facilitation. If the lag is the result of overstretching the repaired tendon, the knee must be kept fully extended without attempts at stretching until the scar tissue can "take hold" and reduce the lag. If the lag occurs secondary to dehiscing and is not detected early, it may be uncorrectable.

■ Estimated Amount of Time Lost

Time lost varies significantly with injury severity and the quality and timing of early treatment. Mild strains may only result in a few days of decreased activity or inactivity. For a moderate strain, 3 to 12 weeks of recovery may be needed. Full recovery from a quadriceps rupture requires 6 to 12 months.

A history of prior strains prolongs the recovery phase, as does a more proximal site of injury. Steroid use, increased age, and poor general health also delay recovery. Failure of an adductor strain to improve in the expected time may merit further investigation for an abdominal sports hernia.

■ Return-to-Play Criteria

If adhesions are present, they should be pliable and not place tension on adjacent muscles or other structures during activity. Hip ROM should be normal compared with the contralateral leg. Agility activities, especially side-to-side maneuvers and sudden changes in direction, should be performed normally, with the athlete showing no hesitation or difficulty using the involved extremity during any explosive or lateral moves.

Functional Bracing

A thigh wrap may feel more secure for the athlete but is not necessary once sport participation is resumed (CT 8-1 and 8-2). Compression shorts may provide some support for high adductor strains (**Figure 8-3**).

Core muscles The muscles closest to the center of the body in the trunk that provide stability of the spine during movement, including the lower internal obliques, transverse abdominis, and multifidus.

Alta An abnormally high position.

Dehiscing Tearing of the repaired tissue.

CT Clinical Technique 8-1

Protective Hip Wrapping for Return to Competition

1. The spica wrap is begun at the proximal thigh.
2. The wrap is angled diagonally, proceeding to the distal lateral aspect of the quadriceps.
3. Above the knee, the wrap is spiraled upward, with each layer overlapping by half of its width.
4. At the proximal end of the thigh, the wrap continues around the waist, pulling laterally and posteriorly.
5. After circling the waist, the wrap is brought downward and around the thigh two or three times.
6. The wrap returns to the waist and back down to the thigh in a figure-of-8 pattern.
7. The wrap ends on the thigh, anchored with a strip of adhesive tape or stretch-elastic tape.

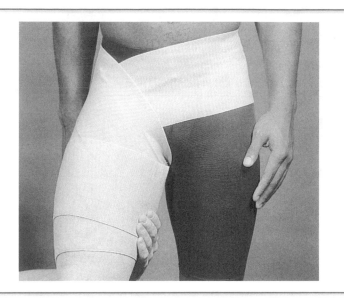

CT Clinical Technique 8-2

Protective Thigh Wrapping for Return to Competition

1. Begin the wrap at the distal portion of the thigh.
2. Angle the wrap diagonally towards the proximal portion of the muscle group.
3. Turn the wrap to begin an upward spiral, overlapping each layer by half its width.
4. End at the proximal portion of the thigh.
5. Secure the wrap using white tape or stretch-elastic tape.

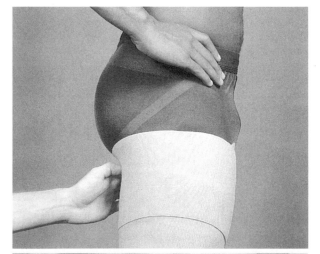

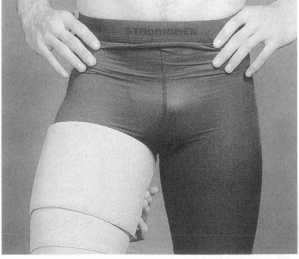

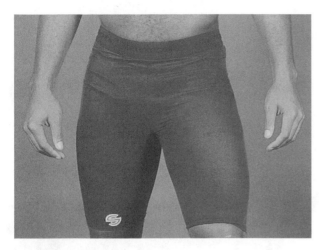

Figure 8-3 Compression shorts.

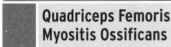

Quadriceps Femoris Myositis Ossificans

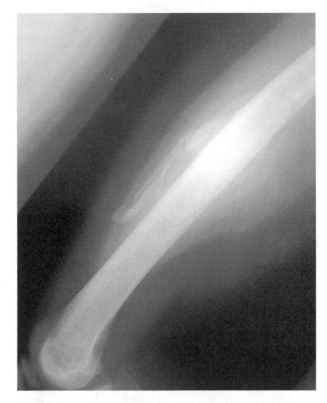

Figure 8-4 Imaging technique for femoral myositis ossificans.

CLINICAL PRESENTATION

History

An unresolved contusion to the anterior thigh
Within 2 to 4 weeks, the ossification can be seen on radiographs.

Observation

Point tenderness and swelling may be apparent over the site.
Knee effusion
If the contusion occurred long ago, discoloration may be absent.

Functional Status

Loss of full knee flexion is common.

Physical Evaluation Findings

A hard, palpable mass is usually noted in the anterior thigh,
Knee-flexion ROM is less than on the contralateral side.

Myositis ossificans occurs as a result of a muscle contusion. Although it can occur anywhere in the body, the lesion is most often found in the quadriceps and brachialis muscles. **Ectopic** bone forms within the muscle as an outgrowth of the hematoma after a contusion. Risk factors for myositis ossificans development include ROM less than 120°, history of a previous quadriceps injury, treatment onset delayed by more than 72 hours, and sympathetic ipsilateral knee effusion.[10]

Differential Diagnosis

Periosteal or bone tumors, muscle spasm, muscle rupture

Imaging Techniques

Radiographs or computed tomography (CT) scans 2 to 4 weeks after injury may show early signs of myositis ossificans (**Figure 8-4**; see also Figure 2-11, p 25). The lateral radiograph merits special attention. Serial films are helpful in documenting mass maturation.

Definitive Diagnosis

The definitive diagnosis is based on the history of trauma and the presence of myositis ossificans on radiographs.

Pathomechanics and Functional Limitations

The mass restricts muscle elongation and decreases the amount of tension that can be generated. Adhesions of the calcific mass within the muscle restrict its ability to contract, thereby limiting the force it can produce. As a result, lower extremity function is inhibited. Reduced knee flexion may result in biomechanical changes during the swing phase of gait, characterized by hip abduction and pelvic elevation to allow the foot to clear the ground. Other functional limitations arise from decreased muscle strength.

■ Immediate Management

To prevent myositis ossificans after a deep quadriceps contusion, treatment consists of ice to minimize hemorrhage, rest, quadriceps stretching, compression, and elevation. Depending on injury severity, this initial treatment may continue until hemorrhage ceases.[10]

Ectopic A structure that is in an anatomically incorrect place.

Medications

Limited evidence suggests that a treatment of iontophoresis using a 2% acetic solution followed by 8 minutes of pulsed ultrasound at 1.5 W/cm^2 can be beneficial in resolving myositis ossificans.[11] NSAIDs or acetaminophen are often used to reduce pain and increase function.

Postinjury/Postoperative Management

Crutches are used until the knee can be flexed to at least 90°, pain is diminished, and the patient can walk normally with good quadriceps control.[10] Ice and quadriceps stretching are continued. When the patient is pain free, additional exercises may begin.

Surgical Intervention

Surgical intervention is not recommended because of the extensive dissection and tissue removal required and the high risk of recurrence.

Injury-Specific Treatment and Rehabilitation Concerns

Specific Concerns
Encourage hematoma resolution. Maintain ROM.

Whirlpool treatments during the first week may promote ROM activities with less discomfort. Other modalities such as electrical stimulation (for pain relief, edema reduction, and muscle facilitation), heat, ice, or ultrasound may also be beneficial.

Gait training for normal ambulation may be required. Along with gait correction, progressive exercises for ROM and strengthening are incorporated early in the program. Before stretching and strengthening exercises, a brief period (10 to 15 minutes) of a cardiovascular activity such as stationary bicycling or upper body ergometry enhances the effects of exercise and joint mobilization. Gentle flexibility exercises should be performed for the first several days. Once the patient resumes full weight bearing, proprioceptive and balance exercises such as Romberg, tandem stance, and stork stand on different surfaces (moving from stable to unstable) can be initiated. From these static exercises, the patient advances to more dynamic exercises that evolve into coordination work and finally agility activities and sport-specific drills.

Idiopathic Of unknown cause or origin.

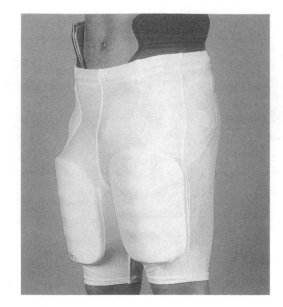

Figure 8-5 Compression girdle with fitted anterior thigh pads and iliac crest protection.

Estimated Amount of Time Lost

A large hematoma can resolve within 3 weeks, but the formation of a large myositis ossificans lesion can significantly increase the amount of time lost.[12]

Return-to-Play Criteria

The patient should be pain free during all activities, and radiographs should show resolution of the hematoma. Strength, ROM, proprioception, agility, and sport performance should all be within normal limits and allow the athlete to perform sport-specific activity at the preinjury level.

Functional Bracing

Bracing, taping, or padding (anterior thigh pad) protects the area from further impact injury and reduces the risk of myositis ossificans (**Figure 8-5**).

Trochanteric Bursitis

Trochanteric bursitis can be caused by friction between the bursa and trochanter or result from direct trauma, such as landing on the lateral hip or a direct blow. **Idiopathic** trochanteric bursitis is often related to other factors, including osteoarthritis of the hip or lumbar spine, degenerative disk disease, obesity, leg-length discrepancy, fibromyalgia, and pes planus.[13] Because bursae form in response to areas of friction, bursitis can occur in a number of possible sites; however, three or four areas around the greater trochanter area are primarily affected.[13]

Proximal Iliotibial Band Syndrome

CLINICAL PRESENTATION

History

Gradual onset of intermittent lateral hip pain aggravated by hip external rotation and abduction

Direct trauma to the area of the greater trochanter

Proximal iliotibial band (ITB) syndrome may result in reports of a "snapping" sensation in the lateral hip during activity.

Observation

No deformity or swelling is usually noted unless trauma has been acute, in which case ecchymosis and swelling may be present.

During static weight bearing, the patient may rotate the femur to clear the ITB from the greater trochanter.

Functional Status

The patient can ambulate, but end ranges of motion may be uncomfortable.

When standing statically, the patient may lean away from the involved leg, placing most of the weight on the uninvolved extremity.

Pain and associated weakness may be described as the ITB passes over the greater trochanter.

Physical Evaluation Findings

Resisted external rotation is often painful.

Deep palpation of the area around the greater trochanter reproduces pain.

Pain is elicited with palpation and during passive stretching.

Pain is elicited if the patient lies on the involved side.

Snapping may be palpated in the hip as the hip is flexed, extended, and rotated.

Symptoms are exacerbated with ITB stretching and passive hip and knee motion.

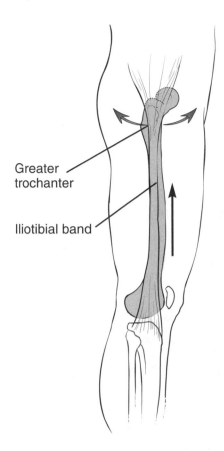

Greater trochanter

Iliotibial band

Figure 8-6   Snapping hip syndrome. The iliotibial band slides anteriorly and posteriorly over the greater trochanter as the hip moves from flexion to extension and back. (Reproduced with permission from Greene WB (ed): *Essentials of Musculoskeletal Care*, ed 2. Rosemont, IL, American Academy of Orthopaedic Surgeons, 2000, p 325.)

Proximal ITB syndrome is a possible cause of "snapping hip" and often occurs concurrently with trochanteric bursitis, although the cause-and-effect relationship is unclear. The snapping results as the ITB moves over the greater trochanter.[14,15]

In other cases, the gluteus maximus snaps over the greater trochanter to produce the symptoms (**Figure 8-6**).[16] Other conditions are also called snapping hip, but they involve either intra-articular factors (eg, loose body) or internal factors (eg, iliopsoas tendon abnormality)[14] (see Iliopsoas Bursitis, p 233).

Differential Diagnosis

Osteoarthritis, femoral head osteonecrosis, femoral neck stress fracture, lumbar disk herniation, lumbar facet syndrome, lumbar spine compression fracture, abductor muscle strain, ischial or iliopectineal bursitis, tendinitis, bursitis, sciatica, tumor[17-19]

Imaging Techniques

Radiographs are negative, and MRI is often not helpful.

Definitive Diagnosis

The definitive diagnosis is based on the clinical examination findings and the exclusion of conditions described in the Differential Diagnosis section.

Pathomechanics and Functional Limitations

Pressure from the greater trochanter and the overlying muscles compresses the bursa into the trochanter, causing irritation and discomfort. Side lying on the hip adds to the pressure against the inflamed bursa, further aggravating the inflammation. If a leg-length discrepancy exists, the longer leg receives increased lateral stress on the soft tissue as the individual stands with a lateral shift toward the longer leg in an attempt to equalize the leg lengths. Pain is the primary limiting factor to activity. Untreated conditions can develop into calcific bursitis.

8

Snapping hip or proximal ITB syndrome is often a pain-free condition.

■ Medications

Acetaminophen or NSAIDs may be used to reduce pain and increase function. Phonophoresis and iontophoresis with anti-inflammatory medications have also been attempted, but the efficacy of these techniques remains controversial. Corticosteroid injections may be necessary in advanced cases.

■ Postinjury Management

Any adaptable causative factors should be identified and corrected. If a leg-length discrepancy is responsible, a heel lift on the unaffected side reduces lateral stress on the affected hip. NSAIDs or corticosteroid injections (or both) help to relieve inflammation. If the condition is not acute or painful, cross-friction massage to loosen adhesions formed secondary to the bursal inflammation may help relieve pain and improve mobility. The condition is self-limiting, but crutches are seldom needed.

■ Surgical Intervention

Surgical excision of the trochanteric bursae or release of the tight ITB (or both) is only indicated in the patient whose symptoms cause disabling pain that is recalcitrant after conservative treatment (**S|T** 8-3).

S|T **Surgical Technique 8-3**

Proximal Release of ITB and Bursectomy

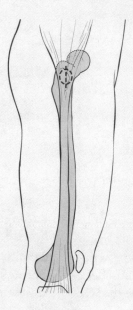

Indications

Disabling pain that fails to improve with conservative treatment

Overview

1. The patient is placed in the lateral decubitus position to permit a direct approach to the greater trochanter laterally.
2. The surgical incision is directly lateral and just anterior or posterior to the landmark of the greater trochanter.
3. Blunt dissection to the ITB is performed.
4. The band is incised, and the bursa is excised.
5. Two techniques have been described to release the ITB:
   A. The band is split such that it separates anterior and posterior to the greater trochanter.
   B. A window is cut in the band, and this window is removed, allowing the greater trochanter to be uncovered by the band.

Functional Limitations

No functional limitations are expected. Full resolution is the rule, and relief of pain is immediate.

Implications for Rehabilitation

Early ROM and weight bearing are allowed to prevent scar tissue from forming in a retracted position.

■ Injury-Specific Treatment and Rehabilitation Concerns

Specific Concerns
Correct biomechanics.
Lengthen the ITB.

Therapeutic modalities are used to provide pain relief. Disability time is rarely prolonged; accordingly, loss of strength and other conditioning is not an issue. When the patient must be reintegrated into activity, early weight-bearing and ROM exercises are instituted with functional progression as tolerated. Exercises are included in the rehabilitation program only if strength and ROM deficiencies are found during the examination. If deficiencies are realized, the same sequence outlined for other injuries is followed. If the bursitis has been present for a while, reduced motion may result from pain and weakness caused by stance and gait deviations.

Stretching exercises for the hip abductors and adductors and ITB reduce the tension stress on the area. Soft-tissue mobilization of the lateral thigh with a foam roller or manual therapy techniques softens and reduces tightness in the lateral thigh and hip (**Figure 8-7**).

■ Estimated Amount of Time Lost

Pain is the primary limiting factor.

■ Return-to-Play Criteria

The athlete should be pain free during all activities, and running gait should be normal.

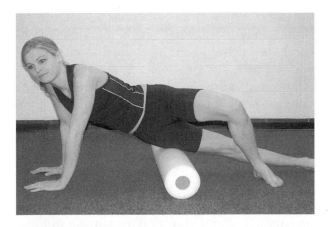

Figure 8-7 Stretching the iliotibial band. To stretch the band, the patient lies on a foam roller and rolls the leg the length of the band.

Functional Bracing

A heel lift for the uninvolved leg helps reduce lateral stress on the hip. If the athlete participates in a collision or contact sport, a protective pad over the bursa may reduce the risk of reinjury from direct contact.

■ Iliopsoas Bursitis

CLINICAL PRESENTATION

History

An insidious, gradual onset of progressive groin or anterior hip pain is described.
Pain, especially during hip extension, may be the only symptom.[20]

Observation

No outward signs

Functional Status

Stride may be shortened during ambulation to reduce hip extension.
In later stages, the hip may be held in flexion, adduction, and external rotation to relieve pressure over the bursa.

Physical Evaluation Findings

Palpation of the bursa just distal to the inguinal ligament and lateral to the femoral artery reveals tenderness.

The iliopsoas bursa is the largest bursa in the body, averaging 6×3 cm.[20] Because of its proximity to the iliopsoas tendon, tendinitis or bursitis can develop secondary to the other, making the conditions difficult to differentiate (**Figure 8-8**). Causes of iliopsoas bursitis include rheumatoid arthritis, acute trauma, and overuse injury.[21] Acute trauma in sports can occur with vigorous hip flexion and extension. Overuse trauma is seen in athletes with hip weakness or tightness who participate in repetitive activities. Individuals involved in uphill running, track and field, rowing, strength training, and ballet are also susceptible to iliopsoas bursitis.

■ Internal Snapping Hip Syndrome

Iliopsoas tendon displacement as it passes the pelvic pectineal eminence, femoral head, or lesser trochanter may be a cause of snapping hip syndrome (see Trochanteric Bursitis, p 230).[15] Chronic pain, snapping, or both in the femoral triangle is reported, especially in the area over the inguinal ligament (**Figure 8-9**). Symptoms develop during exercise and may persist for some time afterward. Passively extending the hip from a position of flexion, abduction, and external rotation reproduces the pain.[15]

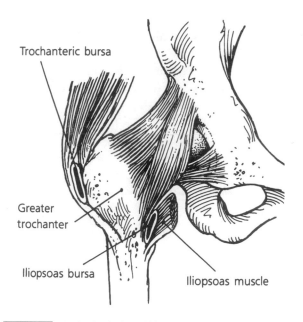

Figure 8-8   The trochanteric and iliopsoas bursae are located around the coxofemoral joint.

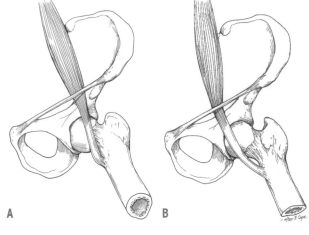

Figure 8-9   The iliopsoas in snapping hip syndrome. **A.** With hip flexion, the iliopsoas tendon shifts laterally in relation to the center of the femoral head. **B.** With hip extension, the tendon shifts medially in relation to the center of the femoral head. (Reproduced with permission from Allen WC, Cope R: Coxa saltans: The snapping hip revisited. *J Am Acad Orthop Surg* 1995;3:303-308.)

Differential Diagnosis

Lymphadenopathy, tumor, inguinal hernia, hematoma, femoral artery aneurysm

Imaging Techniques

Radiographs are negative, and MRI is often inconclusive.

Definitive Diagnosis

The definitive diagnosis is based on bursal inflammation, findings on clinical examination, and the exclusion of conditions described in the Differential Diagnosis section.

Pathomechanics and Functional Limitations

Hip hyperextension is uncomfortable and avoided during gait. Walking and running stride lengths are reduced to avoid hip extension. Sitting is more comfortable than standing, and side lying is more comfortable than lying prone.

■ Immediate Management

Rest with limitation of hip motion, especially limitation of extension by using an elastic wrap, relieves pain. Ice may be used to reduce inflammation.

■ Medications

NSAIDs reduce inflammation. Corticosteroid injections into the bursa have also produced successful results.[15]

■ Postinjury Management

Inflammation is decreased and followed with stretching and strengthening exercises. Any gait or anatomic abnormalities should be corrected to prevent recurrence.

■ Injury-Specific Treatment and Rehabilitation Concerns

> **Specific Concerns**
>
> Limit hip extension early in the program.
> Strengthen hip musculature.

Hip extension is avoided until inflammation and pain are under control. However, during this time and beyond, the hip muscles should be strengthened. Medial and lateral rotator strengthening can begin early.[22] Hip abduction and adduction strengthening are also necessary. Once strength is improved in these motions, combined-plane motions can be performed to strengthen in more functional planes. Hip-flexor stretches should also be included in the program, because tightness of the hip-flexor muscles correlates with the incidence of iliopsoas bursitis.[22]

Deep-tissue, cross-friction massage may be beneficial in relieving adhesions within the bursa if the patient can tolerate the activity. Ultrasound and heat can also be helpful in relieving inflammation.

Proprioceptive and balance exercises such as Romberg, tandem stance, and stork stand on different surfaces (moving from stable to unstable) are initiated when pain is resolved and hip strength is restored. From these static exercises, the patient progresses to more dynamic exercises that evolve into coordination and finally agility activities. Functional activities are started before the final phase of the rehabilitation program, in which sport-specific drills and skill executions are performed.

Estimated Amount of Time Lost

Because pain is the primary limiting factor, time lost varies; activity modification can range from simple modification to complete cessation for several weeks. If the patient has delayed reporting the injury and bursitis is extensive, time lost may be several weeks.

Return-to-Play Criteria

Pain during activities reflects inflammation; consequently, the patient should be pain free in all activities before returning to full participation. If the time away from full participation has been brief, pain relief may be the only requirement for return.

Functional Bracing

Although a hip spica wrap may be used in the early phase, no support is required once the athlete returns to full participation and motion and strength are restored.

Iliac Crest Contusions

CLINICAL PRESENTATION

History

Direct blow to the iliac crest
Immediate debilitation because of pain rather than tissue damage

Observation

Swelling may be localized over the site of injury.
Rapid formation of ecchymosis
Muscle spasm in the abdominal and hip muscles

Functional Status

Hip and trunk ROM are painful and reduced.
Gait may be antalgic.

Physical Evaluation Findings

Point tenderness over the iliac crest
Early onset of a contusion, giving way to widespread ecchymosis
Pain may be reduced when the patient walks backward.

Athletes who participate in contact and collision sports such as football, ice hockey, and soccer, and female gymnasts who compete on the uneven bars are susceptible to iliac crest contusions. Commonly known as a "hip pointer," this condition can be disabling because of the soft-tissue damage and secondary muscle spasm. The abdominal muscles attached to the iliac crest are crushed between the iliac crest and the object, causing the injury. The abdominal muscles and the bone can both be injured by the impacting force. If the contusion occurs just below the crest, the hip muscles can also be affected. Repeated iliac crest trauma or mismanagement of an acute injury to this area can lead to periostitis.

Differential Diagnosis

Stress fracture, muscle strain, iliac crest fracture, iliac crest avulsion fracture, apophysitis, bursitis

Imaging Techniques

Plain radiographs may demonstrate an iliac crest avulsion injury, which can accompany a severe iliac crest contusion (**Figure 8-10**). Generally, MRI is not used to visualize the soft-tissue injury because either the problem is self-limiting or radiographs are adequate.

Definitive Diagnosis

The diagnosis is based on the mechanism of injury, clinical signs, and patient's functional limitations. Clinical evaluation alone may not be sufficient to differentiate an iliac crest contusion

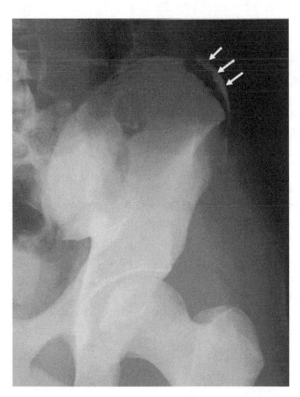

Figure 8-10 Avulsion of the iliac spine with retraction of the fragment indicated by arrows.

from an avulsion of the oblique, latissimus dorsi, or paraspinal muscles or associated fascia.[12]

Pathomechanics and Functional Limitations

Pain and spasm are self-limiting. Spasm makes movement difficult because the abdominal muscles work to stabilize the trunk during extremity movement and work even more during trunk motion. Deep inspirations, coughing, and laughing also cause discomfort as the abdominal muscles are stretched. If the hip abductors are also involved in the injury, ambulation is painful and difficult. A hematoma can form over the femoral or lateral femoral cutaneous nerve, increasing pain and resulting in peripheral motor and sensory dysfunction.[12]

■ Immediate Management

Ice and compression may be applied to the injury site to limit inflammation. Electrical stimulation and mild stretching during icing to the muscles helps to reduce secondary muscle spasm. If tolerable, passive or active-assisted ROM after electrical stimulation may further relax the muscles, and an elastic wrap for support may extend the muscle relaxation after treatment. If gait is not possible without the involved extremity being favored, crutches with partial weight bearing should be used. Prophylactic crutch use is often prescribed for the first 24 hours to limit irritation and muscle spasm.

■ Medications

Analgesic medications for pain and NSAIDs are used in acute injuries. Injection of corticosteroid with an anesthetic is very helpful in the early resolution of pain and spasm. Iontophoresis may also be used to deliver these medications.

■ Postinjury Management

This injury does not usually require long-term disability. The key to reducing disability is limiting the accompanying muscle spasm. Once spasm and pain are relieved and healing is well under way, ROM exercises are initiated to restore lost hip and trunk motion. A brief routine to strengthen the abdominal, hip-flexion, and hip-abduction muscles and restore trunk stabilization is all that is required before the athlete returns to full sport participation. Padding the injured area during participation reduces the risk of reinjury.

■ Injury-Specific Treatment and Rehabilitation Concerns

> **Specific Concerns**
> Control inflammation.
> Encourage pain-free ROM.

Following an iliac crest contusion, recovery is usually rapid with proper management. If muscle spasm is quickly resolved, pain subsides. Strength and motion deficits, if present, are minimal; both are recovered in a few days. However, if spasm is prolonged, recovery is also prolonged. Electrical stimulation can be continued if spasm persists; heat may be used once the acute inflammation has subsided.

■ Estimated Amount of Time Lost

Time lost is 3 days to 1 week, depending on the force of the impact and resulting injury severity. Development of periostitis, however, can significantly delay healing.

■ Return-to-Play Criteria

The athlete should be pain free during all activities, and muscle spasm should be resolved. Normal gait and the ability to run, jump, and perform all sport-specific activities must be demonstrated.

Functional Bracing

A wrap, girdle, or compression shorts with a protective pad over the injured area reduces the risk of reinjury (**CT** 8-3).

Femoral Fracture

■ Acute Fractures

The force required to cause an acute fracture is so great that automobile and motorcycle accidents are the most common causes. The risk of femoral fracture increases in skeletally immature individuals. If a traumatic femoral fracture occurs without significant force in a skeletally mature individual, a precipitating factor such as a bone tumor or osteoporosis should be suspected. Traumatic fractures are often accompanied by shock and neurovascular complications. Because of the extent of possible complications, an acute femoral fracture must be treated as an emergency.

CT Clinical Technique 8-3

Protective Iliac Crest Padding for Return to Activity

1. Begin with vertical anchor strips 4" to 6" anterior and posterior to the trauma site.
2. Create an "X" pattern from anchor-to-anchor using white or elastic tape.
3. Cover the "X" by applying the tape horizontally from anchor-to-anchor.
4. Pad the area using a commercial or custom-built pad.
5. Secure the pad in place using a hip spica (see CT 8-1), crossing the wrap on the lateral portion of the hip.

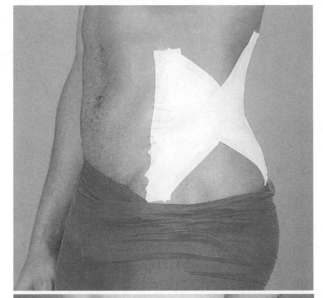

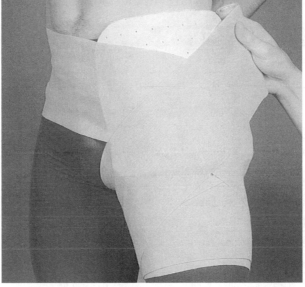

Although the bone is well covered by large muscles, an acute fracture is easily recognized by the patient's severe pain, inability to stand, and deformity. Displaced traumatic femoral fractures are usually hallmarked by exquisite pain and obvious deformity.

Stress Fractures

Femoral stress fractures occur more frequently than acute fractures in athletes, especially among those in distance running sports. Occasionally femoral stress fractures are seen in basketball, baseball, or tennis players. Both adolescents and adults are diagnosed with these fractures.[23] Although the cause of femoral stress fractures is unknown, women experience the injury 4 to 10 times more frequently than men.[24] Female endurance runners, who are often amenorrheic, are more susceptible to stress fractures, possibly because of lower bone mineral densities.[25] Femoral stress fractures may occur secondary to the female athlete triad (disordered eating, amenorrhea, and osteoporosis, see chapter 24).

Stress fractures tend to affect individuals who have been regularly running for at least 2 years and

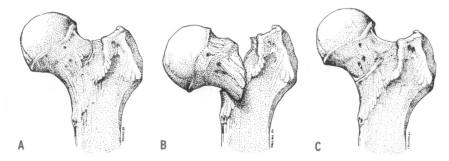

Figure 8-11 Stress fractures of the femoral neck. **A.** Tension-side stress fracture. **B.** Displaced femoral stress fracture. **C.** Compression-side stress fracture. (Reproduced with permission from Fullerton LR, Snowdy HA: Femoral neck stress fracture. *Am J Sports Med* 1988;16:365-377.)

are precipitated by sudden changes in the frequency, intensity, or duration of training.[24] Other factors that predispose to femoral stress fractures are declining fitness levels with age, improperly fitting or worn-out footwear, and poor nutrition.[24]

CLINICAL PRESENTATION

History

Significant increases in the frequency, intensity, or duration of exercise[24]

Gradual, idiopathic onset of symptoms over several weeks' time

The patient may complain of a "pulling" sensation in the anterior thigh.[26]

Pain or tenderness over the rectus femoris muscle or nondescript anterior hip pain

Pain increases with activity and decreases with rest.

Female patients may have a history of amenorrhea.

Observation

Mild swelling without ecchymosis

Functional Status

ROM may be full but uncomfortable in active hip flexion, passive knee flexion, and passive hip extension. No pain is experienced during hip rotation.

Limited ROM may be due to pain rather than physical restriction.

The patient can bear weight but may have an antalgic gait.

Thigh weakness and a slight limp are evident during gait.[26]

Pain may limit running ability.

Physical Evaluation Findings

Normal alignment and neurologic examination

Pain may be experienced when performing a straight-leg raise.

The following special tests may be positive:

- Fist
- Fulcrum
- One-legged hop

Femoral neck stress fractures are classified as tension fractures, displaced fractures, and compression fractures (**Figure 8-11**).[24] Tension fractures form on the superior aspect of the femoral neck.

Displaced fractures are visible on plain radiographs and frequently require surgical fixation. Compression stress fractures occur on the inferior portion of the femoral neck. Three subclasses have been identified—those with no fatigue line, those with a fatigue line less than 50% of the width of the femoral neck, and those with a fatigue line greater than 50% of the width.

Differential Diagnosis

Muscle strain, tendinitis, bursitis, delayed-onset muscle soreness, bone tumor, bone infection, radiculopathy, osteonecrosis, referred pain from the contralateral hip, contusion[24,27]

Imaging Techniques

Traumatic femoral fractures can be diagnosed with radiographs. Anteroposterior (AP) and lateral radiographs are initially negative in 66% of patients with stress fractures. Within the first week of symptoms, the accuracy rate is 10% (**Figure 8-12**).[24] If suspicion is high, a bone scan is often diagnostic within 24 hours of pain onset. MRI can also be diagnostic[24] (**Figure 8-13**).

Definitive Diagnosis

Traumatic fractures are high-energy injuries, and deformity is often obvious. Radiographs or other imaging techniques are positive. Because of the powerful quadriceps and hamstring muscles, femoral shortening is often noted. The patient is unable to ambulate or move the leg without significant pain.

Diagnosing a femoral stress fracture requires a high index of suspicion and is based on positive radiographic studies or the clinical symptoms.

Pathomechanics and Functional Limitations

Frank fractures are usually self-limiting, but improper healing or failed fixation can result in decreased weight-bearing loads, altered gait, and the inability to ambulate.

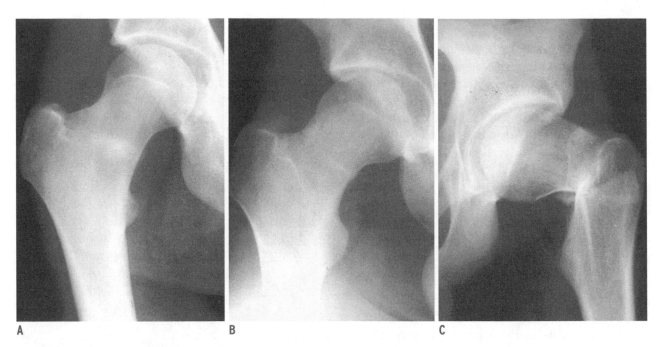

A   B   C

Figure 8-12   Radiographs of femoral neck stress fractures. **A.** A compression-side femoral-neck stress fracture that occurred secondary to overuse (fatigue). Note the periosteal new bone formation on the inferior femoral neck. Callus formation as the result of healing is also present. **B.** A complete, nondisplaced stress fracture of the femoral neck. **C.** A complete, displaced stress fracture of the femoral neck. (Reproduced with permission from Shin AY, Gillingham BL: Fatigue fractures of the femoral neck in athletes. *J Am Acad Orthop Surg* 1997;5:293-302.)

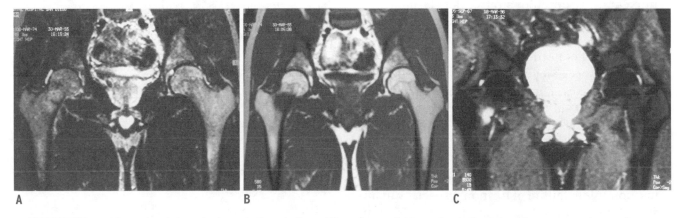

A   B   C

Figure 8-13   MRI of femoral neck stress fractures. **A.** Stress fracture of the posteromedial femoral neck. The darkened area represents a nondisplaced femoral neck fatigue-related stress fracture. **B.** A stress fracture extending from the cortical surface of the compression side of the femoral neck. **C.** Compression-side stress fracture of the right hip. The fatigue line is less than 25% of the femoral neck diameter. Note the brightened area on the femoral neck caused by edema. (Reproduced with permission from Shin AY, Gillingham BL: Fatigue fractures of the femoral neck in athletes. *J Am Acad Orthop Surg* 1997;5:293-302.)

An undiagnosed stress fracture will progress if high-intensity activity is allowed to continue. The compensatory gait redistributes weight-bearing forces along the extremity and increases the possibility of secondary stress fractures and other overuse conditions.

Immediate Management

A traumatic femoral fracture requires stabilization and transport to an emergency room. Shock should be anticipated and appropriate precautions imple-mented. The extremity is not moved until a traction splint can be applied.

Medications

The severe pain associated with a traumatic femoral fracture can only be controlled with narcotic anal-gesics delivered intravenously, intramuscularly, or orally. Toradol and other injectable anti-inflammatory medications may also aid in pain relief. NSAIDs or acetaminophen is usually adequate for pain con-trol of a stress fracture.

■ Postinjury Management

The patient with a stress fracture is placed on crutches with partial or no weight bearing for 1 to 4 weeks.[26,27] The duration of restricted weight bearing is based on the patient's signs and symptoms. Mild analgesics or NSAIDs may assist in pain relief. Surgical intervention is dictated by the fracture location and displacement.

■ Surgical Intervention

Supracondylar (distal femur), intertrochanteric, and subtrochanteric fractures require internal fixation. The surgical approach is usually lateral; the ITB is split, dissection is carried down through muscle tissue to the femur, and the fracture is identified. Stabilization is obtained through plate fixation.

Traumatic femoral fractures require stabilization by various techniques, depending on the fracture location. Midshaft fractures are best treated with an intermedullary (IM) rod fixation using a proximal approach with entry through the piriformis fossa, or distal approach through the intercondylar notch in a retrograde fashion.

IM nailing requires limited dissection, and rehabilitation is faster than that achieved with the lateral approaches needed for plate fixation. Proximal approaches necessitate trunk-stabilization strengthening exercises. Distal retrograde IM nailing involves an **arthrotomy** and patellar mobilization. Rehabilitation includes ROM and quadriceps strengthening exercises.

Complications of traumatic femoral fractures include deep vein thrombosis, pulmonary embolus, nonunion, failure of fixation (especially in unstable comminuted fractures), and infection. Femoral head necrosis can occur if the head is significantly displaced, disrupting the arterial supply. Stress fractures have fewer complications, but nonunion, displacement of femoral neck stress fractures, and recurrence are possible.

Stable compression-side femoral neck stress fractures typically do not require surgery. Patients with compression-side fractures and a fatigue line greater than 50% of the width of the femoral neck are strong candidates for fixation using cannulated screws. Tension-side (superior) stress fractures are stabilized with cannulated screws as well (**Figure 8-14**). Displaced femoral neck fractures require open reduction and internal fixation to prevent further displacement and avoid osteonecrosis.

Arthrotomy The surgical opening of a joint.

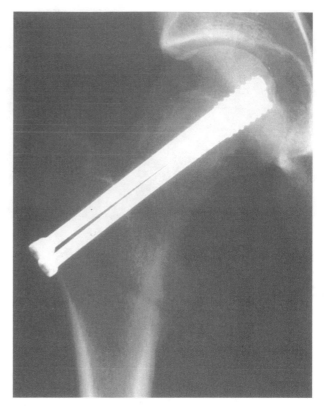

Figure 8-14 Complete, compression-side nondisplaced stress fracture of the femoral neck repaired with three cannulated screws. (Reproduced with permission from Shin AY, Gillingham BL: Fatigue fractures of the femoral neck in athletes. *J Am Acad Orthop Surg* 1997;5:293-302.)

Surgery should be performed as soon as practical after the diagnosis.

■ Postoperative Management

Once an acute fracture is surgically repaired, the patient's postoperative weight-bearing status depends on the stabilization technique used and the fracture condition. The more unstable the construct, the less weight bearing is permitted, and the greater the protection needed with bracing. The IM stabilization generally allows for early weight bearing and ROM exercises; however, if comminution was severe, initial weight-bearing loads must be limited. Once fracture healing can be documented by serial radiographs, the patient is allowed more liberties with weight bearing. ROM and strengthening exercises while weight bearing can also be initiated.

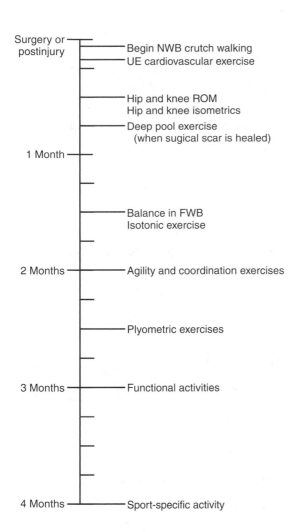

Surgery or postinjury
- Begin NWB crutch walking
- UE cardiovascular exercise

- Hip and knee ROM
- Hip and knee isometrics
- Deep pool exercise (when sugical scar is healed)

1 Month

- Balance in FWB
- Isotonic exercise

2 Months — Agility and coordination exercises

— Plyometric exercises

3 Months — Functional activities

4 Months — Sport-specific activity

Note: Time frames are approximate. Function is the guide.

Injury-Specific Treatment and Rehabilitation Concerns

> **Specific Concerns**
>
> Limit stresses on the healing fracture line.
> Maintain cardiovascular fitness.
> Correct biomechanics (with stress fractures).

Although restricted in activities, the patient can maintain cardiovascular fitness and maintain or develop muscle strength in the uninvolved extremities. Swimming and bicycling are commonly used cardiovascular activities. Open kinetic chain exercises for the hip, knee, and foot of the involved extremity can also be included during the non–weight-bearing phase.

If the thigh fascia or the hip joint capsule is restricted, soft-tissue adhesions and joint mobility in the extremity are assessed. In the first few weeks of treatment, electrical stimulation can be used if muscle spasm is present, and heat can be helpful for relaxation.

Gait training involves progressive advancement from non–weight bearing to full weight bearing, proceeding from two crutches without weight on the involved extremity to two crutches with partial weight bearing, and then one crutch with partial weight bearing before eliminating the crutches and allowing unassisted gait.

Along with gait corrections, progressive exercises for ROM and strength are incorporated early in the program. Before stretching and strengthening exercises, a brief period (10 to 15 minutes) of a cardiovascular activity such as stationary bicycling, swimming, or upper body ergometry enhances the effects of exercise and joint mobilization. Flexibility exercises should address both the area directly involved by the injury and other lower extremity segments that may have been secondarily affected by the reduced activity. If the patient has been bearing no weight or partial weight, strengthening exercises should target the entire lower extremity from the intrinsic toe muscles to the hip muscles. Once full weight bearing has resumed, proprioceptive and balance exercises such as Romberg, tandem stance, and stork stand on different surfaces (moving from stable to unstable) can be initiated.

Estimated Amount of Time Lost

An acute fracture with surgical repair requires a long recovery time, approximately 4 to 6 months. A stress fracture may require 8 to 14 weeks for full recovery. Time lost is related to fracture severity and the amount of healing required. It is common for stress fractures to heal more slowly than traumatic fractures, but stress fractures generally are more stable.

Return-to-Play Criteria

The patient should be pain free during all activities, including running, hopping, and jumping. Radiographs should demonstrate good healing and an obvious maturing callus at the fracture site. Both ROM and strength should be comparable with the contralateral extremity. Proprioceptive ability, including sport-specific activities, must be adequate before return to full activity, especially if the athlete has not been exposed to the stresses of normal activity for a while.

Piriformis Syndrome

CLINICAL PRESENTATION

History

Stair climbing, running, or repetitive squatting and rising

The pain may occur with an acute injury, such as falling and landing on the buttocks, causing the piriformis to go into spasm, or a sudden strain of the piriformis while running and slipping or changing directions unexpectedly.

Pain may be reported when turning in bed from one side to the other.[28]

Observation

No visual deformity may be apparent.

If the patient lies in the relaxed supine position, the involved extremity may rest in greater external rotation than the uninvolved leg.

The involved leg may appear shorter than the uninvolved leg.

Functional Status

Pain may be reported with stair climbing, running, squatting, sitting with legs crossed, or prolonged sitting.

Physical Evaluation Findings

Piriformis palpation reveals tenderness, usually in the junction of either the medial and central third or the central and lateral third of the muscle.

The flexion/adduction/internal rotation position can provoke symptoms.[28,29]

Internal femoral rotation against resistance in the seated position causes pain.

Maximum contraction of the piriformis against resistance (Pace sign) reproduces the pain.

Piriformis syndrome is compression of the sciatic nerve—usually its peroneal portion. Pain along the course of the sciatic nerve may be misdiagnosed as a lumbosacral lesion. Activities that tend to result in piriformis syndrome include prolonged sitting, especially with the leg in external rotation, the shortened position for the piriformis; stair climbing, walking, and running; and a sudden contraction or overstretching of the muscle. Runners, baseball catchers, and softball catchers commonly develop the syndrome.

Differential Diagnosis

Sciatica, gluteal strain, tendinitis, bursitis, herniated lumbar disk, multifidus syndrome

Imaging Techniques

Radiographs eliminate other potential diagnoses. In a patient with recalcitrant symptoms, MRI may be helpful to identify or rule out other conditions.

Definitive Diagnosis

The definitive diagnosis is based on positive physical evaluation findings, negative radiographs, and the exclusion of the conditions described in Differential Diagnosis.

Pathomechanics and Functional Limitations

Motions that stress the piriformis (eg, lateral femoral rotation, squatting, or stair climbing) are limited. Pressure on the sciatic nerve inhibits sensory and nerve function of the distal leg.

■ Medications

NSAIDs or acetaminophen are often used to reduce pain and increase function.

■ Surgical Intervention

Surgery is not normally indicated.

■ Postinjury Management

Relief of muscle spasm and attempts to gain motion in hip internal rotation are initiated. The condition is often accompanied by active trigger points, which can be resolved with myofascial or trigger-point release techniques accompanied by muscle stretching.

■ Injury-Specific Treatment and Rehabilitation Concerns

Specific Concerns

Control muscle spasm.
Increase internal rotation.

Electrical stimulation for pain and spasm relief and muscle facilitation may be used for the first week of treatment. Trigger-point release over the active area, myofascial release, and deep massage may be used to relieve muscle restriction.

Piriformis stretching is important to relax and lengthen the muscle. Once pain and spasm are relieved, the piriformis and other hip-stabilizing muscles, including the lateral and medial hip muscles and hip extensors, should be strengthened.

■ Estimated Amount of Time Lost

Time lost is usually not significant. The pain may be nagging and interfere with performance, forcing the patient to report the problem. Pain is the primary limiting factor; once it is relieved, full activity can resume.

Return-to-Play Criteria

The athlete should be pain free during all activities, and muscle spasm and trigger-point tenderness should be resolved.

Sacroiliac Joint Dysfunction

CLINICAL PRESENTATION

History

Pain or a dull ache in the buttocks
Pain can radiate into the thigh or groin.
Increased pain as the patient attempts to move into the restricted SI motion

Observation

Usually no swelling, discoloration, or deformity is noted.
Close observation may reveal asymmetry of skin creases in the sacral area.
Pelvic levels and leg lengths may be asymmetric.

Functional Status

The patient may sit or stand away from the involved side.

Physical Evaluation Findings

Alignment is assessed by comparing right and left sacral sulci and right and left inferior lateral angles (ILAs). In sacral flexion, the sulci are deeper and the ILA is more posterior, but if the sacrum is extended, the sulci are more posterior.
If sacral torsion is present, one of the ILAs is more posterior and the opposite sulcus is more posterior.
Any of the following special tests may be positive:
- FABER
- Quadrant
- Gaenslen
- SI compression
- SI distraction
- Straight-leg raise

Most "dysfunctions" indicate some loss of mobility. Sacroiliac (SI) dysfunction, also referred to as pelvic dysfunction, occurs when sacral motion is less than normal. Several different restrictions can occur, depending on the forces and torques and where they are applied. For example, one side can become elevated, as when stepping off a curb while running and landing with a sharp jolt on one leg or falling and landing on the buttock, restricting the sacrum in flexion. Trunk flexion and rotation activities can result in torsional joint injuries. Pain is often referred to the lower extremity, groin, buttock, or low back.

Differential Diagnosis

Lumbar spine injury, piriformis syndrome, gluteal strain

Imaging Techniques

Radiographs and CT and MRI scans may all be negative and are usually not helpful; however, they are necessary in working through the differential diagnosis.

Definitive Diagnosis

A definitive diagnosis is based on the physical examination findings and related special tests. To assess SI joint mobility, the patient stands and the clinician's thumbs are on each sulcus. When the patient moves into trunk flexion, the sacrum extends; the normal response is for the sulci to drop. If one does and the other does not, the nonmoving side is the restricted side. Another movement test has the patient standing with the clinician's thumbs over one sulcus and over the midsacrum in line with the sulcus. The patient then raises the leg on that side toward the chest and repeats the lift with the opposite leg. The normal response is for the sacrum to move downward on the side of the lifted leg. If the sacrum does not move down or moves up, motion of that SI joint is restricted.

Pathomechanics and Functional Limitations

In normal mechanics, as the lumbar spine flexes, the sacrum extends; as the lumbar spine extends, the sacrum flexes (**Figure 8-15**). Movement of the sacrum into flexion is called nutation. Movement of the sacrum into extension is termed counternutation. One sacral side moves in the opposite direction from its contralateral side; in ambulation, as the right leg moves forward, the right sacrum rotates posteriorly, and the left sacrum rotates anteriorly. Although the amount of motion allowed in the SI joint is minimal, normal SI mobility during ambulation protects the lower lumbar disks from undue torsional and shearing stresses. If SI motion is restricted, stress applied to the lumbar disks—especially the L5-S1 disk— increases, enhancing the risk of injury.

Several dysfunctions can result from SI joint pathomechanics and are classified according to the malalignment of either the sacrum on the ilium or the ilium on the sacrum. The more common sacrum-on-ilium, or sacroiliac, conditions include sacral flexion, forward torsion, and backward torsion. The more common ilium-on-sacrum, or iliosacral, conditions include pubic subluxation, iliac inflare, iliac outflare, and anterior and posterior up-slips.

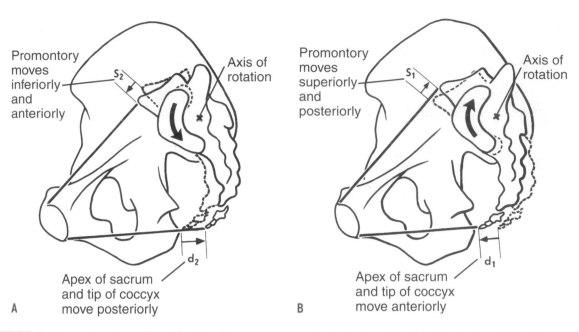

Figure 8-15 Nutation and counternutation. **A.** Nutation of the sacrum occurs when the lumbar spine extends. **B.** Counternutation of the sacrum occurs when the lumbar spine is flexed. (Reproduced with permission from Kapanjii A: *The Physiology of the Joints: Annotated Diagrams of the Mechanics of the Human Joints*, ed 3. New York, NY, Churchill Livingstone, 1974.)

The pathomechanics for each vary, as do their causes and treatments.

◼ Medications

NSAIDs or acetaminophen are often used to reduce pain and increase function.

◼ Surgical Intervention

Surgery is only performed on the SI joint after traumatic injury and is not indicated for conditions with an insidious onset.

◼ Postinjury/Postoperative Management

The restricted SI motions must be identified and resolved. A thorough history of the mechanism of injury and the activities that increase pain as well as a complete physical examination are required to diagnose the underlying ailments.

◼ Injury-Specific Treatment and Rehabilitation Concerns

Specific Concerns

Realign the SI joint and pelvis.
Reeducate the patient in proper posture and biomechanics.

Muscle energy A manual technique that uses voluntary muscle contraction against a resistive force to achieve desired results.

Barrier Restriction of, or resistance to, movement in a joint; the goal of muscle energy is to move the barrier to achieve normal mobility.

If the patient has been unable to participate in sport because of SI pain, progressive exercises for ROM and strength can be incorporated early in the program. Stretching exercises are used to correct the SI dysfunction and are similar to the positions in which the patient was placed to resolve the SI dysfunction. A common treatment technique used to treat SI dysfunction is muscle energy. Techniques for the more common dysfunctions are described below.

Sacroiliac Joint Muscle-energy Techniques

Sacral muscle-energy techniques use light isometric muscle contractions. The patient can control the contracting muscles, but the clinician must ensure that joint position is correct and that the muscle contraction is applied in a specific direction with a very light force ("approximately 2 ounces") that is held for 3 to 10 seconds. At the end of the isometric hold, the patient is instructed to relax, and the clinician moves the joint to the point where a new restriction (barrier) is felt. The process is repeated three to five times.

Pubic Subluxation: The patient is placed in the hook-lying position with the knees positioned together, and the clinician's hands are placed on the knees to maintain the position while the patient gently attempts to move the knees apart (**Figure 8-16**). In the reverse position, the clinician gently resists the patient's pulling the knees together.

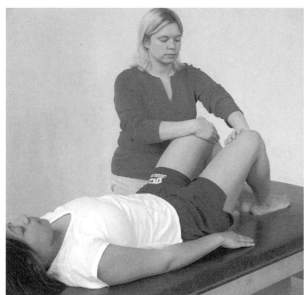 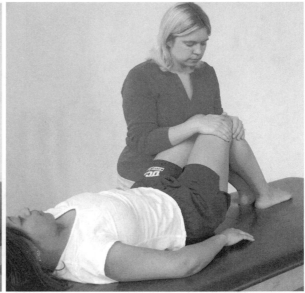

Figure 8-16 Muscle-energy technique for a pubic subluxation. **A.** Adduction. **B.** Abduction.

Right Iliac Inflare: The patient is placed in the supine figure-of-4 position (**Figure 8-17**). A stabilizing hand is placed on the opposite hip and the resisting hand on top of the knee. The patient is instructed to attempt to move the knee across toward the other leg. The applied stretch pushes down on the knee to move it toward the table. In the home exercise for this dysfunction, the patient lies in a figure-of-4 position for several minutes.

Right Iliac Outflare: The patient is supine, and the involved hip is passively moved into internal rotation and adduction with the knee pointed toward the opposite shoulder. The monitoring hand is placed on the patient's sulcus, and the resisting

hand is placed over the anterolateral knee. The patient is instructed to provide resistance into hip external rotation and abduction. The stretch is applied to the barrier of internal rotation (**Figure 8-18**). In the home exercise for this dysfunction, the patient uses a hold-relax self-technique while supine and hugging the knee toward the opposite shoulder.

Left Up-slip: With the patient supine, the clinician grasps the patient's ankle to abduct and flex the hip at 30°. The patient is instructed to take a deep breath in and blow it out slowly. As the patient exhales, the slack in the lower extremity is taken out. The patient is then instructed to perform a couple of quick coughs. The stretch is a sudden thrust per-

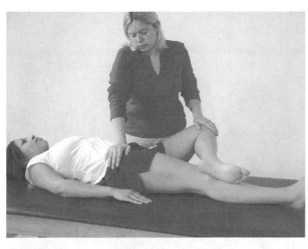

Figure 8-17 Right iliac inflare muscle-energy technique.

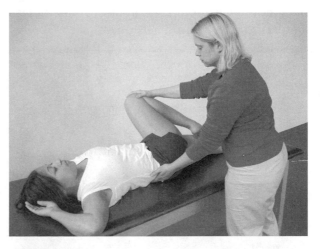

Figure 8-18 Right iliac outflare muscle-energy technique.

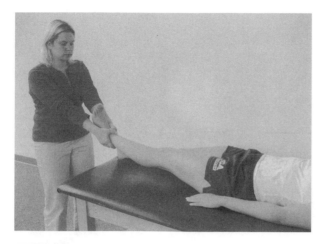

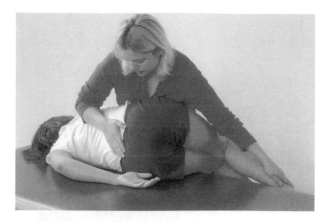

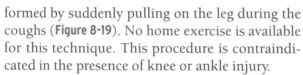

Figure 8-19   Left up-slip muscle-energy technique.

Figure 8-20   Forward torsion muscle-energy technique.

formed by suddenly pulling on the leg during the coughs (**Figure 8-19**). No home exercise is available for this technique. This procedure is contraindicated in the presence of knee or ankle injury.

The same technique is used in a right up-slip except the athlete is positioned prone and the leg is abducted and extended to 30°. The instructions for breathing and coughing are the same.

Forward Torsion: The patient is positioned lying on the involved side. The hips and knees are flexed to 90°, with the knees and legs off the table and the thighs supported on the table. The torso is rotated so that the bottom arm and shoulder are behind the patient, and the top arm is forward and resting comfortably over the table and over its side. The pelvis is monitored by placing one hand over the lumbosacral junction, while the resisting hand grasps the ankles or distal legs. The patient's thighs are supported by the clinician's thigh. The legs are passively rotated downward to the floor until the resistance (barrier) is met. When rotation of the lumbosacral junction is felt, the barrier is met. The patient applies the isometric force, attempting to push the legs and feet to the ceiling. The stretch force is applied downward at the ankles (**Figure 8-20**). In the home exercise for this technique, the athlete lies for several minutes on a couch or bed in the position seen in the figure.

Sacroiliac Joint Mobilizations

A nutated sacrum can be treated using posteroanterior (PA) sacral joint mobilization between the inferior lateral angles. Graded mobilizations over the inferior sacrum are used to obtain a counternutated position (**Figure 8-21, A**). In the case of a counternutated sacrum, PA mobilizations are applied over the superior sacrum (**Figure 8-21, B**).

■ Estimated Amount of Time Lost

Time lost varies depending on the duration of the existing symptoms, the magnitude of pain, and the amount of function lost. Some patients lose no time from activity, but others lose up to 2 months of participation.

■ Return-to-Play Criteria

The athlete should be pain free, and examination of the sacroiliac joint should reveal good alignment.

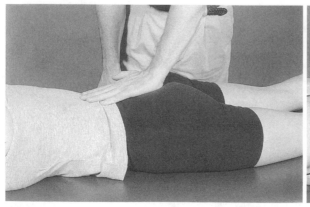

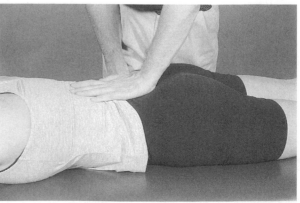

Figure 8-21   Sacral joint mobilizations. **A.** Treatment of a nutated sacrum. **B.** Treatment of a counternutated sacrum.

Rehabilitation

This section includes early rehabilitation exercises for the pelvis, hip, and thigh, including flexibility and early strengthening exercises using isometrics and rubber tubing. Other relevant exercises are presented in chapters 9 and 17.

Flexibility Exercises

Refer to the following exercises in chapter 9:

- Quadriceps stretch
- Alternate quadriceps stretch
- Hamstring stretch
- Alternate hamstring stretch
- Hip flexor stretch
- Adductor stretch
- ITB stretch
- Hip internal rotator stretch
- Hip external rotator stretch
- Piriformis stretch

Strengthening Exercises

Advanced exercises for the hip and lower extremity are presented in chapter 9 (p 251) and chapter 17 (p 551).

Isometrics

Hip abduction   In a seated position, the patient places the opposite hand against the distal lateral thigh and pushes against the thigh with the hand as the hip resists with an abduction force. The position is held for 10 seconds, and repeated 10 times.

Hip adduction   In a seated position, the patient places both fists between the distal thighs and attempts to move the thighs together, holding for 10 seconds. The exercise is repeated 10 times.

Hip extension   Standing with the back to the wall and about 6 inches from the wall, the patient places the heel of an extended leg to the wall and pushes the leg against the wall, holding for 10 seconds. It may be necessary for the patient to hold on to a chair or other secure object for balance. The exercise is repeated 10 times.

Hip internal rotation   Seated on a chair with the legs crossed at the ankles and the involved leg crossed under the uninvolved leg, the patient attempts to pull the ankle of the involved leg away from the uninvolved ankle. The position is held for 10 seconds, and repeated 10 times.

Hip external rotation   Seated on a chair with the legs parallel and the feet touching their medial aspects together, the patient pushes the foot of the involved leg toward the uninvolved extremity, attempting to push the leg into external rotation. The position is held for 10 seconds, and repeated 10 times.

Rubber Tubing Exercises

See Figure 8-22.

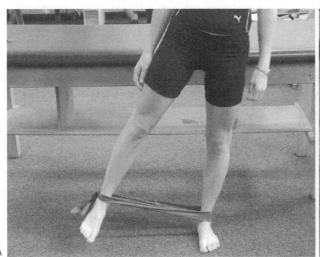
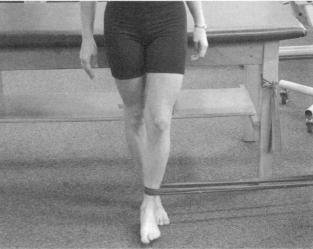

Figure 8-22   Resistive hip strengthening exercises. **A. Hip abduction.** With the patient standing, the tubing is wrapped around both ankles. Using large steps the patient walks sideways toward the involved side. **B. Hip adduction.** With the tubing anchored to a door jamb or an adjacent table, the tubing is wrapped around the patient's involved distal leg. The hip is adducted as far as possible against the tubing.   *Continued*

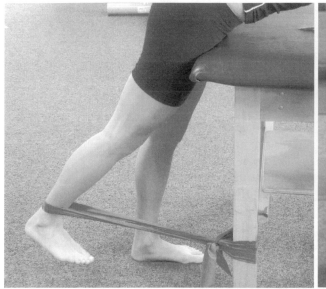

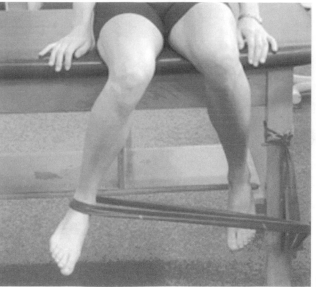

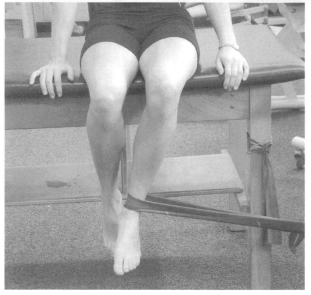

Figure 8-22, *cont'd*   **C. Hip extension.** With the tubing anchored around the ankle and secured to a table leg, the patient stands at the end of the table and leans to place the trunk on the table. The hip is extended while the knee is kept straight. In a variation of this exercise, the patient stands and grasps a chair for stability while the hip is extended from neutral. **D. Hip internal rotation.** With the tubing anchored around a table leg and the patient sitting on the table, the patient attempts to internally rotate the hip against the tubing. **E. Hip external rotation.** With the tubing anchored around a table leg and the patient seated, the patient externally rotates the hip against the tubing.

References

1. Nicholas SJ, Tyler TF: Adductor muscle strains in sport. *Sports Med* 2002;32:339-344.

2. Morelli V, Smith V: Groin injuries in athletes. *Am Fam Physician* 2001;64:1405-1414.

3. Tyler TF, Nicholas SJ, Campbell RJ, Donellan S, McHugh MP: The effectiveness of a preseason exercise program to prevent adductor muscle strains in professional ice hockey players. *Am J Sports Med* 2002;30:680-683.

4. Garrett WE Jr: Muscle strain injuries. *Am J Sports Med* 1996;24(suppl 6):S2-S8.

5. Clanton TO, Coupe KJ: Hamstring strains in athletes: Diagnosis and treatment. *J Am Acad Orthop Surg* 1998;6:237-248.

6. David HG, Green JT, Grant AJ, Wilson CA: Simultaneous bilateral quadriceps rupture: A complication of anabolic steroid abuse. *J Bone Joint Surg Br* 1995;77:159-160.

7. Orchard J, Marsden J, Lord S, Garlick D: Preseason hamstring muscle weakness associated with hamstring muscle injury in Australian footballers. *Am J Sports Med* 1997;25:81-85.

8. Croisier JL, Forthomme B, Namurois M-H, Vanderthommen M, Crielaard JM: Hamstring muscle strain recurrence and strength performance disorders. *Am J Sports Med* 2002;30:199-203.

9. Verrall GM, Slavotinek JP, Barnes PG, Fon GT, Spriggins AJ: Clinical risk factors for hamstring muscle strain injury: A prospective study with correlation of injury by magnetic resonance imaging. *Br J Sports Med* 2001;35:435-440.

10. Ryan JB, Wheeler JH, Hopkinson WJ, Arciero RA, Kolakowski KR: Quadriceps contusions: West Point update. *Am J Sports Med* 1991;19:299-304.

11. Wieder DL: Treatment of traumatic myositis ossificans with acetic acid iontophoresis. *Phys Ther* 1992;72:133-137.

12. Anderson K, Strickland SM, Warren R: Hip and groin injuries in athletes. *Am J Sports Med* 2001;29:521-533.

13. Shbeeb MI, Matteson EL: Trochanteric bursitis (greater trochanter pain syndrome). *Mayo Clin Proc* 1996;71:565-569.

14. Dobbs MB, Gordon JE, Luhmann SJ, Szymanski DA, Schoenecker PL: Surgical correction of the snapping iliopsoas tendon in adolescents. *J Bone Joint Surg Am* 2002;84:420-424.

15. Gruen GS, Scioscia TN, Lowenstein JE: The surgical treatment of internal snapping hip. *Am J Sports Med* 2002;30:607-613.

16. Pelsser V, Cardinal E, Hobden R, Aubin R, Lafortune M: Extraarticular snapping hip: Sonographic findings. *AJR Am J Roentgenol* 2001;176:67-73.

17. Traycoff RB: Pseudotrochanteric bursitis: The differential diagnosis of lateral hip pain. *J Rheumatol* 1991;18:1810-1812.

18. Kagan A II: Rotator cuff tears of the hip. *Clin Orthop* 1999;368:135-140.

19. Jones DL, Erhard RE: Diagnosis of trochanteric bursitis versus femoral neck stress fracture. *Phys Ther* 1997;77:58-67.

20. Toohey AK, LaSalle TL, Martinez S, Polisson RP: Iliopsoas bursitis: Clinical features, radiographic findings, and disease associations. *Semin Arthritis Rheum* 1990;20:41-47.

21. Johnston CAM, Wiley JP, Lindsay DM, Wiseman DA: Iliopsoas bursitis and tendinitis: A review. *Sports Med* 1998;25:271-283.

22. Johnston CAM, Lindsay DM, Wiley JP: Treatment of iliopsoas syndrome with a hip rotation strengthening program: A retrospective case series. *J Orthop Sports Phys Ther* 1999;29:218-224.

23. Davies AM, Carter SR, Grimer RJ, Sneath RS: Fatigue fractures of the femoral diaphysis in the skeletally immature simulating malignancy. *Br J Radiol* 1989;62:893-896.

24. Shin AY, Gillingham BL: Fatigue fractures of the femoral neck in athletes. *J Am Acad Orthop Surg* 1997;5:293-302.

25. Dugowson CE, Drinkwater BL, Clark JM: Nontraumatic femur fracture in an oligomenorrheic athlete. *Med Sci Sports Exerc* 1991;23:1323-1325.

26. Casterline M, Osowski S, Ulrich G: Femoral stress fracture. *J Athl Train* 1996;31:53-56.

27. Brukner P, Bennell K: Stress fractures in female athletes: Diagnosis, management and rehabilitation. *Sports Med* 1997;24:419-429.

28. Beatty RA: The piriformis muscle syndrome: A simple diagnostic maneuver. *Neurosurgery* 1994;34:512-514.

29. Fishman LM, Dombi GW, Michaelsen C, et al: Piriformis syndrome: Diagnosis, treatment, and outcome: A 10-year study. *Arch Phys Med Rehabil* 2002;83:295-301.

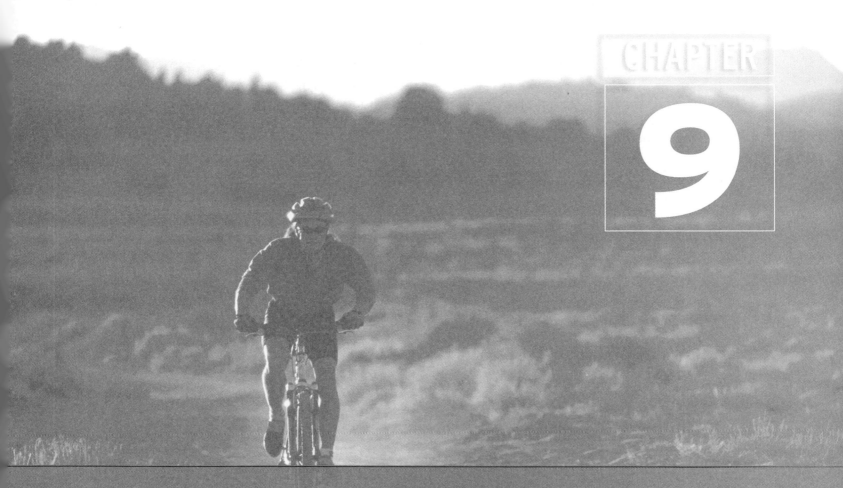

CHAPTER 9

Additional Lower Extremity Therapeutic Exercises

The exercises and techniques presented in this chapter are adjuncts to those presented in chapters 5, 6, 7, and 8. Many other exercises can also be incorporated or substituted for those presented here. In addition, most exercises can be modified based on the patient's needs, equipment on hand, or personal preference. To construct a complete rehabilitation program, cross-referencing among these chapters is required.

Flexibility Exercises

The following stretches are held for 10 to 30 seconds and are repeated three or four times.

Ankle and Lower Leg

> **Cross-references**
>
> Dorsiflexion stretch for the gastrocnemius (p 127)
> Dorsiflexion stretch for the soleus (p 127)
> Prolonged dorsiflexion stretch (p 128)
> Plantar flexion stretch (p 128)

Femoral Muscles

Hamstring Stretch

The patient stands and faces a table about hip height. The foot of the involved leg is placed on the table with the standing foot facing forward. The patient leans from the hips, not the back, to reach toward the elevated foot with the opposite hand until a stretch is felt. Both knees remain straight during the exercise.

Alternate Hamstring Stretch

The patient lies supine with the nonstretched leg extended. The stretched leg is flexed at the hip, with the hands clasped behind the knee to hold the thigh at 90°. The knee is extended until a stretch is felt in the hamstrings (**Figure 9-1**).

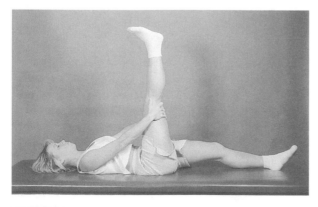

Figure 9-1 Alternate hamstring stretch.

Quadriceps Stretch

The side-lying patient bends the knee and grasps the foot behind the buttock. Keeping the hip and back straight, the patient pulls the heel toward the buttock until tension is felt in the anterior thigh (**Figure 9-2**).

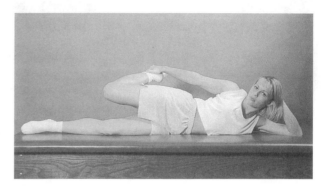

Figure 9-2 Quadriceps stretch.

Alternate Quadriceps Stretch

The patient stands facing a wall, using one hand for support. The opposite hand grasps the foot of the leg being stretched behind the back and, while keeping the knee pointed to the floor and the back straight, the patient pulls the heel toward the buttock until a stretch is felt (**Figure 9-3**).

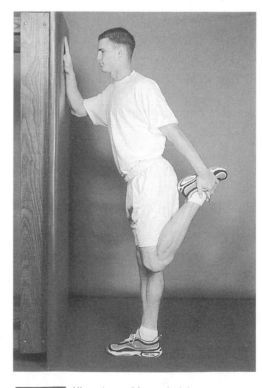

Figure 9-3 Alternate quadriceps stretch.

Cross-references

Hip Muscles

Hip Flexor Stretch

The patient leans forward, extending one leg backward while keeping the opposite knee flexed. The hips are pushed forward until a stretch is felt in the extended hip (**Figure 9-4**).

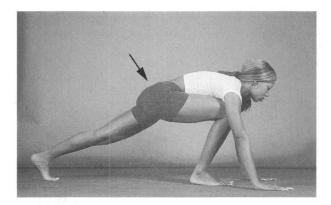

Figure 9-4 Hip flexor stretch.

Adductor Stretch

In the sitting position, the patient flexes both knees and separates the knees to bring the soles of the feet together. With the forearms placed along the legs and the hands at the ankles, the patient pushes the legs down with the forearms until a stretch is felt in the adductors (**Figure 9-5**).

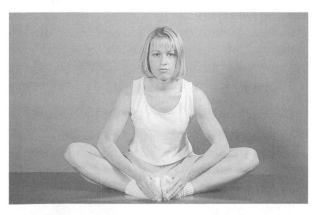

Figure 9-5 Adductor stretch.

Iliotibial Band Stretch

While side lying on a table, the patient places the top leg over the side of the table and relaxes in the position for about 5 minutes. An alternative is to have the clinician apply force to the leg while stabilizing the pelvis (**Figure 9-6**).

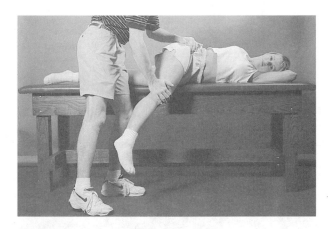

Figure 9-6 Iliotibial band stretch.

Hip Internal Rotator Stretch

The patient sits at the edge of a table. The clinician places one hand distal to the flexed knee and applies external rotational force on the hip until the patient feels a stretch in the internal rotators (**Figure 9-7**).

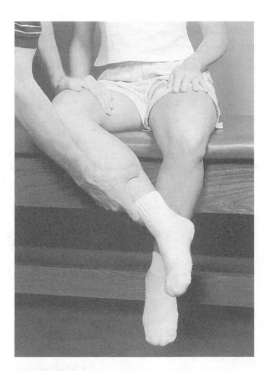

Figure 9-7 Hip internal rotator stretch.

Hip External Rotator Stretch

The patient sits at the edge of a table. The clinician places one hand distal to the flexed knee while the opposite hand stabilizes the femur just proximal to the knee. An internal rotational force is applied on the hip until the patient feels a stretch on the external rotators (**Figure 9-8**).

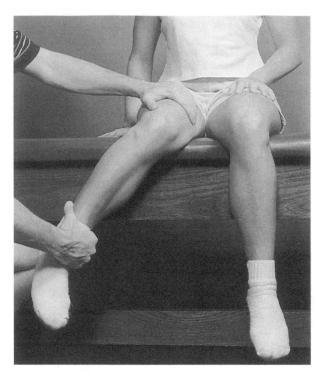

Figure 9-8 Hip external rotator stretch.

Piriformis Stretch

The patient lies supine with the knees and hips flexed and the feet on the floor. The involved leg is crossed over the uninvolved leg. Both knees are

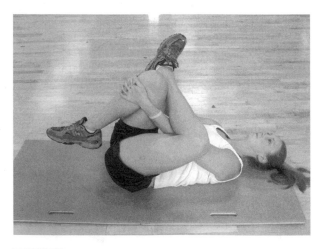

Figure 9-9 Piriformis stretch.

brought toward the chest, and the patient grabs the leg to pull the knees closer. As the knees are brought up, the top knee is angled toward the opposite shoulder (**Figure 9-9**).

Strengthening Exercises

The following are isotonic strengthening exercises used early in the rehabilitation program. When the patient can successfully complete these exercises, weight machines or free weights can be incorporated into the rehabilitation protocol.

■ Ankle and Lower Leg

Cross-references
Isometrics
    Dorsiflexion (p 128)
    Plantar flexion (p 128)
    Inversion (p 128)
    Eversion (p 128)
Rubber-tubing exercises (p 129)
Towel rolls (p 128)
Marble pickups (p 128)
Heel raises (p 128)
Toe raises (p 128)
Ankle weight exercises (p 128)

■ Femoral Muscles

Standing Hamstring Curl

The patient stands with the quadriceps pressed against the table and flexes the knee, bringing the heel toward the buttocks. The position is briefly held and the foot is then lowered to the floor, completely extending the knee. The exercise is repeated, beginning with two to three sets of 10 repetitions and progressing to five sets of 10 repetitions. Weights can be added in increments of 5 lb; however, the patient should begin with two sets of 10 repetitions after any increase.

Standing Hip Extension

The patient stands and leans forward with the upper body supported on the table. Keeping the knee extended, the patient extends the hip by raising the leg toward the ceiling, extending the hip only as far as can be done without externally rotating it. The exercise is repeated, beginning with two to three sets of 10 repetitions and progressing to five sets of 10 repetitions. Weights can be added in increments of 5 lb; however, the patient must begin with two sets of 10 repetitions after any increase.

General Lower Extremity Strengthening

Triceps Surae

The patient is seated with resistance placed over the thigh proximal to the knee as the ankle is plantar flexed against the resistance. An alternate position is for the patient to stand with the weight across the shoulders or held in the hands (**Figure 9-10**). When the knee is extended, the gastrocnemius is emphasized; when the knee is flexed, the soleus is the prime mover.

Step-up and Step-down

These exercises begin at low heights and are advanced as range of motion and strength improve. Forward, lateral, and backward vectors of movement can be used. The patient begins by stepping up on a short stool, first with one foot and then the other, then stepping down in the same order (**Figure 9-11**). The patient should be closely monitored, so that substitutions are not made to assist in performing the exercise.

Squat

The squatting motion can be performed in numerous ways with various devices, including free weights, gym balls, resistive bands, walls, and shuttles. It can be performed in limited range of motion as needed by the individual patient. Hamstring activity is facilitated by trunk flexion.

Single-leg squatting activities can be initiated when the patient is bearing full weight and demonstrates adequate hip and thigh strength to maintain the correct biomechanical position during double leg squats (**Figure 9-12**).

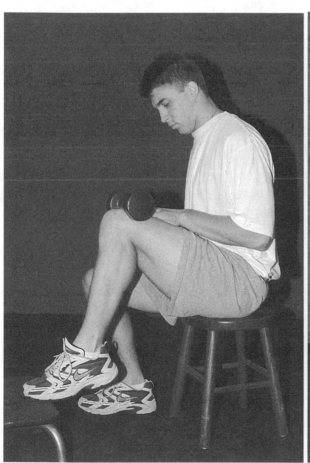
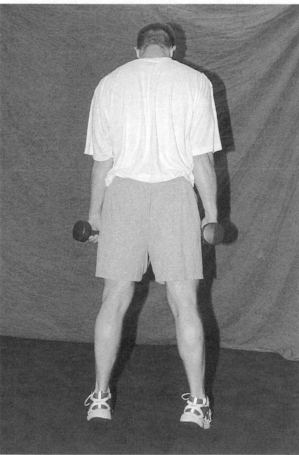

Figure 9-10 Triceps surae.

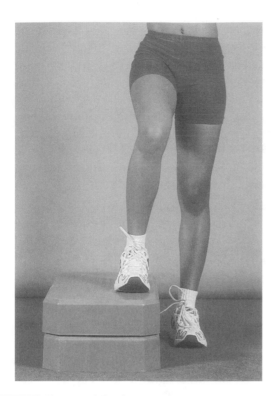

Figure 9-11 Step-up and step-down.

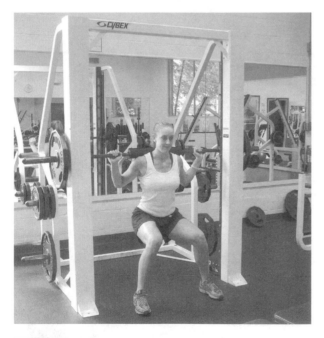

Figure 9-12 Squat.

Hip Muscles

Surgical tubing or TheraBand is looped around the leg, just proximal to the knee. The area may be padded with a towel for patient comfort. While standing on the uninvolved leg, the patient moves the involved leg through sets of abduction, adduction, flexion, and extension (**Figure 9-13**). As the patient advances with this exercise, diagonal motions may be incorporated.

Cross-references

Isometrics
    Hip abduction (p 247)
    Hip adduction (p 247)
    Hip extension (p 247)
    Hip internal rotation (p 247)
    Hip external rotation (p 247)
Rubber-tubing exercises (p 247)

Proprioception and Functional Exercises

Proprioceptive neuromuscular facilitation (PNF) involves mass movement patterns that incorporate spiral and diagonal motions to facilitate selective irradiation (resisting strong muscle groups at specific times in a pattern to facilitate the contractions of weaker muscle groups in the same pattern). These patterns closely resemble sport and work activity movements. Each spiral and diagonal pattern includes a three-component motion with respect to all the joints or pivots of action participating in the movement. The three components are flexion/extension, adduction/abduction, and rotation. The optimal performance of a pattern involves sequential contractions described as a "chain" of muscles moving in synergy. The agonistic pattern involves components of action that are opposite those of the antagonistic pattern.

Improvements in functional output are achieved when proprioceptive, cutaneous, and auditory inputs are used in the rehabilitative setting. The stretch reflex is a neurophysiologic mechanism on which PNF is based. Autogenic inhibition and reciprocal inhibition are two neurophysiologic phenomena used to describe a neuromuscular system's ability to be facilitated and inhibited.

■ Rhythmic Initiation

Rhythmic initiation is used to improve the patient's ability to initiate movement. This technique involves voluntary relaxation, passive movements, and isotonic contractions of major muscle components of the antagonistic pattern.

■ Repeated Contractions

The stretch reflex is facilitated and coupled with repetitive voluntary isotonic contractions to enhance the patient's effort to initiate movement. As the patient's ability to produce an isotonic con-

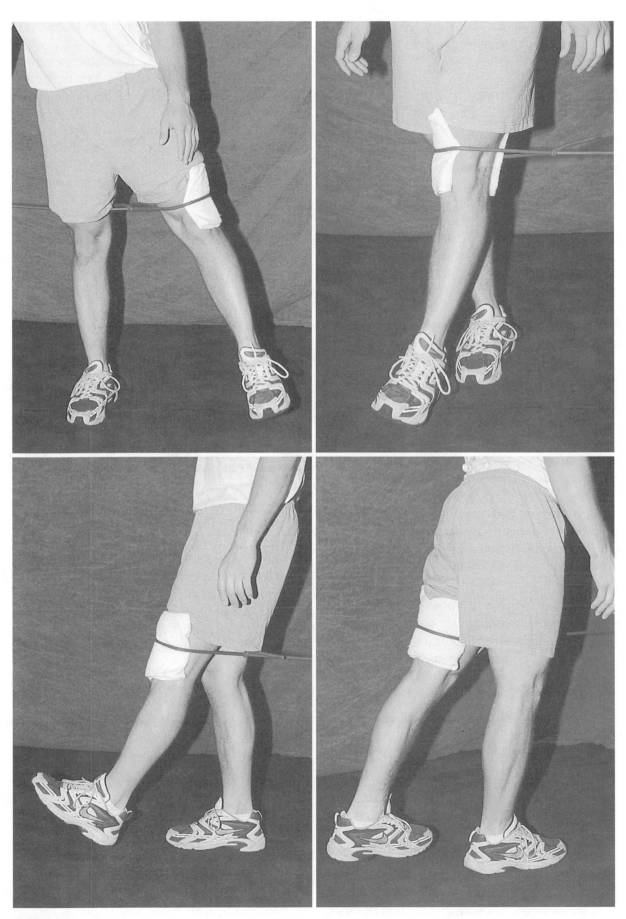

Figure 9-13 Hip muscle exercises.

traction improves, an isometric hold at weaker points in the range may be added to advance the treatment.

Reversal of Antagonists

Stimulation of the agonist contraction occurs when the patient first resists an isometric or isotonic contraction of the antagonist, followed by resistance of the agonist movement as the antagonistic pattern is reversed.

Slow reversal: An isotonic contraction of the antagonist is followed by an isotonic contraction of the agonist.

Slow reversal hold: The antagonist performs an isotonic contraction followed by an isometric contraction; the agonist then performs an isotonic contraction followed by an isometric contraction.

Rhythmic stabilization: An isometric contraction of the antagonist is followed by an isometric contraction of the agonist, resulting in cocontraction.

Relaxation Techniques

Relaxation techniques are used to gain range of motion via the relaxation or inhibition of a pattern's antagonist.

Contract-Relax

The patient's body part is passively moved into the agonistic pattern to the point of limitation, when the patient is instructed to contract ("push" or "pull") isotonically in the antagonistic pattern. As the patient then relaxes, the limb is redirected into the agonistic pattern until the patient again feels limitation.

Hold-Relax

The patient's body part is moved in the same sequence as in the contract-relax technique. At the point of limitation, the patient is instructed to perform a maximal isometric contraction and then to voluntarily relax. As the patient feels the relaxation, the limb is moved into the agonistic pattern to a new point of limitation.

Hold-Contract

The range-limiting (antagonistic) pattern is an isotonic contraction, followed by an isometric contraction of the same pattern against resistance. After a brief, voluntary relaxation, an isotonic contraction of the agonistic pattern is performed.

Lower Extremity PNF Patterns

The two basic PNF patterns for the lower extremity are D1 and D2. These are further divided into two subdivisions: D1 moving into flexion, D1 mov-

ing into extension, D2 moving into flexion, and D2 moving into extension (CT 9-1 and 9-2). These patterns involve diagonal and rotational movements. Each pattern begins when the musculature that will be active is placed in an elongated position and ends when the musculature has obtained a shortened position. Resistance is supplied manually. These patterns incorporate gross muscle activity, not individual or isolated muscle activity. It can be beneficial for patients to learn these patterns before using resistance.

Balance Progression

Proprioception is the term used to define the perception of joint position and limb "heaviness." Kinesthesia is the term used to define the body's ability to detect positional changes. Although the terms are not interchangeable, they are closely related. Articular mechanoreceptors, Golgi tendon organs, muscle spindles, the vestibular system, the visual system, and cerebellar and cerebral functions all contribute to the body's conscious and unconscious positional awareness.

Many proprioceptive and kinesthetic (balance) activities can be performed with very little equipment. The difficulty of the exercises can be changed by several factors.

Standing Tubing Band Kick

The patient stands single legged on the uninvolved extremity. Tubing or a band is wrapped from the involved ankle and foot to the uninvolved ankle and foot or a secure object, and the patient moves the uninvolved extremity against the tension of the tubing or band while attempting to maintain balance. Patterns of hip flexion, adduction, abduction, extension, or diagonals may be used (**Figure 9-14**).

Stork Stand

The patient stands single legged on the involved leg and attempts to maintain balance for as long as possible. The knee can be kept in various angles of flexion depending on the patient's tolerance and restrictions. The patient can perform stork stands while standing on an unstable surface (**Figure 9-15**). The patient should be able to maintain balance without wavering or losing balance for 30 seconds. To further challenge the patient, progress to performing the exercises with the eyes closed to remove visual cues. Functional activities such as tossing and catching a ball, bouncing a ball, setting a ball, or other upper extremity activity is the next progression.

CT Clinical Technique 9-1

D1 Lower Extremity PNF Pattern

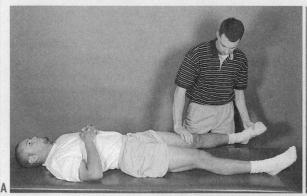
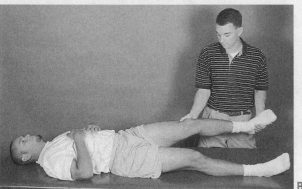
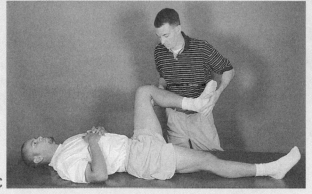

A Starting position; **B** Moving into flexion; **C** Terminal flexion

Body Part	Moving Into Flexion		Moving Into Extension	
	Starting Position	Terminal Position	Starting Position	Terminal Position
Hip	Extended	Flexed	Flexed	Extended
	Abducted	Adducted	Adducted	Abducted
	Internally rotated	Externally rotated	Externally rotated	Internally rotated
Knee	Extended	Flexed	Flexed	Extended
Position of tibia	Externally rotated	Internally rotated	Internally rotated	Externally rotated
Ankle and foot	Plantar flexed	Dorsiflexed	Dorsiflexed	Plantar flexed
	Everted	Inverted	Inverted	Everted
Toes	Flexed	Extended	Extended	Flexed
Hand position*	Right hand on dorsomedial surface of foot		Right hand on lateral plantar surface of foot	
	Left hand on anteromedial thigh near patella		Left hand on posterolateral thigh near popliteal crease	
Verbal command	Pull		Push	

*For patient's right leg.

(Reproduced with permission from Prentice W: *Rehabilitation Techniques in Sports Medicine*, ed 2. St Louis, MO, Mosby-Year Book, 1994.)

CT Clinical Technique 9-2

D2 Lower Extremity PNF Pattern

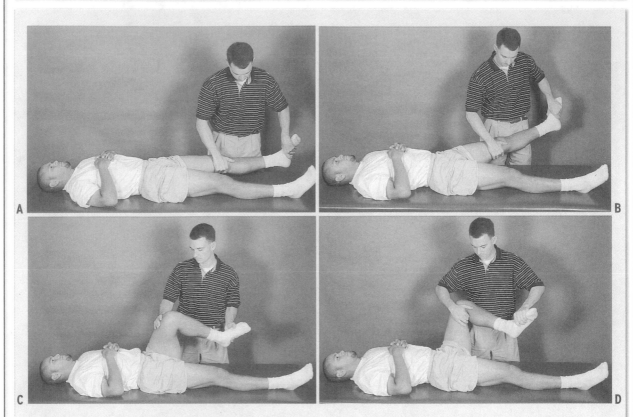

A Movement into extension; **B** Moving into flexion; **C** Hip internal rotation; **D** Hip external rotation

Body Part	Moving Into Flexion		Moving Into Extension	
	Starting Position	Terminal Position	Starting Position	Terminal Position
Hip	Extended	Flexed	Flexed	Extended
	Adducted	Abducted	Abducted	Adducted
	Externally rotated	Internally rotated	Internally rotated	Externally rotated
Knee	Extended	Flexed	Flexed	Extended
Position of tibia	Externally rotated	Internally rotated	Internally rotated	Externally rotated
Ankle and foot	Plantar flexed	Dorsiflexed	Dorsiflexed	Plantar flexed
	Inverted	Everted	Everted	Inverted
Toes	Flexed	Extended	Extended	Flexed
Hand position*	Right hand on dorsolateral surface of foot		Right hand on medial plantar surface of foot	
	Left hand on anterolateral thigh near patella		Left hand on posteromedial thigh near popliteal crease	
Verbal command	Pull		Push	

*For patient's right leg.

(Reproduced with permission from Prentice W: *Rehabilitation Techniques in Sports Medicine*, ed 2. St Louis, MO, Mosby-Year Book, 1994.)

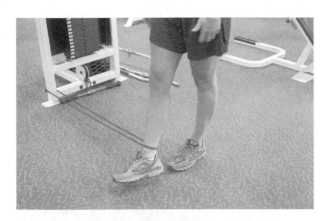

Figure 9-14   Standing tubing band kick.

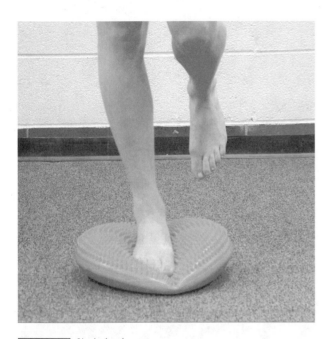

Figure 9-15   Stork stand.

Balance Beam

The balance beam presents the patient with the difficulty of maneuvering on a narrow base of support. Static and dynamic balance can be challenged by variations of the stork stand and by walking forward, backward, and heel to toe and side stepping.

Vestibular Board

The vestibular board typically challenges the patient in two directions: forward-backward and side to side (**Figure 9-16**). Because the board has a larger surface area than other unstable-surface trainers, the patient can perform activities that involve wider stances or kneeling and can focus on controlling two directions of movement.

Proprioception Board

The patient stands on the proprioception or "wobble board" and attempts to balance or trace the edge of the board. Various levels of difficulty can be achieved by changing the height or size of half balls attached to the proprioception board or standing on only one leg. The patient also can perform the exercise using front-to-back or side-to-side motions (**Figure 9-17**). The number of repetitions can vary.

Minitrampoline

Several exercises can be performed on the minitrampoline, including balancing on one foot, stepping on and off the trampoline, hopping on and off the trampoline, and picking up cups positioned from the 3:00 to the 9:00 o'clock positions around the perimeter of the trampoline. Other standard proprioceptive exercises with multiplanar activities and functions such as ball catching while balancing can also be performed. The number of repetitions can vary.

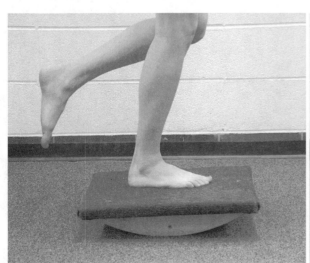

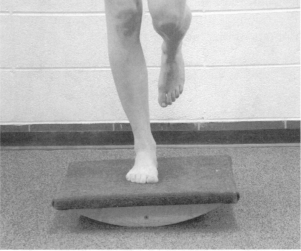

Figure 9-16   Vestibular board.

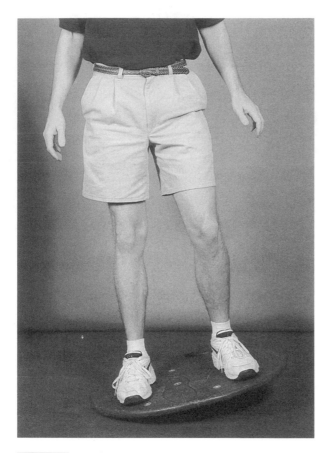

Figure 9-17   Proprioception board.

Single-leg Squat

The patient squats on one leg and balances for 30 seconds, or longer if possible (**Figure 9-18**). This exercise should be performed with the affected leg flexed or extended at various joint angles to change the center of gravity. The number of repetitions can vary.

Wall Squats

The patient assumes a squatting position with the back facing a wall and holding an inflated exercise ball against the wall. The position is held for 30 seconds, or longer if possible (**Figure 9-19**). The number of repetitions can vary.

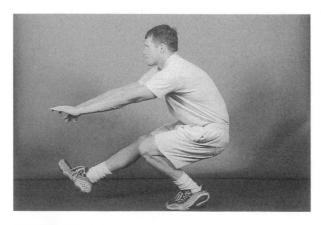

Figure 9-18   Single-leg squat.

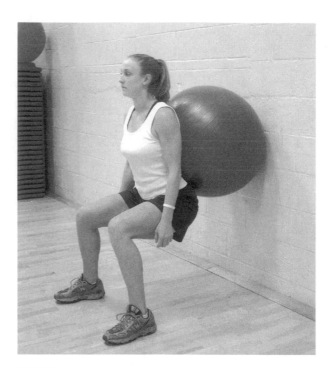

Figure 9-19   Wall squats.

Slide Board

The resistance between the surface of the board and the covering placed on the feet decreases friction, allowing the patient to "skate" glide on the slide board (**Figure 9-20**). Repetitions can be counted as the number of times the patient glides side to side or the number of times the exercise is completed in a specific period.

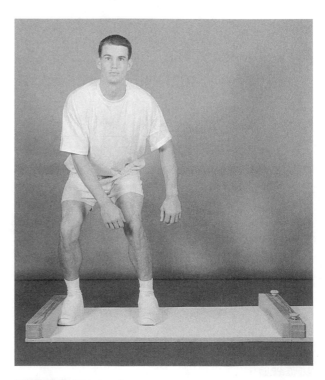

Figure 9-20   Slide board.

Plyometric exercises can be specific for the individual sport demands. Following are examples of plyometric exercises.

Two-Foot Ankle Hop

The patient jumps in place, using only the ankles, jumping as high as possible with only a slight knee bend. As the patient progresses, proprioceptive and kinesthetic challenges can be added by incorporating the hip-twist ankle hop. This is similar to the two-foot ankle hop, but this time the patient twists 90° to the left and then to the right while jumping in place. The sequence is jump with both feet together straight up then land, jump again but twist to the right, jump and twist to the start position, jump and twist to the left, and jump and twist to the start position.

Squat Jump

In this low-intensity plyometric exercise, the patient assumes a half-squat position with hands behind the head, jumps vertically, and, on landing, returns to the half-squat position to repeat the same series without pause (**Figure 9-22**). At least 10 repetitions per set should be performed.

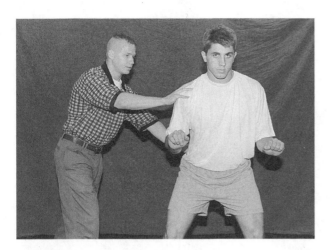

Figure 9-21 Rhythmic stabilization.

Rhythmic Stabilization

Rhythmic stabilization can be performed in functional positions such as in a squat, on stairs, or in a downhill skier's tuck. The patient holds the position while the clinician attempts to move him or her from the position with perturbations (**Figure 9-21**). The force applied is individualized to the patient's tolerance.

Plyometric Exercises

Plyometrics are exercises that enable a muscle to reach maximum strength in as short a time as possible and are useful in improving strength, speed, and kinesthetic ability. Lower extremity plyometrics typically involve jump training. Before starting plyometric exercises, the patient must have adequate muscular strength and endurance. Recovery for plyometrics ranges from 5 to 10 seconds between repetitions and 2 to 3 minutes between sets. The frequency at which the plyometric exercises are performed depends on the patient's level of conditioning and ability and the intensity at which the exercises are performed. High-intensity plyometric exercises should be performed only twice per week to allow adequate recovery.

Plyometric exercises can also be measured by volume, the number of foot contacts made during a workout. Volume for a beginner should be limited to 80 to 100 contacts per session, advancing to 120 to 140 contacts per session. Each activity can be varied in intensity and volume as needed by the patient. Cones, boxes, mats, hurdles, stairs, and medicine balls are used for plyometric activities.

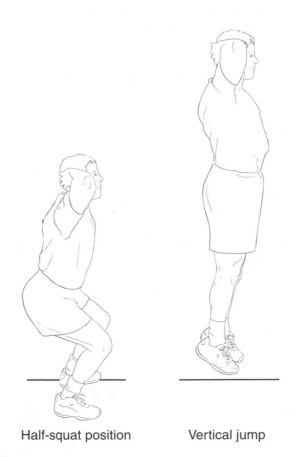

Half-squat position   Vertical jump

Figure 9-22 Squat jump.

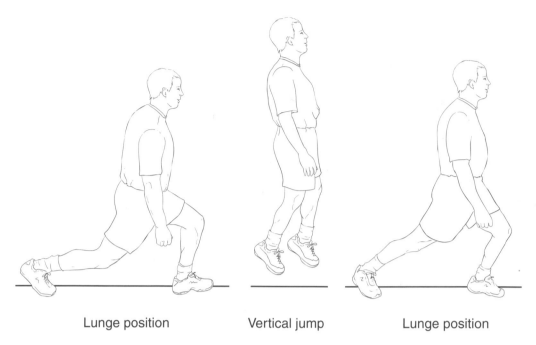

Lunge position   Vertical jump   Lunge position

Figure 9-23   Split-squat jump.

Split-Squat Jump

In this low-intensity plyometric exercise, the patient assumes a lunge position with one foot forward, jumps vertically to land in a lunge position, and repeats the series without pause (**Figure 9-23**). At least 10 repetitions with each foot forward should be performed.

Standing Triple Jump

In this medium-intensity exercise, the patient begins in a partial squat position and jumps horizontally and vertically, using the arms for balance, and lands on one foot. Without pausing, the patient jumps off that foot to land on the opposite foot, and again without pausing, jumps and lands on both feet. Two sets of six jumps each should be performed, with a 30- to 60-second rest period between sets.

Box Jump

In this high-intensity exercise, the patient stands in front of a box in a semisquatting position, jumps up on a box 1 to 2.5 feet high, and immediately on contact, jumps off (**Figure 9-24**). As soon as contact is made with the ground, the patient jumps up or out, using double-arm action. Two to four sets of 5 to 10 repetitions are performed.

Stadium Hop

The patient places the hands on the head and uses both legs to jump stadium steps, one at a time. The movement should be continuous without stopping. The progression can be to jump two steps at a time or increase the number of steps or the speed of the jumps.

Pyramid Box Jump

Three to five boxes are placed from shortest to tallest in series. The patient jumps onto the first one, off and onto the floor, and immediately jumps onto the next box, off and onto the ground, and continues through to the final box.

Depth Jump

The patient stands on a 12-in high box and steps off the box, immediately going into a rapid vertical jump. The arms can be used to assist in the jump, and the patient attempts to jump as high as possible. Taller boxes (up to 18 in) can be substituted as the patient improves.

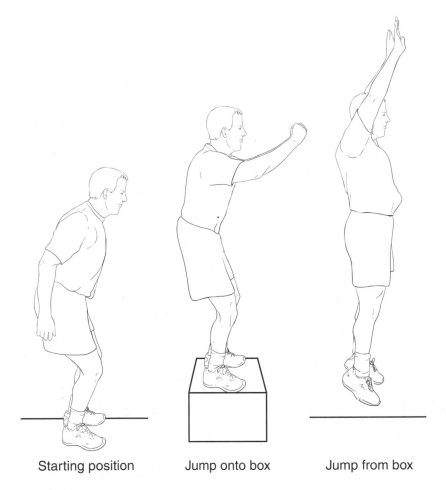

Starting position   Jump onto box   Jump from box

Figure 9-24 Box jump.

9

Functional Agility Exercises

Functional activities are a prelude to sport-specific activities. Some of these functional activities may actually be sport-specific activities, depending on the sport and the functional activity. For example, running and cutting are functional activities but also sport-specific activities for a basketball player or a football running back. Other lower extremity functional activities include activities such as figure-of-eight runs, timed sprints, side shuffles, backward running, run and jump, and other running activities with changes in direction and speed.

Agilities combine speed, power, and skill. The patient should begin with simple, well-controlled tasks such as forward and backward running or side shuffling at low intensities. As the patient improves, the agilities can progress to more com-plex patterns such as figures-of-8, bag drills, or obstacle courses. As with all other rehabilitation programs, agilities should be designed to meet the functional requirements of the individual athlete's sport.

The following are examples of functional agility exercises:

a. The patient jumps over an object on the floor, such as a step stool or box. This exercise can be done in a forward jump or lateral left-to-right jump sequence. The speed, height, and sequence of the jumps can be varied to increase the difficulty.

b. A variety of agility activities can be used to increase performance demands. Examples include running circle-of-eights and running zigzags with sudden changes in running direction (forward, left, right, backward) in response to unpredicted verbal demands, hopping in different directions (eg, forward-left, forward-right, left-right).

Endurance

Muscular endurance is the capacity of a muscle group to perform repeated contractions against a load or sustain a contraction for an extended period. The mechanics of performing an activity often change as the body becomes fatigued. Endurance activities can be performed on treadmills, cycles, skier machines, stair steppers, elliptical runners, and other machines.

Running Progression

Running progressions should begin with low intensities and short distances on smooth, level surfaces such as a treadmill. The degree of activity and the length of rest periods should be determined by the patient's initial fitness level and gradually progress toward the competitive requirements of the individual's sport, whether it be an aerobic activity such as marathon running or an anaerobic activity such as gymnastics. Functional running progressions include everything from walking to sport-specific drills. These are often timed and are limited only by the imagination.

The T-test is a timed functional exercise that uses four cones set in a T formation. Cone A, at the base of the T, is the start and finish. Cone B is 10 yards away at the top of the T, cone C is 5 yards to the right of cone B, and cone D is 5 yards to the left. The patient runs from cone A to touch the base of cone B, then shuffles to touch cone C, shuffles back past cone B to touch cone D, returns to cone B, and races for cone A.

Other functional exercises include jogging, running backward, zigzag running, running circles or figures-of-8, and side shuffles.

Sport-Specific Activities

These activities will depend on the athlete's sport and position within the sport. For example, a basketball forward's activities may include forward sprints the distance of a court length, sprints to a layup or a sudden stop and jump shot, or vertical jumping. A volleyball player's activities would more likely include lateral movements to the left and right with jumps for blocking or hitting, dives, squats for setting, and diagonal sprints for the ball. If the clinician is unfamiliar with the specific sport activities and demands of the athlete's sport and position, he or she should consult with a coach to obtain assistance or instruction in useful activities for this stage of the rehabilitation program. The goal in the final stages of sport-specific activities should be normal performance without signs of favoring or hesitating in using the involved extremity. Observers should not be able to identify which extremity is injured based on the athlete's performance of these tasks.

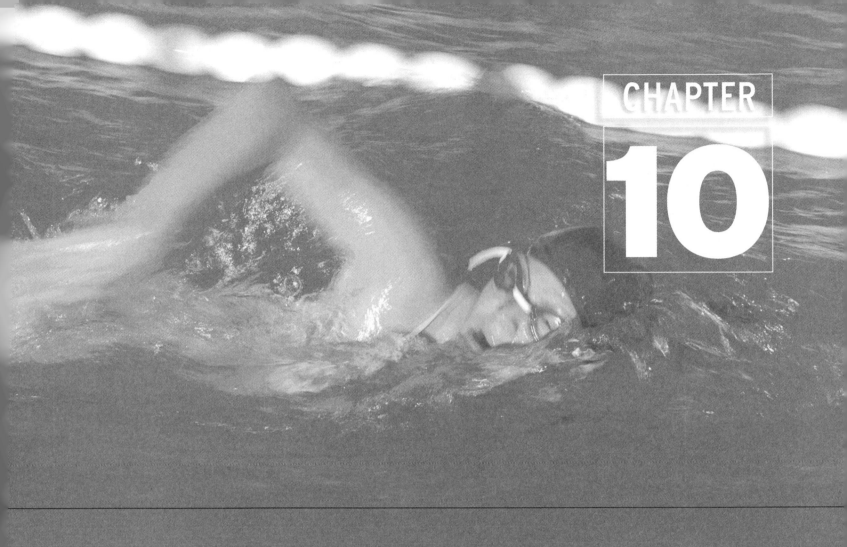

Shoulder Injuries

Ned Bergert, PTA, ATC
Bick Harmon, PT, ATC
Lewis Yocum, MD

Sternoclavicular Joint Sprains

CLINICAL PRESENTATION

History

A direct blow or indirect force to the shoulder girdle

Pain arising from the medial scapular border

The patient complains of increased pain when lying supine.

Observation

In acute injuries, the patient supports the injured arm across the chest.

Dislocations cause the involved shoulder girdle to appear shortened and thrust forward.[1]

Anterior dislocations result in obvious SC joint deformity (see Figure 10-1).

Posterior SC dislocations may produce venous congestion in the neck.

Functional Status

Pain increases with shoulder girdle motion, especially overhead.

Swallowing may be difficult if the SC joint is displaced posteriorly.

Posterior dislocations may obstruct the airway.

Physical Evaluation Findings

SC joint pain increases when the shoulders are pressed together with a lateral force.[1]

During palpation, the medial clavicle may be anterior or posterior to the manubrium.

Posterior dislocations are marked by a palpable manubrium.

Hypomobility or frank instability is noted on glide testing of the medial clavicle.

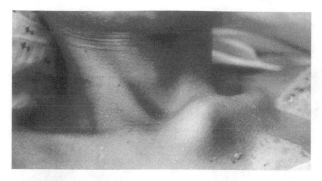

Figure 10-1 Traumatic anterior dislocation of the left sternoclavicular joint. (Reproduced with permission from Wirth MA, Rockwood CA Jr: Acute and chronic traumatic injuries of the sternoclavicular joint. *J Am Acad Orthop Surg* 1996;4:268-278.)

The sternoclavicular (SC) joint is involved in most upper extremity motions. Because of its strong, efficiently designed ligamentous structures, this small joint is one of the least frequently injured joints. Traumatic SC joint dislocation usually occurs only after tremendous direct or indirect forces have been applied to the joint. A direct force to the medial clavicle results in posterior clavicular displacement; an indirect force results in anterior and/or superior clavicular displacement (**Figure 10-1**).

The support structures and disk may be partially disrupted. In a severe SC joint sprain, the capsular and intra-articular ligaments are ruptured. Occasionally, the costoclavicular ligament is intact but stretched, allowing a dislocation to occur. The injury mechanism is usually a force applied indirectly to the SC joint from the lateral or posterolateral shoulder.

Anterior dislocations are the most common SC displacements. The medial end of the clavicle displaces anteriorly or anterosuperiorly relative to the sternal margin. A posterior SC dislocation results when the medial end of the clavicle displaces posteriorly or posterosuperiorly. Although posterior dislocations are uncommon, they can be life threatening because of the potential compromise to the underlying trachea and neurovascular structures.

Differential Diagnosis

Fracture of the medial clavicle, sternum, or hyoid

Imaging Techniques

Plain radiographs of the SC joint are difficult to interpret. Although special views of the chest have been used, interpretation is difficult because of the distortion of one clavicle over the other. Occasionally, routine anteroposterior (AP) or posteroanterior (PA) radiographs of the chest or SC joint suggest clavicular injury because the bone appears to be displaced compared with the normal side. Several views can be used to show the SC joint on plain radiographs (**Figure 10-2**).

Tomograms can be helpful in distinguishing between an SC dislocation and a medial clavicular fracture. They are also helpful in assessing questionable anterior and posterior SC joint dislocation and evaluating the joint for degenerative changes.

A computed tomography (CT) scan is the best imaging technique for all SC joint injuries (see Figure 10-2). It clearly differentiates SC joint injuries from medial clavicular fractures and identifies minor joint subluxations. The orthopaedist will order CT scans of both SC joints and the medial half of both clavicles, so that the injured side can be compared with the normal side.

Definitive Diagnosis

The diagnosis is based on positive radiographic findings (plain films, CT scan) correlated with positive physical findings. The older literature suggests that the diagnosis of SC sprain is best made from clinical examination findings rather than radiographs.

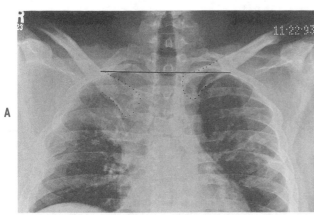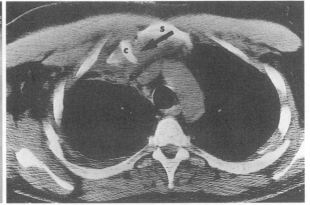

Figure 10-2   Imaging techniques of the sternoclavicular joint. **A.** Serendipity radiographic view. The patient is supine, lying on the film cassette. The x-rays are directed with a 40° cephalic tilt. **B.** CT scan of a right posterior sternoclavicular joint dislocation. Note the degree of posterior displacement of the posterior medial clavicle (arrow). C = medial clavicle; S = sternum. (Reproduced with permission from Wirth MA, Rockwood CA Jr: Acute and chronic traumatic injuries of the sternoclavicular joint. *J Am Acad Orthop Surg* 1996;4:268-278.)

However, CT scans offer more detailed information, often showing small fractures within the joint.

Pathomechanics and Functional Limitations

Shoulder girdle and/or glenohumeral (GH) motions that cause SC joint motion can produce pain and secondary weakness. In overhead throwing athletes, pain and weakness can alter the normal biomechanics and lead to secondary overuse injuries, particularly in the GH joint and elbow.

The original dislocation may go unrecognized, it may be irreducible, or the physician may decide not to reduce certain dislocations. When the initial acute traumatic dislocation does not heal, mild to moderate forces may produce recurrent, possibly painless anterior subluxations or dislocations when the arm is brought through an overhead motion.

■ Immediate Management

Because of potential compromise of the trachea and neurovascular bundle, posterior dislocations are medical emergencies (**Figure 10-3**). The involved arm should be immobilized with a sling and figure-of-8 brace. Anterior dislocations can be stabilized by affixing a compression pad over the joint (**Figure 10-4**). Closed reduction should be performed within 48 hours of the trauma.[1] If a posterior dislocation is suspected, the patient should be transported in a seated position to reduce pressure on the underlying structures.

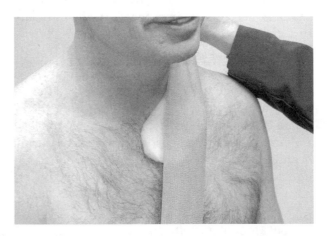

Figure 10-3   CT scan of a posterior sternoclavicular dislocation. The patient was complaining of a "choking sensation" that was increased by lying supine. Note the physeal injury of the medial clavicle and the compression of the trachea (arrow). C = medial clavicle; E = epiphyseal fragment; S = sternum. (Reproduced with permission from Rockwood CA Jr, Green DP, Bucholz RW, et al (eds): *Rockwood and Green's Fractures in Adults*, ed 4. Philadelphia, PA, Lippincott-Raven, 1996, vol 2, p 1448.)

Figure 10-4   Stabilization of anterior sternoclavicular joint dislocations. A pad taped or wrapped over the anterior sternoclavicular joint can maintain joint alignment to allow for healing or to stabilize the joint prior to surgery.

Medications

Nonsteroidal anti-inflammatory drugs (NSAIDs) and narcotic analgesics can be used for pain control.

Postinjury Management

Fractures and dislocations require protective immobilization through either bracing or surgical fixation. Most dislocations can be reduced nonsurgically.

Anterior Dislocations

The patient lies supine on a table with a 3- to 4-in-thick pad between the shoulders. Various forms of local or general anesthetics or muscle relaxants are administered. The physician then manually relocates the medial clavicle; however, in many cases, the SC joint spontaneously redislocates.

Posterior Dislocations

Three closed reduction techniques are commonly used to manage posterior SC dislocations. A general anesthetic or muscle relaxant is usually administered before performing the procedure.

Abduction-Traction Method The patient lies supine with a sandbag between the shoulders and the involved arm near the table edge. The arm is abducted, and traction is applied while the arm is gently extended. In some instances, the medial clavicle must be manually moved from behind the posterior clavicle.

Adduction-Traction Method The patient lies supine with a sandbag between the shoulders. A traction force is applied to the arm as it is moved into adduction and posterior force is applied to both shoulders.

Shoulder Retraction Method The patient is either supine or seated. Both shoulders are then forcefully retracted to realign the SC joint. This technique carries an increased risk of circulatory vessel compromise, nerve tissue impingement, and difficulty swallowing.

Postreduction or Postinjury

Both shoulders are stabilized using a figure-of-8 brace or commercial shoulder harness, and the involved arm is supported with a sling (**Figure 10-5**). A pad can be taped or wrapped over the involved SC joint to prevent anterior displacement during healing. Pain control, rest, and sling immobilization are recommended during the early postoperative or postinjury period.

Surgical Intervention

Surgical reduction is generally indicated only for posterior dislocations, rarely for anterior dislocations. Although closed reduction is often

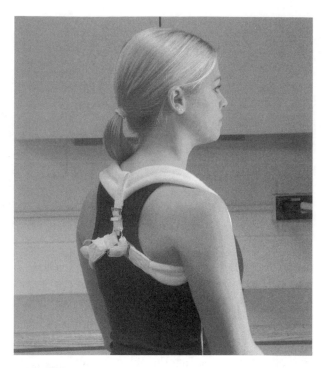

Figure 10-5 Figure-of-8 brace. This brace retracts the scapulae and places a traction force on the clavicles.

unsuccessful, it should be attempted before surgical reduction.[1] If closed reduction fails, open reduction should be performed. Reduction is accomplished with a combination of traction, countertraction, and careful manipulation. If the joint is then stable, it is immobilized for healing. Surgical repair is followed by use of a figure-of-8 brace for 4 to 6 weeks. A sling may also be recommended for the first week.

Injury-Specific Treatment and Rehabilitation Concerns

> **Specific Concerns**
>
> Stabilize the SC joint.
> Reestablish range of motion (ROM) and strength.

Most SC sprains require early symptomatic treatments that focus on pain and edema control. The joint is supported with taping or bracing while ROM is reestablished, and strength is then progressively addressed. Therapeutic modalities such as ice, contrast therapy, and 3-MHz pulsed ultrasound control pain and inflammation.

Once the joint is clinically healed, normal arthrokinematics must be reestablished using joint

CT Clinical Technique 10-1

Kinesio Taping

Kinesio Taping is a taping system that has been developed to treat a range of musculoskeletal, vascular, and neurologic conditions. Using an inelastic and very adherent tape similar to that used for patellofemoral taping, a skilled clinician can correct posture, realign tissues, and prevent improper posture and/or biomechanics. Proponents of this technique also claim that Kinesio Taping can reduce inflammation, minimize the pain inhibition syndrome associated with injury and postoperative inflammation, and assist in the strength recovery phase for both surgical and nonsurgical conditions.

Kinesio Taping can be applied to most areas of the body, including the shoulder, upper and lower extremities, and torso. Certification courses are recommended to develop proficiency in Kinesio Taping.

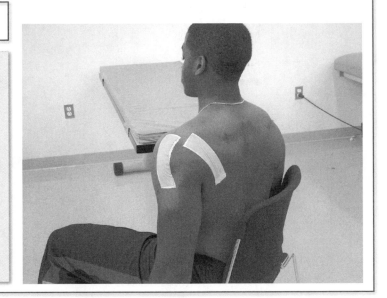

mobilization, therapeutic modalities, and stretching and strengthening exercises. The focus should be on strengthening the muscles attached to the clavicle in a range that does not further stress the joint. The pectoralis muscles are strengthened with the incline press. The sternal fibers of the pectoralis major are strengthened by seated press-ups in limited ROM. The upper trapezius is strengthened by shoulder shrugs. These muscles help control clavicular motion when the scapulohumeral complex moves.

■ Estimated Amount of Time Lost

Stable SC sprains may not result in any time lost if pain does not interfere with sport biomechanics. Dislocations may result in 6 to 8 weeks lost from activity. For posterior SC dislocations, 10 to 12 weeks are required to allow complete ligament healing.

■ Return-to-Play Criteria

Return-to-play criteria include complete physiologic healing; normal ROM, strength, and flexibility; and successful completion of appropriate functional testing demonstrating normal performance of sport-specific tasks.

Functional Bracing

Adhesive taping for SC joint or Kinesio Taping for assistance with pain, swelling reduction, or recapturing of associated muscle strength for function and stability (CT 10-1).

Clavicular Fractures

CLINICAL PRESENTATION

History

A direct force to the clavicle or a force delivered to the clavicle through the humerus
Pain at the fracture site

Observation

To relieve associated sternocleidomastoid spasm, the head and chin are tilted away from the side of the fracture.
The forearm is splinted against the chest, and the opposite arm is used to provide support.
Swelling or gross deformity may be present at the fracture site.
The involved shoulder appears lower and may droop anteriorly and medially.
Possible skin tenting

Functional Status

Upper extremity motion causes pain.

Physical Evaluation Findings

Point tenderness and crepitus at the fracture site
Gentle clavicular palpation produces motion and crepitus.

Clavicular fractures tend to occur in the distal third, particularly distal to the point at which the clavicle begins its posterior curvature. Clavicular fractures are described by their type (**Figure 10-6**), group (fracture location), and resulting displacement (**Table 10-1**).[2]

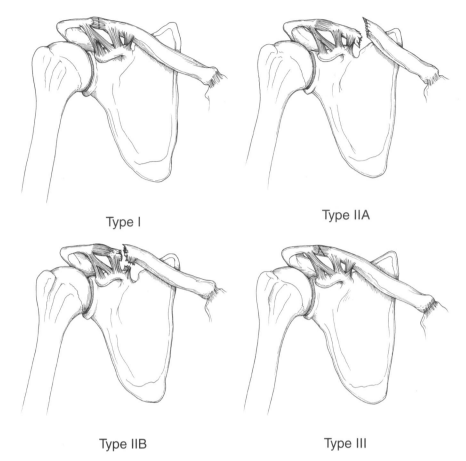

Type I

Type IIA

Type IIB

Type III

Figure 10-6 Types of clavicular fractures. A type I fracture is distal to the coracoclavicular ligaments, with little displacement of the fracture fragments. A type IIA fracture occurs medial to the coracoclavicular ligaments, while a type IIB fracture occurs between the coracoclavicular ligaments. Type III is an intra-articular fracture, frequently without ligament disruption. (Reproduced with permission from Nuber GW, Bowen MK: Acromioclavicular joint injuries and distal clavicle fractures. *J Am Acad Orthop Surg* 1997;5:11-18.)

Injuries related to acute clavicular fractures include (1) associated skeletal injuries, (2) lung and pleural injuries, (3) vascular injuries, and (4) brachial plexus injuries. Associated skeletal injuries include SC and acromioclavicular (AC) joint sprains or fracture-dislocations. Closed reduction of ligamentous injury is more difficult in the presence of a clavicular fracture.

In patients younger than 25 years, medial clavicular fractures may involve the epiphysis and be mistaken for SC dislocations. When the coracoid process is concurrently fractured, open reduction and internal fixation may be required. With displaced distal clavicular fractures, head and neck injuries must be ruled out.

Ipsilateral or contralateral first rib fractures may be associated with clavicular fractures but are easily overlooked. If undetected, these fractures may be directly responsible for traumatizing the lung, brachial plexus, or subclavian vessels. This condition can go unnoticed because it is difficult to identify on standard chest radiographs.

Although nerve or vascular injuries secondary to clavicular fractures are rare, brachial plexus trauma can occur. The neurovascular bundle emerges from the thoracic outlet under the clavicle on top of the first rib.[3] The underlying plexus is somewhat protected by the posterior periosteum, subclavius muscles, and bone, but it may be directly injured by the bone fragments. Accordingly, clavicular fractures should not be manipulated without first obtaining radiographs to determine the position of fragments.

Vascular injuries are rare because the subclavius muscle and the thick, deep cervical fascia act as barriers to direct vessel injury. If the initial fracture displacement has not injured the adjacent vessels, they are unlikely to be injured further because the distal fragment is pulled downward and anteriorly by the limb's weight and the proximal fragment is pulled upward and posteriorly by the trapezius muscle.

Differential Diagnosis

AC sprain, SC sprain, first rib fracture

Table 10-1

Classification of Clavicular Fractures

Group	Location/Structures Involved
I	Fracture of the middle third of the clavicle
II	Fracture of the distal third of the clavicle
	Type I: Minimal displacement (interligamentous fracture)
	Type II: Displaced secondary to a fracture medial to the coracoclavicular ligaments
	Conoid and trapezoid attached
	Conoid torn, trapezoid attached
	Type III: Fractures of the articular surface
	Type IV: Ligaments intact to the periosteum (in children), with displacement of the proximal fragment
	Type V: Comminuted. Ligaments are not attached proximally or distally; ligaments are attached to an inferior, comminuted fragment.
III	Fracture of the proximal third of the clavicle
	Type I: Minimally displaced
	Type II: Displaced (ligaments ruptured)
	Type III: Intra-articular fracture
	Type IV: Epiphyseal separation (in children and young adults)
	Type V: Comminuted

Adapted with permission from Craig EV: Fractures of the clavicle, in Rockwood CA Jr, Matsen FA III (eds): *The Shoulder*. Philadelphia, PA, WB Saunders, 1990, pp 367-412.

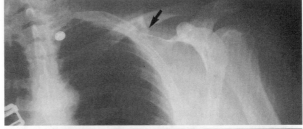
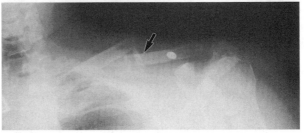

Figure 10-7 Radiographs of a clavicular fracture. **A.** AP view of the left shoulder shows a displaced fracture of the middle third of the clavicle (arrow). **B.** 45° cephalic tilt view demonstrates a comminuted fracture of the midshaft of the clavicle (arrow). (Reproduced with permission from Johnson TR, Steinbach LS (eds): *Essentials of Musculoskeletal Imaging*. Rosemont, IL, American Academy of Orthopaedic Surgeons, 2004, p 181.)

Imaging Techniques

Radiographic views of the clavicle should be obtained from the AP and 45° cephalic tilt view. Two views of the clavicle at right angles to each other—a 45° angle superiorly and a 45° angle inferiorly—have been recommended to assess fracture extent and displacement[4] (**Figure 10-7**). The proximal third of the humerus should also be included in the AP view, and the shoulder girdle and upper lung should be imaged to rule out associated injury.[5] An AP view of the cervical or thoracic spine decreases the chance of overlooking rib fractures.[6] If vessel injury is suspected, an arteriogram should be performed.[7]

Fractures of the proximal third of the clavicle can be difficult to detect in radiographs because of the overlapping of the ribs over the vertebrae and mediastinal shadows. A cephalic tilt view of 40° to 45° often reveals the fracture. In children, medial clavicular fractures are often misdiagnosed as SC dislocations. Tomography or a CT scan can be useful in demonstrating the intra-articular or epiphyseal nature of the injury in this location.

Definitive Diagnosis

The definitive diagnosis is often easily made on the clinical finding of clavicular deformity and displacement. Radiographs are used to confirm the fracture location and type and assist in identifying possible compromise to the underlying neurovascular structures.

Nondisplaced fractures or isolated fractures of the articular surfaces may not cause deformity and may be overlooked. If the diagnosis is in doubt, special radiographs or another radiographic series of the clavicle in 7 to 10 days may be helpful.

Pathomechanics and Functional Limitations

The patient has pain with shoulder and neck motion. Limitations in chest wall expansion are caused by pain from movement of the clavicular fragments. Therefore, exercise may need to be restricted during the early postinjury and postoperative periods because the muscles that attach to the clavicle are also involved in respiration. Upper extremity conditioning may also require restriction to facilitate clinical healing.

■ Immediate Management

Ice is applied to the joint, and a sling is applied for immobilization and protection. The patient should be fitted with a figure-of-8 brace if available to provide traction on the clavicle (see Figure 10-5). If associated lung trauma is suspected, the patient

Cephalic Superior; toward the head.

10

must be checked for symmetric breath sounds. Distal neurovascular function of the involved arm must be assessed to identify trauma to the underlying neurovascular structures.

Medications

NSAIDs and narcotic analgesics are used for pain control.

Surgical Intervention

Open reduction of clavicle fractures is rarely required, but nonunion or vascular damage necessitates open reduction and stabilization. With a large vessel tear, surgical exploration is mandatory. To gain adequate exposure, as much of the clavicle should be excised as is needed to isolate and repair the injured major vessel. Although in some cases the vessel may be ligated, major vessel ligation in the elderly patient may be dangerous because of inadequate remaining circulation to the extremity.[2]

Postinjury/Postoperative Management

The patient should be fitted with a figure-of-8 brace, which maintains a traction force on the clavicle, and placed in a sling. Rest and medications for pain control are initially prescribed, followed by ROM exercises. Once healing is visualized on radiographs, the clavicle brace can be removed, and advanced ROM and strength and conditioning exercises can begin.

Injury-Specific Treatment and Rehabilitation Concerns

Specific Concerns
Maintain longitudinal traction on the clavicle during healing. Avoid stressing the fracture site until healing has occurred. Restore ROM and strength when the fracture is resolved.

If the GH joint and the subacromial bursae have not been surgically violated and are otherwise not diseased, early shoulder ROM exercises are not necessary. Thus the patient may be kept safely supported in a sling or immobilizer until radiographic signs of union occur without risk of developing a frozen shoulder.

Isometric rotator cuff exercises may begin early in the postoperative period. Isometric trapezius and deltoid strengthening are delayed until their suture junction is healed securely (3 to 4 weeks). ROM after surgery is not permitted past 45° of flexion in the scapular plane until clinical signs of union are present, usually at 4 to 6 weeks.

Frozen shoulder A condition characterized by restricted shoulder movement resulting from acute trauma or a periarticular biceps or rotator cuff tendon injury.

When clinical or radiographic union is present, the patient may begin full ROM, particularly in forward elevation using an overhead pulley; external rotation (with a cane or stick) and hyperextension-internal rotation are then added. Resistive exercises of the deltoid, trapezius, rotator cuff, and scapular muscles are also initiated. When radiographic union is present, full active use of the arm is permitted.

The patient is not allowed to return to strenuous work or athletic activities until shoulder ROM is nearly full, strength has returned to near normal, and bone healing is presumed complete.

Estimated Amount of Time Lost

Time lost depends on the amount of collision required in the sport. Athletes participating in noncontact sports may miss 4 to 6 weeks; those in collision sports may lose 6 to 10 weeks.

Return-to-Play Criteria

Fracture union, full and pain-free ROM, and normal strength must be attained for return to sport.

Functional Bracing

For athletes in contact sports, supportive adhesive taping of the distal AC joint may be considered. Bridge padding may also be placed over the AC joint underneath shoulder pads.

Acromioclavicular Joint Sprain

CLINICAL PRESENTATION

History

Direct or indirect trauma to the shoulder
Pain arising from the AC joint, which may migrate proximally

Observation

During ambulation, the patient bends slightly at the waist, leans to the involved side, and holds the involved arm across the chest.
The involved shoulder may be elevated.
Type III AC sprains result in noticeable distal clavicular elevation.

Functional Status

Humeral and shoulder girdle ROM may be limited by pain.

Physical Evaluation Findings

Palpation of the distal clavicle causes pain.
Passive horizontal adduction causes pain.
GH abduction and flexion produce pain.
Piano-key sign may be present during palpation.
AC traction and/or compression tests may be positive.

The AC joint is a diarthrodial joint incompletely divided by a disk. Unlike the SC joint, the AC joint has a large perforation in its center. The capsule is thicker on its superior, anterior, and posterior surfaces than on its inferior surface. The upward and downward movement allows rotation of about 20° between the acromion and clavicle, occurring during the first 20° and last 40° of arm elevation. The AC ligament controls posterior clavicular translation on the acromion. The coronoid and trapezoid ligaments control AP and superior clavicular translation (**Figure 10-8**).

The injury mechanism is commonly a direct blow to the shoulder point with the arm adducted. This occurs most frequently from a fall on the shoulder or a head-on collision with the shoulder lowered and leading the body, driving the scapula caudally. The SC ligaments interlock to prevent caudal clavicular displacement, and the clavicle may impinge on the rib cage. Continued force on the acromion results in stretching or tearing of the AC ligaments (**Figure 10-9**). With more acromial displacement, the coracoclavicular distance increases, stretching or tearing the coracoclavicular ligaments. Other, less common direct injury mechanisms are a posterior blow to the scapula or a lateral blow to the acromion. On rare occasions, a fall on an outstretched hand or elbow may indirectly cause an AC sprain by driving the humerus into the acromion, injuring the AC ligaments.

Complete AC dislocations are rare in children younger than 16 years of age. Visual inspection or palpation may reveal a high-riding clavicle and an apparent AC dislocation that could actually be a transperiosteal distal clavicular fracture or, more commonly, a periosteal rupture and a distal clavicular fracture with the coracoclavicular ligaments remaining attached to the periosteum.

Differential Diagnosis
Distal clavicular fracture, acromial process fracture

Imaging Techniques
The classification of AC sprains is aided by proper radiographic evaluation. Routine radiographs for suspected AC sprains should include an AP 15° tilt (Zanca), axillary lateral, and comparison views of the uninjured shoulder (**Figure 10-10**). An Alexander or "shoulder-forward view" and AP stress views may also be necessary. The AP stress view is performed with 10 to 15 lb of weight tied to both wrists and is compared with the unweighted

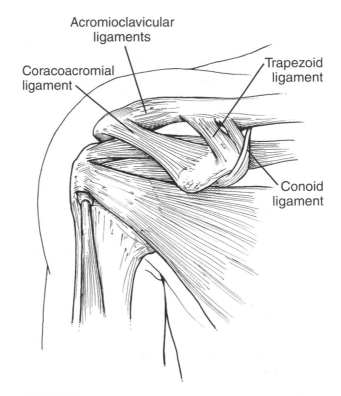

Figure 10-8 The acromioclavicular joint complex is composed of the acromioclavicular ligaments and the coracoclavicular ligaments (conoid and trapezoid). (Reproduced with permission from Shaffer BS: Painful conditions of the acromioclavicular joint. *J Am Acad Orthop Surg* 1999;7:176-188.)

view of both AC joints. With coracoclavicular ligament disruption, the coracoclavicular distance on a weighted view is increased.

Definitive Diagnosis
Positive radiographs and physical examination

Pathomechanics and Functional Limitations
Significant AC ligament disruption causes biomechanical changes to the shoulder girdle. Pain and weakness are described with overhead and cross-chest shoulder motion. Pain and dysfunction occur with lifting activities. The coronoid ligament facilitates much of the superior clavicular rotation as the arm is elevated. AC motion controls cross-chest motion by resisting distraction.

◼ Immediate Management
Ice and sling immobilization are applied for the first 24 to 48 hours in type I injuries; longer treatment is required for more severe injuries. A pad and/or shoulder spica wrap can help stabilize the AC joint (**Figure 10-11**).

◼ Medications
NSAIDs and narcotic analgesics are used for pain control.

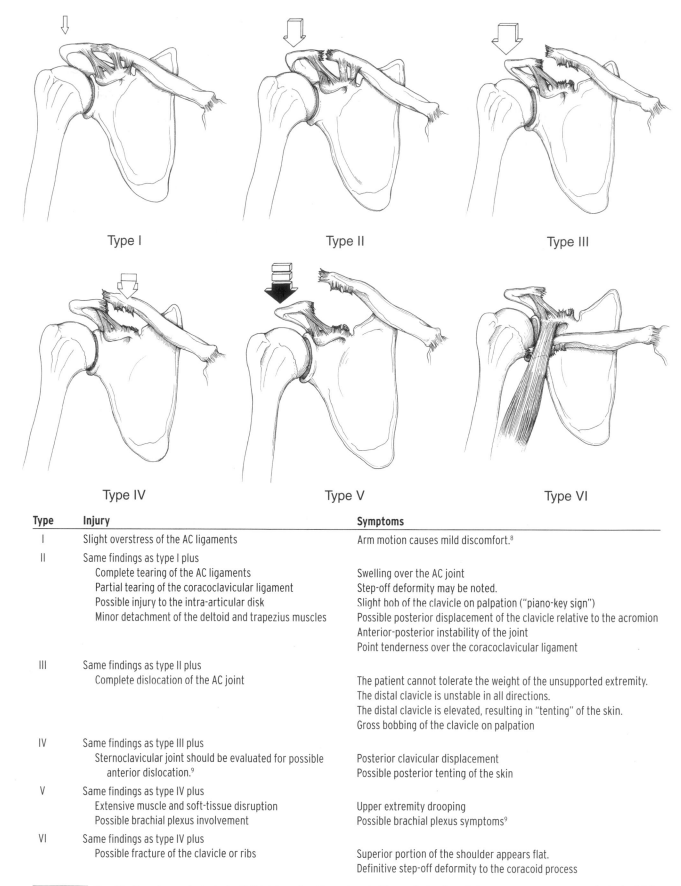

Type	Injury	Symptoms
I	Slight overstress of the AC ligaments	Arm motion causes mild discomfort.[8]
II	Same findings as type I plus	
	Complete tearing of the AC ligaments	Swelling over the AC joint
	Partial tearing of the coracoclavicular ligament	Step-off deformity may be noted.
	Possible injury to the intra-articular disk	Slight bob of the clavicle on palpation ("piano-key sign")
	Minor detachment of the deltoid and trapezius muscles	Possible posterior displacement of the clavicle relative to the acromion
		Anterior-posterior instability of the joint
		Point tenderness over the coracoclavicular ligament
III	Same findings as type II plus	
	Complete dislocation of the AC joint	The patient cannot tolerate the weight of the unsupported extremity.
		The distal clavicle is unstable in all directions.
		The distal clavicle is elevated, resulting in "tenting" of the skin.
		Gross bobbing of the clavicle on palpation
IV	Same findings as type III plus	
	Sternoclavicular joint should be evaluated for possible anterior dislocation.[9]	Posterior clavicular displacement
		Possible posterior tenting of the skin
V	Same findings as type IV plus	
	Extensive muscle and soft-tissue disruption	Upper extremity drooping
	Possible brachial plexus involvement	Possible brachial plexus symptoms[9]
VI	Same findings as type IV plus	
	Possible fracture of the clavicle or ribs	Superior portion of the shoulder appears flat.
		Definitive step-off deformity to the coracoid process

Figure 10-9   Classification of acromioclavicular (AC) joint sprains. (Reproduced with permission from Nuber GW, Bowen MK: Acromioclavicular joint injuries and distal clavicle fractures. *J Am Acad Orthop Surg* 1997;5:11-18.)

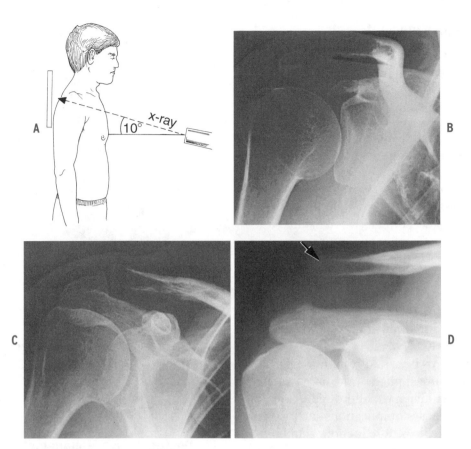

Figure 10-10   Imaging of the acromioclavicular joint. **A.** The Zanca view is obtained by angling the x-ray beam 10° to 15° in the cephalic direction. **B.** AP view of the shoulder demonstrates the glenohumeral anatomy but does not adequately image the acromioclavicular joint. **C.** The Zanca view provides a better image of the acromioclavicular joint but at the expense of the glenohumeral image. **D.** AP radiograph demonstrating a type III acromioclavicular sprain. Black arrow indicates the location of the clavicle above the acromion. (A, B, and C reproduced with permission from Shaffer BS: Painful conditions of the acromioclavicular joint. *J Am Acad Orthop Surg* 1999;7:176-188. D reproduced with permission from Johnson TR, Steinbach LS (eds): *Essentials of Musculoskeletal Imaging.* Rosemont, IL, American Academy of Orthopaedic Surgeons, 2004, p 179.)

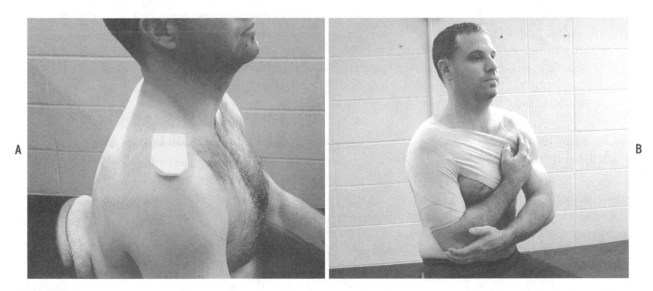

Figure 10-11   Stabilization of acromioclavicular joint sprains. A spica wrap is used to hold a compressive pad over the acromioclavicular joint to maintain alignment. A sling is then applied to reduce traction forces on the joint caused by the weight of the arm.

Postinjury Management

Treatment of a pure posterior clavicular dislocation varies, depending on whether or not the clavicle can be manipulated out of its embedding in the trapezius muscle. Management of AC joint injuries depends on their severity. Type I and II sprains can frequently be successfully managed by applying ice initially and using a sling until discomfort dissipates, usually within 2 to 4 weeks, before a rehabilitation program is begun. Most athletes should have full, painless ROM and no tenderness on direct AC joint palpation or pain when manual traction is applied to the joint before returning to play.

Type III sprains can be managed surgically or nonsurgically. Some athletes can and do function well with complete AC joint dislocations. Nonsurgical treatment can be a sling for comfort or a Kenny-Howard-type AC immobilizer to try to reduce the dislocation (**Figure 10-12**).

The patient must be carefully monitored to ensure that the pressure applied by the harness to the distal clavicle is sufficient to afford reduction but not so great as to cause complications such as poor patient compliance, loss of reduction, skin breakdown, and compression neuropathy. These potential problems necessitate daily examination and readjustment of the device as needed. Patients with type II AC sprains treated by immobilization have better radiographic reduction and fewer residual symptoms, which may justify an attempt at reduction and AC joint immobilization for a type II sprain.

Ice and other modalities are used to decrease initial soreness in an acute AC joint injury. Pain initially limits the patient's ability to perform ROM and strengthening exercises, and full, active ROM must be achieved gently and gradually. Isometric exercises can begin when ROM is still limited, but isotonic strengthening exercises should not be initiated until full ROM is achieved.

Surgical Intervention

Because of the severe posterior distal clavicular displacement in the type IV sprain and the gross displacement in the type V injury, surgical repair is indicated for these situations. Additionally, type V sprains usually require surgical repair due to the severity of clavicular deformity.[9] Surgery is directed at reconstructing the coracoclavicular ligaments and excising the distal clavicle (**ST** **10-1** and **10-2**). Most type VI injuries are surgically repaired because initial attempts at closed reduction fail. The clavicle may be stabilized by suturing the deltoid and trapezius muscle avulsion and repairing the AC joint capsule.

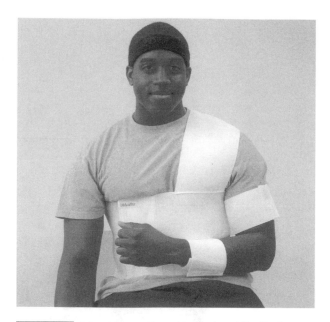

Figure 10-12   A Kenny-Howard-type shoulder immobilization brace used for acromioclavicular joint sprains. This brace decreases the pressure on the joint by supporting the forearm and humerus and providing downward pressure on the distal clavicle to keep the joint structures congruent.

Postoperative Management

Postoperatively, the AC joint may be managed in two ways. Some physicians fit the patient with a sling but allow early motion and activities of daily living within the patient's tolerance. Other physicians do not use a sling and set a goal of obtaining full abduction within 7 to 10 days postsurgery.

For patients undergoing distal clavicular resection, coracoclavicular ligament stability must be assessed. If the joint is stable, the patient can be advanced quickly as pain allows. If the ligaments are unstable and must be repaired, the appropriate protocol is implemented.

Injury-Specific Treatment and Rehabilitation Concerns

> **Specific Concerns**
>
> Maintain approximation of the distal clavicle and acromion.
> Restore GH ROM.
> Ensure proper biomechanics of the shoulder girdle.

Rehabilitation of type I AC sprains includes early active-assisted ROM, then progressive addition of isometric exercises for the clavicular muscles. Progressive resistive exercises for the scapular muscles and GH mechanics are added when pain decreases.

S|T Surgical Technique 10-1

Repair of Coracoclavicular Ligaments (Bosworth Screw)

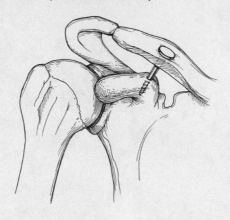

Indications

Extreme clavicular prominence in patients who perform prolonged heavy lifting or repeatedly use the arm with the shoulder abducted or flexed to 90° (eg, throwers)

Overview

1. An incision is made over the AC joint and distal clavicle.
2. The deltoid and trapezius attachments are resected from the area.
3. Using fluoroscopy, a percutaneous guide pin is introduced through the clavicle and into the coracoid process.
4. A cannulated screw is then introduced over the guide pin percutaneously.
5. Position is confirmed with fluoroscopy.

Functional Limitations

The physician may encourage early ROM, delay motion for a short time, or limit activity for 6 to 8 weeks.

Implications for Rehabilitation

Activities of daily living are usually possible 1 week after surgery. Heavy activities are typically restricted for 8 weeks.

Comments

Recommendations regarding screw removal are mixed. Some physicians recommend not removing the screw at all. Others remove the screw under local anesthesia after 6 to 8 weeks.

Other fixation techniques with wires, pins, and Dacron tape have been described but are associated with more complications, such as pin migration and clavicular erosion secondary to pressure necrosis.

Figure reproduced with permission from Nuber GW, Bowen MK: Acromioclavicular joint injuries and distal clavicle fractures. *J Am Acad Orthop Surg* 1997;5:11-18.

Acute type II AC sprains are treated symptomatically with a sling and cryotherapy for 10 to 14 days or until pain subsides. Electric stimulation and exercise may be used to improve or maintain strength in the associated muscles. Active and passive stretching and strengthening exercises are also helpful. The athlete may return to sport when ROM is pain free and strength has returned to normal. Ordinarily this takes 2 weeks; however, individual differences, degree of injury, and therapeutic physiologic response may dictate up to 4 weeks. Athletes also differ in their ability to tolerate pain and carry the involved extremity with the appropriate shoulder posture. Time must be allowed for the soft tissues to heal before beginning exercises that stress the injury; this can take up to 8 to 12 weeks.

More aggressive forms of treatment can be instituted to emphasize reduction of joint deformity and support the joint during healing, including taping and strapping techniques, compressive bandages, harnesses, plaster casts, and traction. Maintaining joint reduction with 3 to 6 weeks of continuous, uninterrupted pressure downward on the distal clavicle and upward on the acromion (indirectly from the elbow through the humerus) is essential for any of these methods to be effective. A modified Kenny-Howard shoulder harness is commonly used (see Figure 10-12).

S|T Surgical Technique 10-2

Excision of the Distal Clavicle

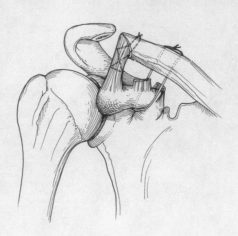

Indications

Chronic pain after the failure of conservative management for an existing AC dislocation with associated degenerative changes

Overview

1. An incision is made over the AC joint and distal clavicle.
2. The distal clavicle is identified.
3. The deltoid and trapezius muscles are resected from the distal clavicle with a cuff of tendinous attachment for later repair.
4. The distal 2 cm of the clavicle are excised back to the costoclavicular ligaments.
5. If the costoclavicular joint is stable, the cuffs of the deltoid muscle and trapezius muscle are repaired and the skin is closed.
6. If the costoclavicular joint is unstable, various techniques are available to stabilize the joint:
   - Weaver-Dunn transferred the ligaments into the intramedullary canal of the remaining clavicle.
   - Others have used the coracoacromial ligaments with an attached small bone block from the acromion affixed to the clavicle with a screw.

Functional Limitations

Decreased strength and performance

Implications for Rehabilitation

If the costoclavicular ligament was intact, passive motion is encouraged immediately. Active ROM and progressive resistance exercises are begun after 2 to 3 weeks. In patients with costoclavicular joint fixation, a longer period of healing is required before beginning rehabilitation.

Figure reproduced with permission from Nuber GW, Bowen MK: Acromioclavicular joint injuries and distal clavicle fractures. *J Am Acad Orthop Surg* 1997;5:11-18.

▨ Estimated Amount of Time Lost

Time lost depends on injury severity and the nature of the sport. Athletes in contact sports may miss more time than those in noncontact sports. Athletes with type I injuries may miss 1 to 2 weeks, whereas those with type III injuries may lose 6 to 8 weeks. Type IV to VI sprains result in an extended amount of time lost, especially with surgery or associated trauma.

▨ Return-to-Play Criteria

Before returning to activity with a mild injury, the athlete should have full and painless ROM, no tenderness on direct AC joint palpation, and no pain when manual traction is applied to the joint. Shoulder strength should be graded as normal on muscle testing. Athletes should be able to perform sport-specific requirements normally on functional testing.

Functional Bracing

An Orthoplast pad or commercially available padding system can speed the return to activity, especially in contact sports (**CT** 10-2).

Scapular Dyskinesis

The scapula is an attachment site for the stabilizing muscles and an origin for the rotator cuff muscles. It is thicker at its superior and inferior angles and lateral border, where the more powerful muscles are attached. The scapula is also thick

CT Clinical Technique 10-2

Orthoplast Padding of the AC Joint

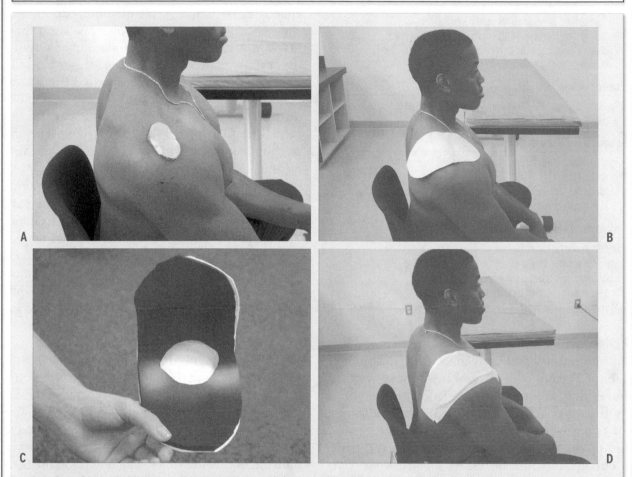

1. A piece of Orthoplast that spans the spine of the scapula to an equal distance down the anterior chest is cut.
2. A form approximately 0.5-in thick is created and affixed to the AC joint. This creates dead air space to further protect the joint (**A**).
3. The Orthoplast is heated and cut to shape, rounding the corners and indenting on the lateral side (to allow for GH motion).
4. While the Orthoplast is still flexible (reheating may be necessary), it is molded to the contour of the torso and the form overlying the AC joint. The material is trimmed as necessary (**B**).
5. Self-adhesive padding is applied to the anterior and posterior portions of the Orthoplast. The indentation made by the form should not be covered. A bridge is created, providing protection to the AC joint (**C**).
6. The pad is affixed to the shoulder using elastic stretch tape and/or a shoulder spica (**D**).

at its processes—the coracoid, scapular spine, acromion, and glenoid. Because they are protected by overlying soft tissue, the processes are fractured by indirect trauma. The scapula also serves as a pulley and lever system for the muscles acting on the humerus.

The scapula performs five specific functions:[10] (1) stabilizes the GH articulation, (2) retracts and protracts along the thoracic wall, (3) elevates the acromion, (4) serves as a base for muscle attachments, and (5) functions as a link in the proximal to distal sequence of energy delivery. A dysfunction in one role or a combination of dysfunctions in several scapular roles puts the throwing athlete at risk.

The shoulder girdle is formed by several articulations that create a complex biomechanical system, increasing overall humeral mobility and improving muscular function. A number of **force couples** are required to move the scapula through its three axes of motion. Upward rotation occurs in the active scapular plane. Posterior tilting occurs in the medial to lateral axes. External scapular rotation occurs around a vertical axis. This arrangement requires less excursion of the muscles that cross the joints, allowing them to maximize their length-tension curves.

Force couple Agonist-antagonist muscle pairs that act in concert to provide a joint compressive force with joint rotation; considered vital to glenohumeral joint stability.

History

Insidious onset
Reports of increased or heavy throwing
Pain over the coracoid process, superior medial aspect of the scapula, AC joint, or subacromial joint
Posterior cervical pain on the dominant side
Radicular pain or symptoms resembling thoracic outlet syndrome may also be reported.

Observation

Scapula is lower, protracted, and abducted relative to the nondominant arm.

Functional Status

Poor GH function with an associated loss of power and endurance
Subsequent biomechanical changes result in a worsening of symptoms and create further dysfunction.

Physical Evaluation Findings

Coracoid process may be tender to palpation.
Tests for rotator cuff impingement may be positive.
Relocation test may be positive.
Scapular winging may be noted.

Normal scapular kinematics are required for optimum upper extremity motion. To maintain a stable GH joint, the glenoid fossa must be continually repositioned to correlate with the moving humerus. A malpositioned scapula increases stress on the anterior capsule. Scapular retraction places the upper extremity in the "full tank of energy" position necessary for throwing (**Figure 10-13**). Scapular protraction in the deceleration phase of throwing is necessary to follow the moving humerus while providing a stable platform. Acromial elevation increases the subacromial space to prevent rotator cuff impingement.

An asymmetric, malpositioned scapula is represented by the acronym SICK:[11] *S*capula, *I*nfera, *C*oracoid, dys*K*inesis. The SICK scapula is a muscular overuse fatigue syndrome that can present clinically with three major components. The scapula drops or is lower than the nondominant scapula; the scapula is protracted or lies further laterally from the spine when compared with the nondominant scapula; and the scapula has increased abduction or a greater angle from the spine to the medial scapular border when compared with the nondominant scapula. Any combination of these components can occur.

Subacromial pain often presents as the inferior position of the SICK scapula, reducing the subacromial space by essentially lowering the acromion. This space reduction hinders rotator cuff function in all phases of the overhand throw. The coinciding lack of posterior scapular tilting with elevation increases the impingement symptoms.[12,13] A scapular relocation test relieves these symptoms and increases the athlete's ability to forward flex, a motion that is often restricted and painful.

The AC joint becomes symptomatic due to altered kinematics of the malpositioned scapula. Because the clavicle is more rigidly secured at the AC joint, scapular protraction and abduction are imposed at the distal clavicular articulation. Thoracic outlet symptoms are present in a small number of individuals due to the "closing down" on the neurovascular structures by the unsupported scapula and clavicle. The challenge is to recognize the subtle changes in scapular position and how those sub-

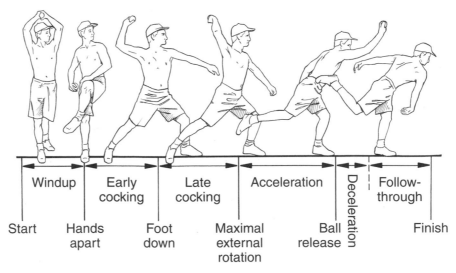

Windup | Early cocking | Late cocking | Acceleration | Deceleration | Follow-through

Start | Hands apart | Foot down | Maximal external rotation | Ball release | Finish

Figure 10-13   Phases of throwing. (Adapted with permission from DiGiovine NM, Jobe FW, Pink M, Perry J: An electromyographic analysis of the upper extremity in pitching. *J Shoulder Elbow Surg* 1992;1:15-25.)

tle changes put the GH joint at risk. Repositioning the scapula is paramount in rehabilitating the overhand throwing athlete.

Differential Diagnosis

Cervical radiculopathy, suprascapular nerve syndrome, thoracic outlet syndrome, brachial plexus neuropathy

Medical Diagnostic Tests

Electromyography and nerve conduction studies may be conducted to rule out palsy of the long thoracic, suprascapular, or other nerves. These tests can also help determine nerve damage location and severity.

Imaging Techniques

The orientation of the scapula and humerus relative to each other and to the thorax is key in obtaining the optimum radiographic studies to best visualize the relationship. Thus the true AP radiograph of the GH joint is taken 30° oblique to the sagittal plane, although a 45° view has also been recommended. The scapular view is taken at a 30° angle to the frontal plane; thus the AP radiograph perpendicular to this view is taken at an angle of about 60° to the thorax.

Definitive Diagnosis

Functional active testing involves visually identifying the scapular malposition as the patient flexes the elbows to 90°, abducts the humerus to 90°, and then externally rotates the shoulder while the clinician views the scapula from behind. The proper (or improper) scapular position is noted.

Pathomechanics and Functional Limitations

Because of the components of a malpositioned scapula (inferiorly located, protracted, and abducted), increased tension is placed on the coracoid by the shortened pectoralis minor tendon and conjoined tendon. With repetitive overhand motions, these shortened tendons encourage a tendinopathy, resulting in a painful medial coracoid. Pain at the superomedial scapula is present at the insertion of the levator scapulae, upper rhomboids, and upper trapezius. These scapular control muscles originate from the spine and are required to function in an overtensioned pattern, referring pain into the muscle belly. The key indicator in this sequence is posterior, dominant-side neck pain. Scapular dyskinesis is the primary cause, and the treatment protocol should be designed to rectify the scapular malposition to resolve the posterior neck symptoms. Any attempt to stretch the injured musculature further exacerbates the condition.

▧ Medications

Analgesics, NSAIDs, and muscle relaxants are helpful in resolving immediate symptoms and facilitating movement into recovery phases.

▧ Surgical Intervention

Surgery is not indicated for scapular dyskinesis. However, associated neurovascular symptoms or conditions relating to the AC joint, GH joint, or rotator cuff may require surgical correction. If the dyskinesis is the result of a neurologic condition, nerve repair or transfer may be performed. If the nerve cannot be repaired, muscle transfers can help improve scapular function.

▧ Injury-Specific Treatment and Rehabilitation Concerns

> **Specific Concerns**
> _____
> Decrease muscle spasm.
> Correct the scapular malposition.
> Avoid stretching the affected musculature.
> Strengthen the spinal and core muscles.

Early rehabilitation incorporates physical agents and medications to reduce pain and inflammation. Soft-tissue mobilization and strengthening of the associated muscles helps to correct the malposition. The initial rehabilitation program should focus on the base of the kinetic chain and correcting lumbar strength and/or flexibility deficits before addressing the scapular component and the upper extremity.[14] See chapters 14 and 17 for lumbar spine rehabilitation exercises.

GH ROM must focus on isolated posterior capsule stretching, including joint mobilization and sleeper stretches (see chapter 13). Stretching the entire upper arm also stretches the scapulothoracic articulation, further exacerbating the patient's symptoms.[14]

Early scapular stability exercises should focus on isometric scapular retraction and scapular elevation. A figure-of-8 brace or scapular taping can assist in scapular control by retracting and elevating the scapula.[14] Once the patient can successfully complete the isometric component, closed chain exercises can be initiated with the arm in 90° of humeral elevation. Muscular cocontractions should be emphasized, with the hand stabilized against a wall, a ball against the wall, or "push-ups with a plus." If the patient has had surgery or experiences pain at 90° of elevation, the amount of elevation can be reduced until pain diminishes.

Open chain and plyometric exercises can be introduced once the patient can complete the closed chain exercises.

Estimated Amount of Time Lost

Frequently, patients are fully functional with scapular dyskinesis, and it is not until further injury occurs that the condition is recognized. The problem oftentimes is self-limiting but can affect shoulder mechanics.

Return-to-Play Criteria

Normal, pain-free ROM and adequate strength with normal performance of sport-specific activities are necessary. Kinesio Taping may be useful in correcting scapular biomechanics early in the rehabilitation process.

Rotator Cuff Pathologies

The rotator cuff controls humeral head movement and is assisted by the deltoid and long head of the biceps during various activities. High-force demands placed on the shoulder may result in muscle fatigue, eccentric overload, inflammation, muscle inhibition, and eventual tissue failure. Once the rotator cuff muscles have been injured, the dynamic stabilizing element is compromised; additional injuries, such as capsular lesions, labral tears, and osseous changes, may arise secondary to excessive humeral head displacement.[14]

Various symptoms suggest cuff injury, including shoulder stiffness, weakness, instability, and crepitus. Stiffness limits passive ROM and causes pain at the motion end point. Stiffness is commonly found with partial-thickness cuff lesions but also can occur with full-thickness cuff lesions (**Table 10-2**). Weakness or pain upon muscle contraction can limit shoulder function. Tendon fibers may become weakened by degeneration and fail without any symptoms or may produce only transient symptoms interpreted as bursitis or tendinitis. A more significant force is required to tear the cuff in younger individuals.

Rotator cuff tears often result from subacromial impingement, but impingement primarily occurs in nonathletic patients. Although primary impingement-related rotator cuff disease may also exist in the athletic population, other causative factors may be more important, including repetitive overuse, GH ligamentous laxity, soft-tissue contracture (especially of the posterior capsule), and poor scapular mechanics. Because of these

Table 10-2

Quantifying Shoulder Stiffness

Motion	Measurement
Internal and external rotation of the humerus in abduction	Degrees from neutral position
Reach up the back	Posterior segment (thoracic spinous process) reached with the thumb
Cross-body adduction	Centimeters from the ipsilateral antecubital fossa to the contralateral acromion or coracoid
Flexion	Degrees from the neutral position

Adapted from Jobe CM: Gross anatomy of the shoulder, in Rockwood CA Jr, Matsen FA III (eds): *The Shoulder,* ed 2. Philadelphia, PA, WB Saunders, 1998, p 781.)

and other mitigating factors, management of rotator cuff disease in athletes can be difficult.

Among athletic patients, overhead throwing athletes are the most susceptible to rotator cuff injuries, exhibiting a high incidence of partial-thickness and small, complete rotator cuff tears. Furthermore, these athletes are often unwilling to modify their activities. Consequently, the persistently high demands on the rotator cuff may predispose them to recurrent episodes of anterior rotator cuff-related shoulder pain. Successful management of these patients requires a thorough knowledge of the relevant pathoanatomy and an accurate and complete diagnosis.

General Imaging Techniques

Evaluation of shoulder injuries has been simplified by advances in imaging techniques. In the past, diagnosis was based on physical examination, plain radiographs, and possibly arthrography; the introduction of CT and MRI, however, has increased the sensitivity and specificity of radiographic studies.

After the clinical evaluation, plain radiographs should be obtained. These basic films assist in evaluating skeletal structures and exclude fractures and dislocations. These films will be reviewed and used later with more complex imaging modalities to confirm the diagnosis.

A complete shoulder series requires at least four views (**Table 10-3**). If clinically indicated, other radiographs should be obtained. To further evaluate the coracoacromial arch, a scapular outlet view can be helpful in demonstrating deformities of the anteroinferior acromion. For the outlet view, the patient is positioned for a true scapulolateral x-ray, and the tube is angled caudally 5° to 10°.

Radiographic visualization of the acromion in a profile view is helpful. With the patient lying

Table 10-3

Radiographic Series for the Shoulder

View	Description/Use
AP	The arm is in maximum internal rotation to demonstrate the general relationship of the bones of the shoulder joint.
External rotation in a true AP view	As in the internal rotation view, the general relationship of the skeletal structures of the shoulder is demonstrated. Patients with a dislocated humerus cannot externally rotate the humerus.[15]
Stryker notch	This view is taken with the patient supine and the cassette under the affected shoulder. The palm of the hand is placed on the top of the head, with the fingers toward the back of the head. The tube is angled 10° cephalad and is centered on the coracoid process. This view shows exostosis formation.[16,17]
West Point	This is a modified axillary view.[18] The patient is prone, and the cassette is placed perpendicular to the table. The affected shoulder is abducted to 90° and the elbow is bent, with the arm hanging over the side of the table. The hand and arm are rotated so that the anterior surface of the humerus faces the floor. The tube is directed at the axilla and angled 25° medially and 25° cephalad and is centered inferior and medial to the AC joint. Bony Bankhart lesions and Hill-Sachs deformities are seen on this examination.

Reproduced with permission from Andrews JR, Zarins B, Wilk KE: *Injuries in Baseball*. Philadelphia, PA, Lippincott-Raven, 1998, 75.

supine on the table, the affected extremity crosses the upper abdomen with the elbows flexed, effectively adducting the humerus and slightly elevating the shoulder girdle. The opposite extremity reaches across the forehead to hold the cassette that presses into the trapezial midpoint, which is parallel to the sagittal plane of the body. The central ray is directed toward the humeral head 20° from perpendicular, and enters 0.75 inches below the humeral head. Immediately before exposure, the patient is asked to depress the cassette into the soft belly of the trapezius.

The glenoid view is a true AP examination, with the patient oblique at approximately 45°. Placing the distal forearm on the abdomen positions the humerus in internal rotation. This view demonstrates the shoulder girdle and the bony glenoid.[15]

Rotator Cuff Impingement/ Rotator Cuff Tendinitis

Rotator cuff impingement occurs when the arm is abducted in forward flexion, creating pressure on the supraspinatus tendon as it is compressed between the greater tuberosity of the humerus and the scapular coracoacromial arch. This condition represents part of a spectrum of rotator cuff disease and degeneration.

Charles Neer first introduced the term impingement in 1972,[19] and paid particular attention to the acromial process. Neer noted bone spurs on the undersurface of the acromial process anteriorly and theorized that they were caused by repeated rubbing of the rotator cuff and humeral head against the acromial undersurface and traction on the cora-

CLINICAL PRESENTATION

History

Repetitive overhead arm motions result in progressive pain and dysfunction.
Discomfort over the anterior and anterolateral shoulder

Observation

Scapular winging, atrophy, and muscle wasting can also be helpful in diagnosing more extensive underlying problems that have manifested as impingement syndrome.

Functional Status

Pain with overhead arm motion
Weakness with lifting overhead
Painful arc (impingement position) when the arm is elevated from 60° to 120°
Pain increases during internal and external humeral rotation.

Physical Evaluation Findings

Painful arc with passive and active motions that reproduce the impingement mechanism
Discomfort to palpation over the impingement interval
Pain increases with flexion when the acromion is manually depressed.
Symptoms increase in patients with concurrent rotator cuff tears or GH instability.
Hawkins and Neer impingement tests are positive.

coacromial ligament. When the arm is in forward elevation, the supraspinatus tendon passes under the anterior acromion and the AC joint. In this position, the rotator cuff and subacromial bursa can become compressed between the coracoacromial arch and the humeral head. This condition can be further differentiated into primary and secondary impingement.

Primary impingement results from repeated compression of the acromial process or coracoacromial arch against the coracoacromial ligament, causing rotator cuff tendon breakdown. Secondary impingement is superior humeral head migration due to supraspinatus tendon weakness, which normally depresses the humeral head. External impingement is another term referring to primary and/or secondary impingement. Internal impingement involves pinching of the rotator cuff against the posterosuperior edge of the glenoid when the arm is abducted, extended, and laterally rotated.

Neer described clinical symptoms that he labeled outlet and nonoutlet impingement in an older, athletic population. However, current understanding of the mechanics of overhead athletes differs considerably. Neer described three stages of impingement syndrome (**Table 10-4**) and suggested that 95% of rotator cuff tendon lesions were due to impingement.

Impingement is the narrowing of the space demarcated by the undersurface of the anterior third of the acromion, distal clavicle, and AC joint superiorly; the proximal humerus inferiorly; and the coracoacromial ligament anteriorly. Impingement refers to the compression of the rotator cuff, biceps tendon, and/or accompanying bursa between these confining structures.

Pure impingement in young athletes is rare. Rather, it is often a manifestation of underlying subtle superior, anterosuperior, or posterosuperior GH instability secondary to a number of causes (**Table 10-5**). In a small number of older athletes (usually over the age of 35 years), primary impingement occurs with overhead activity. In this group, years of repetitive overhead activity can cause excess growth on the acromial undersurface in the AC articulation or a thickening and/or ossification of the AC ligament, which results in space narrowing.

Secondary impingement occurs when the rotator cuff tendon is compressed against the coracoacromial arch as the result of GH instability or functional scapular instability. The supraspinatus

tendon's primary function is to depress the humeral head. During normal shoulder function, the greater tuberosity does not impinge against the acromial process. When the shoulder is static and dynamic restraints can no longer compensate for the forces encountered in overhand athletic activity, the resulting traction on the rotator cuff may produce functional impingement due to rotator cuff or shoulder girdle dysfunction.

An abnormally shaped acromial process can lead to primary impingement syndrome and/or rotator cuff injury (**Figure 10-14**). Rotator cuff tear incidence increases in patients with type III acromial processes or anterior acromial spurs. An unfused acromial apophysis can potentially cause subacromial impingement. Bone spurs associated with AC joint arthritis can also cause rotator cuff injury.

Another impingement-type syndrome, although rare, is diminution of the space between the coracoid process and the anterior humerus caused by a coracoid process anomaly or prior surgery. A contributing factor to impingement is posterior capsular tightness. If the posterior capsule is tight, the humeral head can migrate upward when the shoulder is flexed.

Impingement should be thought of as a symptom if the patient describes pain when the shoulder is abducted, or a sign if the pain is elicited upon examination. The term impingement is losing favor as a diagnosis because many disorders besides rotator cuff disease can cause shoulder pain when the arm is abducted. Impingement may be a result, rather than a cause, of shoulder injury. Evidence supporting this theory includes: (1) most partial-thickness rotator cuff tears occur on the inferior (articular) surface of the supraspinatus tendon rather than on the bursal side; (2) tendons usually fail under tension rather than compression; and (3) if a patient tears the supraspinatus tendon, pain

Table 10-4

Neer Stages of Rotator Cuff Impingement

Stage	Pathology	Typical Age Range
I	Reversible edema and hemorrhage	<25 years old
II	Fibrosis and tendinitis	25 to 40 years old
III	Bone spurs and rotator cuff tendon ruptures	>40 years old

Adapted from Jobe CM: Gross anatomy of the shoulder, in Rockwood CA Jr, Matsen FA III (eds): *The Shoulder*, ed 2. Philadelphia, PA, WB Saunders, 1998, p 756.

Table 10-5

Causes of Subtle Glenohumeral Instability

Thoracoscapular weakness and instability	Rotator cuff or long head of biceps dysfunction
Disruptions of the superior suspensory complex	Lesions of the acromion or distal clavicle
Loss of lower extremity strength	Undersurface AC bony spurs
Faulty lower extremity biomechanics	Displaced AC joint disruptions

Reproduced with permission from Andrews JR, Zarins B, Wilk KE: *Injuries in Baseball*. Philadelphia, PA, Lippincott-Raven, 1998, pp 48-51.

occurs during shoulder abduction and can be relieved by repairing the torn supraspinatus tendons and thereby eliminating the impingement.

Differential Diagnosis

Rotator cuff tear, AC joint injury, GH instability, glenoid labrum lesions, AC arthrosis, proximal biceps tendinitis, nerve entrapment, calcific tendinitis, cervical spine disorders, thoracic outlet syndrome

Medical Diagnostic Tests

The impingement test confirms primary impingement and rotator cuff disease. A single injection of 10 mL of 1% lidocaine (Xylocaine) or bupivacaine (Marcaine) in the subacromial space eliminates the pain of primary impingement and allows full, painless shoulder ROM and strength restoration. If the injection relieves pain but residual strength is limited, a rotator cuff tear is generally indicated. Both passive and active ROM must be assessed before and after the injection. Impingement and isolated rotator cuff disease do not generally limit passive motion. Subacromial scarring and intracapsular and extracapsular contractures limit passive motion when the injection limits impingement-related pain and must to be addressed before the patient can resume activities.

Imaging Techniques

The standard shoulder series (see Table 10-3) is used to identify subacromial spurring or acromial morphology that predisposes the athlete to impingement inflammatory processes. Primary impingement is correlated with an anteroinferior subacromial spur on the 30° caudal-tilt AP radiograph (**Figure 10-15**). The supraspinatus outlet view can help the clinician classify acromial morphology and estimate coracoacromial arch narrowing. Radiographs, especially the scapular outlet view, show acromial beaking and subacromial spur formation.

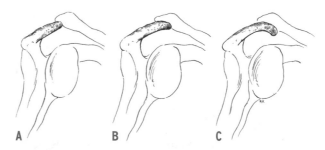

Figure 10-14 Three types (shapes) of acromion processes. **A.** Type I is flat. **B.** Type II is gently curved. **C.** Type III is sharply hooked. (Reproduced with permission from Jobe CM: Gross anatomy of the shoulder, in Rockwood CA Jr, Matsen FA III (eds): *The Shoulder*, ed 2. Philadelphia, PA, WB Saunders, 1998, p 45.)

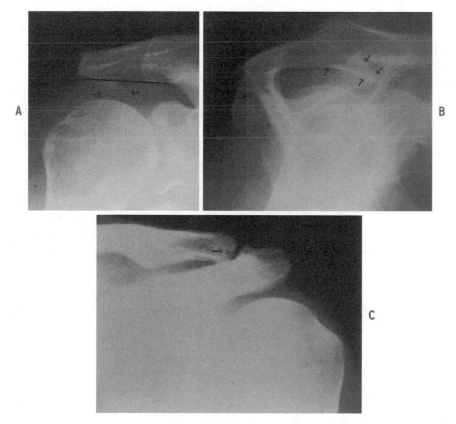

Figure 10-15 Radiographs suggesting impingement syndrome. **A.** An AP 30° caudal tilt (Rockwood tilt) view demonstrating anterior extension of the acromion (arrows) beyond the anterior border of the clavicle (line). **B.** Supraspinatus outlet view showing a large anteroinferior osteophyte (arrows). **C.** Zanca view demonstrating changes in the distal end of the clavicle (arrow). (Reproduced with permission from Iannotti JP: *Rotator Cuff Disorders: Evaluation and Treatment*. Rosemont, IL, American Academy of Orthopedic Surgeons, 1991, p 15.)

MRI may reveal acromial morphology and subacromial bursal inflammation and thickening but is generally more useful in rotator cuff disease. Differentiating partial-thickness tears from rotator cuff tendinitis on MRI can be difficult.

Definitive Diagnosis

Impingement syndrome is a clinical diagnosis based on history and clinical examination. Radiographs may demonstrate subacromial spurs and variations in acromial process morphology. The patient should also be evaluated to identify factors leading to the impingement. Rotator cuff tendinitis is a clinical diagnosis made after rotator cuff tear has been excluded by MRI, medical diagnostic procedures, history, and other radiographic evaluation.

Rotator cuff tendinitis, impingement, and tears are differentiated by a thorough history; detailed physical examination including ROM, joint mobility, and flexibility assessment; and specific tests to indicate functional symptoms related to each type of injury, which are valuable in determining additional imaging. Radiographs and MRI are useful tools in establishing a working differential diagnosis. The clinical response to treatment interventions is also helpful in narrowing the diagnosis.

Pathomechanics and Functional Limitations

Pain and weakness are experienced during overhead activities. Controversy exists as to whether impingement is the cause or result of rotator cuff disease. The concept of cause is that repetitive compression of the rotator cuff tendon against the acromial process and/or coracoacromial arch injures the tendon and eventually leads to rotator cuff breakdown (ie, primary impingement). The concept of secondary impingement is rotator cuff tendon weakness, which causes the humerus to ride upward due to the loss of the depressing effect of the supraspinatus rotator cuff tendons and can result in impingement of the greater tuberosity against the acromial process. With all conditions, scapular muscle atrophy may result (**Figure 10-16**).

■ Medications

Subacromial corticosteroid injections can relieve pain and increase active motion. The corticosteroid injection is an effective short-term intervention for impingement syndrome. However, no more than two injections are recommended. Also, it is common to use NSAIDs as an adjunct to therapeutic exercises.

■ Postinjury Management

The patient is advised to avoid aggravating activities. Ice and NSAIDs (if indicated) are used to control inflammation. Rotator cuff and scap-

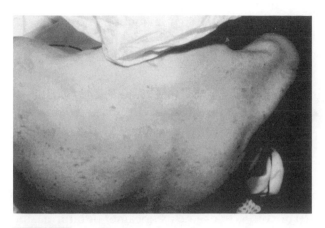

Figure 10-16 Atrophy of the right supraspinatus and infraspinatus muscles. (Reprinted with permission from the *Journal of the American Academy of Orthopaedic Surgeons*, Volume 5 (2), pp 97-108. © 1997 American Academy of Orthopaedic Surgeons.)

ular stabilizer strengthening exercises are instituted during the rehabilitation. Closed chain exercises are implemented for core strength and dynamic scapular stabilization.

■ Surgical Intervention

If conservative treatment fails to return the patient to the preinjury level within 3 to 6 months and painful limitation of motion continues, surgical intervention is recommended. The subacromial space, including the bursa, is debrided, and an acromioplasty is performed. An open approach to this procedure yields similar long-term results. However, arthroscopic subacromial decompression results in less postoperative morbidity, less pain, and an earlier return-to-throwing program (at 6 to 8 weeks).

Neer recommended anterior-inferior acromioplasty to treat the impingement syndrome. Neer's operation consisted of detaching the deltoid muscle from the anterior acromial process and AC joint capsule and splitting the deltoid 5 cm distally. An osteotome was used to remove the anterior edge and undersurface of the acromial process and a portion of the coracoacromial ligament to decompress the subacromial space. If the clavicular joint was arthritic, the distal 2.5 cm of the clavicle was also excised. Neer noted that the anterior acromioplasty operation he described was rarely performed in patients younger than 40 years unless anatomic changes, such as an acromial spur, were present.[15]

Anterior acromioplasty may be accomplished through open or arthroscopic means.[19-21] Arthroscopic acromioplasty is preferred because it is better tolerated in the early postoperative period, has less potential for deltoid morbidity, and allows for management of concomitant, intra-articular injury (ST) **10-3**).

S|T Surgical Technique 10-3

Arthroscopic Subacromial Decompression

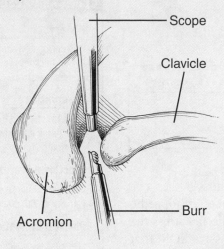

Indications

Many causes of subacromial injury exist. The primary cause should be diagnosed before treating subacromial impingement. Decompression is indicated in patients with subacromial impingement who have failed to improve with conservative treatment and activity modification or radiographic evidence of supraspinatus outlet narrowing.[19]

Overview

1. The affected arm is placed in traction in 15° of abduction with 10 to 15 lb of longitudinal traction.
2. Arthroscopic portals are made on the lateral and/or superior aspects of the joints.
3. Bursectomy is accomplished with a shaver to improve visualization and partially clear the subacromial space.
4. Subacromial decompression and possible distal clavicular resection are accomplished with a burr and shaver if AC joint arthritis is present. The coracoacromial ligament is released and excised. The distal acromial undersurface is shaved to complete the subacromial decompression, taking care to leave the top of the acromial process intact. A distal claviculectomy is indicated if AC arthritis is significant. Care is taken to avoid debriding the rotator cuff.
5. Further arthroscopic evaluation of the GH joint is performed to determine if additional intra-articular injury must be addressed.

Functional Limitations

Few functional limitations occur with arthroscopic subacromial decompression, which is one of the advantages over open debridement.

Implications for Rehabilitation

Rehabilitation after arthroscopic subacromial decompression can proceed relatively quickly after the initial trauma of the arthroscopy has passed. Because no damage was done to the muscular tissues, ROM and strengthening exercises can be initiated soon (3 to 4 days) after arthroscopy. If the debridement was completed through an open procedure, muscle tissues were violated and rehabilitation is a longer process.

Potential Complications

Failure of arthroscopic subacromial decompression can occur if an insufficient amount of the acromial process causing the impingement was removed. Similarly, failure can result from a debridement that was too generous, leading to deltoid muscle damage or acromial fracture. Nerve damage can result from the arthroscopy or from an interscalene block, which is often used to augment the anesthesia.

Comments

Arthroscopic subacromial decompression is preferred because of less morbidity and the ability to visualize the GH joint for possible concurrent injury.

Figure reproduced with permission from Shaffer BS: Painful conditions of the acromioclavicular joint. *J Am Acad Orthop Surg* 1999;7:176-188.

The technical goal of arthroscopic acromioplasty is to smooth the anterior acromial undersurface.[20-23] Although complete anterior acromial flattening relieves rotator cuff impingement, excessive bone removal may result in postoperative acromial stress fracture.[24]

■ Postinjury/Postoperative Management

Appropriate time must be allotted for the tissues to recover from the injury and/or surgery. Initially, this takes the form of rest and elimination of overhead activities, followed by ROM and strengthening exercises that do not stress the joint. As ROM, mobility, and flexibility are restored, the patient can progress from isometric to isotonic, isokinetic, and functional resistive exercises as clinical recovery allows.

■ Injury-Specific Treatment and Rehabilitation Concerns

Specific Concerns
Avoid early overhead activities.
Maintain GH ROM.
Reeducate the rotator cuff muscles.

Atrophic Characterized by atrophy or wasting.

Initial exercises may include saws, cross-bodies, circles and shrugs, and the Kerlan-Jobe Orthopaedic Clinic protocol—all exercises that do not stress the tissues. Pendulum exercises and passive ROM that avoid painful arcs (impingement positions) can also be used to achieve full ROM. Elastic tubing allows the patient to progress with increasing resistance exercises as tolerated. The patient should attempt 5 to 10 repetitions each of external rotation, extension, internal rotation, and flexion. The Jobe position of abduction (abduction in the scapular plane with the arm in internal rotation) should be avoided. Proximal shoulder girdle integrity is fundamental in rehabilitating a rotator cuff tear or impingement. Therefore, strengthening of the periscapular muscles (trapezius, serratus anterior, rhomboids, and levator scapulae) is essential for full recovery. Wall push-ups and shoulder shrugs with low weights are used to isolate these muscles. Joint mobilization, gentle passive ROM, and stretching for motion and flexibility of the entire shoulder girdle should be implemented.

When symptoms are minimal or absent, strength approaches normal, and motion is not restricted, active ROM exercises gradually progress to overhead activities and sport-specific exercises. Sport modification may be necessary to avoid recurrent symptoms (see Rotator Cuff Tear Injury-Specific Rehabilitation Concerns, p 295).

■ Estimated Amount of Time Lost

Time lost varies depending on the degree of injury and structures involved, ranging from a few weeks to several months.

■ Return-to-Play Criteria

The patient should achieve symptom-free normal ROM, strength, and especially function that demonstrates the capacity for resuming unrestricted activity.

Rotator Cuff Tears

CLINICAL PRESENTATION

History

Pain during overhead motions
Partial-thickness tears tend to be more painful than full-thickness tears.

Observation

Atrophic changes in the supraspinatus and infraspinatus may be noted if the dysfunction has been present for more than 1 month.

Functional Status

Decreased ROM, especially for overhead motions
Pain during GH abduction and flexion

Physical Evaluation Findings

Crepitus may be felt or heard during GH motion.
Palpable tendon defects may be noted.
Pain and/or weakness may be found during manual muscle testing of the supraspinatus, subscapularis, and infraspinatus.
The following special tests may be positive:
  Drop arm
  Empty can/full can
  Neer impingement
  Hawkins impingement

The traumatic and degenerative theories of rotator cuff tendon failure can be synthesized into a unified view of pathogenesis. The cuff is subjected to various types of stress—traction, compression, contusion, subacromial abrasion, inflammation, injections, and age-related degeneration. Cuff damage results when the load exceeds the fiber strength, causing immediate or insidious failure. Because these fibers are under load even with the arm at rest, they retract after rupture. Each instance of fiber failure has at least four adverse effects:

1. Load is increased on nearby but unruptured fibers, causing a "zipper" phenomenon.
2. Muscle fibers detach from bone, diminishing the force the cuff muscles can deliver.
3. The tendon fibers' blood supply is compromised as distorted anatomy contributes to progressive local ischemia.
4. Increasing amounts of the tendon are exposed to joint fluid containing lytic enzymes, removing the hematoma that assists in tendon healing.

Even when the tendon heals, its scar tissue lacks the normal tendon resilience and is at increased risk for failure with subsequent loading. These events weaken the cuff substance, impair its function, and diminish its ability to effectively repair itself. A full-thickness rotator cuff tear extends through the tendon from the bursal surface to the articular surface. Partial-thickness tears, more common than full-thickness tears, do not extend through the tendon (**Figure 10-17**).

Tendon fiber failure can be identified by weakness on manual muscle testing, but patients with full-thickness cuff defects may still be able to abduct the arm. Interestingly, those with partial-thickness cuff lesions demonstrate more pain during resisted muscle action than do those with full-thickness lesions. This is analogous to partial tears of the Achilles tendon or patellar tendon being more painful during contraction than when the whole structure is ruptured or surgically released.

Patients with bursal-side tears seem to be more symptomatic than those with deeper tears, due to cuff surface and coracoacromial arch roughness.

Differential Diagnosis
Rotator cuff tendinitis, GH instability, subacromial impingement syndrome, AC joint arthrosis

Medical Diagnostic Tests
The impingement test can be used to confirm a rotator cuff tear (see p 287). If an anesthetic injection relieves pain but strength is low, a rotator cuff tear is likely. In this case, the weakness is caused by the lack of rotator cuff continuity rather than pain.

Imaging Techniques
Suspected rotator cuff tears were once diagnosed via arthroscopy or arthrography; these procedures are invasive, however, and arthrography cannot demonstrate other shoulder soft tissues. Ultrasound has also been used to visualize the rotator cuff, but the interpretations of these findings are inconsistent.[25-27]

MRI is a useful modality for diagnosing rotator cuff injury and is superior to arthrography for demonstrating partial tears and tendinitis.[28-30] MRI can also demonstrate soft-tissue structures not seen on other diagnostic tests (**Figure 10-18**). Classic findings of a complete tear on MRI are a markedly increased signal on the T2-weighted cuff images with subacromial bursal fluid. Some degree of encroachment may or may not be seen. Partial tears show increased cuff signal, although less so than with complete tears. No significant fluid is present in the subacromial space with partial tears. The subdeltoid fat plane is obliterated in complete tears and preserved in partial tears.

Saline or gadolinium-enhanced MRI/arthrography is used in younger patients to diagnose subtle complete tears and partial undersurface tears. The addition of a contrast medium helps to identify the suspected injury because the medium is found in areas where it does not belong or displaces the tissue into an abnormal position. This technique has become very sensitive for this type of injury and has helped with management in these individuals.

Definitive Diagnosis
The definitive diagnosis of rotator cuff tears is based on the clinical findings and imaging results. Tendon defects may be palpated by placing the fingers at the anterior corner of the acromion and rotating the humerus. The defect is often palpated posterior to the anterior groove and anterior to the greater tuberosity of the humerus. Treatment and prognosis differ for individuals with complete tears, partial tears, and tendinitis. Complete tears are usually managed surgically, whereas partial tears and tendinitis are managed conservatively. Any

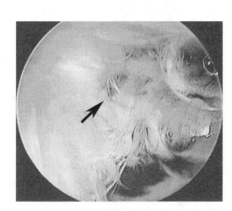
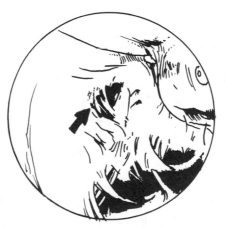

Figure 10-17 Arthroscopic image and accompanying line drawing of a partial-thickness rotator cuff tear (arrow) viewed from the articular surface of the glenohumeral joint. (Reproduced with permission from Gartsman GM: Arthroscopic management of rotator cuff disease. *J Am Acad Orthop Surg* 1998;6:259-266.)

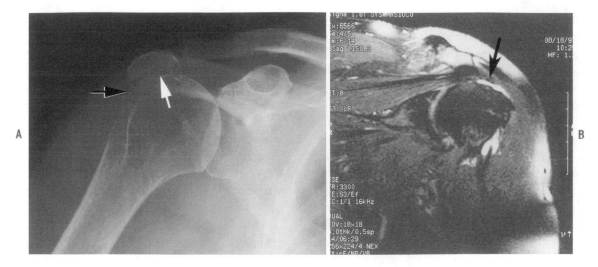

Figure 10-18 Imaging studies of rotator cuff tears. **A.** AP radiograph demonstrating a full-thickness rotator cuff tear. Sclerosis of the greater tuberosity (black arrow) indicates mechanical impaction between the acromion and the humeral head. Decreased space between the acromion and the humeral head is also apparent (white arrow). **B.** Coronal T2-weighted MRI demonstrating a full-thickness rotator cuff tear (arrow). (A is reproduced with permission from Johnson TR, Steinbach LS (eds): *Essentials of Musculoskeletal Imaging.* Rosemont, IL, American Academy of Orthopaedic Surgeons, 2004, p 240. B is reproduced with permission from Gartsman GM: Arthroscopic management of rotator cuff disease. *J Am Acad Orthop Surg* 1998;6:259-266.)

predisposing conditions to shoulder impingement must also be identified and corrected.

Pathomechanics and Functional Limitations

Early identification of rotator cuff defects limits the long-term functional deficits and further cuff deterioration. If the defect is not repaired, the degenerative process tends to contribute through the substance of the supraspinatus' cuff to produce a full-thickness defect in the anterior tendon. This full-thickness defect tends to concentrate loads at its margins, leading to additional fiber failure with smaller loads than those that produced the initial defect. With subsequent loading episodes, this pattern repeats itself, rendering the cuff weaker, more susceptible to additional failure with fewer loads, and less able to heal. Once a supraspinatus defect develops, it typically propagates posteriorly through the remainder of the supraspinatus, then into the infraspinatus.

With progressive cuff tendon dissolution, the spacer effect of the tendon is lost, allowing the humeral head to displace superiorly and increase load on the biceps tendon. As a result, the width of the long head of the biceps tendon (LHBT) is often greater than in the uninjured shoulder in patients with cuff tears. In chronic deficiency, the LHBT is frequently ruptured.

The cuff defect can cross the bicipital groove to involve the subscapularis, beginning at the top of the lesser tuberosity and extending inferiorly. This defect can be associated with transverse humeral ligament rupture and destabilization of the LHBT, facilitating medial displacement.

The concavity compression mechanism of GH stability is compromised by cuff disease. Beginning with the early stages of cuff fiber failure, humeral head compression becomes less effective in resisting the upward pull of the deltoid. Partial-thickness cuff tears cause pain on muscle contraction similar to that seen with other partial tendon injuries (eg, Achilles tendon or extensor carpi radialis brevis). This pain produces reflex inhibition of the muscle action. In turn, this reflex inhibition plus the absolute loss of strength from fiber detachment makes the muscle less effective in balance and stability. However, as long as the glenoid concavity is intact, the compressive action of the residual cuff muscles may stabilize the humeral head. When the weakened cuff cannot prevent the humeral head from rising under the pull of the deltoid, the residual cuff becomes squeezed between the head and the coracoacromial arch. Under these circumstances, abrasion occurs with humeroscapular motion, further contributing to cuff degeneration. Degenerative traction spurs develop in the coracoacromial ligament, which is loaded by humeral head pressure (analogous to the calcaneal traction spur in chronic plantar fascia strains).

Upward humeral head displacement also wears on the upper glenoid lip and labrum, reducing upper glenoid concavity effectiveness. This displacement can lead to cuff deterioration, allowing the tendons to slide down below the center of the humeral head. The cuff tendons become head elevators rather than head depressors. Superior glenoid lip erosion may thwart attempts to keep the humeral head centered after cuff repair. Once the full thickness of the cuff has failed, resultant abrasion of the humeral articular cartilage against the coracoacromial arch may lead to secondary degenerative joint disease.

The cuff muscle deterioration that inevitably accompanies chronic cuff tears is one of the most important limiting factors in surgical cuff repair. Atrophy, fatty degeneration, retraction, and loss of excursion are all commonly found with chronic cuff tendon defects and may be irreversible. Changes increase over time and do not rapidly reverse, even after cuff repair.

Immediate Management

The patient must discontinue aggravating activities. Ice should be applied to the shoulder to control inflammation. The patient may find pain relief using a sling.

Medications

NSAIDs may be prescribed to control inflammation and pain. Patients with acute tears may require narcotic analgesics for immediate pain control.

Postinjury Management

Initial management is supportive and targets pain control. A progressive resistance and ROM exercise routine is implemented, with serial examinations performed to evaluate cuff tension and symptoms. If the improvement plateau is unacceptable, further workup is indicated. Partial tears, as a rule, present a greater diagnostic dilemma and may not be well visualized on further radiologic evaluation.

Surgical Intervention

Some partial-thickness tears can be treated initially nonsurgically, but many physicians recommend arthroscopic subacromial decompression and debridement (see ST 10-3). Others recommend arthroscopic acromioplasty and mini-open (arthroscopically assisted) repairs[31] (ST 10-4). Full-thickness tears are treated surgically with acromioplasty and rotator cuff repair. What constitutes the "best" surgery for rotator cuff repair is controversial, and the procedures have been performed both open and arthroscopically. Open repairs have yielded excellent pain relief for tears of all sizes, but functional results are more variable with the larger tears. The decision to perform an open versus an arthroscopic rotator cuff repair is made after considering severity of pain and dysfunction; symptom duration; tear size and location; and the patient's activity demands, functional limitations, and expectations. A large tear, poor tendon tissue quality, difficulty mobilizing the torn ends, and the presence of a rupture of the long head of the biceps adversely affect postoperative function and patient satisfaction.

Because bursal-side tears may be more symptomatic than articular-side tears of the same size, surgery may be considered more aggressively in athletes with bursal-side partial cuff tears. Partial-thickness rotator cuff tears can be managed with arthroscopic, open, or mini-open techniques.

Diagnostic arthroscopy is helpful in verifying depth of partial tears and assessing quality of the remaining tendon. The rotator cuff insertion must be visualized from both the GH joint and the subacromial bursa. A high-grade partial tear may be present on the bursal surface of the rotator cuff with a normal-appearing articular cuff insertion. In patients with bony supraspinatus outlet impingement, diagnostic arthroscopy is followed by arthroscopic acromioplasty. Articular-side, partial-thickness cuff tears of less than 50% of the tendon thickness and bursal-side tears of less than 25% of the tendon thickness are debrided. All other partial-thickness cuff tears are arthroscopically repaired.

Complete rotator cuff tears in young athletes, particularly athletes in overhead sports, often require surgical repair to enable return to competition. However, a 6- to 12-week trial of rehabilitation and activity modification may be warranted first. If this fails, surgical repair is indicated.

Most complete rotator cuff tears in these athletes are small (1 to 2 cm or 1 tendon), and retraction is minimal. These tears are frequently amenable to arthroscopic or mini-open repair. Conversely, rotator cuff injuries in contact athletes are occasionally larger than 2 cm or 1 tendon and are retracted. Under these circumstances, an open repair is preferable.

In small (2 cm or less), mobile rotator cuff tears, arthroscopic and mini-open techniques are indicated. The purely arthroscopic approach is the least invasive and associated with decreased subacromial and deltoid trauma. Therefore, in young athletes with good bone and tendon quality and small, mobile cuff tears, arthroscopic repairs are preferred. This procedure is combined with arthroscopic acromioplasty for coexistent supraspinatus outlet narrowing.

In larger, less mobile tears (more than 2 cm or 1 tendon), an open repair is frequently performed. Large tears are repaired through a superior, transdeltoid approach. Acromioplasty is only performed

Mini-Open Procedure with Anterior Acromioplasty

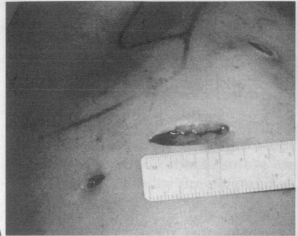
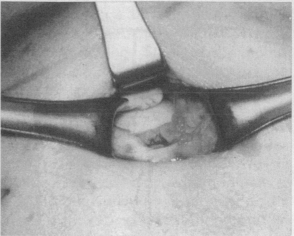
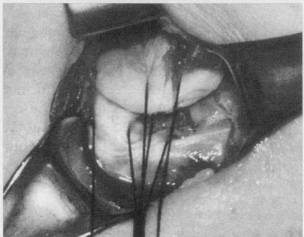

Indications

Patients with full- or partial-thickness tears (<2 cm) of the supraspinatus or infraspinatus tendon who have failed to improve with conservative treatment

Overview

1. The patient is placed in the lateral decubitus or beach-chair position.
2. Arthroscopy portals are made over the superior, anterosuperior, and posterosuperior aspects of the joint.
3. Arthroscopic subacromial decompression is performed (see **S|T** 10-3).
4. Deltoid-splitting procedure is performed through an incision across the lateral acromion (**A**).
5. Dissection is carried out to the cuff bluntly and the tear identified (**B**).
6. The proximal aspect of the tear is mobilized, and the humerus is prepared for reattachment (**C**).
7. Various reattachment techniques are available, including suture anchors and the development of a bony trough and suture reattachment.
8. Tear size, quality of tissue repair, and cuff tension on the repair determine the early postoperative management.

Functional Limitations

Depend on the procedure used, tear size, and the degree of mobilization required to repair the rotator cuff

Implications for Rehabilitation

Rehabilitation speed is determined by the injury and the type of surgical repair. Larger tears require longer healing times.

Potential Complications

Deltoid injury and axillary nerve injury are rare complications.

Comments

The advantage of the mini-open procedure is that it does not require the deltoid origin to be taken down, thereby speeding the rehabilitation process. If the subscapularis is involved in the tear, the more extensive open procedure is more appropriate.

Figure reproduced with permission from Yamaguchi K: Mini-open rotator cuff repair: An updated perspective. *J Bone Joint Surg Am* 2001;83:763-762.

if a subacromial spur is present. Tears that are retracted medial to the midportion of the humeral head are protected in an abduction pillow or brace for 2 to 3 weeks after surgery.

■ Postoperative Management

A support, such as a pillow, is placed under the arm to position it in slight abduction and neutral rotation. A sling is helpful as well. The patient typically returns to the surgeon in 7 to 10 days to have the sutures removed and the shoulder assessed.

Patients undergoing a rotator cuff repair may have an inferiorly subluxated humeral head within 2 weeks of surgery due to postoperative weakness. Proper shoulder position reduces weight on the repair site and discourages an internal rotation contracture. Some physicians may opt for early passive ROM.

■ Injury-Specific Treatment and Rehabilitation Concerns

Specific Concerns
Avoid excessive stresses on the healing cuff tendon.
Maintain normal joint glide.
Restore ROM.
Reeducate biomechanics.

The rehabilitation progression varies with the surgical technique, tear size, and the cuff tension of the repair. The exercises performed are similar to those for nonsurgical treatment, except that soft-tissue healing guidelines are respected. Rehabilitation after arthroscopic surgery that does not involve a rotator cuff repair is identical to rehabilitation after nonsurgical treatment. This protocol is modified slightly after rotator cuff repair to protect the tissues and ensure healing.

Phase I

The goals for this phase are patient education, pain and inflammation control, tendon healing, and maintenance of subacromial gliding and capsuloligamentous complex and tendon pliability. Because the subacromial space has been surgically manipulated, emphasis is placed on preventing subacromial space scarring. Immediate phase I passive ROM exercises are performed to maintain subacromial gliding and capsuloligamentous complex and tendon pliability. Exercises are completed with 20 repetitions, 3 to 6 times a day. Supervised therapy consists of ice and/or heat, joint mobilization, and passive stretching. In the absence of excessive stiffness or pain, the home exercise program is continued.

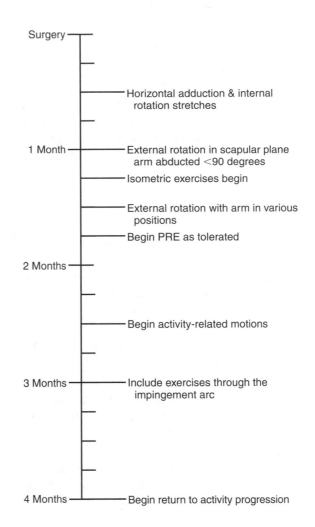

Note: Time frames are approximate. Function is the guide.

The home exercise program includes those exercises within the patient's physiologic tolerance that will assist in maintaining clinically achieved goals as the patient progresses through each rehabilitation phase. These exercises are designed to augment the supervised treatment portion of the rehabilitation, not to supplant it. This approach is useful throughout all phases of rehabilitation.

If an acromioplasty with an intact rotator cuff or a partial rotator cuff debridement was performed, active-assisted ROM exercises, including extension, and phase II stretching (horizontal adduction and internal rotation) are started at 2 to 4 weeks. Phase I strengthening is also begun at 2 to 4 weeks, depending on the patient's tolerance. If arthroscopic repair was performed (ie, a partial-thickness or small full-thickness cuff tear was present), passive ROM and active-assisted ROM exercises into external rotation can be performed at 70° to 90° of scapular plane abduction after 4 weeks if tolerated. If the rotator cuff tear was larger than 1 cm, isometric exercises are delayed until 6 weeks after surgery.

Passive ROM may be purposely restricted during this early rehabilitation phase in patients with large or massive cuff tears who required rotator cuff tissue mobilization and have been placed in an abduction pillow. Capsule and tendon release facilitates tendon repair; however, the prognosis for large tears is not as good as for small tears. Therefore, ROM exercises must be individualized based on repair quality.

Phase II

Phase II extends from 6 to 10 weeks. The patient adds phase II stretches (if not already started) and continues with phase I exercises. If stiffness persists, joint mobilization and gentle, relatively pain-free manual stretching are performed. An effective stretch to improve ROM is to have the patient place the hands anywhere from the forehead to the back of the head (depending on comfort) and let the elbows slowly drop toward the floor. Stretches are maintained for 10 to 20 seconds, and raising the elbows for 5 seconds relieves the discomfort; this sequence is repeated 10 to 20 times. Progressive stretching into external rotation in multiple positions of elevation is emphasized in those patients with an acromioplasty, debridement, or arthroscopic rotator cuff repair. Posterior capsule stretching is also progressed.

If the patient had a large tear repaired, restrictions are expected and should be respected. Progress is slow, and the patient is monitored for excessive stiffness or capsulitis. Slow and gradual return of motion is allowed, avoiding overstretching or disruption of the repair.

The decision to begin resisted exercises is based on the rotator cuff tear size, ease of repair, and tissue quality. In general, however, resistive exercises are restricted for 6 weeks postoperatively in patients who have undergone repair of a full-thickness rotator cuff tear. The exercises performed are the same as those described for conservative treatment. Care is taken to minimize excessive rotator cuff loading by using a bolster when needed and choosing the appropriate resistance level.

The patient begins with yellow Thera-Band and exercises in pain-free ranges. When active elevation is performed, appropriate scapulohumeral rhythm is encouraged. Multiangle isometrics begin at 45° in the scapular plane using manual resistance. The patient performs four directions of submaximal isometric resistance in sequence—abduction and external rotation, adduction and internal rotation, elevation, and extension. This technique assesses the patient's resistance and pain level and continues the neuromuscular GH and scapular muscle training. If pain occurs, the position is modified, resistance level is changed, or the exercise is deferred until another session. The use of this manual-resistance sequence will guide the patient's elastic-band and free-weight program.

Depending on the patient's response to resistive exercise and the time since surgery, the position of resistance is progressed toward 90° in the scapular plane. The motion of individuals who had acromioplasty, rotator cuff debridement, or arthroscopic repair is progressed more quickly. Strengthening may also be initiated 1 to 2 weeks earlier than in patients who underwent open repair of a large or massive defect. However, caution must be exercised that adding or progressing strengthening does not occur too quickly, even after arthroscopic repair of smaller tears. This progression continues to more provocative positions, as tolerated, in all patients regardless of the surgical intervention.

Elevation strength can be compromised because of muscle atrophy, disuse, weakness, or pain reflex inhibition. With a chronic tear, 6 to 12 months could have elapsed since the supraspinatus last translated force from its origin to insertion. This muscle is not only lacking the cross-sectional mass to translate enough force to stabilize and elevate the humerus, it has lost the neuromuscular ability to do so. The supraspinatus tendon is not providing its normal head-depressing force, and the humeral head is potentially migrating superiorly, causing painful compression. This situation emphasizes the need for strengthening in all positions of elevation, starting with those that are less provocative and progressing to those that are more provocative.

To strengthen in elevation, the supine patient is first treated with heat, joint mobilization, and stretching to maximize the elevation range. Multiangle isometrics are performed at different positions of elevation to improve the muscles' ability to contract and centralize the humeral head on the glenoid. The arm is raised to 90°, and the patient is asked to elevate through the pain-free range (90° to 130°). Scapular shrugging is discouraged via verbal and manual cues to reinforce appropriate synergistic scapular muscle activity as the GH muscles are activated. This sequence has proved very effective in safely strengthening the rotator cuff-deltoid-biceps complex in functional ranges while encouraging scapular muscle integration.

In selected patients, a Bodyblade may be used at 8 weeks in nonprovocative positions. As the patient progresses, light free weights (5 to 10 lb) can be used for biceps curls. Triceps isolation exercises are performed on a variable resistance unit or with Thera-Band by placing the arm in a nonprovocative position. Shoulder extension exercises can usually progress without harm to the surgical repair.

Phase III

The patient should have at least 80% to 90% of the normal ROM (100% for those without a rotator cuff repair) in this phase, unless repair of a large rotator cuff tear required lateral tendon mobilization. Patients should be relatively pain free and able to actively elevate above shoulder level with good scapulohumeral rhythm. If the patient continues to shrug with elevation, the cause of the abnormal rhythm should be determined. Is the cause weakness, capsuloligamentous complex tightness, pain, or learned behavior? Depending on the cause, the abnormal rhythm may be expected. However, if full passive ROM is present and the rotator cuff is intact with good strength, further neuromuscular control training is required to improve synchronous recruitment of the GH dynamic stabilizers and scapulothoracic muscles. If pain continues to be an issue, a subacromial or AC joint corticosteroid injection may be helpful to reduce local inflammation.

The patient is progressed to further strengthening exercises and activity-related movements, depending on the symptom level. The progression from nonprovocative to provocative movement is still used, with absolute respect for the rotator cuff repair and the deltoid. The patient may now be moved on to isolated triceps and biceps strengthening with the arm at the side or in slight abduction. Row-type pulls at chest level may be initiated, with progression to latissimus pull-downs (modified to be anterior to the scapular plane). Both exercises move the patient through the impingement zone. However, less rotator cuff recruitment is required and, consequently, less rotator cuff stress is generated. The rotator cuff strengthening exercises are progressed into elevated, sport-specific positions based on signs and symptoms. Manual therapy is performed, attempting to maximize neuromuscular control and integrate scapular muscles in the elevated sport-specific positions. The athlete is progressed with the Bodyblade. In selected patients, a Plyoball progression may be initiated sometime after 10 to 12 weeks postoperatively. Isokinetics may be used in selected patients, but soft-tissue healing requirements must be respected and weighed against the potentially injurious forces encountered during isokinetic exercise. Cardiovascular conditioning is unrestricted during this time.

Phase IV

Phase IV begins at 16 weeks and continues to 6 months. In this phase, lower-demand patients (nonathletes) continue to gradually progress in the home rotator cuff strengthening program and possibly the variable resistance program. Proper lifting technique should be emphasized, particularly to patients with 2- and 3-tendon rotator cuff repairs, because these patients are at great risk of retearing their rotator cuffs. The athlete is progressed in a manner similar to phase IV of the conservatively treated patient but with more consideration for soft-tissue healing requirements and a slower reentry process. As with the conservatively treated athlete, the goal is return to the preinjury level of competition. A sport-specific interval strengthening and throwing program is required to return the athlete to sport.

◼ Estimated Amount of Time Lost

Postsurgical rehabilitation of an athlete with a rotator cuff tear requires 6 to 12 months.

◼ Return-to-Play Criteria

The patient must be symptom free and display normal ROM, strength, and function. This requires satisfactory performance on tests to demonstrate the capacity for resuming normal unrestricted activity—running, sharp turning, jumping, swinging a baseball bat, throwing a baseball, or other sport-specific requirements.

Long Head of the Biceps Brachii Tendinitis

The same mechanism that initiates the impingement syndrome symptoms in rotator cuff injuries can inflame the LHBT as it passes under the acromion. Bicipital tendinitis may also result from subluxation of the tendon from the humeral bicipital groove secondary to transverse ligament rupture or irritation from the subscapularis tendon superiorly (**Figure 10-19**). Pain may also result from LHBT tenosynovitis, which alters the tendon sheath gliding mechanism.

Despite minimal electromyographic activity during throwing, significant traction forces are placed on the biceps brachii and LHBT. In pitching, the biceps muscle functions primarily at the elbow joint. Mild biceps activity occurs during the late cocking phase, when the LHBT is taut (see Figure 10-13). The greatest surge of biceps electromyographic activity occurs during the follow-through phase, when the muscle decelerates the elbow joint.

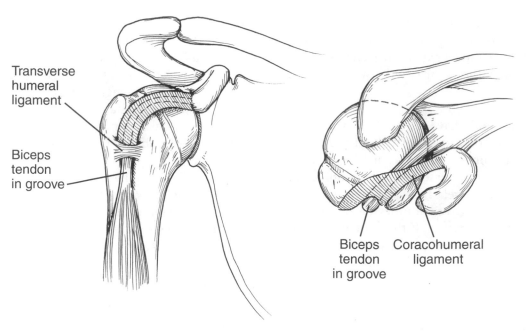

Figure 10-19 Anatomy of the long head of the biceps tendon. As the tendon exits the glenohumeral joint, it proceeds through the rotator interval beneath the coracohumeral ligament. This structure helps to provide stability to the tendon through its thick attachments on either side of the bicipital groove. (Reproduced with permission from Eakin CL, Faber KJ, Hawkins RJ, Hovis WD: Biceps tendon disorders in athletes. *J Am Acad Orthop Surg* 1999;7:300-310.)

CLINICAL PRESENTATION

History

Gradual onset, although acute cases have been reported
Pain arising from the anterior shoulder, possibly radiating to the deltoid tuberosity, cervical spine, and scapula
Crepitation may be described in the shoulder during active motion.
Initially, pain is relieved by rest but becomes more chronic as the condition deteriorates.
Night pain may be described.

Observation

Atrophy may be noted in the biceps brachii and cervical spine.

Functional Status

Pain and weakness increase during the cocking phase of throwing.

Physical Evaluation Findings

Pain increases during active GH joint abduction, rotation, and extension.
Palpable point tenderness and possible crepitus along the LHBT
The patient may have difficulty elevating the arm above shoulder level or placing the dorsum of the hand against the back.
The following special tests may be positive:
- Speed
- Yergason
- Ludington

GH instability increases biceps muscle activity during the late cocking phase. When the humerus is abducted and externally rotated, humeral head force is directed anteriorly. If the shoulder translates excessively anteriorly, biceps muscle activity is facilitated to compensate for this hypermobility.

The biceps brachii also provides GH stability during the acceleration and follow-through phases of throwing. Traction forces are conveyed across the GH joint during the follow-through phase via the LHBT, transmitting the tension to the tendon's origin in the superior glenoid labrum. The biceps also protects the humerus from the high torques experienced as the elbow decelerates during the follow-through phase.

Bicipital tendinitis is the most common biceps tendon lesion seen in the general population and a frequent cause of anterior shoulder pain in throwing athletes of all ages. It is primarily a clinical diagnosis and has been divided into primary and secondary categories. Primary tendinitis, caused by changes within the tendon or the intertubercular sulcus, leads to tendon wearing, synovitis, and groove narrowing and can be a precursor to LHBT rupture.

Most cases of LHBT tendinitis can be related to a pathologic process elsewhere in the shoulder, such as rotator cuff tendinopathy, GH instability, or degenerative joint disease, resulting in secondary tendinitis. Those with bicipital tendinitis often have impingement-type symptoms.

The pain associated with LHBT tendinitis may result from tenosynovitis, which leads to an altered tendon sheath gliding mechanism. Gradual pathologic changes can occur in the tendon, including capillary dilation and tendon edema with progressive cellular infiltration of the tendon sheath and synovium. Filmy adhesions between the tendon and tendon sheath may develop. In the chronic stage, the tendon frays and narrows, and minimal to moderate synovial proliferation and fibrosis develop. Ultimately, the tendon fibers are replaced by fibrous tissue, and dense fibrous adhesions form between the tendon and bicipital groove. Because the LHBT passes directly under the critical zone of the supraspinatus tendon, microscopic changes consistent with an avascular state occur, including irregular atrophic collagen fibers, tendon fiber **fissurization** and shredding, fibroid necrosis, and an inflammatory reaction with an increase in fibrocytes.

The biceps tendon and its synovial sheath can be affected by this GH joint inflammatory process. Tumors can affect the shoulder synovium and may also involve the tendon's sheath. Therefore, LHBT tenosynovitis can facilitate a septic arthritis or rheumatic inflammatory arthritis of the shoulder. The clinical cause in these patients is most likely the articular injury.

Differential Diagnosis

Superior labrum anteroposterior (SLAP) lesion, rotator cuff tendinopathy, AC joint disorders, peripheral nerve entrapment, cervical disk herniation, cervical degenerative disk disease, thoracic outlet obstruction

Medical Diagnostic Tests

A local anesthetic is injected into the bicipital groove. Improved ROM and decreased pain after injection indicate LHBT tendinitis. Other methods for assessing the patient with suspected bicipital tendinitis include selective local anesthetic injections in the subacromial space and biceps tendon sheath to differentiate the primary from the secondary condition. With this technique, the subacromial space is injected first to eliminate confusion due to anesthetic leakage from the biceps tendon sheath into the rotator cuff area.[32]

Imaging Techniques

Radiographs are usually negative in patients who have bicipital tendinitis but are occasionally useful in distinguishing biceps tendon lesions from other causes of shoulder pain. Particular radiographic views of the bicipital groove can be obtained if bony abnormalities are suspected. Although MRI is the most accurate test for evaluating soft-tissue abnormalities about the shoulder, it may not be cost effective when evaluating a patient for bicipital tendinitis.

Arthrography in patients with bicipital tendinitis can show tendon widening and irregularity, loss of the tendon sheath's smooth margin, or groove abnormalities. **False-negative** findings can occur if fluid in the tendon sheath obscures the arthrographic contrast medium or a rotator cuff tear allows the contrast medium to escape and results in failure to fill the sheath.

Ultrasonic imaging can demonstrate fluid collection in the tendon sheath and provides a better image of the tendon than arthrography. Ultrasound is noninvasive, less expensive, and quicker than arthrography but examiner skill is important.

Definitive Diagnosis

The diagnosis of bicipital tendinitis is based on the clinical findings and exclusion of other possible conditions. Bicipital tendinitis is often associated with the presence of other conditions. Therefore, careful consideration of possible rotator cuff tendinopathy is essential in evaluating and managing the patient with bicipital tendinitis.

Pathomechanics and Functional Limitations

Pathologic LHBT changes result from anatomic constraints, force overload, and aging. The tendon and its sheath-gliding mechanism combine to form a delicate structure that can be disturbed by excessive arm activity and cause stress failure. The close anatomic and functional relationships of the biceps tendon to the surrounding shoulder structures facilitate the development of the pathologic processes that affect these tissues. This is particularly true of the rotator cuff, which is commonly injured along with the biceps tendon.

The intertubercular groove configuration may promote pathologic tendon changes. A narrow, sharp-walled canal is more apt to cause traumatic or degenerative changes. A shallow groove or oblique wall may precipitate tendon subluxation. A large supratubercular ridge increases tendon susceptibility to mechanical irritation and subluxation. Congenital variations are particularly significant in younger patients. In older patients, long-standing pathologic biceps tendon changes may result in local soft-tissue and, eventually, osseous changes that further compromise tendon integrity.

A shallow or narrow groove specifically predisposes the athlete to LHBT tendinitis. Spurs in the groove floor may also contribute to pathologic changes. Tendon fraying can occur secondary to LHBT hypermobility in the groove because of a coracohumeral ligament tear. For tendon dislocation to occur, the medial coracohumeral ligament must be ruptured. After repeated dislocations, the groove may fill in with scar tissue and the medial wall may become more worn secondary to attrition, leading to recurrent tendon dislocation.

Fissurization The process of forming long, narrow depressions or cracks in the tissue.

10

False-negative Results incorrectly indicating the absence of trauma or disease.

Medications

Bicipital tenosynovitis may be treated conservatively with two or three 1-mL hydrocortisone injections directly into the tendon sheath (but not into the tendon itself). These injections should be followed by 2 to 3 weeks of rest to protect the tendon from injury. Because corticosteroids may weaken a tendon and have deleterious long-term effects, the number of injections should be limited to 2 or 3.

Postinjury Management

Most cases of LHBT tendinitis are managed nonsurgically. Activities that exacerbate symptoms should be discontinued and motion restricted to a painless arc. Cold therapy, analgesics, anti-inflammatory agents, and immobilization complement the rest program. Cardiovascular fitness, core muscle tone, coordination, and strength should be maintained. When acute symptoms resolve, early supervised therapeutic exercises are performed to maintain ROM to the patient's tolerance. Rotational motion should be emphasized over abduction.

Bicipital tendinitis secondary to impingement may respond to conservative treatment of the rotator cuff injury. Subacromial corticosteroid injections may help a patient with a large rotator cuff tear who does not want surgery. Because the intra-articular and subacromial spaces communicate, there may be little need to inject the biceps tendon area.

Surgical Intervention

Conservative treatment for 4 to 6 months should be attempted before considering surgical repair. Before surgery, the patient should be made aware that postoperative shoulder function might be painless but not normal enough to allow high-level function. Symptoms can recur when the patient resumes hard throwing. Thus, serious consideration should be given to ceasing activity before contemplating surgery.

Biceps tendon tenodesis has been the most common procedure. Various techniques have been promoted, including suturing the tendon to the lesser tuberosity, suturing the tendon to the coracoid process, anchoring the tendon in the humeral head, the keyhole block method, keyhole tenodesis, anchoring the tendon to the groove using a staple, anchoring the tendon to the deltoid muscle insertion, and anchoring the tendon to the pectoralis major muscle[33] (**Figure 10-20**).

Although many physicians advocate tenodesis for treating chronic bicipital tendinitis, the benefits may be short-term. Because tenodesis is not a physiologic procedure, its utility is dubious; it may not adequately address the patient's problem and may actually increase shoulder dysfunction. Long-standing bicipital tendinitis may be the result of other subacromial or rotator cuff injury that must be addressed for symptomatic relief. The LHBT helps stabilize the humeral head; loss of this function can produce GH instability and allow the humeral head to translate superiorly. Analyses of the long-term

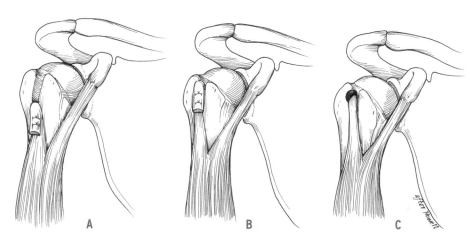

Figure 10-20   Techniques for securing the biceps tendon within its groove. **A.** In the two-pronged staple technique, the tendon is pulled proximally to the appropriate tension and then secured with a staple. The proximal free edge of the tendon is pulled distally over the staple (not shown) and sewn to itself. **B.** In the tunnel technique, a burr is used to create a tunnel approximately 2 cm in length. The tendon is delivered into the distal hole and pulled out the proximal hole to the appropriate tension. The free edge of the tendon is then sewn back onto itself to secure it. **C.** In the keyhole technique, the free edge of the tendon is knotted and sutured. A burr is used to create a keyhole, wider proximally to accommodate the knotted tendon and narrowing distally. The knotted tendon is inserted into the keyhole under slight tension, locking it into place. (Adapted with permission from Hawkins RJ, Bell RH, Lippitt SB (eds): *Atlas of Shoulder Surgery*. St Louis, MO, Mosby, 1996, p 145.)

effects of tenodesis procedures suggest unsatisfactory results in 30% to 50% of patients.

The recent treatment of bicipital tendinitis has focused on the association of this condition with other conditions involving the rotator cuff, acromial process, coracoacromial ligament, and AC joint. Arthroscopy is a useful tool for evaluating the intra-articular course of the biceps tendon. Mild changes in the biceps tendon can be managed by tendon debridement, acromioplasty, or coracoacromial ligament release, with biceps tenodesis reserved for severe changes in a frayed tendon and imminent rupture. Others recommend open acromioplasty anteriorly and inferiorly, coracoacromial ligament resection, and possible coracoid osteotomy. On rare occasions, biceps tendon exploration is indicated if inflammation is severe. Several longitudinal incisions can be placed in the biceps tendon at the site of symptoms in hopes that they will stimulate a healing response. Tenolysis is thought to be helpful. When surgical treatment is chosen, great care should be taken to maintain tendon stability within the groove.

▨ Postoperative Management

The postoperative management depends on the injury encountered and the degree of surgical intervention necessary. Simple tenodesis can be mobilized with early ROM and gradual addition of progressive resistance exercises in 4 to 6 weeks. If rotator cuff damage was addressed or a subacromial decompression was performed, the protocol for this procedure takes precedence.

▨ Injury-Specific Treatment and Rehabilitation Concerns

> **Specific Concerns**
>
> Discontinue pain-causing activities early in the program. Emphasize rotational motions.

Activities that exacerbate symptoms should be discontinued and motion restricted to pain-free ranges. While resting from throwing, the athlete can continue exercises that maintain cardiovascular fitness, muscle tone, coordination, and strength. Cold therapy, analgesics, and anti-inflammatory agents complement the rest program. An upper arm counterforce brace may also be helpful (**Figure 10-21**). As acute symptoms resolve, exercises should be performed to maintain ROM; rotational motion is emphasized over abduction. When ROM is full and pain free,

strengthening exercises are begun. The coaching staff should identify and correct technique errors before the patient resumes unrestricted play.

The best way to address bicipital tendinitis is to prevent its occurrence. Daily stretching and emphasis on strengthening and endurance in the preseason and a maintenance program during the regular season are beneficial, as is a careful warm-up before rehabilitation or participation. Throwing should begin with easy tossing and progress slowly to competitive speed. The shoulder warm-up is the same as that recommended for the rotator cuff. Older pitchers may incur bicipital injuries more often and thus require a longer warm-up than younger pitchers. For any pitcher, the number of innings pitched should be limited, and ice should be applied to the shoulder after pitching.

Tenolysis A surgical procedure performed to remove adhesions from a tendon.

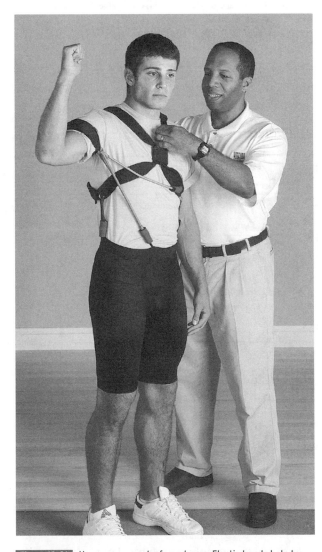

Figure 10-21   Upper arm counterforce brace. Elastic bands help to maintain the humeral head within the glenoid fossa.

▤ Estimated Amount of Time Lost

Time lost ranges from 2 to 4 weeks, depending on the resolution of acute symptoms and full return to normal functional sport-specific activities without pain or weakness.

▤ Return-to-Play Criteria

Normal ROM, strength, and sport-specific function without pain or weakness are necessary before the athlete returns to sport.

Superior Labrum Anteroposterior (SLAP) Lesions

CLINICAL PRESENTATION

History

Pain while throwing, usually with an insidious onset or after a fall on an abducted humerus

In the absence of a traumatic onset, repeated axial traction forces (eg, throwing) may be described.

SLAP lesions may be associated with acute superior labrum lesions.

Deep anterior shoulder pain occurs during overhead motions.

Nonspecific posterior shoulder pain and accompanying "popping" or "catching" sensations may be described while throwing or during similar overhead motions.

Observation

Scapulothoracic dysfunction

Hesitancy and wincing during overhead activities

Functional Status

Pain and weakness with overhead motions

Physical Evaluation Findings

Functional instability may be described, although anatomic instability may not be identified.

The following special tests may be positive:
  Speed (no tenderness in the bicipital groove)
  Superior labral apprehension
  Clunk
  Compression rotation

SLAP lesions and lesions of the LHBT and superior labrum can be caused by two mechanisms: (1) falling onto an abducted upper extremity, pinching the superior labrum between the humeral head and superior glenoid; or (2) excessive and forceful biceps brachii contraction in the deceleration phase of throwing, causing traction and avulsion of the LHBT and superior labral complex in throwers, especially baseball pitchers and quarterbacks. Additionally, SLAP lesion variants have been described in conjunction with complete long head of the biceps ruptures (**Figure 10-22**).

SLAP lesions occur because of the tensile force created by the biceps tendon crossing the elbow and shoulder joints. The biceps brachii's primary function is to supply elbow flexion torque. Eccentric torque, found during both the arm acceleration and deceleration phases, reaches its peak shortly before release. During the deceleration and follow-through throwing phases, the biceps slows elbow extension. The forces generated during this activity are transmitted across the GH joint to the biceps anchor, potentially resulting in biceps-labrum complex avulsion.

A secondary biceps function is to resist humeral distraction. Biceps contraction is particularly efficient in applying a compressive force to the arm at the instant of maximum compressive force; reduced external rotation at this time allows the long head of the biceps to be closely aligned with the compressive direction. Shoulder joint laxity can result in increased shoulder compressive force, further increasing the demand on the biceps-labrum complex and increasing demand in the biceps brachii of shoulders with increased anterior hypermobility.

With improper mechanics, LHBT force is unusually large. Because total force generated by the biceps is a combination of its contribution to elbow flexion torque and shoulder compressive force, evaluating both loads may help explain the relevance of reported increased electromyographic activity. Proper throwing mechanics require maximum elbow flexion torque to occur before maximum shoulder compressive force. Conversely, improper mechanics bring these two loads closer together in time, requiring a greater total force on the biceps.

Differential Diagnosis

Labral tear, osteochondritis dissecans, AC joint sprain, AC arthrosis, rotator cuff tear, GH instability

Imaging Techniques

Magnetic resonance arthrography (MRA) with a contrast medium such as gadolinium injected into the joint enhances visualization of the superior glenoid labrum, particularly when coronal oblique images are obtained.[34] MRA has better diagnostic sensitivity for labral degeneration than MRI and CT arthrography (**Figure 10-23**). Arthroscopy is considered the best method for evaluating this area.

Definitive Diagnosis

Positive magnetic resonance arthrography, MRI studies, and visualization of the lesion during arthroscopy

Pathomechanics and Functional Limitations

The patient experiences pain and weakness with overhead activities. Difficulty may occur with repetitive overhead functions, such as pain during the

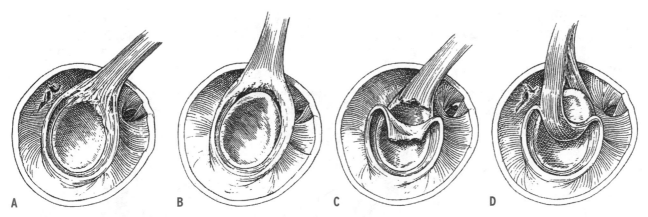

Figure 10-22 SLAP lesions. **A.** Type I lesion of the superior labrum. The edges of the labrum are markedly frayed, whereas the labral attachment to the glenoid is solid. This lesion does not really involve the biceps tendon. **B.** Type II lesion in which the superior labral biceps complex is stripped from the underlying glenoid. The labral biceps anchor is unstable in the portion of the biceps origin that does not insert on the supraglenoid tubercle. **C.** Type III lesions have a bucket-handle tear of the superior labrum without biceps tendon involvement. **D.** Type IV lesions demonstrate a bucket-handle tear with splitting that extends into the biceps tendon. (Reproduced with permission from Snyder SJ, Karzel RP, Del Pizzo W, et al: SLAP lesions of the shoulder. *Arthroscopy* 1990;6:274-279.)

cocking, acceleration, and ball-release phases of throwing. This is a result of the traction stress placed on the biceps-labral complex from functional, sport-specific overhead activities. The patient may also have difficulty with shoulder internal rotation and horizontal abduction, which further stresses the biceps-labral complex.

■ Medications

NSAIDs are used to decrease the initial inflammatory response or for chronic pain relief.

■ Postinjury Management

The initial management focuses on decreasing pain and inflammation with ice, NSAIDs, therapeutic modalities, and brief cessation of aggravating activities. Rehabilitation exercises emphasize posterior capsule stretching and rotator cuff and scapular stabilizer strengthening.

■ Surgical Intervention

The recommended treatment for surgical management of an asymptomatic SLAP lesion depends on its severity:

- Type I: Arthroscopic debridement of unstable and frayed tissue: Care is taken to avoid damaging intact labral tissue and the biceps tendon.
- Type II: Arthroscopic debridement of unstable tissue: Repair of stable tissue to an abraded superior glenoid bed with absorbable tack or suture anchor fixation (ⓈⓉ 10-5)

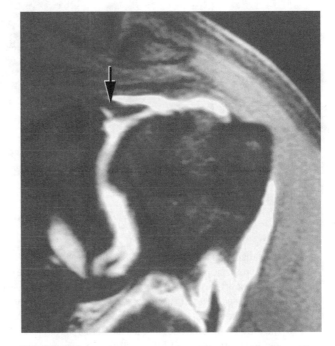

Figure 10-23 Oblique coronal magnetic resonance arthrogram of the left shoulder demonstrates contrast material medial to the labral attachment (arrow), suggesting a SLAP lesion. (Reproduced with permission from Johnson TR, Steinbach LS (eds): *Essentials of Musculoskeletal Imaging.* Rosemont, IL, American Academy of Orthopaedic Surgeons, 2004, p 253.)

- Type III: Arthroscopic debridement of an unstable bucket-handle portion: Similar to debridement of a bucket-handle meniscus tear of the knee
- Type IV: Debridement of small unstable labral/biceps fragments: Repair of larger (>50% thickness) fragments with suture techniques; tenodesis may be considered (see Figure 10-20).

S|T Surgical Technique 10-5

Type II SLAP Lesion Surgery

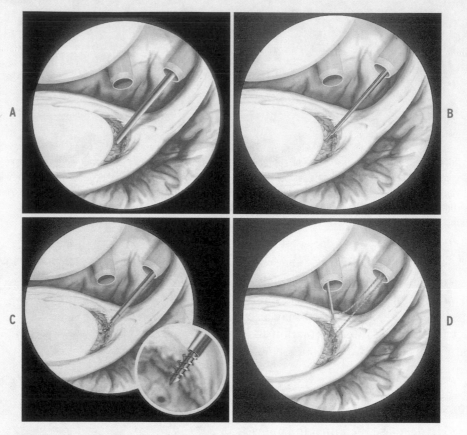

Indications

Patients with SLAP lesions who have failed to improve on a compressive rehabilitation program

Overview

1. The patient is in the lateral decubitus position, and distal traction is applied to the arm.
2. An arthroscopic portal is made posteriorly and two portals are made anteriorly.
3. Diagnostic arthroscopy is performed to confirm the type of SLAP lesion.
4. A burr is used to decorticate exposed bone beneath the superior labrum and the biceps attachment (**A**).
5. A suture anchor is placed directly below the normal biceps tendon insertion (**B** and **C**).
6. The suture is then threaded through the labrum and biceps tendon and reduced into anatomic position and arthroscopically tied by various transport systems (**D**, **E**, **F**, **G**, and **H**).
7. Type IV SLAP lesions may be addressed as a type II with an additional biceps tenodesis for a torn LHBT.

■ Postoperative Management

Patients who are treated surgically will be immobilized in a sling for 3 weeks. Elbow, wrist, and hand exercises are permitted during this time, avoiding stress on the LHBT. After the first week, the patient is allowed to remove the arm from the sling and perform gradual ROM exercises, avoiding external rotation beyond neutral and stretching the biceps tendon insertion with extension of the arm behind the body. After 4 weeks, the patient can begin motion and strengthening exercises with protected biceps strength-

ening. Aggressive biceps strengthening exercises must be avoided for 3 months to protect the repair.

■ Injury-Specific Treatment and Rehabilitation Concerns

Specific Concerns

After surgery, avoid producing undue tension within the biceps brachii muscle or the LHBT.
Avoid early external rotation.

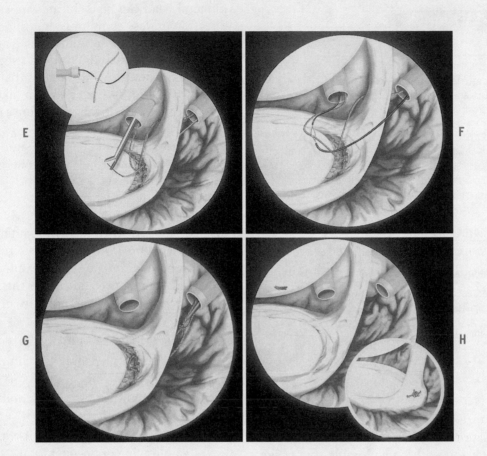

Functional Limitations

Shoulder ROM is limited for 3 to 4 weeks to permit tissue healing if a repair is performed; otherwise, the rehabilitation program is progressive. External rotation beyond neutral and extension of the arm behind the body are avoided for 4 weeks.

Implications for Rehabilitation

Rehabilitation after SLAP debridement can proceed quickly. SLAP repair requires several weeks for tissue healing, followed by progressive ROM and strength exercises. Aggressive biceps muscle contractions should be avoided for 3 months.

Comments

SLAP lesions may be associated with significant damage to the LHBT. If biceps tenodesis is performed, recovery and rehabilitation may be prolonged.

Figures copyright Stephen J. Snyder, MD.

Nonsurgical rehabilitation consists of restoring joint and capsular mobility; joint proprioception and ROM; flexibility of neural, fascial, and muscular tissue; and requisite strength in the involved and related musculature. As proper balances are achieved, return to normal functional capacity is possible, and specific therapy should be included so that the patient can resume normal occupational, athletic, or recreational activities.

For postoperative rehabilitation, these precepts still apply, but in an entirely different timing and sequence, depending on tissue healing.

■ Estimated Amount of Time Lost

The patient treated nonsurgically with rehabilitation may be limited for 2 weeks up to 4 to 6 months. After surgery, 4 to 6 months may be required before returning to sport-specific activities.

■ Return-to-Play Criteria

Before returning to activity, the patient should demonstrate normal, pain-free ROM, strength, flexibility, and sport-specific function.

Traumatic Glenohumeral Dislocation

CLINICAL PRESENTATION

History

Forced humeral abduction and external rotation
A blow to the posterior or posterolateral shoulder
If the neurovascular structures are compromised, radicular
   symptoms are described.

Observation

If the GH joint is still dislocated, the humerus is held in a fixed
   position, usually abducted and externally rotated.
A flattened deltoid may be noted in unreduced dislocations.
In recurrent dislocations, scapular muscle atrophy may occur.
A sulcus above and posterior to the GH joint may be seen.

Functional Status

The patient may be unable or unwilling to move the GH joint.

Physical Evaluation Findings

Decreased or absent external rotation
Guarded or compensated GH joint motion
After reduction, the following tests may be positive:
   Anterior GH glide
   Apprehension
   Relocation
   Surprise

Acute anterior GH dislocation involves the complete dissociation of the joint's articular surfaces, usually associated with considerable soft-tissue injury. The most common mechanism of anterior dislocation is indirect force caused by excessive abduction and external rotation. In rare situations, a direct force from the posterior or posterolateral shoulder causes an anterior dislocation. The humeral head can be dislocated in a subcoracoid direction or, less commonly, in a subclavicular or intrathoracic direction. A dislocated arm is invariably positioned in abduction and slight external rotation. When the shoulder is dislocated, the area just inferior to the acromion takes on a hollow appearance, giving the acromion a more prominent appearance.

Dislocations can result in significant soft-tissue or bony lesions that increase the risk of subsequent dislocations. A Bankart lesion, an avulsion of the anteroinferior labrum with concurrent stretching of the anteroinferior capsule, can predispose the patient to recurrent anterior dislocations (**Figure 10-24**). Although once thought to be the "essential lesion" to produce anterior dislocations, recent evidence contradicts this. Bankart lesions are classified by the integrity of the labrum and glenoid:

- Type I: Intact labrum
- Type II: Simple labral detachment from the glenoid
- Type III: Intrasubstance glenoid labrum tear
- Type IV: Labral detachment with significant fraying or degeneration
- Type V: Complete glenoid labrum degeneration or absence.

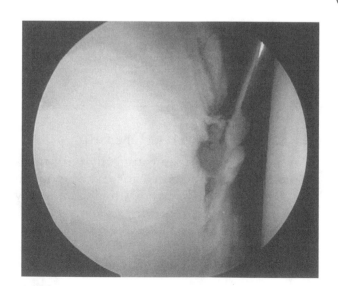

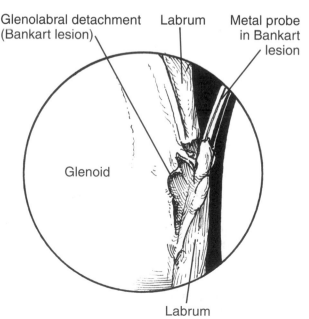

Figure 10-24   Arthroscopic view from the posterior portion of the glenohumeral joint shows a classic Bankart lesion with detachment of the labrum from the underlying glenoid. (Reproduced with permission from Lintner SA, Speer KP: Traumatic anterior glenohumeral instability: The role of arthroscopy. *J Am Acad Orthop Surg* 1997;5:233-239.)

Occasionally the anterior labroligamentous periosteal sleeve is torn from the supporting anteroinferior ligamentous and labral structures. Other lesions, such as a superior labral detachment, may be associated with a Bankart lesion. Arthroscopy may reveal defects in the articular cartilage of the posterolateral humeral head that are not detectable on radiographs. A Hill-Sachs lesion is a posterosuperior humeral head impaction fracture associated with anterior instability[35] (**Figure 10-25**).

Differential Diagnosis
Proximal humeral fracture

Imaging Techniques
The presence and direction of a GH dislocation can be identified radiographically using AP, transscapular, and West Point axillary views (**Figure 10-26**). Hill-Sachs lesions can be identified via the AP, West Point, or Stryker notch axillary views. Bankart lesions are identifiable with MRI or CT scans. MRI is also useful in identifying any associated rotator cuff trauma.

Definitive Diagnosis
Diagnosis is based on a thorough radiographic evaluation supported by clinical examination findings. Additional confounding factors may warrant arthroscopic evaluation of the involved shoulder and establish a more definitive diagnosis of a Hill-Sachs lesion.

Pathomechanics and Functional Limitations
Several factors influence the rate of recurrent shoulder instability after an anterior dislocation. The recurrence rate is greater in patients who suffered atraumatic dislocations than in patients with traumatic dislocations. Athletes have a higher recurrence rate than nonathletes. Interestingly, concomitant greater tuberosity fractures greatly reduce the risk of recurrence. Age at the time of initial dislocation does not appear to influence the recurrence rate.

Dislocation can lead to Hill-Sachs posterolateral humeral fractures or anteroinferior glenoid rim fractures, potentially releasing chondral debris, loose bodies within the joint that can abrade the articular surface and accelerate arthritis. Glenoid rim or posterior humeral head fragmentation can release small particles of bone or chondral surface that the synovial lining attempts to absorb. In the process of absorption, lysosomal enzymes are released, which secondarily affect the joint surface and may cause progressive cartilage thinning and trigger chondrolysis.

Chondrolysis Destruction or atrophy of articular cartilage.

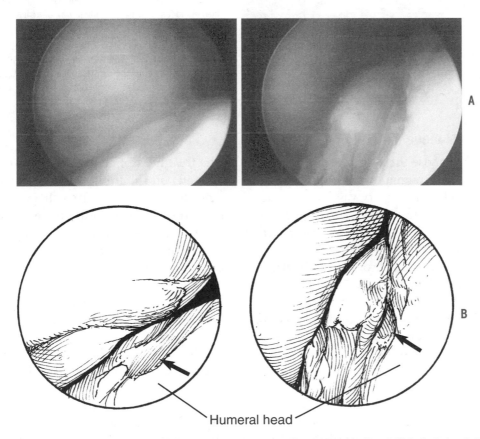

Humeral head

Figure 10-25 Hill-Sachs lesions. **A.** Arthroscopic views of the posterosuperior humeral head demonstrating a Hill-Sachs lesion. **B.** Drawings of same views, with arrows depicting the lesions. (Reproduced with permission from Lintner SA, Speer KP: Traumatic anterior glenohumeral instability: The role of arthroscopy. *J Am Acad Orthop Surg* 1997;5:233-239.)

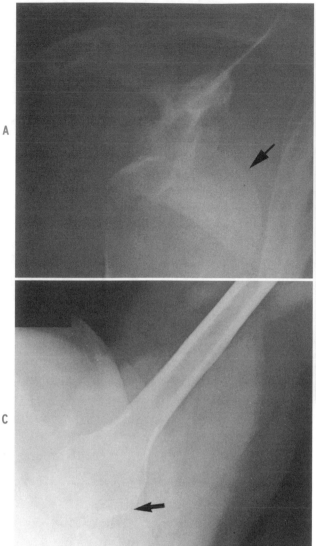

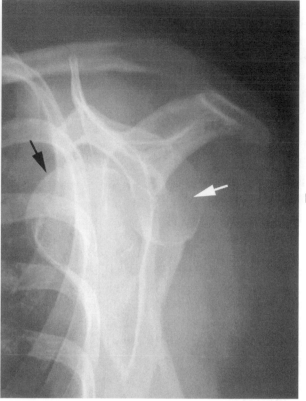

Figure 10-26 Imaging for glenohumeral dislocations. **A.** Antero-posterior view of the right shoulder demonstrating a glenohumeral dislocation (arrow). The humeral head is seen inferior and medial to the glenoid fossa. **B.** Transscapular view of a glenohumeral dislocation. The humeral head (black arrow) is seen medial to the glenoid fossa (white arrow). **C.** Anterior West Point (axillary) view demonstrating an anterior glenohumeral dislocation. (Reproduced with permission from Johnson TR, Steinbach LS (eds): *Essentials of Musculoskeletal Imaging*. Rosemont, IL, American Academy of Orthopaedic Surgeons, 2004, pp 198-199.)

Immediate Management

Dislocations predispose the axillary and musculo-cutaneous nerves to trauma. A thorough physical examination—including sensory, vascular, and motor testing—will indicate whether early surgical intervention is warranted. Once status is determined, the shoulder may be placed in a sling for support and partial immobilization. Ice or medications may be prescribed to manage the initial pain, swelling, and muscle guarding. The patient is then transported for radiographic evaluation and possible reduction.

Recurrent dislocations often spontaneously self-reduce, or the patient may have learned particular maneuvers to reduce the dislocation.

Medications

Narcotic analgesics for acute pain management after traumatic dislocations are prescribed for comfort. Analgesics, anesthetics, or sedatives may be administered to assist in reducing the dislocation.

Postinjury Management

The treatment of acute anterior GH dislocations depends on the injury mechanism and the existence of associated injuries. If a physician is present at the time of dislocation, immediate reduction should be considered. Acutely, the patient usually has no muscle spasm, and reduction is typically easily performed. If reduction is not easily achieved using a gentle maneuver, radiographs should be obtained and the reduction performed in a controlled environment. A sedative or general anesthesia may be required.

To reduce a dislocated shoulder, the arm is first slightly abducted and then internally rotated while longitudinal traction is applied. In the Rowe technique, the patient's arm is placed in neutral rotation and gently elevated. With continued upward and outward traction, the joint is reduced by the clinician's thumb under the humeral head.[36]

If reduction is unsuccessful, a scapular rotation maneuver can be performed.[37] The patient lies prone with the injured arm hanging over the table's edge. The scapula is manipulated so that the glenoid is aligned, allowing the humeral head to relocate. In the Stimson technique, the patient is positioned prone; the arm hangs over the edge of the table with 5 lb of traction applied to the wrist. After the arm has been in traction approximately 10 minutes and the muscles have relaxed, the shoulder is reduced using a gentle internal rotation movement of the arm with simultaneous humeral head compression.[38]

If these maneuvers fail, closed reduction is attempted using the forward elevation maneuver first described by Cooper. With the patient in a semiflexed position, the arm is slowly brought into forward flexion. The humeral head is reduced with mild abduction and pressure on the humeral head.

If all other maneuvers fail, the modified Kocher method can be used for shoulder joint relocation.[39] The supine patient is stabilized with a sheet tied around the patient's chest and placed in an assistant's hands.[39] A second sheet is then placed around the physician's waist and the patient's flexed forearm. Traction is applied to the shoulder via the flexed forearm. The arm is flexed, abducted, and then internally and externally rotated. Care is taken to avoid injury to the brachial plexus, vascular structures, bone, and soft tissue around the shoulder due to excess traction.

The shoulder of a young patient who has had a traumatic anterior dislocation should be immobilized for 6 weeks. An alternate approach is to immobilize the humerus in abduction and external rotation with a brace for 3 weeks. MRI studies have shown better reduction with external rotation than internal rotation.[40]

Surgical Intervention

Surgical intervention is required to retrieve the avulsed supraspinatus, infraspinatus, and teres minor from their interposition between the humeral head and the glenoid (**ST** 10-6). Persistent GH joint subluxation and glenoid rim fracture are additional considerations for early surgical intervention. Surgery may also be appropriate for patients who require absolute and complete shoulder stability before returning to occupation or sport. Early study data suggest that a Bankart lesion repaired arthroscopically after initial dislocation reduces recurrent instability from 80% with nonsurgical management to 14% with early repair.[41,42]

Postoperative Management

The patient is placed in an immobilizer for the first 2 to 3 weeks, and a sling is used for the first 4 weeks. Active-assisted ROM is started 2 to 3 weeks after surgery. At 4 weeks postoperatively, ROM is increased to within 20° to 30° of normal motion. Aggressive stretching exercises begin at 8 weeks postoperatively to establish full ROM. Return to noncontact sports is possible 3 to 4 months after surgery; contact sports require 5 to 6 months' recovery.

Injury-Specific Treatment and Rehabilitation Concerns

> **Specific Concerns**
>
> Avoid early motion into extreme internal or external rotation.
> Avoid early activity above 90° of abduction.
> Reestablish full ROM.
> Develop proprioception.

Motions that exacerbate joint instability must be restricted so these tissues can heal. Therapeutic agents are needed to reduce pain and swelling and maintain the strength and proprioception of the involved joint. The associated uninvolved structures must be maintained to prevent compensatory adaptive shortening later, which can complicate the progressive stretching and strengthening phase.

The patient is then instructed in a 6-week rehabilitation program, including active-assisted ROM and rotator cuff and scapular strengthening exercises. Next, external rotation ROM exercises are initiated. Care is taken not to place the patient's shoulder in the extremes of motion. This period is followed by a regimen that employs rotator cuff and scapular rotator strengthening exercises (see exercise protocols described in the Recurrent Instability section). External rotator strengthening exercises receive particular emphasis. Terminal abduction and external rotation are avoided for 2 months.

Estimated Amount of Time Lost

The injured tissue requires 3 to 6 weeks to heal, depending on the injury and resulting damage. As healing occurs, the tissues need to be mobilized and stretched, the related musculature strengthened, and the involved area put through a functional exercise regimen in preparation for return to activity. This process can take 1 to 3 months, depending on how vigorously the patient maintains physical conditioning for return to sport.

S|T Surgical Technique 10-6

Glenohumeral Dislocation: Open Capsular and Bankart Repair

A   B   C

Indications

Recurrent dislocations or irreducible dislocation

Overview

1. The patient is placed supine in the modified beach-chair position and anesthetized.
2. Physical examination is performed to confirm the diagnosis.
3. Diagnostic arthroscopy is performed to determine the full extent of the injury.
4. A vertical incision is made just inferior to the coracoid process, extending to the anterior midaxillary crease.
5. Full-thickness skin flaps are developed to expose the deltoid and pectoralis fascia.
6. Two choices exist to manage the subscapularis tendon (**A**):
   - A tendon-splitting technique splits the fibers in the line of the muscle fibers. This technique offers limited access to the lateral and superior capsule but is useful in overhead throwing athletes because of quicker rehabilitation.
   - A tendon-separating technique divides the tendon laterally 1 cm medial to its insertion.
7. The anterior capsule is incised with a "T" incision beginning at the superior rotator cuff interval, extending inferiorly to the 6:00 position. The capsule is then split horizontally just superior to the inferior GH ligament and extending medially to the labrum.
8. A retractor is used to retract the humeral head.
9. The bony surface of the anterior glenoid rim and glenoid neck is decorticated.
10. Three or four drill holes are made on the glenoid articular surface, just posterior to the articular margin. Another option is to use suture anchors for the repair.
11. Drill holes are developed into the prepared glenoid surface.
12. Nonabsorbable sutures are passed through the drill holes and tied to restore the anatomic position of the capsule and labrum.
13. Suture anchors are used to repair the Bankart lesion (**B**).
14. Closure and repair of the capsule are customized to the patient and injury. Care must be taken to avoid overtensioning the repair (**C**).
15. If ROM testing reveals that the capsule is under too much tension, the sutures in the capsule are removed and the closure is repeated, changing the arm position during closure.

Functional Limitations

Limitations are determined by the tension of the capsule repair.

Implications for Rehabilitation

The shoulder is immobilized for the first 2 to 3 weeks and placed in a sling for 4 weeks.

Figure reproduced with permission from Altcheck DW, Dines DM: Shoulder injuries in the throwing athlete. *J Am Acad Orthop Surg* 1995;3:159-165.

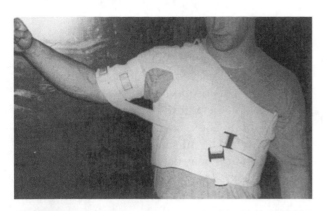

Figure 10-27 An adjustable shoulder brace used to help prevent the glenohumeral joint from reaching provocative positions leading to a dislocation or subluxation. (Reprinted with permission from Griffin LY (ed): *Orthopaedic Knowledge Update: Sports Medicine.* Rosemont, IL, American Academy of Orthopaedic Surgeons, 1994, p 102.)

■ Return-to-Play Criteria

Normal, pain-free ROM, strength, and functional capacity for sport-specific activities are required for return to regular sport activities. A shoulder brace may reduce the risk of subsequent dislocations (**Figure 10-27**).

Glenohumeral Instability

Traumatic instability arises from an injury of sufficient magnitude to tear the GH capsule, ligaments, labrum, or rotator cuff or to fracture the humerus or glenoid. A typical injury mechanism for recurrent anterior GH instability begins with a fall on an abducted, externally rotated arm. Avulsion of the anteroinferior capsule and ligaments from the glenoid rim is the most common condition associated with traumatic instability. Although this load may be applied directly to the proximal humerus, an indirect loading mechanism is more common. Chronically, the inability to keep the head centered in the glenoid may be the result of cuff disease. Acute subscapularis tears can also contribute to recurrent anterior instability.

■ Anterior-Posterior Instability

The anterior band of the inferior GH ligament (AIGHL) is the primary static restraint against anterior humeral head translation when the arm is abducted, extended, and externally rotated. The AIGHL is also a checkrein for external humeral rotation with the arm abducted and extended. In the late cocking phase of throwing, the humerus is markedly externally rotated, significantly stressing the AIGHL. Repeated AIGHL stress may cause lig-

ament elongation and allow excessive humeral external rotation. In the presence of AIGHL laxity, repeated external hyperrotation can traumatize the supraspinatus tendon and result in significant undersurface partial tears, causing internal glenoid impingement.

The relationship between excessive humeral external rotation and symptomatic internal glenoid impingement is not thoroughly understood. Increased external rotation in the throwing arm of asymptomatic athletes is not uncommon. Decreased humeral retrotorsion, when combined with AIGHL laxity and excessive external rotation, contributes to internal impingement.

Retrotorsion Posterior displacement or angulation.

■ Multidirectional Glenohumeral Instability

Multidirectional instability (MDI) involves symptomatic GH instability in more than one direction and most frequently occurs in three patterns: (1) anteroinferior dislocation with posterior subluxation, (2) posteroinferior dislocation with anterior subluxation, or (3) dislocation in all three directions (anterior, posterior, and inferior). Although excessive laxity may be exhibited in asymptomatic individuals, MDI represents excessive symptomatic multiplanar translations.

A number of factors have been implicated in MDI, including inherent laxity, recurrent macrotrauma, and cumulative, repetitive microtrauma. Patients experiencing MDI often demonstrate hyperextension at the elbows.[43] Frequently, these athletes repeatedly stress the shoulder capsule with overhead sport activities, such as throwing, gymnastics, or swimming, which selectively stretch the shoulder ligaments. "Positional dislocators" can reproduce the instability by placing the shoulder in a provocative position.

Chronic loss of the normal compressive effect of the cuff mechanism and the stabilizing effect of the superior cuff tendon interposed between the humeral head and the coracoacromial arch may contribute to superior GH instability. This instability is magnified when the upper glenoid rim is worn and the normal supportive function of the coracoacromial arch is lost to erosion or surgical removal.

Differential Diagnosis

Impingement syndrome, rotator cuff tear, AC joint arthrosis

Imaging Techniques

The "thrower's series" is helpful in demonstrating problems in athletes, such as Bankart and Hill-Sachs lesions. A full radiographic evaluation should

10

CLINICAL PRESENTATION

History

Pain may be experienced when carrying objects, especially in the presence of inferior instability.[44]

Inferior humeral head translation can produce paresthesia secondary to traction on the brachial plexus.[45]

The patient may describe a "dead arm."

History of traumatic shoulder injury with dislocation/subluxation

Easily fatigued shoulder muscles

Pain with abduction and external rotation (cocking phase)– anterior instability

Pain during pitch follow-through–posterior instability

Observation

Muscle mass and tone may appear normal.

Nerve inhibition can result in atrophy.

Sulcus sign may be present.

Functional Status

The patient may describe shoulder subluxation during activities of daily living, especially when the GH joint is flexed, internally rotated, and adducted.

Subtle subluxation may occur during the follow-through phase of throwing.

Loss of throwing velocity

Recurrent pain and weakness with shoulder motion and function

Physical Evaluation Findings

Decreased ROM during internal and/or external rotation

The following special tests may be positive:

Drawer (Bankart lesion)

Sulcus

Push-pull

Jerk

Neer-Hawkins

Apprehension

Relocation/surprise

Posterior apprehension

Posterior apprehension in the scapular plane

Hypermobile joint glide

include a true AP view in the plane of the scapula, a lateral scapular view (Y view), and an axillary view. An oblique axillary view (West Point) may show an anteroinferior glenoid fracture more readily than a routine axillary lateral view. A Stryker notch view may demonstrate a Hill-Sachs lesion. CT arthrogram and MRI demonstrate soft-tissue lesions (**Figure 10-28**, see also Figure 10-26).

Definitive Diagnosis

The diagnosis is based on a positive history of dislocations, radiographs, or physical examination demonstrating instability patterns or the ability of the joint to subluxate or dislocate. For MDI, the clinical diagnosis is made based on instability in more than one direction. A 2-cm sulcus sign is considered pathognomonic of MDI.

Pathognomonic
Specifically distinctive for some disease or disease process; absolutely diagnostic.

Pathomechanics and Functional Limitations

Anterior instability is expressed with the arm abducted and externally rotated—the position of risk for anterior dislocation. Shoulders with more than five recurrent dislocations demonstrate anterior articular cartilage erosion; in 20% of patients, subchondral bone is exposed.[46] Adaptive shortening of the surrounding musculature, such as restricted internal rotation, may occur to compensate against instability.

Atraumatic instability arises without the trauma necessary to tear the stabilizing soft tissues or to create a humeral head defect, tuberosity fracture, or glenoid lip fracture. Certain anatomic configurations may predispose the patient to atraumatic instability. A small or functionally flat glenoid fossa may jeopardize the concavity compression, adhesion-cohesion, and glenoid suction cup stability mechanisms. Thin, excessively compliant capsular tissue may invaginate into the joint when traction is applied, limiting the effectiveness of stabilization from limited joint volume. An excessively large capsule may allow humeroscapular positions outside the range of balance stability. Weak rotator cuff muscles may provide insufficient compression for the concavity compression stabilizing mechanism. Poor neuromuscular control may fail to position the scapula to balance the net humeral joint reaction force. Voluntary or inadvertent humeral malpositioning in excessive anterior or posterior scapular planes may cause the net humeral joint reaction force to be outside balance stability angles. Once initiated, the instability may be perpetuated by glenoid rim compression resulting from chronically poor humeral head centering. Excessive labral compliance may predispose to this loss of effective glenoid depth.

Because malposition usually results from loss of midrange stability, atraumatic instabilities are more likely to be multidirectional. Pathologic factors such as a flat glenoid, weak muscles, and a compliant capsule may produce instability anteriorly, inferiorly, posteriorly, or in a combination of directions.

■ Immediate Management

Immediate management consists of immobilization and ice with transport for radiographic evaluation and possible reduction. In recurrent dislocations, the shoulder often reduces itself spontaneously, or the patient has learned to perform maneuvers that reduce the dislocation. In chronic instability with no dislocation, ice, NSAIDs, and limited sling use are employed.

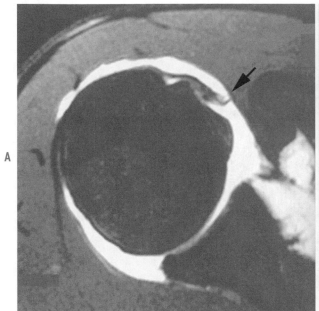

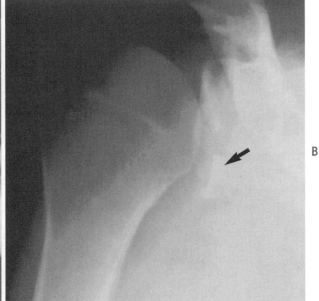

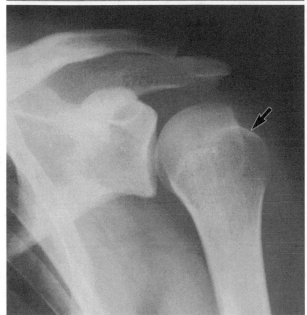

Figure 10-28 Multidirectional glenohumeral instability. **A.** Axial MRI demonstrating a Bankart lesion. The arrow identifies an avulsion of the anterior glenoid labrum. **B.** AP view of the glenohumeral joint demonstrating a fracture of the glenoid (arrow) associated with a Bankart fracture. **C.** AP internal rotation view depicting a Hill-Sachs lesion (arrow). (Reproduced with permission from Johnson TR, Steinbach LS (eds): *Essentials of Musculoskeletal Imaging.* Rosemont, IL, American Academy of Orthopaedic Surgeons, 2004, pp 199-201.)

Medications

NSAIDs, iontophoresis, or phonophoresis may be used to control inflammation. Selective therapeutic and diagnostic injections can help in the case of a diagnostic dilemma. AC, subacromial, and GH injections may be given to better differentiate the source of symptoms.

Postinjury Management

The risk of recurrent dislocations is directly related to activity level and inversely related to age. Treatment and immobilization for up to 6 weeks has had little effect on the natural history. Swelling is controlled with appropriate compression and cryotherapy. Initial instability treatment is nonsurgical and combines activity modification (avoiding provoca-

tive activities) with a prolonged exercise program. Deltoid and rotator cuff muscle strengthening below the horizon are initiated, as well as periscapular muscular conditioning to stabilize the scapula. Rehabilitation is generally successful in patients with involuntary atraumatic MDI treated by conservative measures. In rare instances, subacromial inflammation develops in a patient with MDI. A subacromial corticosteroid injection to reduce symptoms allows the patient to continue the exercise program.

Surgical Intervention

Anterior-Posterior Instability

Surgical intervention for initial dislocators is a relatively new concept. It is being performed in active young adults and adolescents with high recurrence

S|T Surgical Technique   10-7

Posterior-Inferior Capsular Shift

Indications

Failure to reduce posterior dislocation or recurrent posterior instability

Overview

1. The patient is placed in the lateral decubitus position.
2. A vertical incision is made from the lateral edge of the acromion toward the axillary crease.
3. A skin flap is developed, exposing the deltoid fascia.
4. The deltoid is split the length of the fibers from the spine of the scapula inferiorly, exposing the infraspinatus and teres minor and avoiding the axillary nerve.
5. The posterior capsule is identified through the intramuscular division
6. Beginning at the glenoid edge, a T-shaped capsulotomy is performed with a horizontal extension directly lateral.
7. A posterior capsulorrhaphy is accomplished by reattaching the capsule to the glenoid. If the labrum is detached or posterior Bankart lesions are present, they are repaired as in the anterior Bankart lesion. Suture anchors can also be used.
8. If the posterior labrum is intact, the capsulorrhaphy can be completed by passing suture through the labrum.
9. The capsule is advanced medially and superiorly and tensioned with the arm in 20° of abduction and neutral rotation.
10. If inferior laxity is marked, the capsule can be shifted superiorly and laterally at the glenoid.
11. If the bony rim of the posterior glenoid is deficient, a bone block can be placed to augment the bony anatomy.

Capsulotomy Cutting of the joint capsule.

Functional Limitations

Restrictions of internal rotation past neutral are important to avoid tensioning the repair.

Implications for Rehabilitation

Slow progression with rotational motions and strengthening must be implemented to ensure adequate healing.

Comments

Contraindications to the posterior approach are: (1) significant humeral head involvement of 20% to 50%, which necessitates a subscapular transfer; and (2) total head destruction requiring hemiarthroplasty. These procedures use the anterior approach previously described.

rates, with little change in the natural history using conservative management. In these high-risk individuals, visualization and repair of the acute injury dramatically reduce the recurrence rates.[47]

Various surgical techniques have been used to stabilize the shoulder (see **ST** 10-6). Arthroscopic approaches with transglenoid sutures, stapling, and open capsular shift have been successful. Although surgical treatment for recalcitrant anterior instability is well accepted, posterior stabilization is more controversial. Posterior-inferior capsular shift is recommended as the standard surgical approach for posterior instability (**ST** 10-7).

Multidirectional Instability

Surgical repair is indicated for traumatic events that lead to MDI and in patients who have been compliant with rehabilitation but whose shoulders remain unstable. An inferior capsular shift with Bankart repair (if needed) yields good results. The goal of surgical intervention is to correct traumatic lesions and decrease capsular volume through open soft-tissue capsular shift procedures. Open inferior capsular shift with capsuloligamentous injury repair is the recommended treatment when nonsurgical management has failed. The inferior capsular shift is approached through the most symptomatic site (**Figure 10-29**). Tensioning the opposite side of the joint by overlapping the capsular flaps on the symptomatic side reduces volume and helps reduce recurrence.

Capsular shrinkage can also be performed by electrothermal-assisted capsulorrhaphy and laser-assisted capsular shift techniques. Although they initially showed some promise, these techniques are probably not indicated in the young, high-demand athlete.

■ Postoperative Management

The patient is placed in an immobilizer to maintain the arm in neutral rotation and slight extension or slightly abducted with the humerus in neutral position for 6 weeks (**Figure 10-30**). The brace

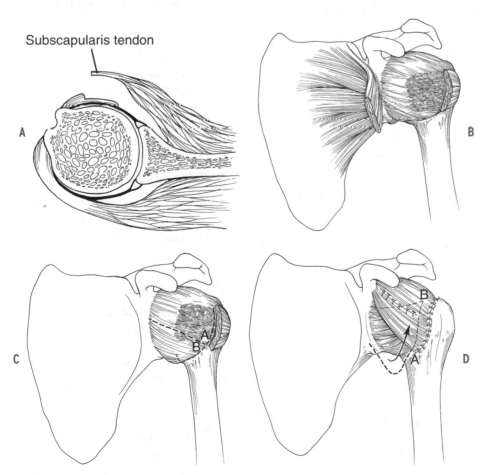

Figure 10-29 Inferior capsular shift. **A.** The anterior two thirds of the subscapularis tendon is dissected medially, leaving the posterior portion of the tendon to reinforce the anterior capsule. **B.** The subscapularis muscle belly and the anterior portion of the tendon are retracted medially. **C.** The capsule is incised in a "T" fashion, creating superior and inferior leaflets. **D.** The capsule is advanced and shifted; the superior flap overlaps the inferior flap. (Reproduced with permission from Schenk TJ, Brems JJ: Multidirectional instability of the shoulder: Pathophysiology, diagnosis, and management. *J Am Acad Orthop Surg* 1998;6:65-72.)

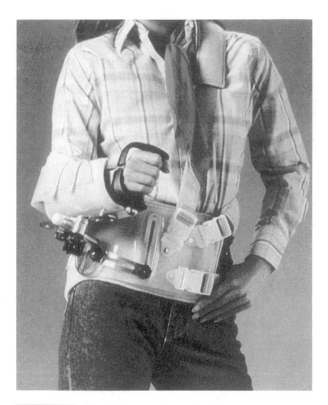

Figure 10-30 Brace used in the early postoperative period in patients with multidirectional instability and associated posterior dislocations. (Reproduced with permission from Cordasco FA: Understanding multidirectional instability of the shoulder. *J Athl Train* 2000;35:278-285.)

is then removed, and ROM and progressive resistance exercise programs are initiated. Passive external rotation is not limited; however, internal rotation is only allowed to neutral. Internal and external rotation strengthening exercises using Thera-bands are initiated at week 7. Light weights can be used at week 12, progressing to higher demands by week 20. Noncontact sports are allowed after 5 months, and contact sports are 6 to 9 months after surgery. Repetitive overhead or throwing sports are not initiated until after 9 months.

Injury-Specific Treatment and Rehabilitation Concerns

Specific Concerns

Avoid internal rotation past neutral.
Avoid provocative motions early in the rehabilitation program.
Encourage joint mobilization and tissue stretching as healing allows.
Reestablish normal neuromuscular control.

Restriction of motions that exacerbate joint instability allows the repaired tissues to heal. Limiting specific directions of movement, using therapeutic agents to reduce pain and swelling, and maintaining strength and proprioception of the involved joint are important. The length of the associated uninvolved structures must be maintained to prevent compensatory adaptive shortening.

As healing progresses, the tissue needs to be mobilized and stretched. Progressive stretching and strengthening reestablish normal motion, mobility, and joint kinematics. SC, AC, and scapulothoracic joint mobilities need to be achieved and maintained. The shoulder girdle and shoulder joint musculature are progressively strengthened. Exercise schemes are included to develop the functional requirements for return to sport-specific activities as clinical healing occurs.

Coordinated, strong muscle contraction is key to stabilizing the humeral head in the glenoid. Optimal neuromuscular control is required of the rotator cuff, deltoid, pectoralis major, and scapular musculature. These dynamic stabilizing mechanisms need muscle strength, coordination, and training. Such a program is likely to be of particular benefit in patients with atraumatic instability, because loss of neuromuscular control is a major feature of this condition. Nonsurgical management is also an attractive option for children, patients with voluntary instability, those with posterior GH instability, and those requiring a supranormal ROM (eg, baseball pitchers and gymnasts) in whom surgical management often does not permit return to a competitive level of function.

Estimated Amount of Time Lost

Recovery and rehabilitation can take up to 3 to 6 months to achieve the required tissue healing and maturation and reestablish joint mobility, motion, strength, and flexibility.

Return-to-Play Criteria

Normal, pain-free ROM, strength, and functional capacity for sport-specific activities are required for return to regular sport. Braces have been used with limited success to maintain joint stability (see Figure 10-27).

Humeral Fractures

The most common mechanism of injury for proximal humeral fractures is a fall on the outstretched hand from standing height or lower. In younger patients, high-energy trauma is more frequently involved, resulting in a more serious fracture. These

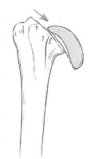
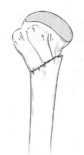
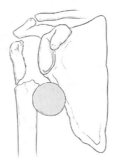
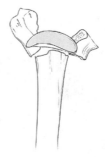

Two-Part Fracture
Anatomic neck

Two-Part Fracture
Surgical neck

Three-Part Fracture
Surgical neck
Greater tuberosity
Shaft

Four-Part Fracture
Humeral head
Greater tuberosity
Lesser tuberosity
Shaft

Figure 10-31 The Neer classification of proximal humeral fractures. (Reproduced with permission from Neer CS II: Displaced proximal humeral fractures. I: classification and evaluation. *J Bone Joint Surg Am* 1970;52:1077-1089.

CLINICAL PRESENTATION

History

Falling on the shoulder, elbow, or outstretched arm
Blow to the arm
Immediate pain and dysfunction

Observation

Deformity and swelling are usually noted.

Functional Status

Inability to move the arm without significant pain

Physical Evaluation Findings

Pain with any motion of the shoulder, elbow, and arm (may be
    minimal with proximal humeral fractures)

patients usually have fracture-dislocations with significant soft-tissue disruption and multiple injuries. Another cause of injury is excessive arm rotation, especially in the abducted position, when the humerus locks against the acromion in a pivotal position, a mechanism seen in older patients with osteoporotic bone. Proximal humeral fractures can also occur from a direct lateral blow and may result in a greater tuberosity fracture.

A fracture-dislocation may occur anteriorly or posteriorly. Metastatic disease may significantly weaken the bone; thus, a pathologic fracture can occur in an otherwise trivial activity. Whenever a trivial event results in a fracture, a pathologic cause should be considered.

The force produced during the acceleration phase of throwing can lead to humeral fatigue injuries. Bony and soft-tissue structures hypertrophy when subjected to gradually increasing loads. If the applied load is greater than the surrounding structures can withstand, a fatigue fracture occurs.

A spontaneous humeral fracture from ball throwing can have the characteristics of a stress fracture. This is due, in part, to the torque developed during the power phase of throwing, which can exceed the fracture torque of the humerus. The throwing force can result in widening, demineralization, and fragmentation of the proximal humeral epiphysis and subsequent osteochondrosis of the proximal humeral epiphysis in growing athletes.

Severely displaced proximal humeral fractures are typical of high-velocity blunt trauma and rarely occur during athletics but are prevalent in elderly people. The evaluation and treatment of two-part proximal humeral fractures, including those through the proximal humeral growth plate in young athletes, must be identified and treated.

A four-segment classification of proximal humeral fractures has been developed in which any segment displaced more than 1 cm or angulated more than 45°, regardless of the number of fracture lines, is considered a part. One-part fractures make up approximately 80% of all proximal humeral fractures and include those in which none of the major segments is displaced 1 cm or more or rotated 45° or more (**Figure 10-31**). This section will only consider two-part fractures, which include surgical neck fractures and greater or lesser tuberosity fractures.

Differential Diagnosis

GH dislocation

Imaging Techniques

In addition to the standard radiographic views, scapular Y views or axillary views are important to rule out an associated dislocation, which is particularly common with greater and lesser tuberosity fractures (**Figure 10-32**). Routine radiographs alone may be inadequate to judge displacement of

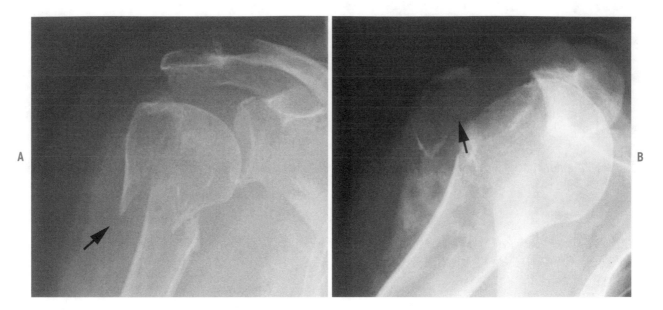

Figure 10-32 | Imaging of proximal humerus fractures. **A.** AP radiograph of the right shoulder showing a comminuted fracture of the surgical neck (arrow) and head. **B.** AP radiograph demonstrating a displaced fracture of the greater tuberosity (arrow). (Reproduced with permission from Johnson TR, Steinbach LS (eds): *Essentials of Musculoskeletal Imaging.* Rosemont, IL, American Academy of Orthopaedic Surgeons, 2004, pp 189-191.)

proximal humeral fractures, particularly those involving the tuberosities. For this purpose, CT scan of the proximal humerus is useful.

Definitive Diagnosis

Although the history and examination are helpful in making the diagnosis, radiographic examination is more important. Patients who suffer relatively low-energy fractures may also need to be evaluated for low bone mineral density and the possibility of metastases.

Pathomechanics and Functional Limitations

By definition, if the greater tuberosity is fractured, a full-thickness rotator cuff tear is present. Posterior greater tuberosity displacement can result in limited external rotation, whereas superior displacement can lead to impingement difficulties and restricted abduction. In rare instances, a symptomatic nonunion may occur. Surgical treatment is necessary and involves an anatomic reduction and internal fixation of the displaced tuberosity and repair of the rotator cuff tear. Isolated, displaced lesser tuberosity fractures are rare and are associated with subscapularis tendon damage. Some internal rotation loss may occur, and, theoretically, a nonunion may develop. In general, however, these fractures are not functionally important and require only symptomatic care.

The greater the separation between the segments, the greater the risk of a nonunion. Fractures angulated more than 45° and/or rotated fractures may heal but with significant limitation of GH motion in one or more directions. Nonsurgical treatment involves closed reduction to correct the

angulation, rotation, and impaction of the fracture surfaces and immobilization of the arm in a sling and swathe dressing or a shoulder splint, brace, or spica designed to relax the deforming pull of the surrounding soft tissues.

■ Immediate Management

Immediate management entails immobilization of the elbow, humerus, and GH joint and transport to a medical facility for radiographs. A careful neurovascular examination should be conducted, paying specific attention to radial nerve function.

■ Medications

Narcotic analgesics are used in the early postinjury period to control pain. NSAIDs are helpful during rehabilitation to decrease inflammation in the surrounding tissues.

■ Postinjury Management

Management of one-part fractures consists of immobilizing the arm in a sling and swathe dressing until the entire humerus moves as a unit (approximately 2 weeks), followed by progressive ROM exercises during the subsequent 4 weeks (dependent circular and pendulum ROM exercises, as well as external rotation to neutral during weeks 3 and 4, and more aggressive ROM exercises in all directions during weeks 5 and 6). At the 6-week point, bony healing is usually clinically solid, and active use can be allowed.

For surgical neck fractures, absolute immobilization continues until the entire humerus moves as a unit (approximately 2 weeks), followed by progressive passive ROM exercises during the subsequent 4 weeks. At the 6-week point, bony healing is usually sufficient, and active use can be allowed. Therapy continues until ROM and strength are maximized. Percutaneous pinning of the fracture after the closed reduction can also be considered, especially if the fracture is unstable. Overhead olecranon pin traction may be of use in patients with multiple injuries and those with extensive comminution in the surgical neck region (seen in the most violent sports, such as auto racing). If the fracture remains in an unacceptable position despite all attempts, surgical open reduction and internal fixation must be considered.

In young athletes, particularly pitchers who have pain in the proximal humerus of the throwing arm, the possibility of "Little League shoulder" should be considered. This condition is usually described as pain in the throwing shoulder of the skeletally immature athlete. Radiographs may demonstrate an irregularity of the proximal humeral growth plate, probably resulting from traction or stress on the physis, or a subacute Salter-Harris fracture from repetitive microtrauma to the growth plate. This injury usually responds well to rest.

Surgical Intervention

The trend in management of proximal humeral fractures is reduction and percutaneous pin fixation using a fluoroscope to visualize the fracture site. An advantage of this procedure is the ability to perform early ROM. In pediatric patients, angulation limits are approximately 50% apposition and 45° angulation. Acceptable alignment becomes more precise in older age groups, and the possibility of surgical intervention has increased as the acceptable limits of displacement have been reduced. In the 10- to 12-year-old age group, the least acceptable reduction is 50% displacement and 30° angulation, and in the age 12 years to maturity group, the least acceptable reduction is 30% displacement and 25° angulation. If the position is unsatisfactory, closed reduction should be attempted. If closed reduction is not obtainable, then open reduction is indicated. If closed reduction is obtained but unstable, percutaneous pin fixation should be considered.

Displaced proximal humeral fractures are difficult to manage, and a wide spectrum of complications has been reported after both closed and open treatment. Complications include osteonecrosis, nonunion, malunion, hardware failure, frozen shoulder, infection, neurovascular injury, pneumothorax, and pneumohemothorax.

Greater Tuberosity Fractures

In displaced greater tuberosity fractures, the supraspinatus, infraspinatus, and teres minor muscles cause superior, posterior fragment displacement. This fracture is associated with a rotator cuff tear. A significantly displaced fracture is best treated surgically with rotator cuff repair and fracture fixation. Such a fracture may also be associated with anterior GH dislocation.

Lesser Tuberosity Fractures

Surgical fixation is recommended for displaced, isolated lesser tuberosity fractures. The usual injury mechanism is a strong external rotation force with the arm in maximal external rotation at 90° of abduction. In young adolescents, lesser tuberosity fractures may result from traction on the apophyseal plate of the lesser tuberosity. In adults, these fractures are commonly mistaken for pronounced calcific tendinitis. Lesser tuberosity fractures are associated with posterior GH dislocations.

Subscapularis muscle pull is responsible for lesser tuberosity displacement. Surgical treatment is usually not required unless the fragment is large enough to prevent internal rotation. In this case, open reduction and internal fixation should be performed.

Postoperative Management

The postoperative management is determined by the extent of the injury and fixation stability (if applicable). Once healing has been documented or a stable contruct is demonstrated, ROM and early progressive resistance exercises can be initiated. These are gradually advanced as healing is documented radiographically and clinically. In general, ROM exercises can be initiated with Codman pendulum exercises in the first 3 weeks. Healing is usually accomplished in 6 to 8 weeks, and more aggressive exercises can be performed.

Injury-Specific Treatment and Rehabilitation Concerns

Specific Concerns

Maintain stability of the fracture site.
Restore ROM.
Restore muscle function.

Rehabilitation of proximal humeral fractures must restore adequate motion for optimal function. If a fracture or fracture repair is stable, then rehabilitation should be started by day 7 to 10. After surgical repair, passive exercises can be started within 24 to 48 hours. The most useful proximal humeral fracture rehabilitation protocol is a three-phase system. Phase I consists of passive-assistive exercises. Three weeks after fracture, assisted forward elevation exercises may begin. Pulley exercises should be avoided until there is radiographic evidence of tuberosity healing, usually after 6 weeks. Isometric exercises are generally started at 4 weeks. In phase II, active- and early-resistive exercises are initiated. Phase III is a maintenance program of advanced stretching and strengthening exercises and is usually started at 3 months. Application of this approach varies with the fracture type, fracture or fracture repair stability, and the patient's ability to comprehend the exercise program.

Estimated Amount of Time Lost

Four to six months are usually required before returning to activity.

Return-to-Play Criteria

Normal, pain-free ROM, strength, and satisfactory demonstration of normal capacity for sport-specific activity requirements, including a clinical orthopaedic evaluation, are required for complete clearance to return to sport activities.

Rehabilitation

The rehabilitation progression for most types of injuries follows a consistent sequence (**Table 10-6**).[48-52] This chapter provides ROM and early strengthening exercises for the shoulder. Also refer to chapter 13 for upper extremity therapeutic exercises (including proprioceptive and plyometric activities) and chapter 17 for spinal and core muscle group exercises.

Joint Mobilization Techniques

The following joint mobilization techniques are used to treat pain, stiffness, and reversible joint hypomobility. These exercises are indicated to reestablish the joint-play motion necessary for restoring shoulder complex movement.

◼ Clavicular Glide

Inferior Glide

Inferior glide of the clavicular head is indicated as a component motion for shoulder elevation. The patient is supine, and the clinician stands above the patient's head. The thumb pad contacts the most superior/proximal surface of the clavicle. The opposite thumb is placed on top, and inferior force is exerted diagonally away from the patient's midline.

Posterior Glide

Posterior glide of the clavicular head is indicated as a component motion for shoulder retraction and horizontal abduction. The patient is supine, with the clinician standing to the side of the patient. The thumb pad contacts the anterior/proximal surface of the clavicle. The opposite thumb is placed on top, and posterior force is exerted (**Figure 10-33**).

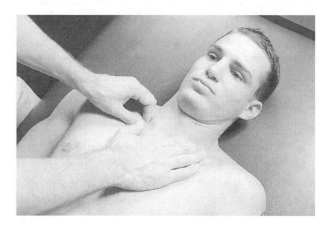

Figure 10-33 Sternoclavicular joint mobilization technique: posterior glide.

Posterosuperior and Anteroinferior Glide of the Clavicle on the Acromion

The patient is supine, and the clinician stands facing the patient. The anterior humeral surface is grasped with one hand while the opposite thumb contacts the anterolateral surface of the clavicle. A force is then exerted in a posterior/superior/medial direction through the thumb, followed by an anterior/inferior/lateral directional force (**Figure 10-34**).

Table 10-6

Phases of Shoulder Rehabilitation

Phase I

Rest from painful activity

Anti-inflammatory therapy

Passive and active-assisted ROM exercises

Joint mobilization

Scapulothoracic strengthening (submaximal to maximal), aerobic conditioning

Phase II

Progress ROM and flexibility

Strengthening (submaximal to maximal) manual, elastic band, and isotonic multiangle isometrics

Short-arc to full-arc excursion

Aggressive scapulothoracic strengthening and integration, aerobic conditioning

Phase III

Prophylactic stretching

Strengthening and endurance (to full range with emphasis on eccentrics, then progress to sport-specific positions)

Variable and/or free-weight resistance

Bodyblade

Isokinetics

Plyometrics

Phase IV

Return to sport

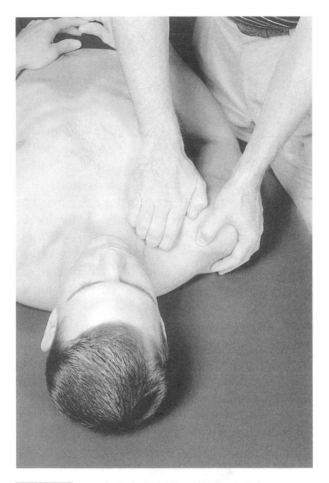

Figure 10-34 Acromioclavicular joint mobilization technique: posterosuperior and anteroinferior glide of the clavicle on the acromion.

■ Scapular Mobilization

Distraction

The patient is prone, and the clinician stands facing the patient. The anterior surface of the humerus is grasped with one hand, pulling posteriorly. The opposite second proximal phalanx rests on the thoracic wall, squeezing under and gently lifting the inferior angle of the scapula (**Figure 10-35**).

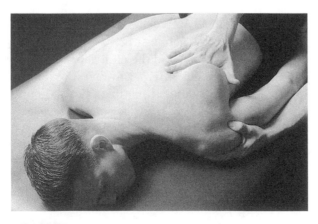

Figure 10-35 Scapular mobilization technique: distraction.

Superior and Inferior Glide

The patient lies on the side, and the clinician stands facing the patient. The humerus is maintained against the clinician's torso as the scapula is moved superiorly and inferiorly (**Figure 10-36**).

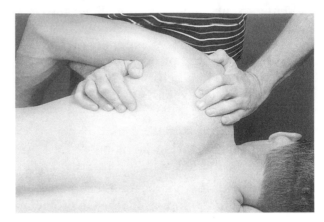

Figure 10-36 Scapular mobilization technique: superior and inferior glide.

Lateral and Medial Rotation

The patient lies on the side, and the clinician stands facing the patient. The humerus is maintained against the clinician's trunk as the scapula is rotated medially and laterally (**Figure 10-37**).

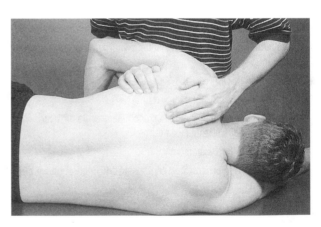

Figure 10-37 Scapular mobilization technique: lateral and medial rotation.

■ Glenohumeral Joint Mobilization

Anterior Humeral Glide

Anterior humeral glide is indicated as a component motion for GH external rotation, extension, and abduction. The patient is prone, and the clinician stands facing the patient, holding the patient's arm in a loose-packed position. One hand holds the proximal humerus, while the other hand is distal to the acromion. Force is applied in an anterior direction (**Figure 10-38**).

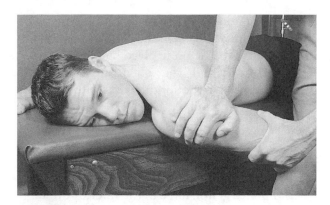

Figure 10-38 Glenohumeral joint mobilization technique: anterior humeral glide.

Inferior Humeral Glide

Inferior humeral glide is indicated as a component motion for flexion and abduction. The patient is supine, and the clinician stands at the patient's side. The proximal phalanx index finger is positioned against the neck of the scapula, while the other hand contacts the lateral/distal surface of the humerus. An inferior force is exerted through the contact on the distal humerus (**Figure 10-39**).

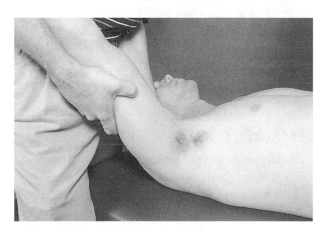

Figure 10-39 Glenohumeral joint mobilization technique: inferior humeral glide.

Lateral Distraction of the Humeral Head

Lateral humeral head distraction is indicated as a joint-play motion for shoulder complex movement. The patient is supine, and the clinician stands at the patient's side. The outside hand grasps the anterior/distal part of the humerus, and the hand nearest the patient is placed so that the proximal phalanx of the index finger and the first web space contact the medial/proximal surface of the humeral neck. A lateral force is exerted with the inside hand's index finger and web space (**Figure 10-40**).

Figure 10-40 Glenohumeral joint mobilization technique: lateral distraction of the humeral head.

Posterior Glide of the Humeral Head

Posterior humeral head glide is indicated as a component motion for internal rotation and flexion. The patient is supine, and the clinician stands at the patient's shoulder facing the patient. The anterior/distal surface of the humerus is grasped with one hand, while the opposite hand contacts the proximal anterior humeral surface, exerting a posterior force (**Figure 10-41**).

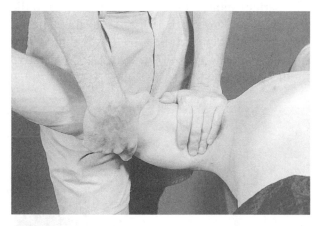

Figure 10-41 Glenohumeral joint mobilization technique: posterior glide of the humeral head.

Self-Mobilization Techniques

■ Lateral Glide

The patient is seated in a chair at the side of the table, with the involved extremity resting in the scapular plane on the table. The uninvolved hand is placed on the medial humerus just below the axilla. The patient applies gentle force in the lateral direction with the uninvolved hand (**Figure 10-42**).

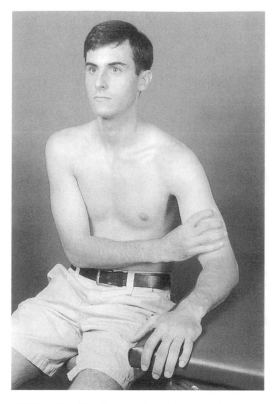

Figure 10-42   Self-mobilization technique: lateral glenohumeral glide.

Inferior Glide

The patient stands at the edge of the table, and the involved hand grasps the edge of the table. The patient leans away from the edge of the table while maintaining the grasp (**Figure 10-43**). Alternative methods include the following:

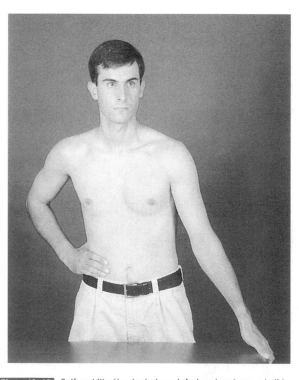

Figure 10-43   Self-mobilization technique: inferior glenohumeral glide.

- The patient sits in a chair with the involved extremity resting in the coronal plane on the table. The uninvolved hand is placed on the deltoid. The patient applies gentle force in the inferior direction with the uninvolved hand.

- The patient stands with the involved upper extremity in neutral position, and the uninvolved hand grasps the humerus just above the epicondyles. The patient then applies gentle force in the inferior direction with the uninvolved hand.

Posterior Glide

The patient is prone on the table and rests on the elbows before allowing the body weight to shift downward (**Figure 10-44**).

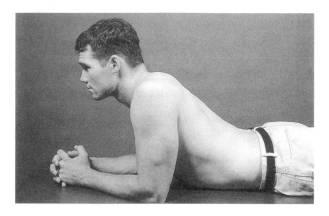

Figure 10-44   Self-mobilization technique: posterior glenohumeral glide.

Anterior Glide

The patient is supine on the table with shoulders extended and rests on flexed elbows before allowing the body weight to shift downward (**Figure 10-45**).

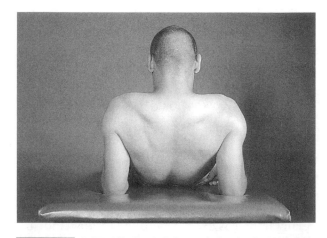

Figure 10-45   Self-mobilization technique: anterior glenohumeral glide.

Range-of-Motion Exercises

■ Passive Range-of-Motion Exercises with a Wand

The following ROM exercises are performed using a wand or cane.

Shoulder Flexion

The patient stands or is supine, holding the wand at waist level with palms pronated. Both upper extremities are lifted directly overhead in the sagittal plane, guiding the involved extremity with the uninvolved extremity (**Figure 10-46**).

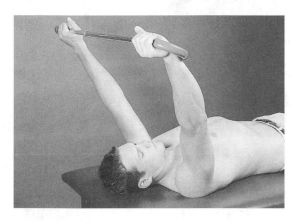

Figure 10-46 Range-of-motion exercise: shoulder flexion.

Shoulder Abduction

The patient stands or is supine, holding the wand at waist level with the involved hand supinated and the uninvolved hand pronated. The patient guides the involved upper extremity with the uninvolved extremity and moves it overhead in a lateral direction in the coronal plane (**Figure 10-47**).

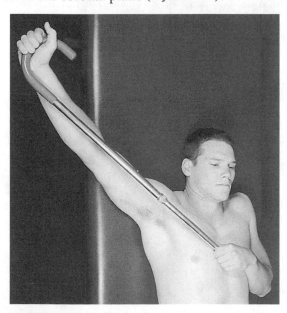

Figure 10-47 Range-of-motion exercise: shoulder abduction.

Shoulder Internal Rotation

The patient stands or is supine, holding the wand at the umbilical level with elbows flexed to 90°. The involved arm is guided medially (**Figure 10-48**).

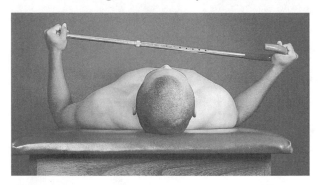

Figure 10-48 Range-of-motion exercise: shoulder internal rotation.

Shoulder External Rotation

The patient stands or is supine, holding the wand at chest level with shoulders abducted to 90° and elbows flexed to 90°. The patient guides the involved hand with the uninvolved hand to move it inferiorly and superiorly from the waist to the overhead position, with the forearm moving in the sagittal plane (**Figure 10-49**).

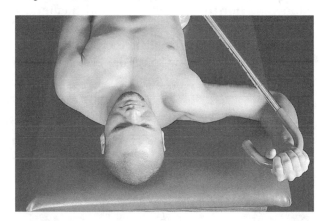

Figure 10-49 Range-of-motion exercise: shoulder external rotation.

Shoulder Horizontal Abduction

The patient stands or is supine and holds the wand at chest level with the involved hand supinated. The patient guides the involved hand with the uninvolved hand to move it laterally and medially in the transverse plane.

Shoulder Extension

The patient sits or stands, holding the wand on the involved side at waist level with the hand in neutral position. The uninvolved hand is held in horizontal adduction with the hand at waist level. The patient guides the involved hand with the uninvolved hand to move it posteriorly in the sagittal plane (**Figure 10-50**).

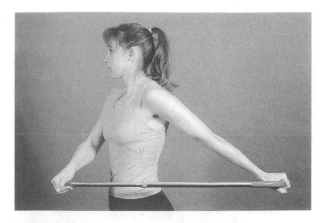

Figure 10-50 Range-of-motion exercise: shoulder extension.

Shoulder Pendulum Exercises (Codman Exercises)

The patient stands flexed at the waist and supports the uninvolved side by leaning on the table. The involved extremity is allowed to hang in a relaxed position free from support. Using a rocking motion of the entire body, the patient oscillates the involved extremity through flexion, extension, horizontal adduction, horizontal abduction, and circumduction (**Figure 10-51**). This exercise should not be performed with weights because the resulting joint distraction stretches the static stabilizers.

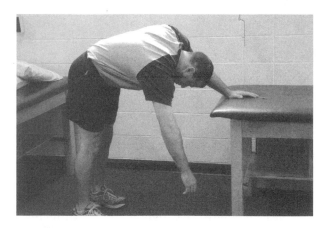

Figure 10-51 Shoulder pendulum exercise: Codman exercises.

Wall Exercises

Shoulder Flexion

The patient stands facing the wall and, with the palm facing the wall, moves toward the wall, sliding the involved hand upward along the wall (**Figure 10-52A**).

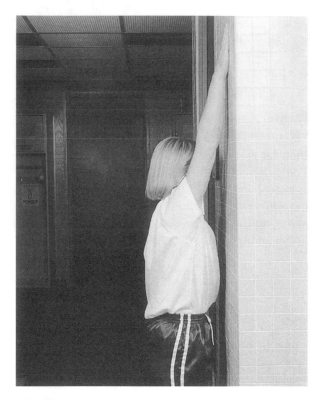

Figure 10-52A Wall exercise: shoulder flexion.

Shoulder Abduction

The patient stands with the involved upper extremity nearest the wall and, with the palm facing the patient, moves toward the wall, sliding the hand upward along the wall (**Figure 10-52B**).

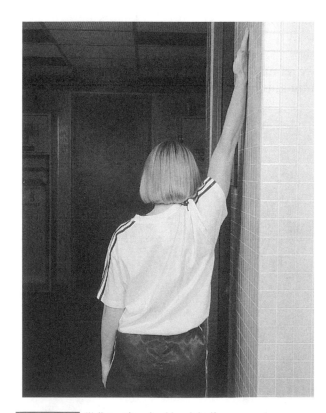

Figure 10-52B Wall exercise: shoulder abduction.

Shoulder Horizontal Abduction

The patient stands facing the wall with the involved shoulder abducted to 90° and the palm flat against wall. The patient then turns the trunk away from the shoulder until he or she feels a stretch (**Figure 10-52C**).

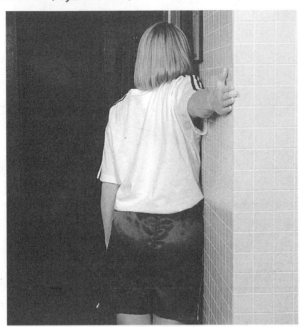

Figure 10-52C   Wall exercise: shoulder horizontal abduction.

Shoulder External Rotation

The patient stands facing a corner or door frame with the involved elbow flexed 90° and the hand against the wall. The patient turns the trunk away from the wall until a stretch is felt (**Figure 10-52D**).

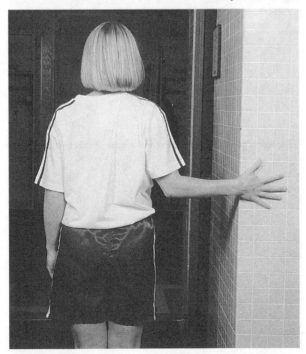

Figure 10-52D   Wall exercise: shoulder external rotation.

▦ Inflated Ball Exercises

Shoulder Flexion

The patient stands facing the wall, holding the ball on the wall with the involved shoulder flexed to 90°. The patient then rolls the ball up the wall by stepping closer to the wall as the upper extremity moves along the ball superiorly in the sagittal plane (**Figure 10-53**).

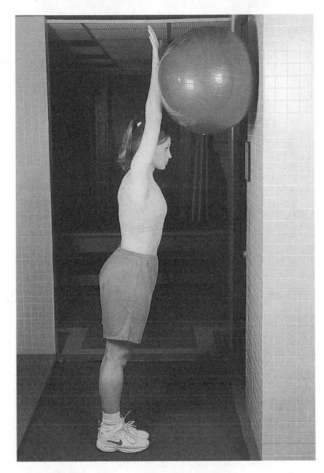

Figure 10-53   Inflated ball exercise: shoulder flexion.

Alternatively, the patient can stand facing a ball that is lying on a table and rest the involved hand low on the ball. The patient then rolls the ball away by leaning the trunk forward, allowing the involved hand to move superiorly as the ball rolls forward.

Shoulder Abduction

The patient stands with the involved shoulder holding the ball to the wall at 90° of abduction. The patient rolls the ball up the wall by stepping closer to the wall, allowing the involved extremity to move superiorly in the coronal plane (**Figure 10-54**).

Alternatively, the patient can stand at the side of the table with the involved upper extremity resting on the ball, which is on the table surface. The patient rolls the ball laterally by leaning the trunk, allowing the involved hand to move along the ball superiorly in the coronal plane.

10

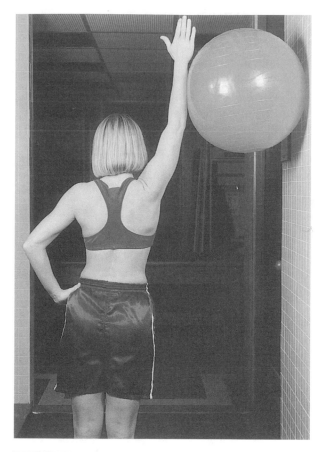

Figure 10-54 Inflated ball exercise: shoulder abduction.

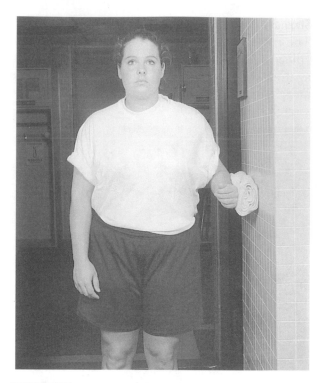

Figure 10-55 Isometric shoulder exercise: abduction.

Strengthening Techniques

Strength is developed through progressive resistance exercises, which can be isolated movements or combined movement patterns. An isolated movement is used to strengthen a particular weak muscle. A common isolated movement is the "empty can," which isolates the supraspinatus muscle. Combined patterns such as proprioceptive neuromuscular facilitation D2 flexion and extension exercises are used to reestablish, encourage, and strengthen a specific functional movement (see chapter 13).

All exercises can be performed with limb weight, body weight, manual resistance, dumbbells, elastic bands, barbells, or machines. They should be performed in the pain-free ROM or as allowed by precautions.

Isometric Shoulder Exercises

Abduction

The patient stands with the involved upper extremity next to a wall, with the elbow flexed to 90°. The patient presses a pillow or rolled towel into the wall with the elbow held away from the body in the coronal plane (**Figure 10-55**).

Adduction

The patient stands with a pillow or rolled towel held between the trunk and involved elbow with the elbow flexed to 90°. The patient presses the elbow toward the trunk in the coronal plane (**Figure 10-56**).

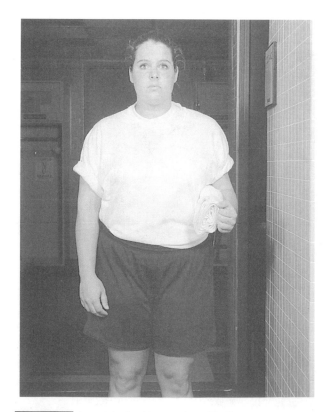

Figure 10-56 Isometric shoulder exercise: adduction.

Flexion

The patient stands facing the wall with the involved elbow flexed to 90° and presses the fist anteriorly in the sagittal plane into a pillow or rolled towel held against the wall (**Figure 10-57**).

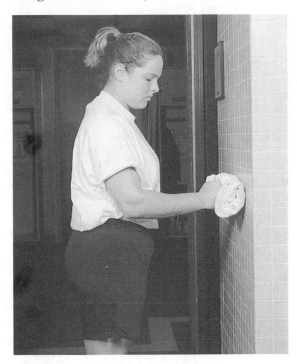

Figure 10-57   Isometric shoulder exercise: flexion.

Extension

The patient stands facing away from the wall with the involved elbow flexed to 90° and presses the elbow posteriorly in the sagittal plane against a pillow or rolled towel held against the wall (**Figure 10-58**).

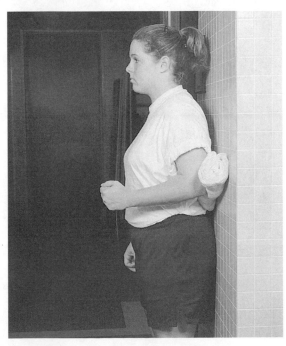

Figure 10-58   Isometric shoulder exercise: extension.

Internal Rotation

The patient stands facing the corner of the wall with the involved elbow flexed to 90° and presses the fist medially in the transverse plane into a pillow or rolled towel held against the wall (**Figure 10-59**).

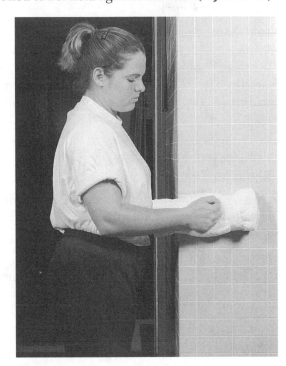

Figure 10-59   Isometric shoulder exercise: internal rotation.

External Rotation

The patient stands facing the corner of the wall with the involved elbow flexed to 90° and presses the dorsum of the hand or fist laterally in the transverse plane into or a rolled towel held against the wall (**Figure 10-60**).

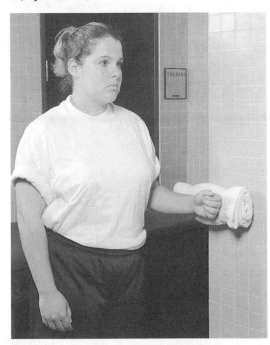

Figure 10-60   Isometric shoulder exercise: external rotation.

10

Horizontal Adduction

The patient stands facing the corner of the wall with the involved shoulder and elbow flexed to 90° and presses the medial forearm medially in the transverse plane into a pillow or rolled towel held against the wall.

Horizontal Abduction

The patient stands facing the corner of the wall with the involved shoulder and elbow flexed to 90° and presses the lateral forearm laterally in the transverse plane into a pillow or rolled towel held against the wall.

Progressive Resistance Shoulder Exercises

Progressive resistance exercises can be performed using surgical tubing, Thera-Band, free weights, or weight machines.

Flexion

The patient stands or sits with the upper extremity in a neutral position at the side and lifts the upper extremity in the sagittal plane forward from the body in a pain-free arc (**Figure 10-61**).

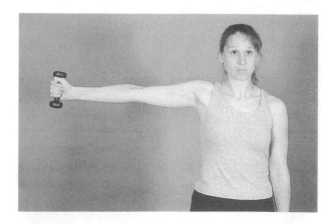

Figure 10-62   Progressive resistance shoulder exercise: abduction.

Extension

The patient stands or sits with the upper extremity in neutral position at the side. The patient then lifts the upper extremity in the sagittal plane backward from the body (**Figure 10-63**).

Alternatively, the patient can lie prone on the table with the upper extremity in a relaxed position over the edge of the supporting surface. The patient lifts the upper extremity in the sagittal plane toward the midline of the body and continues beyond the neutral position if possible.

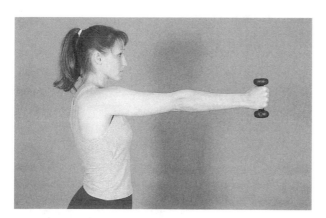

Figure 10-61   Progressive resistance shoulder exercise: flexion.

Abduction

The patient stands or sits with the upper extremity in the neutral position. The patient abducts the upper extremity in the coronal plane away from the body (**Figure 10-62**).

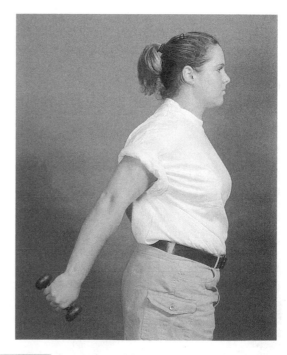

Figure 10-63   Progressive resistance shoulder exercise: extension.

External Rotation

The patient stands or sits with the upper extremity at the side and the elbow flexed to 90° (**Figure 10-64**). The patient pulls the tubing by moving the hand away from the midline of the body in the transverse plane.

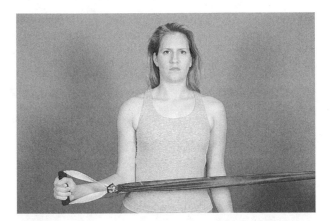

Figure 10-64   Progressive resistance shoulder exercise: external rotation.

Alternative methods include the following:

- The patient lies on the uninvolved side, with the involved upper extremity at the side and the elbow flexed to 90°. The patient lifts a weight by moving the hand away from the midline of body in the transverse plane.

- The patient lies on the involved side with the involved upper extremity in a relaxed position over the edge of the supporting surface. While holding a weight in the involved hand, the patient turns the upper extremity outward as a unit in the transverse plane of the limb.

- The patient stands or sits with the upper extremity abducted to 90° and the elbow flexed to 90° and stabilized in this position by a supporting surface. The patient pulls the tubing by moving the hand posteriorly in the sagittal plane.

Internal Rotation

The patient stands or sits with the upper extremity at the side and the elbow flexed to 90° (**Figure 10-65**). The patient pulls the tubing by moving the hand toward the midline of the body in the transverse plane.

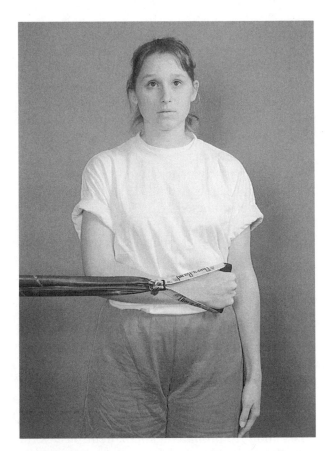

Figure 10-65   Progressive resistance shoulder exercise: internal rotation.

Alternative methods include the following:

- The patient lies on the involved side of the body with the involved upper extremity at the side and the elbow flexed to 90°. The patient lifts a weight by moving the hand toward the midline of the body in the transverse plane.

- The patient lies on the involved side with the involved upper extremity in a relaxed position over the edge of the supporting surface. The patient holds a weight and turns the upper extremity inward as a unit in the transverse plane of the limb.

- The patient stands or sits with the upper extremity abducted to 90° and the elbow flexed to 90°. This position is stabilized by a supporting surface. The patient pulls the tubing by moving the hand anteriorly in the sagittal plane.

Seated Rows

The patient sits with the trunk in neutral, the shoulders flexed between 70° and 90° the elbows fully extended, and the hands holding the tubing with a neutral grip. The patient pulls the tubing to the umbilicus by retracting the scapulae, extending the shoulders, and flexing the elbows.

Latissimus Pull-Downs

The patient sits with the shoulders in full flexion and the elbows fully extended and holds the resistance with a supinated grip. The patient pulls the resistance downward to chest level by retracting and depressing the scapulae, extending the shoulders, and flexing the elbows.

Alternatively, the patient can sit with the shoulders flexed to 90° and the elbows flexed to 90° and hold the resistance with a supinated grip. The patient pulls the resistance downward to chest level by retracting and depressing the scapulae, extending the shoulders, and flexing the elbows.

Shoulder Press

The patient stands or sits while holding weights at shoulder height, with the hands shoulder width apart and grip pronated. The patient pushes the weights upward to a position of shoulder abduction, flexion, and elbow extension (**Figure 10-66**).

Supraspinatus Open Can ("Full Can")

The patient stands with the involved extremity at the side in a neutral position and holds a weight with a neutral grip, thumbs up (**Figure 10-67**). The patient abducts the upper extremity in the scapular plane approximately 30° anterior to the coronal plane (military salute).

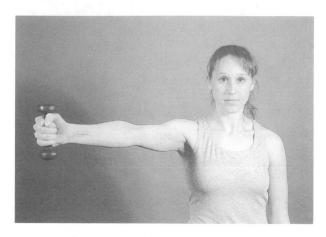

Figure 10-67 Progressive resistance shoulder exercise: supraspinatus open can ("full can").

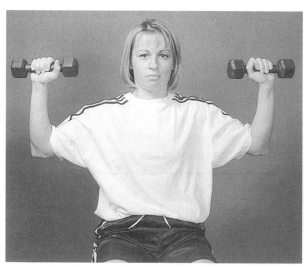
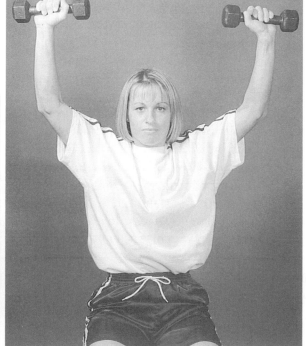

A   B

Figure 10-66 Progressive resistance shoulder exercise: shoulder press.

Push-Up with a Plus

The patient performs a push-up in the standard or modified position. On reaching the top position of the movement, the patient protracts the scapulae to push beyond the normal stopping position (the "plus") (**Figure 10-68**).

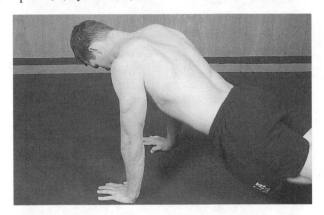

Figure 10-68 Progressive resistance shoulder exercise: push-up with a plus.

Hughston Prone Series

The Hughston Clinic protocol includes exercises performed with the patient prone. The patient begins the exercise by performing 10 repetitions with no weight in the hand. Each week (or at another interval determined by the physician or clinician), the number of repetitions is increased by 10 until 60 continuous repetitions can be performed. The motion is held for 2 seconds and then repeated. One pound of weight is added, and the sequence is repeated until the patient can perform 60 repetitions with 2 or 3 lb of weight. The only rest period occurs when changing position (**Figure 10-69**).

10

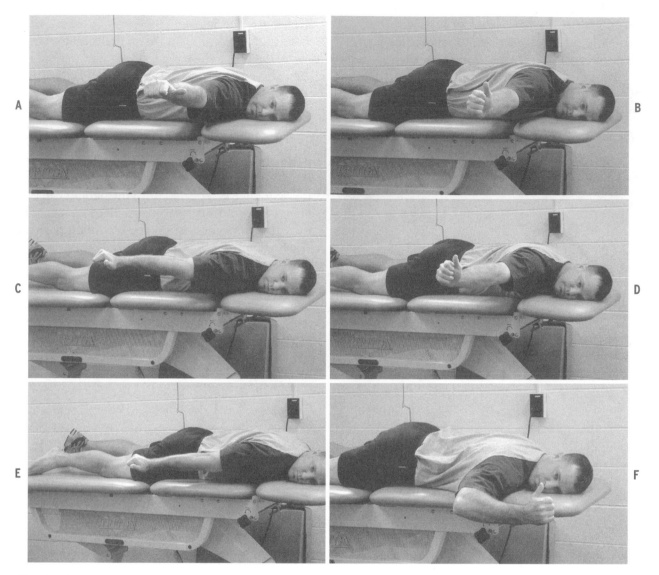

Figure 10-69 Hughston prone series. **A.** The involved extremity is abducted to 90° and the thumb pointed parallel to the floor. The patient lifts the extremity away from the floor. **B.** The involved extremity is abducted to 90° with the thumb pointed toward the ceiling. The patient lifts the extremity away from the floor, pauses for 2 seconds, lowers the arm to the starting position, and repeats the movement. **C.** The humerus is abducted to 45° with the thumb parallel to the floor. The arm is lifted away from the floor. **D.** The humerus is abducted to 45° with the thumb pointing toward the ceiling. The arm is lifted away from the floor. **E.** The humerus is at the side with the palm parallel to the floor. The arm is lifted away from the floor. **F.** The humerus is abducted to 90° and the elbow flexed 90°. The humerus is externally rotated.

■ References

1. Wirth MA, Rockwood CA: Acute and chronic traumatic injuries of the sternoclavicular joint. *J Am Acad Orthop Surg* 1996;4:268-278.

2. Craig EV: Fractures of the clavicle, in Rockwood CA Jr, Matsen FA III (eds): *The Shoulder*. Philadelphia, PA, WB Saunders, 1990, pp 367-412.

3. Reid J, Kennedy JK: Direct fracture of the clavicle with symptoms simulating a cervical rig. *Br Med J* 1925;2:608-609.

4. Quesana F: Technique for the roentgen: Diagnosis of fractures of the clavicle. *Surg Gynecol Obstet* 1926;42:4261-4281.

5. Rowe CR: An atlas of anatomy and treatment of mid-clavicular fractures. *Clin Orthop* 1968;58:29-42.

6. Weiner DS, O'Dell HW: Fractures of the first rib associated with injuries to the clavicle. *J Trauma* 1969;9:412-422.

7. Yates DW: Complications of fractures of the clavicle. *Injury* 1976;7:189-193.

8. Grana WA, Kalenak A: *Clinical Sports Medicine*, ed 2. Philadelphia, PA, WB Saunders, 1998, pp 143-199.

9. Rockwood CA Jr, Matsen FA III: The acromioclavicular joint, in *The Shoulder*, ed 2. Philadelphia, PA, WB Saunders, 1998, pp 480-529.

10. Kibler WB: The role of the scapula in athletic shoulder function. *Am J Sports Med* 1998;26:325-337.

11. Burkhart SS, Morgan CD, Kibler WB: The disabled throwing shoulder: Spectrum of pathology. Part III: The SICK scapula, scapular dyskinesis, the kinetic chain, and rehabilitation. *Arthroscopy* 2003;19:641-661.

12. Lukasiewicz AC, McClure P, Michener L, Pratt N, Sennett B: Comparison of 3-dimensional scapular position and orientation between subjects with and without shoulder impingement. *J Orthop Sports Phys Ther* 1999;29:574-583.

13. Ludewig PM, Cook TM: Alterations in shoulder kinematics and associated muscle activity in people with symptoms of shoulder impingement. *Phys Ther* 2000;80:276-291.

14. McMullen J, Uhl TL: A kinetic chain approach for shoulder rehabilitation. *J Athl Train* 2000;35:329-337.

15. Andrews JR, Zarins B, Wilk KE: *Injuries in Baseball*. Philadelphia, PA, Lippincott-Raven, 1998, p 452.

16. Cooper A: On the dislocation of the os humeri upon the dorsum scapula and upon fractures near the shoulder joint. *Guys Hosp Rep* 1839;4:265.

17. Hovelius L, Thorling J, Fredin H: Recurrent anterior dislocation of the shoulder: Results after the Bankhart and Putti-Platt operations. *J Bone Joint Surg Am* 1979;61:566-569.

18. Rokous JR, Feagin JA, Abbott HG: Modified axillary roentgengram: A useful adjunct in the diagnosis of recurrent instability of the shoulder. *Clin Orthop* 1972;82:84-86.

19. Neer CS II: Anterior acromioplasty for the chronic impingement syndrome in the shoulder: A preliminary report. *J Bone Joint Surg Am* 1972;54:41-50.

20. Ellman H, Kay SP: Arthroscopic subacromial decompression for chronic impingement: Two- to five-year results. *J Bone Joint Surg Br* 1991;73:395-398.

21. Ellman H: Arthroscopic subacromial decompression: Analysis of one- to three-year results. *Arthroscopy* 1987;3:173-181.

22. Gartsman GM, Blair ME Jr, Noble PC, Bennett JB, Tullos HS: Arthroscopic subacromial decompression: An anatomical study. *Am J Sports Med* 1988;16:48-50.

23. Gartsman GM: Arthroscopic acromioplasty for lesions of the rotator cuff. *J Bone Joint Surg Am* 1990;72:169-180.

24. Matthews L, Burkhead W, Gordon S, Racanelli J, Ruland L: Acromial fracture: A complication of arthroscopic subacromial decompression. *J Shoulder Elbow Surg* 1994;3:256-261.

25. Soble MG, Kaye AD, Guay RC: Rotator cuff tear: Clinical experience with sonographic detection. *Radiology* 1989;173:319-321.

26. Brandt TD, Cardone BW, Grant TH, Post M, Weiss CA: Rotator cuff sonography: A reassessment. *Radiology* 1989;173:323-327.

27. Vick CW, Bell SA: Rotator cuff tears: Diagnosis with sonography. *Am J Roentgenol* 1990;154:121-123.

28. Zlatkin MB, Iannotti JP, Roberts MC, et al: Rotator cuff tears: Diagnostic performance of MR imaging. *Radiology* 1989;172:223-229.

29. Rafii M, Firooznia H, Sherman O, et al: Rotator cuff lesions: Signal patterns at MR imaging. *Radiology* 1990;177:817-823.

30. Kjellin I, Ho CP, Cervilla V, et al: Alterations in the supraspinatus tendon at MR imaging: Correlation with histopathologic findings in cadavers. *Radiology* 1991;181:837-841.

31. Weber SC: Arthroscopic debridement and acromioplasty versus mini-open repair in the treatment of significant partial-thickness rotator cuff tears. *Arthroscopy* 1999;15:126-131.

32. Burkhead WZ: The biceps tendon, in Rockwood CA Jr, Matsen FA III (eds): *The Shoulder*. Philadelphia, PA, WB Saunders, 1990, pp 791-886.

33. Waugh RE, Hathcock TA, Elliott JL: Rupture of muscles and tendons, with particular reference to rupture (or elongation of long tendon) of biceps brachii with report of fifty cases. *Stugert* 1949;15:370-378.

34. Guidi EJ, Zuckermann JD: Glenoid labral lesions, in Andrews JR, Wilk KE: *The Athlete's Shoulder*. New York, NY, Churchill Livingstone, 1994, pp 231-240.

35. Hill H, Sachs M: Grooved defect of the humeral head: A frequently unrecognized complication of dislocation of the shoulder joint. *Radiology* 1940;35:690-700.

36. Rowe CR: *The Shoulder*. New York, NY, Churchill Livingstone, 1988, p 187.

37. Anderson D, Zvirbulis R, Ciullo J: Scapular manipulation for reduction of anterior shoulder dislocation. *Clin Orthop* 1982;164:181-183.

38. Stimson L: An easy method of reducing dislocation of the shoulder and the hip. *NY Mecl Rec* 1900;57:356-357.

39. Kocher E: Eine neue rcductionsmethodc fur schulterverrenkung. *Bert Klin Wbcherrschr* 1870;7:101-105.

40. Itoi E, Sashi R, Minagawa H, Shimizu T, Wakabayashi I, Sato K: Position of immobilization after dislocation of the glenohumeral joint. *J Bone Joint Surg Am* 2001;83:661-667.

41. Arciero RA, Taylor DC, Snyder RJ, Uhorchak JM: Arthroscopic bioabsorbable tack stabilization of initial anterior shoulder dislocations: A preliminary report. *Arthroscopy* 1995;11:410-417.

42. Arciero RA, Wheeler JH, Ryan JB, McBride JT: Arthroscopic Bankhart repair versus nonoperative treatment for acute, initial anterior shoulder dislocations. *Am J Sports Med* 1994;22:589-594.

43. Schenk TJ, Brems JJ: Multidirectional instability of the shoulder: Pathophysiology, diagnosis, and management. *J Am Acad Orthop Surg* 1998;6:65-72.

44. Cordasco FA: Understanding multidirectional instability of the shoulder. *J Athl Train* 2000;35:278-285.

45. Satterwhite YE: Evaluation and management of recurrent anterior shoulder instability. *J Athl Train* 2000;35: 273-277.

46. Harryman DT II: Common surgical approaches to the shoulder. *Instr Course Lect* 1992;41:3-11.

47. Arciero RA, Wheeler JH, Ryan JB, McBride JT: Arthroscopic Bankart repair versus nonoperative treatment for acute, initial anterior shoulder dislocations. *Am J Sports Med* 1994;22:589-594.

48. Harryman DT, Mack LA, Wang KY, Jackins SE, Richardson ML, Matsen FA III: Repairs of the rotator cuff: Correlation of functional results with integrity of the cuff. *J Bone Joint Surg Am* 1991;73:982-989.

49. Payne LZ, Altchek DW, Craig EV, Warren RF: Arthroscopic treatment of partial rotator cuff tears in young athletes: A preliminary report. *Am J Sports Med* 1997;25: 299-305.

50. Miniaci A, MacDonald PB: Open surgical techniques in the athlete's shoulder. *Clin Sports Med* 1991;10:929-954.

51. Tibone JE, Jobe FW, Kerlan RK, et al: Shoulder impingement syndrome in athletes treated by an anterior acromioplasty. *Clin Orthop* 1985;19R:134-140.

52. Penny JN, Welsh RP: Shoulder impingement syndromes in athletes and their surgical management. *Am J Sports Med* 1981;9:11-15.

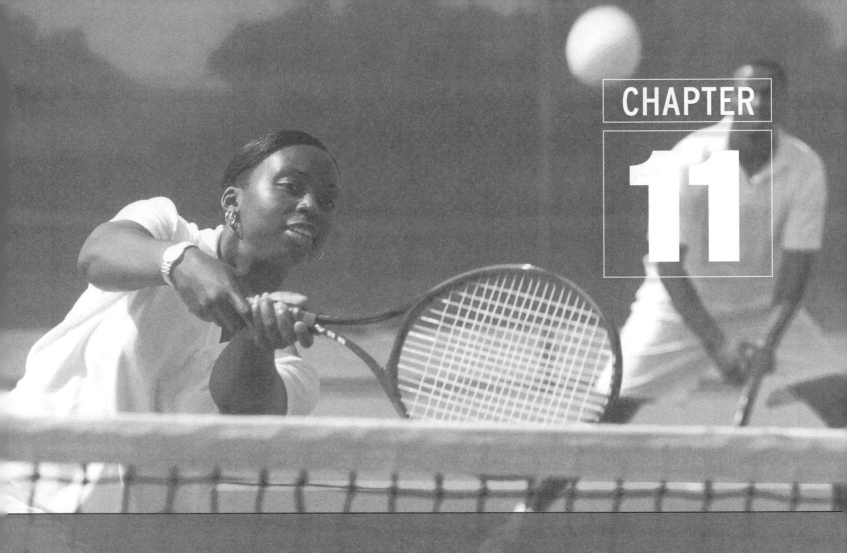

Elbow Injuries

Jeff Ryan, PT, ATC
John P. Salvo, MD

Distal Biceps Tendon Rupture

CLINICAL PRESENTATION

History

Acute pain in the antecubital fossa while lifting a heavy object
A "pop" may be reported.

Observation

Marked deformity in the antecubital fossa
The biceps brachii is retracted proximally.
Elbow and forearm ecchymosis

Functional Status

Decreased range of motion (ROM), especially during elbow extension, which stretches the unattached tendon
Marked pain and weakness during elbow flexion and forearm supination

Physical Evaluation Findings

Palpable biceps tendon defect; the tendon may be absent from the antecubital fossa.
Resisted elbow flexion is weak or absent.
Resisted forearm supination is weak or absent.

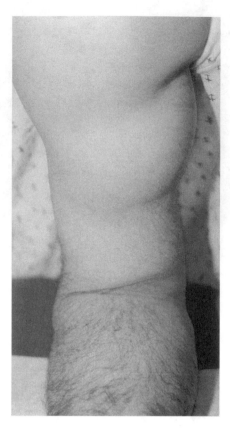

Figure 11-1 Proximal retraction of the biceps muscle belly with attempted elbow flexion. (Reproduced with permission from Ramsey ML: Distal biceps tendon injuries: Diagnosis and management. *J Am Acad Orthop Surg* 1999;7:199-207.)

Complete rupture of the distal biceps brachii tendon represents approximately 3% of all biceps injuries. Usually involving the dominant arm, rupture occurs when the patient lifts a heavy object.[1] Most patients are males in their 40s and 50s. Although many injuries are work related, sport-related injuries also occur in activities such as weightlifting.

The patient usually reports sudden pain and weakness while lifting a heavy object. Antecubital fossa palpation reveals a loss of tendon continuity (**Figure 11-1**). Weakness with supination is demonstrated. With a partial rupture or a long delay between injury and examination, the diagnosis may be less clear; magnetic resonance imaging (MRI) can be useful.

Most surgeons recommend early reattachment of complete distal biceps tendon ruptures. The goal is stable reattachment to allow for early rehabilitation.

Differential Diagnosis

Biceps brachii strain

Imaging Techniques

The standard elbow radiographic series—anteroposterior (AP), lateral, and oblique—reveals tuberosity avulsion. MRI or ultrasonography can identify a partial rupture or, if the diagnosis is delayed, a ruptured and retracted biceps (**Figure 11-2**).

Definitive Diagnosis

The definitive diagnosis is based on the clinical findings and supported by MRI findings.

Pathomechanics and Functional Limitations

Pain and loss of mechanical function of the biceps brachii cause difficulty with elbow motion extremes. Resisted elbow flexion with the forearm in neutral results in discomfort, but resisted elbow flexion with the forearm supinated produces frank pain and deformity.

Pain with active elbow motion may decrease after a few days, but pain and weakness persist with resisted and weight-loaded flexion and supination. Manual laborers, weightlifters, and other athletes have difficulty returning to their previous activities without surgical intervention.

■ Immediate Management

The elbow in flexion should be immobilized and ice applied to decrease local inflammation and muscle spasm.

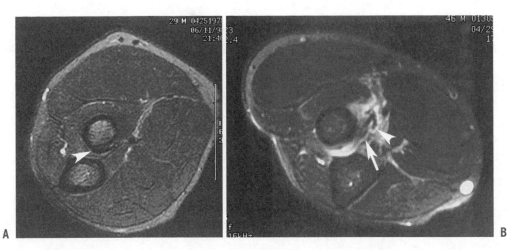

Figure 11-2   MRI of a biceps tendon rupture. **A.** Normal biceps tendon insertion (arrowhead). **B.** Partial rupture at the insertion (arrowhead) with degeneration of the distal biceps insertion (arrow). (Reproduced with permission from Ramsey ML: Distal biceps tendon injuries: Diagnosis and management. *J Am Acad Orthop Surg* 1999;7:199-207.)

Medications

Narcotic analgesics may be prescribed for acute pain management. Nonsteroidal anti-inflammatory drugs (NSAIDs) may be avoided with ruptures because of possible platelet dysfunction and the urgent need for tendon repair.

Postinjury Management

Early diagnosis allows repair within 3 weeks of injury and produces the best surgical results. The patient is placed in a posterior splint or a hinged ROM brace for comfort, and palliative care is provided until surgical repair is performed. Patients with partial ruptures or medical contraindications to surgery should start on a rehabilitation program as soon as swelling decreases.

Surgical Intervention

Most patients benefit from surgical reattachment of the distal biceps tendon to the radial tuberosity (**ST** 11-1). The most common surgical procedures are the two-incision technique and a one-incision technique through an anterior approach.[2-4] The two-incision technique is less likely to result in radial nerve injury but has an increased incidence of heterotopic bone formation. This risk can be minimized by copious irrigation of the surgical sites and by using a drill and osteotome instead of a burr to excavate the radial tuberosity.

Although the one-incision technique is more likely to cause radial nerve injury from overzealous traction, the incidence of heterotopic bone formation is lower. Using a single anterior incision to reach the radial tubercle is technically more demanding because of radial nerve proximity. Advances in the suture anchors used for tendon fixation have limited the need for extensive dissection to expose the cubital fossa.[5,6] An Achilles tendon allograft may be required to repair a chronic distal biceps tendon rupture.[7]

Postoperative Management

After surgical repair, the elbow is splinted in 90° of flexion with the forearm supinated or in neutral position for 7 to 10 days. The sutures are then removed and the patient placed in a hinged flexion-assist splint with a 30° extension block for another 7 weeks.

Injury-Specific Treatment and Rehabilitation Concerns

Specific Concerns

Protect the healing repair.
Prevent excessive stress on the biceps brachii tendon based on the healing stage.
Encourage early ROM to decrease scar tissue formation and prevent functional shortening.

Conservative treatment of distal biceps tendon ruptures can result in considerable, permanent loss of strength and endurance of elbow flexion and supination and typically is not recommended.[8]

With advances in secure surgical fixation techniques, postoperative rehabilitation has become more aggressive, leading to better outcomes with

Palliative Relief of the symptoms without correcting the underlying cause.

Heterotopic The formation of lamellar bone within soft tissues as the result of osteoblastic activity, similar to myositis ossificans.

S|T **Surgical Technique   11-1**

Repair of a Distal Biceps Tendon Rupture

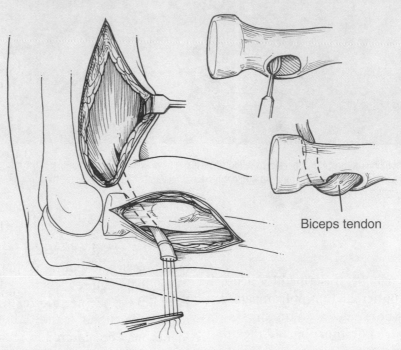

Biceps tendon

Indications

Acute rupture of the distal biceps tendon

Overview

Two-Incision Technique (pictured)
1. A transverse incision is made along the anterior cubital crease.
2. The distal end of the biceps tendon is located.
3. Sutures are placed through the tendon.
4. A second incision is made along the ulnar border of the dorsal forearm to expose the radial tuberosity, where sutures will be secured.
5. A trough with suture tunnels is made in the radial tuberosity.
6. Sutures are passed through the bone tunnels, the tendon is pulled down into the trough, and the sutures are tied, fixating the tendon.
7. The repair is tested in gentle pronation, supination, flexion, and extension.
8. The elbow is placed in a posterior splint in flexion.

One-Incision Technique
1. An anterior incision is made along the cubital crease.
2. The distal end of the biceps tendon is located.
3. Sutures are placed through the tendon.
4. With the forearm supinated, the radial tuberosity is identified in the depth of the anterior cubital exposure.
5. Using two or three suture anchors, the tendon is reattached to the radial tuberosity.
6. The repair is tested in gentle pronation, supination, flexion, and extension.
7. The elbow is placed in a posterior splint in flexion.

Functional Limitations

Radial nerve complications can occur with either procedure but more frequently result from the one-incision technique. Early protected ROM is important to attaining functional outcomes. Long-term strength deficits may occur in elbow flexion and supination but usually are not functionally limiting. Soft-tissue healing of the tendon to a bony bed requires avoiding traction (elbow extension) on the repair in the early postoperative period.

Implications for Rehabilitation

Protected return of motion and strength is necessary to ensure healing of the repair. Initially, the patient's arm is splinted or casted in neutral forearm position and 90° of elbow flexion.

Figure adapted with permission from the Mayo Clinic.

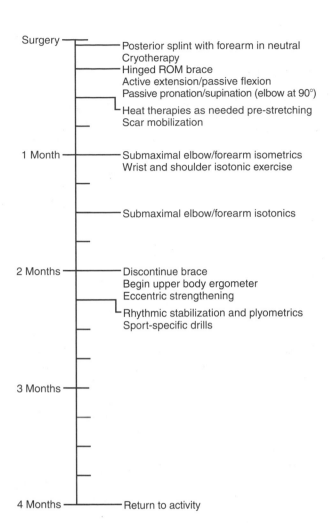

Surgery — Posterior splint with forearm in neutral
Cryotherapy
Hinged ROM brace
Active extension/passive flexion
Passive pronation/supination (elbow at 90°)
Heat therapies as needed pre-stretching
Scar mobilization

1 Month — Submaximal elbow/forearm isometrics
Wrist and shoulder isotonic exercise

— Submaximal elbow/forearm isotonics

2 Months — Discontinue brace
Begin upper body ergometer
Eccentric strengthening
Rhythmic stabilization and plyometrics
Sport-specific drills

3 Months

4 Months — Return to activity

Note: Time frames are approximate. Function is the guide.

fewer complications.[9] ROM is performed within the passive limits so the patient feels no tension at the repair site. The brace is then set to allow this motion. The brace ROM is incrementally advanced as the patient gains motion and healing progresses. The patient can discontinue brace use when ROM is full but no sooner than 8 weeks after surgery in order to protect the repair from reinjury.

Initially, self-ranging (to tolerance) exercises of active extension and passive flexion are performed with the arm supported on a table. Passive pronation and supination are conducted with the elbow in 90° of flexion. The brace is worn while performing the exercises for the first 2 weeks. Properly educating the patient in maintaining motion within pain-free limits is essential, and self-ranging exercises are continued until 6 weeks after surgery. If the patient has not obtained full ROM, passive ROM is instituted. If a contracture appears to be developing, motion is lost, or a plateau lasts longer than a week, passive ROM may begin sooner.

Moist heat or a warm whirlpool bath may be helpful before ROM exercises to promote relaxation and increase tissue extensibility. Scar massage and mobilization are helpful to minimize excessive scar formation in the cubital crease. Use of an upper body ergometer to actively warm the joint can be initiated 8 weeks after surgery.

Strengthening exercises commence at 4 weeks postoperatively. Initially these consist of submaximal isometric activities for elbow extension, flexion, pronation, and supination. Shoulder and wrist isotonic exercises are performed by attaching cuff weights around the wrist during the shoulder exercises. Submaximal isotonic exercises to strengthen the elbow musculature begin 6 weeks after surgery. At 8 weeks, tissue healing to bone is sufficient to allow strengthening to progress to patient tolerance. The eccentric phase of strengthening is emphasized, because this is usually the muscle-contraction phase during which the rupture occurred.

At 12 weeks, more functional activities focus on the patient's needs. Proprioceptive and plyometric exercises, such as tossing a ball against a back stop or tossing a medicine ball to develop power, occupational activities, and sport-specific drills can be initiated.

■ Estimated Amount of Time Lost

Return to full activities can be achieved after 4 to 6 months of postoperative rehabilitation. Secure tendon fixation to the radial tuberosity allows early rehabilitation. Patients with partial ruptures may return to full activities after 4 to 6 weeks of rehabilitation.

The elbow is prone to stiffness from scar formation within the cubital fossa. Heterotopic ossification has been reported with distal biceps repair. Early recognition and treatment of these conditions should limit their effects on outcomes and return to activity, but any increased joint stiffness postoperatively increases the time lost. Delayed surgical repair also delays the return to play.

■ Return-to-Play Criteria

The patient must have ROM and strength within functional limits to return to activity. Full restoration of ROM and strength is possible after surgical repair. Typically the dominant arm is injured, which must be considered when comparing progress with the contralateral extremity.

Functional Bracing
No bracing is required upon return to activity.

Ulnar Collateral Ligament Sprain

CLINICAL PRESENTATION

History

Pain during activities that apply a valgus load to the elbow (eg, throwing)

Chronic instability can occur with repetitive, long-term valgus loading of the elbow.

The patient is often unable to continue with the activity.

A past history of elbow pain may be reported.

Possible radicular symptoms along the ulnar nerve distribution

Observation

Medial elbow swelling may be noted.

Functional Status

ROM is usually full.

Athletes report pain during throwing and decreased throwing velocity and distance.

Physical Evaluation Findings

Pain during UCL palpation posterior to the medial epicondyle

Positive valgus stress test with the elbow flexed to 30° and 90°

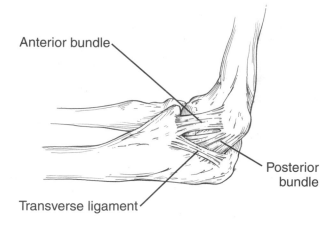

Figure 11-3   The UCL complex consists of the anterior bundle (functionally the most important for valgus stability), the posterior bundle, and the transverse ligament (oblique bundle). The anterior bundle is further subdivided into anterior and posterior bands, which perform reciprocal functions. (Adapted with permission from Kvitne RS, Jobe FW: Ligamentous and posterior compartment injuries, in Jobe FW [ed]: *Techniques in Upper Extremity Sports Injuries.* Philadelphia, PA, Mosby-Year Book, 1996, p 412.)

Injury to the ulnar collateral ligament (UCL) is most commonly encountered in athletes who participate in throwing and overhead sports. The injuries result from tremendous valgus stress at the elbow during the throwing motion, especially the late cocking and early acceleration phases.

The restraining contribution of bony and soft tissues in valgus stress depends on the elbow position.[10-12] The articulating surfaces, joint capsule, and UCL complex provide almost equal amounts of restraint against valgus stress in elbow extension. The UCL complex has three parts—anterior and posterior bundles and the transverse ligament (**Figure 11-3**). As the joint flexes, the UCL complex assumes more of the restraining role. The anterior bundle, in both extension and flexion, provides almost all of the medial ligament complex's contribution in restraining valgus stress.[10-12]

Medial elbow biomechanics are often described relative to the pitching motion. Peak angular velocities and valgus stress are greatest during the late cocking and early acceleration phases. These forces can exceed the tensile strength of the medial ligamentous and tendinous structures, at which point the force must be absorbed by the other medial elbow structures. The stresses are initially transmitted to the flexor pronator musculature (especially the pronator teres) and then to the deeper UCL. When the ligamentous and musculature tensile strength is ex-

ceeded, injury occurs. With continued repetitive valgus stress, ligament attenuation or frank rupture can occur. Improper mechanics, poor flexibility, and inadequate conditioning can worsen symptoms and lead to frank ligament rupture. Valgus stress also causes compressive forces on the lateral elbow.

Differential Diagnosis

Medial epicondylitis, ulnar neuropathy, cervical radiculopathy

Imaging Techniques

Radiographs reveal any traction osteophytes or avulsion fractures. Stress radiographs can reveal the amount of valgus laxity (**Figure 11-4**). MRI is excellent for UCL imaging.

Definitive Diagnosis

The definitive diagnosis is based on the clinical findings and MRI studies.

Pathomechanics and Functional Limitations

Patients with UCL injuries are unable to continue with activities that place a valgus stress on the elbow, such as throwing or swinging a golf club. Many lose significant velocity or distance, and the golf swing is affected by the valgus stress placed on the dominant extremity (ie, right arm for right-handed golfers). They usually do not have difficulty with any other activities.

■ Immediate Management

In acute ruptures, ice is applied, and the extremity is splinted or placed in a sling as needed for comfort.

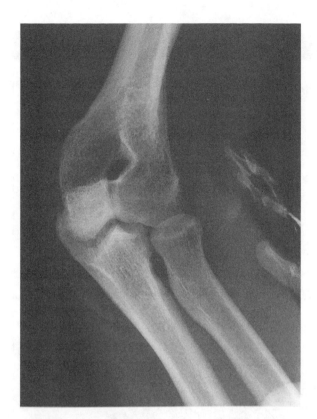

Figure 11-4 Stress radiograph demonstrating UCL deficiency during the application of a valgus load. (Reproduced with permission from Morrey BF: Acute and chronic instability of the elbow. *J Am Acad Orthop Surg* 1996;4:117-128.)

Medications

NSAIDs may be prescribed to control pain and inflammation.

Postinjury Management

Postinjury management consists of rest, NSAIDs, and early rehabilitation aimed at regaining full motion and strength in the first 2 to 4 weeks. Any ulnar nerve symptoms that may be presented must be documented. Once the patient has full motion and strength, a well-supervised throwing program is initiated. Up to 50% of patients may be able to return to their previous level of activity with non-surgical management.

Surgical Intervention

Those who fail to regain function through a well-supervised exercise program, who do not or cannot modify their activities, who have a complete UCL tear, or who want to return to throwing at a high level are prime candidates for surgical correction.[13,14]

Multiple techniques are available for surgical repair or reconstruction, but the results of repair have been inferior to those of reconstruction. Typically, the patient does not present during the acute

stage of injury, making repair more difficult. The ligament is reconstructed using the palmaris longus tendon, if present, or the plantaris or Achilles tendon.[14,15]

The most common surgical procedure—the Jobe technique—is commonly referred to as "Tommy John" surgery, after the major-league baseball pitcher who returned to high-level pitching. The technique has since undergone several adaptations (ST 11-2).[14,16]

Postoperative Management

A brief period (3 to 7 days) of postoperative immobilization is followed by early rehabilitation. The patient is typically immobilized in a posterior splint and then placed in a hinged ROM brace, which allows immediate wrist and hand movement, including active wrist and hand ROM and squeezing a sponge ball. Valgus stress is avoided for 4 months after surgery.

Injury-Specific Treatment and Rehabilitation Concerns

> **Specific Concerns**
> Protect the healing graft from valgus stress.
> Maintain grip strength.
> Allow flexion-extension ROM as tolerated to reduce the formation of scar tissue and other adhesions.

Conservative Treatment

In most cases of UCL injury and especially in the absence of an acute injury, the patient should pursue a 3- to 6-month course of conservative treatment, especially rest from aggravating activities. If needed, a hinged ROM brace is applied to limit the patient to pain-free ROM. The brace's ROM limits can be increased as symptoms abate.

Conservative management focuses on a well-rounded rehabilitation program including all aspects of the kinetic chain. Posterior shoulder capsule tightness must be addressed. Over time, a tight capsule limits internal rotation and leads to a compensatory increase in external rotation, which increases stress along the medial elbow while throwing. All throwers with medial elbow pain should perform stretching exercises for the posterior capsule and musculotendinous tissues. The "sleeper stretch" isolates these tissues (see chapter 13).

A complete strengthening program is instituted, including leg and pelvic exercises emphasizing gluteal muscles; trunk strengthening emphasizing rotational activity; scapulothoracic control exercises; and

S|T Surgical Technique 11-2

Jobe Technique for UCL Reconstruction ("Tommy John" Surgery)

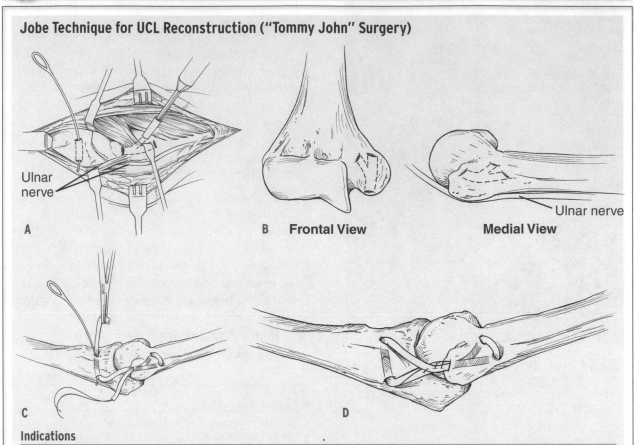

A

B **Frontal View** **Medial View**

Ulnar nerve

Ulnar nerve

C

D

Indications

Surgical intervention is indicated for those patients who have failed to improve on a proper course of conservative treatment, who cannot or do not wish to modify their activities, who have a complete tear, or who wish to return to throwing at a high level.

Overview

1. A 10-cm incision is made over the medial epicondyle.
2. The flexor-pronator muscle group is split to provide access to the underlying tissues, and the anterior portion is released from the medial epicondyle (**A**). The ulnar nerve is not exposed unless it is symptomatic.
3. The attachment sites of the UCL are identified.
4. The isometric point of the ligaments is identified, and three tunnels are drilled to form a "lazy Y" in the medial epicondyle (**B**).
5. Anterior and posterior holes are drilled into the proximal ulna near the coronoid tubercle (**C**).
6. A graft approximately 15 cm long is harvested from the contralateral palmaris longus, plantaris, or Achilles tendon (see Comments section below).
7. The graft is weaved in a figure-of-8 and reattached to itself; the graft is tensioned with the elbow flexed to 45° (**D**).
8. Ulnar or medial antebrachial cutaneous nerve transposition is performed only if electromyographic and nerve conduction tests are positive.

Functional Limitations

Postoperative flexion contractures are possible.

Implications for Rehabilitation

Approximately 70% to 85% of athletes who undergo UCL reconstruction can return to their previous level of activity and velocity.

Potential Complications

Ulnar nerve injury

Comments

Results of reconstruction are superior to those of primary repair. If ulnar nerve symptoms exist preoperatively, then a transposition should be performed. Multiple techniques are documented in the literature. Typically the surgeon subcutaneously transposes the nerve anteriorly; the nerve is then held in place by flaps created with the flexor pronator fascia.

Figure reproduced with permission from Chen FS, Rokito AS, Jobe FW: Medial elbow problems in the overhead-throwing athlete. *J Am Acad Orthop Surg* 2001;9:99-113.

exercises targeting rotator cuff function, elbow flexion and extension, pronation and supination, and wrist strengthening.[13,17,18] This program decreases valgus elbow stress. Increased trunk kinetic energy alleviates the need to compensate at the extremity and place valgus stress on the elbow.

Strengthening begins with isolated isometric exercises for the elbow, wrist, and hand to decrease muscle atrophy. Strengthening using isotonics, proprioceptive neuromuscular facilitation (PNF) exercises, and functional activities develops coordinated synergistic activity.

Activities to attain functional dynamic stabilization include PNF, rhythmic stabilization, and plyometrics. Functional stabilization exercises begin with nonprovocative positions, such as two-handed activities with the elbow close to the body. Increasingly provocative positioning with the shoulder and elbow in more functional positions mimicking throwing is incorporated as tolerated.

Most athletes with UCL injuries are throwers, and many different throwing programs exist.[18] Typical progressions initially incorporate an interval program from flat surfaces, building on the distance, intensity, and number of pitches. As the patient progresses, throwing from a mound is started, and the focus is on a return to normal activity. Advancement during the interval throwing program is highly individualized. The patient must successfully complete the present level and be symptom free before advancing to the next program level.

Postoperative Rehabilitation

During postoperative rehabilitation, symptoms related to ulnar nerve function should be carefully evaluated and documented. Deteriorating symptoms are cause for concern and warrant referral back to the physician.

After surgery, the patient is guided through a very specific rehabilitation routine. When the hinged ROM brace is applied, motion is set from 30° to 100°. The brace stops are moved to 15° and 110° at week 3 and progress by 5° into extension and 10° into flexion every week after that. This protocol may vary slightly from surgeon to surgeon, but in general, movement into the extremes of motion is a progression.

Initially, the patient performs pain-free wrist and elbow isometrics and shoulder isometrics, except for external rotation. At week 4, light isotonic exercises for the shoulder, wrist, and elbow begin. Shoulder external rotation is not started until at least 6 weeks after surgery. The patient initially avoids full external rotation but can progress to that point at 8 weeks postoperatively. Exercise resis-

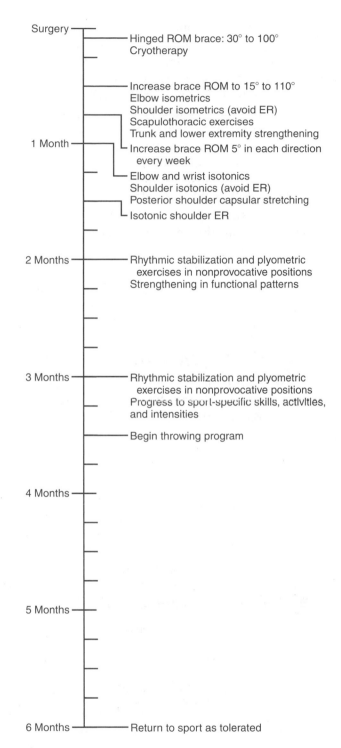

Surgery	Hinged ROM brace: 30° to 100° Cryotherapy
	Increase brace ROM to 15° to 110° Elbow isometrics Shoulder isometrics (avoid ER) Scapulothoracic exercises Trunk and lower extremity strengthening
1 Month	Increase brace ROM 5° in each direction every week
	Elbow and wrist isotonics Shoulder isotonics (avoid ER) Posterior shoulder capsular stretching
	Isotonic shoulder ER
2 Months	Rhythmic stabilization and plyometric exercises in nonprovocative positions Strengthening in functional patterns
3 Months	Rhythmic stabilization and plyometric exercises in nonprovocative positions Progress to sport-specific skills, activities, and intensities
	Begin throwing program
4 Months	
5 Months	
6 Months	Return to sport as tolerated

Note: Time frames are approximate. Function is the guide.

tance steadily advances after week 8, when functional strengthening exercises begin.

As with the conservative treatment of UCL injuries, functional strengthening incorporates a program for the legs, trunk, shoulder girdle, and upper extremity to maximize proper mechanics and alleviate compensatory stress at the medial elbow. Exercises in the form of PNF techniques, isotonics, or resistance tubing are applied in functional activities and incorporated into sport-specific activities. The program emphasizes concentric function of the flexor-pronator group and eccentric function of the scapular stabilizers, posterior rotator cuff, and elbow flexors. Dynamic stabilization exercises using rhythmic stabilization in multiple angles, medicine ball tosses, and Plyoball tosses are incorporated. Initially, the patient should protect the elbow from valgus stress by keeping the arm close to the trunk. Potentially provocative drills with the shoulder in abduction and external rotation are started 3 to 4 months after surgery, before the throwing program begins.

Estimated Amount of Time Lost

Three to 6 weeks are required for recovery from a partial UCL tear. If ligament reconstruction is required, rehabilitation takes 9 to 12 months.[13,19]

Return-to-Play Criteria

A throwing program may begin when the patient has full motion and full shoulder and elbow strength, usually 4 to 6 months after surgery. Return to full activity can occur when ROM, strength, and mechanics throughout the trunk and upper extremity are normal and the elbow is symptom free.

Functional Bracing

No brace is used after UCL injury in a thrower. Wrestlers or football players sustaining an acute injury may use a hinged functional brace.

Posterolateral Rotatory Instability

CLINICAL PRESENTATION

History

Possible prior elbow dislocation
A "clunk" and/or catching as the elbow moves from extension to flexion or, less commonly, from flexion to extension is described.
Pain may be noted arising from the posterolateral elbow.

Observation

No swelling or deformity

Functional Status

ROM is within normal limits.

Physical Evaluation Findings

Positive pivot-shift test
Positive PLRI test
Negative varus stress test

Posterolateral rotatory instability (PLRI), a deficiency of the lateral ligament complex that produces a subtle instability pattern, is most often the result of a prior acute elbow dislocation.[20] PLRI may also result from an iatrogenically induced instability after soft-tissue release for lateral epicondylitis,[20] when the lateral ligament complex and a portion of the annular ligament are cut during the procedure (**Figure 11-5**).[21] PLRI is characterized by a rotatory subluxation of the ulna from the humeral trochlea with concurrent posterolateral dislocation of the radial head from the capitellum.

Clinical findings may be subtle. Patients with PLRI most commonly report a catching sensation as the elbow moves from full extension to flexion and possibly from flexion to full extension.[16] Pain at the lateral and posterolateral aspects of the elbow during activity may be a more dominant complaint, because the instability is masked by pain.

Differential Diagnosis

Radial collateral ligament sprain, synovitis, lateral epicondylitis, osteochondral defect, arthritis

Imaging Techniques

A standard elbow series (AP, lateral, and obliques) should be obtained to rule out bony injuries. MRI may demonstrate an attenuated or torn lateral UCL, or a stress radiograph may reveal radial collateral ligament laxity (**Figure 11-6**).

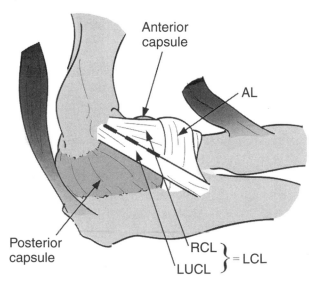

Figure 11-5   The lateral collateral ligament complex consists of the radial collateral ligament (RCL), lateral ulnar collateral ligament (LUCL), and annular ligament (AL). The LCL consists of the radial collateral ligament and the LUCL. The dashed line indicates the dividing line used to distinguish the RCL from the LUCL. (Reproduced with permission from Dunning CE, Zarzour ZDS, Patterson SD, Johnson JA, King GJW: Ligamentous stabilizers against posterolateral rotatory instability of the elbow. *J Bone Joint Surg Am* 2001;83:1823-1828.)

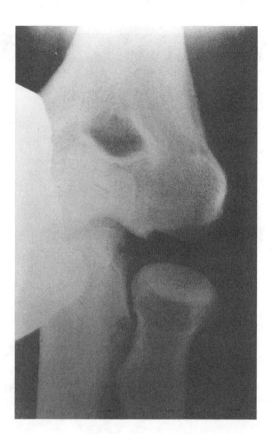

Figure 11-6 Lateral collateral ligament insufficiency demonstrated with varus stress. (Reproduced with permission from Morrey BF: Acute and chronic instability of the elbow. *J Am Acad Orthop Surg* 1996;4:117-128.)

Definitive Diagnosis

The definitive diagnosis of PLRI is often based on a positive pivot-shift or PLRI test.

Pathomechanics and Functional Limitations

Patients usually have limitations due to pain from the chronic instability. As the elbow moves from flexion to extension, instability occurs, and the patient is unable to generate forces through the joint distally to the hand.

■ Medications

NSAIDs have been tried routinely, but they do not help instability symptoms. However, if synovitis is present, NSAIDs may decrease the inflammatory response.

■ Surgical Intervention

Lateral UCL reconstruction, the treatment of choice, is performed to stabilize the elbow (⑤T 11-3).[16,22] Because of the rotational nature of this injury, most individuals and certainly throwing athletes do not respond favorably to conservative management.

■ Postoperative Management

The limb is immobilized for 2 weeks, and then a hinged elbow ROM brace is used for 4 to 6 more weeks. To decrease stress on the lateral ligaments, the brace holds the forearm pronated, and motion in the brace is set with a 30° extension block. Extension past 30° is begun after 6 weeks. The elbow is protected against varus stress for 4 to 6 months.[16]

■ Injury-Specific Treatment and Rehabilitation Concerns

Specific Concerns

Avoid stress on the lateral ligaments.
Encourage gentle, passive ROM within 30° of extension as soon as possible.

Active and active-assisted ROM within 30° of extension to full flexion is permitted. After 6 weeks, motion into extension can be progressed. Passive ROM is performed into extension only out of necessity.

Pain-free isometrics for the shoulder, elbow, and wrist muscles are started during the second week. To decrease elbow stress, the resistance is placed proximal to the elbow for shoulder exercises and wrist and elbow exercises are performed with the forearm pronated. At week 4, light isotonic exercises can be steadily progressed.

At 8 weeks, more functional exercises are initiated. Rhythmic stabilization, Plyoballs, and tubing at multiple angles are recommended to attain dynamic stabilization. The joint should be protected from varus stress, and progression to more provocative drills is necessary. Early in the functional exercises, the patient performs drills with elbow flexion past 30°. At 6 months, the patient may perform all tolerated activities but should avoid varus stress until 9 to 12 months, when all restrictions are lifted.

■ Estimated Amount of Time Lost

After surgery, 9 to 12 months of rehabilitation are required.

■ Return-to-Play Criteria

Full, pain-free ROM without any sensation of instability as well as normal strength and function of the trunk, shoulder, elbow, and wrist musculature are required before return to sport.

Functional Bracing

No bracing is used on return to activity.

S|T Surgical Technique 11-3

Reconstruction of the Lateral UCL

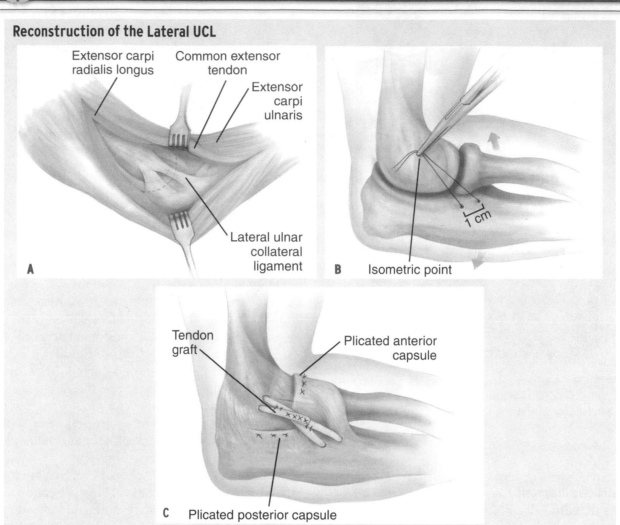

A Extensor carpi radialis longus — Common extensor tendon — Extensor carpi ulnaris — Lateral ulnar collateral ligament

B Isometric point — 1 cm

C Tendon graft — Plicated anterior capsule — Plicated posterior capsule

Indications

Demonstrated PLRI by positive pivot shift or MRI demonstrating a ruptured lateral UCL

Overview

1. Lateral incision is made through the Kocher interval between the anconeus and extensor carpi ulnaris muscle. A subperiosteal reflection of the anconeus muscle distally and the exposure of the lateral epicondyle proximally exposes the lateral ligament complex (**A**).
2. Two bone tunnels are drilled in the ulna at the lateral UCL insertion site and at the point of isometry of the ligament origin on the lateral column of the humerus. A suture marks the isometric point (**B**).
3. A palmaris longus or other tendon graft is then harvested.
4. The graft is passed through the bone tunnels in a figure-of-8 manner (**C**).
5. The graft is sutured to itself in approximately 30° of flexion.
6. The elbow is immobilized in flexion.

Functional Limitations

Flexion contractures may be or become permanent.

Implications for Rehabilitation

Extension is limited for 6 weeks. Gentle advancement of ROM and progressive resistance exercise is then instituted.

Potential Complications

Elbow flexion contractures can result from the surgery and may already be present in a throwing athlete. Repair failure can occur with early return to activities or continued prolonged lateral trauma.

Comments

This procedure is approximately 90% effective in restoring stability when no other injuries to the elbow are present.[22]

Figure reproduced with permission from Morrey BF: Acute and chronic instability of the elbow. *J Am Acad Orthop Surg* 1996;4:117-128.

Valgus Extension Overload

CLINICAL PRESENTATION

History

Repetitive hyperextension and/or valgus stress to the elbow
Pain increases during throwing or similar activities.
Acute symptom onset can frequently be linked to a specific
point in time.
Chronic UCL injuries have an insidious onset but may progress
to frank rupture.

Observation

Medial elbow swelling

Functional Status

Throwing activities are limited by pain and instability.
Osteophyte formation may limit full extension.

Physical Evaluation Findings

UCL point tenderness
Pain with valgus testing of the elbow while the forearm is
pronated

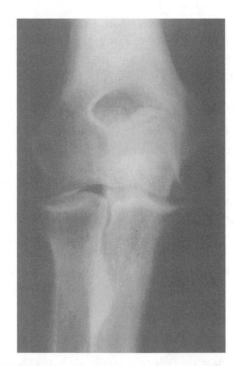

Figure 11-7 Large traction spur on the medial aspect of the ulnar notch. Note the osteophyte formation on the medial trochlea. (Reproduced with permission from Miller CD, Savoie FH: Valgus extension injuries of the elbow in the throwing athlete. *J Am Acad Orthop Surg* 1994;2:261-269.)

Valgus extension overload syndrome results from medial elbow laxity with repetitive hyperextension. The patient has a history of throwing or some other activity requiring forceful hyperextension. A wide spectrum of valgus extension injuries affect the elbow, including muscle inflammation, UCL microtearing, frank UCL rupture, and bony changes such as osteophytes, chondromalacia, and osteochondritis (see p 360).[23] The repetitive valgus load leads to impingement of the posteromedial olecranon. As the condition progresses, osteophytes and subsequent loose bodies may form.

Chronic valgus overload results in medial elbow pain due to olecranon osteophyte formation. Lateral pain can result from lateral compression injury to the radial head and capitellum, including osteochondral lesions. Over time, the patient loses the ability to effectively perform athletic activities.

Differential Diagnosis

Olecranon osteophyte, radiocapitellar arthritic changes, osteochondral defect, medial elbow instability

Imaging Techniques

A full elbow series including AP, lateral, and oblique views should be obtained. Radiographs may reveal a posteromedial osteophyte extending off the olecranon (**Figure 11-7**). MRI (with gradient echo sequence) should be obtained with acute UCL injury.

Definitive Diagnosis

The definitive diagnosis is based on the findings of the physical examination and radiographic studies. MRI (with gradient echo sequence) is excellent for revealing acute UCL injury.

Pathomechanics and Functional Limitations

Symptoms include possible valgus instability, resulting in decreased ROM and loss of throwing velocity. Throwing is not possible with an acute injury.

■ Immediate Management

Acute ruptures are treated with cessation of activity, ice, and a sling for comfort.

■ Medications

Narcotic analgesics may be prescribed for acute ligament rupture, and oral NSAIDs are usually recommended. Corticosteroid injection directly into the joint is not advised because of the detrimental effects on the joint cartilage and attenuated structures around the joint capsule.[23]

■ Postinjury Management

Conservative care includes therapeutic treatments for the inflammatory condition and rest from aggravating activities. Once the inflammation is controlled, exercises to restore ROM and strength are started. Joints inflamed from valgus extension overload can be managed with a simple sling for several days to a week for comfort.

■ Surgical Intervention

When UCL insufficiency is the underlying cause, consideration should be given to ligament reconstruction. The section on UCL injuries covers ligament reconstruction in detail (see p 347).

A posteromedial olecranon osteophyte can be excised via an open or arthroscopic procedure.[24] For an experienced arthroscopist, elbow arthroscopy is an excellent choice, allowing removal of loose bodies and inflamed synovium and excision of olecranon osteophytes. Pain is usually relieved with osteophyte removal.

■ Postoperative Management

After removal of olecranon osteophytes, no immobilization is necessary. Early rehabilitation is aimed at restoring ROM and strength. Refer to the section on UCL injuries for the postoperative management of ligament reconstruction (see p 343).

■ Injury-Specific Treatment and Rehabilitation Concerns

Specific Concerns
Protect postsurgical tissue (if applicable).
Decrease inflammation.
Restore forearm muscle strength.
Increase forearm muscle flexibility.
Reeducate dynamic control of the elbow musculature.

Treatment includes rest; NSAIDs; ROM exercises for the shoulder; strengthening of the shoulder, elbow, and wrist musculature; dynamic stabilization exercises; and a gradual return to throwing. The shoulder should be assessed for any internal rotation deficit, which increases valgus stress on the elbow with throwing. Internal rotation should be increased through passive and self-stretching techniques.

The strengthening and stabilization program focuses on control of rapid elbow extension and valgus forces. Emphasis is placed on the concentric function of the flexor-pronator group and eccentric function of the scapular stabilizers, posterior rotator cuff, and elbow flexors. Dynamic stabilization exercises with manual techniques or rubber tubing and a Plyoball are used to attain control of the elbow extension and valgus forces.

Postoperative Rehabilitation

Postoperative care after either arthroscopic or open debridement focuses on relief of pain and inflammation and restoration of motion. Active ROM begins as soon as tolerable. No restrictions are placed on motion, except those necessary for surgical wound healing. The clinician may perform gentle, passive extension as necessary, and full motion should be obtained 3 to 4 weeks after surgery. The shoulder should be continually reevaluated in order to identify and correct any deficits in internal rotation that have occurred over time. Stretching to ensure full internal shoulder rotation must be undertaken to decrease valgus stress upon return to activity.

The patient may perform pain-free isometric exercises for the shoulder, elbow, and wrist during the first 2 weeks. Isotonic exercises begin at week 4. At 6 weeks, more functional strengthening exercises are started for the legs, trunk, shoulder girdle, and extremity. As with conservative treatment, the program focuses on developing control of the rapid elbow extension and valgus forces experienced during throwing.

The patient may begin to return to throwing 10 to 12 weeks after surgery. Throwing athletes should undergo a progressive routine involving incremental increases in duration, frequency, and intensity. Many throwing programs are available that can be adapted to the specific needs of the patient. Return to full activity may take 3 to 4 months.

If surgical reconstruction of the medial elbow ligamentous complex was performed, the rehabilitation guidelines in the section on UCL injuries should be followed (see p 343).

■ Estimated Amount of Time Lost

Time lost ranges from 3 to 6 weeks for partial ligamentous tears and overuse inflammatory conditions. Surgical osteophyte excision may require 6 to 8 weeks before full return to activity. Ligament reconstruction requires 9 to 12 months of rehabilitation.

■ Return-to-Play Criteria

The patient should have a pain-free joint with functional ROM and strength of the shoulder, elbow, and wrist before beginning a sport-specific training or throwing program. A progressive training or throwing program must be successfully completed before full return to play is possible.

Functional Bracing

No braces are typically used to treat valgus extension overload.

Elbow Fractures

Elbow fractures result in a wide spectrum of injuries and subsequent treatment and management techniques. This section focuses on the more common fracture types and general acute fracture treatment.

The elbow joint depends on its bony architecture for stability. Approximately half the elbow's stability is provided by soft tissues and half by bony architecture. Consequently, elbow fractures are likely to affect joint stability. The section on elbow dislocations covers fractures combined with instability (see p 356). The objective in treating any elbow fracture is to provide a stable joint that allows early motion.

The Müller system classifies fractures of the distal humerus (**Figure 11-8**).[25] Distal humeral fractures carry an increased risk of secondary trauma to the neurovascular structures that cross the elbow. Dealing with intra-articular fractures (types B and C) is particularly difficult. The objective of any treatment is a stable, anatomic reduction of the joint surface to allow early motion.

The radial head provides stability against valgus stress along with the UCL and affords longitudinal stability to the elbow. Fractures to this structure are classified using the Mason system (**Figure 11-9**). Posterior ulnar translation on the humerus is restricted by the coronoid process, which is frequently fractured during elbow dislocations.[26] The olecranon prevents anterior ulnar translation on the humerus. By virtue of anatomy, olecranon fractures are intra-articular; they are described using the Schatzker classification system (**Figure 11-10**).[27]

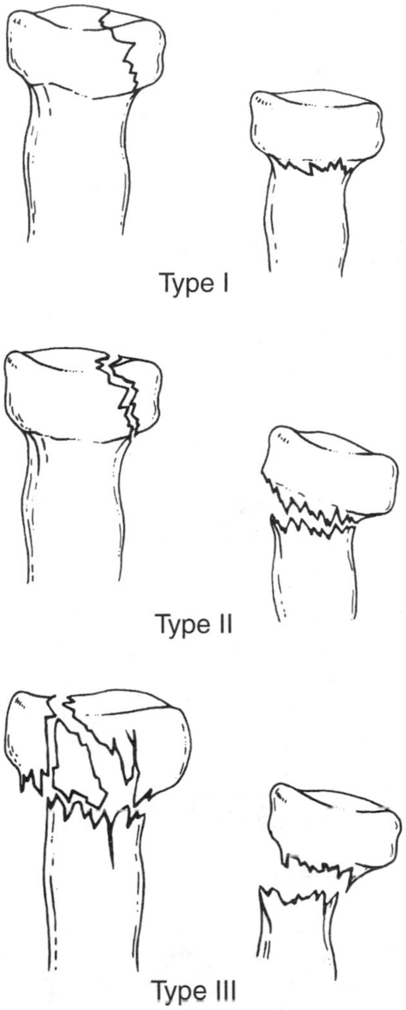

Type I

Type II

Type III

Type	Displacement	Symptoms
I	Minimally displaced (<2 mm)	Forearm pronation/ supination is limited by pain.
II	Displaced >2 mm	Motion has a mechanical block secondary to displacement.
	Fracture is angulated, but minimal or no comminution	
III	Displaced >2 mm	Gross deformity
	Severe comminution	Not amenable to surgical repair and requires resection of the radial head

Figure 11-9 Modified Mason classification for radial head fractures.[28] (Adapted with permission from Browner BD, Jupiter JB, Levine AM, Trafton PG [eds]: *Skeletal Trauma*. Philadelphia, PA, WB Saunders, 1992, p 1137.)

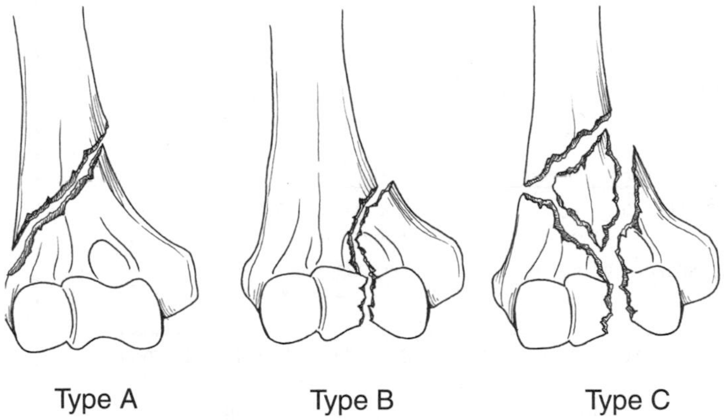

Type A   Type B   Type C

Figure 11-8 Müller's classification of distal humeral fractures. Type A is nonarticular, type B is articular with one articular fragment being continuous with the shaft, and type C is articular with the shaft separated from the articular fragments. (Reproduced with permission from Webb LX: Distal humerus fractures in adults. *J Am Acad Orthop Surg* 1996;4:336-344.)

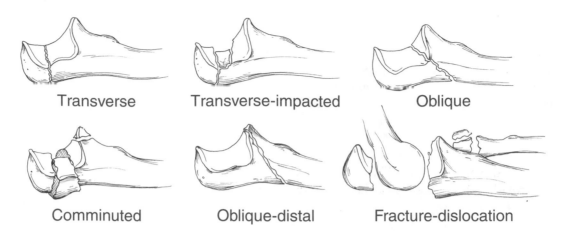

Transverse   Transverse-impacted   Oblique

Comminuted   Oblique-distal   Fracture-dislocation

Figure 11-10   Schatzker classification of olecranon fractures. (Adapted with permission from Browner BD, Jupiter JB, Levine AM, Trafton PG [eds]: *Skeletal Trauma*. Philadelphia, PA, WB Saunders, 1992, p 1137.)

Differential Diagnosis

Elbow dislocation, radial collateral ligament sprain, posterolateral complex trauma

Imaging Techniques

AP, lateral, and oblique radiographs are obtained to show the fracture pattern (**Figure 11-11**).

Definitive Diagnosis

Radiographs demonstrating a fracture

Pathomechanics and Functional Limitations

Elbow biomechanics are disrupted differently for each type of fracture. Radial head fractures result in decreased strength during pronation and supination and pain during flexion and extension. Unrecognized proximal radius instability can lead to chondromalacia of the radial head and capitellum.[29] Elbow extension strength is decreased in the pres-

CLINICAL PRESENTATION

	Radial Head Fractures	Olecranon Fractures	Humeral Fractures
History	Valgus stress applied to the elbow Axial load applied through an outstretched hand with the forearm in pronation Pain is reported along the lateral aspect of the elbow.	A direct blow to the elbow Elbow hyperextension Pain arising from the posterior elbow	A forceful injury such as a fall Pain just proximal to the elbow
Observation	Swelling along the lateral elbow	Posterior elbow swelling Olecranon deformity	Medial and/or lateral swelling Deformity above the elbow
Functional Status	Pain with elbow motion Pronation and supination are limited by a mechanical block.	Pain during elbow flexion and extension Active elbow extension may be absent.	Pain with elbow motion Inability to actively move the elbow secondary to pain
Physical Evaluation Findings	Point tenderness and possible crepitus over the radial head Decreased strength during resisted ROM for forearm pronation and supination Possible increased varus laxity noted on stress testing	Point tenderness over the olecranon process The subcutaneous location of the olecranon often makes the fracture line easily palpable. The strength of resisted ROM is decreased because of the unstable insertion of the triceps brachii on the olecranon process.	Point tenderness and possible crepitus over distal humerus Palpable deformity in distal humerus Pain with any resisted ROM testing

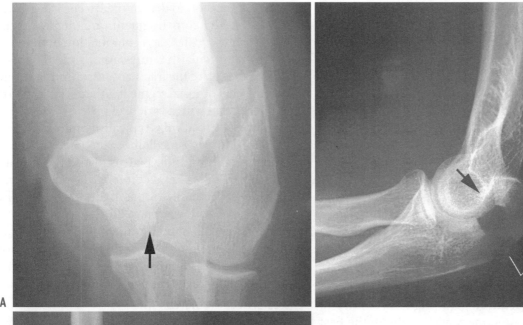

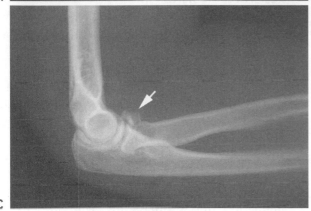

Figure 11-11 Imaging of fractures about the elbow. **A.** AP view of an intercondylar fracture of the distal humerus. The arrow illustrates the fracture line extending into the articular surface. **B.** Lateral view demonstrating an olecranon fracture (arrows). Traction caused by the triceps displaces the proximal fragment. **C.** Lateral view demonstrating a radial head fracture (arrow). (Reproduced with permission from Johnson TR, Steinbach LS (eds): *Essentials of Musculoskeletal Imaging.* Rosemont, IL, American Academy of Orthopaedic Surgeons, 2004, p 270, 274, 278.)

ence of even minor olecranon process fractures, because the triceps lacks a stable insertion on which to pull. If not properly treated, intra-articular distal humeral fractures lead to reduced ROM, pain, and dysfunction. Epicondylar fractures reduce the strength of wrist flexion (medial epicondyle) or extension (lateral epicondyle). Pronation and supination are also impaired.

■ Immediate Management

If a fracture is suspected, the extremity should be immobilized and the patient transported for radiographs. Neurovascular status should be evaluated before the joint is immobilized and regularly monitored during patient transport.

■ Medications

Narcotic analgesics may be prescribed to control pain. NSAIDs may be avoided with fractures because of the possibility of platelet dysfunction and the urgent need for fracture fixation.

■ Postinjury Management

Distal Humeral Fractures

Stable fractures can be managed nonsurgically. The physician can reduce a displaced fracture by gently applying axial traction while the arm is in the neutral position. The fracture is then immobilized with a cast or rigid splint for 2 weeks, followed by a hinged brace to allow early, controlled ROM.[25] Nonsurgical management requires frequent follow-up radiographs, and when a hinged brace is used, it must be regularly adjusted. A less than optimal alignment is a common result of conservative management of type A distal humeral fractures.[25]

Radial Head Fractures

Loss of motion, especially terminal extension, is a common result of radial head fracture, even after surgery. However, the amount of motion lost rarely causes functional disability. With conservative treatment, the amount of fracture healing that has occurred must be known. Adequate healing permits more aggressive pursuit of motion and the start of strengthening.

Olecranon Fractures

Nondisplaced olecranon fractures in which the extensor mechanism is still intact may be managed nonsurgically. To improve reduction in displaced fractures, the arm is immobilized with the elbow fully extended; however, this technique can result in a loss of flexion ROM. If the fracture is nondisplaced, the elbow is immobilized in 45° to 90° of flexion for 3 weeks. ROM is limited to 90° until healing is seen on radiographs.[27] Most olecranon fractures are intra-articular and require surgical fixation.

■ Surgical Intervention

Distal Humeral Fractures

Extensive preoperative planning is necessary to ensure an efficient surgery and to obtain the best long-term results.[30] Radiographs are obtained to identify the fracture lines and determine the amount of displacement. Views of the uninvolved elbow are also taken and flipped, to provide a silhouette of the expected anatomic alignment.[25] Computed tomography (CT) scans can be helpful in elucidating fracture configurations during preoperative planning.

Surgical management of nonarticular fractures may involve an inverted-V turndown of the triceps brachii tendon, but this technique can result in residual triceps weakness. This risk can be avoided with a medial incision to detach the triceps from the periosteum. The bony fragments are then reattached using screws, plates, or a combination of these.[25]

Intra-articular fractures are managed by using screws to replace the fragments that form the articular surface. The distal segment is then stabilized to the humeral shaft with a variety of plates (**Figure 11-12**). A double-plate fixation is typically employed. A plate is fixated directly medially to stabilize the medial humeral column and a plate is placed posterolaterally to fixate the lateral column. The posterolateral placement decreases the possibility of contact of the ulnar nerve with the plate. If plate placement encroaches on the cubital tunnel, ulnar nerve transposition is required. Other potential complications include stiffness, fibrosis, heterotopic ossification, and nonunion or malunion.[31]

Radial Head Fractures

Indications for surgical fixation of radial head fractures include displaced fractures (>2 mm) and comminution (types II and III, see Figure 11-9).[24] In recent years, more attention has been given to open reduction and internal fixation (ORIF) of radial head and neck fractures.[29] This technique is difficult and should be performed only by surgeons who are very familiar with elbow anatomy. Specific small screw-and-plate sets are excellent for radial head or neck ORIF. A lateral Kocher approach exposes the fracture, and the fragments can be preliminarily reduced with K-wires. The type of fixation (screws or plates) depends on the fracture pattern

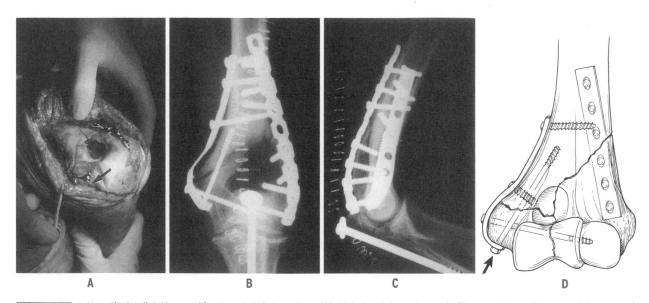

| A | B | C | D |

Figure 11-12 Intra-articular distal humeral fracture. **A.** A flattened one-third tubular plate contoured to fit around the medial epicondyle was used for fixation. Instrumentation imposed on the cubital tunnel (arrow) necessitated transposition of the ulnar nerve. AP (**B**) and lateral (**C**) radiographs depict arrangement of the plates at right angles to each other. **D.** Illustration of the repairs involved. (Reproduced with permission from Webb LX: Distal humerus fractures in adults. *J Am Acad Orthop Surg* 1996;4:336-344.)

and is beyond the scope of this chapter. The objective is stable fixation that allows early motion. In rare instances, the radial head is excised, although this procedure is not recommended for young, active patients and is contraindicated with an accompanying elbow dislocation.[28]

Olecranon Fractures

A displaced or comminuted olecranon fracture requires ORIF to restore elbow function. A straight posterior approach to the elbow is used.[24] The triceps and anconeus are brought over as a subperiosteal sleeve to expose the fracture fragments. Fixation choices include a large intramedullary screw, tension band, K-wires, plate and screw, or a combination of these (**Figure 11-13**). The objective is a stable, anatomic reduction of the olecranon and articular surface to allow early motion. Patients with thin arms may be able to feel the plate and screws postoperatively. In some instances, this hardware must be removed after healing has been accomplished.[27]

Postoperative Management

A short course (5 to 10 days) of immobilization with a posterior splint for comfort is indicated postoperatively. Early motion is begun as soon as the patient is comfortable. A ROM brace may be used early in the course for patient comfort.

Distal Humeral Fractures

The elbow and arm are supported in a sling. Active or active-assisted ROM should be initiated as soon as possible to maintain motion and prevent joint adhesions. A hinged ROM brace may be worn at the physician's discretion. Resisted ROM is not begun until the fracture has healed, usually at 8 to 12 weeks.

Radial Head Fractures

After ORIF, the fracture site should be stable enough to allow early passive motion. Typically after about 4 weeks, strengthening and more aggressive motion can be started as needed.

Olecranon Fractures

Extra caution is needed to identify postoperative wound-healing issues. The superficial nature of the fixation hardware can create problems with healing. Once stabilized, the olecranon fracture does well with rehabilitation. After an initial 1- to 2-week period to allow adequate wound healing, motion exercises can commence. At about 3 to 4 weeks, isometric exercises may begin; at 6 to 8 weeks, more aggressive strengthening may be started.

■ Injury-Specific Treatment and Rehabilitation Concerns

Specific Concerns

Protect the healing fracture.
Restore functional ROM.
Restore strength to the surrounding musculature.

Distal Humeral Fractures

Any posterior incision must be thoroughly evaluated for closure problems. The small amount of soft tissue between the bone and plates and the skin can lead to healing difficulties. At about 1 week, placing the arm in a hinged ROM brace allows active and active-assisted motion to begin without placing stress along the incision. When the incision is completely closed, ROM progresses unimpeded. Passive range of motion begins with radiographic evidence of bone healing at approximately 4 to 6 weeks.

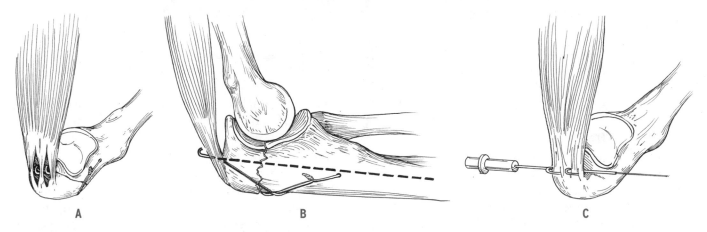

A   **B**   **C**

Figure 11-13 Technique for tension-band wiring after an olecranon fracture. **A.** Fibers of the triceps tendon should be split or moved to allow the bent end of the K-wires to be impacted firmly against bone. **B.** If the ends of the K-wires are left superficial to the triceps tendon, elbow extension may cause migration or fatigue failure of the wires. **C.** A 16-gauge or larger intravenous catheter is used to pass the tension-band wire deep to the triceps fibers. (Reproduced with permission from Hak DJ, Golladay GJ: Olecranon fractures: Treatment options. *J Am Acad Orthop Surg* 2000;8:266-75.)

Strengthening exercises for the entire extremity begin with isometrics at 2 to 3 weeks. If the surgical procedure requires triceps tendon release and reattachment to gain exposure to the fracture, elbow extension should not commence until 4 weeks. Light isotonic exercises may start at 6 weeks and the patient can strengthen the arm without restrictions after radiographic evidence of adequate healing is present, usually around 8 weeks after surgery.

Radial Head Fractures

For a type I radial head fracture, active elbow motion begins immediately. The patient can remain in a sling for comfort. Patients with type II fractures treated without surgery undergo a short period of immobilization. In both cases, formal rehabilitation can start about 3 weeks after injury.

For type I radial head fractures, active motion is begun and progressed as tolerated. Passive motion, if needed, is not used until adequate fracture healing is demonstrated on radiographs. Isometric exercises start at 3 weeks and isotonic exercises at 5 to 6 weeks. Heavy resistance is not incorporated until 8 weeks—later if adequate healing is not yet evident in radiographs.

For a type II radial head fracture, the patient performs active wrist and hand ROM immediately, but elbow ROM begins after the joint has been in a splint for 3 to 5 days. Strengthening exercises follow a schedule similar to that of conservative treatment for type I injuries.

ROM is started after 3 to 5 days of immobilization for type II fractures managed with ORIF. All motions are accomplished actively or actively assisted, with passive ROM performed only if necessary and then only after adequate fracture healing. Strengthening begins at about 3 weeks with submaximal isometric exercises and progresses to isotonic exercises at 6 weeks. Heavy resistance is not initiated until after 8 weeks.

Patients with type III fractures treated with radial head excision begin active motion after 3 to 5 days of immobilization. If other tissues were repaired, the repair takes precedence, and rehabilitation follows the course dictated by that procedure.

Olecranon Fractures

The patient may undergo conservative treatment for nondisplaced or minimally displaced type IA and IB fractures.[24] The elbow is immobilized in the flexion midrange for 7 to 10 days. Radiographs are then repeated; if no further displacement is demonstrated, gentle active flexion with passive extension is attempted. Any increased displacement requires surgical fixation.

Surgical fixation of the olecranon fracture should allow early, protected motion. Because of the superficial nature of the olecranon and the hardware, skin-healing problems may dictate a prolonged period of immobilization. To protect the skin, the patient uses a posterior splint at 90° but can still begin active motion as soon as the first day.[24] The exception is patients with comminuted or type III fractures, who may require a less aggressive approach. Active and active-assisted motions are used, especially for flexion, but the patient is closely monitored.

Isometric exercises to strengthen the shoulder, elbow, and wrist can begin at 4 weeks. Isotonic exercises can start at 6 to 8 weeks if stable fixation and adequate healing are present.

■ Estimated Amount of Time Lost

Time lost is based on the fracture pattern and whether surgical fixation was required. Generally, the patient needs at least 8 to 12 weeks before returning to full activity.

■ Return-to-Play Criteria

The patient can return to sports and physical activities when adequate fracture healing is demonstrated radiographically and clinically. Clinically, patients must have functional ROM of the elbow and superior radioulnar joints and adequate strength compared with the contralateral extremity.

Functional Bracing

No braces, taping, or padding are needed. An athlete with a healed olecranon fracture may find an elbow pad useful for comfort to soften blows to the area.

Elbow Dislocations

Elbow dislocations account for 10% to 25% of all elbow injuries and are second only to the shoulder in upper extremity dislocations among adults.[32] The elbow is the most frequently dislocated upper extremity joint in children. More than 90% of elbow dislocations occur posteriorly or posterolaterally.

By definition, all dislocations involve ligament trauma. Simple elbow dislocations do not involve a fracture, whereas complex dislocations do involve fractures. When a fracture does occur, the radial head and coronoid process are most commonly involved, but the epicondyles and olecranon can also be involved. A shallow olecranon fossa and a prominent olecranon process may increase the risk of a dislocation.[33]

CLINICAL PRESENTATION

History

Application of a high-energy force to the elbow
A fall on an outstretched hand while the forearm is supinated
Exquisite pain

Observation

Obvious elbow deformity
Gross elbow swelling develops rapidly.

Functional Status

Elbow ROM is not possible.
Decreased or absent grip strength

Physical Evaluation Findings

Distal neurovascular function may be compromised.
Point tenderness throughout the elbow
Once the joint is relocated, valgus, varus, and posterolateral in-
    stability may be present.

Differential Diagnosis

Distal humeral fracture, proximal ulnar fracture, proximal radial fracture, radial head dislocation

Imaging Techniques

Radiographs confirm the diagnosis and direction of dislocation. AP, lateral, oblique, and true lateral are the most important views (**Figure 11-14**). Oblique views or CT are especially helpful to identify peri-articular fractures (**Figure 11-15**). MRI evaluation is useful in planning surgical intervention.

Definitive Diagnosis

The definitive diagnosis is based on the clinical findings and radiographic images.

Pathomechanics and Functional Limitations

Most patients are unable to move the elbow until it is relocated. Once the displacement is reduced, joint stability must be determined. Many patients can restore full, stable motion and functional elbow use with conservative care.

Simple dislocations resulting in continued instability and complex dislocations may require surgical intervention to restore stability and repair the fractures. Heterotopic ossification can occur after a dislocation and result in a debilitating loss of ROM, especially for athletes.

Although radiographs have revealed periarticular fractures in 12% to 60% of all dislocations, surgical exploration revealed a nearly 100% incidence of unrecognized osteochondral injuries in elbow dislocations.[34] Most of these injuries do not require fixation.

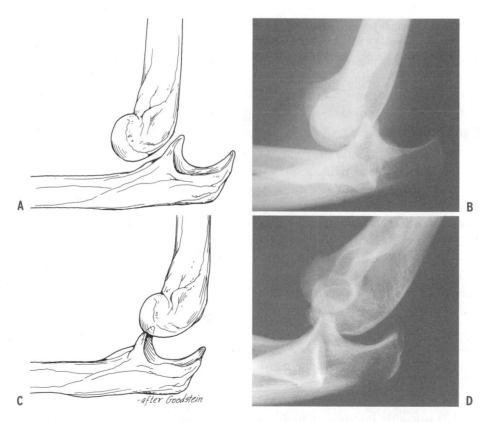

Figure 11-14 **A** and **B**, Illustration and radiograph of complete posterior dislocation. **C** and **D**, "Perched" posterior dislocation. (Reproduced with permission from Morrey BF: Acute and chronic instability of the elbow. *J Am Acad Orthop Surg* 1996;4:117-128.)

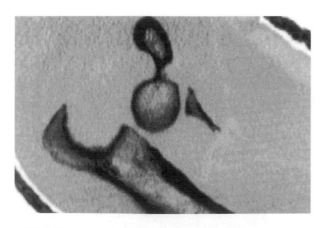

Figure 11-15   A sagittal CT image of a coronoid fracture. (Reproduced with permission from Ring D, Jupiter JB, Zilberfarb J: Posterior elbow dislocation with radial head and coronoid fractures. *J Bone Joint Surg Am* 2002;84:547-551.)

Immediate Management

The elbow is splinted in the position in which it is found and distal neurovascular status monitored regularly. The shoulder and wrist must be examined to rule out concomitant injury, which occurs in 10% to 15% of elbow dislocations.[33] The distal radioulnar joint is also examined, to rule out interosseous membrane injury.

Medications

Appropriate analgesia, sedation, and muscle relaxants are required for reduction. Minimal sedation is required if the reduction is attempted early, before spasm and swelling develop. Narcotic analgesics may be prescribed after reduction.

Medical Management

Complete neurovascular examination is required before and after reduction. Timely reduction is essential but should be performed in an emergency room or office setting. Sedation and muscle relaxation are the keys to reduction. Medial-lateral displacement must be corrected first, followed by forearm traction with the elbow flexed to 20° to unlock the coronoid by application of gentle pressure on the olecranon to bring it distal and anterior. An appreciable "clunk" is a favorable sign for stability.[33]

Surgical Intervention

Although surgical intervention for acute elbow dislocation is rarely needed, two indications exist: (1) the elbow remains unstable in extension between 0° and 50°; and (2) unstable fractures, which require fixation.[34] The goal of surgical fixation is stability to allow early motion.

Elbows that are chronically unstable after reduction may require an additional surgical procedure, such as that described in the section on PLRI (see p 346). Complex dislocations need appropriate fracture fixation in the operating room, and sometimes surgical repair of ligamentous structures (**Figure 11-16**). An associated coronoid process or radial head fracture can cause inherent instability and increase the risk of complications.[26]

Postinjury/Postoperative Management

Postreduction assessment of neurovascular status and stability in extension is critical. Instability in extension after reduction signifies a problematic joint that will likely remain unstable. If the joint is stable after reduction, the elbow is immobilized in 90° of flexion for about 7 days. Positioning of the proximal radioulnar joint depends on collateral ligament stability.[35] Injury to the lateral ligaments requires splinting in pronation to tighten any intact medial ligaments and lateral musculotendinous structures. Injury to the medial ligaments requires splinting in supination to tighten any intact lateral ligaments and medial musculotendinous structures. If both collateral ligamentous structures are compromised, the forearm is left in neutral.

Once the elbow is relocated and neurovascular status is determined to be satisfactory, the elbow is placed in a posterior splint or hinged ROM brace and the extremity in a sling. A hinged brace can either be locked or allow limited ROM within a stable, pain-free range. The wrist and hand should be free to move. Regular follow-up radiographs ensure that reduction has been maintained.

Wrist and hand ROM exercises are initiated as soon as possible. Flexion-extension elbow ROM exercises can begin at approximately 1 week, when the patient is fitted with an extension block (**Figure 11-17**).[33,36] Extension is gradually increased over the next 3 to 6 weeks.

Injury-Specific Treatment and Rehabilitation Concerns

Specific Concerns
Protect the joint from any forces that would cause further instability.
Maintain grip strength.
Encourage wrist ROM while the elbow is immobilized.
Introduce passive pronation-supination and flexion-extension ROM as allowed.
Determine UCL stability and take corrective measures if necessary.

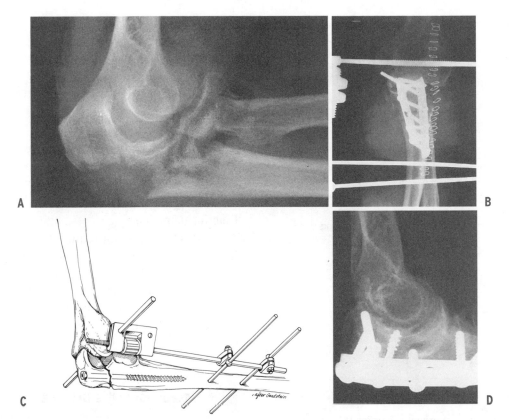

In uncomplicated dislocations, immobilization for 3 to 7 days is followed by a rehabilitation program aimed at regaining motion while preserving stability. Patients begin rehabilitation 3 to 7 days after injury. Early in rehabilitation, the patient's complaints of elbow instability may increase as the amount of extension is increased. A hinged ROM brace with an extension block can be used to limit

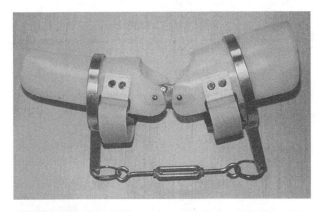

the elbow to the stable ranges of motion during activities of daily living (see Figure 11-17).

UCL instability can increase posterolateral elbow instability.[37] If the patient demonstrates UCL laxity, UCL rehabilitation should be incorporated into the program (see p 343).

Active and active-assisted ROM exercises begin 7 days after injury for the elbow that was easily reduced, remains reduced, and is stable throughout a full ROM. A stable joint need not be protected during activities of daily living, but a sling may be used for comfort for another 1 or 2 weeks. A patient whose elbow was reduced but is unstable in extension begins guarded, active ROM about 1 week after injury. ROM limits increase as joint stability increases. The goal is to attain full, stable motion by about 6 weeks.

As inflammation decreases, modalities such as moist heat packs and whirlpool therapy promote relaxation and increase tissue viscoelasticity before ROM exercises. An upper body ergometer may be used, with low loads and within stable ROMs, after 3 weeks or as soon as tissue inflammation decreases.

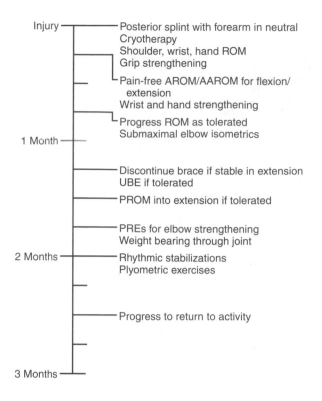

Injury — Posterior splint with forearm in neutral
Cryotherapy
Shoulder, wrist, hand ROM
Grip strengthening

Pain-free AROM/AAROM for flexion/
extension
Wrist and hand strengthening

Progress ROM as tolerated
Submaximal elbow isometrics

1 Month —

Discontinue brace if stable in extension
UBE if tolerated

PROM into extension if tolerated

PREs for elbow strengthening
Weight bearing through joint

2 Months — Rhythmic stabilizations
Plyometric exercises

Progress to return to activity

3 Months —

Note: Time frames are approximate. Function is the guide.

Passive motion, especially into extension, is performed only out of necessity in the first 3 to 6 weeks. A progressive loss of ROM is an indication to begin passive motion but only within the stable ROMs. In addition to the elbow, early cervical spine, shoulder, wrist, and hand ROM exercise is performed.

The patient begins squeezing a sponge ball or putty immediately. Submaximal isometrics for the shoulder, elbow, and wrist musculature commence at 2 to 3 weeks. Isotonic strengthening starts at 4 to 5 weeks within stable ranges. About 6 weeks after injury, the patient can progress strengthening exercises as tolerated.

At 4 to 6 weeks, more functional positioning and movements are initiated. Weight bearing through the joint, initially with minimal weight, promotes proprioception and joint stability. Rhythmic stabilization and Plyoball exercises are useful to improve joint dynamic stability.

Postoperative rehabilitation of the unstable joint generally follows the guidelines in the section on PLRI. Surgical intervention for complex fractures follows the guidelines in the section on fractures (p 354).

Estimated Amount of Time Lost

Many athletes return to sports activity in 5 to 10 weeks, depending on the exact nature of the dislocation. Dislocations requiring surgical intervention for instability and complex dislocations can be debilitating. Time lost varies depending on the amount and type of ligamentous and bony injury. Complex dislocations require a longer recovery period, and full motion may not be regained.

Return-to-Play Criteria

The joint must remain stable throughout the full ROM. The patient must have a pain-free joint and full strength and be able to perform all functional activities.

Functional Bracing

A brace is typically not required to return to activity. For some athletes attempting a quick return to activity, a brace limiting extension may be helpful. However, these athletes must be able to perform their activities safely in this type of brace. For example, a football lineman may be able to return more quickly with a brace that limits full extension.

Osteochondritis Dissecans

CLINICAL PRESENTATION

History

Elbow pain during throwing or similar activities
Popping and catching may be described.
Loose bodies in the joint can result in elbow locking.

Observation

Mild swelling may be noted on the lateral elbow.

Functional Status

ROM may be notably decreased.
The patient may describe grating or crunching during elbow motion.

Physical Evaluation Findings

Crepitus may be noted during elbow palpation during flexion and extension.
Valgus stress test may be positive or increase pain.

Osteochondritis dissecans occurs in younger throwing athletes and usually involves the capitellum of the distal humerus.[38] Increased valgus stress across the elbow during throwing increases contact pressures between the capitellum and radial head. These contact pressures can also lead to secondary radial head degenerative changes. The sections on UCL and valgus extension overload describe the throwing motion and valgus stress across the elbow in detail. Patients are usually males, age 13 to 16 years, involved in throwing activities.[39]

Differential Diagnosis

Valgus extension overload, isolated ligament sprain, overuse tendinitis, arthritis

Imaging Techniques

Radiographs may reveal the capitellar lesion and any radial head changes. MRI can be used to obtain images of capitellar lesions and loose bodies, but several views with the elbow in various degrees of flexion may be required to identify the defect (**Figure 11-18**). Ultrasound imaging has also been used successfully to identify capitellar osteochondritis.[38]

Definitive Diagnosis

The definitive diagnosis is based on radiographic findings.

Pathomechanics and Functional Limitations

During throwing, contact pressure increases in the capitellum and the radial head laterally. Articular cartilage changes can result and lead to early degenerative changes laterally. Loose bodies can form, causing further biomechanical problems.

Athletes have throwing limitations secondary to pain and may subsequently change their throwing mechanics. Other than throwing or similar overhead motions, athletes may not have any functional limitations.

■ Immediate Management

A short course (3 to 5 days) of immobilization for acute pain may be necessary. Throwing and other aggravating activities should be discontinued until symptoms resolve.

■ Medications

NSAIDs may be prescribed to control pain and inflammation.

■ Postinjury Management

Most patients respond to conservative treatment. The main focus is complete compliance with rest from aggravating activities. NSAIDs and ice constitute the initial treatment. In patients whose pain persists even with everyday activities, splinting or casting for 3 to 4 weeks followed by active and active-assisted ROM may be recommended. The patient must continue to restrict activity for 6 to 8 weeks after symptoms are fully relieved. Before the patient attempts to return to activity, radiographic findings should be stable or improving but need not be normal, which may take years.[39] The return to activity should progress cautiously. Although most athletes return to sport, baseball pitchers have a guarded prognosis.[40]

Educating the patient, coaches, and often parents about avoidance of aggravating activities is essential. Any activity that causes pain results in a prolonged course of treatment and increases the likelihood of an unfavorable outcome.

■ Surgical Intervention

Surgery is indicated in those patients who have failed to improve in an appropriate conservative course of rest, rehabilitation, and a throwing program. Arthroscopy is an excellent tool for visualizing

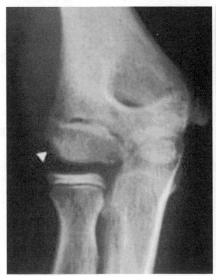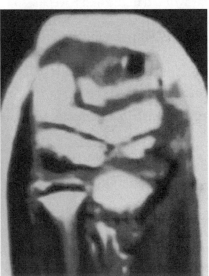

A   B

Figure 11-18 Imaging techniques to identify elbow osteochondritis. **A.** AP radiograph with the elbow flexed to 45°. Slight flattening and sclerosis of the lateral surface of the capitellum (arrowhead) are seen. **B.** T1-weighted MRI view showing low-signal intensity in the superficial aspect of the capitellum. (Reproduced with permission from Takahara M, Shundo M, Kondo M, Suzuki K, Nambu T, Ogino T: Early detection of osteochondritis dissecans of the capitellum in young baseball players: Report of 3 cases. *J Bone Joint Surg Am* 1998;80:892-897.)

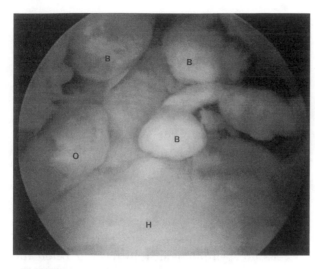

Figure 11-19 Intraoperative photograph demonstrating the presence of loose osteochondral fragments (B) in the posterior elbow compartment of a throwing athlete secondary to valgus extension overload (H = humerus, O = olecranon). (Reproduced with permission from Williams RJ, Altcheck DW: Atraumatic injuries of the elbow in athletes, in Arendt EA (ed): *Orthopaedic Knowledge Update: Sports Medicine*, ed 2. Rosemont, IL, American Academy of Orthopaedic Surgeons, 1999, p 226.)

the elbow and removing loose bodies (**Figure 11-19**). Lesions may be debrided, drilled, repaired, or excised. Results in the literature vary with regard to return to throwing. Open techniques also have successful results but do not allow easy visualization of the rest of the joint.

Postoperative Management

Postsurgically, the healing lesion must be respected. Joint motion is beneficial, because it brings fresh synovial fluid to the lesion. Shearing and compressive loading must be avoided in the first 8 weeks, so that the healing fibrocartilage clot or osteochondral fragment is not dislodged from the injury site.

Injury-Specific Treatment and Rehabilitation Concerns

Specific Concerns

Protect the capitellum and other load-bearing structures from stress.
After surgery, protect the incision site.
Correct poor biomechanics.

The nonsurgical rehabilitation program is based completely on symptoms. ROM and strengthening exercises can progress in intensity as tolerated. If symptoms abate for 6 to 8 weeks and the patient has full ROM and strength, a supervised throwing program may be attempted.

After surgery, the elbow is placed in a soft dressing for 1 week. Continuous passive motion stimulates the delivery of nutrition to the area from the synovial fluid. Shearing and heavy compressive forces across the joint must be avoided for at least 8 weeks. With fragment removal, the treatment is once again based completely on symptoms. ROM and strengthening exercises can progress in intensity as tolerated.

If the fragment is reattached, early motion is used to stimulate healing. Strengthening begins at about 3 weeks with submaximal isometrics and progresses to isotonics at about 6 weeks. Heavy resistance should not be applied for at least 8 weeks. After 12 weeks and once the patient has full ROM and strength, a supervised throwing program may begin.

Estimated Amount of Time Lost

Time lost is highly variable. Patients with moderate osteochondritis dissecans may lose 4 weeks of activity. Those with severe damage to the articular surface may never return to throwing activity. After surgery, return to full activity can take up to 6 months.

Return-to-Play Criteria

The patient can return to sports and physical activities when adequate healing is demonstrated clinically. Compared with the contralateral extremity, the athletes must have functional ROM and adequate strength and successfully complete a supervised throwing program.

Osteoarthritis

Although pain is the most common complaint with arthritis of the elbow, patients can also complain of stiffness, weakness, instability, or deformity.[32] Treatment and outcome depend on the type of arthritis, severity and duration of symptoms, amount of contracture, and age.

Osteoarthritis is becoming more frequently recognized, and most cases are in males. Patients usually have a history of heavy labor, weightlifting, or throwing and present in the third to eighth decades. Radiographs reveal osteophytes (olecranon, coronoid) and loose bodies (see Figure 11-19).

Posttraumatic arthritis is the result of injury to the elbow articulation, most commonly an intra-articular fracture of the distal humerus. Stiffness is common after these injuries, and nonunions can lead to chronically unstable, painful elbows.

History

History of heavy labor, weightlifting, and/or throwing
The patient may describe catching during joint motion.
Pain is noted during joint motion and increases when the joints are loaded (eg, while weightlifting).
Pain may be most intense in terminal extension.

Observation

A flexion contracture may be noted.
Outward joint deformity may be present in the late disease stages.

Functional Status

The patient is unwilling to use the involved extremity secondary to pain and/or decreased ROM.

Physical Evaluation Findings

Pain during joint palpation
Crepitus may be felt during elbow motion.

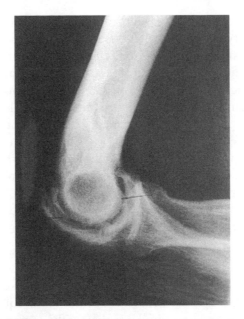

Figure 11-20 Lateral radiograph of an elbow with arthritis. (Reproduced with permission from Norberg FB, Savoie FH III, Field LD: Arthroscopic treatment of arthritis of the elbow. *Instr Course Lect* 2000;49:247-253.)

Differential Diagnosis

Rheumatoid arthritis, osteochondritis, osteochondritis dissecans, medial epicondylitis, lateral epicondylitis

Medical Diagnostic Tests

A blood test may be ordered to rule out rheumatoid arthritis.

Imaging Techniques

The standard elbow series of AP, lateral, and oblique views is ordered to identify possible decreased joint space, osteophytes, and/or loose bodies (**Figure 11-20**).

Definitive Diagnosis

Radiographs demonstrate decreased joint space.

Pathomechanics and Functional Limitations

Patients have gradual onset of pain and loss of motion. If loose bodies are present, the patient has mechanical symptoms, which may include frank locking. Osteophyte formation may present as decreased ROM with a hard end feel. Pain increases when carrying something at the side with the elbow terminally extended. Patients who are heavy laborers or weightlifters have increased pain with these activities.

■ Medications

A trial of NSAIDs may be prescribed. If NSAIDs are tolerated and beneficial, the patient may try an over-the-counter NSAID on a long-term basis. Chondroitin sulfate and glucosamine may also be used (see chapter 4). Corticosteroid injections may be administered to help relieve pain in early stages. Further discussion regarding arthritis medications can also be found on pp 49 and 179.

■ Postinjury Management

Typically patients are treated conservatively. Initial treatment includes NSAIDs, rehabilitation, and rest from aggravating activities. A corticosteroid injection may be useful in the early disease stages. A carefully designed rehabilitation program should follow.

■ Surgical Intervention

Surgery is indicated in those patients who fail to improve with conservative measures and whose symptoms persist. Options include arthroscopy (with loose body removal, synovectomy, and osteophyte excision as appropriate), resection or interposition arthroplasty, **arthrodesis**, and total elbow arthroplasty. The procedure depends upon the severity of arthritis and deformity and patient age, activity level, and expectations.

Elbow arthroscopy should be performed by a surgeon who is familiar and comfortable with the intricate elbow anatomy, because the portals can be within 3 to 5 mm of a nerve branch. The skilled arthroscopist can address loose bodies and osteophytes and perform a complete synovectomy and capsular releases as necessary. These procedures can all be helpful in the early to midstages of arthritis, especially in younger, active patients.

When deformity or stiffness is severe, arthroscopic procedures are not indicated. Osteotomy or interposition arthroplasty are viable options. Total

Arthrodesis Fusion of bones across a joint space that limits or restricts joint motion.

elbow arthroplasty is indicated when pain and deformity are significant, conservative and other surgical measures fail, or laxity with deformity is chronic. Most surgeons recommend a semiconstrained design. The patient must have a good understanding of the realistic functional levels after these procedures. The primary goal is to provide pain relief. Although ROM increases after surgery, postoperative ROM is usually not full.[41] The patient will still be limited in activities that require greater degrees of extension and flexion.

■ Postinjury/Postoperative Management

Postsurgical treatment of arthroscopic conditions requires a soft dressing for about 1 week, followed by rehabilitation. The patient can perform ROM exercises during this time. After the wounds are adequately healed, a program similar to that for the conservative treatment of arthritis should be followed.

After osteotomy or joint replacement surgery, wound care is of the utmost importance. Elbow flexion places stress across most surgical exposures. To assist with incisional healing, the surgeon splints the elbow until the wound is well healed. Semiconstrained implants are splinted in extension, whereas resurfacing implants require a more stable 90° position.

■ Injury-Specific Treatment and Rehabilitation Concerns

Specific Concerns

Protect the joint surfaces (after arthroscopic procedures).
Protect the healing osteotomy or joint replacement.
Restore function.
Restore functional ROM.
Restore pain-free strength to the surrounding musculature.

Conservative care focuses on controlling pain and inflammation, restoring motion, and strengthening the trunk and entire extremity. ROM is usually best attempted with active or active-assisted exercise to minimize joint irritation. The clinician should be mindful of the end feels with ROM exercises and never force ROM with a hard end feel. Trunk and upper extremity strengthening decreases joint stress. Joint compression should be minimized when the patient with arthritis is pursuing strengthening.

After arthroscopic procedures, ROM and strengthening exercises are based completely on symptoms. These exercises can progress in intensity as tolerated, but excessive joint loading should be avoided. Both the patient and clinician should have realistic expectations for return to activity.

In rehabilitation after arthroplasty, active ROM begins as soon as the third postoperative day. A splint protects the joint between sessions. More aggressive active-assisted exercises and passive ROM are performed only if necessary. Once again, expectations after surgery must be realistic. The primary goal is to attain pain relief and have adequate ROM and strength for activities of daily living. The patient typically needs adequate reach for objects during everyday activities, including the head for grooming; approximately 20° of extension and 100° of flexion accomplishes this goal in most individuals.

Although it is important to strengthen the upper extremity after surgery, a permanent lifting restriction of 5 to 10 lb is typically imposed.[42] The patient must understand this restriction before the treatment plan is developed. With a semiconstrained prosthesis, isometric exercises can begin about 3 weeks after surgery, with light isotonic exercises starting at 6 weeks. A resurfacing arthroplasty may require a 2- to 3-week delay in initiating these exercises. Strength progression is highly individualized and must be determined in consultation with the surgeon.

■ Estimated Amount of Time Lost

Time lost depends on the patient's activities and the amount of contracture and deformity. Patients usually modify activities rather than stopping them completely.

■ Return-to-Play Criteria

The patient can return to sports and physical activities when tolerated. Clinically, the patient must have functional ROM and adequate strength compared with the contralateral extremity. Because of the chronic, progressive nature of this condition, the patient usually modifies activities as needed.

After surgical joint replacement, the patient is advised to avoid any activities that may place heavy shear or compressive forces through the joint.

Synovitis

Elbow synovitis can be caused by an inflammatory arthritic process or overuse. In athletes, synovitis almost always results from overuse and is usually self-resolving. The condition is common in overhead athletes, weightlifters, and heavy laborers and can occur concomitantly with medial or lateral epicondylitis.

History

Generalized elbow pain with an insidious onset
History of repetitive motion or overuse

Observation

Swelling may be noted.

Functional Status

ROM limited by pain and swelling
Decreased strength secondary to pain

Physical Evaluation Findings

The elbow may be warm to the touch.

Rheumatoid arthritis, an inflammatory process of the joint's synovial lining, is the most common cause of the inflammatory arthritides. However, it affects the elbow less often than other joints. Patients present with pain and deformity and may have laxity. Unlike patients with primary osteoarthritis, those with rheumatoid arthritis can lose bone stock (and eventually develop periarticular destruction), which can lead to joint laxity. The ulnohumeral articulation is most frequently involved.

Differential Diagnosis

Osteoarthritis, rheumatoid arthritis, tendinitis

Medical Diagnostic Tests

Laboratory analysis of aspirated synovial fluid identifies rheumatologic disorders.

Imaging Techniques

Radiographs may show bony destruction on both sides of the articulation if the condition has rheumatologic origins. MRI can reveal synovitis, especially in the earlier stages.

Definitive Diagnosis

The definitive diagnosis is based on the patient's history, physical examination, and radiographic findings.

Pathomechanics and Functional Limitations

Synovitis causes pain, swelling, and an inability to function in sport. The athlete may also have loose bodies and/or osteophytes in conjunction with the synovitis, which leads to increased pain and swelling and decreased ROM.

■ Immediate Management

Immediate management consists of rest from aggravating activities, as well as application of ice, compression, and elevation.

■ Medications

NSAIDs may be prescribed to control inflammation and swelling. Corticosteroid injections can temporarily relieve symptoms; however, active joint infection should be ruled out before a corticosteroid is injected.

■ Postinjury Management

Conservative medical management initially consists of avoiding aggravating activities, NSAIDs, and application of ice to decrease the inflammatory process. As the inflammatory process abates, therapeutic exercise is beneficial to restore normal motion. Corticosteroid injection is indicated in patients who do not improve on oral NSAIDs.

After injury, the patient is treated with relative rest. Aggravating activities must be avoided. The extremity can be used for activities requiring very low joint loads, but repetitive motions should be eliminated. Therapeutic modalities and gentle ROM exercises with low-load, prolonged stretches are instituted. As inflammation subsides, resistance exercises are initiated.

■ Surgical Intervention

Surgery is indicated in patients whose symptoms persist despite conservative measures. The procedure depends on the severity of the condition and patient age, activity level, and expectations. The most common surgical approach is the arthroscopic removal of loose bodies and excision of osteophytes. Severe cases with associated arthritis may require resection or interposition arthroplasty, arthrodesis, or total elbow arthroplasty.

■ Postoperative Management

After surgery, the elbow is placed in a compressive bandage for several days. After this is removed, the wounds are bandaged as needed. Movement within tolerable limits is encouraged to limit stiffness. The patient must not use the elbow in the motion extremes, which stress the healing wounds. Sutures are removed about 1 week after surgery, and rehabilitation is started.

■ Injury-Specific Treatment and Rehabilitation Concerns

Specific Concerns

Maintain pain-free ROM.
Control inflammation.

Conservative and postoperative rehabilitation protocols are similar. The initial focus is on decreasing inflammation. ROM exercises can be initiated with low-load, prolonged stretches to decrease stiffness and stimulate the synovial lining. Short, intense stretches and repetitive motions may increase inflammation and must be avoided. ROM should be performed with self-ranging exercises; passive ROM activity is included only out of necessity.

Trunk, shoulder, elbow, and wrist strengthening should be added as the patient attains pain-free, full, active motion. Strengthening the entire kinetic chain minimizes repetitive elbow stresses. Strengthening begins with light resistance and increases as tolerated.

Because synovitis is typically caused by repetitive overuse, a sport-specific program of functional activities is instituted. Low repetitions of drills and activities are initiated. Inflammation is closely monitored and activity durations increased as tolerated. Throwing athletes should be placed on a progressive routine involving incremental increases in duration, frequency, and intensity. Many throwing programs are available that can be adapted to meet the patient's needs. For instance, an outfielder focuses on longer, less frequent throws. A pitcher focuses on more frequent, high-intensity throws, while a catcher focuses on frequent, low-intensity throws with intermittent, high-intensity throws.

■ Estimated Amount of Time Lost

Overuse synovitis can resolve in days to weeks. The ability to truly rest the joint and allow pharmacologic and therapeutic modalities to reduce inflammation has the greatest influence on decreasing time lost to synovitis. Athletes can return to their sports about 8 weeks after surgery; however, if the condition existed for a long time before surgery, return may be delayed.

■ Return-to-Play Criteria

The athlete should have a pain-free, swelling-free elbow with full ROM and strength and must complete a sport-specific program of functional activities working up to the normal routine.

■ Lateral Epicondylitis

Lateral epicondylitis ("tennis elbow") is an inflammatory process of the common extensor tendons at their origin on the lateral epicondyle and is most commonly found in golfers and tennis players. Electromyographic studies indicate that the greatest amount of elbow muscle activity during tennis ground strokes is in the wrist-stabilizing muscles, specifically the extensor carpi radialis longus and brevis and extensor digitorum communis. As the

---

CLINICAL PRESENTATION

History

Insidious onset of pain arising from the lateral epicondyle
Pain may radiate into the forearm.
The patient usually has a history of repetitive elbow activity or overuse.

Observation

Mild swelling may be noted over the lateral epicondyle.

Functional Status

Active ROM is not restricted except in extreme cases.
Pain and weakness with lifting or other load-bearing wrist extension
Possible decreased grip strength

Physical Evaluation Findings

Point tenderness and possible crepitus 2 cm distal to the lateral epicondyle
Pain during lateral epicondyle palpation while resisting wrist extension
Pain arising from the lateral epicondyle during resisted second and third finger extension while the wrist and elbow are extended

---

racquet makes contact with the ball or the golf club makes contact with the ball and/or ground, torque increases and is transmitted through the tendons.[43]

The common extensors of the wrist originate on the lateral epicondyle. These include the extensor carpi radialis longus and brevis, extensor digitorum communis, and extensor carpi ulnaris. The extensor carpi radialis brevis is most commonly involved in lateral epicondylitis.[44] Although not a wrist extensor, the brachioradialis may be inhibited during elbow flexion. Lateral epicondylitis begins as microtears of the extensor carpi radialis brevis tendon,[44] but the other extensor tendons may also be involved. Lateral epicondylitis typically appears in the fourth and fifth decades and occurs equally in men and women.[45,46] Most cases involve the dominant arm.

In surgery, the tissue appears grayish and friable; tendon fibrillation and a sinus tract into the elbow joint may be seen. Characteristic microscopic angiofibroblastic dysplasia of the involved tissue is also noted.[45]

Differential Diagnosis

Radial tunnel syndrome, posterior interosseous nerve syndrome, lateral complex ligament injury, C7 radiculopathy

Imaging Techniques

Standard elbow radiographs (AP, lateral, and oblique) may be ordered to rule out soft-tissue calcification. Irritation of the lateral epicondyle and the tendinous attachment may be noted on MRI (**Figure 11-21**).

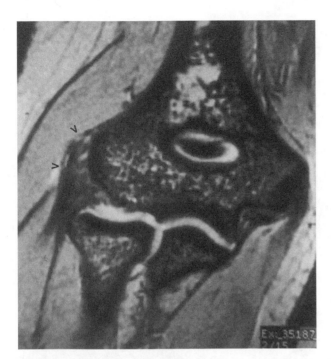

Figure 11-21 Coronal MRI demonstrating lateral epicondylitis (arrowheads). (Reproduced with permission from Williams RJ, Altchek DW: *Atraumatic injuries of the elbow in athletes, in Arendt EA (ed): Orthopaedic Knowledge Update: Sports Medicine,* ed 2. Rosemont, IL, American Academy of Orthopaedic Surgeons, 1999, p 228.)

Definitive Diagnosis

The definitive diagnosis is based on the clinical evaluation findings and the exclusion of ligament injury, nerve entrapment, and cervical radiculopathy.

Pathomechanics and Functional Limitations

Activities involving loaded wrist extension or grip strength are affected. Although grip is primarily provided by the flexors, to attain a strong grip the wrist extensors extend the wrist, thus creating better length-tension development within the flexor group. Overhand activities also create pain as the wrist extensors hold the wrist in neutral or extension. Repetitive activities exacerbate the condition and further increase pain. Some sport and work activities may be precluded by pain and weakness.

■ Immediate Management

Lateral epicondylitis is initially managed by applying ice and avoiding activities that load the wrist during extension.

■ Medications

A 2-week course of oral NSAIDs may be prescribed, with instructions for the patient to take the medication as needed thereafter. If the patient fails to respond to conservative treatment and NSAIDs, the physician may opt to inject a corticosteroid

deep to the extensor carpi radialis brevis. No more than three injections should be given to control this condition.

■ Postinjury Management

Most patients respond to conservative treatment in the form of rest, NSAIDs, and therapeutic exercise. Nighttime wrist-neutral splinting may reduce tension on the lateral epicondylitis and extensor group.

■ Surgical Intervention

Surgical treatment involves a small skin incision to expose the common extensor tendons. Any tendon defect is repaired, but the surgeon must take care not to imbricate the tissue, which could lead to decreased elbow extension. Any pathologic tissue is then excised; usually this includes most of, or the entire origin of, the extensor carpi radialis brevis. The extensor group is then reattached and repaired (**ST** 11-4).

■ Postoperative Management

Soft-tissue dressings are applied after surgery. Some surgeons prefer a posterior splint for 5 to 7 days. The patient can begin moving the elbow within a tolerable ROM at 3 days, and a formal exercise program may begin at 1 week if skin closure is adequate.

■ Injury-Specific Treatment and Rehabilitation Concerns

Specific Concerns
Protect the healing extensor group.
Control inflammation.
Correct improper biomechanics.

Initial attempts to reduce pain and inflammation involve patient education, treatment, and avoidance of aggravating activities. Typically such activities include gripping or using the hand in a pronated position requiring wrist extensor activity. Use of the extremity for nonaggravating activities is encouraged.

The mechanism of injury can typically be related to poor technique during activities or the improper use of equipment. A careful assessment, correction of poor techniques, and evaluation of all equipment must be performed. Close communication with a knowledgeable coach is helpful in directing the patient in proper techniques, which may include modifications such as a two-handed backhand stroke.

Use of inappropriate equipment may also be common in this patient population. Most often in

S|T Surgical Technique   11-4

Correction of Lateral Epicondylitis

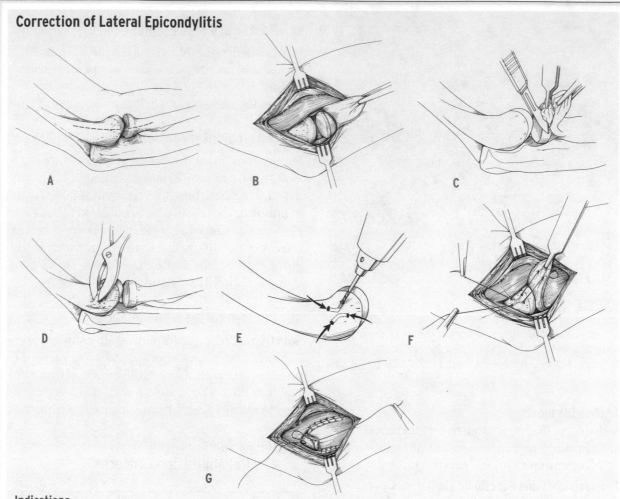

Indications

Pain and symptoms unresponsive to 6 to 12 consecutive months of adequate conservative treatment when other causes have been ruled out

Overview

1. An incision is made over the lateral epicondyle (**A**).
2. The common extensor tendon insertion on the lateral epicondyle is identified (**B**).
3. The extensor mechanism is reflected distally.
4. The pathologic tissues are excised from the extensor mechanism (**C**).
5. The lateral epicondyle is decorticated (**D**).
6. V-shaped tunnels are drilled into the epicondyle (**E**).
7. The common extensor tendon origin is reattached to the lateral epicondyle (**F**).
8. The extensor mechanism is reoriented to the surrounding structures using sutures (**G**).

Functional Limitations

No long-term functional limitations are expected.

Implications for Rehabilitation

These surgical procedures tend to be painful, and early ROM is encouraged. As pain resolves, ROM continues and early progressive resistance exercises are initiated.

Potential Complications

Failure to control symptoms and pain

Comments

Identification of offending biomechanics or activities and subsequent modification help to prevent recurrence.

Figure is reproduced with permission from Jobe FW, Ciccotti MG: Lateral and medial epicondylitis of the elbow. *J Am Acad Orthop Surg* 1994;2:1-8.

Decorticated The surgical removal of the outer layer of a structure.

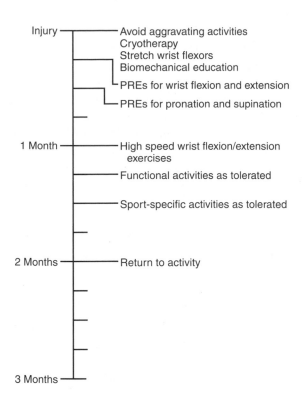

Injury — Avoid aggravating activities
Cryotherapy
Stretch wrist flexors
Biomechanical education
└ PREs for wrist flexion and extension
└ PREs for pronation and supination

1 Month — High speed wrist flexion/extension exercises

Functional activities as tolerated

Sport-specific activities as tolerated

2 Months — Return to activity

3 Months —

Note: Time frames are approximate. Function is the guide.

racquet sports, the racquet grip size is too big. The recommended grip size is measured from the proximal palmar crease to the tip of the ring finger, along the radial side of the finger.[44,47] Other racquet modifications may include an increased head size (increases "sweet spot"), a lighter racquet (offers better control), and decreased string tension (reduces impact forces).

Many patients use a computer workstation that may add to elbow inflammation. Proper workstation design allows the arms to be relaxed at the side and the hands to sit easily on the keyboard.

Initial attempts to reduce pain and inflammation focus on ice application. Phonophoresis or iontophoresis with anti-inflammatory agents may be attempted. Soft-tissue, deep, or cross-friction massage can help decrease pain and promote blood flow. Continuous ultrasound may be used to increase the tissue's viscoelastic properties before deep friction massage is applied.

The patient should begin flexibility exercises for the wrist extensor group within a pain-free range. Initial attempts may require keeping the elbow in some degree of flexion. Ultimately, the patient pro-gresses to performing flexibility exercises with the elbow extended.

Resistance exercises strengthen the extensor mechanism and should be performed in a pain-free manner. Initial strengthening consists of isometric or light isotonic exercises, with the resistance increased as tolerated. A comprehensive strengthening program for the entire trunk and upper extremity is also started.

As the patient progresses, more functional activities are included to prepare for the return to full activity. Use of rubber tubes or bands in short concentric and eccentric bursts mimic the forces placed on the elbow during sport activities. The patient can also practice functional motions with a racquet or club. Resistance can be added by using heavier tubing. The patient performs sport-specific drills and activities, progressing to a gradual return to full activity.

The postoperative rehabilitation program follows a course similar to conservative treatment after initial tissue healing occurs. The patient may perform gentle, active ROM exercises 3 days after surgery. The wrist extensors are gently stretched after suture removal. Strengthening exercises are added at 3 to 4 weeks. A counterforce brace is used with strengthening and activities for 2 to 3 months after surgery. After 3 months, the brace is only used with sport and work activities that require prolonged, repetitive use of the extensor mechanism. The patient begins a gradual return to sport and work activities 2 to 3 months after surgery and progresses to full activity as tolerated.

■ Estimated Amount of Time Lost

Time lost is based on symptom severity and duration. Acute conditions can resolve quickly (2 to 3 days) after short-term treatment. Chronic lateral epicondylitis may have a waxing and waning symptom course, depending on the patient's activity level. Surgical intervention may prolong return to activity to about 4 months.

■ Return-to-Play Criteria

The patient must have full, pain-free ROM and strength to progress to more functional activities. Return to full sport participation occurs when functional activities can be performed without pain during or after the activity.

Functional Bracing

A counterforce "tennis elbow strap" may help control symptoms by altering force distribution at the elbow (**Figure 11-22**).

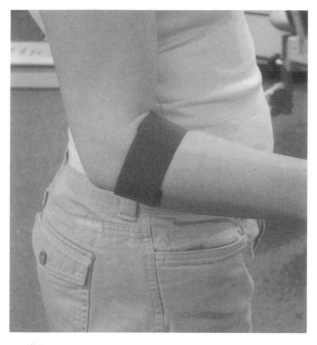

Figure 11-22 Lateral epicondylitis brace. The strap helps reduce tension on the wrist extensor muscles, thereby decreasing symptoms.

Medial Epicondylitis

CLINICAL PRESENTATION

History

Insidious onset of pain in the medial elbow
Pain increases during activities that increase valgus stress on the elbow (eg, golf or throwing).

Observation

Mild swelling of the medial elbow

Functional Status

Active ROM may not be noticeably limited.
Pain and weakness may be reported during functional activities.
Grip strength may be decreased.

Physical Evaluation Findings

Medial tenderness over the pronator teres and flexor carpi radialis muscles just distal to the medial epicondyle
Pain occurs during resisted wrist flexion and pronation.

Medial epicondylitis ("golfer's elbow") is less common than lateral epicondylitis.[44] It can occur in patients who are involved in sports or occupations that create valgus forces about the elbow. The muscles originating from the medial epicondyle include the pronator teres, flexor carpi radialis, palmaris longus, flexor digitorum superficialis, and flexor carpi ulnaris. The pronator teres and flexor carpi radialis are most commonly involved in medial epicondylitis.

Although termed "golfer's elbow," the condition can occur with any active endeavor that places valgus force on the elbow.[48-50] Medial elbow biomechanics have been well described with regard to the pitching mechanism. Peak angular velocity and valgus stress are greatest during the acceleration phase, exceeding the tensile strength of the medial ligamentous and tendinous structures. The stresses are initially transmitted to the flexor pronator musculature (especially the pronator teres) and then to the deeper medial collateral ligament.

Medial epicondylitis typically appears in the fourth and fifth decades and occurs equally in men and women.[44,50] Improper technique, inadequate warm-up, fatigue, and poor conditioning can lead to medial elbow inflammation.

Differential Diagnosis

UCL sprain, medial elbow instability

Imaging Techniques

Standard elbow (AP, lateral, and oblique) radiographs are taken to rule out soft-tissue calcification, osteophytes, and intra-articular conditions.

Definitive Diagnosis

The definitive diagnosis is based on the findings of the clinical evaluation and the exclusion of ligamentous injury.

Pathomechanics and Functional Limitations

Activities requiring wrist flexion may be affected, and the patient increases elbow flexion to compensate for the deficit. Activities that apply a valgus force to the elbow may be diminished secondary to pain. Grip may be affected secondary to flexor group pain.

■ Immediate Management

Medial epicondylitis is initially managed by avoiding activities that require repetitive wrist flexion. Ice application controls inflammation.

■ Medications

A 2-week course of an oral NSAID may be prescribed, with instructions to take the medication as needed thereafter.

■ Postinjury Management

Most patients with medial epicondylitis respond to conservative treatment. Rest from the aggravating activity, local modalities, rehabilitation, and night wrist-neutral splinting may reduce tension on the tissues.

S|T Surgical Technique 11-5

Surgical Correction of Medial Epicondylitis

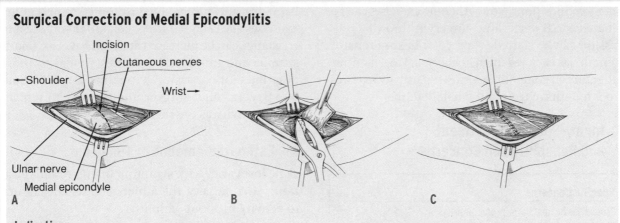

Indications

Pain and symptoms unresponsive to 12 consecutive months of adequate conservative treatment when other causes have been ruled out

Overview

1. A 3- to 7-in incision is centered over the medial epicondyle.
2. The medial epicondyle, flexor pronator group, and cutaneous nerves are identified (**A**).
3. The common flexor origin is incised and reflected.
4. The ulnar nerve is identified and protected.
5. Any pathologic tissue is identified and excised.
6. The medial epicondyle is debrided of soft tissue, and a vascular bed is created by drilling several small holes in the epicondyle (**B**).
7. The common flexor group tendons are reattached to the medial epicondyle (**C**).

Functional Limitations

No functional limitations are expected, but the ulnar nerve should be protected posterior to the medial epicondyle.

Implications for Rehabilitation

These surgical procedures tend to be painful, and early ROM is encouraged. As pain resolves, ROM continues and early progressive resistance exercises are initiated.

Potential Complications

Surgery may fail to relieve pain.

Comments

Identifying and modifying offending biomechanics or activities help to prevent recurrence.

Figure reproduced with permission from Jobe FW, Ciccotti MG: Lateral and medial epicondylitis of the elbow. *J Am Acad Orthop Surg* 1994;2:1-8.

■ Surgical Intervention

Surgery is indicated for medial epicondylitis if 1 year of conservative management fails, but it is possible the surgery will not enable return to the desired functional level. In patients who are not expected to experience considerable valgus load after surgery, debridement and segmental resection of the medial conjoined tendon yield good results. However, in patients who are expected to subject the surgical tissues to significant and continued valgus load, such as throwing athletes, debridement with anatomic repair (instead of resection) of the medial conjoined tendon is performed to reestablish the dynamic valgus stability provided by the flexor pronator mass (S|T 11-5). The loss of innervation to the flexor-pronator group can produce debilitating strength deficits.

■ Postoperative Management

The elbow is immobilized in a posterior splint for 5 to 10 days to allow wound healing. Elbow motion is allowed from 45° to 120° for the next 2 weeks. At the end of week 3, the splint is removed and replaced with a neutral wrist splint. Elbow ROM is then performed with the forearm pronated and the wrist flexed. Forearm and wrist ROM is done with the elbow flexed to 90°. No tension is placed on the repair because tendon relaxation at one joint allows ROM exercises at the other joint. This protocol is maintained for 3 weeks and then full ROM of all joints is allowed with little regard to the other joint positions. Strengthening exercises can be initiated 6 to 8 weeks after surgery. A throwing progression can be started when good flexor pronator strength has been regained, usually at 3 to 4 months. Full return to competitive throwing usually requires 6 to 9 months of time and rehabilitation.

Injury-Specific Treatment and Rehabilitation Concerns

Specific Concerns

Protect the healing flexor pronator group.
Control inflammation.
Correct poor biomechanics.

In the early stages of medial epicondylitis, pain and inflammation are controlled as for lateral epicondylitis. Avoiding aggravating activities, altering technique and equipment, using counterforce bracing, and applying ice can be beneficial. Phonophoresis or iontophoresis with anti-inflammatory agents may be helpful.

Flexibility exercises are initiated for the pronator teres muscle and wrist flexor group. Initially the elbow may need to be positioned in slight flexion, but it should be extended for flexibility exercises as soon as possible. The shoulder should be assessed for any internal rotation deficit, which increases valgus stresses on the elbow with throwing. Internal rotation is increased through passive (with the clinician) and self-stretching techniques.

Strengthening focuses on the flexor pronator muscle group and includes the trunk and entire extremity.

As the patient progresses, more functional activities are incorporated to prepare for the return to full activity. Use of rubber tubes or bands in short concentric and eccentric bursts mimic elbow forces during sport activities.

The patient can also practice functional motions with a racquet or club, adding resistance with rubber tubing. Sport-specific drills and activities are included, progressing to a gradual return to full activity. Functional training usually focuses on endurance activities, because these tissues usually perform many short bursts of activity that lead to fatigue.

Postoperative care is similar to that for lateral epicondylar release. Early treatment includes a removable posterior splint for about 1 week, with gentle wrist and hand ROM exercises beginning about 3 days after surgery. Squeezing a sponge can also begin at about 3 days, emphasizing submaximal contraction rather than a maximal squeeze. Isometric and submaximal isotonic strengthening exercises start about 3 to 4 weeks after surgery, and resistance can be increased at about 6 weeks. Sport-specific and functional activities similar to those described for conservative treatment begin about 6 to 8 weeks after surgery, and the patient returns to full activity as tolerated.

Estimated Amount of Time Lost

Time lost varies with symptom intensity and duration. After surgery, the athlete can usually return to activity in about 4 months.

Return-to-Play Criteria

The patient must have full, pain-free ROM and strength to progress to more functional activities. Return to full sport activities is permitted when all activities can be performed without pain during or after the activity.

Functional Bracing

Although a counterforce brace can be used with medial epicondylitis, it is typically not as helpful as with lateral epicondylitis. Braces are usually not used after surgery.

Elbow Neuropathies

Because of the relatively subcutaneous location of the nerves crossing the elbow, the muscular and ligamentous architecture, and the risk of compromise secondary to other trauma, elbow neuropathies are a frequent occurrence. These neuropathies can produce symptoms in the forearm, wrist, hand, and fingers.

Ulnar Neuropathy

Ulnar nerve compression is second only to the carpal tunnel in the frequency of upper extremity compressive neuropathies. The two most common sites of compression are the epicondylar groove and between the heads of the flexor carpi ulnaris (**Figure 11-23**). Less common sites of compression include the arcade of Struthers, medial intermuscular septum, medial epicondyle, and cubital tunnel (**Figure 11-24**).[51,52]

Compressive neuropathies of other peripheral nerves at the elbow are less common. Neurologic inhibition at the elbow can cause abnormal hand postures (see chapter 12).

CLINICAL PRESENTATION

Ulnar Neuropathy	Radial Tunnel Syndrome	Posterior Interosseous Nerve Syndrome	Anterior Interosseous Nerve Syndrome
History			
Pain and paresthesia in the ring and little fingers Medial elbow pain	Pain in the radial tunnel No numbness is reported.	Pain and weakness in the finger extensors and thumb abductors	Pain and weakness in the thumb flexors, medial flexor digitorum profundus, and pronator quadratus
Observation			
Wasting of the intrinsic hand muscles (late stages)	No deformity or muscle wasting	No deformity or muscle wasting	No deformity or muscle wasting
Functional Status			
Weakness of the intrinsic hand muscles Decreased grip strength	Function limited by pain and weakness	Function limited by pain and weakness	Inability to flex the thumb interphalangeal joint Inability to flex the second dorsal interphalangeal joint
Physical Evaluation Findings			
Point tenderness over the ulnar nerve Symptoms are exacerbated when the elbow is flexed. Positive Tinel sign Positive cubital tunnel compression test	Point tenderness over the anterior radial neck Pain with elbow extension, forearm pronation, wrist flexion	Extended wrist deviates ulnarly secondary to the unopposed action of the extensor carpi radialis longus.	During attempted circumduction of the thumb and index finger, the interphalangeal joint (thumb) and dorsal interphalangeal joint (index finger) remain extended.

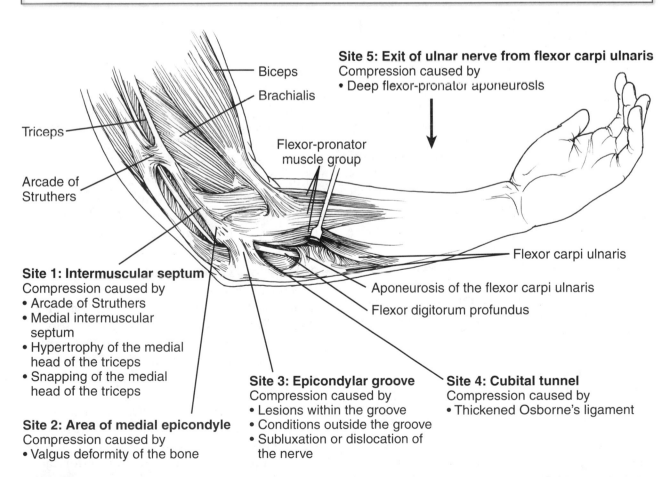

Site 5: Exit of ulnar nerve from flexor carpi ulnaris
Compression caused by
• Deep flexor-pronator aponeurosis

Biceps
Brachialis
Triceps
Flexor-pronator muscle group
Arcade of Struthers
Flexor carpi ulnaris
Aponeurosis of the flexor carpi ulnaris
Flexor digitorum profundus

Site 1: Intermuscular septum
Compression caused by
• Arcade of Struthers
• Medial intermuscular septum
• Hypertrophy of the medial head of the triceps
• Snapping of the medial head of the triceps

Site 2: Area of medial epicondyle
Compression caused by
• Valgus deformity of the bone

Site 3: Epicondylar groove
Compression caused by
• Lesions within the groove
• Conditions outside the groove
• Subluxation or dislocation of the nerve

Site 4: Cubital tunnel
Compression caused by
• Thickened Osborne's ligament

Figure 11-23 Five sites for potential ulnar nerve compression and their associated causes. (Adapted with permission from Amadio PC: Anatomical basis for a technique of ulnar nerve transposition. *Surg Radiol Anat* 1986;8:155-161.)

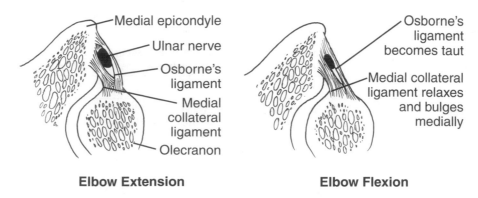

Figure 11-24 Anatomy of the cubital tunnel with the elbow in extension and flexion. (Adapted with permission from Adelaar RS, Foster WC, McDowell C: The treatment of the cubital tunnel syndrome. *J Hand Surg Am* 1984;9:90-95.)

Radial Tunnel Syndrome

Radial tunnel syndrome causes radial nerve compression. The radial tunnel is between the radiohumeral joint and supinator muscle. Compression sites include the fibrous margin of the extensor carpi radialis brevis, fibrous bands at the radiocapitellar joint, radial recurrent artery, arcade of Frohse, and a fibrous band at the distal margin of the supinator muscle. Radial tunnel syndrome should be considered in patients with recalcitrant lateral epicondylitis.

Posterior Interosseous Nerve Syndrome

Posterior interosseous nerve syndrome results from compression of the posterior interosseous nerve (PIN) and causes loss of motor function without sensory deficits. The PIN is a branch of the radial nerve (becoming the PIN as it exits the supinator muscle) and innervates the extensor carpi ulnaris, extensor digiti quinti, extensor digitorum communis, abductor pollicis longus, extensor pollicis longus and brevis, and extensor indicis proprius. PIN syndrome can coexist with, and be confused with, lateral epicondylitis.

Anterior Interosseous Nerve Syndrome

With anterior interosseous nerve compression in the forearm, pain and swelling occur, but no sensory deficits are noted. The anterior interosseous nerve innervates the flexor pollicis longus, radial two-flexor digitorum profundus (thumb and index finger), and pronator quadratus.

Differential Diagnosis

Lateral epicondylitis, medial epicondylitis, cervical abnormality, thoracic outlet syndrome, other neuropathies

Medical Diagnostic Tests

Electromyographic studies and nerve conduction velocity testing help pinpoint the location of any compressive lesion. Electromyography can map out the affected musculature and thus identify the affected nerves. Nerve conduction velocity testing can better determine the location and extent of nerve compression.

Imaging Techniques

Radiographs are usually normal in neuropathies but can confirm the presence of a supracondylar process, a potential site for nerve compression. In the event of posttraumatic neuropathy, radiographs can aid in ruling out nerve injury secondary to bony trauma.

Cervical spine radiographs and MRI may be warranted to rule out cervical involvement.

Definitive Diagnosis

The definitive diagnosis is based on the patient's history and the clinical examination findings. The diagnoses of ulnar neuropathy and anterior interosseous nerve syndrome are assisted by the electromyographic findings. Negative findings in the distal humerus and elbow warrant cervical spine and shoulder evaluation for compressive or occlusive neuropathies. **Table 11-1** presents the effects of neuropathy specific to the involved nerve.

Pathomechanics and Functional Limitations

Functional deficits occur along the distribution of the involved nerves and distal branches (**Figure 11-25**). With careful assessment of motor and sensory status, a more accurate diagnosis of neuropathy can be made and possible causes identified. The pattern of deficits can vary widely, but most are exhibited in specific areas of the hand.

Ulnar Neuropathy Compressive ulnar neuropathy results in numbness and weakness of the hand intrinsic muscles, which can affect grip and fine motor activities and thus the athlete's performance. The pain can cause functional limitations and is usually exacerbated when the elbow is flexed.

Table 11-1

The Effects of Injury to Specific Peripheral Nerves

Musculocutaneous nerve (C5, C6, C7)

Sensory supply

- Lateral half of the anterior surface of the forearm from the elbow to the thenar eminence

Effect of injury

- Severe weakness of elbow flexion
- Weakness of supination
- Loss of biceps deep tendon reflex
- Loss of sensation, cutaneous distribution

Radial nerve (C5, C6, C7, C8, T1)

Sensory supply

- Back of the arm, forearm, wrist, radial half of the dorsum of the hand, back of the thumb, index finger, and part of the middle finger

Effect of injury

- Loss of triceps reflex
- Weakness of elbow flexion
- Loss of supination (when the elbow is extended)
- Loss of wrist extension
- Weakness of ulnar and radial deviation
- Loss of extension at the metacarpophalangeal joints
- Loss of extension and abduction of the thumb

Median nerve (C5, C6, C7, C8, T1)

Sensory supply

- Radial half of the palm; palmar surface of the thumb; index, middle, and radial half of the ring finger; and dorsal surfaces of the same fingers

Effect of injury

- Loss of complete pronation (brachioradialis can bring the forearm to midpronation but not beyond)
- Weakness with flexion and radial deviation (ulnar deviation with wrist flexion)
- Loss of flexion at the metacarpophalangeal joints
- Loss of thumb opposition or abduction, loss of flexion at the interphalangeal or metacarpophalangeal joints

Ulnar nerve (C7, C8, T1)

Sensory supply

- Dorsal and palmar surfaces of the ulnar side of the hand, including the little finger and ulnar half of the ring finger

Effect of injury

- Weakness of wrist flexion and ulnar deviation (radial deviation with wrist flexion)
- Loss of flexion of dorsal interphalangeal joints of ring and little fingers
- Inability to abduct or adduct fingers
- Inability to adduct thumb
- Loss of flexion of fingers, especially ring and little fingers at the metacarpophalangeal joints
- Loss of extension of fingers, especially ring and little fingers at the interphalangeal joint

---

Radial Tunnel Syndrome Functional limitations are secondary to pain. Activities requiring repetitive elbow and/or wrist motion are also affected. Radial nerve compression is most common with passive elbow extension, forearm pronation, and wrist flexion.

Posterior Interosseous Nerve Syndrome Compression may result in loss of motor function, depending on the specific area of nerve involvement. Although commonly thought of as affecting only motor function, the syndrome produces pain that mimics that of lateral epicondylitis. Most PIN compressions resolve spontaneously.

Anterior Interosseous Nerve Syndrome The patient experiences difficulty pinching with the thumb and index finger (**Figure 11-26**). Fine motor skills may also be affected.

■ Immediate Management

With any compressive neuropathy, patients are encouraged to avoid provocative maneuvers that exacerbate symptoms. This restriction is especially important in acute compressive neuropathies.

■ Medications

If the neuropathy is extremely painful, narcotic analgesics may be warranted. The patient may also respond positively to a course of NSAIDs.

Patients with neuropathies refractory to initial management can be considered for corticosteroid injection. The medication should be carefully injected immediately adjacent to, and not directly into, the nerve.

■ Postinjury Management

Ulnar Neuropathy

Initial treatment is nonsurgical. Modifying the patient's activities to avoid prolonged elbow flexion, valgus elbow stress, and other offensive activities can relieve symptoms in acute compressive neuropathy. A short course of NSAIDs in addition can speed recovery.

Radial Tunnel Syndrome

Initial treatment is modification of activities to avoid provocative maneuvers.

Posterior Interosseous Nerve Syndrome

Initial treatment for PIN syndrome is supportive care, as most cases resolve spontaneously.

Anterior Interosseous Nerve Syndrome

Anterior interosseous nerve syndrome is typically related to a neuritis or acute **demyelinization** within the brachial plexus. Thus most episodes resolve spontaneously.

Demyelinization
Erosion of a nerve's myelin layer, resulting in decreased nerve function.

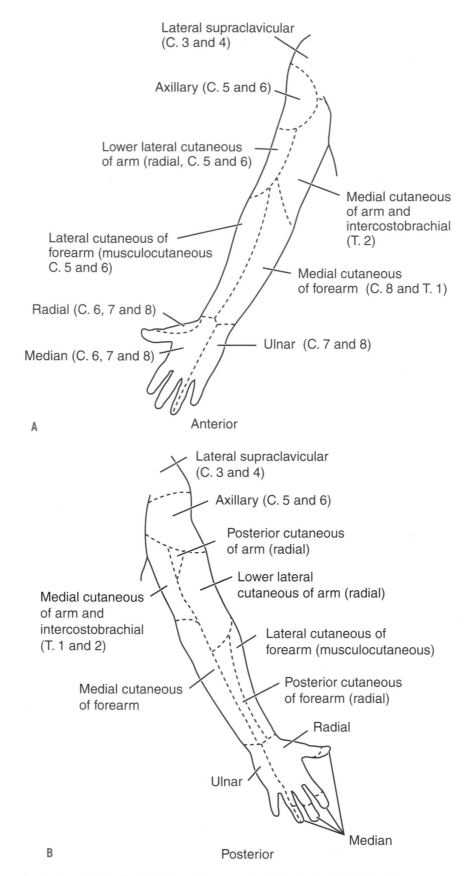

Figure 11-25 Sensory function is provided by the C5, C6, T1, and T2 nerve roots. **A.** Anterior view. **B.** Posterior view.

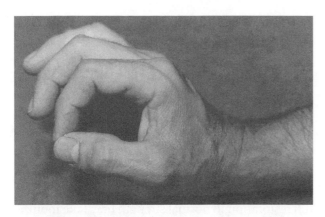

Figure 11-26 Patients with anterior interosseous nerve syndrome are asked to position the hand as shown. Those with absent profundus and flexor pollicis longus activity flex only the interphalangeal joint of the index finger and the metacarpophalangeal joint of the thumb. (Reproduced with permission from Lubahn JD, Cermak MB: Uncommon nerve compression syndromes of the upper extremity. *J Am Acad Orthop Surg* 1998;6:378-386.)

Surgical Intervention

Ulnar Neuropathy

Surgery is indicated for those patients whose symptoms progress despite, or are refractory to, conservative management. Surgical release of Osborne's ligament at the cubital tunnel can relieve symptoms. Medial epicondylectomy has been used in the past but is usually not effective for throwing athletes. Decompression with transposition is the most common procedure performed for ulnar neuropathy at the elbow. This procedure has the advantage of removing the nerve from the compressive bed and also effectively lengthens the nerve by transposing it anteriorly. Subcutaneous transposition is the most common type, although some surgeons still perform submuscular transpositions. Proximal and distal nerve release must accompany the nerve transposition from its original bed.

Radial Tunnel Syndrome

Before committing to surgery, the physician should make every attempt to confirm that the symptoms are truly due to radial tunnel compression. During a radial tunnel release, care should be taken to ensure that all potential areas of compression are released, including the entire supinator and the distal tissue edge.

Posterior Interosseous Nerve Syndrome

If no clinical evidence of recovery occurs within 90 days, spontaneous recovery is unlikely and surgery should be performed. By 18 months, muscle fibrosis can be irreversible and muscle transfers are necessary. If surgical treatment is attempted, the surgeon must obtain adequate nerve exposure, identify all areas of compression, and release as needed. The extent of decompression varies widely.

Anterior Interosseous Nerve Syndrome

If no improvement occurs with 3 to 6 months of conservative treatment or a space-occupying lesion is present, surgery is indicated. Exposure through an S-shaped incision over the forearm is proximal to the elbow. The median nerve is exposed and traced distally. The most common entrapment area is under the ulnar head of the pronator teres, which is taken down for exposure and later reattached. Possible areas of entrapment that may need to be released include the pronator teres, lacertus fibrosus, fibrous fascial arches in the pronator teres, and flexor digitorum superficialis.

Postinjury/Postoperative Management

A splint is used for 3 to 7 days after surgery for comfort, and then rehabilitation begins.

Injury-Specific Treatment and Rehabilitation Concerns

> **Specific Concerns**
> Restore neurologic function.
> Restore patient to full activity.

Typical conservative treatment focuses on avoiding activities that cause symptoms. Flexibility exercises are performed for any musculature that may be compressing the affected nerve.

Prolonged neuropathy may lead to wasting of the innervated muscles. Neuromuscular electric stimulation may be useful to prevent or manage disuse atrophy. Therapeutic exercises for gaining active motor function and strengthening should also be performed. A general strengthening program is instituted for the trunk, shoulder girdle, elbow, and wrist muscles, with a more specific program targeting areas affected by the compression.

Functional activities involving fine motor skills should be included. A progressive sport-specific program is instituted once the patient is symptom free. Functional training should be closely monitored for any return of the patient's neurologic symptoms, which necessitates activity cessation. A biomechanical evaluation of the athlete's activities is essential to determine any improper mechanics that may contribute to the compression neuropathy.

After surgery, ROM exercises are started at about 1 week. Nerve-gliding exercises are essential. Strengthening involving isometrics can begin at 2 to 3 weeks, with light resistance started at 3 to 4 weeks. If any musculature was detached to gain exposure to the nerve and then reattached, strengthening begins with submaximal exercises of that muscle at 4 to 5 weeks. Resistance should not be increased until after 6 weeks.

Functional activities involving fine motor tasks can begin as soon as motor function is demonstrated in the previously affected musculature. However, the clinician should be mindful that the musculature may fatigue very quickly.

Functional training in sport-specific activities commences at 8 weeks.

■ Estimated Amount of Time Lost

Estimated time lost is highly variable. Symptoms can persist for days to months.

■ Return-to-Play Criteria

Functional strength should be completely restored before the athlete returns to full activity. However, full restoration to normal strength may take months and is not an absolute requirement for return to activity.

Rehabilitation

Refer to chapter 13 for additional therapeutic exercise techniques.

Soft-Tissue Mobilization

The skin, fascia, muscle, tendons, and ligaments around the elbow may be shortened or postsurgical tissues may be adhered, resulting in decreased ROM. Standard massage and myofascial release techniques can be used to increase soft-tissue mobility.

Extensor Group Tendon Cross-Friction Massage

The patient sits with the arm at the end of a table. Using either the thumb or a combination of the index and middle fingers, cross-friction massage is applied to the common extensor tendon approximately 1 to 2 cm distal to the lateral epicondyle.

Range-of-Motion Exercises

Stretching of the shoulder girdle should be emphasized during elbow flexibility routines (see chapters 10 and 13).

Passive Range of Motion

Obtaining full ROM in the restricted elbow can be difficult. The greatest increases will occur with passive ROM performed for 10 to 15 minutes. The patient is positioned seated or supine with the affected arm supported with toweling. The clinician slowly moves the patient's arm into the extreme of ROM being treated and holds for 20 to 30 seconds. Wrist flexion and extension can be alternately incorporated into every other extension phase of the exercise (**Figure 11-27**).

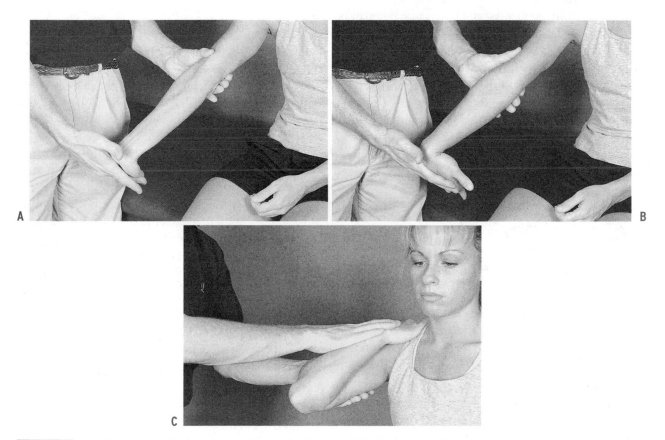

Figure 11-27 The patient stretches the injured extremity against resistance for 10 to 12 minutes. **A.** Elbow extension, wrist extension. **B.** Elbow extension, wrist flexion. **C.** Elbow flexion.

■ Alternative Active-Assisted/ Passive Range of Motion

Flexion

The patient sits with the upper arm supported on a table with the elbow just off the edge. The opposite extremity is used to flex the elbow.

Extension

The patient sits with the upper arm supported on a table with the elbow just off the edge. Using the opposite extremity, the elbow is extended. A small weight (heavy enough to create stretch but not a reflexive muscle contraction) is placed around the wrist to produce passive ROM. The upper extremity is stabilized, and the position is held for a low-load, prolonged stretch.

An alternative stretch for extension can be obtained by strapping the weight to the wrist, and having the patient stand against a wall so the upper arm is stabilized. A towel is placed between the arm and the wall, allowing the elbow to rest in extension.

Pronation and Supination

Seated or standing, the patient holds the end of a 1-foot dowel. The elbow is flexed to approximately 90° and stabilized against the body. The forearm is slowly moved into pronation, held, and then moved into supination and held. For slightly more pressure, the patient can use the opposite hand on the upper end of the dowel to apply more force, or a weight can be strapped to the end of the dowel (or a hammer). The patient then controls the upper end with the free hand as the forearm moves in and out of the extremes of motion. The exercise can be performed in various degrees of elbow flexion.

Strengthening Techniques

■ Isometric Elbow Exercises

Flexion

Standing with the elbow flexed to the desired angle, the patient provides matching resistance to elbow flexion with the opposite hand placed on the forearm.

Extension

Standing with the elbow flexed to the desired angle, the patient provides matching resistance to elbow extension with the opposite hand placed on the forearm.

Pronation and Supination

Grasping a bar or handle affixed to a wall, the patient attempts to supinate or pronate the forearm.

■ Progressive Resistive Elbow Exercises

Flexion

Standing with the arm at the side and forearm in a neutral position, the patient flexes the elbow and supinates the forearm in a pain-free arc. Free weights, tubing, or a weight machine designed for elbow flexion can be used for this exercise.

Extension

Lying supine, the patient flexes the shoulder to 90°. The elbow is taken from extension into flexion. Using tubing attached overhead, the patient can stand and pull down, extending the elbow. Resistance can also be applied through the use of a machine.

Pronation and Supination

Standing, the patient holds the lower end of a dowel with a cuff weight attached. The elbow is flexed to 90° and stabilized against the body. The forearm is moved slowly into pronation and then into supination. Resistance can be adjusted by grasping the dowel closer to the weight (decreasing resistance) or closer to the end (increasing resistance). A hammer is a good substitute for a weighted dowel early in the strengthening process.

Proprioceptive Neuromuscular Facilitation Exercise

Refer to chapter 13 for other upper extremity proprioceptive neuromuscular facilitation exercises.

■ Extension Control Exercises

Patients with extension overload injuries must develop dynamic control in the elbow to limit stress to the posterior structures. Standing and facing tubing that is attached to a wall at about shoulder height, the patient grasps the tubing with the shoulder flexed to about 90°. The elbow is concentrically flexed and then extended in a controlled motion through an eccentric flexor contraction. Before the elbow is fully extended, the patient flexes the elbow again, never letting the olecranon process make contact with the olecranon fossa.

Plyometric Exercises

Refer to chapter 13 for other upper extremity plyometric exercises.

■ Medicine Ball Exercises

Initially, these exercises are performed with the elbow close to the body in a nonprovocative position. A basketball or weighted medicine ball can be

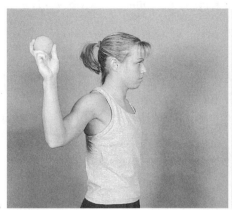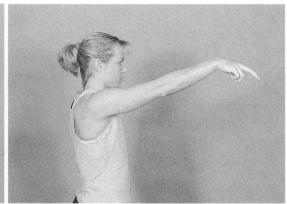

A   B

Figure 11-28 These drills can be used to replicate the throwing motion. **A.** Overhead throw. **B.** Ball release.

used to perform a two-handed passing motion, throwing to a partner or a trampoline.

Weighted Ball Exercises

As the patient progresses, the arm can be moved out to the side, so that more provocative stresses are placed upon the elbow and control is developed.

Using a small weighted ball, the patient cocks the arm (Figure 11-28) and tosses the ball at the trampoline using proper throwing mechanics. As the ball returns, the patient catches it, controlling the valgus stress placed upon the elbow. As the patient progresses, the full throwing motion is replicated in the exercise.

11

■ References

1. D'Alessandro DF, Shields CL Jr, Tibone JE, Chandler RW: Repair of distal biceps tendon ruptures in athletes. *Am J Sports Med* 1993;21:114-119.

2. Boyd MM, Anderson LD: A method of reinsertion of the distal biceps brachii tendon. *J Bone Joint Surg Am* 1961;43:1041-1043.

3. Morrey BF: Injury of the flexors of the elbow: Biceps in tendon injury, in Morrey BF (ed): *The Elbow and Its Disorders*. Philadelphia, PA, WB Saunders, 2000, pp 468-478.

4. Norman WH: Repair of avulsion of insertion of biceps brachii tendon. *Clin Orthop* 1985;193:189-194.

5. Rantanen J, Orava S: Rupture of the distal biceps tendon: A report of 19 patients treated with anatomic reinsertion, and a meta-analysis of 147 cases found in the literature. *Am J Sports Med* 1999;27:128-132.

6. Ramsey ML: Distal biceps tendon injuries: Diagnosis and management. *J Am Acad Orthop Surg* 1999;7:199-207.

7. Sanchez-Sotelo J, Morrey BF, Adams RA, O'Driscoll SW: Reconstruction of chronic ruptures of the distal biceps tendon with use of an Achilles tendon allograft. *J Bone Joint Surg Am* 2002;84:999-1005.

8. Baker BE, Bierwagen D: Rupture of the distal tendon of the biceps brachii: Operative versus non-operative treatment. *J Bone Joint Surg Am* 1985;67:414-417.

9. D'Arco P, Sitler M, Kelly J, et al: Clinical, functional, and radiographic assessments of the conventional and modified Boyd-Anderson surgical procedures for repair of distal biceps tendon ruptures. *Am J Sports Med* 1998;26:254-261.

10. Sisto DJ, Jobe FW, Moynes DW, Antonelli DJ: An electromyographic analysis of the elbow in pitching. *Am J Sports Med* 1987;15:260-263.

11. Morrey BF, An KN: Articular and ligamentous contributions to the stability of the elbow joint. *Am J Sports Med* 1983;11:315–319.

12. King GJW, Morrey BF, An KN: Stabilizers of the elbow. *J Shoulder Elbow Surg* 1993;2:165-170.

13. Conway JE, Jobe FW, Glousman RE, Pink M: Medial instability of the elbow in throwing athletes: Treatment by repair or reconstruction of the ulnar collateral ligament. *J Bone Joint Surg Am* 1992;74:67-83.

14. Jobe FW, El Attrache NS: Diagnosis and treatment of ulnar collateral ligament injuries in athletes, in Morrey BF (ed): *The Elbow and Its Disorders*. Philadelphia, PA, WB Saunders, 2000, pp 549-555.

15. Chen FS, Rokito AS, Jobe FW: Medial elbow problems in the overhead-throwing athlete. *J Am Acad Orthop Surg* 2001;9:99-113.

16. Morrey BF: Acute and chronic instability of the elbow. *J Am Acad Orthop Surg* 1996;4:117-128.

17. Wilson FD, Andrews JR, Blackburn TA, McCluskey G: Valgus extension overload in the pitching elbow. *Am J Sports Med* 1983;11:83-88.

18. Azar FM, Wilk KE: Nonoperative treatment of the elbow in throwers. *Oper Techniq Sports Med* 1996;4:91-99.

19. Wilk KE, Arrigo CA, Andrews JR, Azar FM: Rehabilitation following elbow surgery in the throwing athlete. *Oper Techniq Sports Med* 1996;4:114-132.

20. O'Driscoll SW, Bell DW, Morrey BF: Posterolateral rotatory instability of the elbow. *J Bone Joint Surg Am* 1991;73:440-446.

21. Dunning CE, Zarzour ZDS, Patterson SD, Johnson JA, King GJW: Ligamentous stabilizers against posterolateral rotatory instability of the elbow. *J Bone Joint Surg Am* 2001;83:1823-1828.

22. Nestor BJ, O'Driscoll SW, Morrey BF: Ligamentous reconstruction for posterolateral rotatory instability of the elbow. *J Bone Joint Surg Am* 1992;74:1235-1241.

23. Miller CD, Savoie FH 3rd: Valgus extension injuries of the elbow in the throwing athlete. *J Am Acad Orthop Surg* 1994;2:261-269.

24. Bennet JB, Mehlhoff TL: Articular injuries in the athlete, in Morrey BF (ed): *The Elbow and Its Disorders*. Philadelphia, PA, WB Saunders, 2000, pp 563-576.

25. Webb LX: Distal humeral fractures in adults. *J Am Acad Orthop Surg* 1996;4:336-344.

26. Ring D, Jupiter JB, Zilberfarb J: Posterior dislocation of the elbow with fractures of the radial head and coronoid. *J Bone Joint Surg Am* 2002;84:547-551.

27. Hak DJ, Golladay GJ: Olecranon fractures: Treatment options. *J Am Acad Orthop Surg* 2000;8:266-275.

28. Hotchkiss RN: Displaced fractures of the radial head: Internal fixation or excision? *J Am Acad Orthop Surg* 1997; 5:1-10.

29. Ring D, Quintero J, Jupiter JB: Open reduction and internal fixation of fractures of the radial head. *J Bone Joint Surg Am* 2002;84:1811-1815.

30. Kuntz DG, Baratz ME: Fractures of the elbow. *Orthop Clin North Am* 1999;30:37-61.

31. Helfet DL, Kloen P, Anand N, Rosen HS: Open reduction and internal fixation of delayed unions and nonunions of fractures of the distal part of the humerus. *J Bone Joint Surg Am* 2003;85:33-40.

32. O'Driscoll SW: Elbow dislocations, in Morrey BF (ed): *The Elbow and Its Disorders*. Philadelphia, PA, WB Saunders, 2000, pp 409-420.

33. Cohen MS, Hastings H 2nd: Acute elbow dislocation: Evaluation and management. *J Am Acad Orthop Surg* 1998;6:15-23.

34. Durig M, Muller W, Ruedi TP, Gauer EF: The operative treatment of elbow dislocation in the adult. *J Bone Joint Surg Am* 1979;61:239-244.

35. Hildebrand KA, Patterson SD, King GJW: Acute elbow dislocations: Simple and complex. *Orthop Clin North Am* 1999;30:63-79.

36. Jupiter JB, Ring D: Treatment of unreduced elbow dislocations with hinged external fixation. *J Bone Joint Surg Am* 2002;84:1630-1635.

37. Uhl TL, Gould M, Gieck JH: Rehabilitation after posterolateral dislocation of the elbow in a collegiate football player: A case report. *J Athl Train* 2000;3:108-110.

38. Takahara M, Shundo M, Kondo M, Suzuki K, Nambu T, Ogino T: Early detection of osteochondritis dissecans of the capitellum in young baseball players: Report of 3 cases. *J Bone Joint Surg Am* 1998;80:892-897.

39. Shaughnessy WJ: Osteochondritis dissecans, in Morrey BF (ed): *The Elbow and Its Disorders*. Philadelphia, PA, WB Saunders, 2000, pp 255-260.

40. Tivnon MC, Anzel, SH, Waugh TR: Surgical management of osteochondritis dissecans of the capitellum. *Am J Sports Med* 1976;4:121-128.

41. Kozak TK, Adams RA, Morrey BF: Total elbow arthroplasty in primary osteoarthritis of the elbow. *J Arthroplasty* 1998;13:837-842.

42. Lee DH: Posttraumatic elbow arthritis and arthroplasty. *Orthop Clin North Am* 1999;30:141-162.

43. Morris M, Jobe FW, Perry J, Pink M, Healy BS: Electromyographic analysis of elbow function in tennis players. *Am J Sports Med* 1989;17:241-247.

44. Jobe FW, Ciccotti MG: Lateral and medial epicondylitis of the elbow. *J Am Acad Orthop Surg* 1994;2:1-8.

45. Nirschl RP, Pettrone FA: Tennis elbow: The surgical treatment of lateral epicondylitis. *J Bone Joint Surg* 1979; 61:832-839.

46. Gruchow HW, Pelletier D: An epidemiologic study of tennis elbow: Incidence, recurrence, and effectiveness of prevention strategies. *Am J Sports Med* 1979;7:234-238.

47. Nirschl RP: Elbow tendinosis/tennis elbow. *Clin Sports Med* 1992;11:851-870.

48. Leach RE, Miller JK: Lateral and medial epicondylitis of the elbow. *Clin Sports Med* 1987;6:259-272.

49. Glousman RE, Barron J, Jobe FW, Perry J, Pink M: An electromyographic analysis of the elbow in normal and injured pitchers with medial collateral ligament insufficiency. *Am J Sports Med* 1992;20:311-317.

50. Plancher KD, Halbrecht J, Lourie GM: Medial and lateral epicondylitis in the athlete. *Clin Sports Med* 1996;15:283-305.

51. Posner MA: Compressive ulnar neuropathies at the elbow: I. Etiology and diagnosis. *J Am Acad Orthop Surg* 1998;6:282-288.

52. Posner MA: Compressive ulnar neuropathies at the elbow: II. Treatment. *J Am Acad Orthop Surg* 1998;6:289-297.

11

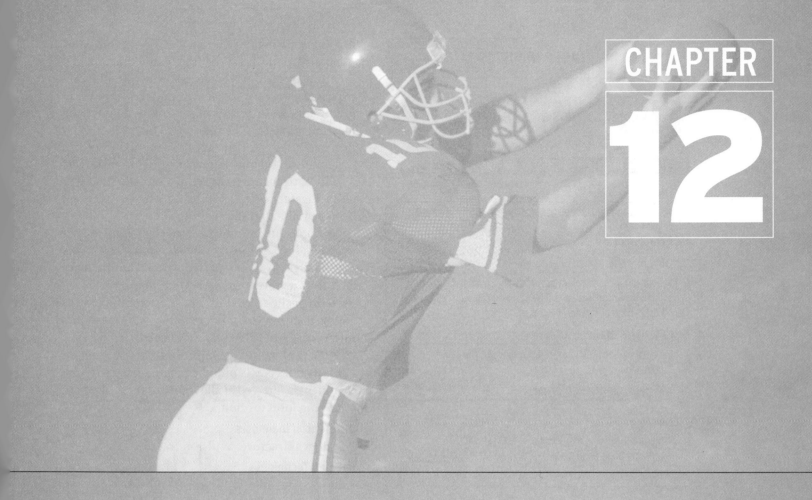

Wrist, Hand, and Finger Pathologies

Susan Saliba, PhD, PT, ATC
Frank C. McCue III, MD

FINGER INJURIES

Finger Sprains and Dislocations

CLINICAL PRESENTATION

History

An axial, valgus, varus, or rotational force to the interphalangeal joint

Pain localized to the involved joint

Observation

With an unreduced dislocation, deformity is obvious.

A sprain results in joint swelling and possible discoloration.

A flexion contracture may be present.

Functional Status

Range of motion (ROM) is decreased secondary to pain and swelling.

Physical Evaluation Findings

Joint palpation produces pain.

ROM produces pain.

Anterior-posterior joint glide may reveal instability.

Valgus and/or varus stress testing of the joint may result in pain and laxity.

The fingers are easily injured in athletics. They are struck by balls, twisted by opponents, and smashed by objects. Most athletes are able to participate despite the pain of a finger sprain, also termed "coach's

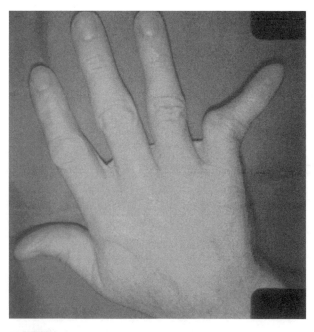

Figure 12-1 An interphalangeal collateral ligament sprain can cause chronic instability, leading to repetitive injury and dysfunction.

finger" or a "jammed finger."[1,2] The coach or another athlete pulls on the finger to reduce the dislocation or realign the finger, and the player is expected to return to the game. Often there is no follow-up care or proper treatment because the dislocation appears to be reduced. This lack of attention can result in contractures, missed fractures, instabilities, and malaligned, dysfunctional fingers.

The fingers are designed for mobility and dexterity. Ligaments that stabilize the finger joints can become injured, resulting in sprains. Each joint has collateral ligaments and a volar plate to provide palmar stability. The most severe sprain is a dislocation that requires closed or open reduction. The phalangeal architecture can cause a fracture, either from the dislocation or the reduction. The most common dislocation is either dorsal or palmar at the proximal interphalangeal (PIP) joint (**Figure 12-1**).

Once a ligament is injured, instability can occur if its integrity cannot be regained. Appropriate treatment is directed at allowing proper healing and regaining joint motion.

Differential Diagnosis

Phalangeal fracture, avulsion fracture

Imaging Techniques

Anteroposterior (AP), lateral, and oblique plain radiographs help to rule out fractures and ensure proper reduction. Subluxated interphalangeal joints can be identified by the "V" arrangement of the joint surfaces (**Figure 12-2**). Images obtained from unreduced dislocations assist in determining the best reduction method and identifying intra-articular fractures.

Definitive Diagnosis

The definitive diagnosis is based on pain or instability with ligamentous stress tests and the absence of a fracture on radiographs.

Normal

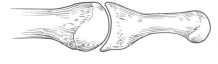

Subluxated

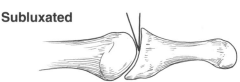

Figure 12-2 A dorsal "V" sign on lateral radiographs can indicate a joint subluxation. The "V" illustrates that the articular surfaces are not congruent or parallel. (Reproduced with permission from Blazar PE, Steinberg DR: Fractures of the proximal interphalangeal joint. *J Am Acad Orthop Surg* 2000;8:383-390.)

Pathomechanics and Functional Limitations

A tear in a collateral ligament causes lateral instability and may result in recurrent dislocations.[3] Repeated joint trauma causes damage to the articular cartilage and degenerative joint disease. Osteophytes form, reducing ROM and giving the joint a gnarled appearance.

If not adequately treated, injury to the volar plate on the palmar aspect of the joint results in a flexion contracture. The volar plate contracts, and the PIP joint appears to have a boutonnière deformity; this is commonly termed a pseudoboutonnière deformity (see boutonnière deformity, p 389) because the extensor tendons are intact (**Figure 12-3**).

■ Immediate Management

After the initial evaluation, ice, compression, and elevation are instituted. The patient is referred for radiographs and reduction if necessary.

■ Medications

Generally pharmacologic agents are unnecessary. However, an athlete taking narcotic pain medicine should not be permitted to participate.

■ Postinjury Management

When a collateral ligament is injured, a splint should be applied with the PIP joint in 30° of flexion for 2 weeks. The distal interphalangeal (DIP) joint should be splinted in full extension.[1-3] Buddy taping should continue for an additional 2 to 4 weeks (**Figure 12-4**). When the volar plate is injured, the PIP joint is splinted in full extension for 4 weeks. Joint protection is continued with tape for a total of 6 to 8 weeks.

Taping the injured finger to the adjacent finger helps to protect and further splint the injury from excessive movement, especially rotation.

■ Surgical Intervention

A torn volar plate can lodge within the joint, requiring an open reduction.[4,5] Recurrent collateral ligament sprains, especially of the fifth finger, may also require surgery. Surgery is indicated if joint instability results in repeated dislocations or if closed reduction is impaired by soft-tissue interposition.[5]

The reduction is made through a midlateral incision over the involved joint. After reduction, the ligament is reconstructed. A wire may be used to provide further stability by replicating the ligament course, then running through the skin where it is fixated to a button. Once the injury is healed, approximately 3 weeks after surgery, the button and wire are removed.

After surgery, the joint is often stiff. ROM exercises should be initiated within the limits set by the physician to keep scarring to a minimum. Once activity is resumed, the finger should be buddy taped for protection.

■ Injury-Specific Treatment and Rehabilitation Concerns

12

> **Specific Concerns**
> ────────────────────
> Reduce the dislocation.
> Decrease pain and swelling while protecting the joint.
> Provide support to the affected joint during activity.
> Institute early ROM exercises emphasizing flexion and extension.
> Avoid valgus and varus joint loading during the early stages of rehabilitation.

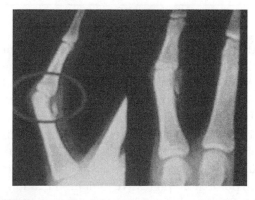

Figure 12-3 An avulsion fracture on the palmar aspect of the interphalangeal joint indicates a volar-plate injury.

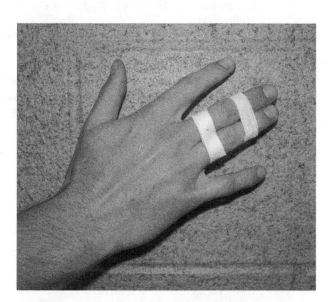

Figure 12-4 Buddy taping. The injured finger is taped to one or both of the neighboring fingers for support and protection.

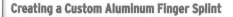

CT **Clinical Technique** 12-1

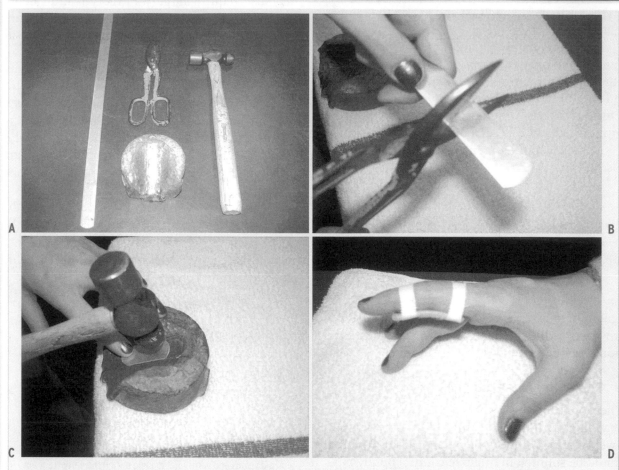

Creating a Custom Aluminum Finger Splint

A. Supplies needed: raw aluminum, lead block (or other form), tin snips, ball-peen hammer.
B. A thin piece of nonpadded aluminum is cut to the appropriate length, and any sharp edges are filed down.
C. The ball-peen hammer is used to make a trough in the splint. The appropriate angle of flexion or extension is pounded in. A block of lead helps to mold the splint when using the hammer. The splint is covered with a thin layer of moleskin to absorb moisture and is taped to the finger.
D. Nonadhesive elastic tape can also secure the splint to help reduce edema. Further protection is offered by buddy taping to the adjacent finger. The splint can be applied dorsally or to the palmar surface of the finger.

This type of custom splint is preferred to foam-backed aluminum, which is bulkier and permits more finger movement.

If no intra-articular fracture is disrupting joint function, conservative therapy is indicated. A splint should be applied for 4 weeks. After 2 weeks, the splint can be removed for active ROM and gripping exercises at least twice daily. The patient is taught to flex and extend each joint independently by blocking the other joints. The splint can be shortened to incorporate only the injured joint at this time. Passive ROM and aggressive stretching can cause further inflammation. During this time, ice, compression, and elevation are helpful in controlling inflammation.

After 4 weeks, the splint may be removed for daily activities but may be required during athletics if the patient is vulnerable to reinjury. Gentle passive stretching may begin, as well as soft-tissue mobilization if motion is limited. Buddy taping should continue for approximately 8 weeks, at which point more aggressive joint mobilization may begin. Such mobilization is often necessary with volar-plate injuries, which tend to scar more on the palmar aspect and restrict extension.

Estimated Amount of Time Lost

Many times, an athlete can participate with a splint or buddy taping for protection. If a dislocation is open or open reduction is required, participation should be limited until the wound has closed to prevent infection.

Return-to-Play Criteria

Participation is permitted when pain is controlled sufficiently to allow good function. A splint or tape is used for protection until adequate healing is achieved.

Functional Bracing

An aluminum splint can be customized to immobilize only the affected joint (**CT** 12-1). Tape secures the finger to the adjacent one for added protection (see Figure 12-4). Nonadherent elastic tape helps to control swelling. The splint, brace, or tape support may be discontinued when joint stability and strength are at the preinjury level and active ROM has been restored.

Extensor Tendon Rupture

CLINICAL PRESENTATION

History

An axial load resulting in forced flexion of the PIP joint, and possibly the DIP joint
Pain is along the finger length but concentrated around the PIP joint.

Observation

The finger is held in a semiflexed position.

Functional Status

Inability to actively extend the PIP joint
Decreased DIP joint flexion

Physical Evaluation Findings

Positive Haines-Zancolli test: Flexion of the DIP joint is not possible with the PIP joint extended. If passive flexion of the DIP joint is possible with the PIP joint extended, then conservative intervention may be possible.

The boutonnière, or "buttonhole," injury is a rupture of the central slip of the extensor tendon at the PIP joint. The lateral slips of the tendon form a buttonhole, and the joint slides through into a fixed, flexed position. Classically, the PIP joint is flexed and the DIP joint becomes hyperextended because of the pull of the lateral bands of the extensor mechanism.

The extensor tendons in the fingers have a central slip that attaches to the proximal aspect of the middle phalanx, whereas the lateral bands continue to the distal aspect of the finger. Trauma causes a central slip rupture, which disrupts the delicate balance of the extensor mechanism over the intrinsic muscles of the fingers. Central-slip disruption allows the lateral bands of the extensor tendon to migrate volarly to the axis of rotation of the PIP joint, resulting in flexion (Figure 12-5).

A boutonnière deformity can be caused by trauma or rheumatoid arthritis. The tendon can rupture when the finger is jammed by forced flexion or axial loading; a laceration can injure the central slip of the extensor tendon. In rheumatoid arthritis, the PIP joint is slowly forced into flexion by chronic synovitis, which elongates the central slip of the tendon, ultimately rupturing it.[6-8]

The classic deformity does not present until 2 to 3 weeks after the initial injury. If a collateral sprain is misdiagnosed and a splint is applied in 30° of flexion, the deformity is accentuated. At this point, the PIP joint has a flexion contracture, and surgical management is often necessary.[9-12]

Differential Diagnosis

PIP joint sprain, pseudoboutonnière deformity, phalangeal fracture

Imaging Techniques

AP, lateral, and oblique radiographs of the finger are obtained to rule out fracture.

Definitive Diagnosis

Inability to actively extend the PIP joint and the findings on imaging studies indicate a longitudinal tear of the extensor tendon.[9]

Pathomechanics and Functional Limitations

When the central portion of the extensor tendon is avulsed, the lateral bands continue to exert their force on the DIP joint, causing a flexion deformity at the PIP joint and extension at the DIP joint.[9,11] The lumbrical and interosseous muscles lose their insertion into the middle phalanx due to the incompetent central slip, and their force of action is diverted through the lateral bands. This causes DIP joint hyperextension, accentuated by secondary shortening of the oblique retinacular ligaments. The deformity prevents proper finger function because the PIP joint becomes contracted in the flexed position.

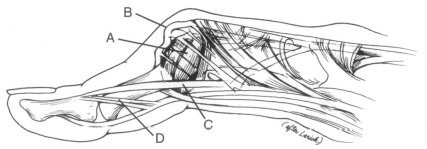
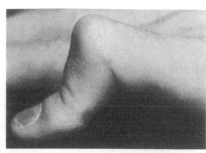

Figure 12-5 A boutonnière deformity. Left, Primary synovitis of the proximal interphalangeal (PIP) joint (**A**) may lead to attenuation of the overlying central slip (**B**) and dorsal capsule and increased flexion at the joint. Lateral-band subluxation volar to the axis of rotation to the joint (**C**) may lead to hyperextension. Contraction of the oblique retinacular ligament (**D**), which originates from the flexor sheath and inserts into the dorsal base of the distal phalanx, may lead to extension contracture of the distal interphalangeal (DIP) joint. Right, Photograph illustrates flexion posture of the PIP joint and hyperextension posture of the DIP joint. (Reproduced with permission from *J Am Acad Orthop Surg* 1999;7:92-100. © 1999 American Academy of Orthopaedic Surgeons.)

Immediate Management

The digit should be splinted with the PIP and DIP joints extended and treated with ice to reduce inflammation. The patient is referred for physician evaluation and radiographs.

Medications

Nonsteroidal anti-inflammatory drugs (NSAIDs) and analgesics may help with symptom management.

Postinjury Management

The PIP joint must be splinted in extension to approximate the central tendon to the dorsal aspect of the distal phalanx.[8] The splint should allow active DIP joint ROM, and exercise of this joint is encouraged. Splinting should be strictly adhered to for 6 weeks and continued at night for 2 to 4 more weeks. Dynamic or safety-pin splints are often used to apply a long-duration, low-load force to extend the PIP joint (**Figure 12-6**). These are helpful in treating a PIP joint flexion contracture.

> **Tenotomy** Surgical cutting or division of a tendon.

Surgical Intervention

If conservative management fails to produce good PIP joint function, surgical reattachment of the central slip should be considered. Surgical outcome depends on the severity of the preoperative joint contracture. Surgery is indicated for a chronic boutonnière deformity with a fixed PIP joint flexion contracture and a DIP joint extension contracture.[12,13] Late diagnosis can cause joint contracture, hindering efforts to regain full ROM.

The most common surgical procedure is an extensor tenotomy with a release and shift of the lateral bands.[14] A tendon graft may be necessary to reattach the central slip.[12] After surgery, the PIP joint is held in extension with a K-wire for at least 10 days, followed by splinting in extension for an additional 2 weeks, after which the splint may be removed for activities of daily living; however, the joint must be protected during athletics for at least 8 weeks.

Procedures that incorporate a tenotomy require early motion. Efforts should be made to avoid extensor tendon stress while mobilizing the finger to prevent lateral band adherence. Possible surgical complications include infection, deformity from contracture, edema, and scar tissue formation.

Injury-Specific Treatment and Rehabilitation Concerns

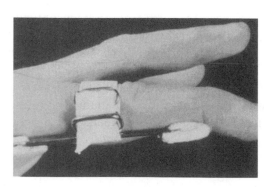

Figure 12-6 A safety-pin splint dynamically loads the finger so that the proximal interphalangeal joint is extended. The tension should be a low-level, long-duration stretch. The distal interphalangeal joint should be free.

Specific Concerns

Reduce the contracture while allowing the central slip to reattach in an acute injury.

Reduce swelling.

Encourage lateral band mobility.

Achieve independent control of the PIP and DIP joints.

For an acute injury, the finger should be splinted continuously in extension for 6 weeks to allow healing of the extensor tendon central slip. The patient should be taught to block the other joints to isolate the DIP joint and encourage active DIP joint ROM throughout the immobilization period. After 6 weeks, active and assisted DIP joint flexion allows mobilization of the lateral bands and helps to prevent their volar migration. If the PIP joint is allowed to flex or if primary healing is not possible, a surgical consult should be obtained after 6 weeks. Grip exercises can be initiated, and functional stresses may be added. Because of the long immobilization time, the patient should expect the PIP joint to be thick and stiff for several weeks. PIP joint active motion is encouraged, but the finger should be protected during athletic participation for at least 10 weeks.

If surgical management is required, the outcome expectation is for full ROM and function. Stiffness should be anticipated for several months as the soft tissue remodels and often depends on the degree of preoperative contracture.

Postoperative rehabilitation focuses on independent DIP joint function. Active DIP joint ROM exercises with the PIP joint blocked may begin at 2 weeks. At 4 weeks, the splint may be removed and gentle, active PIP joint flexion and extension may begin, but the DIP joint should continue to be blocked. When the wounds are well healed, gentle soft-tissue mobilization may be initiated. Passive ROM and joint mobilization can be incorporated at 6 to 8 weeks, watching for tissue reaction and edema. The splint can be discontinued after 6 weeks if there is no flexion contracture. If extension is limited, then a dynamic splint can be applied to encourage ROM. The finger should be protected during athletics for at least 8 weeks. Gradually progressive grip, pinch, and dexterity activities are added after 6 weeks and should continue until function plateaus.

■ Estimated Amount of Time Lost

When the injury is managed conservatively, strict splinting is required for 6 weeks, and the joint should be protected in extension for an additional 4 weeks. The athlete may be able to participate with the splint, but this can be difficult with the extended PIP joint.

A concomitant avulsion of the dorsal phalanx or irreducible dislocation of the PIP joint requires primary surgical management. Time lost from the injury is increased if the diagnosis is delayed.

■ Return-to-Play Criteria

Participation is permitted when the patient understands the consequences of the ruptured tendon and splinting is used. When surgical management is required, the patient must not compete for at least 2 weeks after surgery while the K-wire is in place.

Functional Bracing

PIP joint protection should continue for at least 8 weeks during activity. Buddy taping can be used with an aluminum or spring-loaded safety-pin splint, which should be padded during athletic participation (see Figure 12-6).

Extensor Tendon Avulsion

CLINICAL PRESENTATION

History

Forced flexion of an extended DIP joint
A popping sensation in the fingertip may be reported.
Pain is localized to the distal finger.

Observation

Distal phalanx swelling
The DIP joint remains in a flexed position.

Functional Status

The patient is unable to actively extend the DIP joint.

Physical Evaluation Findings

Little to no tension is produced during resisted ROM testing of the DIP joint.
The joint can be passively extended.

The extensor tendon of the finger attaches to the proximal aspect of the distal phalanx. When the finger is extended and struck by an object on the tip, forceful DIP joint flexion can avulse or rupture the extensor tendon. A mallet finger results, and the patient is unable to actively extend the DIP joint (**Figure 12-7**).

Differential Diagnosis

Phalangeal fracture, extensor tendon rupture

Imaging Techniques

Standard radiographs include AP, lateral, and posteroanterior (PA) views (**Figure 12-8**).

Definitive Diagnosis

The definitive diagnosis is based on the inability to actively extend the DIP joint and radiographic findings indicating an extensor tendon avulsion.

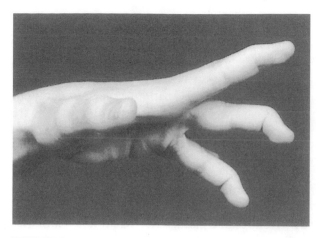

Figure 12-7 The distal interphalangeal joint cannot actively extend with a mallet finger.

Pathomechanics and Functional Limitations

Rapid tendon loading can rupture the extensor tendon or avulse the bony attachment. When the extensor tendon is no longer attached to the distal phalanx, the patient cannot extend the DIP joint. Except for swelling, passive motion is initially unaffected. Permanent disability, including arthritis, can result when the joint is not kept extended to allow tendon reattachment. When treatment is delayed, the splinting time is much longer because of less inflammation and much slower and less effective fibroplasia.[15]

Function is limited because the patient is unable to actively extend the DIP joint. This limitation rarely precludes sports activities, but initially pain limits function. The inability to extend the DIP joint causes more functional deficits in manual dexterity and fine motor skills than in gross sports skills.

■ Immediate Management

The finger is splinted with the DIP joint in extension or slight hyperextension. Ice controls swelling and reduces pain. The extensor mechanism must be evaluated, and radiographic images assist in differentiating between bony and tendinous involvement. Tendon reattachment to the distal phalanx is required for healing. This generally occurs with strict DIP joint splinting in extension for 8 to 9 weeks. Surgical management is usually not necessary. However, disrupting healing by allowing the DIP joint to flex can cause a permanent extension lag. Inconsistent splinting also results in poor long-term outcomes.

■ Medications

NSAIDs may be prescribed to reduce pain and swelling.

Fibroplasia Development of fibrous tissues during wound healing.

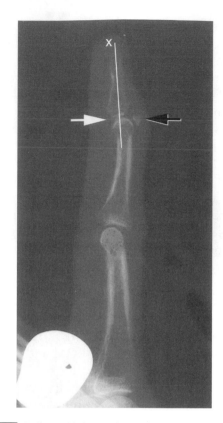

Figure 12-8 Radiographic image of an extensor tendon avulsion. A bone fragment avulsed from the distal phalanx (black arrow) is clearly visible. In this case, the avulsion fracture is intra-articular. The joint space is reduced (white arrow), demonstrated by line X intersecting the midportion of the condyle and proximal middle phalanx. (Reproduced with permission from Johnson TR, Steinbach LS (eds): *Essentials of Musculoskeletal Imaging*. Rosemont, IL, American Academy of Orthopaedic Surgeons, 2004, p 369.)

■ Postinjury Management

With conservative management, most mallet finger injuries heal with relatively good outcomes. Mallet-finger treatment requires strict splinting of the DIP joint in full extension. With a bony avulsion, splinting should continue for 4 to 5 weeks. If the injury involves a tendon rupture, splinting should continue for 8 weeks. Patient education is essential to prevent DIP joint flexion and skin maceration from excessive moisture.[16] Dorsal and volar splints can be alternated to relieve the constant contact of the splint with the skin. The dorsal splint allows the tactile stimulation that is important in some sport skills.[15] When changing the splint, the patient should hold the finger extended and not let the distal aspect drop into flexion. Stack splints can also be used to maintain DIP joint extension (**Figure 12-9**).

■ Surgical Intervention

Surgery for an extensor tendon avulsion is indicated if the patient cannot, or will not, continuously wear a splint for 8 to 9 weeks.[17] A K-wire can

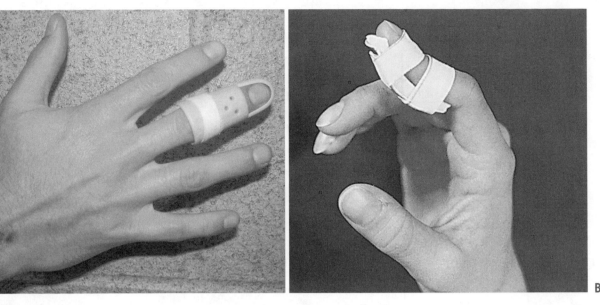

A   B

Figure 12-9 Mallet finger splints. **A.** Stack splint. These commercial splints are used to keep the distal interphalangeal joint in extension. They also provide protection to the tip of the finger. **B.** Volar splint for the management of an extensor tendon avulsion. Because padding on splints holds moisture and can prevent the joint from full extension, the padding may be removed.

be placed transarticularly to maintain DIP joint extension, but this is usually only necessary for vocational reasons.[18,19]

Surgically, a **percutaneous** K-wire is inserted to hold the DIP joint extended. The pin is inserted under fluoroscopy and maintains full joint extension while the tendon heals. A cork or padding is attached to the tip of the K-wire to minimize injury from the protruding wire. The DIP joint is often stiff after the immobilization, but active extension is the goal.

Fingertip pressure that forces the DIP joint into flexion must be avoided for 3 months after surgery. Postoperative complications can include infection, secondary injury from the protruding pin, and loss of DIP joint motion. Patients treated nonsurgically often have better DIP joint motion than those treated surgically.

Athletes cannot participate with K-wires in place; consequently, surgical treatment does not expedite the healing process and return to competition. Extensor tendon ruptures can be directly repaired (**Figure 12-10**).

Injury-Specific Treatment and Rehabilitation Concerns

Specific Concerns

Control flexion ROM to allow healing to occur.
Obtain full DIP joint extension.

The primary goal in managing a mallet finger is to achieve full DIP joint extension. Arthritic changes may occur over time when good DIP joint function is not restored with initial immobilization. Compliance with continual splinting is imperative for 9 weeks to ensure good extensor tendon scarring. Because only DIP joint immobilization is necessary, PIP joint motion is unrestricted. Thus, PIP joint stiffness is rare.

Once the immobilization period has ended, active DIP joint ROM is encouraged. The patient should be taught how to isolate each joint's function by blocking other joints. Generally most patients regain function without supervised therapy.

Estimated Amount of Time Lost

Many athletes can participate with the DIP joint splinted in full extension. The PIP joint is not immobilized, increasing function, but care should be taken to prevent the DIP joint from flexing. Poor or inconsistent splinting increases the time for healing.

Return-to-Play Criteria

The athlete can participate with a splint in place if function is not compromised. Full healing must occur before sports are permitted without splint protection.

Functional Bracing

Either a dorsal or volar splint should be applied in full DIP joint extension. Padding should be minimized, however, because it retains moisture and

Percutaneous
Through the skin.

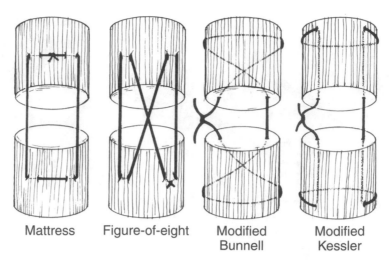

Mattress   Figure-of-eight   Modified Bunnell   Modified Kessler

Figure 12-10   Four commonly used repair techniques for extensor tendon lacerations. (Reproduced with permission from Newport ML: Extensor tendon injuries in the hand. *J Am Acad Orthop Surg* 1997;5:59-66.)

prevents the splint from maintaining full extension. Stack splints can be used but should fit well; splints that are too loose allow DIP joint flexion, while those that are too tight can cause skin breakdown (see Figure 12-9).

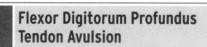

Flexor Digitorum Profundus Tendon Avulsion

CLINICAL PRESENTATION

History

Forced extension of the fingers while grasping
The patient may report hearing or feeling a "pop" as the tendon avulsed.
Pain is reported at the distal phalanx and DIP joint.

Observation

DIP joint swelling
Ecchymosis may be present.
There may be no obvious deformity.

Functional Status

ROM is initially limited by pain.
The patient is unable to actively flex the DIP joint, which is evident when the patient is asked to make a fist.

Physical Evaluation Findings

The retracted tendon may be felt at the PIP joint or in the palm.
Passive DIP joint ROM is normal; active and resisted ROM is absent.

An avulsion of the flexor digitorum profundus (FDP) tendon can occur with forced DIP joint extension while the athlete is grasping. This entity is commonly termed "jersey finger," because it most often results when a player grabs an oppo-

nent's jersey or uniform. The fifth finger slides off the jersey and the force is directed to the fourth finger, which has the highest incidence of FDP injury. The tendon rupture site is frequently the bone-tendon attachment at the distal phalanx. The patient is unable to fully flex the DIP joint; however, PIP joint motion is unaffected because the flexor digitorum superficialis (FDS) is still intact (**Figure 12-11**).

Jersey finger is commonly missed; in a cursory evaluation, inability to flex the DIP joint may be assumed to be caused by swelling or pain in the fingertip. When the FDP is avulsed, it retracts to the PIP joint or into the palm if diagnosis is delayed. If retraction is extensive, the tendon can lose blood supply from the vinculae.[20,21] When tendon nutrition has been compromised, direct repair may not be possible. All FDP avulsions should be surgically repaired within 2 weeks.

Differential Diagnosis

Phalangeal fracture, DIP joint sprain or dislocation

Imaging Techniques

Lateral radiographs are used to determine the location of the tendon end. A small piece of bone usually avulses with the tendon (**Figure 12-12**).

Definitive Diagnosis

A lateral radiograph revealing an avulsion fracture near the middle phalanx and the patient's inability to actively flex the DIP joint indicate a rupture of the FDP.

Pathomechanics and Functional Limitations

The FDS and FDP control flexion of the finger interphalangeal joints. The FDS inserts on the middle phalanx and is responsible only for flexing the

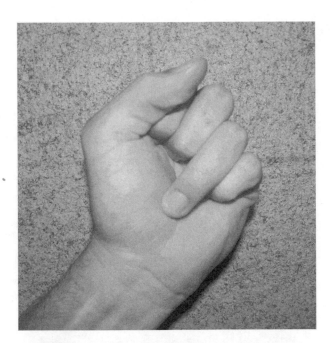

Figure 12-11 Presentation of "jersey finger." The patient is able to flex all fingers except the distal interphalangeal joint of the affected finger.

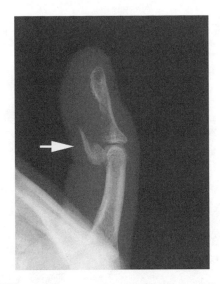

Figure 12-12 Radiographs help determine the presence of an avulsion fracture of the flexor tendon. The site of the bone fragment aids in localizing the tendon end. (Reproduced with permission from Johnson TR, Steinbach LS (eds): *Essentials of Musculoskeletal Imaging.* Rosemont, IL, American Academy of Orthopaedic Surgeons, 2004, p 318.)

PIP joint. The FDP extends to the fingertip and inserts on the distal phalanx. Because of the vinculae, this tendon flexes both the PIP and DIP joints.

When the finger is forced into extension while the flexors are contracting, the stress causes the FDP to rupture, most commonly at the distal insertion site. If tendon retraction has not occurred, the avulsed tendon end may be located at the DIP joint. However, the tendon may retract, either to the level of the FDS hiatus at the middle phalanx or into the palm. The tendon's blood supply may be compromised with retraction, placing a time limit on the possibility of direct repair.[21]

The outcome depends on the initial management, good surgical skills, management of scarring, and adherence to a rehabilitation program to restore tendon gliding and joint mobility.

■ Immediate Management

A complete examination should be done to determine the whether the tendon is still attached to the distal phalanx. Immediate referral to a hand surgeon is necessary to determine the best course of treatment. If either the referral or the surgery is delayed, a tendon graft is necessary because the FDP retracts.

■ Medications

NSAIDs may be prescribed to reduce pain and swelling.

■ Surgical Intervention

Surgical reattachment of the FDS tendon is necessary with jersey finger (**ST** 12-1). The method is determined by the level of tendon retraction, which is usually a function of the time elapsed since the injury. If the retraction is at the level of the FDS hiatus, the tendon can be reattached if treated within 3 to 6 weeks. If retraction is at the level of the palm, surgery must be performed within 7 to 10 days. If direct repair is not possible, a tendon graft must be used to restore DIP joint function. This can be done with the palmaris longus tendon or with a Hunter rod.[20,21]

■ Postoperative Management

Postoperatively, the finger is splinted in a functional position (**Figure 12-13**). Once healing has begun, active ROM is encouraged to assist in restoration of tendon gliding. Passive motion is delayed for 6 weeks to ensure that the repair has healed. The athlete is not permitted to participate in sports until the tendon has healed.

■ Injury-Specific Treatment and Rehabilitation Concerns

Specific Concerns
Regain ROM of the affected finger.
Prevent contracture.
Control edema.

12

S|T Surgical Technique 12-1

Repair of a Flexor Tendon Avulsion

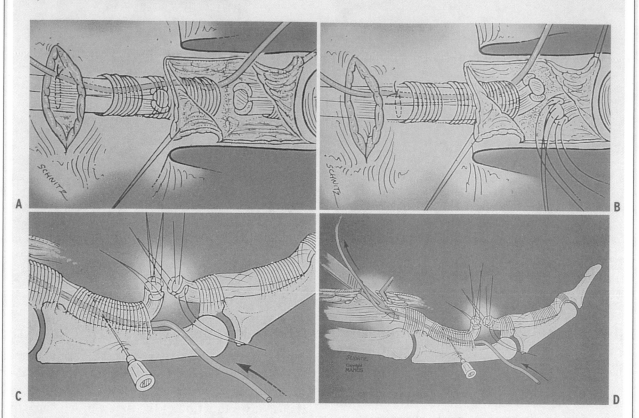

Indications

An avulsed FDP tendon

Overview

Depending on the level of retraction of the injured tendon and its viability, the tendon may be directly reattached. This is the best option, but the diagnosis and treatment course must be defined early.

1. A midlateral or volar zigzag incision is used, depending on the location of the retracted flexor tendon.
2. The tendon sheath is exposed from the area of the profundus insertion to a point just proximal to the PIP joint. The end of the tendon is identified (**A**).
3. A small catheter is placed retrograde from distal to proximal, passing under the sheath and pulleys to the retraction point of the tendon (**B**).
4. A hypodermic needle is used to temporarily "pin" the proximal tendon in place (**C**).
5. The tendon is drawn up to its attachment site.
6. Using various fixation techniques, the FDP is reattached to the distal phalanx (**D**).
7. If tendon viability has been lost, the tendon must be replaced with either a graft or a Hunter rod. The graft is prepared and pulled through the space the FDP occupied.

Functional Limitations

Tendon retraction can cause necrosis, requiring the use of a tendon graft or Hunter rod to restore active DIP joint flexion. Delayed repair can cause finger stiffness and contracture, making rehabilitation arduous. Digit dexterity and flexibility may be affected.

Implications for Rehabilitation

Tendon stress should be minimized. Passive flexion is encouraged but not forced, because the tissues react to excessive forces by swelling. The hand should be protected from grasping or using the flexors with resistance until the tendon is well healed. It may take 4 to 6 weeks for the tendon to regain sufficient tensile strength. Gentle active motion is encouraged to aid tendon gliding.

Potential Complications

Tendon retraction into the palm, stiffness, failure of the tendon graft, rerupture

Figures reproduced with permission from Strickland JW: Flexor tendon injuries: II. Operative technique. *J Am Acad Orthop Surg* 1995;3:55-62.

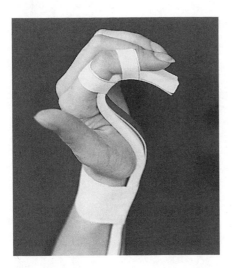

Figure 12-13 Splitting the finger in a functional position. Note the slight extension of the wrist and the slight amount of flexion at the metacarpophalangeal, proximal interphalangeal, and distal interphalangeal joints.

Postoperatively, the goals are to allow tendon gliding while minimizing stress on the repair. Gentle ROM is encouraged after 2 weeks of immobilization. The patient is taught to actively extend the fingers, then flex each joint with no resistance by blocking other joints. Active motion should be performed at least twice a day for 6 weeks. At that time, increased stress can be applied with massage and soft-tissue and joint mobilization. Grasping with the fingers or stress such as carrying a plastic grocery sack should be avoided for 8 to 10 weeks. At 10 to 12 weeks, more aggressive activities to regain motion can be tolerated.

■ Estimated Amount of Time Lost

Surgical repair is necessary to regain DIP joint function. The repair should be protected with splinting for 6 weeks for normal activities and for an additional 4 to 6 weeks during sports activities.

Delayed diagnosis causes the retracted tendon to lose its blood supply, making it unsuitable for reattachment. Furthermore, delayed treatment causes the joint to become stiff from disuse; the DIP joint loses ROM and can become fibrotic. If a tendon graft is required, sports activities are generally restricted for at least 12 weeks.

■ Return-to-Play Criteria

Once the tendon has healed, the athlete may return to sports. A protective splint should be worn for 4 to 6 weeks after the tendon has healed to reduce DIP and PIP joint stress.[2]

Functional Bracing

The finger should be splinted with a customized aluminum splint in a functional position. The finger is buddy taped for additional support (see Figure 12-4).

Finger Fractures

CLINICAL PRESENTATION

History

Trauma to the involved finger, usually involving a twisting force or direct impact
Pain

Observation

Swelling may be observed.
Ecchymosis is common.
Malalignment may be noted with the fingers flexed or extended.
The nail of the involved finger may be malaligned.

Functional Status

ROM is limited by pain.

Physical Evaluation Findings

Point tenderness over the fracture site
Crepitus may be present.
Positive percussion and bump tests

Some finger fractures heal well without treatment; however, intra-articular fractures can cause stiff and painful joints, and spiral fractures can cause deformities. Proper evaluation and treatment help to ensure good alignment and function.

The fingers can be fractured in many ways. The distal phalanx is most commonly fractured with a direct, crushing force and often has a subungual hematoma. The middle phalanx is often fractured with either a direct force or twisting of the finger.[22-24] The proximal phalanx is usually fractured with torsion and may have a spiral or angular fracture. The tendinous attachment of the muscles that control the phalanges can cause dynamic instability of some finger fractures (**Figure 12-14**). The fracture location and direction must be considered to determine whether conservative or surgical management is needed to prevent deformity and dysfunction.[24-26]

Differential Diagnosis

Metacarpal fracture, interphalangeal joint dislocation, metacarpophalangeal (MCP) joint dislocation, finger sprain

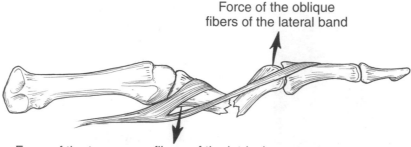

Force of the oblique
fibers of the lateral band

Force of the transverse fibers of the intrinsic apparatus

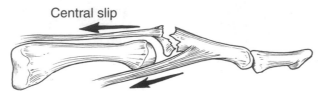

Central slip

Flexor digitorum superficialis

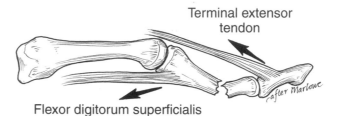

Terminal extensor
tendon

Flexor digitorum superficialis

after Marlowe

Figure 12-14   Deforming forces on phalangeal fractures. (Modified with permission from J. Marlowe.)

Imaging Techniques

AP, PA, lateral, and oblique radiographs should be obtained to confirm the diagnosis and identify the presence of an intra-articular fracture (**Figure 12-15**).

Definitive Diagnosis

The definitive diagnosis is based on radiographic and clinical findings (**Figure 12-16**).

Pathomechanics and Functional Limitations

Phalangeal fracture stability depends on the location, fracture orientation, and degree of initial displacement. Distal phalanx fractures are usually stable, even though they may be comminuted. Fractures within the diaphyses of the proximal and middle phalanges are typically stable when there is no initial displacement. These fractures generally have good outcomes, especially when the patient complies with splinting.[22]

When an intra-articular interphalangeal fracture involves the condyles, the fracture is inherently unstable. Similarly, displaced fractures involving the diaphyses of the proximal and middle phalanges are also unstable secondary to the pull of the intrinsic muscles and flexor tendons. These fractures require greater care and often surgical management to prevent deformity and regain joint function.[25-27]

Most fractures heal well with the use of a splint for 3 to 6 weeks.[22] Some fractures require surgical management to prevent deformation or allow a joint to function properly.[25,28]

■ Immediate Management

Treatment should focus on minimizing pain and swelling. Buddy taping and a splint should be applied, and the patient should be referred to a physician for radiographs.

■ Medications

NSAIDs may be prescribed for pain relief.

■ Surgical Intervention

Nondisplaced, stable phalangeal fractures typically heal well with splinting and nonsurgical treatment. Indications for surgical management include open fractures, irreducible fractures, unstable fractures, failed closed reductions, fractures involving more than 25% of the articular surface, and displaced intra-articular fractures. Treatment of avulsion injuries, such as mallet finger (p 392) or jersey finger (p 395), should focus on the soft tissue. All finger surgery should be performed with minimal

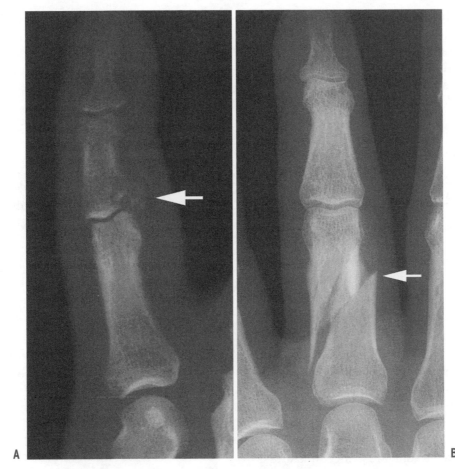

Figure 12-15 Radiographs of phalangeal fractures. **A.** Posteroanterior view demonstrating an intra-articular fracture of the proximal interphalangeal joint (arrow) caused by an avulsion of the radial collateral ligament. **B.** Posteroanterior view showing an oblique fracture of the proximal phalanx (arrow). Clinically, the finger would appear shortened. (Reproduced with permission from Johnson TR, Steinbach LS (eds): *Essentials of Musculoskeletal Imaging.* Rosemont, IL, American Academy of Orthopaedic Surgeons, 2004, pp 350-351.)

incisions and a concerted effort to reduce scar formation between the tendons and bones.

An intra-articular unicondylar and bicondylar fracture is unstable and requires fixation. The fracture is reduced and fixated using screws or minicondylar plates with intraosseous wiring.[25,27] Unstable shaft fractures of the middle and proximal phalanges can be fixated with longitudinal K-wires. With longer spiral fractures, percutaneous minifragment screws can be used.

Postoperatively, interposition of periosteum within the fracture can cause nonunion, pain, and deformity. Poor follow-up or noncompliance with splinting can also result in deformity. Neglect of intra-articular fractures causes deformity, pain, and degenerative joint disease.

■ Postinjury/Postoperative Management

Most displaced finger fractures can be treated conservatively with closed reduction and immobilization. Displaced intra-articular fractures require anatomic reduction of the joint surface and some-

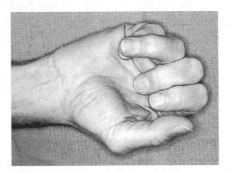

Figure 12-16 Active finger flexion produced overlap, indicating malrotation associated with a spiral fracture of the proximal phalanx of the ring finger. Alignment appeared normal when the fingers were extended. (Reproduced with permission from Kozin SH, Thoder JJ, Liberman G: Operative treatment of metacarpal and phalangeal shaft fractures. *J Am Acad Orthop Surg* 2000;8:111-121.)

times open reduction and internal fixation (ORIF). Once the fracture has been stabilized, early ROM is recommended to prevent adhesions. The splint can be removed up to 6 times per day to allow passive motion. Generally, K-wires are removed after 4 weeks and active motion is encouraged.

Most finger fractures heal well with time and protection. The clinician should emphasize that the splinting is not necessarily for pain reduction but to ensure good alignment and function later. Many athletes use the splint as long as the finger hurts but discard the device soon afterward.[22,28,29]

Injury-Specific Treatment and Rehabilitation Concerns

> **Specific Concerns**
>
> Rotational fractures should be followed up to monitor healing.
> Ensure compliance with splinting.
> Restore ROM.

The time required for immobilization depends on the type of fracture but generally is 3 to 6 weeks. Once the immobilization period has ended, attempts to restore mobility begin. Gentle active motion is encouraged at each joint independently. If digital stiffness or thickening exists, soft-tissue mobilization may begin. Aggressive joint mobilization and passive stretching should start only when the fracture is well healed. Again, this time period is dictated by the type of fracture present. Most finger fractures do not require a supervised strengthening program.

Estimated Amount of Time Lost

An athlete may be able to participate with a nondisplaced, extra-articular fracture if splinting and buddy taping are used. If the fracture is intra-articular or displaced, sport participation may be prohibited for 2 weeks to avoid the need for surgery.[22]

Finger fractures require 3 to 6 weeks to heal. If the athlete is unable to participate using a pro-

tective splint or taping, then return to competition should be delayed until the fracture is healed. Complicated fractures, especially spiral fractures of the proximal phalanx, can rotate and displace, increasing the amount of time lost from the injury.

Return-to-Play Criteria

Return to play is dictated by the physician because unstable fractures may require surgery if they are displaced during activity. Many athletes with finger fractures can participate using a splint. All open fractures preclude participation until the wound has healed.

Functional Bracing

An aluminum splint can be cut to the correct size so that the joints above and below the fracture are stabilized (see **CT 12-1**). If no other soft-tissue injury is present, the interphalangeal joints should be flexed to 30°. Nonadherent elastic tape helps to control edema. The finger can be buddy taped to the adjacent finger for added stability (see Figure 12-4). Proximal phalanx fractures can be immobilized with a moldable thermoplastic splint that covers the injured and adjacent fingers (**Figure 12-17**).

Trigger Finger

CLINICAL PRESENTATION

History

Patients tend to be over 30 years old; most are 55 to 60 years old.
Complaints of locking, snapping, or catching during finger flexion and extension
Pain may be in the distal palm, possibly radiating into the finger.
Trigger finger often affects multiple digits.

Observation

Hesitation may be noted during active motion.
Audible snapping may be heard.
Possible flexion contracture

Functional Status

ROM is limited secondary to pain.
Nodules may restrict ROM.

Physical Evaluation Findings

The A1 pulley is tender to palpation.
A nodule may be felt in the FDS tendon.
Triggering or snapping of the fingers may be noted.

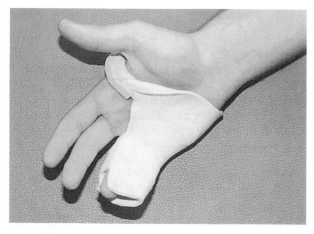

Figure 12-17 Thermoplastic splint used in the treatment of a proximal phalanx fracture.

Trigger finger occurs when the flexor tendon becomes caught in the A1 retinacular pulley (**Figure 12-18**). The tendons are attached to the bones and volar plates by pulleys that prevent the tendons from bowstringing. When the tendon sheath becomes thickened or swollen, it pinches the tendon and prevents it from gliding smoothly (**Figure 12-19**). With trigger finger, the finger snaps as it goes through flexion and extension; in the late stages, the patient may need to manipulate the digit to achieve extension. Although trigger finger may be caused by a collagen vascular disease, such as rheumatoid arthritis, or diabetes, most cases are idiopathic.[30,31] The occurrence of trigger finger correlates with activities that require pressure in the palm and a high-load power grip. The thumb is most commonly affected, followed by the ring, long, little, and index fingers.

Differential Diagnosis

Dupuytren contracture, sesamoiditis

Imaging Techniques

Radiologic studies are rarely needed, but views of the hand may help to rule out sesamoiditis.

Definitive Diagnosis

The diagnosis of trigger finger is based on the clinical findings.

Pathomechanics and Functional Limitations

Repetitive activities that require digital flexion and extension are affected. Finger mobility is reduced because of pain.

Medications

A corticosteroid may be injected into the tendon sheath[31-35] (**Figure 12-20**). The patient is encouraged to actively move the digit to disperse the medication. In many cases, the triggering is relieved.

Postinjury/Postoperative Management

Patients who decline a corticosteroid injection may be splinted with the MCP joint in 15° of flexion. This alternative may be moderately effective.

Surgical Intervention

When one or two corticosteroid injections fail to relieve symptoms, surgical management is recommended to release the A1 pulley. Care is taken to maintain hemostasis and to avoid disrupting the A2 pulley, which may cause tendon bowstringing.[31] The procedure requires a small incision over the metacarpal head of the affected digit and is frequently performed under local anesthesia. The A1 pulley is divided at the midline to release the restriction. The patient is asked to flex and extend the finger to confirm the release.

Active finger ROM is encouraged the day of surgery, and the wound is protected for approximately 2 weeks. Edema should be managed, but the patient can generally perform many activities of daily living soon after surgery. Sutures are removed in 10 days, and most sports activities can resume.

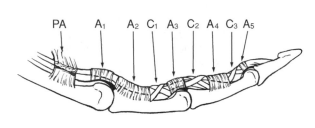
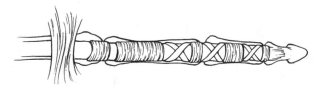

Figure 12-18 Lateral (top) and dorsal (bottom) views of a finger illustrating the components of the digital flexor sheath. The sturdy annular pulleys (A1, A2, A3, A4, and A5) are important biomechanically in keeping the tendons closely applied to the phalanges. The thin, pliable cruciate pulleys (C1, C2, and C3) collapse to allow full digital flexion. A recent addition to the nomenclature is the palmar aponeurosis pulley (PA), which adds to the biomechanical efficiency of the sheath system. (Reproduced with permission from Strickland JW: Flexor tendon injuries: I. Foundations of treatment. *J Am Acad Orthop Surg* 1995;3:44-54.)

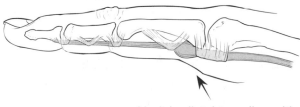

Nodule distal to pulley with finger in extension

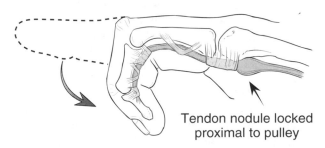

Tendon nodule locked proximal to pulley

Figure 12-19 The trigger-finger phenomenon. A nodule or thickening develops in the flexor tendon and strikes the proximal pulley, making finger flexion difficult. (Reproduced with permission from Greene WB (ed): *Essentials of Musculoskeletal Care*, ed 2. Rosemont, IL, American Academy of Orthopaedic Surgeons, 2000, p 282.)

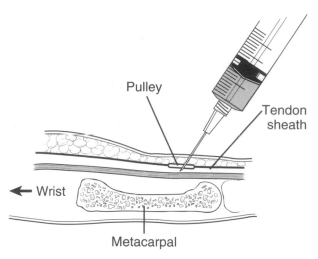

Figure 12-20   Injection site for trigger finger. The needle is carefully passed through the pulley before the medication is injected. (Reproduced with permission from Greene WB (ed): *Essentials of Musculoskeletal Care*, ed 2. Rosemont, IL, American Academy of Orthopaedic Surgeons, 2000, p 285.)

■ Injury-Specific Treatment and Rehabilitation Concerns

Specific Concerns

Reduce edema and inflammation.
Allow tendon gliding to reduce loss of ROM.

Conservative management involves reducing inflammation and reestablishing function. Night splinting, NSAIDs, and even corticosteroid injections can be used. Early postoperative ROM ensures smooth tendon gliding. Protection of the surgical incision is necessary.

■ Estimated Amount of Time Lost

The finger may be tender for 2 to 3 days after the corticosteroid injection. Patients treated surgically generally require 2 to 4 weeks of protection, although most sports activities may resume after 10 to 14 days. Extra padding over the incision may be necessary for golf, as an example. Excessive scarring after surgery may increase the duration of dysfunction.

■ Return-to-Play Criteria

Patients treated conservatively may return to play when the finger has full ROM. After surgery or an injection, the athlete may return once pain is controlled and no swelling is present.

Functional Bracing

A silicone-padded glove can be used for golf or other activities that put pressure on the metacarpal heads, which may be sensitive after treatment.

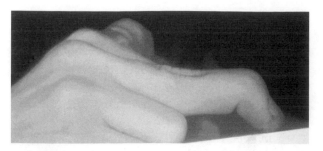

Figure 12-21   A swan-neck deformity is characterized by proximal interphalangeal (PIP) joint hyperextension and distal interphalangeal joint flexion. (Image © 1999 American Academy of Orthopaedic Surgeons. Reprinted from the *Journal of the American Academy of Orthopaedic Surgeons*, Volume 7 (2), pp 92-100 with permission.)

The glove is padded in the palm with a shock-absorbent material to relieve pressure from the bony prominences.[29]

Swan-Neck Deformity

CLINICAL PRESENTATION

History

An axial force applied to the finger, resulting in forced PIP joint flexion
An associated PIP joint dislocation may have occurred.

Observation

PIP joint hyperextension or dorsal dislocation
PIP joint swelling
With time, the finger assumes a posture of PIP joint hyperextension and DIP joint flexion.

Functional Status

Decreased PIP and DIP joint ROM
Decreased grip strength

Physical Evaluation Findings

Decreased resisted ROM for finger flexion and extension
Joint instability may be noted.

A dorsal dislocation of the PIP joint can rupture the volar plate. The volar plate stabilizes the PIP joint and helps to prevent hyperextension. When the PIP joint loses volar stability, the finger hyperextends at the PIP joint, disrupting the balance of the intrinsic muscles' pull on the DIP joint and causing flexion. When finger extension is attempted, the DIP joint drops into flexion (**Figure 12-21**).

The volar plate is a thick, fibrocartilaginous structure with a firm attachment on the middle phalanx, where it becomes continuous with the articular cartilage. The volar plate limits PIP joint extension beyond 0°. Proximally, the volar plate is thinner, which allows the base of the middle phalanx to glide along the articular surface of the prox-

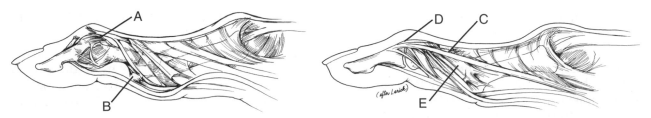

Figure 12-22 Swan-neck deformity. Left, Terminal tendon rupture may be associated with synovitis of the distal interphalangeal (DIP) joint, leading to DIP joint flexion and subsequent proximal interphalangeal (PIP) joint hyperextension (**A**). Flexor digitorum superficialis tendon rupture may occur due to infiltrative synovitis, which may lead to decreased volar support of the PIP joint and subsequent hyperextension deformity (**B**). Right, Lateral-band subluxation dorsal to the axis of rotation of the PIP joint (**C**), contraction of the triangular ligament (**D**), and attenuation of the transverse retinacular ligament (**E**) are depicted. (Reproduced with permission from *J Am Acad Orthop Surg* 1999;7:92-100.)

imal phalanx as the finger flexes. Thus the volar plate is both a static stabilizer, limiting hyperextension beyond 0°, and a dynamic stabilizer, influencing the position of the flexor tendons at initiation of PIP joint flexion.[36]

A swan-neck deformity can also result from an unrepaired FDP rupture, intrinsic muscle contracture, or extensor-mechanism disruption at the DIP joint (**Figure 12-22**). Swan-neck deformities are seen in rheumatoid arthritis, but the mechanism is not the same as with traumatic injuries. Normal laxity in some individuals may result in a swan-neck deformity if the PIP joint can hyperextend, but this need not be immediately repaired if the individual has good finger function.

Differential Diagnosis

PIP joint dislocation, boutonnière deformity, mallet finger

Imaging Techniques

AP, lateral, and oblique plain radiographs should be obtained to rule out other trauma.

Definitive Diagnosis

PIP joint hyperextension and DIP joint flexion are characteristic of a swan-neck deformity. With a volar plate injury, the PIP joint is unstable.

Pathomechanics and Functional Limitations

When the volar plate is ruptured (most often pulled from the distal attachment), the PIP joint loses the ability to prevent hyperextension. As the PIP joint hyperextends, the lateral bands of the extensor mechanism displace dorsally, disrupting the extensor force on the DIP joint. Furthermore, the pull of the spiral oblique retinacular ligament becomes volar to the DIP joint axis, causing flexion rather than extension.

■ Immediate Management

The finger should be evaluated for soft-tissue and bony injury, treated with ice to minimize inflammation, and splinted with the PIP joint in exten-

sion and the DIP joint in slight flexion. The patient should then be referred to a physician for radiographic evaluation.

■ Medications

NSAIDs may be prescribed to reduce pain and swelling.

■ Surgical Intervention

In the athletic population, this injury rarely requires surgery because splinting facilitates adequate healing. Furthermore, the volar plate often shortens, causing a pseudoboutonnière deformity and a PIP joint flexion contracture. When indicated in chronic cases or if aesthetics are an issue, surgical management targets reattachment of the volar plate to regain PIP joint stability. The repair is generally secured with thin wires that can be removed percutaneously after 4 to 6 weeks.[36]

■ Postoperative Management

Wires are removed after 4 weeks, and gentle active ROM can be initiated. Joint protection should continue while the patient is active until healed.

■ Injury-Specific Treatment and Rehabilitation Concerns

> **Specific Concerns**
> Reduce pain and edema.
> Prevent PIP joint flexion contracture.

During the immobilization period, efforts should focus on reducing edema. After the K-wires are removed, gentle ROM should begin. The athlete should flex and extend each joint independently at least twice daily. Because of the volar-plate disruption, the PIP joint tends to become thickened.

Depending on wound healing, soft-tissue mobilization is initiated at 4 to 6 weeks. If the PIP joint shows early signs of contracture, a safety-pin or dynamic splint can be used to help regain extension. Joint mobilization and aggressive ROM techniques should not begin before 8 weeks, and the clinician should be cautious of tissue reaction with passive stretching.

■ Estimated Amount of Time Lost

Surgical repair of the volar plate is necessary to restore volar integrity of the PIP joint. The joint should be protected for 4 weeks for all activities, and then splinting is continued for another 4 weeks while athletics are permitted. Wound healing from surgery can increase the time lost, as can prolonged swelling and stiffness.

■ Return-to-Play Criteria

The surgeon dictates when the athlete is allowed to participate after surgery, typically at 4 to 6 weeks. Splinting and buddy taping are required during sports while the athlete is rehabilitating the finger (see Figure 12-4).

Functional Bracing

A customized aluminum splint can be fabricated to protect the PIP and DIP joints (see **CT** 12-1). The injured finger should be taped to the adjacent finger for added stability.

THUMB INJURIES

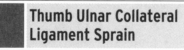

Thumb Ulnar Collateral Ligament Sprain

CLINICAL PRESENTATION

History

Forceful thumb abduction while the MCP joint is extended
Pain arising from the ulnar side of the joint
The patient may demonstrate functional thumb instability.

Observation

MCP joint swelling and ecchymosis

Functional Status

Decreased grip and pinch strength

Physical Evaluation Findings

Valgus stress test reveals pain and instability.
Pain and swelling may prohibit a thorough evaluation of the thumb.

A sprain of the thumb's ulnar collateral ligament (UCL) is commonly known as gamekeeper thumb. The injury occurred as gamekeepers sacrificed rabbits by breaking their necks using the ground and their thumbs and index fingers. The thumb is injured as a result of the valgus force on an abducted MCP joint, spraining the UCL.[37-39] If the force is sufficient, MCP joint dislocation occurs (**Figure 12-23**). Falling while holding a ski pole with the band improperly wrapped around the wrist (skier thumb)[40] or striking an opponent or object with an open hand can result in a UCL sprain or dislocation. Because thumb stability is important for prehension, treatment is directed to optimize ligament healing to restore full ligament function.

A Stener lesion occurs when the adductor aponeurosis becomes interposed between the ruptured UCL and its insertion site at the base of the proximal phalanx, and either the distal portion or the ligament retracts superficially and proximally.[39] The UCL is no longer in contact with the insertion area and cannot heal. Therefore, the ligament must be reattached to provide joint stability.

Differential Diagnosis

Bennett's fracture, UCL avulsion fracture, phalangeal fracture

Imaging Techniques

AP, lateral, and oblique radiographic views of the thumb are taken. Magnetic resonance imaging (MRI) can be used to determine the presence of any intact fibers. A stress radiograph may also be performed (**Figure 12-24**). The joint is anesthetized and imaged while a valgus force is applied. However, this technique may encourage a partial tear to become complete.[41,42]

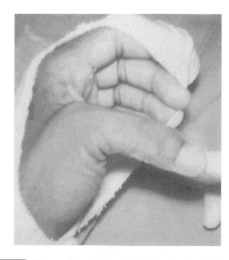

Figure 12-23 Ulnar collateral stress test shows laxity at the metacarpophalangeal joint with valgus stress. The test is applied in 0° and 30° of flexion, and the results are compared bilaterally.

Definitive Diagnosis

The definitive diagnosis is based on clinical findings and/or MRI demonstrating a UCL tear and the absence of bony injury.

Pathomechanics and Functional Limitations

A UCL injury causes MCP joint instability, resulting in disability in grasp. Pinch strength and grip strength with the thumb abducted are also weakened. As long as a few fibers of the ligament remain intact, the ligament can heal. However, if a complete tear occurs, the intrinsic aponeurosis lies between the ends of the UCL ligament and blocks healing[37,39,42,43] (**Figure 12-25**).

▓ Immediate Management

For grade I and II injuries, the thumb should be splinted with an ulnar gutter splint or thumb spica splint.

▓ Medications

NSAIDs may be prescribed to control postinjury or postoperative pain and inflammation.

▓ Postinjury Management

Valgus stress to the thumb with an empty end feel indicates a complete ligament tear, and the patient should be referred to a physician. Grade I and II sprains can be treated with splinting. Grade III sprains usually require surgical correction.[37]

At rest, the splint should include the thumb interphalangeal joint and extend onto the forearm for greater pain control. The athlete may participate with the thumb MCP joint immobilized with a thermoplastic splint and tape. In a grade III injury, the UCL tear is complete, and surgical repair is necessary.

▓ Surgical Intervention

The torn UCL may retract under the adductor aponeurosis. With an acute injury, the ligament ends may be reapproximated with a direct repair, or the ligament may be reattached to the periosteum (ⓢⓣ 12-2). Chronic injuries may require a ligament reconstruction, usually with the abductor pollicis longus (APL) tendon.

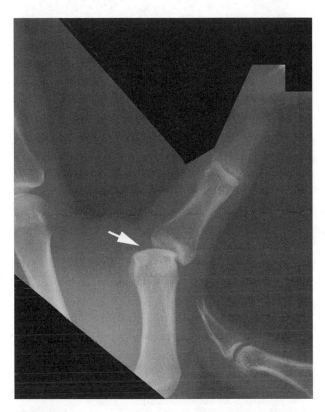

Figure 12-24 Stress radiograph demonstrating a grade III sprain of the ulnar collateral ligament. The metacarpophalangeal joint opens on the ulnar side when stress is applied (arrow). A Stener lesion may also be present. (Reproduced with permission from Johnson TR, Steinbach LS (eds): *Essentials of Musculoskeletal Imaging.* Rosemont, IL, American Academy of Orthopaedic Surgeons, 2004, p 378.)

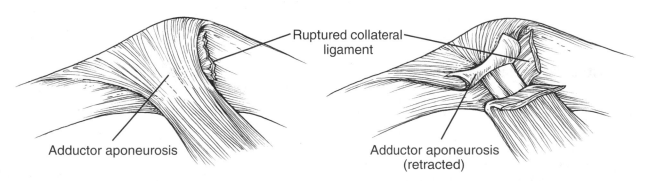

Ruptured collateral ligament

Adductor aponeurosis

Adductor aponeurosis (retracted)

Figure 12-25 Left, When a complete rupture of the ulnar collateral ligament occurs, the distal end of the torn ligament is usually displaced proximal and superficial to the proximal edge of the intact adductor aponeurosis. Right, Division of the adductor aponeurosis is required for repair of the ligament. (Reproduced with permission from Heyman P: Injuries to the ulnar collateral ligament of the thumb metacarpophalangeal joint. *J Am Acad Orthop Surg* 1997;5:224-229.)

S|T Surgical Technique   12-2

Repair of a UCL Sprain/Dislocation

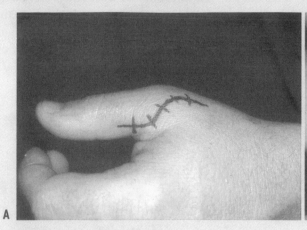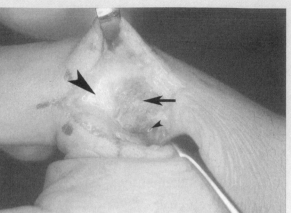

A   B

Indications

Complete tear of the UCL (Stener lesion)

Overview

1. A chevron, straight, or S-shaped incision is made over the dorsal MCP joint with the apex directed toward the UCL and the broad base toward the thumb's dorsal aspect (**A**).
2. The adductor aponeurosis is identified and detached from the extensor pollicis longus and reflected to be repaired at closing.
3. The injury is identified (**B**).
4. If the stump is adequate, the ligament is prepared.
5. If the stump will not hold a suture, the avulsed ligament is reattached using a pull-out wire technique. The wire reinforces the attachment and is removed percutaneously after 4 weeks. If the ligament has been torn in its midportion, sutures are placed with the MCP joint flexed to 15° to 20° and the area is immobilized in a thumb-spica cast for 5 weeks.
6. For chronic instability, a reconstruction can be done using a slip of the APL tendon. The surgical approach is the same as above.
7. The tendon graft is fed through drill holes about the joint and secured.

Functional Limitations

No limitations are anticipated.

Implications for Rehabilitation

Partial tears should be protected to allow closed healing. Efforts should be made to minimize ligament stress, even with examination, to prevent a complete tear. If a Stener lesion exists, surgical management is required for adequate stability.

Potential Complications

Early stress can cause instability. Immobilization after repair is required, and protection during athletic activity is necessary to prevent reinjury. Sensory nerve loss at the incision site may occur.

Figures reproduced with permission from Heyman P: Injuries to the ulnar collateral ligament of the thumb metacarpophalangeal joint. *J Am Acad Orthop Surg* 1997;5:224-229.

■ Postoperative Management

After surgery, the thumb is placed in a spica splint or cast for 3 to 4 weeks. The patient may begin carefully monitored interphalangeal and MCP joint ROM exercises. At 4 weeks, the patient can progress to a removable thumb spica splint. The splint should only be removed for exercises and hygiene for an additional 2 weeks. At that point, a decision can be made regarding athletic participation with a protective splint. The joint should be protected during sports activities for 3 months after surgery.[37]

■ Injury-Specific Treatment and Rehabilitation Concerns

Specific Concerns

Protect the joint from stress to allow healing.
Restore full ROM and attain equal grip and pinch strength.

When the immobilization period has ended, efforts focus on regaining wrist and grip strength. Resistive exercise is initiated 6 weeks after surgery. Multiplanar wrist curls are performed with dumbbells. Grip exercise begins with light therapeutic putty or a sponge and progresses to thicker putty.

Thumb ROM is usually regained by allowing normal daily activities, but the range should be compared by placing both hands palm up on a hard surface. Flexion, abduction, adduction, extension, and opposition are evaluated. Any deficiency is noted and addressed. Dexterity of the involved thumb can also be restored with handheld computer games, because most games require extensive thumb use.

■ Estimated Amount of Time Lost

Depending on the injury grade, the ligament may require up to 4 weeks to heal. After surgical repair, the athlete may be able to participate with the thumb immobilized.

■ Return-to-Play Criteria

The thumb should be protected until full, pain-free ROM is attained. All swelling and tenderness should be resolved, and valgus stress must not reproduce pain. Grip strength should be equal bilaterally. Reinjury causes chronic MCP joint instability, resulting in pain and dysfunction.

Functional Bracing

Thumb-spica taping or a thermoplastic, removable splint can be used (**CT** 12-2). Full interphalangeal joint motion should be allowed, and the splint should not cause pinching at the wrist.[29] Nonadherent tape can be applied to secure the splint.

To protect the joint after injury, a thumb-spica wrist splint is often used. This device immobilizes the wrist and carpometacarpal (CMC) and MCP joints, rendering it ideal for healing. However, the splint makes it difficult for the athlete to participate in sports. When sufficient healing has taken place, a smaller splint only on the MCP joint can be used.

Bennett's Fracture

A Bennett's fracture occurs at the first CMC joint and results from axial and abduction forces to the thumb. The fracture is associated with a subluxation of the metacarpal on the trapezium from the pull of the APL tendon (**Figure 12-26**). Early diagnosis and treatment are imperative to prevent loss of function of this highly mobile joint.[44-46] Unless properly recognized and

---

CLINICAL PRESENTATION

History

An axial load and forced abduction of the thumb, causing CMC joint subluxation
Intense pain arising from the CMC joint

Observation

Swelling and possible deformity may be observed.

Functional Status

Abduction and flexion ROM are decreased or absent.
Decreased grip strength

Physical Evaluation Findings

Crepitus over the CMC joint
Resisted ROM produces pain and weakness.
The following special tests are positive:
  Bump test
  Teeter-totter test, in which pressure is applied to the distal metacarpal, and the clinician feels the metacarpal sublux when pressure is released

---

treated, this intra-articular fracture-subluxation can result in an unstable, arthritic joint with secondary loss of motion and pain.[47] Because the thumb CMC joint is critical for pinch and opposition, Bennett's fractures may severely affect thumb function.

Differential Diagnosis

CMC joint sprain, carpal fracture, metacarpal fracture, phalangeal fracture

Imaging Techniques

Standard PA, lateral, and oblique radiographs should be obtained in patients with suspected thumb fractures or dislocations. Traction radiographs may be used to assess the degree of comminution (**Figure 12-27**).

Computed tomography (CT) or tomograms can help define both the degree of comminution within a fracture and suspected impaction of the articular surface.

Definitive Diagnosis

The definitive diagnosis is based on radiographic findings.

Pathomechanics and Functional Limitations

The fracture is unstable because the APL tendon places tension on the fractured bone fragment. The CMC joint becomes dysfunctional, and all thumb motions are affected.[46,47]

■ Immediate Management

The thumb is splinted; ice is applied to control swelling; and the athlete is immediately referred to a hand or orthopaedic surgeon.

CT Clinical Technique 12-2

Constructing a Moldable Thermoplastic Splint

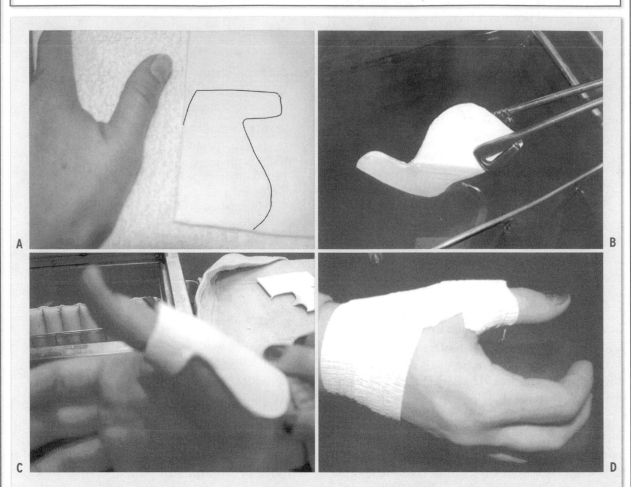

This technique demonstrates construction of an ulnar-side CMC thumb splint for a UCL injury. Because the splint minimizes the amount of material in the palm, skill players are more likely to use the device during sport. The mold shape and location of splint application vary with the injury being treated. Several different types of thermoplastic splinting materials are available in varying thicknesses.

   A. A pattern is drawn onto the material, which is heated for cutting.
   B. The splint is heated in warm water until malleable.
   C. The plastic is then dried to prevent a burn to the athlete during molding, applied to the injured part, and positioned correctly.
   D. Nonadhesive elastic tape is used to secure the splint and apply even pressure during molding. The athlete can hold a sport implement, such as a bat or stick, during molding and must maintain the correct position until the splint cools and hardens. Any rough edges can be reheated with a heat gun or padded with moleskin.

During athletic participation, the splint is held in place with athletic tape; during daily activities, the splint can be secured with a hook-and-loop strap glued to the plastic.

■ Medications

Narcotic analgesics may be required to control acute pain. NSAIDs may be prescribed to control postinjury or postoperative pain and inflammation.

■ Postinjury Management

Closed reduction followed by thumb-spica cast immobilization can be effective in treating some Bennett's fractures, especially those characterized by small avulsion fractures and minimal articular incongruity and instability. These patients must be followed with serial radiographs to monitor reduction. However, the strong pull of the APL frequently leads to displacement; consequently, open or closed reduction combined with internal fixation is frequently required.[45]

A thumb-spica cast is applied for 2 to 6 weeks, depending on the stability achieved at surgery. A

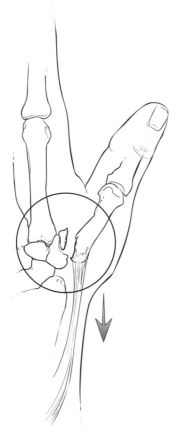

Figure 12-26 A Bennett's fracture causes a retraction of the first metacarpal (arrow). This fracture is unstable and requires surgical management. (Reproduced with permission from Greene WB (ed): *Essentials of Musculoskeletal Care*, ed 2. Rosemont, IL, American Academy of Orthopaedic Surgeons, 2000, p 259.)

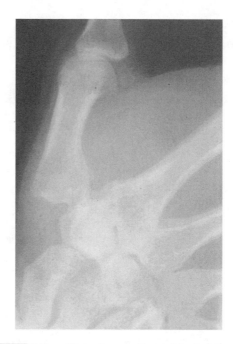

Figure 12-27 A Bennett's fracture usually consists of a triangular piece from the first metacarpal, which remains in its anatomic position, while most of this bone tends to draw proximally.

thermoplastic splint can be used after the cast is removed, and rehabilitation may begin (see **CT** 12-2).

Surgical Intervention

The strong pull of the APL frequently causes displacement, which requires ORIF or closed reduction with percutaneous pinning (**S T** 12-3). Generally, closed reduction followed by percutaneous K-wire fixation is successful in maintaining reduction. Wires are drilled through the dorsal radial thumb metacarpal base into the reduced volar ulnar fragment. If the fragment is very small, reduction may be maintained by placing the K-wire from the thumb metacarpal into the trapezium or the index metacarpal.

Injury-Specific Treatment and Rehabilitation Concerns

Specific Concerns

Stabilize the CMC joint.
Reduce edema.
Regain thumb ROM.
Increase grip strength.

Gentle mobility of the thumb interphalangeal joint begins within 2 weeks of surgery to help manage edema and prevent adhesion formation. Depending on fracture stability, immobilization using a thumb-spica cast may last from 2 to 6 weeks. When the immobilization period ends and all pins have been removed, wrist strengthening may begin with multiplanar dumbbell curls. Grip strength may also be addressed with a sponge at first, gradually increasing resistance with therapeutic putty. Active motion is encouraged for the first 8 weeks and then passive motion and joint mobilization if needed. Dexterity is regained using coordination drills or handheld video games.

Estimated Amount of Time Lost

Fracture healing requires 4 to 6 weeks, depending on the amount of stability achieved. Surgical management will affect time lost from sport. The athlete may not participate with percutaneous pins in place.

Return-to-Play Criteria

Full thumb strength and flexibility are required for participation without a protective device. Early participation may be authorized if bone healing is complete and function with a splint is good.

Functional Bracing

Thumb-spica taping improves stability, and a thermoplastic splint can be worn during play (**CT** 12-3).

S|T Surgical Technique 12-3

Repair of a Bennett's Fracture

A

B

Outrigger

Cast

Indications

When articular incongruity is more than 1 mm after closed reduction, surgical intervention is indicated.

Overview

1. The procedure may be performed under local or general anesthesia.
2. Efforts are made to pin percutaneously under fluoroscopy; this is usually very successful.
3. Fracture reduction is accomplished under fluoroscopy with traction on the thumb in palmar abduction. The subluxated metacarpal is reduced medially toward the palm.
4. K-wires are drilled through the dorsal radial thumb metacarpal base into the reduced volar ulnar fragment. If the fragment is very small, reduction may be maintained by placing the K-wire from the thumb metacarpal into the trapezium or the index metacarpal (**A**).
5. Splinting may also be performed to help protect the K-wire stabilization (**B**).

Functional Limitations

Degenerative joint disease and loss of motion after immobilization can affect the outcome.

Implications for Rehabilitation

Percutaneous pins should be removed before activity is accelerated. Thumb abduction should not be stressed too early to help stabilize the CMC joint.

Potential Complications

Displaced intra-articular fractures predispose the patient to arthritis and loss of motion within the affected joints. Unfortunately, even after restoration of articular congruity, some patients develop posttraumatic arthritis secondary to the osteocartilaginous injury sustained in the initial trauma. Loss of motion also occurs after prolonged immobilization. Other complications can include thumb infection and instability.[45,47]

Figures reproduced with permission from Soyer AD: Fractures of the base of the first metacarpal: Current treatment options. *J Am Acad Orthop Surg* 1999;7:403-412.

de Quervain Tenosynovitis

In de Quervain tenosynovitis, the tendons of the APL and extensor pollicis brevis (EPB) become thickened, restricting tendon gliding within their sheath (**Figure 12-28**). The APL and EPB are held against the radial styloid process by the extensor retinaculum. Acute trauma or repetitive motion can cause swelling, and thumb motion causes pain, especially when the wrist is ulnarly deviated.[48,49]

The patient reports pain with thumb and wrist motion. This injury is frequently seen in baseball players who have increased their batting-practice

CT **Clinical Technique** 12-3

Thumb-Spica Taping

1. Prewrap is applied to the wrist, hand, and thumb.
2. Anchors are placed just proximal to the wrist and across the hand using 1- or 1.5-in tape (**A**).
3. Two or three figure-of-8 strips are placed over the MCP and CMC joints (**B**).
4. Either individual or continuous spicas are made around the base of the thumb, metacarpal, and CMC joint.
5. "U" strips are used around the metacarpal, and the wrap is finished with closing anchors (**C**).
6. An optional checkrein may be used to further limit mobility by buddy taping to the index finger (**D**).

repetitions, but can occur in a variety of sports in which repetitive wrist motion is common, eg rowing and tennis.

Differential Diagnosis
CMC joint arthritis

Imaging Techniques
Radiographic evaluation of the CMC joint and wrist helps to rule out other joint abnormalities.

Definitive Diagnosis
The definitive diagnosis is based on a positive Finkelstein test as demonstrated by pain over the APL and EPB, but the rate of false-positive results is high.

Pathomechanics and Functional Limitations
de Quervain syndrome is an overuse injury that is exacerbated by repetition. When the tenosynovitis is in an acute inflammatory stage, the patient has functional limitations due to pain with all thumb and wrist motions. As the syndrome becomes chronic, functional problems increase. If the tenosynovitis remains untreated, the edema within the tendon sheath becomes exudative and eventually can become calcific.[49] The longer the inflammatory process is allowed to cycle due to repeated injury, the longer it will take to resolve once rest and rehabilitation have begun.

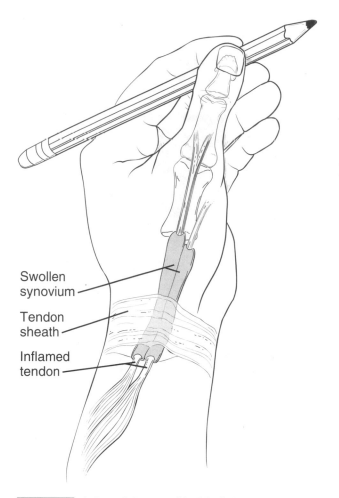

Swollen synovium

Tendon sheath

Inflamed tendon

Figure 12-28 de Quervain tenosynovitis of the first extensor compartment. (Reproduced with permission from Greene WB (ed): *Essentials of Musculoskeletal Care*, ed 2. Rosemont, IL, American Academy of Orthopaedic Surgeons, 2000, p 232.)

Medications

NSAIDs control the inflammatory process and are effective when used in conjunction with splinting and restricted activities. A corticosteroid injection into the sheath of the first dorsal compartment may reduce tendon thickening and improve gliding.

Postinjury Management

A resting splint is used to reduce the inflammation. Once pain has subsided during nonstressful activities, the splint can be removed for strengthening exercises. Active ROM should be performed daily.

Surgical Intervention

If conservative management fails, the first dorsal compartment can be surgically released. An incision is made over the thickened area, and blunt dissection is performed to release the compartment.[50] Care is taken to avoid the superficial radial nerve. Tendon gliding must be regained to prevent the structures from scarring down.

CLINICAL PRESENTATION

History

Pain arising from the thumb during thumb and wrist motion

Observation

APL or EPB tendon swelling may be noted on the radial side of the wrist.

Functional Status

Thumb motion becomes painful and restricted.

Physical Evaluation Findings

On palpation, thickening and crepitus may be noted in the tendons.
Tendon palpation causes pain.
Positive Finkelstein test (poor reliability)
Passive CMC joint manipulation does not produce pain.

Postoperative Management

After surgery, postoperative splinting is used for 10 to 14 days. Patients are encouraged to undertake normal activities and active thumb exercises to improve tendon gliding.

Injury-Specific Treatment and Rehabilitation Concerns

Specific Concerns

Reduce swelling within the tendon sheath that can cause stenosis.
Improve tendon gliding by maintaining ROM.

Because this is an overuse injury, therapy can begin immediately after the evaluation. Modalities may help relieve the pain and inflammation. Splinting during activities of daily living can protect the tendons, but controlled activity and active ROM help to keep the tendons gliding.

The time required for splinting depends on the patient's response. If the symptoms are not relieved with splinting, removing the patient from the aggravating position, and using modalities and NSAIDs, then reevaluation may be necessary. If the first dorsal compartment must be surgically released, continual splinting is used for 10 to 14 days. At that time, the splint may be removed for gentle wrist, hand, and thumb active ROM twice daily. At 6 weeks, the splint may be removed for daily activities, and wrist strengthening may begin. Multiplanar curls, pronation, supination and grip exercise can be taught. Exercises should be well tolerated and continue until all symptoms resolve.

Estimated Amount of Time Lost

Limitations are due to pain, and the athlete should not participate if the ability to perform is decreased. Consequently, no strict prohibition on participating with de Quervain syndrome exists. In an acute flare-up, the tenosynovitis may require 2 to 3 days of protected rest.

Return-to-Play Criteria

The athlete can participate when pain, swelling, and crepitus are controlled. Splinting during participation may allow an early return to sports.

Functional Bracing

An ulnar gutter splint reduces thumb and wrist motions (see Figure 12-26). Commercial braces, as well as tape, offer protection by restricting wrist ulnar and radial deviation and thumb mobility.

HAND AND WRIST PATHOLOGIES

Metacarpophalangeal Joint Dislocation

CLINICAL PRESENTATION

History
Hyperextension of the MCP joint
Pain arising from the knuckles

Observation
Obvious MCP joint deformity
Alteration of the palmar crease
Marked swelling

Functional Status
Inability to move the knuckles

Physical Evaluation Findings
The metacarpal head can be palpated in the palm.
ROM tests cannot be performed.

Forced hyperextension disrupts the volar plate and palmar stability of the MCP joint. The dislocation is typically in the dorsal direction, and can be complex or simple. With a complex dislocation, the metacarpal head becomes buttonholed between the palmar fascia and lumbrical and flexor tendons, making closed reduction impossible (**Figure 12-29**).

The palmar fascia tightens around the metacarpal head when the lumbrical and flexor muscles are active. This tightening tends to strangle the metacarpal head, making it impossible to reduce

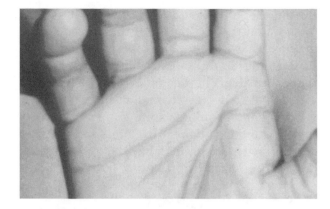

Figure 12-29 Metacarpophalangeal joint dislocation. The patient has immobility, pain, and deformity in the palm.

the dislocation. The problem is referred to as a "Chinese finger puzzle" because the more it is manipulated, the tighter the palmar fascia becomes around the metacarpal head.[29,51] Open reduction is recommended if the initial closed attempt fails.

Differential Diagnosis
Phalangeal fracture, metacarpal fracture

Imaging Techniques
AP and lateral radiographs of the hand are used to rule out fractures and to confirm proper relocation following closed reduction.

Definitive Diagnosis
The definitive diagnosis is made from joint observation, but radiographs are needed to rule out associated fracture.

Pathomechanics and Functional Limitations
Forced MCP joint hyperextension can cause a dislocation. The joints are typically very stable, but when a force is applied while the intrinsic muscles are contracting, the proximal phalanx may be pried from the metacarpal head. The affected joint is unable to function properly, and any movement tightens the palmar fascia around the metacarpal head.

Immediate Management

Neurovascular function should be monitored, the proximal and distal joints splinted, and the patient immediately referred for evaluation and reduction.

Medications

NSAIDs and analgesics are used after injury and/or surgery.

Postinjury Management

If the dislocation is treated immediately, the reduction technique involves manipulating the MCP joint to slide the phalanx back into place and then flexing and applying pressure to the MCP joint. Traction on the MCP joint during attempted reduction tends to entrap the ruptured palmar plate between the joint surfaces and make closed reduction impossible. If closed reduction fails, immediate open reduction is recommended.

The hand should be splinted in an intrinsic-plus position where the MCP joints are in flexion and the fingers are straight. Early, active finger motion is encouraged.[51]

Surgical Intervention

If closed reduction is not possible, open reduction is necessary because the palmar fascia tightens around the metacarpal head. A volar approach is most commonly used. A retractor is inserted to manipulate the soft tissue, and the surgeon can then move the structures to reduce the dislocation. Once reduced, the joint is often very stable. Care must be taken to minimize scar formation in the palm. Scar-tissue formation from an incision through the palmar fascia can cause pain and decrease MCP joint extension.

Postoperative Management

After surgery, scar tissue should be minimized with compression. Hyperextension is avoided for 5 weeks. A splint is used for 2 weeks, and then rehabilitation may begin.

Injury-Specific Treatment and Rehabilitation Concerns

> **Specific Concerns**
>
> Maintain active interphalangeal joint ROM during immobilization.
> Reduce scar-tissue formation in the palm.

Good functional outcomes are obtained in most patients. Rehabilitation is directed at maintaining finger ROM, minimizing scar formation in the palm, and preventing MCP joint hyperextension.

The hand is immobilized for 2 weeks after injury or surgery. At this time, the patient is taught gentle active motion of all fingers, incorporating light gripping. Hyperextension is avoided, and protection may be necessary during athletics to prevent this stress. If needed, soft-tissue mobilization may begin at 3 weeks. Generally passive mobility and joint mobilization are not necessary to gain function. Grip strength is emphasized about 6 weeks after surgery.

Estimated Amount of Time Lost

The athlete can generally return to play 3 to 4 weeks after a closed reduction or 6 to 8 weeks after an open reduction.[51] When open reduction is required, return to play is delayed for 6 to 8 weeks, depending on wound healing, scar management, and the return of strength and motion. Minimizing scarring merits special attention because scar-tissue formation in the palm can restrict function.

Return-to-Play Criteria

The patient should demonstrate the functional ROM required for sport-specific skills. In some cases, the patient can return to competition earlier if the joint can be protected with bracing and/or padding. If an open reduction was performed, the wound and underlying tissue should be healed.

Functional Bracing

The finger should be taped to the adjacent finger for stability (see Figure 12-4); most athletes are unable to tolerate a splint at the MCP joint. Silicone padding or a gel-filled glove can reduce the pressure at the metacarpal head if this area is sensitive to pressure.

Metacarpal Fractures

CLINICAL PRESENTATION

History

An axial force being delivered to the metacarpals, such as improper punching
A rotational or crushing force to the hand
Pain localized to the involved metacarpals

Observation

Deformity, swelling, and discoloration may be present.
Knuckle asymmetry may be observed, and the knuckle may appear to be missing.
The fingernail of the involved metacarpal may be rotated relative to the other nails.
Finger malalignment may be noted. During metacarpal and PIP joint flexion, the fingers should point to the scaphoid.

Functional Status

Decreased finger ROM secondary to pain and possible deformity
Decreased grip strength

Physical Evaluation Findings

Metacarpal palpation may reveal crepitus, tenderness, and deformity along the injured part of bone.
Pain radiates through the affected finger.

Hand trauma often results in a fracture to one of the metacarpals. The first and fifth metacarpals are most commonly injured, the fifth because of the increased mobility of these bones. First metacarpal fractures and fracture-dislocations are covered in the section on thumb injuries (p 404). The second and third metacarpals are rigidly fixed at their bases and stable, with little motion at the CMC joints. The fourth and fifth metacarpals move more freely, with 15° and 25° of motion in the CMC joints, respectively.[52-54]

Metacarpal fractures account for 30% to 40% of all hand fractures and result from either a direct force or indirect trauma through axial loading.[55,56] Torsional stress on the digits can also produce a metacarpal fracture. A "boxer fracture" is the most common type, occurring at the neck of the fifth metacarpal from a compressive force as the fist makes contact with another object.

The metacarpal fracture pattern often describes the mechanism of injury. Direct or axial trauma leads to transverse or oblique fractures, whereas torsional injury leads to spiral fractures. The fractures can be stable or unstable, depending on whether shortening, rotation, or angulation is present.[52,53,55] Malrotation can cause the fingers to overlap when the hand is made into a fist. Efforts should be made to prevent even small amounts of rotation, which can cause permanent disability. Most metacarpal fractures can be treated conservatively with immobilization of the hand, wrist, and involved fingers. However, articular fractures of the fifth metacarpal between the metacarpal ligament insertion and the insertion of the extensor carpi ulnaris (ECU) tendon may cause migration of the proximal fractured portion and often require ORIF.[56]

Differential Diagnosis
MCP joint dislocation, CMC dislocation, phalangeal fracture, carpal dislocation

Imaging Techniques
AP, lateral, and oblique radiographs should be obtained (**Figure 12-30**). A CT scan is helpful when an intra-articular fracture is present.

Definitive Diagnosis
Radiographs are used to definitively diagnose a metacarpal fracture.

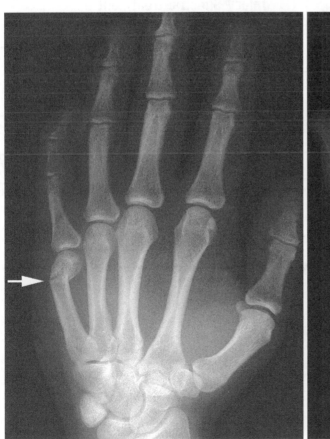
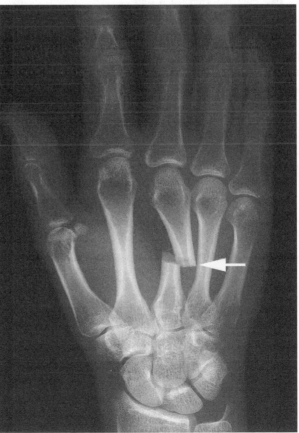

Figure 12-30   Radiographs of metacarpal fractures. **A.** Fracture of the fifth metacarpal ("boxer fracture"). **B.** Fracture of the third metacarpal. The fracture displacement warrants closed reduction before casting. (Reproduced with permission from Johnson TR, Steinbach LS (eds): *Essentials of Musculoskeletal Imaging.* Rosemont, IL, American Academy of Orthopaedic Surgeons, 2004, pp 346-347.)

Pathomechanics and Functional Limitations

Metacarpal fractures usually heal without consequence. However, neglect or improper immobilization can result in a nonunion or malunion and subsequent decreased grip strength.

◼ Immediate Management

A suspected metacarpal fracture should be immobilized with a splint and the patient referred for radiographs. Taping the fingers also prevents rotation and displacement of a spiral fracture.

◼ Medications

Analgesics may provide relief from pain in the acute or postoperative period.

◼ Postinjury Management

The fracture is reduced (if necessary) and a cast applied. The bone is difficult to immobilize; although a short arm cast effectively restricts wrist and hand ROM, the metacarpal bone moves when the finger moves. Accordingly, the generally accepted treatment is to apply a cast and tape the fingers together to restrict metacarpal motion.

The cast is worn for 4 weeks, after which gradual hand and wrist ROM and strengthening exercises are implemented. Active finger motion is encouraged early to prevent stiffness and help reduce edema. Rehabilitation is started when the immobilization phase has ended. Efforts are made to regain ROM and strength in the wrist, hand, and fingers.

◼ Surgical Intervention

Surgical treatment of metacarpal fractures is indicated with intra-articular disruption, severe angulation that cannot be reduced by a closed method, and multiple fractures. Most often, the closed re-duction can be stabilized using percutaneous pinning that minimizes the disruption of normal tissue. Depending on the orientation, rotation, and stability of the fracture, small screws may be necessary to facilitate proper healing. These are inserted through a dorsal incision over the fracture site.

Percutaneous pinning with K-wires may help stabilize the fracture. Comminution of the metacarpal shaft can be treated with pinning, minifragment screws, plate-and-screw fixation, or a tension band (**Figure 12-31**).[53,57] Percutaneous pins are left in place for 4 to 6 weeks, when healing is confirmed by radiography.

Functional limitations may arise with metacarpal malrotation. If fracture fixation and stability are lost, the bone's tendency is to return to its original deformity. Open reduction of a metacarpal shaft fracture can compromise the bone's blood supply or cause fibrosis of the interosseus muscles, adherence of the extensor tendons, or a local infection.

With closed reduction, up to 40° of angulation is acceptable in the fourth or fifth metacarpal. It is not necessary to hold the MCP or PIP joints flexed because this often results in excessive stiffness.

◼ Injury-Specific Treatment and Rehabilitation Concerns

Specific Concerns
Maintain stability of the fracture site.
Promote and restore ROM.

Rehabilitation is initiated as soon as the immobilization period ends. Generally, active ROM of all fingers should be normal if the cast was applied properly. If the cast extended beyond the distal palmar crease in the hand, motion may be impaired

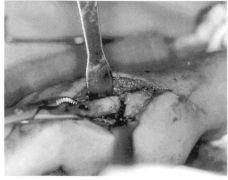
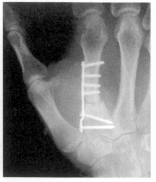

Figure 12-31 Plate-and-screw fixation of a displaced metacarpal fracture. **A.** Exposure of nonunion site in preparation for curettage, bone grafting, and internal fixation. **B.** Internal fixation accomplished with a minicondylar blade-plate device to achieve skeletal stability. (Reproduced with permission from Kozin SH, Thoder JJ, Lieberman G: Operative treatment of metacarpal and phalangeal shaft fractures. *J Am Acad Orthop Surg* 2000;8:111-121.)

until the MCP joints can be stretched. Wrist strength is addressed with multiplanar dumbbell curls, pronation, and supination. Grip exercise is gradually increased in intensity using therapeutic putty. All exercise progresses at the patient's tolerance. Sport-specific tasks such as palming a basketball can be employed for hand strengthening.

■ Estimated Amount of Time Lost

The fracture requires 4 to 6 weeks to heal, after which a gradual return to participation is permitted. A displaced fracture requires a longer healing time and possibly ORIF. Hand weakness and pain may restrict participation.

■ Return-to-Play Criteria

The fracture should be healed before the athlete returns to participation in sports in which playing with a padded cast or splint on the hand is prohibited (eg, wrestling). However, early return to athletics is possible when the fracture is stable and adequate protection is provided in the form of thermoplastic materials, padding, and casts. The athlete may participate without protection when the fracture is healed and full strength and mobility have returned to the upper extremity.

Functional Bracing

Fractures to the second through fourth metacarpals can often be padded and protected with thermoplastic materials and gel padding. The fingers should remain taped together to prevent rotation. Depending on the fracture location and stability, the physician may permit play with a custom-fabricated silicon splint (**CT** 12-4).

Lunate Dislocations

The lunate is the most commonly dislocated of all the carpal bones. Perilunate dislocations result from a dislocation of the distal carpal row. In a lunate dislocation, the space between the distal and proximal carpal bones is forced open. The lunate cup is commonly directed volarly in dislocation because of the mechanism of injury, which is a fall on an outstretched hand.[58,59] Because of the stresses involved, a scaphoid fracture often accompanies a perilunate dislocation.[60,61] The intercarpals supinate, stressing the carpals and causing either a lunate or perilunate dislocation. If the scapholunate ligament remains intact, the scaphoid may be fractured.[62]

Carpal instability can take many forms and represents a spectrum of injury, including scapholunate

CLINICAL PRESENTATION

History

A fall or other mechanism that results in forceful hand rotation or wrist hyperextension and/or ulnar deviation
Pain arising from the palmar or dorsal aspect of the hand, proximal to the wrist

Observation

When the patient makes a fist, the third metacarpal is at the same level as the other knuckles (Murphy sign).
Diffuse swelling can occur.
In some patients, lunate displacement is observed.

Functional Status

Pain occurs with all wrist motions.
Wrist and finger flexion may be limited by swelling.

Physical Evaluation Findings

Pressure on the median nerve can result in flexor muscle numbness or paralysis.
Diffuse pain during palpation
The displaced lunate may be detected during palpation.

dissociation, lunate and perilunate dislocations, scaphoid fracture, and other intercarpal instabilities (**Figure 12-32**). This injury is often misdiagnosed as a wrist sprain and may lead to chronic wrist pain and instability.

Differential Diagnosis

Scapholunate sprain, scaphoid fracture, triangular fibrocartilage complex (TFCC) tear

Imaging Techniques

AP and lateral radiographs of the wrist are required to diagnose a lunate dislocation or other carpal instability (**Figure 12-33**). On the AP view, 2 arcs should be identified. The first proximal arc is the radiocarpal row, which should be smooth and continuous; disruption suggests a lunate dislocation.[63,64] The second arc is the midcarpal row, which also should be smooth and continuous; disruption suggests a perilunate dislocation. The lunate is normally quadrangular; when dislocated, however, it appears triangular on the AP view—an additional clue to dislocation.

On the lateral view, the column formed by the radius, lunate, and capitate in a series of "C" shapes provides evidence of a lunate dislocation. The lunate should lie within the radius cup, and the capitate should rest within the lunate cup. Loss of this normal column implies lunate or perilunate dislocation.

Stress radiographs of the wrist may be necessary to demonstrate intercarpal ligamentous instability when no evidence of wrist dislocation is

CT Clinical Technique 12-4

Constructing a Removable Silicone Playing Cast

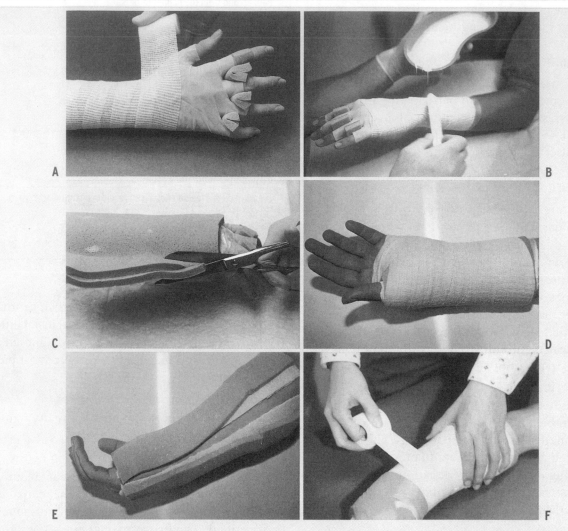

Although most secondary school and collegiate athletic conferences permit athletes to participate with padded silicone casts or hard casts with padding, certain sport situations or environmental conditions call for the use of a silicone playing cast. Because league rules vary, an official should always be consulted before an athlete wearing any type of cast or splint enters into participation.

Materials Needed

Disposable drape	Disposable bowl
Latex surgical gloves	Tongue depressors
Foam to place between the fingers	Polyurethane foam padding (optional)
Prewrap	3 to 4 rolls of gauze bandage
Elastic wrap	1-lb can of RTV-11 with catalyst
Scissors	

A. A latex surgical glove is placed over the area to be splinted, ensuring that the proximal and distal joints are supported. The glove is wrapped with one layer of gauze.

B. The silicone is spread over the gauze surface with a tongue depressor. The process is repeated, adding roll gauze and silicone until the desired thickness is obtained. Increasing the silicone thickness increases the splint's rigidity.

C. The final layer of gauze and silicone may be covered with another latex glove. If indicated, adhesive foam padding is wrapped around the cast and secured, and excess foam is cut off.

D. The entire cast is wrapped with a 2- or 5-in elastic wrap while the silicone dries (see label for drying time).

E. After the cast has been allowed to dry, the cast is cut off along the seam of the foam padding.

F. For practice or competition, the cast may be applied using prewrap and athletic tape.

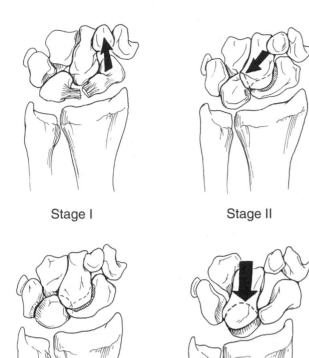

Stage I   Stage II

Stage III   Stage IV

Figure 12-32 Stages of progression of perilunar instability. Stage I: Disruption of the scapholunate ligamentous complex. Stage II: The force propagates through the space of Poirier and interrupts the lunocapitate connection. Stage III: The lunotriquetral connection is violated, and the entire carpus separates from the lunate. Stage IV: The lunate dislocates from its fossa into the carpal tunnel, the lunate rotates into the carpal tunnel, and the capitate becomes aligned with the radius. (Reproduced with permission from Kozin SH: Perilunate injuries: Diagnosis and treatment. *J Am Acad Orthop Surg* 1998;6:114-120.)

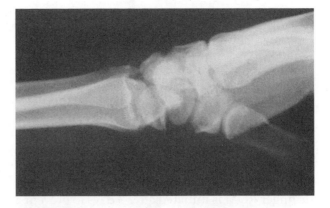

Figure 12-33 Lateral radiograph depicts a dorsal perilunate dislocation, with the capitate and scaphoid dorsal to the lunate. (Reproduced with permission from Kozin SH: Perilunate injuries: Diagnosis and treatment. *J Am Acad Orthop Surg* 1998;6:114-120.)

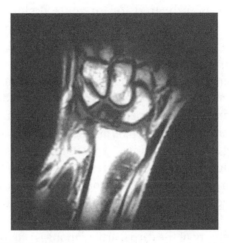

Figure 12-34 T1-weighted MRI reveals decreased signal intensity of the lunate in the wrist of a patient with Kienböck's disease. (Reproduced with permission from Allan CH, Lichtman DM: Kienböck's disease: Diagnosis and treatment. *J Am Acad Orthop Surg* 2001; 9:128-136.)

apparent on plain films. Stress radiographs obtained with radial and ulnar deviation of the hand may demonstrate scapholunate dissociation (see Scapholunate Dissociations, p 425).

Definitive Diagnosis
The definitive diagnosis is based on the radiographic findings.

Pathomechanics and Functional Limitations
Carpal dislocations often result in carpal instability, which causes chronic pain and loss of function. Failure to diagnose and treat the injury promptly contributes to this problem. Median nerve inhibition can lead to signs and symptoms similar to carpal tunnel syndrome (CTS) (see p 433).

If the dislocation is not identified early, the lunate may deteriorate to the point that it must be surgically removed. The lunate may also rotate around the dorsal ligament, interfering with the

blood supply and resulting in Kienböck's disease (**Figure 12-34**).[63-65] Early reduction prevents these complications.

■ Immediate Management
The wrist should be assessed for the entire spectrum of injuries. If a carpal dislocation is suspected, the wrist, forearm, and hand should be splinted. Attempts to reduce a dislocation should not be made without a radiograph, even with symptoms of median nerve compromise during the on-field evaluation. The injury may be mistaken for a distal radius fracture, which is difficult to reduce.

A patient with a lunate dislocation should be referred to a hand specialist or a physician trained in carpal instabilities. A hand surgeon may decide to immobilize the elbow to reduce pronation and supination.

12

Medications

Pain medication may be needed to allow closed reduction.

Postinjury Management

Carpal instability can exist even in the presence of negative radiographs; consequently, immobilizing the wrist in a cast for 2 weeks and then reevaluating is often advised. Cast immobilization is required after both surgical and nonsurgical reduction. Gentle finger ROM is initiated after 3 days to prevent a contracture. Once the cast is removed, aggressive ROM tactics and strengthening are initiated.

Surgical Intervention

Surgery is indicated for an acute dislocation if scapholunate instability exists. Surgical management is also necessary in Kienböck's disease, which is a progressive collapse of the lunate from osteonecrosis. Maintaining scapholunate function is the goal of surgical management for a lunate dislocation. Generally, percutaneous K-wires are used to manipulate the carpals and secure their location during immobilization.[65] In Kienböck's disease, a leveling procedure that entails shortening the radius or lengthening the ulna is useful in decompressing the lunate and allowing a return of function (**Figure 12-35**).

Stability of the carpal articulations is often traded for mobility. The midcarpal joints frequently are stiff, and ROM is limited. Because of the complexity of the carpal biomechanics and the potential for osteoarthritic changes, this injury should be managed by a hand surgeon. Wrist ROM is often limited, especially in extension, but a pain-free outcome is anticipated.

Injury-Specific Treatment and Rehabilitation Concerns

> **Specific Concerns**
>
> Reduce the dislocation and remove pressure from the median nerve.
> Prevent osteonecrosis and lunate collapse (Kienböck's disease).

Rehabilitation may be extensive with carpal dislocations, because a long immobilization period is often necessary. Wrist flexion and extension and ulnar and radial deviation, pronation, and supination are often limited. When the pins have been removed, aggressive ROM techniques may begin. The clinician should direct passive stress and joint mobilization to both the radiocarpal joints and the midcarpal joints. Long-duration, low-load stretches to promote supination can be applied by the patient sitting on his or her own hand.

Hand and wrist strengthening is done with resistive exercise. Wrist curls, grip exercise, and upper body strengthening apply this stress to the involved hand. Resistance exercise should be performed after mobility exercise to take advantage of any newly gained range. Therapeutic exercise is generally done 4 to 5 times per week.

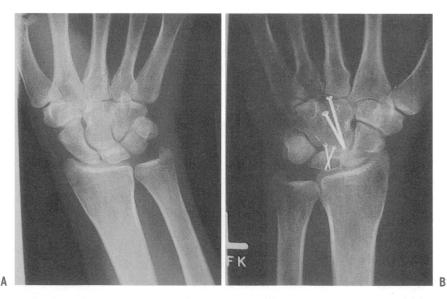

Figure 12-35 **A.** Preoperative anteroposterior wrist radiograph of a patient with stage IIIA Kienböck's disease. **B.** Postoperative radiograph shows lunate fracture fixation and vascularized bone grafting, in addition to capitate shortening. (Reproduced with permission from Allan CH, Lichtman DM: Kienböck's disease: Diagnosis and treatment. *J Am Acad Orthop Surg* 2001;9:128-136.)

Estimated Amount of Time Lost

Cast immobilization is usually required for 6 weeks. The disability length depends on the presence of concomitant injury and carpal instability. Lunate and perilunate dislocations can cause significant time lost from athletics, especially when weight bearing on the hand is required. Brace support or taping is often needed as the athlete is reintroduced to sport.

Return-to-Play Criteria

Return to play is permitted when ROM and strength are good and healing is complete. If ROM is affected, modifications in technique or the use of a brace may be necessary.

Functional Bracing

Athletic tape or a commercially available brace can be used for sport participation (**Figure 12-36**).

Scaphoid Fractures

CLINICAL PRESENTATION

History

Forced extension of the wrist, such as falling on an outstretched arm

Pain originating from the "anatomic snuffbox"

Observation

Little deformity from the scaphoid fracture is noted.

Secondary swelling from contusive forces may be observed.

Functional Status

Decreased grip strength

Decreased ROM in all directions, but most notably during flexion, extension, and ulnar deviation

Physical Evaluation Findings

Pain, point tenderness, and possible crepitus during palpation of the anatomic snuffbox

Pain is significantly increased during active and passive radial deviation.

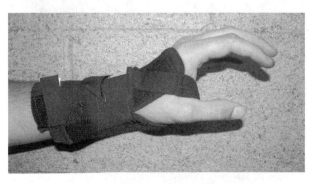

Figure 12-36 Commercially available braces often provide enough support for daily activities and participation in some sports.

The wrist comprises an intricate network of eight carpal bones arranged in two rows that articulate with the radius and fibrocartilaginous end of the ulna proximally and the metacarpals distally. The carpal frame stabilizes the wrist and allows the hand and fingers to move. The hand muscles primarily originate in the forearm and pass over the wrist. The flexor carpi ulnaris, which inserts into the pisiform bone, is the only muscle that inserts into the wrist complex.

The carpal bones move in concert during flexion, extension, ulnar and radial deviation, and pronation and supination. With wrist extension and radial deviation, the scaphoid is impinged by the radius; because of its narrow midportion (waist), the scaphoid is predisposed to injury[66,67] (**Figure 12-37**). A carpal fracture can occur with compression and shearing of the bone, as when falling on an outstretched hand, compressing the scaphoid between the radius and the second row of carpal bones, particularly the capitate. Inline skating falls account for most of the scaphoid fractures seen in emergency departments.[66] The scaphoid can also be injured in a weight-bearing position, eg, in gymnasts, when the hand is stabilized and the forearm rotates abruptly.

The scaphoid bone is the most frequently fractured carpal bone. Because healing depends on blood supply and the blood enters the scaphoid along the dorsal surface near its midportion, the bone is prone to osteonecrosis.[63,68,69] A scaphoid fracture is often missed and mistaken for a wrist sprain on an early radiograph.

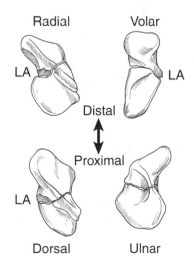

Figure 12-37 Four views of a right scaphoid demonstrate its complex shape. The surface is predominantly articular, and most of the blood supply enters through the nonarticular dorsal ridge (LA = lateral apex of the dorsal ridge). The fracture line depicts the pattern of so-called waist fractures. (Adapted with permission from Compson JP: The anatomy of acute scaphoid fractures: A three-dimensional analysis of patterns. *J Bone Joint Surg Br* 1998;80:218-224.)

Differential Diagnosis

Wrist sprain, radial or ulnar fracture, thumb sprain, metacarpal fracture

Imaging Techniques

A scaphoid fracture can be diagnosed with high-quality AP and lateral radiographic images. A PA view of the scaphoid with the wrist in ulnar deviation may distract the fragments and make the fracture more apparent. Many times, however, the fracture cannot be visualized on initial plain films (**Figure 12-38**).

A bone or CT scan may be necessary to detect an occult fracture that is not visible on plain films (**Figure 12-39**).

Definitive Diagnosis

The definitive diagnosis is based on positive findings on plain radiographs or MRI. If the initial radiograph does not show the fracture when there is a strong clinical suspicion, the wrist should be placed in a thumb-spica cast for 2 weeks and reevaluated. Positive clinical findings and a mechanism of forced wrist extension may warrant the initial diagnosis of a scaphoid fracture until it can be definitively ruled out.[66,67,70] MRI or radiographs repeated after 2 weeks should identify the fracture.

Pathomechanics and Functional Limitations

Most scaphoid fractures occur at the narrow midpoint of the waist. This aspect of the scaphoid can be impinged by the styloid process of the radius during forced radial deviation. This fracture is usually associated with a force applied to the distal pole of the scaphoid, often with wrist hyperextension. The radial styloid process functions as a fulcrum against the center of the scaphoid, resulting in the predominance of fractures at the waist. The mechanism of injury usually is a fall on an outstretched hand. On clinical examination, pain is elicited when pressure is exerted on the distal pole or on the scaphoid at the anatomic snuffbox on the radial aspect of the wrist.

A gap or fracture offset of 1 mm or more indicates instability, with the potential for nonunion or malunion, and internal fixation should be considered.[63,70,71] Internal fixation may also be considered routinely for proximal-pole fractures, regardless of the degree of displacement, in view of the long healing time and high risk of nonunion despite cast treatment.

■ Immediate Management

If a scaphoid fracture is suspected, ice should be applied immediately to prevent edema. A splint should be applied to immobilize the wrist, el-bow, and thumb. Given the mechanism of injury (wrist hyperextension) and pain over the scaphoid, care should proceed as if a scaphoid fracture is present.

■ Medications

Analgesic medication or NSAIDs may be prescribed to control the athlete's pain and inflammation.

■ Surgical Intervention

In managing acute scaphoid fractures, the fracture stability, ease of reduction, associated ligamentous injury, and risk of impaired blood supply must be considered, rather than the direction of the fracture line or location of the fracture within the scaphoid. Nonunion and osteonecrosis are common sequelae of acute fractures. Because the risk of impaired vascularity is greater with fractures located in the proximal third, stable internal fixation may be indicated to provide mechanical stability and fracture-surface contact to enhance revascularization. Faster healing rates and earlier rehabilitation with percutaneous techniques of internal fixation have produced a clear shift from classic conservative treatment to internal fixation. Although the rates of union for well-vascularized nonunions have not been dramatically improved with the use of internal fixa-

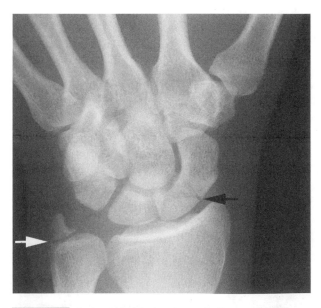

Figure 12-38 Posteroanterior view demonstrating a scaphoid fracture (black arrow). Note the associated fracture of the ulnar styloid process (white arrow). (Reproduced with permission from Johnson TR, Steinbach LS (eds): *Essentials of Musculoskeletal Imaging*. Rosemont, IL, American Academy of Orthopaedic Surgeons, 2004, p 356.)

tion compared with inlay bone grafting, restoring scaphoid anatomy and preventing malunion and associated carpal collapse with interpositional bone-grafting techniques may reduce the risk of osteoarthritis[63] (**ST** 12-4). The fracture location may be a poor prognosticator of the outcome, because the architecture of the blood supply can be variable and unpredictable.

Postinjury/Postoperative Management

Conservative management is the first option in treating a presumed scaphoid fracture. The wrist and thumb should be immobilized for 2 weeks using a short or long arm cast, even if a fracture is not definitively identified. Follow-up radiographs help to determine whether to continue immobilization. Once union has been established, wrist strengthening exercises may begin, but additional protection should be provided against impact loading for another 3 months. Postoperative management of a scaphoid fracture with bone graft also requires extensive healing time. A thumb-spica cast is used for 6 to 8 weeks, and then strengthening exercises are initiated.

Injury-Specific Treatment and Rehabilitation Concerns

> **Specific Concerns**
>
> Promptly diagnose and treat with immobilization to allow primary bone healing.
> Maintain immobilization during participation in athletics if possible.
> Achieve full, pain-free ROM of the affected wrist and hand.

After the immobilization period for scaphoid fractures, wrist and hand ROM and strengthening may begin. Because of the extensive casting, joint mobilization and stretching techniques may be implemented right away. Wrist flexion, extension, pronation, and supination are addressed.

Wrist strengthening is done with multiplanar dumbbell curls and gripping exercise. Weight bearing through the involved wrist for closed chain upper body exercise should be performed with the wrist in a neutral position. Push-ups are performed in a "knuckle" position or using handles. Support should be provided to the wrist with tape or bracing for this activity.

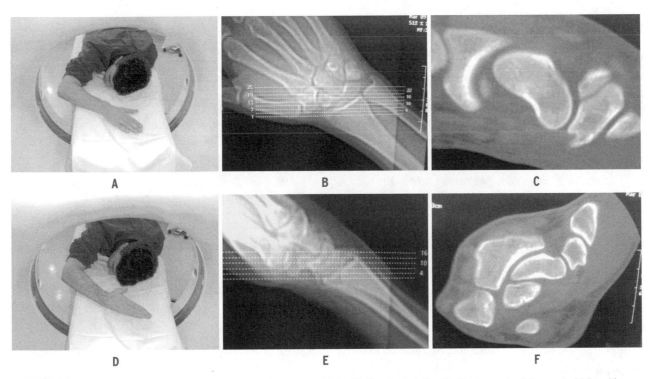

Figure 12-39 CT of the scaphoid is easier to interpret if the images are obtained in the planes defined by the long axis of the scaphoid. To achieve this, the patient lies prone on the table with the arm overhead. **A.** For sagittal-plane images, the forearm is held pronated, and the hand lies flat on the table. The forearm crosses the gantry at an angle of approximately 45° (roughly in line with the abducted thumb metacarpal). **B.** Scout images are obtained to confirm appropriate orientation and to ensure that the entire scaphoid is imaged. Sections are obtained at 1-mm intervals. **C.** Images obtained in the sagittal plane are best for measuring the intrascaphoid angle. **D.** For coronal-plane images, the forearm is in neutral rotation. **E.** Scout images demonstrate the alignment of the wrist through the gantry of the scanner. **F.** Interpretation of images obtained in the coronal plane is straightforward. (Copyright 1999 by Jesse B. Jupiter, MD.)

S|T Surgical Technique 12-4

Repair of the Scaphoid: Inlay Technique

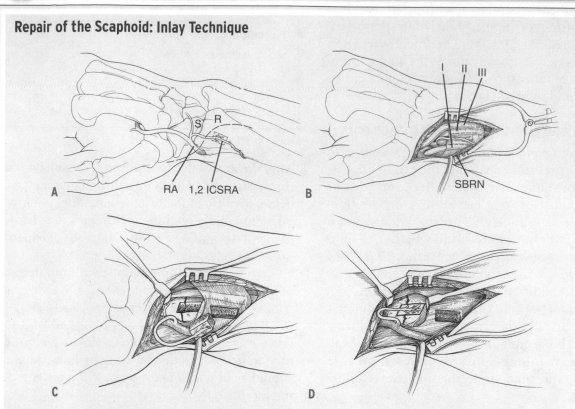

RA = radial artery; S = scaphoid; R = radius; 1, 2 ICSRA = first and second vessels, intercompartmental supraretinacular artery; I, II, III = superficial branches of the radial nerve

Indications

Unstable, displaced scaphoid fractures need primary ORIF and sometimes primary grafting. Fractures at the proximal pole or waist of the scaphoid require long immobilization periods, and if nonunion or osteonecrosis occurs, surgical intervention is indicated.

Overview

1. A curvilinear incision is made over the dorsolateral scaphoid (**A**).
2. The arteries 1, 2 ICSRA and the superficial branches of the radial nerve (I, II, III) are identified and protected (**B**).
3. The bone graft is harvested with an intact arteriole, and the graft-site vascularity is confirmed (**C**).
4. A notch is made in the two halves of the scaphoid to accept the graft.
5. The graft bone (with its arterial blood supply) is fitted into the notch in the scaphoid (**D**).
6. Additional fixation using K-wires or scaphoid screws may be performed at this time.

Functional Limitations

Surgical intervention with bone grafts may cause midcarpal stiffness, resulting in a permanent loss of wrist motion. Generally, the athlete can adapt to the loss of motion, even in a skill position. However, an athlete who bears weight on the upper extremity, such as a gymnast, may not be able to gain enough pain-free wrist extension to perform.

Implications for Rehabilitation

The patient is fitted with a long arm thumb-spica splint for 10 to 14 days, followed by a long arm thumb-spica cast for up to 6 weeks. The long immobilization period required for bone healing causes wrist and hand weakness and stiffness.

Potential Complications

Nonunion of the scaphoid, scapholunate dissociation, and instability

Comments

Osteogenic ultrasonic or electromagnetic bone stimulators can be used to assist healing (see p 32).

Figures adapted with permission from the Mayo Foundation, Rochester, MN.

Estimated Amount of Time Lost

Depending on the sport's requirements, an athlete may be incapacitated from 6 to 12 weeks, barring complications. Cast immobilization of the wrist with a thumb-spica cast for 6 weeks remains the treatment of choice for stable fractures of the scaphoid midportion and distal pole. If a fracture is suspected but plain films are negative, the wrist should be immobilized for 2 weeks. Reevaluation and more extensive diagnostic testing such as MRI may be performed at that time. If rules permit and the athlete is functional, participation in athletics can proceed with cast immobilization and appropriate padding.

Many scaphoid fractures require 8 weeks of immobilization for union to occur. Follow-up radiographs should be taken to monitor signs of nonunion or osteonecrosis.

Return-to-Play Criteria

The key to treating a scaphoid fracture is to obtain primary healing. Many scaphoid fractures are missed on initial evaluation and result in nonunion or osteonecrosis. Treatment requires extensive immobilization, which can result in wrist and hand weakness. Rehabilitation should focus on increasing upper extremity strength. Protection should be used for wrist support and to prevent stress when the bone has healed enough for the athlete to return to play.

Functional Bracing

The athlete may be able to participate while immobilized if a cast is permitted with appropriate padding. A wrist brace that incorporates the thumb can be used in transition, and tape can offer support in the later stages of healing. Once the bone has healed, the wrist should be protected for at least another 2 weeks, especially if the athlete is participating in a contact sport. Gentle strengthening and flexibility exercises can be initiated during this period.

Scapholunate Dissociations

The wrist is an intercalated segment based on the configuration of multiple joint segments and ligamentous stabilizing elements. The carpal bones shift in concert when the wrist moves from flexion, extension, and radial and ulnar deviation. The scapholunate articulation creates a stable column for wrist function, thus even a partial ligament tear can result in instability[72] (**Figure 12-40**). The most common pattern of carpal instability is the dorsal intercalated segment instability (DISI), in which

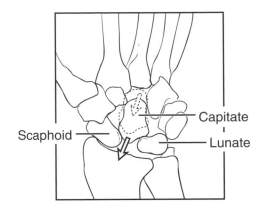

Figure 12-40 Compression of the capitate between scaphoid and lunate can rupture the scapholunate ligament and/or the lunotriquetral ligament, causing instability.

the lunate is displaced volarly and flexed dorsally. The volar intercalated segment instability (VISI) pattern occurs when the lunate is displaced dorsally and flexed into the volar position.[72,73]

The scaphoid bone is important to wrist stability because it bridges both the radiocarpal and midcarpal joints. The carpal bones flex and rotate to produce wrist extension, flexion, and radial and ulnar deviation. The carpal bones function at two primary articulations—the radiocarpal joint between the distal radius and proximal carpal row and the midcarpal joint between the proximal and distal carpal rows. The strongest and most important wrist ligaments are located intracapsularly on the palmar side. These ligaments are configured in a double "V" with the apex pointing distally.[29] A site of potential weakness exists between the "V" formations near the lunate-capitate articulation at the space of Poirier, where carpal dislocations occur most commonly.[72]

CLINICAL PRESENTATION

History

Forced wrist extension
Forced wrist rotation
Pain and crepitus may be described.

Observation

Swelling may be present.

Functional Status

Decreased grip strength
Decreased ROM in all planes secondary to pain

Physical Evaluation Findings

A "pop" and pain may be experienced during pronation and ulnar deviation, indicating midcarpal instability.
The following special tests may be positive:
    Watson test for scapholunate instability[73]
    Lunotriquetral ballottement test

A scapholunate dissociation generally occurs after wrist trauma, such as a fall on the hand, forcing the wrist into extension; rotational forces may cause shearing. Pain and inability to use the wrist are usually immediate.

Differential Diagnosis

Lunate dislocation, scaphoid fracture, wrist sprain

Imaging Techniques

AP and lateral views are taken first, and additional images in ulnar and radial deviation and clenched views are ordered as necessary to determine carpal instability, especially the DISI and VISI patterns (**Figure 12-41**). The clenched-fist view is helpful in accentuating a scapholunate gap. MRI can distinguish tears in the scapholunate ligament and determine the presence of occult fractures.

Definitive Diagnosis

The normal scapholunate angle is 30° to 60°; an angle greater than 70° is diagnostic for carpal instability. A capitolunate angle greater than 20° also suggests carpal instability. A scapholunate space of more than 3 mm is abnormal.[72,74]

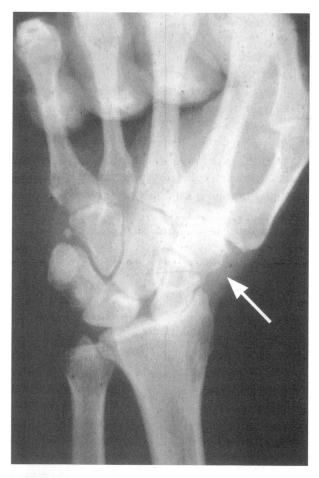

Figure 12-41 Scapholunate dissociation. Radiographs are taken with the fist clenched. The space between the scaphoid and lunate indicates a ligament disruption.

Pathomechanics and Functional Limitations

Wrist instability occurs when the scapholunate ligament stabilizing the proximal scaphoid pole or the interosseous ligament between the individual carpal bones are torn. The scaphoid may subluxate in a rotational manner, and the lunate may flex or dorsiflex with wrist motion. Pain and weakness ultimately limit the athlete's function.

■ Immediate Management

Neurovascular status should be monitored and a splint used to immobilize the wrist in a position of comfort.

■ Medications

Narcotic pain medicine is used after surgery.

■ Surgical Intervention

Carpal instability is treated with reduction and immobilization in radial deviation and extension. The scapholunate gap should be closed, and the lunate and capitate must be realigned. In acute injuries, closed reduction is obtained and percutaneous K-wires are used to fixate the joints under fluoroscopy.[75,76] A short-arm cast is worn for 6 to 8 weeks, followed by a removable splint for an additional 4 weeks. When scapholunate instability is complete, both dorsal and volar incisions are necessary to repair the anterior ligamentous complex and decompress the median nerve. The dorsal interosseous ligaments are repaired by reattaching the ligaments directly or by roughening the bone and attaching the ligaments through drill holes with a reefing of the dorsal capsule. The immobilization period is similar with both open and closed reductions.

■ Postinjury/Postoperative Management

After injury, the wrist is splinted in a position of function until proper clinical and radiologic evaluation can be made. If the injury warrants surgical management, a short-arm cast is used postoperatively for 6 to 8 weeks. Percutaneous K-wires can then be removed, and active motion begins. Joint mobilization is often necessary because of the lengthy immobilization period.

■ Injury-Specific Treatment and Rehabilitation Concerns

Specific Concerns

Protect the healing bone during healing.
Restore wrist ROM.
Restore thumb ROM, especially in opposition.

Rehabilitation is begun after the immobilization period, when the percutaneous K-wires are removed. Active wrist ROM in all planes is encouraged, and strengthening of the entire upper extremity is incorporated as indicated. Generally, finger ROM is unaffected, but the thumb may be stiff, especially in opposition.

Passive motion and aggressive joint mobilization of the wrist may begin after 8 weeks. The patient may have difficulty achieving full supination. Grip, all planes of wrist activity, and supination and pronation should be strengthened in addition to the elbow and shoulder.

Full strength and flexibility are the goals, but a functional, pain-free result is ideal. The athlete is generally advised to avoid excessive stresses and weight bearing on the involved wrist for several months to a year after the injury.

■ Estimated Amount of Time Lost

The wrist requires 8 to 12 weeks of immobilization after reduction. Further protection is required for sports activities while rehabilitating. The patient may be able to participate in athletics while immobilized, but not if percutaneous pins are in place. Once the pins are removed, conditioning exercises and limited participation with a cast are permitted. The time lost is influenced by the type of surgical reconstruction and whether the rules of the athlete's sport allow participation while wearing a cast.

■ Return-to-Play Criteria

The wrist should be protected from falls and excessive stress until ROM and strength are similar to the contralateral side; this may take several months. Again, the ability to participate in athletics is generally dictated by the acceptance of and ability to perform using a protective device.

Functional Bracing

A commercial wrist splint is often used to protect the wrist from excessive stress during sports. Athletic tape can also be used, either circumferentially to help stabilize the wrist or through the hand to help control motion.

Hamate Fractures

The hamate can be injured in a variety of ways in athletes. The body of the hamate is fractured less frequently than its "hook," which projects into the

<table>
<tr><td colspan="2">CLINICAL PRESENTATION</td></tr>
<tr><td colspan="2">History</td></tr>
<tr><td colspan="2">Reports a fall on the hand or an impact while holding an implement such as a racquet or bat
Generalized wrist and hand pain</td></tr>
<tr><td colspan="2">Observation</td></tr>
<tr><td colspan="2">Outward deformity is rarely noted.</td></tr>
<tr><td colspan="2">Functional Status</td></tr>
<tr><td colspan="2">Pain is produced during abduction and adduction of the fifth finger.
Decreased grip strength</td></tr>
<tr><td colspan="2">Physical Evaluation Findings</td></tr>
<tr><td colspan="2">Pain during resisted flexion and/or abduction of the fifth finger
Pain is produced during palpation of the hook of the hamate.</td></tr>
</table>

palm. Fractures of the body of the hamate are usually associated with fourth and fifth CMC fracture-dislocations. The hook of the hamate serves as a muscular attachment for the flexor digiti minimi brevis and the opponens digiti minimi and as a ligamentous attachment for the transverse carpal and pisohamate ligaments (**Figure 12-42**). A fracture of

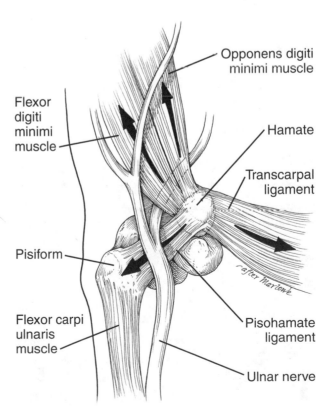

Figure 12-42　Intrinsic forces acting on the hook of the hamate. (Modified with permission by J. Marlowe.)

the hamate body or hook causes grip instability, and excessive movement can result in ulnar nerve motor and sensory deficits.[77,78]

Fractures of the body of the hamate can result from an axial force through the metacarpals or a direct blow to the ulnar aspect of the wrist. Although the hook of the hamate can be fractured by a fall, fractures are more common in sports that require holding an implement, such as a softball or baseball bat, golf club, hockey or lacrosse stick, or tennis racket. The fracture can also occur from repetitive stress or a direct blow when the club or racquet strikes the ground.

The hook of the hamate is located by identifying the pisiform and then palpating along a line from the pisiform to the head of the second metacarpal. Although firm pressure over a fractured hook generally causes discomfort, mild to moderate pressure may cause little pain. As a consequence, many fractures are overlooked.

Differential Diagnosis
CMC fracture, CMC dislocation, false aneurysm of the ulnar artery

Imaging Techniques
Radiographs should include the carpal-tunnel view and a view with the wrist supinated to visualize the hook of the hamate and pisiform. CT should be considered when clinical findings suggest a fracture not visible on routine radiographs[79,80] (**Figure 12-43**).

Definitive Diagnosis
Imaging studies are performed to identify the presence or absence of a hamate fracture. Follow-up studies are used to determine whether a nonunion has occurred.

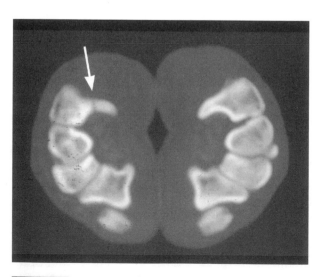

Figure 12-43 CT scan of bilateral hands showing a fracture of the hook of the hamate.

Pathomechanics and Functional Limitations
If the diagnosis is not made promptly, the ulnar nerve within the Guyon canal can be damaged, resulting in palsy, or the fifth flexor digitorum profundus tendon can rupture.[79,80] Over time, a definite protrusion over the hamate becomes sensitive during gripping (**Figure 12-44**). The athlete may have a functional disability because of grip weakness and pain when using the sport implement.

■ Immediate Management
Immediate management consists of immobilization, application of ice, and referral for radiographs.

■ Medications
Pain medications are not often needed, but NSAIDs can be used to control inflammation.

■ Surgical Intervention
Fractures of the hamate hook and body are usually nondisplaced and can be treated with cast immobilization. Intra-articular fractures with displacement of more than 1 mm are best treated with ORIF. Displaced fractures that involve the distal aspect of the hook often result in nonunion if they are not treated with ORIF. The simplest procedure that allows an early return to athletics is to remove the fractured portion of the bone.[80] This is often done with painless nonunions to prevent a later tendon rupture. Surgical intervention generally does not affect long-term hand strength or motion.

■ Postinjury/Postoperative Management
Compression is applied to the hand to minimize edema formation in the palm. Finger ROM is initiated after 3 days. Power grips that stress the flexor tendons are avoided for 2 weeks.

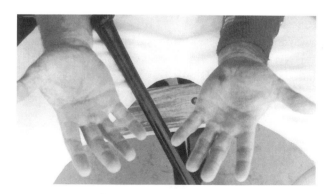

Figure 12-44 Mark over the hook of a hamate in a professional baseball player. (Reproduced with permission from *J Am Acad Orthop Surg* 2001;9:389-400. © 2001 American Academy of Orthopaedic Surgeons.)

■ Injury-Specific Treatment and Rehabilitation Concerns

Specific Concerns
Protect the hamate from pressure.
After surgery, avoid gripping activities.

Treatment focuses on reducing pain while allowing surgical incisions to heal (if applicable). A supervised rehabilitation program is not generally required after this procedure. Efforts should target decreasing edema formation, which may lead to scar formation in the palm. Active finger ROM is encouraged early, and grip and wrist exercises may begin at 2 to 4 weeks, when the immobilization period has ended.

When the patient is ready to participate in athletics, excessive pressure on the Guyon canal must be avoided; this pressure can cause ulnar nerve symptoms. Gloves with silicone padding can reduce stress on this area.

■ Estimated Amount of Time Lost

After 4 weeks of cast immobilization, the patient may be able to return to sport with the hook of the hamate padded. Early diagnosis influences the time lost, because the severity of soft-tissue damage increases if the hand is not immobilized.

■ Return-to-Play Criteria

Return to sport is allowed when the athlete can grasp the stick, bat, or racket without pain and has pain-free function of the fifth finger.

Functional Bracing
A donut or relief pad can be used over the sensitive area. Silicone or gel-padded gloves can be worn to minimize the amount of restrictive material in the palm.

Triangular Fibrocartilage Complex Injuries

The TFCC describes the ligamentous and cartilaginous structures that suspend the distal radius and ulnar carpus from the distal ulna. The TFCC is the primary ligamentous stabilizer of the distal radioulnar joint (DRUJ) and the articulation of the ulna and carpal bones. The TFCC provides a continuous gliding surface that allows 3 degrees of freedom in the wrist (flexion/extension, ulnar/radial deviation,

CLINICAL PRESENTATION

History
_____
Wrist hyperextension and ulnar deviation
Repetitive stress
Pain increases with wrist extension and ulnar deviation.
Grinding, clicking, and/or general wrist weakness may be described.

Observation
_____
On rare occasions, the distal ulna is diffusely swollen.

Functional Status
_____
Decreased wrist active, passive, and resistive ROM, especially in extension
Load bearing on the hands, such as performing a push-up or bench press, is limited by pain.

Physical Evaluation Findings
_____
Wrist crepitus, popping, locking, or clicking may be felt during active ROM.
Decreased wrist and grip strength
Piano-key sign of the distal ulna
Point tenderness on the medial wrist
Possible tenderness of the UCL
UCL stress testing produces pain, but no laxity is noted.
Ulnar deviation and compression of the wrist produce pain.
---

supination/pronation).[81-83] Similar to the knee menisci, the TFCC is a shock absorber that absorbs about 40% of the force applied to the wrist; the other 60% is absorbed by the radius. Also similar to the meniscus, the TFCC can be injured with a shearing force, impact to the hand, or repetitive stress.[83,84] Acute TFCC tears are difficult to diagnose and are often associated with wrist sprains.

A DRUJ fracture should raise suspicion for a TFCC injury. TFCC tears are present in 35% of intra-articular fractures and 53% of extra-articular fractures, but there is no correlation between ulnar styloid fractures and TFCC injuries.[81,85] The TFCC can be degenerative, especially if the athlete is more than 30 years old and the area has been chronically stressed. Degenerative injuries are difficult to treat because fibrocartilage heals poorly, and activity modifications may be required to reduce pain.[83,84] A TFCC injury can be debilitating for some athletes, and surgical intervention may be needed after an acute injury if function is limited despite efforts to facilitate proper healing and rehabilitation.[86,87]

Differential Diagnosis
Ulnar fracture, carpal fracture

Imaging Techniques
Radiographs help to rule out fractures and other carpal instabilities. Patients with a torn TFCC display average ulnar variance (radial shortening) of

4.6 mm versus 2.5 mm for those with no tear and dorsal angulation of 24° versus 12° for no tear.[83,84] MRI is beneficial in diagnosing TFCC tears, although degeneration may be difficult to identify. An arthrogram can also be used to diagnose a TFCC tear (**Figure 12-45**).

Definitive Diagnosis

The piano-key sign, a prominent and ballotable distal ulna with full forearm pronation, may be present. Lunotriquetral ballottement and extensor carpi ulnaris tendon subluxation may also be demonstrated. The definitive diagnosis can be made arthroscopically if surgical intervention is indicated.

Pathomechanics and Functional Limitations

The TFCC helps to absorb shock and provide stability at the wrist. Degenerative disease or shearing of the joint can cause a tear, resulting in pain and loss of motion. Pain and weakness may reflect DRUJ instability. Gymnasts and weightlifters who bear weight on the upper extremities are affected. Basketball shooting may cause pain because of the hyperflexed and pronated position during follow-through.

■ Immediate Management

Immediate management includes rest, ice, compression, and elevation; the patient may engage in nonpainful activity with the wrist protected.

■ Medications

NSAIDs can be used to decrease pain and swelling.

■ Postinjury Management

If a TFCC injury is suspected without an associated fracture, cast immobilization should be applied in slight flexion for 4 to 6 weeks. Failure to treat the injury appropriately can lead to degeneration, ulnar chondromalacia, impingement, or calcification. Conservative management should be attempted before surgical intervention, because the patient will continue to require protection and will probably have pain with many activities, even after surgery.

■ Surgical Intervention

Surgical treatment is indicated if the DRUJ is unstable or if a Galeazzi fracture-dislocation is present.[85,87] In addition to repairing the TFCC using sutures, K-wire stabilization just proximal to the DRUJ is recommended for 4 to 6 weeks.

Some surgeons prefer wrist arthroscopy to an open procedure, although visualization is difficult and the instruments are large in relation to the joint size. General principles include debriding to a stable, smooth rim of tissue; maintaining a 2-mm peripheral rim; and limiting the debridement to less than two thirds of the central TFCC. Variations on the procedure, including stabilization, can be performed, depending on the findings during arthroscopy and the involvement of the ECU tendon.

An ulnar-shortening osteotomy may be considered for patients with ulnar-positive variance or a failed debridement. Arthroscopic techniques have become more common for the treatment of TFCC

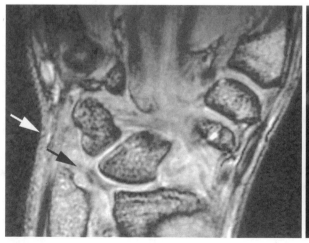
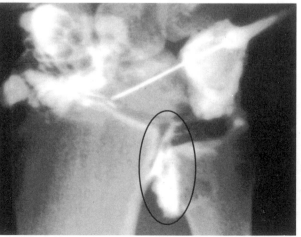

Figure 12-45   Imaging of triangular fibrocartilage complex trauma. **A.** Coronal MRI showing disruption of the complex (black arrow) and the area of maximum tenderness on palpation (white arrow). **B.** Arthrogram demonstrating a complex tear. (Figure A reproduced with permission from Johnson TR, Steinbach LS (eds): *Essentials of Musculoskeletal Imaging.* Rosemont, IL, American Academy of Orthopaedic Surgeons, 2004, p 333. Figure B reproduced with permission from Nagle DJ: Evaluation of chronic wrist pain. *J Am Acad Orthop Surg* 2000;8:45-55.)

injuries. Debriding only the degenerative tissue while leaving most of the tissue can alleviate the pain in some patients.[87-90]

An open procedure requires a longer immobilization period postoperatively, but the surgeon can usually visualize and debride the area better. Activity should be minimized when the K-wire is in place. Wrist pronation and supination are affected by this injury, and stabilization procedures can result in further loss of motion. Degenerative disease of the TFCC and DRUJ can also affect the outcome, producing continued pain and loss of motion, especially with weight-bearing functions.

Injury-Specific Treatment and Rehabilitation Concerns

> **Specific Concerns**
>
> Stabilize and protect the wrist during healing.
> Encourage ROM.

The athlete is encouraged to rest the wrist and to reduce stress by using a brace or tape during everyday activities and athletics. Any modality that is indicated for an inflamed condition can also be used.[86] Specific exercises include active and passive wrist ROM. Long-duration stretches with the elbow extended help to lengthen the wrist flexors and extensors. Strengthening is done in all wrist planes and for grip and the elbow. Pronation and supination are also resisted, but these exercises should be within pain-free limits.

Postoperative rehabilitation mirrors the preoperative phase, while respecting the acute phase in the 2 to 4 weeks after surgery. This time period for immobilization varies, depending on the presence of a fracture and the degree of damage. The surgeon dictates the aggressiveness of the early rehabilitation phase, because the surgical procedure may range from an endoscopic debridement to an open repair.

Estimated Amount of Time Lost

Depending on the severity and whether an associated fracture is present, immobilization ranges from 4 to 10 weeks, with a gradual adaptation to stress through rehabilitation. The amount of damage and the demands of the sport dictate the time lost with a TFCC injury. Some athletes, depending on their sport position, may participate during the immobilization period if adequately protected. Treatment

should not be compromised to permit participation, although an interior lineman in football, for example, may be able to play with a fiberglass cast. If symptoms do not improve with immobilization and rehabilitation, some patients may require arthroscopic or open surgical intervention.

Return-to-Play Criteria

The athlete may return to play using a protective brace or tape if he or she can participate without pain. Full ROM and strength are long-term goals that must be met before participation without protection is permitted.

Functional Bracing

Commercial wrist braces offer protection and limit ROM. Athletic tape applied circumferentially can also protect the wrist with a TFCC injury.

Colles' Fractures

CLINICAL PRESENTATION

History

Fall on an outstretched arm or other forceful wrist extension
Exquisite pain

Observation

Obvious dorsal wrist displacement
The wrist and forearm may have a "dinner-fork" appearance.

Functional Status

The involved wrist and arm are incapacitated.

Physical Evaluation Findings

Wrist motions are impaired.

Fractures of the distal third of the forearm and wrist are common in both elderly and youth populations. These fractures, involving the radius and/or ulna, are termed Colles' fractures. Compression and torsion across the articular surfaces result in a variety of patterns of intra-articular displacement.[91] Typically, the fracture occurs in the distal end of the radius, where it widens. The displaced portion is wider than the rest of the bone, making it difficult to fit together. Improper reduction can cause early degenerative wrist changes and deformity.

A strong force, such as a hard fall on an outstretched hand, can push the hand into the forearm, causing a Colles' fracture. This injury is common among inline skaters because of higher fall velocity.

Differential Diagnosis
Carpal ligament disruption

Imaging Techniques
Lateral and AP radiographs are obtained to identify a transverse fracture of the distal radius about 2.5 cm from the wrist. The fragment is commonly tilted and shifted backward and radially, with proximal impaction[91-93] (**Figure 12-46**). Occasionally, the distal fragment is severely comminuted or crushed. An ulnar styloid fracture may also be present.

Definitive Diagnosis
The findings on the clinical evaluation are confirmed by radiographs.

Pathomechanics and Functional Limitations
While the fracture is healing, wrist, hand, and finger motions are limited. The fracture may also impair the median, radial, and/or ulnar nerves.

■ Immediate Management
The forearm should be splinted as found with the hand in a functional position. Neurovascular function should be checked before and after splinting. Ice may be applied, and the extremity should be elevated with a sling (**Figure 12-47**).

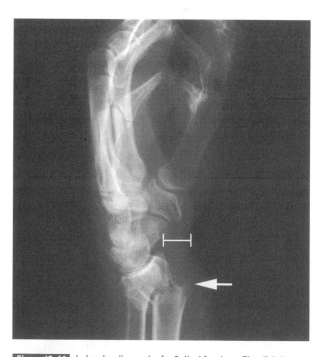

Figure 12-46 Lateral radiograph of a Colles' fracture. The distal radius is displaced dorsally approximately 50% of the metaphyseal diameter (lines) and is dorsally angulated approximately 30° (arrow). (Reproduced with permission from Johnson TR, Steinbach LS (eds): *Essentials of Musculoskeletal Imaging.* Rosemont, IL, American Academy of Orthopaedic Surgeons, 2004, p 340.)

■ Surgical Intervention
The fracture should be reduced to anatomic alignment. Colles' fracture reduction is achieved with longitudinal traction, palmar tilt, and ulnar deviation. If adequate reduction is not possible, ORIF with a plate is necessary to achieve a good outcome. Generally, if the DRUJ is in good alignment, wrist ROM and strength are expected to return to normal.

■ Postinjury/Postoperative Management
A short arm cast is applied for 6 weeks. Early finger motion is encouraged, and elbow and shoulder strengthening may begin as pain subsides. Rehabilitation commences when the cast is removed.

■ Injury-Specific Treatment and Rehabilitation Concerns

> **Specific Concerns**
> Obtain suitable reduction, fixation, and stabilization.
> Maintain upper extremity strength and ROM during the wrist immobilization period.
> Maintain general cardiovascular conditioning.

Immediately after surgery, the extremity is immobilized in a splint. Efforts should be undertaken to reduce edema formation. Active finger ROM is encouraged early during this phase. Once the immobilization has been removed, wrist ROM and strengthening may begin. Wrist ROM may be slow to return and, depending on the reactivity of the tissues, aggressive joint mobilization may be used. Supination is most difficult to achieve. Long-duration stretches may be accomplished by having

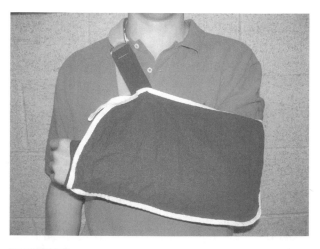

Figure 12-47 Postinjury management of forearm fracture. The wrist should be splinted and placed in a sling that elevates the hand.

the athlete sit on his or her hand with the palm up. Wrist curls and pronation and supination resistance can be performed, as well as grip exercises.

■ Estimated Amount of Time Lost

Short arm cast immobilization for at least 6 weeks is required for healing. If closed reduction is not adequate, ORIF may be necessary.[92] After immobilization, regaining strength and flexibility may take an additional 4 weeks.

Radial shortening causes malunion. Associated DRUJ injury further incapacitates the patient. Concomitant injury to the median nerve or excessive swelling results in carpal tunnel syndrome.

■ Return-to-Play Criteria

The athlete should have full strength and ROM compared with the uninjured side. Bracing during participation may allow an early return once the fracture is healed and the athlete has demonstrated good functional skills.

Functional Bracing

A wrist brace can be used. Circumferential tape around the wrist may provide some functional support.

Carpal Tunnel Syndrome

CLINICAL PRESENTATION

History

Repetitive stress to the wrist and hand
Recent other trauma to the wrist and hand
Numbness or paresthesia in the median nerve distribution (thumb, index, and middle fingers; palm of the hand).
Symptoms may increase at night.
The patient may report dropping items.

Observation

Chronic CTS may lead to thenar eminence atrophy.

Functional Status

Pain or paresthesia increases during wrist extension or hyperflexion.
Wrist strength and ROM are usually within normal limits.
Grip strength, especially thumb opposition, may be decreased.

Physical Evaluation Findings

Sensory and motor deficits in the median nerve distribution
The following special tests may be positive:
   Phalen test
   Tinel sign
   Carpal-compression test

CTS is the most common entrapment neuropathy and is characterized by pain, weakness, and paresthesia in the median nerve distribution of the hand. The carpal tunnel is located on the anterior wrist. The floor of the carpal tunnel is forward by the carpal bones, and the roof is by the transverse carpal ligament. Eight finger flexor tendons, their synovial sheaths, and the median nerve course through this limited space (**Figure 12-48**). If the median nerve is compressed under the flexor retinaculum at the wrist, CTS results.[94-96]

CTS may have an acute onset after wrist trauma, but it is more commonly associated with repetitive stress that results in inflammation of the tendons and synovial sheaths within this space, leading to median nerve compression. Compression can follow trauma (for example, a Colles' fracture or lunate dislocation), and decompression should be performed as soon as possible to reduce the potential for permanent nerve damage. The tightness of splints should always be checked and vascular function monitored after an acute injury of the wrist, hand, or arm to avoid nerve damage.

Flexor tendon tenosynovitis, a ganglion, and osteoarthritis or rheumatoid arthritis can be associated with CTS. The condition can occur in athletes who perform repeated wrist-flexion activities and most frequently is unilateral, affecting the dominant hand. It is also commonly seen in younger patients who use their wrists a great deal in repetitive manual labor or are exposed to vibration.[95]

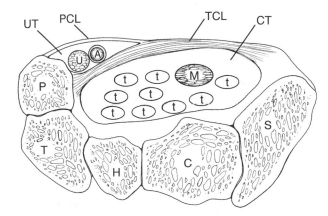

Figure 12-48 Cross-section of the wrist demonstrating the relationship of the carpal tunnel (CT) and the ulnar tunnel (UT). A = ulnar artery, C = capitate, H = hamate, M = median nerve, P = pisiform, PCL = palmar carpal ligament, S = scaphoid, t = flexor tendon, T = triquetrum, TCL = transverse carpal ligament, U = ulnar nerve. (Reproduced with permission from Szabo RM, Steinberg DR. Nerve entrapment syndromes in the wrist. *J Am Acad Orthop Surg* 1994; 2:115-123.)

Differential Diagnosis

Cervical spine trauma; C5, C6, or C7 nerve-root impingement trauma along the path of the median nerve

Medical Diagnostic Tests

Electromyography or nerve conduction tests can be performed on the median nerve distribution (**Figure 12-49**).

Imaging Techniques

Radiographs are used to rule out bony changes in the wrist.

Definitive Diagnosis

Electromyography is used to determine median nerve function. However, most diagnoses are based on the clinical findings.

Pathomechanics and Functional Limitations

Repetitive finger activity, especially when the wrist is not supported in a slightly extended position, causes mild swelling within the tendon compartments.[96,97] Any volume change in the area constrained by the transverse carpal ligament can place pressure on its contents. The structure most vulnerable to the subtle increase in pressure is the median nerve. The nerve becomes demyelinated, causing the symptoms associated with CTS. In severe cases, secondary axonal loss may occur.

■ Medications

A corticosteroid is injected into the tendon sheath to decrease inflammation.[97]

■ Postinjury/Postoperative Management

Initially, CTS is treated conservatively with rest, immobilization, and NSAIDs. The wrist is immobilized in 10° of extension using a commercial or thermoplastic cock-up splint, which is worn throughout the day and night. If symptoms persist, corticosteroid injection and surgical decompression of the transverse carpal ligament may be necessary.

■ Surgical Intervention

Surgery for CTS is directed at releasing the transverse carpal ligament. Endoscopic techniques are available, but most patients undergoing open procedures heal quickly. The median nerve is more easily visualized with an open procedure.[98-101]

■ Injury-Specific Treatment and Rehabilitation Concerns

Specific Concerns
Encourage extension activities. Limit early flexion posture.

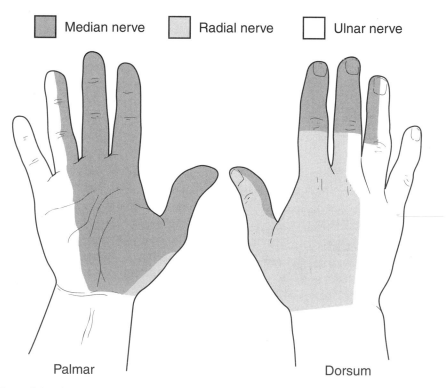

Median nerve   Radial nerve   Ulnar nerve

Palmar   Dorsum

Figure 12-49 The median, radial, and ulnar nerve distributions in the hand.

Pressure is applied to control edema, and the hand is splinted for 10 days to 2 weeks. Finger ROM is encouraged early. Gentle wrist ROM is initiated at 2 weeks, and progressive strengthening is begun at 3 weeks. A night splint or a functional brace is used during activity to help support the wrist. This is generally a commercial device and should be used during the precipitating activity, such as keyboard use. Supervised rehabilitation programs are often unnecessary after surgical procedures for CTS. Unless there is actual damage to the median nerve, full function should return in 6 to 8 weeks, when the soft tissue heals.

■ Estimated Amount of Time Lost

Because CTS is a chronic inflammatory condition, efforts are made to change the biomechanics to reduce pressure on the wrist. The athlete may continue to participate in athletics while altering techniques, using splints, and beginning a rehabilitation program. If the symptoms cannot be controlled, the precipitating activity must be ceased. Generally, the longer the patient has had the condition, the longer it will take for the symptoms to resolve.

If surgical management is necessary, the athlete typically needs 4 to 6 weeks of healing before protected return to activity is tolerated.[100]

■ Return-to-Play Criteria

The athlete is permitted to participate when the neurologic symptoms have subsided. Postoperatively, athletic participation is allowed when wrist strength and flexibility are normal.

Supports can help to reduce symptoms. However, if symptoms persist, activity should be discontinued. Once the nerve has healed, the athlete may return to sport when the progressive addition of stressful activities can be tolerated.

Functional Bracing

Braces are used to help support the wrist in a functional position, minimize pressure, and aid posture.

Ulnar Nerve Injuries in the Hand

The hand is innervated by three distinct nerves—ulnar, radial, and median (see Figure 12-49). Each has a sensory and a motor component. The ulnar nerve is the most commonly injured nerve in the upper extremity. Nerve injury results in weak-

---

CLINICAL PRESENTATION

History

Compression along the ulnar nerve, especially at the Guyon canal

Bicyclists may report weakness and numbness after a long ride, particularly on a bumpy surface.

Fracture of the radius, ulna, or carpal bones, especially the pisiform or hamate, which compresses the nerve

Numbness and/or paresthesia over the ulnar nerve distribution

Observation

The fourth and fifth fingers are flexed (bishop's palsy).

Functional Status

Inability to extend the fourth and fifth fingers
Decreased grip strength

Physical Evaluation Findings

Paresthesia or other neurologic impairment over the ulnar nerve distribution.

Positive Tinel sign over the Guyon canal

---

ness, paralysis, and sensory dysfunction. The site of the nerve injury must be identified and may be at the cervical spine, thoracic outlet, elbow region, wrist, or hand.

Anatomically, the Guyon canal is divided into three zones. Zone 1 is the area proximal to the ulnar nerve bifurcation. Compression in zone 1 causes combined motor and sensory loss and is most commonly caused by a fracture of the hook of the hamate (see p 427) or a ganglion. Zone 2 encompasses the motor branch of the nerve after it has bifurcated. Compression causes pure loss of motor function to all of the ulnar-innervated muscles in the hand. Ganglion and fracture of the hook of the hamate are the most common causative factors. Zone 3 encompasses the superficial or sensory branch of the bifurcated nerve. Compression here causes sensory loss to the hypothenar eminence, the small finger, and part of the ring finger, but no motor deficits. Common causes are an ulnar artery aneurysm, thrombosis, and synovial inflammation.[29]

Ulnar-nerve entrapment in an athletic population is usually due to compression in the Guyon canal, which is formed by the hook of the hamate and the pisiform.[102,103] The median nerve is often injured in the carpal tunnel, and the radial nerve is typically injured in the shoulder or upper arm. The presentation is often that of a motor lesion, due to isolated involvement of the deep motor branch as it courses around the hook of the hamate. Nerve compression, either from swelling or body weight, can cause injury. At the hand and wrist, repetitive stress or compression can injure the nerve. Such an injury is often termed "bishop's palsy," because the motor involvement causes an inability to extend the fourth and fifth fingers (**Figure 12-50**). The resultant hand posture resembles that of a clergyman giving a blessing. Bicyclists often develop bishop's palsy caused by ulnar nerve compression from the weight on the handlebars. The pressure may be relieved by wearing cycling gloves and using thickly padded handlebars.[104]

Differential Diagnosis

Nerve entrapment syndrome in the upper extremity or cervical spine

Medical Diagnostic Tests

Electromyographic and nerve conduction studies are used to identify the site of the nerve compression.

Imaging Techniques

To determine the presence of a carpal fracture, hand radiographs are taken. The carpal tunnel view is helpful in visualizing the hook of the hamate and pisiform. If the condition does not resolve, MRI is used to determine the presence of scar tissue or edema in the canal of Guyon.

Definitive Diagnosis

The definitive diagnosis is based on the nerve conduction study and clinical findings.

Pathomechanics and Functional Limitations

Generally when pressure is reduced, nerve function returns. If a neurapraxia is caused by chronic or repetitive stress, the nerve may require several weeks to regain full function. However, if rest does not relieve nerve pressure, the ligament overlying the Guyon canal can be surgically released.[105]

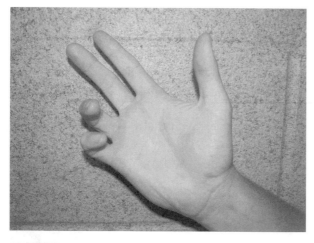

Figure 12-50 Presentation of motor involvement of ulnar nerve compression in the hand. Wasting and inability to extend the fourth and fifth fingers are seen.

■ Immediate Management

The hand is splinted in a functional position that relieves pressure from the proximal palm.

■ Medications

To reduce swelling that puts pressure on the nerve, 0.5 cc of Kenalog is injected into the canal.

■ Surgical Intervention

If a fracture of the hook of the hamate is noted, cast immobilization or splinting is required for 4 to 6 weeks. The Guyon canal is decompressed by releasing the retinaculum.[106] The surgeon should minimize the palm dissection, because scar tissue can produce similar symptoms. Scarring can restrict flexor tendon function, especially in the fourth and fifth fingers. Early active ROM helps to prevent adhesion formation.

■ Postoperative Management

The postoperative dressing should apply even pressure in the palm to minimize swelling. Pressure dressings are applied immediately after surgery and removed after 3 to 4 days.

■ Injury-Specific Treatment and Rehabilitation Concerns

Specific Concerns

Support the wrist during healing.
Encourage early finger ROM.

Smaller dressings are applied to cover the wound, and a commercial wrist brace can support the hand and reduce use of the affected upper extremity during the acute healing phase. Wrist and finger ROM is encouraged early and often. After 2 weeks, the patient may discard the brace and resume normal activities. If there is pressure on the palm, the area should be padded to distribute and absorb the force. Generally no supervised rehabilitation program is required after this procedure.

■ Estimated Amount of Time Lost

When the acute nerve pressure is eliminated, the deformity resolves in 24 to 72 hours. If equipment can be modified, the problem may resolve and participation can resume. However, if the injury is due to chronic stress and the development of scar tissue within the canal, symptom resolution will require more time. A neurapraxia may require 2 to 6 weeks to resolve.[100] Similarly, if the nerve injury is caused by a carpal fracture, immobilization and healing time are affected by the fracture.

The time lost from sport increases if scar tissue forms within the Guyon canal or if a fracture of the pisiform or the hook of the hamate occurs concomitantly.

■ Return-to-Play Criteria
Participation is permitted when motor and sensory nerve functions return.

Functional Bracing
Shock-absorbing gloves should be worn to reduce pressure on the palm. If the injury occurred from bicycling, padding may also be applied to the handlebars.

Rehabilitation

Wrist and Hand Rehabilitation

The goal of wrist and hand rehabilitation is to restore complete extremity function, but return to sport is always secondary to long-term recovery. For many patients, early return to sport may be safely accomplished with a protective brace, cast, or tape; however, certain leagues and sports have restrictions on protective equipment, especially for the hand. These rules must be consulted before clearing the athlete for sport participation. Ultimately, the umpire or referee decides whether to allow use of a protective device in competition. The clinician should also be knowledgeable about the functional requirements of the specific sport and should ensure that the athlete and, in the case of minors, the parents understand the consequences of an early return to activity.

The functional goals of wrist rehabilitation vary with the demands of the individual's sport. For example, a gymnast bears weight on the upper extremity, placing increased stress on the wrist's supportive structures, and requires increased ROM. This situation is in sharp contrast to that of a football lineman, who can participate with minimal limitations despite wrist immobilization. The athlete can generally return to sport when strength and ROM are adequate to participate effectively and enough tissue healing has occurred to prevent reinjury, pain, and a poor outcome. Young athletes should be protected from early degenerative changes, and older athletes must accept that longer healing times, loss of motion, and prolonged discomfort are the result of acute injury compounded by normal degeneration. Some injuries cause a permanent loss of motion and reduced function. Expectations should be explained, activities modified, and therapeutic exercises prescribed while the patient is in the healing phase to maximize functional outcome.

Rehabilitation for the wrist can be divided into four phases: (1) acute management, (2) rehabilitation with activity restriction, (3) progressive rehabilitation, and (4) sport reintegration. The general rehabilitation goals include decreasing pain; minimizing the inflammatory response; reducing swelling; increasing ROM and strength; improving general conditioning; and maximizing muscle control, coordination, and sport-specific skills to allow a safe return to activity. Guidelines and timelines for protection and immobilization should always be clearly dictated by the physician, so that this information is understood by the athletic trainer, physical therapist, coach, parent, and athlete.

■ Objective Evidence of Rehabilitation Goals

Goniometric measurement determines wrist ROM. Normal ROM is the goal of rehabilitation, but this outcome is not always possible due to the complex nature of many wrist injuries. Depending on the nature of the injury, an estimation should be made of the expected ROM. For example, scapholunate injuries cause changes in the intercalated motion of the carpals and a loss of motion; therefore, motion may be limited to 60% to 80% of normal. Furthermore, because normal variances may exist due to sport stress or genetics, motion should be compared with the opposite side and expectations adjusted accordingly.

Normal wrist ROM is characterized by:

- Flexion = 80°
  (32° = radiocarpal, 48° = midcarpal)
- Extension = 70°
  (47° = radiocarpal, 23° = midcarpal)
- Radioulnar deviation = 50°
  (20° = radiocarpal, 30° = midcarpal)
- Pronation = 80°
- Supination = 90°

Functional motion can be measured according to the activity requirement of the sport. For example, is motion adequate for push-ups, follow-through in basketball, or batting a ball? If not, modifications are necessary to prevent injury when the athlete is ready to reintegrate these activities.

The athlete should have normal strength compared with the opposite side. Strength can be measured by manual muscle testing in flexion, extension, pronation, and supination. Grip strength can be measured using a dynamometer. Most people normally have greater strength on the dominant side, and rehabilitation goals should take this fact into consideration. Functional strength and endurance can be measured by weight bearing and tolerance to repetitive activities, such as throwing and catching balls of different sizes and weights.

■ Therapeutic Exercises

Therapeutic exercises are designed to meet the rehabilitation goals, depending on the healing phase. Generally, exercises are prescribed to increase ROM, strengthen the extremity, and promote function.

Phase 1 of wrist rehabilitation—acute management—may involve immobilization with a fiberglass or plaster cast, splint, or brace. The physician should clearly dictate the immobilization period, especially with removable appliances. Casts should be used for athletes who require strict immobilization, and the athlete should be taught finger ROM exercises and edema precautions. Removable appliances should be reserved for injuries that need rest from daily activities and for patients who perform gentle, therapeutic exercise at certain times during the day. During the acute management phase, therapeutic exercise is directed at pain and edema reduction and tissue healing. All activity should be pain free, and ROM should be active or done by the patient. Passive motion at this stage could cause increased swelling or pain.

Phase 2 of wrist rehabilitation incorporates strengthening exercises and more aggressive ROM therapy. The wrist may continue to require protection from stress of daily activity in the form of a supportive brace, which should be removed for exercise. Resistance can be added with weights or resistive bands. Although weights are more easily controlled by the patient and help prevent substitution patterns, bands are portable and easy to use.

Exercises:

- Passive and active stretching. This is done first to warm up the joint and to ensure that resistance is performed over a greater ROM.
- Wrist extension
- Wrist flexion
- Radial deviation
- Biceps curl
- Triceps elbow extension
- Pronation/supination with hammer
- Grip exercise

All exercise should be pain free, and the weight chosen should cause fatigue at the end of the set but not result in a substitution pattern. The joint should be isolated as much as possible. Joint mobilization may begin in this stage but is limited to grade 1 and 2 mobilization forces.

Phase 3 of wrist rehabilitation incorporates progressive functional training. Strength-training exercises similar to phase 2 should be done, but sport-specific drills may be added. Polyurethane-covered medicine balls can be used in a traditional throw-and-catch exercise. Additionally, balls can be used for weight bearing. Traditional strength-training exercises can be integrated into the program, but the wrist should be supported with taping or bracing to minimize motion and increase stability. Joint mobilization can be more aggressive, and efforts should be made to increase motion to full range. The patient should sit on the hand, both in pronated and supinated positions, for a long-duration stretch.

Phase 4 of wrist rehabilitation is sport reintegration. By this time, the tissues have healed enough to withstand the rigors of sports participation. The patient should continue to perform maintenance exercises for isolated upper extremity strengthening. Both active and passive ROM exercises should continue, and the clinician should pay close attention to tissue reaction from overexertion or stress.

Finger Rehabilitation

Injuries to the fingers are often overlooked or neglected with respect to rehabilitation. Sprains and some fractures go untreated because the injury rarely prevents the athlete from competing. However, poor care often leads to the crooked, contracted knuckles that are the war wounds of old injuries. Proper treatment with protection and rehabilitation can prevent deformities while improving function.

The fingers are highly innervated and produce a tremendous amount of pain when injured. Despite this, most athletes can participate with splints and tape on the fingers, even if the sport requires the use of the hands. Yet some injuries and surgical interventions preclude sport participation, even with adequate protection. Restrictions on the return to competition should be clearly outlined.

The goal of rehabilitation for the fingers is to reduce edema and pain while promoting full ROM. Full PIP joint extension is difficult and can be compared with the opposite side. Flexion is measured by goniometry or by the proximity of the fingertip to the distal palmar crease. Finger flexion should also be checked with the MCP joint extended by having the patient attempt to touch the fingertip to the point where the finger meets the hand.

The fingers are very reactive to stress, and strict attention should be paid to increased swelling and pain after passive therapies and therapeutic exercise. The network of tendons and ligaments is intricate, and the joint capsules are very vascular.

12

Aggressive joint mobilization can be more detrimental than helpful in some patients.

Although the goals of rehabilitation are swelling control and full ROM, most athletes are able to participate early. Splinting is in positions of function, and often an injured finger is buddy taped to another for added support. Once the immobilization phase has ended, protection should continue during sports activities.

Therapeutic Exercises

Therapeutic exercises for the fingers should concentrate largely on active rather than passive exercise. Active exercise causes the tendons to slide within their sheaths, decreases swelling, and is limited by patient tolerance, resulting in less tissue reaction. The patient should emphasize full ROM, and the clinician should teach the patient to block other joints to isolate DIP and PIP joint function. Long-duration passive stretching can be done with splints or gentle joint mobilization.

Thumb Rehabilitation

The goal of thumb rehabilitation is to restore compete function. Although the athlete's goal is to return to sport as quickly as possible, the clinician must consider the safety of sport participation during injury healing and the consequences of secondary injury. Return to sport is always secondary to long-term recovery. Early return to sport may be safely accomplished with protective braces, casts, or tape in many patients.

The functional goals of thumb rehabilitation are for the athlete to effectively use the hand in the sport. The thumb should have good interphalangeal, MCP, and CMC joint motion. Flexion, extension, abduction, adduction, and opposition should be exercised. The clinician often must teach the patient to move in each direction and block unwanted motion to isolate joint function and allow the ap-

propriate tendons to glide. Creative techniques, including the use of handheld games, can promote good thumb mobility and strength.

Thumb rehabilitation begins after a protective phase during acute inflammation or when immobilization is required for proper healing. Many immobilization devices are easily removed, but this should be done only on the advice of the physician directing the patient's care. Too many splints are discarded, resulting in a poor outcome. As with the fingers, active exercise is preferred because the tissues in the small joints react to stress, and increased swelling and pain may result from overly aggressive exercise.

Objective Evidence of Rehabilitation Goals

Goniometric measurement determines thumb ROM. The patient is encouraged to touch the thumb tip to each finger to promote and measure thumb opposition. Strength can be determined using a grip dynamometer and by manual muscle testing of individual motions and comparing these with the uninvolved side. Function can be determined by the patient's ability to perform complex tasks.

Therapeutic Exercises

Therapeutic exercises are designed to meet the rehabilitation goals, depending on the phase of healing. Generally, exercises are prescribed to increase ROM, strengthen the thumb, and promote function.

Exercises:

- Interphalangeal flexion/extension
- MCP and CMC flexion, extension, abduction, adduction, and opposition

The final phase of thumb rehabilitation is sport reintegration. The patient should continue to perform maintenance exercises for isolated upper extremity strengthening. Ball skills and use of sports implements such as sticks and bats are addressed during this phase.

■ References

1. McCue FC, Andrews JR, Hakala M, Gieck JH: The coach's finger. *J Sports Med* 1974;2:270-275.

2. McCue FC, Garroway RY: Sports injuries to the hand and wrist, in Schneider RC, Kennedy JC, Plant ML, eds: *Sports Injuries: Mechanisms, Prevention and Treatment.* Baltimore, MD, Williams & Wilkins, 1985, pp 743-763.

3. Lairmore JR, Engber WD: Serious, often subtle, finger injuries: Avoiding diagnosis and treatment pitfalls. *Physician Sportsmed* 1998;26:57-73.

4. Harrison BP, Hilliard MW: Emergency department evaluation and treatment of hand injuries. *Emerg Med Clin North Am* 1999;17:793-822.

5. McCue FC, Honner R, Johnson MC, Gieck JH: Athletic injuries of the proximal interphalangeal joint requiring surgical treatment. *J Bone Joint Surg Am* 1970;52:937-956.

6. Souter WA: The problem of boutonnière deformity. *Clin Orthop* 1974;104:116-133.

7. Aronowitz ER, Leddy JP: Closed tendon injuries of the hand and wrist in athletes. *Clin Sports Med* 1998; 17:449-467.

8. Coons MS, Green SM: Boutonnière deformity. *Hand Clin* 1995;11:387-402.

9. Hurlbut PT, Adams BD: Analysis of finger extensor mechanism strains. *J Hand Surg Am* 1995;20: 832-840.

10. Massengill JB: The boutonnière deformity. *Hand Clin* 1992;8:787-801.

11. Palmer RE: Joint injuries of the hand in athletes. *Clin Sports Med* 1998;17:513-531.

12. Urbaniak JR, Hayes MG: Chronic boutonnière deformity: An anatomic reconstruction. *J Hand Surg Am* 1981; 6:379-383.

13. Hester PW, Blazar PE: Complications of hand and wrist surgery in the athlete. *Clin Sports Med* 1999;18:811-829.

14. Wehbe MA, Schneider LH: Mallet fractures. *J Bone Joint Surg Am* 1984;66:658-669.

15. McCue FC III, Meister K: Common sports hand injuries: An overview of aetiology, management and prevention. *Sports Med* 1993;15:281-289.

16. Rayan GM, Mullins PT: Skin necrosis complicating mallet finger splinting and vascularity of the distal interphalangeal joint overlying skin. *J Hand Surg Am* 1987; 12:548-552.

17. Garberman SF, Diao E, Peimer CA: Mallet finger: results of early versus delayed closed treatment. *J Hand Surg Am* 1994;19:850-852.

18. Lubahn JD: Mallet finger fractures: a comparison of open and closed technique. *J Hand Surg Am* 1989;14:394-396.

19. Stern PJ, Kastrup JJ: Complications and prognosis of treatment of mallet finger. *J Hand Surg Am* 1988;13:329-334.

20. Leddy JP, Packer JW: Avulsion of the profundus tendon insertion in athletes. *J Hand Surg Am* 1977;2:66-69.

21. McCue FC III, Wooten SL: Closed tendon injuries of the hand in athletes. *Clin Sports Med* 1986;5:741-755.

22. McCue FC III, Meister K. Common sports hand injuries: An overview of aetiology, management and prevention. *Sports Med* 1993;15:281-289.

23. Lubahn JD, Hood JM: Fractures of the distal interphalangeal joint. *Clin Orthop* 1996;327:12-20.

24. Strickland JW, Steichen JB, Kleinman WB: Phalangeal fractures: Factors influencing performance. *Orthop Rev* 1982;1:39.

25. Baratz ME, Divelbiss B: Fixation of phalangeal fractures. *Hand Clin* 1997;13:541-555.

26. Creighton JJ Jr, Steichen JB: Complications in phalangeal and metacarpal fracture management: Results of extensor tenolysis. *Hand Clin* 1994;10:111-116.

27. Freeland AE, Benoist LA, Melancon KP: Parallel miniature screw fixation of spiral and long oblique hand phalangeal fractures. *Orthopedics* 1994;17:199-200.

28. Schenck RR: Dynamic traction and early passive movement for fractures of the proximal interphalangeal joint. *J Hand Surg Am* 1986;11:850-858.

29. McCue FC III, Mayer V: Rehabilitation of common athletic injuries of the hand and wrist. *Clin Sports Med* 1989;8:731-776.

30. Freiberg A, Mulholland RS, Levine R: Nonoperative treatment of trigger fingers and thumbs. *J Hand Surg Am* 1989;14:553-558.

31. Green DP, Wolfe SW: Tenosynovitis, in Green DP, Hotchkiss RN, Pederson WC (eds): *Green's Operative Hand Surgery,* ed 4. New York, NY, Churchill Livingstone, 1999, vol 2, p 2029.

32. Carlson CS Jr, Curtis RM: Steroid injection for flexor tenosynovitis. *J Hand Surg Am* 1984;9:286-287.

33. Murphy D, Failla JM, Koniuch MP, et al: Steroid versus placebo injection for trigger finger. *J Hand Surg Am* 1995;20:628-631.

34. Marks MR, Gunther SF: Efficacy of cortisone injection in treatment of trigger fingers and thumbs. *J Hand Surg Am* 1989;14:722-727.

35. Rhoades CE, Gelberman RH, Manjarris JF: Stenosing tenosynovitis of the fingers and thumb: Results of a prospective trial of steroid injection and splinting. *Clin Orthop* 1984;190:236-238.

36. Boyer MI, Gelberman RH: Operative correction of swan-neck and boutonniere deformities in the rheumatoid hand. *J Am Acad Orthop Surg* 1999;7:92-100.

37. McCue FC III, Hakala MW, Andrews JR, Gieck JH. Ulnar collateral ligament injuries of the thumb in athletes. *J Sports Med.* 1974;2:70-80.

38. Campbell CS: Gamekeeper's thumb. *J Bone Joint Surg Br* 1955;37:148-149.

39. Stener B: Displacement of the ruptured ulnar collateral ligament of the metacarpophalangeal joint. *J Bone Joint Surg Br* 1962;44:869-879.

40. Gerber C, Senn E, Matter P: Skier's thumb: Surgical treatment of recent injuries to the ulnar collateral ligament of the thumb's metacarpophalangeal joint. *Am J Sports Med* 1981;9:171-177.

41. Heyman P: Injuries to the ulnar collateral ligament of the thumb metacarpophalangeal joint. *J Am Acad Orthop Surg* 1997;5:224-229.

42. Kozin SH, Bishop AT: Gamekeeper's thumb: Early diagnosis and treatment. *Orthop Rev* 1994;23:797-804.

43. Glickel SZ, Malerich M, Pearce SM, Littler JW: Ligament replacement for chronic instability of the ulnar collateral ligament of the metacarpophalangeal joint of the thumb. *J Hand Surg Am* 1993;18:930-941.

44. Green DP, Stern PJ: Fractures of the metacarpals and phalanges, in Green DP, Hotchkiss RN, Pederson WC (eds): *Green's Operative Hand Surgery,* ed 4. New York, NY, Churchill Livingstone, 1999, vol 2, pp 711-772.

45. Soyer AD: Fractures of the base of the first metacarpal: Current treatment options. *J Am Acad Orthop Surg* 1999;7:403-412.

46. Metacarpal and carpometacarpal trauma, in Peimer CA, Wolfe SW, Elliot AJ: *Hand and Upper Extremity.* New York, NY, McGraw-Hill, 1996, pp 883-920.

47. Rockwood CA, Green DP, Butler TE Jr: Fractures and dislocations of the hand, in Rockwood CA Jr, Green DP, Bucholtz RW, Heckman JD (eds): *Rockwood and Green's Fractures in Adults*. Philadelphia, PA, Lippincott-Raven, 1996, pp 607-744.

48. Arons MS: de Quervain's release in working women: A report of failures, complications, and associated diagnoses. *J Hand Surg Am* 1987;12:540-544.

49. Weiss AP, Akelman E, Tabatabai M: Treatment of de Quervain's disease. *J Hand Surg Am* 1994;19:595-598.

50. Louis DS: Incomplete release of the first dorsal compartment: A diagnostic test. *J Hand Surg Am* 1987;12:87-88.

51. Kahler DM, McCue FC III. Metacarpophalangeal and proximal interphalangeal joint injuries of the hand, including the thumb. *Clin Sports Med* 1992;11:57-76.

52. Stern PJ: Fractures of the metacarpals and phalanges, in Green DP, Hotchkiss RN, Pederson WC (eds): *Green's Operative Hand Surgery*, ed 4. New York, NY, Churchill Livingstone, vol 1, 1999, pp 711-771.

53. Green DP, Butler TE: Fractures and dislocations in the hand, in Rockwood CA Jr, Green DP, Bucholtz RW, Heckman JD (eds): *Rockwood and Green's Fractures in Adults*, ed 4. Philadelphia, PA, Lippincott Williams & Wilkins, vol 1, 1996, pp 607-744.

54. Ashkenaze DM, Ruby LK: Metacarpal fractures and dislocations. *Orthop Clin North Am* 1992;23:19-33.

55. Axelrod TS: Metacarpal fractures. *Hand Surg Update* 1999;2:11-17.

56. de Jonge JJ, Kingma J, van der Lei B, Klasen HJ: Fractures of the metacarpals: A retrospective analysis of incidence and aetiology and a review of the English-language literature. *Injury* 1994;25:365-369.

57. Maruyama T, Saha S, Mongiano DO, Mudge K: Metacarpal fracture fixation with absorbable polyglycolide rods and stainless steel K wires: A biomechanical comparison. *J Biomed Mater Res* 1996;33:9-12.

58. Berger RA: The gross and histologic anatomy of the scapholunate interosseous ligament. *J Hand Surg Am* 1996;21:170-178.

59. Campbell RD Jr, Lance EM, Yeoh CB: Lunate and perilunate dislocations. *J Bone and Joint Surg Br* 1964; 46:55-72.

60. Cooney WP, Linscheid RL, Dobyns JH: Fractures and dislocation of the wrist, in Rockwood CA Jr, Green DP, Bucholtz RW, Heckman JD (eds): *Rockwood and Green's Fractures in Adults*. Philadelphia, PA, Lippincott Williams & Wilkins, 1996, vol 1, pp 745-867.

61. Herzberg G, Comtet JJ, Linscheid RL, Amadio PC, Cooney WP, Stalder J: Perilunate dislocations and fracture-dislocations: A multicenter study. *J Hand Surg Am* 1993; 18:768-779.

62. Kobayashi M, Berger RA, Linscheid RL, An KN: Intercarpal kinematics during wrist motion. *Hand Clin* 1997; 13:143-149.

63. Redler MR, McCue FC III: Injuries of the hand in athletes. *VA Med* 1988;115:331-336.

64. Minami A, Kaneda K: Repair and/or reconstruction of scapholunate interosseous ligament in lunate and perilunate dislocations. *J Hand Surg Am* 1993;18:1099-1106.

65. Sotereanos DG, Mitsionis GJ, Giannakopoulos PN, Tomaino MM, Herndon JH: Perilunate dislocation and fracture dislocation: A critical analysis of the volar-dorsal approach. *J Hand Surg Am* 1997;22:49-56.

66. Barnaby W: Fractures and dislocations of the wrist. *Emerg Med Clin North Am* 1992;10:133-149.

67. Calandra JJ, Goldner RD, Hardaker WT Jr: Scaphoid fractures: Assessment and treatment. *Orthopedics* 1992; 15:931-937.

68. Adolfsson L, Lindau T, Arner M: Acutrak screw fixation versus cast immobilisation for undisplaced scaphoid waist fractures. *J Hand Surg Br* 2001;26:192-195.

69. Geissler WB: Carpal fractures in athletes. *Clin Sports Med* 2001;20:167-188.

70. Seitz WH, Papandrea RF: Fractures and dislocations of the wrist, in Bucholz RW, Heckman JD (eds): *Rockwood and Green's Fractures in Adults*, ed 5. Phliadelphia, PA, Lippincott Williams & Wilkins, 2001, pp 749-799.

71. Simank HG, Schiltenwolf M, Krempien W: The etiology of Kienbock's disease: A histopathologic study. *J Hand Surg* 1998;3:63-69.

72. Taleishik J: Scapholunate dissociation, in Strickland JW, Steichen JB (eds): *Difficult Problems in Hand Surgery*. St Louis, MO, CV Mosby, 1982, pp 341-348.

73. Watson HK, Weinzweig J: Physical examination of the wrist. *Hand Clin* 1997;13:17-34.

74. Mayfield JK, Johnson RP, Kilcoyne RK: Carpal dislocations: pathomechanics and progressive perilunar instability. *J Hand Surg Am* 1980;5:226-241.

75. Lavernia CJ, Cohen MS, Taleisnik J: Treatment of scapholunate dissociation by ligamentous repair and capsulodesis. *J Hand Surg Am* 1992;17:354-359.

76. Watson HK, Ryu J: Evolution of arthritis of the wrist. *Clin Orthop* 1986;202:57-67.

77. Rettig AC: Athletic injuries of the wrist and hand: Part I. Traumatic injuries of the wrist. *Am J Sports Med* 2003; 31:1038-1048.

78. Aldridge JM III, Mallon WJ: Hook of the hamate fractures in competitive golfers: results of treatment by excision of the fractured hook of the hamate. *Orthopedics* 2003;26:717-719.

79. David TS, Zemel NP, Mathews PV: Symptomatic, partial union of the hook of the hamate fracture in athletes. *Am J Sports Med*. 2003;31:106-111.

80. McCue FC III, Faltaous AA, Baumgarten TE: Bilateral hook of the hamate fractures. *Orthopedics* 1997; 20:470-472.

81. Palmer AK, Werner FW: The triangular fibrocartilage complex of the wrist: anatomy and function. *J Hand Surg Am* 1981;6:153-162.

82. Cooney WP, Linscheid RL, Dobyns JH: Triangular fibrocartilage tears. *J Hand Surg Am* 1994;19:143-154.

83. Nakamura T, Yabe Y, Horiuchi Y: Functional anatomy of the triangular fibrocartilage complex. *J Hand Surg Br* 1996;21:581-586.

84. Palmer AK: Triangular fibrocartilage complex lesions: A classification. *J Hand Surg Am* 1989;14:594-606.

85. Bowers WH: The distal radioulnar joint, in Green DP, Hatchkiss RN, Pederson WC (eds): *Green's Operative Hand Surgery*. New York, NY, Churchill Livingstone, 1999, pp 989-995.

86. Nguyen DT, McCue FC III, Urch SE: Evaluation of the injured wrist on the field and in the office. *Clin Sports Med* 1998;17:421-432.

87. Adams BD: Partial excision of the triangular fibrocartilage complex articular disk: A biomechanical study. *J Hand Surg Am* 1993;18:334-340.

88. Bednar JM: Arthroscopic treatment of triangular fibrocartilage tears. *Hand Clin* 1999;15:479-488.

89. Lucey SD, Poehling GG: Arthroscopic treatment of triangular fibrocartilage complex tears. *Techniq Hand Upper Extrem Surg* 1997;1:228-236.

90. Minami A, Ishikawa J, Suenaga N, Kasashima T: Clinical results of treatment of triangular fibrocartilage complex tears by arthroscopic debridement. *J Hand Surg Am* 1996;21:406-411.

91. Dekkers M, Soballe K: Activities and impairments in the early stage of rehabilitation after Colles' fracture. *Disabil Rehabil* 2004;26:662-668.

92. Raisbeck CC: Closed reduction of Colles fractures. *J Bone Joint Surg Am*. 2003;85:1614.

93. Fernandez DL, Palmer AK: Fractures of the distal radius, in Green DP, Hatchkiss RN, Pederson WC (eds): *Green's Operative Hand Surgery*. New York, NY, Churchill Livingstone, 1999, pp 930-933.

94. Pfeffer GB, Gelberman RH, Boyes JH, Rydevik B: The history of carpal tunnel syndrome. *J Hand Surg Br* 1988; 13:28-34.

95. Atroshi I, Gummesson C, Johnsson R, Ornstein E, Ranstam J, Rosen L: Prevalence of carpal tunnel syndrome in a general population. *JAMA* 1999;282:153-158.

96. Bindra RR, Evanoff BA, Chough LY, Cole RJ, Chow JC, Gelberman RH: The use of routine wrist radiography in the evaluation of patients with carpal tunnel syndrome. *J Hand Surg Am* 1997;22:115-119.

97. Dammers JW, Veering MM, Vermeulen M: Injection with methylprednisolone proximal to the carpal tunnel: Randomised double blind trial. *BMJ* 1999;319:884-886.

98. Bozentka DJ, Osterman AL: Complications of endoscopic carpal tunnel release. *Hand Clin* 1995;11:91-95.

99. Cook AC, Szabo RM, Birkholz SW, King EF: Early mobilization following carpal tunnel release: A prospective randomized study. *J Hand Surg Br* 1995;20:228-230.

100. Lundborg G, Dahlin LB: The pathophysiology of nerve compression. *Hand Clin* 1992;8:215-227.

101. Palmer AK, Toivonen DA: Complications of endoscopic and open carpal tunnel release. *J Hand Surg Am* 1999; 24:561-565.

102. Posner MA: Compressive ulnar neuropathies at the elbow: I. Etiology and diagnosis. *J Am Acad Orthop Surg* 1998;6:282-288.

103. Edmonson AS, Crenshaw AH: Ulnar nerve, in Canale ST (ed): *Campbell's Operative Orthopaedics*, ed 6. St Louis, MO, Mosby, 1980, pp 1679-1684.

104. Sicuranza MJ, McCue FC III: Compressive neuropathies in the upper extremity of athletes. *Hand Clin* 1992; 8:263-273.

105. Kleinman WB: Cubital tunnel syndrome: anterior transposition as a logical approach to complete nerve decompression. *J Hand Surg Am* 1999;24:886-897.

106. Szabo RM, Steinberg DR: Nerve entrapment syndromes in the wrist. *J Am Acad Orthop Surg* 1994;2:115-123.

12

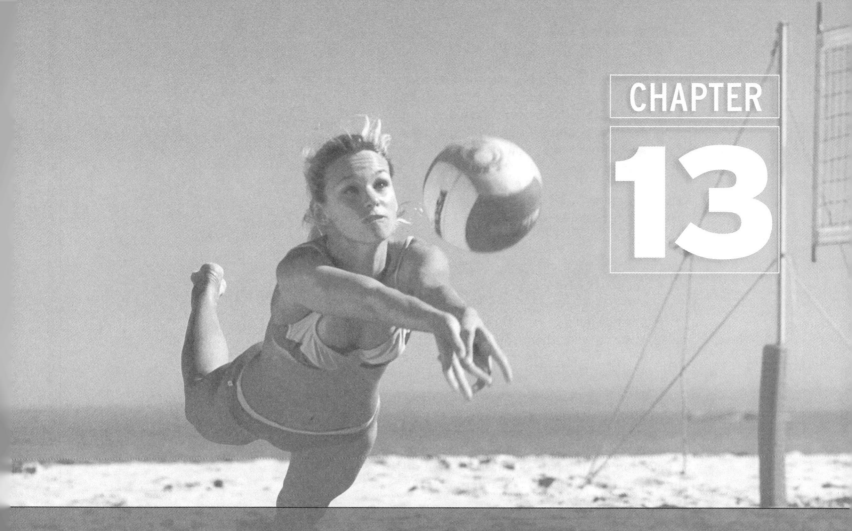

Additional Upper Extremity Therapeutic Exercises

The exercises and techniques presented in this chapter are adjuncts to those presented in chapters 10, 11, and 12. Many other exercises can also be incorporated or substituted for those presented here. In addition, most exercises can be modified based on the patient's needs, equipment on hand, or personal preference. To construct a complete rehabilitation program, cross-referencing among these chapters may be required.

Flexibility Exercises

The following stretches are held for 10 to 30 seconds and are repeated three or four times.

Shoulder

Sleeper Stretch

The patient lies on the involved side with the humerus and elbow flexed to 90° (a pillow may be placed under the patient's head for comfort). The opposite hand is used to internally rotate the humerus (**Figure 13-1**).

Cross-references

Clavicular mobilization:
    Inferior glide (p 321)
    Posterior glide (p 321)
    Posterosuperior and anteroinferior glide (p 321)
Scapular mobilization:
    Distraction (p 321)

Elbow and Forearm

Cross-references

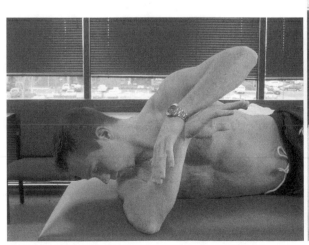
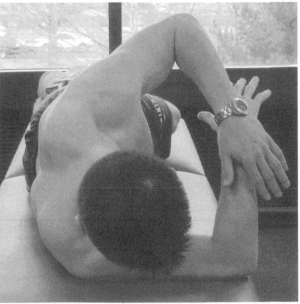

Figure 13-1   Sleeper stretch.

Arm, Wrist, and Hand Flexibility

With the elbow extended, passively flexing the wrist and fingers stretches the posterior forearm muscles (wrist and finger extensors); passively extending the wrist and fingers stretches the anterior forearm muscles (wrist and finger flexors).

Strengthening Exercises

Each exercise should be performed in 3 sets of 5, progressing to 3 sets of 10 with the same weight before increasing weight. The weight should be easy to lift and cause no discomfort or radiculopathy. Be certain to slowly lower the weights against resistance, and always release air (breathe) when performing the concentric phase of the exercise. Proper posture is essential to enable the target muscles to work most effectively.

Chapter 10 presents progressive resistance exercises for the shoulder and upper extremity using surgical tubing or elastic bands (see pages 330 to 334). Most strengthening exercises presented in this chapter can be performed with bands before moving to free weights or machines.

Shoulder Girdle and Arm Exercises

Prone Horizontal Abduction
The patient lies prone on a table with the involved extremity hanging off the side and holding a dumbbell parallel to the body. The arm is brought level with the tabletop, held for 2 seconds, and slowly lowered to the starting position. The exercise is then repeated with the humerus externally rotated.

Prone Row
The patient lies prone on the table with the involved arm holding a dumbbell off the edge of the table. The weight is lifted by horizontally adducting the shoulder and flexing the elbow, raising the weight as high as possible while keeping the chest on the table. The ending position is held for 2 seconds and slowly lowered to the starting position.

Lateral Raise
The patient stands with the feet shoulder width apart and the knees slightly bent, abducting the arms to raise the weights from the thighs to shoulder height (**Figure 13-2**).

Bent Lateral Raise
The patient bends forward, with knees slightly flexed and feet shoulder width apart, raising each weight to nearly shoulder height laterally and then slowly lowering the weight to the front of the body (**Figure 13-3**). An incline bench may be used to support the trunk if needed. This exercise should not be performed with a patient in the early stages of lumbar disk disease.

Supraspinatus Press
The patient stands with the shoulders abducted in the scapular plane to 90°, externally rotated to 90°, and the elbows flexed to 90° and holds a weight in each hand. The patient moves the weights in a short arc from chin height to head height.

Upright Row
The patient stands with the feet shoulder width apart and the knees slightly bent, gripping a barbell using an overhand grasp. The bar is raised to the chin, lifting the elbows as high as possible (**Figure 13-4**).

13

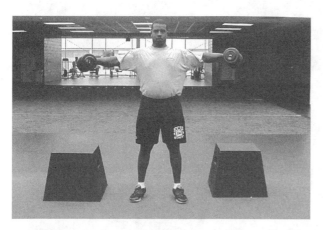

Figure 13-2 Lateral raise.

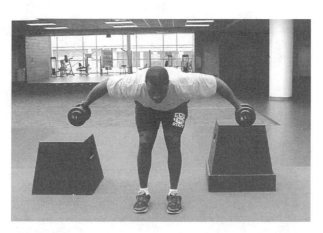

Figure 13-3 Bent lateral raise.

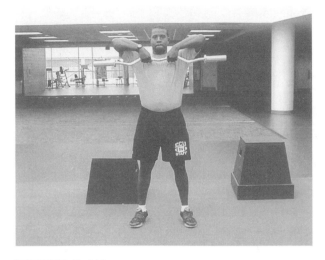

Figure 13-4 Upright row.

Seated Row

The patient is seated with the feet braced on the floor shoulder width apart. The hands are placed in an overhand grip to work the upper trapezius, rhomboids, and latissimus dorsi. The bar is raised to the chest and then slowly returned to the starting position (**Figure 13-5**).

Bent Row

The patient stands with the feet shoulder width apart and the knees slightly flexed, bending the trunk to approximately 45° with the spine straight. Using an overhand grip, the patient pulls the barbell to the chest by raising the elbows laterally away from the body and moving the scapulae together. The abdominal muscles are contracted during the lift and the subsequent return to the starting position (**Figure 13-6**).

Shrug

The patient stands with the feet shoulder width apart. Using an overhand grip on the bar, the patient shrugs the shoulders to lift the weight, holds for 3 seconds, and then slowly returns to the starting position. Proper posture should be maintained during the lift.

Bench Press

The bench press can be used in the standard form or in limited (elbows do not go behind shoulder) ranges of motion. Range limits can be set using spotting racks or padded rolls on the bar itself. Chest-press machines or dumbbells can be used for unilateral motions.

Cross-references

Shoulder isometric exercises:
  Abduction (p 328)
  Adduction (p 328)
  Flexion (p 328)
  Extension (p 328)
  Internal rotation (p 328)
  External rotation (p 328)
  Horizontal adduction (p 328)
  Horizontal abduction (p 330)
Shoulder isotonic exercises:
  Flexion (p 330)
  Abduction (p 330)
  Extension (p 330)
  External rotation (p 330)
  Internal rotation (p 331)
  Seated rows (p 332)
  Latissimus pull-downs (p 332)
  Shoulder press (p 332)
  Open can (p 332)
  Push-up with a plus (p 333)
  Hughston prone series (p 333)

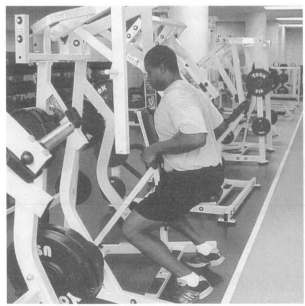
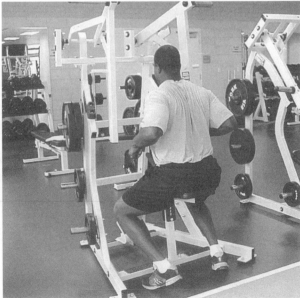

Figure 13-5 Seated row.

Elbow Exercises

Biceps Curl

There are several different patient positions for performing biceps curls, including standing, sitting, or reclining. The position of the forearm and hand affects the primary elbow mover:

- Pronated: moving into supination during flexion: biceps brachii
- Neutral: brachioradialis
- Supinated: brachialis

Although these exercises primarily focus on the muscles acting on the forearm, wrist, and finger flexors, extensors are also strengthened.

Triceps Extension

The patient sits or stands holding a dumbbell overhead by abducting the humerus to 180° and internally rotating it. The opposite hand can be used to support the arm just proximal to the elbow. The weight is slowly lowered by flexing the elbow and then returned to the starting overhead position.

Cross-references

Elbow isometric exercises:
    Flexion (p 380)
    Extension (p 380)
    Pronation/Supination (p 380)
Elbow isotonic exercises:
    Flexion (p 380)
    Extension (p 380)
    Pronation/Supination (p 380)

Wrist and Hand

Putty Exercises

Commercial putty such as TheraPutty can be used to strengthen the finger, hand, and forearm muscles. Putty is available in various viscosities, each providing different resistance to deformity. Depending on the grip, isolated finger flexion, abduction, adduction, and gripping exercises can be performed. The amount of putty used should be adequate for the size of the patient's hand and the particular exercise being performed.

Rubber-Band Exercises

Standard office rubber bands can be used to reeducate the intrinsic muscles of the hand and fingers. For finger abduction and adduction exercises, loop the band around the contiguous fingers.

Grip Strength

Putty, spring-loaded hand grips, or dynamometers can be used to restore the patient's grip strength. Initially, putty (see "Putty Exercises") should be used to restore neuromuscular control as it does not entail an eccentric component. The patient can then progress to isotonic exercises using the grips. Progress can be quantified by using the dynamometer.

Wrist Flexion and Extension

The pronated forearm is supported on a table, holding the weight off the edge of the table. The forearm and hand are pronated for wrist extension exercises and supinated for flexion exercises.

Pronation and Supination

The forearm is supported on a table with the forearm and wrist in the neutral position. The patient holds one end of a dumbbell, alternately slowly lowering and raising the weight by pronating and supinating the forearm and returning to the starting position.

Towel Roll/Wrist Roll

The patient grasps a rolled towel with both hands. One wrist is extended and the other flexed as if wringing out the towel (**Figure 13-7**). The position is held for 5 seconds and then repeated in the

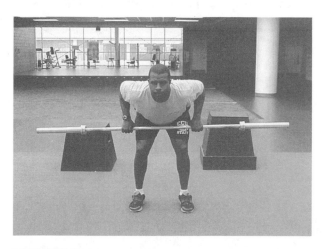

Figure 13-6 Bent row.

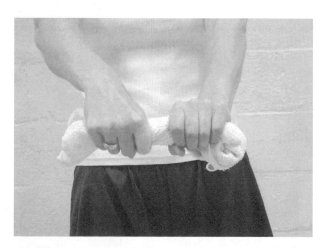

Figure 13-7 Towel roll/wrist roll.

opposite direction. An alternate method is to tie a weight to the center of a 2-ft dowel using a 2- or 3-ft rope or strap. With the shoulders flexed to 90° and the elbow straight, the patient winds the dowel to lift the weight.

Proprioception and Functional Exercises

■ Drop/Catch Ball

The patient stands and uses the involved upper extremity to drop and catch a ball or weighted medicine ball as quickly and with as little motion as possible while maintaining a stable position (**Figure 13-8**). To increase the difficulty, the patient progresses from positions of 0° of flexion and abduction into flexion and abduction.

■ Inflated Exercise-Ball Walkout

The patient lies prone over an inflated exercise ball. The patient walks forward and backward using his or her hands, maintaining balance and stability as the body rolls across the ball. To increase stability, the patient should hold the lower extremities and trunk rigid (**Figure 13-9**).

■ Minitrampoline Push-Up

The patient performs standard or modified push-ups while his or her hands are supported on the surface of the miniature trampoline or other unstable surface. The mobility of the supporting surface increases the stabilization demand on the shoulders. When the hands are spread shoulder width or more apart, the shoulder muscles are emphasized. When the hands are close together, the triceps are emphasized.

■ Inflated Exercise-Ball Push-Up

The patient performs standard or modified push-ups while the hands are supported on the inflated exercise ball (**Figure 13-10**). The mobility of the ball increases the stabilization demand on the shoulders.

■ Slide-Board Movements

The patient is in a quadruped position with the involved extremity bearing weight as tolerated on the slide board. While wearing a slide board slipper on the involved hand, the patient performs rapid, small circles in clockwise and counterclockwise directions (**Figure 13-11**). The initial position of the exercise is below shoulder level (<90° of flexion) and progresses by increasing time, weight bearing, circle circumference, and positions (to beyond 90° of flexion).

■ Upper Extremity Proprioceptive Neuromuscular Facilitation Patterns

The two primary proprioceptive neuromuscular facilitation (PNF) patterns for the upper extremity are the D1 (**CT** 13-1) and D2 (**CT** 13-2). These exer-

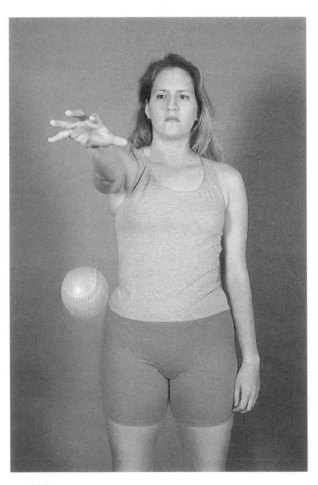

Figure 13-8 Drop/catch ball.

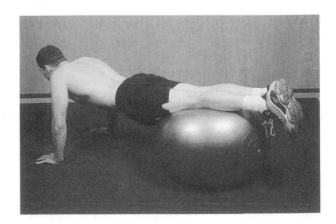

Figure 13-9 Inflated exercise-ball walkout.

cises are particularly useful because they move the extremity across the cardinal planes in a functional manner.

Plyometrics

Plyometrics are exercises that enable a muscle to reach maximum strength in as short a time as possible. Implements such as weighted balls, basketballs, elastic bands, and rebounders can be used for various catching or throwing drills. Exercises such as power drops, backward throws, overhead throws, pullover passes, and side throws can increase the shoulder girdle response to functional demands. Sport-specific programs are recommended, and patterns can be mixed with jumping and catching drills. Some of these programs include interval throwing, mound pitching, golf, tennis, and swimming.

Cross-references
Medicine ball exercises (p 380)
Weighted-ball exercises (p 381)

Throwing Protocol

The patient is allowed to initiate a throwing program if the following criteria are met:

- Full range of motion with no pain
- Satisfactory results on the clinical examination with no neurologic symptoms and with adequate medial stability
- Satisfactory muscular performance
- Proper throwing mechanics

Once the patient fulfills these criteria, the throwing program can be initiated. **Table 13-1** presents the first phase of an interval throwing program. Throwers are started on an interval long-toss program beginning with light tossing from 45 feet. Progression of the throwing program is based on the distance, intensity, and number of throws that are increased gradually during the next several weeks. Once the thrower successfully completes step 8 of phase 1, phase 2, which is throwing from the pitching mound, can be initiated.

Table 13-2 presents the second phase in the interval throwing program. During this return-to-activity phase, the thrower begins the strengthening program referred to as the "thrower's 10 program." Once the throwing program is successfully completed, the patient may gradually return to play.

A complete throwing rehabilitation program focuses on the entire kinetic chain. Throwers develop power from their legs and pelvis and transmit it through the trunk and scapulothoracic complex to the upper extremity. The thrower with a decreased ability to generate power from below compensates by attempting to generate the power within the upper extremity, creating increased stresses throughout the joints. A well-rounded rehabilitation program focuses on all aspects of the kinetic chain, including the legs, hips, and trunk.

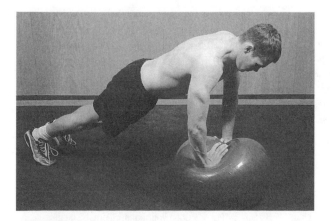

Figure 13-10 Inflated exercise-ball push-up.

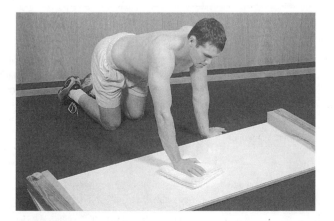

Figure 13-11 Slide-board movements.

CT Clinical Technique 13-1

D1 Upper Extremity PNF Pattern

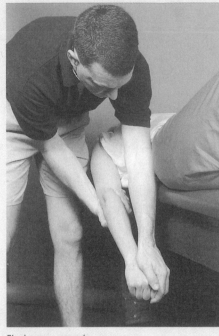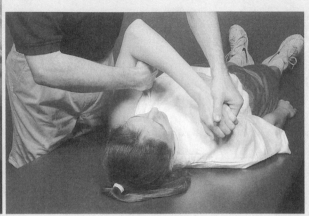

A   Flexion component

B   Extension component

Body Part	Moving Into Flexion		Moving Into Extension	
	Starting Position	Terminal Position	Starting Position	Terminal Position
Fingers	Flexed and adducted toward ulna	Extended and abducted toward radius	Extended and abducted toward radius	Flexed and adducted toward ulna
Thumb	Flexed, abducted, and internally rotated toward ulna	Extended, adducted, and externally rotated toward radius	Extended, adducted, and externally rotated toward radius	Flexed, abducted, and internally rotated toward ulna
Wrist	Pronated and flexed toward ulna	Supinated and extended toward radius	Supinated and extended toward radius	Pronated and flexed toward ulna
Elbow	Extended	Flexed	Flexed	Extended
Shoulder	Extended, adducted, and internally rotated	Flexed, abducted, and externally rotated	Flexed, abducted, and externally rotated	Extended, adducted, and internally rotated
Scapula	Abducted at medial angle, depressed anteriorly	Adducted at medial angle, posterior elevation	Adducted at medial angle, posterior elevation	Abducted at medial angle, depressed anteriorly
Clavicle	Rotates and depresses anteriorly toward the sternum	Rotates and elevates anteriorly away from the sternum	Rotates and elevates anteriorly away from the sternum	Rotates and depresses anteriorly toward the sternum
Hand position	The clinician's left hand is in the palm of the patient's right hand so that the patient may grasp it with the fingers and thumb to resist wrist flexion toward the radial side. To control external rotation and proximal components of motion, the clinician's right arm and hand are placed on the elbow and distal humerus.		The clinician's left hand cups the dorsal ulnar aspect of the patient's left hand, wrist, and fingers. To control internal rotation and the proximal components of motion, the clinician places the right hand on the posterolateral surface of the patient's arm.	
Timing/sequence	Movement is distal to proximal: first at the fingers, thumb, wrist/forearm, then at the shoulder, scapula, and clavicle.		Movement is distal to proximal: first at the fingers, thumb, wrist/forearm, then at the shoulder, scapula, and clavicle.	
Verbal command	Initial instructions: "Squeeze my hand, turn it, and bend your elbow, then pull my hand up across your face."		Initial instructions: "Open your hand, turn it, and push it down and away from your face."	
	Verbal cues: "Pull," "Squeeze my hand," "Turn it," "Bend your elbow," "Pull up across your face."		Verbal cues: "Push," "Open your hand," "Turn it," "Keep your elbow straight," "Push it down toward me."	

CT **Clinical Technique** 13-2

D2 Upper Extremity PNF Pattern

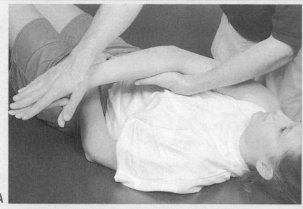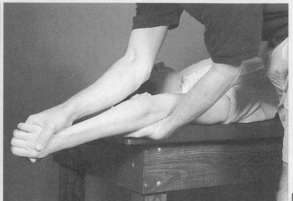

A   B

Starting position   Terminal extension

	Moving Into Flexion		Moving Into Extension	
Body Part	**Starting Position**	**Terminal Position**	**Starting Position**	**Terminal Position**
Fingers	Extended and abducted toward ulna	Flexed and adducted toward radius	Flexed and adducted toward radius	Extended and abducted toward ulna
Thumb	Internally rotated, extended, and abducted toward ulna	Externally rotated, flexed, and adducted toward radial side	Externally rotated, flexed, and adducted toward radial side	Internally rotated, extended, and abducted toward ulna
Wrist	Pronated and extended toward ulna	Supinated and flexed toward radius	Supinated and flexed toward radius	Pronated and extended toward ulna
Elbow	Extended	Slightly flexed	Slightly flexed	Extended
Shoulder	Extended, abducted, and internally rotated	Flexed, adducted, and externally rotated	Flexed, adducted, and externally rotated	Extended, abducted, and internally rotated
Scapula	Rotates and adducts at inferior angle, depressed anteriorly	Rotates and abducts at inferior angle, elevated anteriorly	Rotates and abducts at inferior angle, elevated anteriorly	Rotates and adducts at inferior angle, depressed anteriorly
Clavicle	Rotated and depressed anteriorly away from sternum	Rotated and elevated posteriorly to approximate sternum	Rotated and elevated posteriorly to approximate sternum	Rotated and depressed anteriorly away from sternum
Hand position	Using the right hand, the clinician grasps the dorsoradial aspect of the patient's right fingers, hand, and wrist. To control external rotation and proximal components of motion, the clinician places the left hand on the anterolateral surface of the patient's right arm.		The patient grasps the clinician's right hand with the fingers and thumb so that the wrist can flex toward the ulna. To control internal rotation and proximal motion, the clinician's left hand and arm are placed on the posterolateral surface of the patient's arm.	
Timing/sequence	Movement is from distal to proximal: first at the fingers, thumb, and wrist/forearm and then at the shoulder, scapula, and clavicle.		Movement is from distal to proximal: first at the fingers, thumb, and wrist/forearm and then at the shoulder, scapula, and clavicle.	
Verbal command	Initial instructions: "You are going to open your hand, turn it, and lift it up and out toward me, keeping your elbow straight."		Initial instructions: "You are going to squeeze my hand, turn it, and pull it down toward your left hip, keeping your elbow straight."	
	Verbal cues: "Lift," "Open your hand," "Turn it," "Keep your elbow straight," "Lift it toward me."		Verbal cues: "Pull," "Squeeze my hand," "Turn it," "Keep your elbow straight," "Pull it down toward your left hip."	

13

Table 13-1

Interval Throwing Program: Phase 1

45' Phase

Step 1: A. Warm-up throwing
B. 45 ft (25 throws)
C. Rest 15 minutes
D. Warm-up throwing
E. 45 ft (25 throws)

Step 2: A. Warm-up throwing
B. 45 ft (25 throws)
C. Rest 10 minutes
D. Warm-up throwing
E. 45 ft (25 throws)
F. Rest 10 minutes
G. Warm-up throwing
H. 45 ft (25 throws)

60' Phase

Step 3: A. Warm-up throwing
B. 60 ft (25 throws)
C. Rest 15 minutes
D. Warm-up throwing
E. 60 ft (25 throws)

Step 4: A. Warm-up throwing
B. 60 ft (25 throws)
C. Rest 10 minutes
D. Warm-up throwing
E. 60 ft (25 throws)
F. Rest 10 minutes
G. Warm-up throwing
H. 60 ft (25 throws)

90' Phase

Step 5: A. Warm-up throwing
B. 90 ft (25 throws)
C. Rest 15 minutes
D. Warm-up throwing
E. 90 ft (25 throws)

Step 6: A. Warm-up throwing
B. 90 ft (25 throws)
C. Rest 10 minutes
D. Warm-up throwing
E. 90 ft (25 throws)
F. Rest 10 minutes
G. Warm-up throwing
H. 90 ft (25 throws)

120' Phase

Step 7: A. Warm-up throwing
B. 120 ft (25 throws)
C. Rest 15 minutes
D. Warm-up throwing
E. 120 ft (25 throws)

120' Phase, cont'd

Step 8: A. Warm-up throwing
B. 120 ft (25 throws)
C. Rest 10 minutes
D. Warm-up throwing
E. 120 ft (25 throws)
F. Rest 10 minutes
G. Warm-up throwing
H. 120 ft (25 throws)

150' Phase*

Step 9: A. Warm-up throwing
B. 150 ft (25 throws)
C. Rest 15 minutes
D. Warm-up throwing
E. 150 ft (25 throws)

Step 10: A. Warm-up throwing
B. 150 ft (25 throws)
C. Rest 10 minutes
D. Warm-up throwing
E. 150 ft (25 throws)
F. Rest 10 minutes
G. Warm-up throwing
H. 150 ft (25 throws)

180' Phase

Step 11: A. Warm-up throwing
B. 180 ft (25 throws)
C. Rest 15 minutes
D. Warm-up throwing
E. 180 ft (25 throws)

Step 12: A. Warm-up throwing
B. 180 ft (25 throws)
C. Rest 10 minutes
D. Warm-up throwing
E. 180 ft (25 throws)
F. Rest 10 minutes
G. Warm-up throwing
H. 180 ft (25 throws)

Step 13: A. Warm-up throwing
B. 180 ft (25 throws)
C. Rest 10 minutes
D. Warm-up throwing
E. 180 ft (25 throws)
F. Rest 10 minutes
G. Warm-up throwing
H. 180 ft (25 throws)

Step 14: Begin throwing off the mound or return to respective position

*Pitchers progress to flat ground throwing from windup at 60 ft, then progress to phase 2 of the interval throwing program.

Table 13-2

Interval Throwing Program: Phase 2, Throwing Off the Mound

Stage 1: Fastball only	Stage 2: Fastball only
Step 1: Interval throwing 15 throws off mound at 50%	Step 9: 45 throws off mound at 75% 15 throws in batting practice
Step 2: Interval throwing 30 throws off mound at 50%	Step 10: 45 throws off mound at 75% 30 throws in batting practice
Step 3: Interval throwing 45 throws off mound at 50%	Step 11: 45 throws off mound at 75% 45 throws in batting practice
Step 4: Interval throwing 60 throws off mound at 50%	**Stage 3: Fastballs and breaking balls**
Step 5: Interval throwing 30 throws off mound at 75%	Step 12: 30 throws off mound at 75% 15 throws off mound at 50% with breaking balls 45 to 60 throws off mound at 75%
Step 6: 30 throws off mound at 75% 45 throws off mound at 50%	Step 13: 30 throws in batting practice (fastball only) 30 breaking balls at 75% 30 throws in batting practice
Step 7: 45 throws off mound at 75% 15 throws off mound at 50%	Step 14: 30 throws off mound at 75% 60 to 90 throws off mound at 75%
Step 8: 60 throws off mound at 75%	Step 15: Simulated game: progressing by 15 throws per workout (use interval throwing to 120 ft as warm-up). All throwing off the mound should be done in the presence of the pitching coach to stress proper throwing mechanics (use of a speed gun may aid in effort control).

13

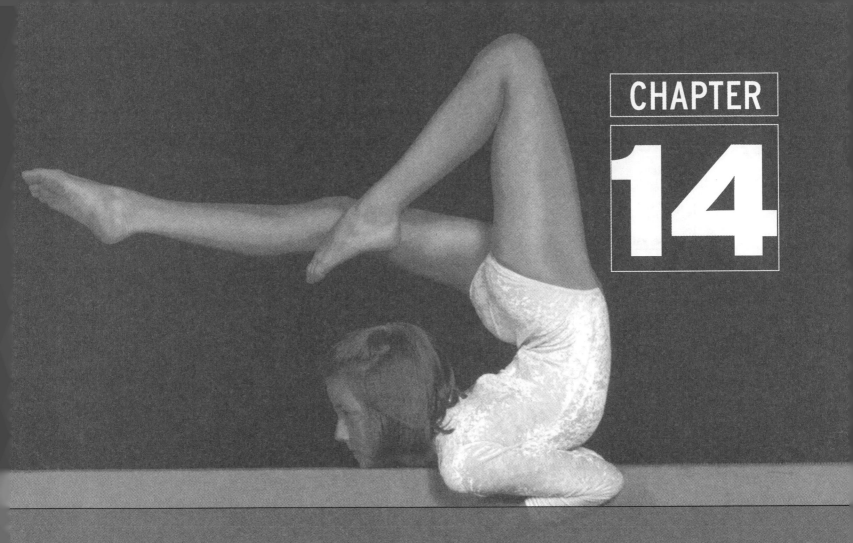

Lumbar Spine Injuries

Peggy A. Houglum, PhD, ATC, PT

Brett A. Taylor, MD

Facet Joint Dysfunction

CLINICAL PRESENTATION

History

Sudden lumbar extension, lateral bending, and/or rotation

Sciatic-like symptoms in the lower extremity may be described, although no sciatic impingement is present.

Observation

Secondary muscle spasm is common.

Swelling may be noted.

The patient may stand in the position producing the least discomfort, eg, lateral bending away from the impingement. Rotation is not always as obvious as lateral bending.

Functional Status

Loss of normal lumbar motion

Lumbar motion is restricted in side bending to the opposite side and rotation to the same side of the injury.

Physical Examination Findings

Loss of lateral bending with loss of rotation to the opposite side

Pain with extension and rotation and moving from flexion to extension

Point tenderness over the involved joint

The quadrant test may be positive.

Tests for sciatic nerve involvement are negative.

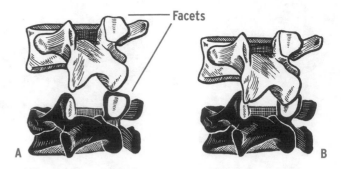

Figure 14-1 Articulation of facet joints. **A.** Vertebrae shown separated illustrate how the articular surfaces fit together. **B.** Normal appearance of the vertebrae. (Reproduced with permission from Kapanji A: *The Physiology of the Joints: Annotated Diagrams of the Mechanics of Human Joints*, ed 3. New York, NY, Churchill Livingstone, 1974.)

"Dysfunction" is a term used to identify the existence of an abnormal condition. Facet joint dysfunction describes the loss of normal function caused by either hypermobility or hypomobility of the facets. Hypomobility is the most common cause of facet joint pain.

Facet joint dysfunction is common after trauma; other causes include inflammation and facet joint degeneration. During facet trauma, the richly innervated facet capsule may be impinged between the two facet surfaces. Facet joint impingement falls on the same continuum as facet joint sprain, but sprains are more severe injuries, produce more severe symptoms, and are managed with extended nonoperative care.

Facet joints, also known as zygapophyseal joints, Z joints, apophyseal joints, and posterior intervertebral joints, are synovial diarthrodial articulations with a rich supply of various nerve endings, including proprioceptive and nociceptive receptors. As such, the surrounding capsule can become inflamed and produce pain during motion. Because the joint surfaces are covered with hyaline cartilage, repetitive stress and osteoarthritic degeneration can produce facet hypertrophy, degeneration, inflammation, and pain with joint movement.

Each vertebra has four facet surfaces that form two inferior and two superior facet joints. One superior and one inferior facet joint are on each side, posterior and lateral to the vertebral body (**Figure 14-1**). One facet joint is created by the posterolateral articulation between the inferior articular process of a vertebra and the superior articular process of the vertebra immediately below it. The superior articular process is slightly concave and faces anterolaterally. The inferior articular process is slightly convex and faces posteromedially. In the upper lumbar spine, the facets are aligned in a sagittal arrangement, but the alignment gradually changes to a frontal plane orientation. The facets are interdependent with the intervertebral disks and vertebral bodies between which they are aligned.

Because of their positions, the facets resist both axial and vertical stress and shearing forces directed at the spine. If the disk between the vertebrae becomes narrowed, the facet's ability to withstand vertical forces is decreased. If loads on the facets become greater than the joints can tolerate, the inferior facet rotates posteriorly and the joint's neurally enriched capsule is stretched, causing facet pain.

Although facet pain can occur from many causes—including degenerative changes, nerve irritation, nerve root entrapment, and frank joint and capsule injury—facet "locking" is a more common source of facet pain. A locked segment is quite possibly a hypomobile facet. The mechanism of injury for this dysfunction can be extension, side bending, rotation, or some combination of these. A locked facet is typically more painful at rest and becomes less painful with movement. Pain and restricted range of motion (ROM) may be significant in the acute stages.[1] The patient may be able to point to the exact spot of the facet pain, usually about a thumbwidth lateral to the spinous processes. Decreased motor function and radiating pain are not normally considered facet symptoms, but the joint has been implicated in radiculopathy. Radiating sensory symptoms during a straight-leg–raise test do not necessarily indicate that intervertebral disk material is pressing on a nerve root; some clinicians require motor involvement in the extremity to implicate the nerve root.[1]

Facet joint syndrome is associated with articular cartilage damage characteristic of chondromalacia. Because other clinical studies have been unable to determine a clear pathoanatomic cause, however, this diagnosis is questionable.

Differential Diagnosis

Herniated disk, spondylolysis or spondylolisthesis, arthritis, stress or compression fracture, lumbar disk disease, spinal stenosis, hip conditions, sacroiliac conditions

Medical Diagnostic Tests

Facet joint diagnostic blockade is indicated for painful lumbar disorders.[2] A facet diagnostic injection is accomplished with the aid of fluoroscopy. The symptomatic facet is approached and visualized fluoroscopically, and the joint is injected with a long-acting anesthetic such as bupivacaine HCl. Pain relief is temporary, and recent studies show limited long-term therapeutic benefits.

Several clinical characteristics are useful in identifying patients whose low back pain will be relieved by facet joint anesthesia: age over 65 years; pain not exacerbated by coughing, hyperextension, flexion, rising from flexion, or extension rotation; and pain relieved by recumbency.[2]

Imaging Techniques

Although an anteroposterior (AP) radiographic projection shows the facet joints, they are best profiled with oblique views that are obtained if specific conditions are suspected. The oblique views best profile the facet joints and the pars interarticularis. In the oblique views, the facet joints can be examined for asymmetry or degenerative changes (**Figure 14-2**).

Definitive Diagnosis

No specific diagnostic criteria or pathognomonic sign exists for facet-related pain. In fact, the facet is likely an overlooked source of pain in the lumbar spine. Facet joint syndrome is diagnosed primarily on the mechanism of injury, patient reports of pain location, and movements.

Pathomechanics and Functional Limitations

Because the coupled motions of lateral bending and rotation occur to opposite sides in the lumbar spine, the patient usually has restricted lateral bending to

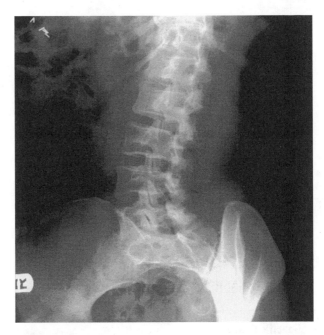

Figure 14-2 Oblique view of the lumbar vertebral facet joints and the pars interarticularis. Note the characteristic "Scotty dog" shape formed by these structures. (Image © Neil Borden/Photo Researchers, Inc.)

Spinal stenosis
Developmental narrowing of the spinal canal that can affect either the spinal cord or peripheral nerve roots.

the side opposite the involved facet and restricted rotation to the same side. A left facet impingement presents with a loss of motion in right side bending and rotation to the left. The restricted side bending is on the side opposite the locked facet because the pain with impingement stops motion from occurring. Although this presentation is not always the case in the lumbar spine, it is the most common.

■ Immediate Management

Immediate ice and reduced stress on the involved facet minimize the effects of the injury. The patient often feels the injury is minor and may not report it right away. Significant time may elapse before the clinician is informed of the injury, often when the pain interferes with performance.

■ Medications

Medications should play a secondary role in the treatment of facet joint disorders. Aspirin, acetaminophen, and nonsteroidal anti-inflammatory drugs (NSAIDs) are useful for analgesic and anti-inflammatory effects. Opioids and muscle relaxants should not be routinely used for this injury.

■ Postinjury Management

Aggressive rehabilitation with active treatment is indicated and should include aerobic training.

■ Surgical Intervention

Surgical intervention is rarely indicated for facet joint dysfunction in chronic lower back pain or degenerative conditions. In acute trauma, facet joint disruption combined with an anterior column injury may suggest 3-column instability and require surgical intervention (see p 466).

Radiofrequency neurotomy may be used to treat chronic low back pain by interrupting the pain pathways. Few controlled studies to date indicate efficacy, but limited evidence suggests that radiofrequency facet joint denervation can provide short-term improvement.[3]

■ Injury-Specific Treatment and Rehabilitation Concerns

> **Specific Concerns**
>
> Avoid extension early in the rehabilitation process.
> Alleviate spasm if present.
> Increase mobility of hypomobile segment.

If the facet joints are hypomobile, grade I and II joint mobilizations should be performed. Grade III and IV mobilizations are contraindicated for hypermobile joints; consequently, each joint must first be carefully examined (see p 482). Finding a hypermobile joint adjacent to a hypomobile joint is common; therefore, mobility at each spinal level must be evaluated before using joint mobilization. Once pain and spasm are under control, the more aggressive grade III and IV mobilizations can facilitate increased motion gains if the joints are still restricted.

Therapeutic modalities are used in the early phases of rehabilitation to relieve pain and spasm. These can include gentle traction with lateral bending to open the facet joint and a variety of thermal modalities based on the clinician's preference.

Gentle rotation and side bending in the pain-free ROM can be followed by progressive exercises into the less comfortable ROM to tolerance. Extension motions are initially avoided to eliminate high compressive forces on the recovering tissue. Strengthening exercises are incorporated as early as tolerated in the program once ROM is normal. The next course of exercises follows the routine for extremity injuries. Because the capsule and its neural structures are likely damaged, proprioception must be restored using static balance activities when the patient can move freely without pain. The patient then progresses to more dynamic exercises, evolving into more complex proprioceptive coordination and, finally, agility activities. Functional activities are initiated before the final

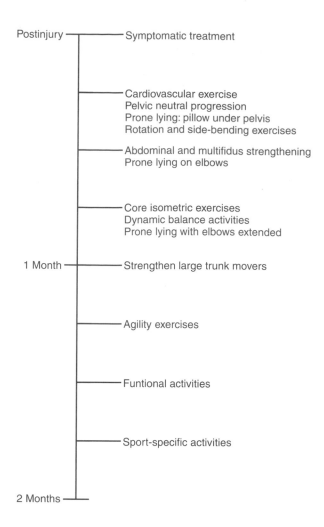

Postinjury — Symptomatic treatment

Cardiovascular exercise
Pelvic neutral progression
Prone lying: pillow under pelvis
Rotation and side-bending exercises

Abdominal and multifidus strengthening
Prone lying on elbows

Core isometric exercises
Dynamic balance activities
Prone lying with elbows extended

1 Month — Strengthen large trunk movers

Agility exercises

Funtional activities

Sport-specific activities

2 Months —

Note: Time frames are approximate. Function is the guide.

phase of the rehabilitation program, in which sport-specific drills and skill executions are performed.

After any lumbar injury, the patient should be instructed in pelvic-neutral positioning, pelvic stabilization, and proper body mechanics. In order to perform these activities, the patient may first need to improve proprioception and body awareness, flexibility, strength, and endurance; any deficiencies in these areas, including muscle imbalances, should be addressed with exercises in the rehabilitation program.

A strength and endurance program for the transverse abdominis, lower internal obliques, and multifidus muscles should be included in all lumbar injury rehabilitation programs because these are the lumbar spine stabilizers.

■ Estimated Amount of Time Lost

Time lost varies, depending on whether the injury is an impingement or a sprain. Sprains resolve more slowly. Secondary effects such as pain, muscle spasm, and weakness may delay the recovery time.

Return-to-Play Criteria

The patient should be pain free during all activities. Full lumbar spine ROM, especially extension with rotation, should be restored before return to full participation. Core-muscle strength (especially the transverse abdominis, multifidus, and trunk rotators) and sufficient muscle endurance are necessary to allow the patient to maintain proper trunk position and movement throughout the sport's specific requirements. Because strength and flexibility muscle imbalances (eg, tight hip flexors, tight paraspinals, weak hip extensors, and weak core abdominals) are often found in patients with lumbar spine injuries, they should be corrected before return to full sport participation. Trunk proprioception should be restored to preinjury levels as required by body position and movement during agility and sport-specific activities.

Lumbosacral Sprains and Strains

CLINICAL PRESENTATION

History

Sudden flexion, twisting, or lifting mechanism
Sudden impact force
Sudden onset of pain
Muscle spasm may prevent normal posture or motion. Finding a comfortable position is difficult because of pain, which can radiate into the buttock.

Observation

The patient is in obvious discomfort, frequently changing positions or standing or sitting in an abnormal posture to either guard or relieve the pain.
Paraspinal muscle spasm

Functional Status

ROM is limited by pain and spasm.
Forward flexion is often reduced, whereas extension is less painful.
If the injury is unilateral, lateral bending to the uninvolved side is more painful as the muscle on the injured side is stretched.
Extension ROM is often normal and painless.

Physical Evaluation Findings

Neurologic tests for sensory and motor function and reflexes are normal.
Although straight-leg-raise test may be painful as the lumbar muscles are stretched during the maneuver, there is no radiating neurologic pain.
Palpation reveals local tenderness at the injured site and in the muscles affected by spasm.
Muscles in spasm may feel rigid and thick.

Sprains and strains are among the most common low back injuries and involve injury to the inert back support structures. A low back strain is an injury to the paraspinal muscles traversing the spinal column (**Figure 14-3**). Despite the distinct difference in definitions, the terms "sprain" and "strain" are commonly misused. A sprain or strain has come to describe a soft-tissue injury of the back that does not involve the intervertebral disks or spinal nerves.

Differential Diagnosis

Herniated disk, ankylosing spondylitis, nondisplaced vertebral fracture, arthritis

Imaging Techniques

Radiographs are negative. In patients older than 30 years, some intervertebral disk-space narrowing is normal and expected.

Definitive Diagnosis

Lumbar sprain or strain is frequently a diagnosis of exclusion based on the physical examination and normal radiographs.

Pathomechanics and Functional Limitations

Pain and spasm restrict the patient's movements and abilities, but first-time events are self-limiting. A patient who experiences repeated episodes may develop chronic low back pain. Poor posture and body mechanics, combined with muscle imbalances, especially in the trunk and hip muscle groups, often predispose the patient to the initial injury, and if not corrected, can be sources of repeated episodes of low back pain.

Immediate Management

Immediate management consists of ice; splinting with a brace (**Figure 14-4**), tape, or elastic wrap; rest; and mild stretching to reduce spasm.

Medications

Aspirin, acetaminophen, and NSAIDs are useful for analgesic and anti-inflammatory effects. Opioids and muscle relaxants should not be used routinely for this condition.

Postinjury Management

Once pain and spasm are controlled, treatment includes various techniques to regain pain-free ROM. Posture and biomechanics must be evaluated so that dysfunctions can be corrected before the patient returns to activity to reduce the risk of recurring injury.

Ankylosing (Ankylosis)
Immobility of a joint, often progressive in nature.

14

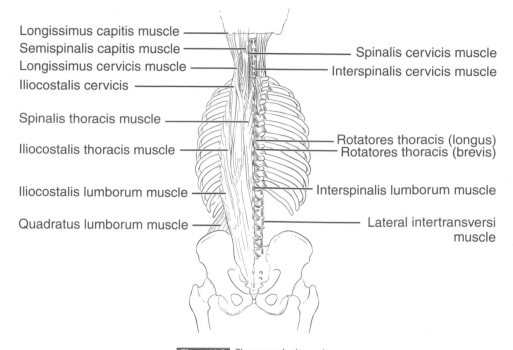

Longissimus capitis muscle
Semispinalis capitis muscle
Longissimus cervicis muscle
Iliocostalis cervicis

Spinalis thoracis muscle

Iliocostalis thoracis muscle

Iliocostalis lumborum muscle

Quadratus lumborum muscle

Spinalis cervicis muscle
Interspinalis cervicis muscle

Rotatores thoracis (longus)
Rotatores thoracis (brevis)

Interspinalis lumborum muscle

Lateral intertransversi muscle

Figure 14-3 The paraspinal muscles.

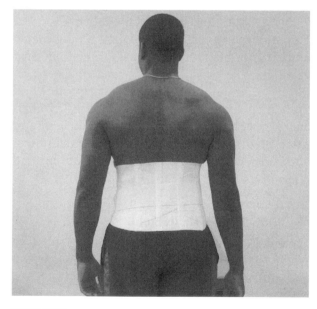

Figure 14-4 Lumbar brace used to stabilize the lumbar spine and sacroiliac joint.

■ Injury-Specific Treatment and Rehabilitation Concerns

Specific Concerns

Relieve pain and muscle spasm.
Regain ROM, soft-tissue mobility, strength, endurance, and proprioception.
Restore functional abilities to preinjury levels.

All lumbar injury recovery programs should include cardiovascular exercise, which is an important aspect of total recovery in patients with low back disability.[4] Before stretching and strengthening exercises, a brief period (10 to 15 minutes) of cardiovascular activity, such as stationary bicycling or upper body ergometry, enhances the effects of exercise and joint mobilizations.

Soft-tissue restriction and joint mobility in the back and hips should be assessed, especially if the patient has a history of back injuries or pain; soft-tissue scarring and restricted movement contribute to the risk of future injuries. Grade I and II joint mobilizations can help to relieve pain and spasm in the very early days of treatment. Other modalities, such as electrical stimulation for pain and swelling relief and muscle facilitation, may provide early symptomatic relief.

Balance of the trunk and hip muscles, in particular the abdominals (including the transverse abdominis, obliques, hip flexors, hip extensors, multifidus, and erector spinae), must be emphasized because both tight and lengthened muscles display weakness. The transverse abdominis, lower internal obliques, and multifidus are especially important for pelvic and spinal stabilization and should be emphasized early in the rehabilitation program.

Flexibility exercises should address the area directly involved in the injury and other segments that influence trunk stability and activity. If facet joint restriction is present between the vertebrae, grade III

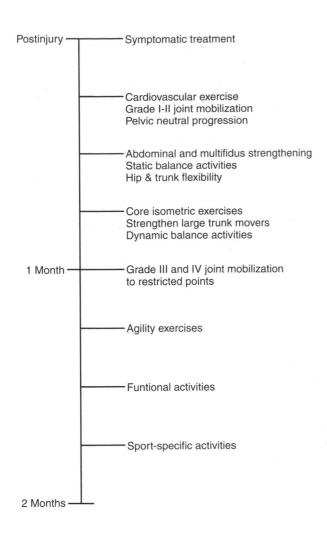

Postinjury — Symptomatic treatment

Cardiovascular exercise
Grade I-II joint mobilization
Pelvic neutral progression

Abdominal and multifidus strengthening
Static balance activities
Hip & trunk flexibility

Core isometric exercises
Strengthen large trunk movers
Dynamic balance activities

1 Month — Grade III and IV joint mobilization
to restricted points

Agility exercises

Funtional activities

Sport-specific activities

2 Months —

Note: Time frames are approximate. Function is the guide.

and IV mobilizations can improve mobility. Standing static exercises increase trunk and hip strength and stability and also provide early proprioceptive and balance activities. From these static exercises, the patient progresses to more dynamic exercises that evolve into coordination and, finally, agility activities. The patient then moves to functional activities before beginning the final phase of the rehabilitation program, in which sport-specific drills and skills are performed.

Estimated Amount of Time Lost

Time lost can vary from a few days to 4 weeks or more. It is influenced by injury severity, whether the injury is initial or chronic, the patient's age and physical condition, and the specific stress applied to the back during sport participation.

Return-to-Play Criteria

The patient should be pain free in all lumbar motions—flexion, extension, lateral flexion, and rotation—both actively and with overpressure. All functional and sport-specific activities should also be pain free, and soft-tissue mobility should be sufficient. Good balance in flexibility and strength of the opposing muscle groups (lumbar muscles and hip flexors, abdominal muscles and hip extensors) is necessary. Appropriate endurance and strength of the multifidus, lower internal obliques, and transverse abdominis stabilize the lumbar spine throughout all activities. Proprioception, agility, and sport performance should all be within normal limits and allow the patient to execute any sport-specific activity in a manner equivalent to the preinjury performance.

Vertebral Fractures and Dislocations

CLINICAL PRESENTATION

History

A sudden flexion force
Unstable fractures can impinge on the spinal cord, causing numbness, weakness, or paralysis.
If only the bone and/or its ligaments are affected and paralysis is not present, the patient may report severe back pain that increases with movement and decreases with rest.

Observation

Pain and muscle spasm
Discoloration may not be visible immediately, but swelling or deformity may be evident.

Functional Status

ROM is severely restricted by pain and muscle spasm.
The patient may not be able to walk secondary to pain.
If the spinal cord has been affected, motor, sensory, and reflex deficiencies may exist.

Physical Evaluation Findings

Palpation may reveal spasm, swelling, or deformity.
Tenderness to palpation over the fracture site is present.
A step-off deformity or a gap between the spinous processes may be present.
Appropriate neurologic tests are performed to identify associated spinal cord injury.
The patient is questioned regarding difficulty with urination or bowel evacuation or reduced perianal sensations.

Vertebral fractures can involve the vertebral body or the posterior structures (**Figure 14-5**). Vertebral body fractures most often occur from axial loading or compression. Body fractures are usually stable, without fragment displacement. They are seen more often in older individuals with osteoporosis, in younger individuals with a history of steroid use, or after high-energy trauma. Posterior vertebral

Axial loading A load directed vertically along the axis of the spine creating a compression force.

14

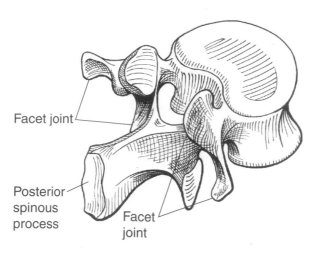

Figure 14-5 The posterior division of the vertebral column includes the facet joints on either side of the arch and the posterior spinous process. (Reproduced with permission from Kapanji A: *The Physiology of the Joints: Annotated Diagrams of the Mechanics of the Human Joints*, ed 3. New York, NY, Churchill Livingstone, 1974.)

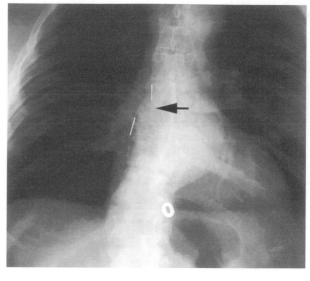

Figure 14-6 Anteroposterior view of a comminuted fracture-dislocation of T9. (Reproduced with permission from Johnson TR, Steinbach LS (eds): *Essentials of Musculoskeletal Imaging.* Rosemont, IL, American Academy of Orthopaedic Surgeons, 2004, p 697.)

fractures occur during high-impact flexion injuries. They can disrupt bony alignment and result in fracture fragment dislocation, ligamentous instability, and secondary spinal cord injury. Stress fractures can also occur in the spine, usually affecting older individuals and females whose health is influenced by the female athlete triad.

Differential Diagnosis
Herniated lumbar disk, muscle strain, internal organ injuries

Medical Diagnostic Tests
Patients with vertebral fractures should also be evaluated for their risk of osteoporosis. If the mechanism of injury is low energy, the physician should consider bone-density evaluation with dual-energy x-ray absorption scanning. If osteoporosis is detected, a treatment protocol should be initiated.

Imaging Techniques
Lateral, AP, and oblique lumbar spine radiographs are obtained to identify fractures and dislocations (**Figure 14-6**). Compression and burst fractures reveal decreased anterior-border vertebral body height, especially on lateral views (**Figure 14-7**). A kyphotic deformity may also be noted. Increased space between spinous processes may indicate an unstable flexion-distraction injury.

Computed tomography (CT) best visualizes the bony architecture of the fracture. CT imaging allows coronal and sagittal reconstructed images to identify overall spinal alignment. MRI is best suited for identification of marrow changes consistent with early fracture, ligamentous and other soft-tissue injury, and neural element impingement.

Active dynamic radiographs (flexion-extension) should be avoided during the acute postinjury phase if a fracture has been identified. Muscle guarding in the acute postinjury phase may obscure evidence of instability. Passive dynamic images are not indicated.

Definitive Diagnosis
A fracture may be suspected after signs and symptoms are investigated but can only be confirmed with radiographic evaluation.

Pathomechanics and Functional Limitations
The location of the trauma can be classified based on the columnar anatomy of the spinal column[5,6] (**Figure 14-8**). Trauma involving the middle or posterior column has the greatest risk of neurologic problems. After a fracture or dislocation, the patient may experience persistent back pain, especially if the fracture is unstable. If nerve damage has also occurred, paralysis or sensation loss persists.

■ Immediate Management
The emergency medical plan is enacted, with immobilization and transport to an emergency facility via a backboard for further medical evaluation.

■ Medications
NSAIDs and opioid analgesics are effective in pain management. However, patients undergoing fusion surgery should avoid NSAIDs, which may inhibit bone fusion.

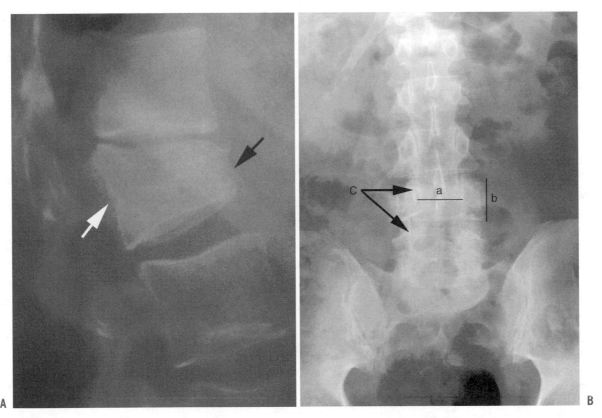

Figure 14-7 Radiographs of compression and burst fractures. **A.** Lateral radiograph of a compression fracture. Note that the anterior aspect of the vertebral body (black arrow) is less than the posterior aspect (white arrow). **B.** AP view of a burst fracture of a lumbar vertebra shows the characteristic widening of the interpedicular distance (A) associated with the loss of vertebral height (B). The facet joints appear to be normally aligned (C). (Reproduced with permission from Johnson TR, Steinbach LS (eds): *Essentials of Musculoskeletal Imaging.* Rosemont, IL, American Academy of Orthopaedic Surgeons, 2004, pp 691, 711.)

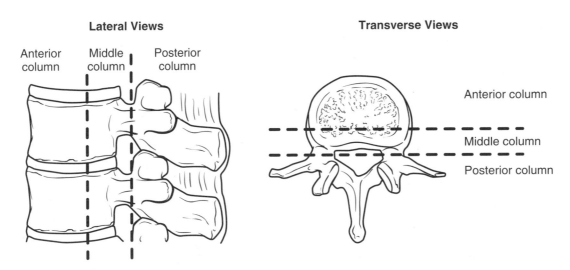

Figure 14-8 Three-column theory of spinal anatomy. The anterior column consists of the anterior two thirds of the vertebral body and annulus fibrosus and the anterior longitudinal ligament. The middle column is formed by the posterior third of the vertebral body and the annulus fibrosus and the posterior longitudinal ligament. The posterior column is formed by the neural arch, the ligamentum flavum, intraspinous ligament, and the supraspinous ligament. (Reproduced with permission from Spivak JM, Vaccaro AR, Cotler JM: Thoracolumbar spine trauma: I. Evaluation and treatment. *J Am Acad Orthop Surg* 1995;3:345-352.)

Although results from the National Acute Spinal Cord Injury Study trials support the use of methylprednisolone for acute spinal cord injury, this issue is controversial. Corticosteroid use after spinal cord injury should be weighed against the known side effects of these medications (see p 55).

Postinjury Management

The initial postinjury management goal is to assess the extent of injury and plan for stabilization of the involved structures. Transverse spinous process fractures may only need bracing, whereas a burst fracture requires surgical stabilization. The immediate management is designed to relieve pain and spasms associated with the injury while providing protection from further injury.

Lumbar fractures involving the posterior elements or transverse processes without instability can be treated with bracing and mobilization. Lumbar burst fractures are high-energy injuries. Treatment options include nonoperative bracing, casting, or surgical intervention. Surgical treatment is considered in patients with neurologic deficits, canal compromise, and instability. Nonoperative treatment may be selected for neurologically intact patients with burst fractures.

Surgical Intervention

Surgery is indicated for instability, progressive neurologic dysfunction, persistent pain despite nonoperative management, and unstable spinal fractures. These techniques, often referred to as "fusions" can be performed from a posterior (ⓢⓣ 14-1) or anterior (ⓢⓣ 14-2) approach. Brace or cast immobilization can be effective for some stable fractures, but a fracture-dislocation often requires reduction and surgical fixation. Posterior segmental instrumentation provides fixation of the anterior, middle, and posterior columns using pedicle screw constructs. The pedicle screw can stabilize all three columns via a posterior approach. A short construct using pedicle screw fixation maintains lordosis, avoiding more complication–inducing long distraction constructs such as hooks and rods.

A patient with a lumbar burst fracture without neurologic deficit initially treated with nonoperative management who now has the onset of neurologic deficits, including increased canal impingement may require surgical correction. Anterior decompression with instrumentation is indicated when the anterior column has failed and the middle-column fragments have retropulsed into the canal.

Adequate decompression in the subacute time frame often requires exposure of the anterior and middle columns with direct decompression via a retroperitoneal approach.

Postoperative Management

Functional limitations are related to injury severity and whether or not neurologic involvement is present. Limitations are influenced by the extent of the surgical intervention required to stabilize the condition. Once in place, treatment includes provisions to ensure no further neurologic compromise and maximize functional outcomes. Rehabilitation concerns and implications are determined by the injury extent, subsequent surgery required, and the patient's neurologic status. A postoperative bracing regimen limits trunk flexion; a gradual progressive rehabilitation is instituted. Compression fractures may be immobilized in a brace with restricted flexion and rotation. During this time, cardiovascular activities and exercises to maintain extremity strength may be employed, pending a physician's clearance.

Injury-Specific Treatment and Rehabilitation Concerns

Specific Concerns

Limit spinal flexion.
Relieve pain, muscle spasm, and soft-tissue restrictions.
Restore muscle balance, trunk and hip flexibility and strength, and muscle endurance.
Establish core-stabilization strength with application for functional activities.

Symptomatic relief of muscle spasm and pain can begin while the patient is still wearing the brace. The physician may permit brace removal for such passive treatments. Because stability with minimal joint movement is desired, joint mobilization is contraindicated, but thermal modalities and electrical stimulation for symptomatic relief and strengthening may be employed.

The physician may permit mild exercises during the later stages of the brace period. Although trunk and hip exercises may be difficult, open chain strengthening exercises for the extremities can be used. The patient must be instructed to isometrically contract the core muscles to aid in stabilizing the trunk during these exercises, placing less stress on the injury site and preparing the trunk muscles

S|T Surgical Technique 14-1

Posterior Stabilization (Fusion) of the Lumbar Spine

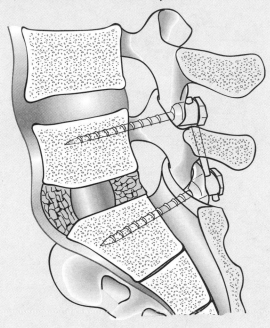

Indications

Unstable fractures involving the anterior and middle column with neurologic involvement (radicular symptoms)

Overview

1. The patient is positioned prone on a lumbar spine table.
2. The posterior elements are exposed using subperiosteal dissection. The capsules of the facets above and below the fusion are not violated.
3. The transverse processes are cleared of muscular attachments and the transverse process and pars are identified, providing the landmarks for pedicle screw placement.
4. Pedicle screws are directed along the pedicle using a probe to palpate all five quadrants of the pedicle to ensure there are no pedicle wall violations.
5. The pedicle path is tapped, and a pedicle screw is placed. Triggered electromyographic (EMG) testing of pedicle screws will improve the accuracy of screw placement.
6. After the pedicle screw is inserted appropriately into the pedicle, a bone graft is placed over the decorticated facet and transverse process, providing the posterolateral fusion.
7. The fracture fragments are indirectly decompressed with distraction during the acute posttraumatic period.

Functional Limitations

Limitations are determined by the degree and level of neurologic function. Trunk flexion must be restricted in the early postoperative phase. Functional limitations created by this surgical approach affect trunk- and core-stabilization musculature. Many spine surgeons discourage contact athletics after an instrumented lumbar fusion.

Implications for Rehabilitation

Postoperative bracing protects the stable construct during the healing phase (3 to 6 months). Trunk- and core-stabilization strengthening exercises are initiated.

Potential Complications

There is a slight risk of rod or screw failure or nerve root damage. EMG monitoring can help prevent nerve damage during the pedicle screw fixation. Other complications include damage to nerves and vessels; malalignment of the hardware resulting in neurologic impingement; failure or loosening of hardware; and adjacent segment disease, which is degeneration of the segment above and/or below a fusion.

14

S|T **Surgical Technique** **14-2**

Anterior Stabilization (Fusion) of the Lumbar Spine

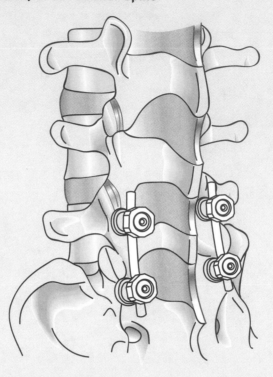

Indications

Unstable fractures involving the anterior and middle columns without neurologic involvement

Overview

1. The patient is positioned on the surgical table in a lateral position for a thoracic or thoracolumbar approach. The table is flexed to facilitate exposure to the target structures.
2. An incision is made lateral to the body's midline.
3. The muscles, internal organs, inferior vena cava, and abdominal aorta are retracted to expose the anterior vertebral body.
4. The disk's superior and inferior vertebral endplate attachment are dissected, and the disk is removed.
5. If applicable, displaced bony fragments are reduced.
6. The endplates are scarified to cause bleeding in the subchondral bone.
7. Notches are made in the superior and inferior vertebral bodies to accept the graft.
8. The graft is harvested from the donor site (typically the iliac crest).
9. The disk space is spread, and the graft is inserted between the vertebrae. A shim may be inserted to hold the graft in place.
10. A fixation plate (rod) is positioned over the anterior surface of the fractured vertebra, extending one or two segments above and below.
11. Holes are drilled into the vertebrae, and the plate is fixated.
12. The incision site is closed.

Functional Limitations

Limitations are ultimately determined by the degree and level of neurologic function. Trunk flexion must be restricted in the early postoperative period. Functional limitations created by this surgical approach affect trunk- and core-stabilization musculature.

Implications for Rehabilitation

Postoperative bracing is instituted to protect the stable construct during the healing phase. Trunk- and core-stabilization strengthening exercises are initiated.

for later exercises. Once the patient is out of the brace, mild flexibility exercises and early strengthening exercises can be initiated. Flexibility exercises should be accompanied by soft-tissue mobilization to restore motion, especially of the back. Strengthening exercises begin as isometrics, progressing to early stabilization with upper and lower extremity motion activities and then to active motion exercises for the back extensors, abdominal, and oblique muscles.

Special attention should be paid to developing strength and muscle endurance in the transverse abdominis, lower internal obliques, and multifidus muscles (primary stabilizers of the trunk) in addition to the larger, more peripheral trunk muscle groups. The hip extensors, abductors, and adductors also contribute to trunk stabilization and can be rehabilitated once the patient is ambulating in the brace. Standing balance activities for proprioception can begin in the brace and continue in a more aggressive progression once the brace is removed. From these static exercises, the patient advances to more dynamic exercises that evolve into coordination and finally agility activities. Functional activities begin before the final phase of the rehabilitation program, in which sport-specific drills and skill executions are performed.

■ Estimated Amount of Time Lost

Without neural involvement, disability can last up to 3 to 6 months. Neural damage, general health, and degree of fracture instability or dislocation all affect the amount of time lost. After spinal fusion, many surgeons do not allow return to contact athletics.

■ Return-to-Play Criteria

With no permanent neurologic damage, the patient may return to full sport participation provided there is no pain during motion and activity, appropriate core stability is maintained throughout all activities, functional motion and strength are adequate to meet the sport stresses, performance of functional and sport-specific activities is normal, and the physician provides a release to participate.

Functional Bracing

Initial back bracing may be required (see Figure 14-4), but is no longer needed once the patient has completed a full rehabilitation course.

Disk Pathologies and Nerve-Root Impingement

CLINICAL PRESENTATION

History

A single incident that produces an acute onset of pain, usually a bending and/or twisting motion, is often described, but the actual degeneration is more insidious.

Low back pain and/or unilateral referred leg pain may be reported.

The patient may have difficulty finding a position of comfort, especially if the disk is herniated.

The hook-lying position may be assumed to relieve pain.

Sleep is disturbed and prolonged positioning is not possible because of the pain.

Observation

A lateral shift of the spine away from the site of pain may be observed in standing.

Loss of lordosis

Muscle spasm secondary to pain

The patient uses guarded movements.

The patient must change positions frequently during the evaluation.

Functional Status

Lumbar ROM is restricted, especially in trunk flexion.

Straight-leg raising is usually limited by pain to less than 45°.

The patient changes positions frequently.

Physical Evaluation Findings

Pain may lessen when the back is extended or the patient lies prone on the elbows.

Neurologic testing for motor and sensory function and reflexes identifies deficiencies according to the neural level involved.

The following special tests may be positive:

  Well-leg straight-leg raise

  Straight-leg raise

  Milgram

The intervertebral disks lie between the vertebrae and function to separate them, permitting motion and absorbing shock. The central area, the nucleus pulposus, is surrounded by a fibrous outer shell of several layers, the annulus fibrosis (**Figure 14-9**).

Lumbar disk injury is also known as lumbar disk disease. The various levels of disk disease lie along a continuum from pressure of the nucleus pulposus without annulus fibrosis rupture to annulus fibrosis fragmentation with portions of the nucleus pulposus lying outside the intervertebral disk (**Figure 14-10**).

Although the cause of disk disease is not completely known, any activity that affects inherent

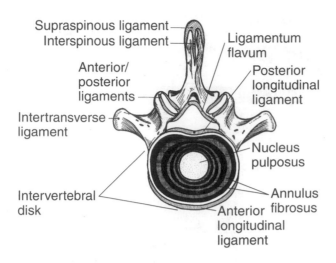

Figure 14-9 Anatomy of an intervertebral disk. (Reproduced with permission from Kapanji A: *The Physiology of the Joints: Annotated Diagrams of the Mechanics of the Human Joints*, ed 3. New York, NY, Churchill Livingstone, 1974.)

segment stability may affect the disk. Possible results of instability include facet synovitis, annulus breakdown, and nuclear material migration beyond the confines of the disk and surrounding ligaments. These developments may produce a mechanical or chemical irritation of the nerve roots or spinal cord.[5] When the nucleus pulposus herniates into the spinal column, the spinal nerves experience both mechanical pain and chemical irritation from the nucleus pulposus. This condition is more severe and causes intractable pain.

The most common sites for disk bulges and herniations in the lumbar spine are at L4-L5 and L5-S1, the locations of the greatest stress on the lumbar spine in forward bending and rotation.

Differential Diagnosis

Muscle spasm, active trigger points, fracture, facet syndrome, spinal stenosis (in older patients)

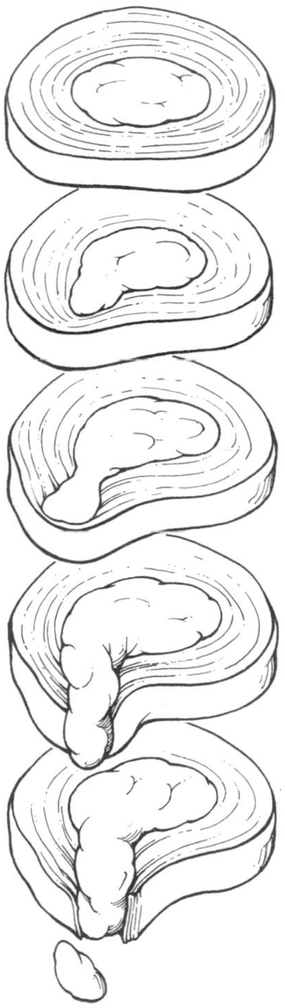

Illustration	Classification	Description
	A. Normal	
	B. Protrusion	Some of the fibers of the annulus fibrosus are damaged. The nucleus pulposus bulges into the annulus fibrosis.
	C. Prolapse	Pressure from the nucleus pulposus pushes the outer annulus fibrosis fibers toward the spinal canal.
	D. Extrusion	Tearing of the outer layers of the annulus fibrosis; the intact nucleus pulposus moves into the spinal canal
	E. Sequestration	Fragments of the annulus fibrosus and/or the nucleus pulposus break off and are outside the disk in the spinal canal, or in the intervertebral foramen, where pressure on the nerve roots may result.

Figure 14-10 Classifications of disk pathology. (Reproduced with permission from Gill K: Percutaneous lumbar diskectomy. *J Am Acad Orthop Surg* 1993;1:33-40.)

Medical Diagnostic Tests

Neurophysiologic EMG testing can be helpful in determining chronicity or permanent nerve injury. These tests are also helpful in differentiating polyneuropathy and other systemic neurologic disorders from radiculopathy.

Imaging Techniques

AP and lateral radiographs may demonstrate intervertebral space narrowing, indicating reduced height of the intervertebral disks. Sagittal and axial MRI can indicate a herniated or ruptured intervertebral disk. Compression on the spinal cord, lumbar nerve root, and cauda equina may also be noted (**Figure 14-11**). A myelogram identifies spinal cord impingement caused by a herniated lumbar disk (**Figure 14-12**).

Diskography, the injection of an opaque contrast medium into an intervertebral disk, has been used to characterize small tears in the annulus fibrosis (**Figure 14-13**). However, the use and reliability of diskography remain controversial.[7]

Definitive Diagnosis

Clinical findings are not always accurate in diagnosis of disk disease. The traditionally accepted symptom is radiating sensory and/or motor symptoms within a dermatomal distribution. Motor findings can include weakness in foot dorsiflexion and great toe extension and flexion, indicating impairment of the nerves that exit the intervertebral foramen at L4 to L5 and L5 to S1, the levels most commonly affected by lumbar disk disease. The significance of radicular symptoms as a diagnostic tool has diminished in importance. Asymptomatic individuals often have disk changes identified on MRI, suggesting that radiographic impingement does not indicate the presence of clinical symptoms.[5]

Diskography is not indicated to diagnose lumbar disk herniation with radiculopathy. Its reliability is disputed in the diagnosis of diskogenic low back pain. Even after the diagnosis is certain, traditional conservative rehabilitation measures are effective in 95% of patients.[8,9]

Polyneuropathy
A disease that affects a number of peripheral nerves.

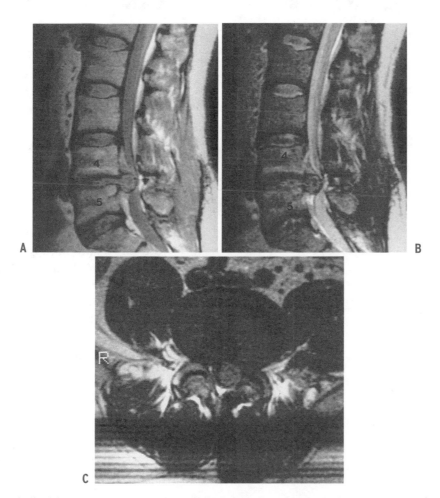

Figure 14-11   MRI demonstrating intervertebral disk lesions. **A.** Sagittal T1-weighted image demonstrating a herniation at L4-L5 with cauda equina compression. **B.** Sagittal T2-weighted image demonstrating the herniated disk and decreased disk signal intensity at several lumbar levels. **C.** Axial image demonstrating a large disk fragment that could be misinterpreted as the thecal sac. (Reproduced with permission from Boden SD, Wiesel SW: Lumbar spine imaging: Role in clinical decision making. *J Am Acad Orthop Surg* 1996;4:238-248.)

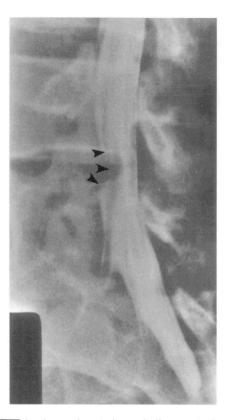

Figure 14-12 Lumbar myelogram demonstrating an extradural defect around the exiting nerve root and a curved or deflected path of the exiting root secondary to a herniated disk. (Reproduced with permission from Boden SD, Wiesel SW: Lumbar spine imaging: Role in clinical decision making. *J Am Acad Orthop Surg* 1996;4:238-248.)

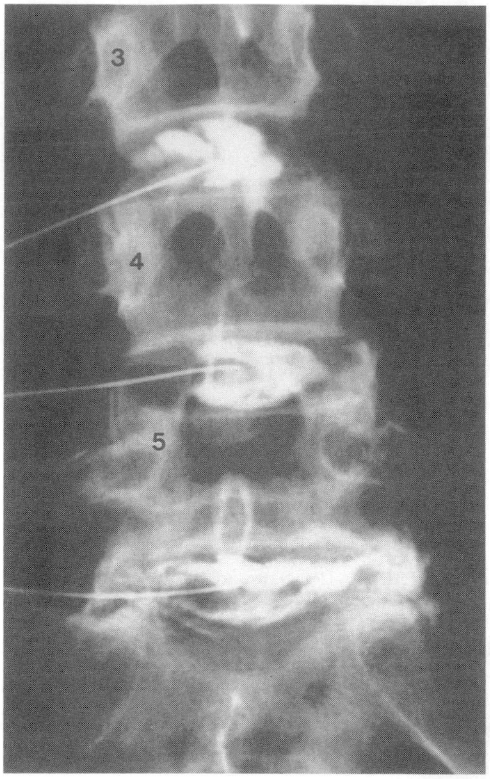

Figure 14-13 Lumbar diskogram. The L4-L5 disk demonstrates an annular fissure on the left side without external extravasation. The L5-S1 disk has a posterolateral tear that communicates with the epidural space. (Reproduced with permission from Boden SD, Wiesel SW: Lumbar spine imaging: Role in clinical decision making. *J Am Acad Orthop Surg* 1996;4:238-248.)

Pathomechanics and Functional Limitations

Pain is the primary factor restricting function and can be debilitating until it resolves. Patients should avoid positions that place increased pressure on the irritated disk. Forward bending, flexion, and rotation substantially increase posterior disk pressure. Rotation also increases pressure on the weakened and irritated disk. The symptoms of disk injury, unless at the sequestration stage, can often be resolved with appropriate conservative care.

■ Immediate Management

This situation is not emergent unless evidence of cauda equina syndrome exists (see p 476). The patient should initially be treated symptomatically, and then the extent of the injury should be determined.

■ Medications

NSAIDs and oral corticosteroids are standard pharmacologic treatments for radiculopathy. Selective nerve root blocks are both diagnostic and therapeutic. Narcotics and muscle relaxants have not been shown to improve the long-term outcome of patients with lumbar radiculopathy. These medicines should be judiciously used in this condition.

■ Postinjury Management

To determine the extent of the disk disease, physician referral for MRI is often required. Pain relief is an immediate concern and can frequently be accomplished in the short term with electric stimulation to relieve muscle spasm and by placing the patient in a supine, hook-lying position or prone in conjunction with medications. If the injury is recent, the supine, hook-lying position will probably be more comfortable; if the injury is subacute with distal referral symptoms, however, more relief may be obtained by brief periods of prone lying.

Surgical Intervention

Surgical intervention is indicated for patients whose intractable pain persists despite 4 to 6 weeks of nonoperative treatment. Decompressive laminectomy is the standard surgical procedure for spinal stenosis that causes radicular symptoms. In this procedure, the lamina and ligamentum flavum are removed on both sides of the vertebra (bilateral laminectomy) or unilaterally (hemi-laminectomy) (ST 14-3). Lumbar disk herniations may be corrected using the microdiskectomy technique, especially if radicular symptoms are present (ST 14-4).

Some physicians suggest that the optimal time for surgical intervention is during the first 3 to 4 months of symptoms. Surgery should be performed sooner if muscle weakness is significant or bowel or bladder dysfunction is present. In the case of bowel or bladder dysfunction, emergency surgery is indicated (see Cauda Equina Syndrome, p 476).

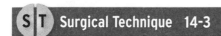

S|T Surgical Technique 14-3

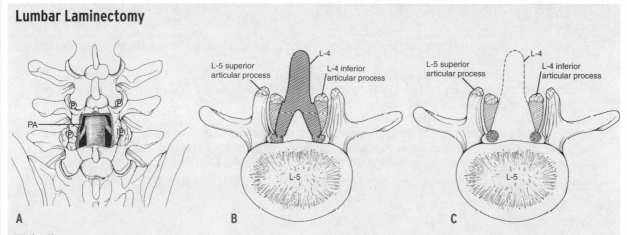

Lumbar Laminectomy

A   **B**   **C**

Indications

Failure of conservative management for 4 to 6 weeks; cauda equina syndome with bowel and bladder dysfunction

Overview

1. The patient is positioned prone on a frame to maximize lumbar flexion and increase the space between the laminae.
2. The lamina is exposed using subperiosteal dissection (**A**).
3. The lamina is thinned with a high-speed burr and removed with a punch, protecting the underlying dural tissues (**B**).
4. The integrity of the facet capsules and pars interarticularis must be maintained to avoid iatrogenic postdecompressive instability (**C**).

Functional Limitations

Postsurgical hospitalization may be required for up to 72 hours. Walking is encouraged as soon as possible. Lumbar flexion and rotation are limited to protect the healing tissues.

Implications for Rehabilitation

Heavy lifting and exertional activities may be restricted for up to 6 weeks.

Figures reproduced with permission from Frymoyer JW: Degenerative spondylolisthesis: Diagnosis and treatment. *J Am Acad Orthop Surg* 1994;2:9-15.

14

> ## S|T Surgical Technique 14-4
>
> ### Microdiskectomy
>
>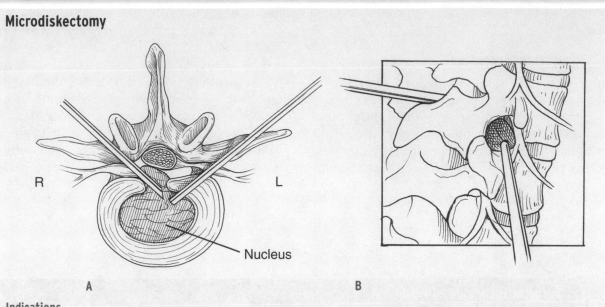
>
> A   B
>
> #### Indications
>
> Failure of conservative management for 4 to 6 weeks; unilateral radicular symptoms with foot pain greater than back pain
>
> #### Overview
>
> 1. The patient is positioned prone on a frame to maximize lumbar flexion and increase the space between the laminae, allowing access to the ligamentum flavum.
> 2. A small (approximately 1-in) incision is made over the spinous process(es).
> 3. A high-speed burr is used to thin the lamina inferiorly and superiorly at the affected level. A small portion of the facet joint may be removed to relieve pressure on the nerve root.
> 4. The ligamentum flavum is dissected free from the dura.
> 5. The nerve root is identified and gently retracted, allowing access to the disk herniation (**A**).
> 6. The disk herniation is removed using minimal annular incisions to decrease the incidence of disk reherniation. The endplates of the intervertebral disk are not violated during the removal of the herniated disk fragment (**B**).
>
> #### Functional Limitations
>
> Sitting, bending, and lifting are restricted for the first 1 to 2 weeks.
>
> #### Implications for Rehabilitation
>
> Formal rehabilitation focusing on abdominal and core strengthening does not begin until 3 to 4 weeks after surgery.
>
> #### Comments
>
> Microsurgical technique using a microscope or loupe and headlight offers decreased postoperative pain because of smaller surgical incisions. The use of tubular retractors also offers decreased postoperative pain with less subperiosteal dissection of muscles to access the affected intervertebral disk.
>
> Figures reproduced with permission from Mathews HH, Long BH: Minimally invasive techniques for the treatment of intervertebral disk herniation. *J Am Acad Orthop Surg* 2002;10:80-85.

▪ Postoperative Management

Postoperative management depends on the surgery performed. Bed rest may be recommended for 1 to 3 days following surgery. Provocative positions, especially lumbar flexion and rotation should be avoided while the tissues are healing. An advantage of the microdiskectomy is a faster rehabilitation progression, allowing rehabilitation to begin at 3 to 4 weeks.

■ Injury-Specific Treatment and Rehabilitation Concerns

Specific Concerns

Centralize the patient's pain.

Improve the patient's posture, body mechanics, and general fitness level.

Teach the patient to move into and maintain pelvic-neutral position.

Restore muscle balance, flexibility, endurance, and strength, especially the muscles controlling the trunk, pelvis, and hips.

Relieve pain and muscle spasm.

Exercises can be used initially to relieve pain from the disk protrusion if surgery is not performed. These exercises may consist of prone positioning of the patient to "centralize" the pain from the lower extremity to the central low back. In theory, this positioning reduces the posterior disk pressure by allowing gravity to pull the bulge back toward the disk's center. (Refer to Williams' flexion and McKenzie extension exercises on p 484.)

If the patient is unable to lie flat in the prone position, one or more pillows can be placed under the low back and hips, gradually reducing the pillow height as the patient's tolerance improves. From a flat, prone position, the patient progresses to lying prone on elbows and then to performing a prone press-up.

A standing trunk-extension exercise is performed as a home exercise throughout the day. The patient is instructed in finding a pelvic-neutral position, and then exercises to improve the flexibility and strength of the muscles required to hold this position are gradually introduced according to tolerance. Once the pain has become more centralized, the patient may advance to flexibility exercises for the hips and other lower extremity joints and then to strengthening exercises. These strengthening exercises must include the abdominals, especially the transverse abdominis and obliques, hip and back extensors (particularly the hip extensors and abductors and the multifidus), and the lower extremities if weakness has developed secondary to the injury.

Hip- and trunk-stabilization exercises should be a part of the strengthening program and are presented at the end of this chapter. Static balance activities beginning with a stork stand, first with eyes open and then with eyes closed, are also incorporated. The patient then proceeds to more dynamic exercises that evolve into coordination and agility activities. Functional activities are started before the final phase of the rehabilitation program, in

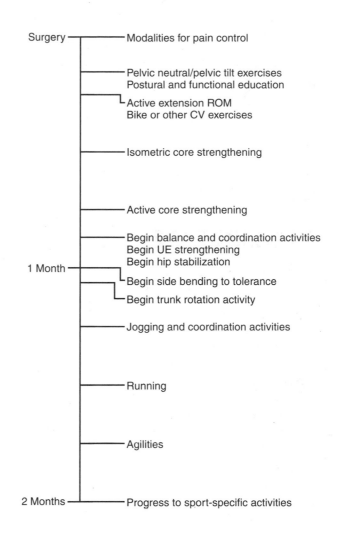

Surgery — Modalities for pain control

— Pelvic neutral/pelvic tilt exercises
Postural and functional education
Active extension ROM
Bike or other CV exercises

— Isometric core strengthening

— Active core strengthening

— Begin balance and coordination activities
Begin UE strengthening
Begin hip stabilization

1 Month — Begin side bending to tolerance
Begin trunk rotation activity

— Jogging and coordination activities

— Running

— Agilities

2 Months — Progress to sport-specific activities

Note: Time frames are approximate. Function is the guide.

which sport-specific drills and skill executions are performed.

■ Estimated Amount of Time Lost

Time lost varies but can range from 2 weeks to 2 months. If surgery has been performed, the size of the herniation, intensity and prolongation of pain, neural deficits, degree of motor deficiency (if neural innervation has been impaired), and extent of the surgery all affect the disability time.

Single-level microdiskectomy allows 90% of elite athletes to return to competitive sports. Unfortunately, athletes who undergo surgical intervention for multilevel disk herniations are less likely to resume high-level activity.

■ Return-to-Play Criteria

The patient should be pain free during all activities. Soft-tissue and joint mobility should be normal, and the patient should be strong enough to tolerate all stresses applied to the lumbar spine. The patient should have good pelvic (trunk) stability and be able to maintain pelvic-neutral position during sport activities. Hip, abdominal, and back strength and endurance should be sufficient to provide adequate support during sport performance.

Cauda Equina Syndrome

CLINICAL PRESENTATION

History

A prior lumbar fracture, central disk herniation, epidural hematoma, or other compressive trauma to the low back
Symptoms can occur immediately or gradually after injury.
Saddle anesthesia, difficulty or lack of control of urination or bowel function, sexual dysfunction, and reduced sensation or weakness in both legs may be described.

Observation

Motor weakness may make walking difficult (drop-foot gait). Walking on the heels or toes may be impossible.
The patient may not be able to rise from a chair without upper extremity assistance.

Functional Status

Difficulty walking
Balance may be affected secondary to loss of sensation and strength bilaterally.

Physical Evaluation Findings

Bilateral lower extremity weakness and reduced sensation
The patient's history, complaints of bladder and/or bowel dysfunction, and bilateral lower extremity involvement are key to the diagnosis.
Cauda equina syndrome is a medical emergency.

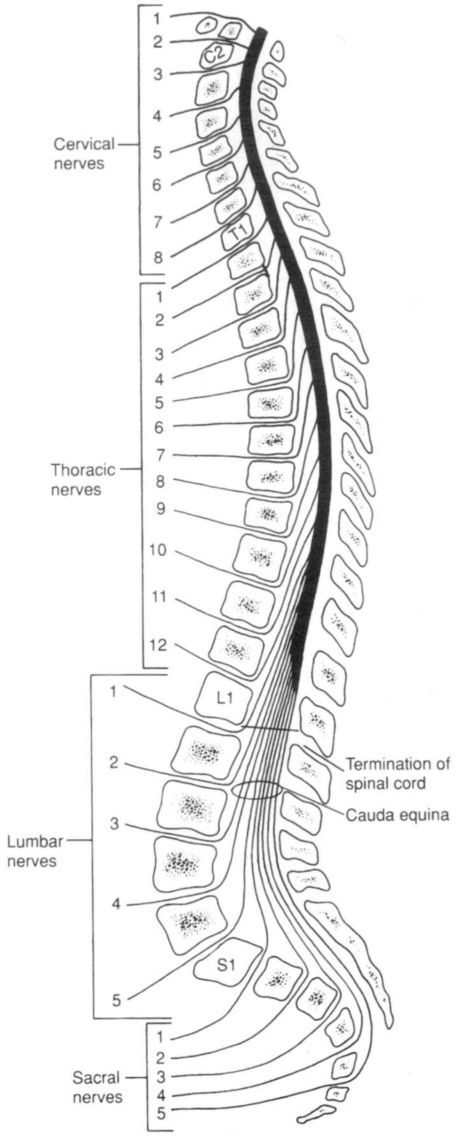

Figure 14-14 Nerve roots exiting the spinal column. The cauda equina is formed by the L2 to S4 nerve roots.

Compression of the spinal nerve roots innervating the bladder and bowel is known as cauda equina syndrome. The spinal cord terminates at the L1-L2 level. Below this point, the spinal canal is filled with the L2 to S4 nerve roots (the cauda equina) (**Figure 14-14**). Cauda equina compression results in paralysis without muscle spasticity and is a medical emergency.

Cauda equina compression may result from a herniated disk or other condition that reduces the volume of the spinal foramen. Sensory deficits or saddle anesthesia, urinary and bowel incontinence or retention, and sexual dysfunction can occur and become permanent if surgery is not performed within 48 hours to relieve the pressure on the cauda equina.[10,11] Signs and symptoms demand immedi-

ate referral to a surgeon because the condition is a medical emergency.

Differential Diagnosis

Guillian Barré syndrome, tumor, multiple sclerosis

Imaging Techniques

Sagittal MRI can identify a disk bulge or other space-occupying lesion that compresses the cauda equina (see Figure 14-11).

Definitive Diagnosis

Presenting symptoms, including bladder and bowel dysfunction, saddle anesthesia, and motor loss in the lower extremities, are key elements. The pres-

Saddle anesthesia Numbness in the groin and upper inner thighs.

Guillian Barré syndrome An inflammatory disorder of the peripheral nervous system characterized by weakness or paralysis of the extremities, face, and respiratory muscles.

ence of any of these symptoms demands immediate medical referral. The diagnosis also requires imaging tests, in particular MRI studies showing a space-occupying lesion.

Pathomechanics and Functional Limitations

This medical emergency must be surgically corrected with a decompressive maneuver if permanent damage is to be prevented. Beyond 48 hours after neural compromise, the surgical success rate is dramatically reduced. Because nerve roots from the left and right of the spinal cord emerge in the cauda equina below L2, symptoms include bilateral loss of sensation and motor innervation. Autonomic retroperineal nerves innervating the bladder, bowel, and sexual organs also pass through the cauda equina and are at risk for permanent damage if surgical decompression is not performed soon after symptom onset.

If the patient's signs and symptoms are recognized early and medical treatment is provided, the patient may suffer minimal or no lasting pathologic results.

Immediate Management

If bladder and bowel dysfunction are present, immediate referral to a surgeon is required. Emergency radiographic evaluation (MRI) is conducted to determine the level of compromise and assist the surgeon in planning the surgery.

Surgical Intervention

Surgical decompression is the only treatment indicated for cauda equina syndrome. Surgical decompression for cauda equina can be performed using standard microsurgical laminotomy-foraminotomy techniques (see $\boxed{\text{S T}}$ 14-4). However, many surgeons feel that with true cauda equina a subtotal laminectomy is the preferred treatment allowing more aggressive decompression of the region in question. The lamina over the affected region is carefully removed to protect the facet capsules, avoiding iatrogenic postdecompressive instability. The pars is maintained intact to avoid postoperative fracture.

Postinjury/Postoperative Management

The speed of referral and subsequent surgical intervention will determine the degree of neurologic compromise. The patient should be restricted from lumbar flexion and rotation and other provocative positions. If surgery was performed early, full restoration of function should be anticipated. Severe compromise of the cauda equina may necessitate extensive neurologic rehabilitation.

Injury-Specific Treatment and Rehabilitation Concerns

> **Specific Concerns**
>
> Relieve pressure on the cauda equina immediately.
> Establish rehabilitation goals once surgical treatment has been successfully completed.
> Alleviate pain and muscle spasm.
> Restore ROM, strength, proprioception, balance, and agility.

After a successful surgical release, the patient undergoes a routine rehabilitation program. Flexibility exercises to restore ROM are initiated early in the postoperative period. Early activities can also include awareness of pelvic-neutral position and isometric exercises to facilitate and maintain that position. Strengthening exercises for the pelvic floor muscles, trunk (especially the transverse abdominis, obliques, and multifidus), and hips in addition to other muscles affected by the nerve compression can be added after about 2 weeks. Balance exercises begin with static activities such as a stork stand or tandem stand with eyes open and eyes closed, and can commence when the patient is allowed to stand. The patient progresses to more dynamic exercises that evolve into coordination and agility activities. Functional activities are started before the final phase of the rehabilitation program, in which sport-specific drills and skill executions are performed.

Estimated Amount of Time Lost

The recovery from decompressive procedures for cauda equina syndrome is related only to the magnitude of neurologic dysfunction prior to surgery and the duration of compression prior to decompression.

Return-to-Play Criteria

The patient should be pain free and able to locate and maintain pelvic-neutral position and perform proper body mechanics during all activities. The muscles vital to supporting the spine, the larger muscles that move the spine, and the hip muscles should all have normal strength. Joint and soft-tissue mobility, especially around the surgical site, is important. Full and functional ROM and sufficient proprioception and agility are also necessary.

14

Spondylolysis and Spondylolisthesis

CLINICAL PRESENTATION

History

Participation in activities where the lumbar spine is repeatedly hyperextended

The patient may present with back pain radiating into the buttocks or down to the knee, but the pain is usually localized along the belt line, either unilaterally or bilaterally.

Pain is dull, aching, and/or cramping in the low back.

Pain is aggravated with standing, trunk extension, and trunk rotation.

Observation

The patient often demonstrates an excessive lumbar lordosis.

To relieve the low back pain, the patient may stand with the hips and knees flexed and the pelvis tilted posteriorly, creating flattened buttocks.

Functional Status

Hamstrings and paraspinal muscle tightness and spasm may occur. ROM is usually full, but painful in lumbar extension and rotation.

Physical Evaluation Findings

Passive straight-leg raising may reproduce the patient's symptoms.

If the patient stands on the ipsilateral leg and extends the trunk, pain during the maneuver constitutes a positive test.

Table 14-1

Classification of Spondylolysis and Spondylolisthesis

Type	Onset	Description
I	Dysplastic	Congenital abnormalities
II	Isthmic	Fatigue fracture of the pars interarticularis
III	Degenerative	Associated with long-term instability
		Occurs more in women older than 40 years of age
IV	Traumatic	Acute fracture of the neural arch other than the pars
V	Pathologic	Associated with bone disease

Spondylolysis is a defect in the pars interarticularis of the vertebral arch, usually at the L5-S1 level in athletes. In older patients, the L4-L5 level is most affected secondary to a degenerative process. When the vertebral body below the lesion slips anteriorly, this more severe condition is called spondylolisthesis. Both conditions can cause low back pain, particularly in adolescent athletes.[12] Of the five classifications of these conditions (**Table 14-1**), types I and II occur only in children and adolescents.[13]

Significant slippage can narrow the spinal canal and increase the possibility of spinal cord damage.[14,15] These conditions can occur at any lumbar level, but defects and possible impingement as a result of slippage are most common at the L4 and L5 levels. Although the cause of these conditions is unknown, some believe that a stress fracture may result, at least in part, from the repetitive hyperextension common in sports such as gymnastics, weight lifting, football, and hockey.[14,16]

The clinical evaluation of patients with these conditions is frequently unremarkable. Nonspecific low back pain is often the major complaint. The pars defect itself has been implicated in producing pain.[16] Passive intervertebral motion findings should indicate significant hypermobility at the segment in question. Imaging studies such as a bone scan may be indicated.[14]

Differential Diagnosis

Ankylosing spondylitis, herniated nucleus pulposus, tumor

Imaging Techniques

To establish the diagnosis, AP and weight-bearing lateral radiographs of the lumbar spine are obtained. The weight-bearing views increase the anterior displacement of the vertebral body as identified by their posterior alignment (**Figure 14-15**). Sufficient anterolisthesis can compress the associated nerve roots and/or cauda equina (see p 476).

Single-photon emission computed tomography (SPECT) can be used to detect injury of the pars that may not be detectable on plain radiographs. Serial SPECT evaluations may be recommended after therapeutic treatment or resolution of uptake with brace therapy. A CT myelogram may be performed to verify the diagnosis of a pars defect based on SPECT scanning (**Figure 14-16**).

Definitive Diagnosis

For spondylolisthesis, lateral radiographs will demonstrate the malignment. In the case of spondylolysis, the diagnosis is made with various radiographic techniques already described.

Pathomechanics and Functional Limitations

In the early phases of treatment, back hyperextension and twisting motions should be eliminated or modified as much as possible, especially in spondylolisthesis. Over time, slippage of the vertebra can compress the caudal sac or compress the lumbar nerve roots[17] (**Figure 14-17**).

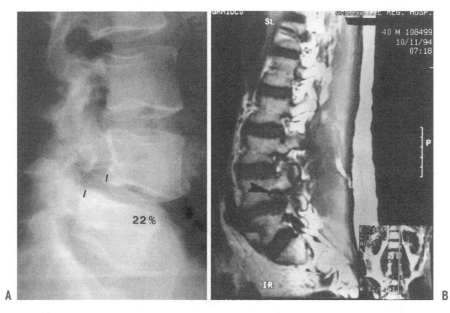

Figure 14-15 Imaging of spondylolisthesis. **A.** Lateral radiograph demonstrating anterior slippage of L4 on L5. **B.** Sagittal MRI revealing stenosis of the foramen (arrow) and flattening of the nerve root. (Reproduced with permission from Lauerman WC, Cain JE: Isthmic spondylolisthesis in the adult. *J Am Acad Orthop Surg* 1996;4:201-208.)

Medications

NSAIDs or acetaminophen may be prescribed to control pain and inflammation.

Postinjury Management

Limiting extension is key in controlling pain with either condition. Rest and an extension-limiting brace may be used for 3 to 6 weeks or even longer to facilitate healing. In severe cases, a rigid brace may

be used for 6 months; however, this treatment method is not universally accepted by orthopaedic surgeons.[12] Most surgeons do agree that bracing is important for pain control and activity restriction.

Surgical Intervention

Surgery is indicated in the presence of intractable pain, neurologic deficits, instability of the segment, or patients who have failed to improve with non-operative management (including bracing).[12]

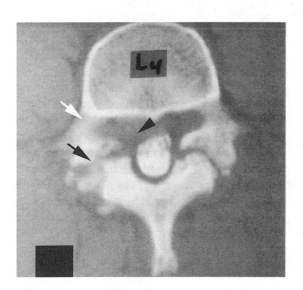

Figure 14-16 CT myelogram of the L4 pars interarticularis. The left black arrow indicates a pars interarticularis defect at the level of the pedicle (white arrow). Nerve root compression is identified by the right black arrow. (Reproduced with permission from Johnson TR, Steinbach LS (eds): *Essentials of Musculoskeletal Imaging*. Rosemont, IL, American Academy of Orthopaedic Surgeons, 2004, p 687.)

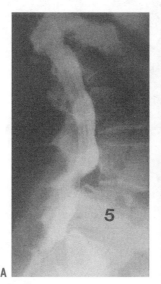
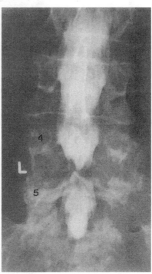

Figure 14-17 Typical lateral (**A**) and anteroposterior (**B**) myelographic appearance of degenerative spondylolisthesis. Significant constriction is apparent on the caudal sac at L4-L5. (Reproduced with permission from Frymoyer JW: Degenerative spondylolisthesis: Diagnosis and treatment. *J Am Acad Orthop Surg* 1994;2:9-15.)

For an isolated pars defect without significant neurologic deficits, a surgical option is repair of the pars defect with bone grafting and instrumentation. This is not a fusion procedure. The pars defect is grafted with bone and secured with either screw fixation or a pedicle screw rod-hook construct. If neurologic symptoms are present and decompression is indicated, however, a fusion is also warranted because decompression alone is associated with poor outcomes in comparison to decompression and fusion (**Figure 14-18**). Although the fusion procedure can be performed with or without instrumentation, instrumentation is thought to improve fusion rates (see Vertebral Fractures and Dislocations, Surgical Intervention, p 466). However, instrumentation also increases surgical complication rates and costs of the procedure. The fusion options include posterolateral fusion with bone placed over the decorticated transverse process and a combined posterior fusion with transforaminal or posterior lumbar interbody fusion. These techniques allow anterior interbody fusion from a posterior approach.

■ Postoperative Management

Patients are often braced depending on the technique used for fusion. When bony fusion is confirmed using radiographic criteria, the patients are allowed to increase their activity without limitations.

■ Injury-Specific Treatment and Rehabilitation Concerns

Specific Concerns

Limit lumbar extension and rotation in the early stages of rehabilitation.
Restore normal lumbar mobility.
Regain normal trunk and extremity strength, balance, and agility.
Achieve adequate strength and endurance of the trunk and hip stabilizers during functional activities.
Properly perform functional and sport-specific activities in the posterior pelvic-tilt position.
Obtain pain-free lumbar extension and rotation.

In young athletes with spondylolisthesis, surgical repair may be the treatment of choice. Older athletes and those with spondylolysis are generally treated conservatively, with instruction in proper positioning (posterior pelvic tilt), cardiovascular exercises, and strength and muscle endurance exercises. Williams' flexion exercises can be initiated early, and the importance of maintaining a posterior pelvic tilt must be stressed. Exercises may need to be performed in the brace (for postoperative patients), especially in the early phases of rehabilitation. During the healing phase, symptoms will dictate the need for the brace during exercises. Flexibility of the hips (including the hamstrings and hip flexors) and the back, along

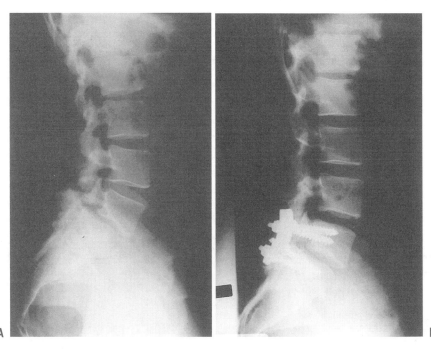

Figure 14-18   L5-S1 spondylolisthesis. **A.** Lateral radiograph demonstrating vertebral displacement. **B.** Following resection of the arch, bilateral foraminotomies, and decompression of the L5 nerve roots, the vertebrae were fused and fixated with pedicle screw instrumentation at L5-S1. (Reproduced with permission from Lauerman WC, Cain JE: Isthmic spondylolisthesis in the adult. *J Am Acad Orthop Surg* 1996;4:201-208.)

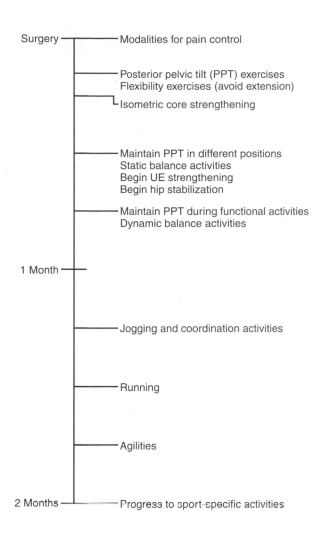

Surgery — Modalities for pain control

Posterior pelvic tilt (PPT) exercises
Flexibility exercises (avoid extension)
Isometric core strengthening

Maintain PPT in different positions
Static balance activities
Begin UE strengthening
Begin hip stabilization

Maintain PPT during functional activities
Dynamic balance activities

1 Month —

Jogging and coordination activities

Running

Agilities

2 Months — Progress to sport-specific activities

Note: Time frames are approximate. Function is the guide.

with strengthening of the abdominal (especially the transverse abdominis and obliques) and the paraspinal muscles (especially the multifidus), is important to establish a good base for subsequent stability during functional activities and exercises. Balance activities begin in the brace with static stork standing or tandem standing, and advance to performance out of the brace. From these static exercises, the patient progresses to more dynamic exercises that evolve into coordination and, finally, agility activities.

The duration of the rehabilitation process depends on the length of time activity is restricted; the loss of flexibility, strength, and muscle endurance during the immobilization period; and the amount of general deconditioning that has occurred. If the patient is required to maintain restricted activity in the brace for 6 months, rehabilitation may take at least that long.

◼ Estimated Amount of Time Lost

Time lost is influenced by a number of factors. Recovery time from spondylolisthesis, the more severe injury, can be prolonged, with severe cases extending into months of time lost. Athletes with minor cases of spondylolysis may lose only a few days, with minimal or no interference with activity. The physician is likely to place restrictions on participation until both signs and symptoms are resolved and radiographs no longer indicate a need for activity restriction.

◼ Return-to-Play Criteria

Patients with asymptomatic spondylolisthesis may participate in competitive sports. A patient whose symptoms have subsided may practice in the brace but should avoid activities that overstress the lumbar spine. If pain continues for 9 months after the injury (at which point results are unlikely to improve), the patient is allowed to resume full sport participation if able to perform despite pain. If full sport participation is not possible because of pain, surgery and reduced activity are the available options.[18]

Functional Bracing

A slip between the vertebrae is most likely in patients 9 to 15 years of age, and females are twice as likely to experience a slip as males.[18] If the patient is not a surgical candidate, bracing is advantageous. Rigid bracing to limit trunk mobility entirely or limit only trunk extension is likely to be used during the first 3 to 6 weeks up to 6 months, depending on the amount of slippage and the physician's recommendation. A brace may also be worn during the first half of rehabilitation and perhaps even after the patient has returned to activity. The physician's instructions and the patient's symptoms are the key guiding elements.

14

Rehabilitation

Bed rest was once the primary treatment for low back injuries. Recently, however, the routine care of patients with low back injuries has changed dramatically. Treatment has become dynamic, starting exercises early in the program, restricting rest to extreme cases only, and creating more aggressive protocols. The favorable results are longer lasting, with less residual disability.

Exercises for ROM and strength are incorporated early in a low back injury rehabilitation program. Before stretching and strengthening exercises, a brief period (10 to 15 minutes) of cardiovascular activity, such as a stationary bicycle or upper body ergometer, enhances the effects of exercise and joint mobilization.

Lumbar Spine Mobilization Techniques

Manual therapy interventions focus on facilitating normal joint motion and are used to treat the hypomobile segment (**Figure 14-19**). Mobilizations are typically graded from I through IV.[19] (Grade V represents a high-velocity thrust, a manipulation, and is not covered here.) The mobilization grade is selected based on the desired amount and range of passive motion to be gained at the segment. Grades I and II are helpful for the more acute conditions to relieve pain, and grades III and IV are for chronic conditions, in which the goal is to increase mobility.

Central posteroanterior (PA) glides are used to treat facet hypomobility. This technique is simply the spring test in which PA pressure is applied to the spinous process using various grades of mobilization. Unilateral PA glides promote rotation in a hypomobile segment. Using the pisiform, pressure is applied over the opposite facet, typically one thumb-width lateral to the spinous process in a PA direction. Transverse glides are applied with the thumbs over the spinous process to rotate the segment.

Patients can be instructed in self-mobilization techniques to help relieve facet pain. The patient lies in the supine, hook-lying position with knees together and then rocks the hips to the side, rolling the knees from one side to the other, while the shoulders remain on the surface.

Additional facet joint motion may be obtained through passive rotation of the involved joints. With the patient side lying, the clinician positions the fingers on the superior and inferior aspects of the spinous process of the involved level and gently rocks it back and forth to introduce motion to the segment (**Figure 14-20**).

The Maitland technique employs specific degrees of oscillation or sustained holds to eliminate reproducible signs of pain (**Figure 14-21**). Graded oscillations of I through IV are directed at pain relief or ROM gains; grades I and II focus solely on reducing pain, and grades III through IV are used to

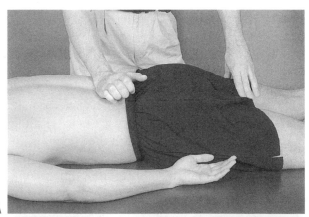
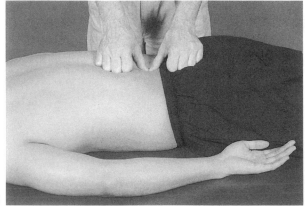

Figure 14-19 Lumbar spine mobilization techniques. **A.** Unilateral PA glide. **B.** Transverse glide. Central PA glide not shown.

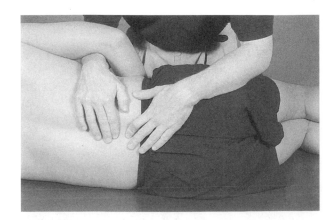

Figure 14-20 Passive rotation of the dysfunctional facet may increase motion and decrease pain.

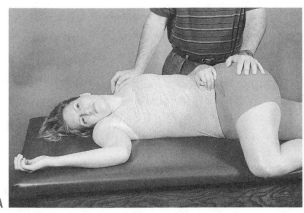
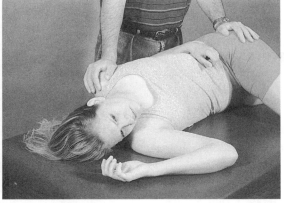

Figure 14-21   The Maitland technique. **A.** The left hand rotates the pelvis forward and indirectly applies an axial torque to the thoracic and lumbar spine. The right hand steadies the thorax. **B.** The same procedure seen from a different angle.

increase mobility. The oscillations fire both type I postural and type II dynamic mechanoreceptors (position- or pressure-sensitive neurons) to reduce pain and muscle guarding.

Flexibility Exercises

Because the hip and thigh muscles originate in the back and pelvis, flexibility exercises that target these muscles are just as important as those for the lumbar muscles. Any hip or thigh muscle with restricted motion that attaches to the pelvis or spine should be included in a lumbar spine rehabilitation program.

Also see chapter 9:
Hamstring stretch (p 252)
Quadriceps stretch (p 252)
Hip flexor stretch (p 253)
Adductor stretch (p 253)
Iliotibial band stretch (p 253)

Active Lumbar Rotation Stretch

In the supine position, the patient bends both knees and hips with the feet flat. The knees are then rotated to the same side, while the shoulders remain in contact with the surface (**Figure 14-22**). A stretch should be felt in the low back on the side opposite the knees. The position is held for about 20 seconds. The stretch is relaxed and repeated 3 to 4 times on the same side, then repeated on the opposite side.

Cat-Cow Stretch

In a quadruped position, the patient arches the back upward as high as possible (**Figure 14-23A**), and then sinks the low back down toward the floor as low as possible (**Figure 14-23B**).

Stabilization Exercises

The patient must be able to stabilize the pelvis to reduce lumbar spine stresses and allow lower extremity forces (rather than back forces) to produce power during sport activity (**Table 14-2**). These exercises should be incorporated early in the program

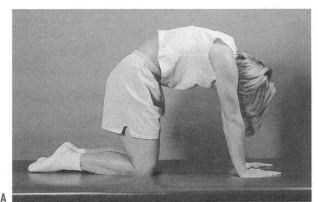

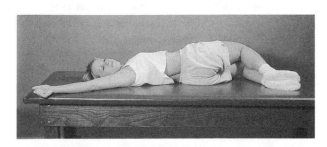

Figure 14-22   Active lumbar rotation stretch.

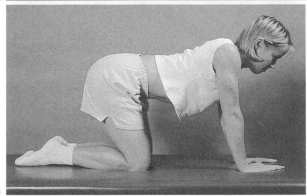

Figure 14-23   Cat-cow stretch (back press and release).

Table 14-2

Basic Progression of Lumbar Stabilization Exercise

1. Determine the full excursion of lumbar-pelvic motion.
2. Identify and maintain pelvic-neutral position.
3. Practice extremity motions in pelvic-neutral position.
4. Superimpose mass body movements.
5. Maintain stabilization during functional and sport-specific activities.

and be mastered before the patient progresses to agility, functional, or sport-specific activities. The exercises range from simple to complex. The early exercises primarily focus on body awareness and pelvic positioning. Later exercises emphasize maintenance of the correct pelvic position while performing upper and lower extremity activities.

Pelvic-Neutral Position

The patient is instructed in finding and maintaining pelvic-neutral position, a midmotion position between the extremes of full anterior and full posterior pelvic tilt. This is the least stressful and most desirable position for the pelvis throughout any activity. The patient rocks the pelvis between anterior and posterior tilts, slowly diminishing the excursion until the pelvis settles into the midposition.

The patient can be instructed in how to find pelvic-neutral position in supine, seated, and standing position. A supine or seated position may be easier for the patient at first. Once comfortable in locating pelvic-neutral in one position, however, the patient should be instructed in finding pelvic-neutral in the other positions. Once the pelvic-neutral position is found, it should be maintained while performing all activities (**Figure 14-24**).

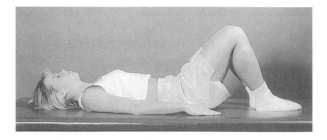

Figure 14-24 Finding the pelvic-neutral position while supine. The neutral position is the midpoint between full anterior pelvic tilt and posterior pelvic tilt.

Arm and Leg Motions

These exercises include a series of stabilization activities to increase trunk stability and control the core muscles during upper and lower extremity movement through reeducation (**Figure 14-25**). The pelvic-neutral position must be maintained throughout the exercise, simplified by use of a mirror. The patient should not be allowed to perform any of these exercises unassisted until pelvic-neutral position can be maintained without either verbal cueing or tactile feedback. The first series of exercises is performed in the supine, hook-lying position.

The second series of stabilization activities is performed in a quadruped position (**Figure 14-26**). As in the supine, hook-lying exercises, pelvic-neutral position must be maintained throughout the activity. If pelvic-neutral is lost or the patient rolls the hips to the side, the clinician should use verbal and tactile cueing to correct the position. This exercise should be performed on a firm surface; a soft tabletop requires excessive movement of the body.

A further progression of these stabilization activities can be performed while sitting on a Swiss ball. The erect position and the unstable surface of the Swiss ball increase the difficulty.

If additional progression is desired, the same sequence of exercises can be performed in a standing position. Once the patient can perform these exercises, the next advance is to simple functional activities, such as kicking or throwing a ball while maintaining pelvic-neutral position.

Williams' Flexion and McKenzie Extension Exercises

During the 1950s, Williams' flexion exercises were introduced for the treatment of low back pain. These exercises were the predominant choice for exercise treatment of low back pain until the 1980s, when McKenzie presented his approach to back pain. Although they both used exercise to relieve back pain and believed that such pain resulted from stress on the intervertebral disks, their theories, philosophies, and approaches differed radically.

Current trends reflect an individualized program based on a patient's examination findings. Neither Williams' flexion exercises nor McKenzie's program currently predominate. In fact, specific references to Williams' flexion exercises or McKenzie exercises are now uncommon. Many clinicians find these exercises to be rather low level and advance patients to other exercises.

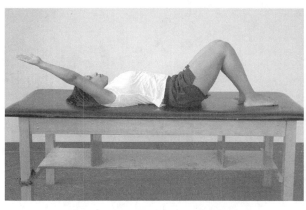

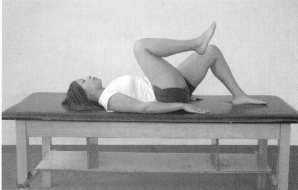

A. Upper extremity movement. The arms start at the sides. One arm is raised overhead, then returned to the start position; the opposite arm is raised overhead, then returned to the start position in alternating windmill fashion.

B. Lower extremity movement. The legs start in the hook-lying position. The patient raises one knee toward the chest and then returns it to the start position. The exercise is repeated in an alternating manner with the opposite leg.

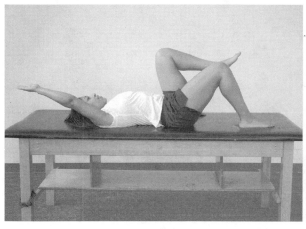

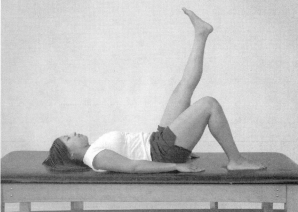

C. Upper and lower extremity movement. As the left leg is brought toward the chest, the right arm is simultaneously raised overhead. Both extremities are then returned to the start position, and the exercise is repeated with the opposite extremities.

D. Once these activities have been mastered without losing pelvic-neutral position, a further progression in the hook-lying position can include extending one leg fully, then returning it to the start position, and repeating the exercise on the opposite side.

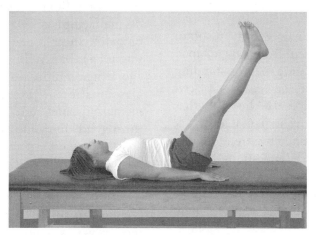

E. The next exercise can include extension of both legs simultaneously, followed by return to the start position. Caution must be exercised with each progression to ensure that the patient does not lose the pelvic-neutral position and arch the back.

Figure 14-25 Stabilization activities to increase trunk stability.

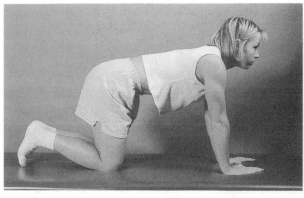

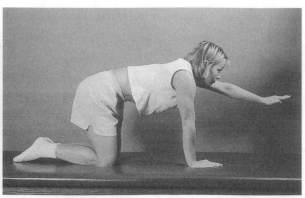

A. In the proper quadruped position, the shoulders are directly over the hands, which are spread about shoulderwidth apart, and the knees are directly under the hips.

B. While the patient maintains pelvic-neutral position, one arm is raised overhead and returned to start position. The exercise is repeated with the opposite arm.

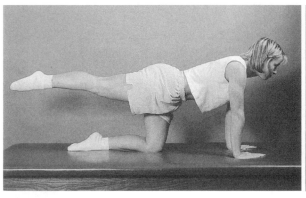

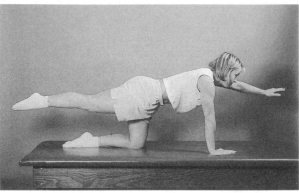

C. One leg is extended off the surface and behind the body, then returned to the start position. The exercise is repeated with the opposite leg.

D. The left leg and right arm are lifted simultaneously, then returned to the start position. The exercise is repeated with the opposite extremities.

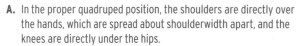

Figure 14-26 Quadruped stabilization exercises.

■ Williams' Flexion Exercises

Williams believed that back pain was the result of human evolution in movement from a quadruped to an upright position, proposing that the standing position was the cause of back pain because it placed the low back in a lordotic curve. He theorized that this increased lordosis was the source of low back pain and relief could be obtained by stretching the hip flexors and erector spinae and strengthening the abdominal and gluteal muscles. Williams advocated seven exercises to minimize the lumbar curve—pelvic tilt exercises, partial sit-ups, single knee-to-chest and bilateral knee-to-chest, hamstring stretching, standing lunges, seated trunk flexion, and full squat (**Figure 14-27**).

■ McKenzie Exercises

McKenzie professed that people spent too much time in a lumbar-flexed position, a primary cause of low back pain. Although McKenzie incorpo-

rated some flexion exercises into his programs, his main emphasis was extension. McKenzie's approach to lumbar pain was more flexible (no pun intended) than Williams', and was based on categorizing an individual's pain into three primary classifications—postural syndromes, derangement syndromes, and dysfunction syndromes. Postural syndromes are the mildest of the lumbar conditions and essentially represent soft-tissue–related lumbar pain that remains localized. Numbness and tingling are absent, and pain is intermittent. Derangement syndromes involve some changes in the intervertebral disk and exhibit more severe symptoms, with possible pain referral into the lower extremity. Changes in motion are seen, and the pain can be either constant or intermittent. A dysfunction is the most severe condition, with the patient demonstrating vertebral position changes that increase disk pressure. McKenzie advocated six different exercises—prone lying flat for 5 minutes, prone lying on elbows,

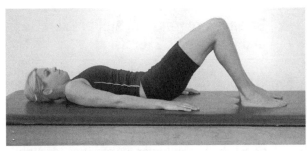

A. Pelvic tilt

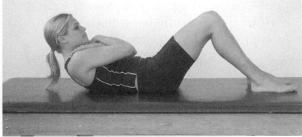

B. Sit-up in knee flexion

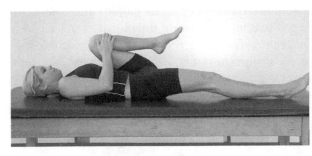

C. Single knees to chest and double knees to chest to stretch the erector spinae

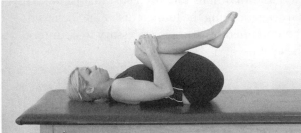

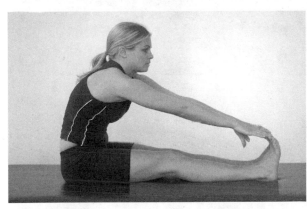

D. Seated reach to toes to stretch the hamstrings and erector spinae

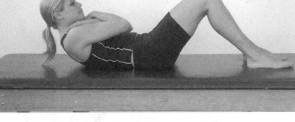

E. Forward crouch to stretch the iliofemoral ligament

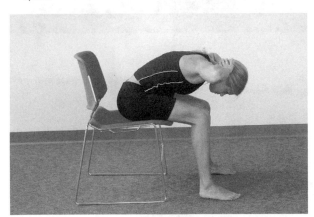

F. Seated flexion

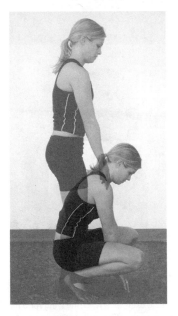

G. Standing squat to strengthen quadriceps

Figure 14-27 Williams' flexion exercises.

prone press-ups, standing trunk extensions, seated lumbar flexion-extensions, and both knees to chest in supine position (**Figure 14-28**). The precise regimen is based on the patient's pain complaints.

These exercises emphasize trunk-extension activities. McKenzie theorized that with a disk bulge or herniation, gravity could pull the fragment into proper position, thereby relieving the symptoms and reducing the bulge or herniation. He also proposed that individuals too often sustained a flexed position, aggravating the lumbar disks, and believed that an extended position is necessary to counteract these abuses.

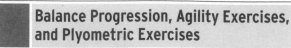

Balance Progression, Agility Exercises, and Plyometric Exercises

Chapter 9 provides a progression of proprioception, balance, coordination, agility, and plyometric exercises. At the outset, they may not appear to be balance activities for the trunk, but because the trunk depends on the lower extremities for stability, the activities are appropriate for low back rehabilitation (**Table 14-3**). The patient must maintain a pelvic-neutral position during all exercises. Verbal cueing for this activity may be necessary, especially as the patient starts a new activity.

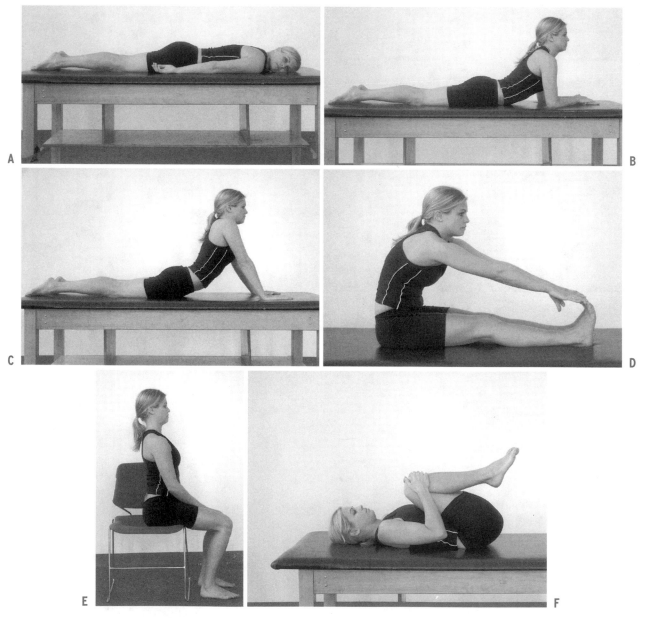

Figure 14-28   McKenzie exercises. **A.** Prone lying for 5 minutes. **B.** Prone lying on elbow for 5 minutes. **C.** Prone press-ups (10 repetitions, 6 to 8 times per day). **D.** Trunk extension in standing (10 repetitions, 6 to 8 times a day). The hands are placed in the low back area and extended backward from the trunk. Knees are not flexed. **E.** Seated lordosis (15 to 20 repetitions, 3 times a day). The lumbar spine is moved from flexion to extension. **F.** Both knees to chest (10 repetitions). One knee is brought to the chest at a time, and one knee is lowered at a time. This prevents excessive lumbar lordosis during the exercise.

Table 14-3

Sample Early Lumbar Stabilization Program

The patient advances to higher levels if he or she can complete a predetermined number of repetitions in lower levels without difficulty.

Supine Progression

Start position: The patient is supine with knees bent and feet flat on support surface. The patient finds and maintains a neutral spine position throughout the exercise.

Levels	Action
1	Contract abdominal muscles*–hold and release
2	Contract gluteal muscles†–hold and release
3	Cocontract gluteal and abdominal muscles–hold and release
4	Cocontract muscles, alternate sides: raise and lower heels
5	Cocontract muscles, alternate sides: raise and lower toes
6	Cocontract muscles, lift both legs off surface and alternately extend knees
7	Cocontract muscles, lift both arms together over head and back down
8	Cocontract muscles, alternate sides: lift arms up over head and back down
9	Cocontract muscles, lift both legs together, combine arm motions from level 8 with alternating knee extension

Prone Progression

Start position: The patient is prone with a pillow placed for support under the pelvis and abdomen and arms resting overhead. The patient finds and maintains a neutral spine position throughout the exercise.

Levels	Action
1	Contract abdominal muscles–hold and release; contract gluteal muscles–hold and release
2	Cocontract abdominal and gluteal muscles–hold and release
3	Cocontract abdominal and gluteal muscles, contract adductors–hold and release
4	Cocontract abdominal and gluteal muscles, first contract adductors and then hip extensors to alternately raise legs
5	Cocontract abdominal and gluteal muscles, first contract adductors and then bilateral hip extensors to raise both legs at once
6	Cocontract abdominal and gluteal muscles, alternate sides: lift one arm up overhead and lower, then the other arm
7	Cocontract abdominal and gluteal muscles, combine levels 5 and 6–the arm and leg on opposite sides are raised and lowered together (raise left arm and right leg and lower, then raise right arm and left leg and lower)

Quadruped Progression

Start position: The patient is on hands and knees and finds and maintains a neutral spine position throughout the exercise.

Levels	Action
1	Contract abdominal muscles–hold and release
2	Contract gluteal muscles–hold and release
3	Cocontract gluteal and abdominal muscles–hold and release
4	Coontract abdominal and gluteal muscles, shift weight anterior and posterior
5	Cocontract abdominal and gluteal muscles, alternate sides: straighten and extend one leg and return to start position, then the other leg
6	Cocontract abdominal and gluteal muscles, alternate sides: straighten and extend one arm in front, then the other
7	Cocontract abdominal and gluteal muscles, alternate sides: extend and straighten opposite arm and leg simultaneously

Bridging Progression

Start position: The patient is supine with knees bent and feet flat on support surface. The patient lifts the pelvis off the surface (the abdomen and pelvis should form a "flat" surface) and finds and maintains a neutral spine position throughout the exercise.

Levels	Action
1	Contract abdominal muscles–hold and release
2	Contract gluteal muscles–hold and release
3	Cocontract abdominal and gluteal muscles–hold and release
4	Cocontract abdominal and gluteal muscles, alternate sides: lift heels off surface and lower
5	Cocontract abdominal and gluteal muscles, alternate sides: lift toes off surface and lower
6	Cocontract abdominal and gluteal muscles, alternate sides: lift foot off surface and lower
7	Cocontract abdominal and gluteal muscles, alternate sides: extend knee, lower leg to surface, slide heel back to start position
8	Same as for Level 7, but without letting the leg touch the floor

Reproduced with permission from Dynamic Lumbar Stabilization Program, The San Francisco Spine Institute, Daly City, CA 1989.

14

Table 14-3

Sample Early Lumbar Stabilization Program (Continued)

Standing Progression

Start position: The patient stands with the feet shoulder width apart and finds and maintains a neutral spine position thoughout the exercise.

Levels	Action
1	Contract abdominals—hold and release
2	Contract gluteals—hold and release
3	Cocontract abdominal and gluteal muscles—hold and release
4	Maintain cocontraction in walking
5	Maintain cocontraction while performing semisquats (no more than 30° to 40° of hip flexion)

Note: When alternating sides, the patient performs the action first on one side and then on the other.

* Use the command "Pull your navel to your spine."

† Use the command "tighten your muscles as if stopping urination midflow"

Adapted with permission from the Dynamic Lumbar Stabilization Program, The San Francisco Spine Institute, 1989.

References

1. Mooney V, Robèrtson J: The facet syndrome. *Clin Orthop* 1976;115:149-156.

2. Revel M, Poiraudeau S, Auleley GR, et al: Capacity of the clinical picture to characterize low back pain relieved by facet joint anesthesia: Proposed criteria to identify patients with painful facet joints. *Spine* 1998; 23:1972-1976.

3. Leclaire R, Fortin L, Lambert R, Bergeron YM, Rossignol M: Radiofrequency facet joint denervation in the treatment of low back pain: A placebo-controlled clinical trial to assess efficacy. *Spine* 2001;26:1411-1417.

4. Feuerstein M, Berkowitz SM, Huang GD: Predictors of occupational low back disability: Implications for secondary prevention. *J Occup Environ Med* 1999;41:1024-1031.

5. Spivak JM, Vaccaro AR, Colter JM: Thoracolumbar spine trauma: II. Principles of management. *J Am Acad Orthop Surg* 1995;3:353-360.

6. Spivak JM, Vaccaro AR, Colter JM: Thoracolumbar spine trauma: I. Evaluation and classification. *J Am Acad Orthop Surg* 1995;3:345-352.

7. Boden SD, Wiesel SW: Lumbar spine imaging: Role in clinical decision making. *J Am Acad Orthop Surg* 1996;4: 238-248.

8. Young JL, Press JM, Herring SA: The disc at risk in athletes: Perspectives on operative and nonoperative care. *Med Sci Sports Exerc* 1997;29(suppl 7):S222-S232.

9. Wheeler AH: Diagnosis and management of low back pain and sciatica. *Am Fam Physician.* 1995;52:1333-1341, 1347-1348.

10. Ahn UM, Ahn NU, Buchowski JM, Garrett ES, Sieber AN, Kostuik JP: Cauda equina syndrome secondary to lumbar disc herniation: A meta-analysis of surgical outcomes. *Spine* 2000;25:1515-1522.

11. Shapiro S: Medical realities of cauda equina syndrome secondary to lumbar disc herniation. *Spine* 2000;25:348-352.

12. Standaert CJ, Herring SA, Halpern B, King O: Spondylolysis. *Phys Med Rehabil Clin N Am* 2000;11:785-803.

13. Lonstein JE: Spondylolisthesis in children: Cause, natural history, and management. *Spine* 1999;24:2640-2648.

14. Skinner HB: *Diagnosis and Treatment in Orthopedics.* Norwalk, CT, Appleton & Lange, 1995.

15. Schneiderman GA, McLain RF, Hambly MF, Nielsen SL: The pars defect as a pain source: A histologic study. *Spine* 1995;20:1761-1764.

16. Letts M, Smallman T, Afanasiev R. Gouw G: Fracture of the pars interarticularis in adolescent athletes: A clinical-biomechanical analysis. *J Pediatr Orthop* 1986;6:40-46.

17. Frymoyer JW: Degenerative spondylolisthesis: Diagnosis and treatment. *J Am Acad Orthop Surg* 1994;2:9-15.

18. Hambly MF, Wiltse LL, Peek RD: Spondylolisthesis, in Watkins RG, ed: *The Spine in Sports.* St. Louis, MO, Mosby-Year Book, 1996, pp 157-163.

19. Edmond SL: *Manipulation and Mobilization: Extremity and Spinal Techniques.* St. Louis, MO, Mosby-Year Book, 1993.

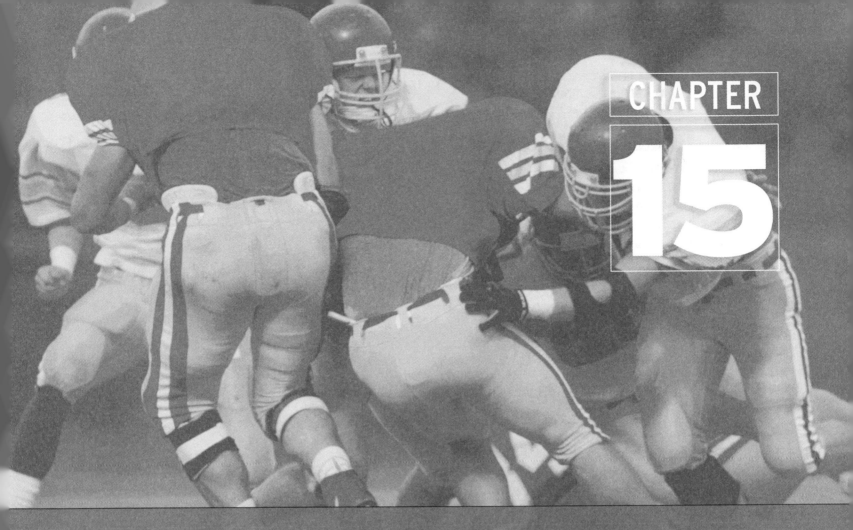

Abdominal and Thorax Injuries

Allen Mathieu, PAC, MS, ATC
L. Michael Brunt, MD

Cardiac Tamponade

CLINICAL PRESENTATION

History

Blunt trauma to the chest
Feeling of impending doom

Observation

Distended neck veins
Severe agitation
Anxiety

Functional Status

The patient may display the signs and symptoms of shock.

Physical Evaluation Findings

Distant or muffled heart sounds
Tachycardia
Hypotension
Paradoxical pulse

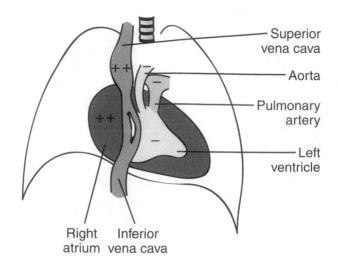

Figure 15-1 Cardiac tamponade. As effusion develops, both atria and ventricles are compressed. Inflow pressure in the superior and inferior vena cavae and right atrium rises, but inspite of this ventricular volume falls and arterial pressure is reduced. (Reproduced with permission from Henry MM, Thompson JN (eds): *Clinical Surgery*. Philadelphia, PA, WB Saunders, 2001.)

Cardiac tamponade is most commonly the result of a penetrating torso wound, which is exceedingly rare in athletics. However, it also can be caused by blunt trauma. Injury to the inelastic pericardium allows blood to fill the pericardial cavity; as the pressure builds, the heart muscle becomes compressed. The thin walls of the atria collapse, causing decreased end-diastolic volume.[1] Further increases in pressure affect the ventricular wall, increasing end-diastolic pressure. With reduced blood volume entering and leaving the heart, cardiac output falls, and hypotension and shock occur. A lethal condition can rapidly develop. Adults can accommodate only about 100 mL of pericardial blood without experiencing shock.

Penetrating trauma causes pericardial bleeding due to a hole in the pericardium that is too small to vent blood. Blunt trauma disrupts epicardial vessels or ruptures the heart. The signs and symptoms of cardiac tamponade can be delayed for days to weeks after injury. Symptoms then develop as a result of rebleeding or effusions from pericarditis (**Figure 15-1**).

Differential Diagnosis

Myocardial contusion, pulmonary contusion, rib or sternal fracture

Medical Diagnostic Tests

The pressure within the superior vena cava, the central venous pressure, is greater than 15 mm Hg. A paradoxical pulse also suggests tamponade.

Imaging Techniques

Cardiac ultrasound enables rapid and accurate diagnosis. Echocardiography can reveal features of tamponade, such as right atrial compression and right ventricular diastolic collapse. Rapid-imaging spiral computed tomography (CT) scans are accurate in diagnosing tamponade.

Definitive Diagnosis

The definitive diagnosis is based on clinical evaluation followed by cardiac ultrasound or CT scans revealing a fluid-filled pericardial cavity.

Pathomechanics and Functional Limitations

Once the patient begins to demonstrate the signs and symptoms of cardiac tamponade, signs of shock and a rapid decline in vital signs rapidly occur. Immediate definitive treatment is necessary to save the patient's life.

■ Immediate Management

The patient is treated for shock and immediately transported for medical care.

■ Medical Management

A patient in severe shock with suspected tamponade requires immediate pericardial decompression. This can best be completed through a subxiphoid pericardial window, thoracotomy, or sternotomy. Controversy exists regarding therapeutic pericardiocentesis. Aspiration may be warranted

---

Paradoxical pulse
The pulse becomes weaker during inspiration and stronger during expiration.

Pericardiocentesis
A diagnostic procedure in which a needle is used to draw fluid from the pericardium.

in those patients with urgent signs of severe tamponade. Aspiration and pericardial windows increase the patients' viability, but surgical decompression of the thorax is necessary.

In those individuals whose conditions appear nonemergent, IV fluids are begun with close cardiac and hemodynamic monitoring. The need for intubation and oxygenation is assessed. Small changes in pericardial blood volume can result in significant hemodynamic changes.

■ Estimated Amount of Time Lost

Time lost from sport depends on the severity of the heart-muscle damage, which is determined by a thorough cardiac evaluation. The patient may have a complete recovery or long-term disability.

■ Return-to-Play Criteria

Recovery from surgery and return to physical activity are closely monitored. Upon complete recovery from the surgical decompression, physical activity is progressed gradually under close medical supervision.

Myocardial Contusion

CLINICAL PRESENTATION

History

Blunt impact to the sternum
Mild to severe chest pain

Observation

Pallor

Functional Status

Shock is possible.
The patient may be unconscious.

Physical Evaluation Findings

Tachycardia
Irregular heart rate
Hypotension

Myocardial contusion occurs when blunt trauma creates forces that compress the heart between the sternum and the thoracic vertebrae. It can also occur from rapid chest-wall deceleration. The heart rebounds against the sternum, and the ensuing cardiac-muscle damage can cause death. Life-threatening ventricular dysfunction or ventricular arrhythmia may develop. Myocardial

contusions can occur in contact sports; baseball (being hit by a pitched ball); lacrosse; and activities such as cycling, skiing, rock climbing, and motor sports.[2]

Most cases of myocardial contusion are minor. Severe contusions are unusual in contact sports and most often result in sudden death. These individuals die of heart-muscle laceration, valve disruption, transmural hematoma, or, in rare situations, main coronary artery occlusion. Death occurs from hemodynamic decompensation.

Differential Diagnosis

Cardiac tamponade, pulmonary contusion, rib or sternal fracture

Imaging Techniques

Echocardiography provides an image of ventricular hypokinesis.

Definitive Diagnosis

Along with echocardiography, 24-hour cardiac rhythm monitoring, serial troponins, and creatine phosphokinase enzyme monitoring confirm the diagnosis.[2]

Pathomechanics and Functional Limitations

Patients with minor contusions do very well, typically with no long-term problems. Patients with severe contusions have high death rates.

■ Immediate Management

If the signs and symptoms of cardiac involvement are present (eg, tachycardia, irregular heart rate, hypotension), the patient must be immediately transported for medical care.

■ Medications

Ionotropic agents, peripheral vascular drugs, and volume expanders are used for emergent care.

■ Medical Management

The primary goal in minor cardiac injury is to monitor cardiac function and intervene appropriately to prevent hemodynamic collapse. In severe injury, hemodynamic support is necessary during and after surgical intervention.

Hospitalization with cardiac monitoring is necessary for mild contusions. Most dysrhythmias occur within the first 24 hours of trauma.[2] Cardiac monitoring (electrocardiogram) and hemodynamic monitoring of blood pressure, pulse, and neck venous distension are important and may signal more serious injury. After 24 hours of normal results, the patient may be discharged.

Volume expanders
Benign IV agents that allow temporary restoration of blood volume without having to wait for blood type matching.

15

■ Estimated Amount of Time Lost

Time lost depends on cardiac-muscle damage and recovery as demonstrated by cardiac function. Mild contusion is expected to result in little time loss. Severe cardiac-muscle damage may result in permanent cardiac-muscle dysfunction and long-term participation loss.

■ Return-to-Play Criteria

Progressive aerobic exercise and strengthening are permitted, with progression to full sport participation as tolerated by the cardiovascular system.

Pulmonary Contusion

CLINICAL PRESENTATION

History
Blunt blow to the chest
Severe chest pain
Dyspnea

Observation
Cough
Hemoptysis

Physical Evaluation Findings
Tachypnea
Diminished breath sounds
Rales
Respiratory distress

Hemoptysis Coughing up blood.

Parenchyma The internal functional tissues of an organ.

A pulmonary contusion involves a bruise of the lung that is associated with hemorrhage and edema into the lung parenchyma.[2] This occurs from blunt trauma, which results in rib fractures that displace and penetrate the lung parenchyma. Pulmonary contusions also occur with rapid chest-wall deceleration. The lung rebounds against the chest wall, resulting in a contusion. Children are more prone to pulmonary contusion because their chest walls are compressed and less force is dissipated by the ribs.

The lung insult results in interstitial bleeding, followed by edema and alveolar thickening. The injured lung develops decreased blood flow with increased pulmonary vascular resistance. Ventilation-perfusion mismatch occurs from edema and pulmonary pressure changes. Depending on the contusion size, respiratory distress is mild to severe. Symptoms may not become significant until 24 to 48 hours after injury.

Differential Diagnosis

Myocardial contusion, cardiac tamponade, rib or sternal fracture, pneumothorax

Imaging Techniques

Chest radiography remains the imaging modality of choice. Findings range from fluffy, patchy infiltrates to pulmonary consolidation. A CT scan is rarely necessary but in stable patients may help to reveal additional underlying injury.

Definitive Diagnosis

Diagnosis is based on physical findings and confirmed by chest radiographs.

Pathomechanics and Functional Limitations

Shortness of breath and chest pain can be debilitating. In addition, symptom onset can be delayed after initial injury. Failure to recognize progressive respiratory compromise can result in loss of respiratory function and death.

■ Immediate Management

The first priority is to ensure an open airway, breathing, and circulation. Immediate transport to the hospital should be arranged.

■ Medications

Aggressive pain control is initiated using oral or injectable narcotic analgesics.

■ Medical Intervention

Hospitalization is necessary for observation when lung contusion is suspected or diagnosed. Observation with monitoring of vital signs and serial chest radiographs may be all that is necessary. However, with significant respiratory distress, intensive care unit admission is necessary. Large-bore IV lines are required for fluid resuscitation and tissue perfusion in the presence of shock. Because the lung damage is very sensitive to fluid balance, judicious fluid management is necessary, including the possible use of diuretics once the patient's tissue perfusion and urine output are restored.

Intercostal anesthetic blocks for rib fractures are helpful. Epidural catheters may be used for prolonged pain control. A chest tube may need to be placed if hemothorax or pneumothorax exists. Aggressive pulmonary drain with vigorous suctioning, chest physiotherapy, and postural drainage is important in order to maintain the patient's airway and remove secretions. Intubation and ventilatory support are necessary in patients with severe respiratory distress and ventilatory failure.

■ Injury-Specific Treatment and Rehabilitation Concerns

The gradual return to exercise training involves an aerobic program, weight training, and functional training.

■ Estimated Amount of Time Lost

Return to activity is anticipated in 3 to 4 weeks.

■ Return-to-Play Criteria

Return is based on exercise tolerance and the ability to progress exercises.

Spontaneous Pneumomediastinum

CLINICAL PRESENTATION

History

Retrosternal chest pain
Neck pain

Observation

Patient often appears anxious.

Functional Status

Shortness of breath
Dysphagia
Dysphonia

Physical Evaluation Findings

Subcutaneous emphysema over the supraclavicular area
Hoarseness
Hamman sign (precordial crackles or crunching sounds with each heartbeat)

In spontaneous pneumomediastinum, free air enters the mediastinum as a result of alveolar rupture, which occurs because of elevated alveolar pressure. This pressure may result from decompression diving, coughing, vomiting, or sudden exertion. The condition is often associated with the Valsalva maneuver.[3]

Differential Diagnosis

Pneumothorax, hemothorax, lung contusion, rib fracture, myocardial contusion, pleural effusion

Imaging Techniques

Chest and cervical spine radiographs are typically diagnostic, revealing free air within the mediastinal tissue. Lateral cervical spine films may demonstrate free air in the deep cervical tissues and behind the trachea and larynx. CT may be helpful in the diagnosis, but the priority is to identify the underlying cause, such as a pneumothorax. Imaging with a Hypaque swallow may be necessary to exclude an esophageal injury.

Definitive Diagnosis

Diagnosis is confirmed by a chest radiograph showing mediastinal air.

Pathomechanics and Functional Limitations

The condition is typically self-limiting, with no long-term functional deficits.

Immediate Management

Activity is discontinued, and medical attention sought immediately. The patient's airway is maintained, and respiration and circulation are regularly monitored. Associated injuries are excluded (see Differential Diagnosis).

■ Medications

Pain medications may be necessary.

■ Medical Management

Medical management includes rest and pain management. No evidence-based medical guidelines exist; therefore, treatment varies.[3] Some advocate hospitalization because of potential complications (eg, pneumothorax). Others believe that no restrictions are necessary. A CT scan may be prudent to evaluate for occult pneumothorax, which occurs in 18% of patients with spontaneous pneumomediastinum.

Occult Hidden or not readily detectable by laboratory tests or physical examination.

■ Injury-Specific Treatment and Rehabilitation Concerns

Progression to aerobic activities and weight training are permitted as tolerated. The patient must be counseled against performing the Valsalva maneuver.

■ Estimated Amount of Time Lost

Full activity can usually be resumed 7 to 10 days after injury.

■ Return-to-Play Criteria

The patient must demonstrate symptom-free, sport-specific training levels.

Pneumothorax

CLINICAL PRESENTATION

History

Sudden, unrelieved shortness of breath
Mild to severe chest pain localized to the affected lung, which is
   often pleuritic

Observation

Dyspnea, especially on exertion
Dry cough
Asymmetric chest-wall expansion

Functional Status

Altered breathing pattern

Physical Evaluation Findings

Possible chest-wall tenderness
Tachypnea
Tachycardia
Decreased **fremitus**
Hyperresonance
Diminished breath sounds
Patient complaints can vary greatly.

Fremitus Palpable vibration, as felt when placing the hand on the chest or throat during speaking.

Embolus Solid, liquid, or gaseous mass blocking a passageway.

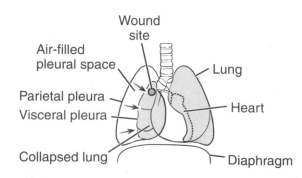

Figure 15-2 Pneumothorax occurs when air enters the pleura from an opening in the chest wall and causes intraplueral pressure to increase.

Pneumothorax is the result of air leakage from the lung into the pleural space, usually from lung parenchyma disruption. Greater air pressure in the pleural cavity than in the lung causes lung collapse and respiratory compromise. The degree of compromise depends on the air volume in the pleural cavity. Pneumothorax can be either spontaneous or traumatic (**Figure 15-2**). Spontaneous pneumothorax occurs predominantly in men 20 to 40 years old.

Spontaneous Pneumothorax

Spontaneous pneumothorax typically occurs without trauma. The cause is not clearly understood, but the most accepted explanation is rupture of subpleural blebs.[4] The origin of these blebs is unknown. They are thought to be congenital, but associated factors such as a tall and thin body build, tobacco smoking, or abusing substances such as "ecstasy" may increase the risk of occurrence. Activities that increase intrathoracic pressure have also been postulated as a contributing factor. Most cases, however, are unrelated to exercise and sports. Recurrence rates vary from 20% to 50%.[4]

Traumatic Pneumothorax

Traumatic pneumothorax can result from either blunt or penetrating trauma and is the most common intrathoracic injury after blunt trauma.[2] Pneumothorax may result from a rib fracture penetrating the lung, a decelerating injury resulting in a lung tear, a crush injury disrupting alveoli, or a sudden increase in intrathoracic pressure.[5] Multiple injury mechanisms warrant a high index of suspicion.

Differential Diagnosis

Hemothorax, spontaneous pneumomediastinum, rib fracture, myocardial contusion, pulmonary embolus

Imaging Techniques

Posteroanterior and lateral chest radiographs are obtained.

Definitive Diagnosis

Clinical findings are confirmed with chest radiographs that reveal loss of lung volume and air in the pleural space.

Pathomechanics and Functional Limitations

Loss of usable lung volume results in diminished oxygen exchange and shortness of breath. Tension pneumothorax can occur if left untreated, with resultant shock and death (see p 498).

■ Immediate Management

Airway, breathing, and circulation must be monitored and vital signs checked every 5 minutes. Oxygen should be administered if the patient is experiencing shortness of breath or is tachypneic. If the patient is unstable and a tension pneumothorax is suspected, qualified personnel may perform needle decompression via the second intercostal space at the midclavicular line. If onsite facilities are available and the patient is stable, a chest radiograph should be obtained. The patient should be transported to the hospital (via ambulance if markedly symptomatic) for appropriate definitive diagnostic evaluation and management.

Immediate care is important, but emergent care is not always necessary. Patients with suspected pneumothorax should not be left unattended and should be continually monitored until the medical evaluation is complete.

Individuals with a suspected pneumothorax should not be allowed to travel by airplane. Changes in cabin pressure increase the risk of acutely exacerbating the pneumothorax.

■ Medications

Oral, intramuscular, or IV analgesics are required during and for a short period after hospitalization with chest-tube placement. Nonsurgical treatment requires little or no medications.

■ Medical Management and Surgical Intervention

Pneumothorax is typically managed with placement of a chest tube (ST 15-1). However, a small, asymptomatic pneumothorax can occasionally be managed with serial chest radiographs and close observation. Daily chest radiographs are recommended until resolution.

■ Injury-Specific Treatment and Rehabilitation Concerns

Advancement through aerobic activities, strength training, and sport-specific functional progression is permitted as tolerated.

■ Estimated Amount of Time Lost

Return to play is allowed 3 to 4 weeks after symptoms resolve.

■ Return-to-Play Criteria

The patient must delay normal sport activities until the pneumothorax has completely resolved on chest radiographs.

Tension Pneumothorax

Tension pneumothorax is characterized by the rapid development of large air volumes trapped in the pleural space. This can occur from blunt trauma, a penetrating chest wound, or a spontaneous pneumothorax.

The defect in the lung parenchyma or bronchus may act as a flap valve, allowing air to enter the pleural space with each breath but not escape back through the lung or tracheobronchial tree. As intrapleural pressure increases, the lung collapses and the mediastinal structures shift away from the side of the pneumothorax. The large veins (vena cava) in the mediastinum collapse, venous return to the

---

CLINICAL PRESENTATION

History

Blunt trauma and/or penetrating chest wound that may involve the lung itself

Observation

Difficulty breathing

Bulging of the chest-wall intercostal muscles and supraclavicular area

Neck-vein distension

Cyanosis

Tracheal deviation to the side opposite the pneumothorax

Functional Status

Severe, rapid, progressive respiratory distress

Increasing air hunger

Physical Evaluation Findings

Weak pulse

Drop in blood pressure

Chest hyperresonance on the side of the pneumothorax but with decreased breath sounds

These findings vary and are not consistently present.

---

heart is compromised, and hemodynamic instability ensues (**Figure 15-3**).

Sucking Chest Wound (Open Chest Injury)

An open chest-wall injury may allow air to enter the pleural space directly due to negative intrathoracic pressure; this occurs most commonly after a shotgun blast or impalement injury. Pneumothorax or hemothorax may also be present. Immediate treatment consists of placement of an occlusive dressing taped on three sides. This allows air to es-

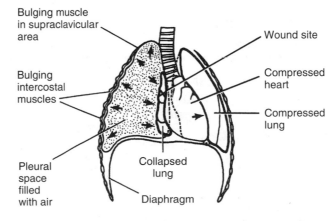

Figure 15-3 Tension pneumothorax. When air enters the pleural space but cannot exit, a tension pneumothorax develops. Continued leaking of air from the lung into the pleural space causes the lung to collapse until it is reduced to 2″ to 3″ in diameter.

S|T Surgical Technique 15-1

Chest-Tube Placement

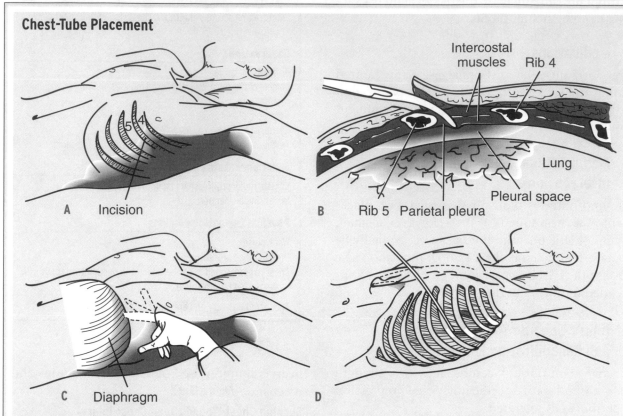

Indications

Greater than 20% pneumothorax with respiratory distress

Overview

1. A local anesthetic is administered.
2. A 20- to 22-French diameter tube or 16-French Thal tube is inserted in the fifth intercostal space at the anterior or midaxillary line. The tube is passed through the skin and subcutaneous tissue and over the top of the rib. It is then passed through the intercostal muscle and into the pleural space.
3. The opposite end of the tube is connected to an underwater seal with negative suction.
4. Negative pressure (suction) should be maintained at a water level of approximately 20 cm to obtain adequate drainage.
5. The chest tube is maintained until the air leak has sealed (no water-level fluctuation with inspiration) and no air is leaking, with fluid drainage less than 100 mL per 24 hours.
6. A chest radiograph is taken at the end of the procedure to evaluate lung reexpansion and tube location.

Functional Limitations

While the tube is in place, hospitalization is required. The tube is removed when it has stopped functioning (no water-level fluctuation). Daily radiographs document improvement. Upon discharge, the patient rests and follows up with radiographs to confirm progressive resolution.

Implications for Rehabilitation

Because of the significant recurrence rate, the patient and athletic trainer must be educated in recurrent signs and symptoms. Slow, conservative return to activity is suggested.

Potential Complications

Unilateral pulmonary edema from rapid reexpansion, lung injury, chest-wall bleeding, air leak, tube occlusion, persistent pneumothorax, subcutaneous emphysema, diaphragm laceration, infection, extrapleural tube positioning, cardiac arrhythmia

Comments

Tube placement and size vary with respect to the diagnosis. For example, to treat a hemothorax, a 36-French diameter tube is placed in the fifth or sixth intercostal space at the midaxillary line.

Figures reproduced with permission from Pearson FG, Cooper JD, et al: *Thoracic Surgery*, ed 5. New York, NY, Churchill Livingstone, 2002.

cape through the open side but prevents air from being sucked back into the chest with inspiration. A full, four-sided occlusion dressing may exacerbate or increase the pneumothorax. This is a medical emergency that can result in death if untreated.

Differential Diagnosis

Pneumothorax, hemothorax, myocardial injury, pulmonary embolus, cardiac tamponade

Definitive Diagnosis

Clinical findings, response to emergency treatment, and chest radiographs indicate the diagnosis.

Pathomechanics and Functional Limitations

Rapid respiratory and circulatory collapse occurs because of increased intrathoracic pressure on the lung, heart, and major vessels. If function is restored, no long-term functional loss typically occurs. However, failure to recognize and treat the condition is life threatening.

▣ Immediate Management

A partially sealed occlusive dressing allows air to exit through the unsealed dressing side, while preventing air from reentering during breathing (**Figure 15-4**). Complete occlusion may increase the pneumothorax.

Qualified personnel can decompress the pleural space with a large-bore (14-gauge) needle inserted through the anterior chest wall in the second intercostal space at the midclavicular line.[5]

This is a quick method of decompressing the pleural space by allowing trapped air to flow out through the needle and can be lifesaving. It must be followed by formal chest-tube placement.

▣ Medications

Oral, intramuscular, or IV analgesics are required during and for a short period after hospitalization with chest-tube placement.

▣ Medical and Surgical Intervention

When the patient reaches the emergency room, a large-bore chest tube (24 French) is placed into the fifth or sixth intercostal space at the midaxillary line. A larger tube (36 to 40 French) should be placed if there is an associated hemothorax. The tube is connected to an underwater seal with

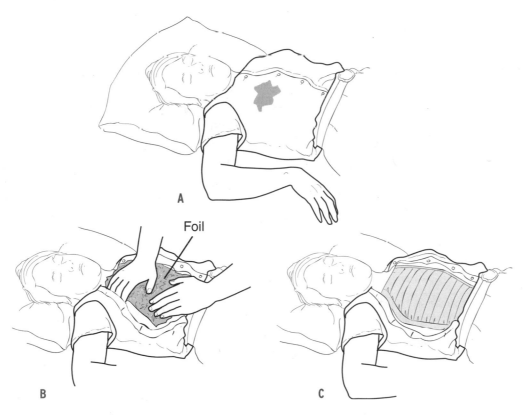

Foil

A

B

C

Figure 15-4 In an open chest injury, air moves in and out of the wound, remaining in the pleural space and causing a tension pneumothorax. **A.** This partially sealed occlusive dressing allows air to exit through the unsealed side, while preventing air from reentering during breathing. Complete occlusion potentially increases the pneumothorax. **B.** One side of the dressing should be left untaped so that air can exit the wound during breathing; however, the dressing should be snug enough so that air does not enter the wound from the untaped side (**C**).

negative suction. A chest radiograph is obtained to ensure adequate lung expansion, and vital signs and blood oxygen levels are closely monitored.

■ Postinjury/Postoperative Management

Once the patient is stabilized, serial chest radiographs are taken to monitor pneumothorax resolution. Chest-tube removal criteria are the same as for a pneumothorax.

■ Injury-Specific Treatment and Rehabilitation Concerns

Advancement through aerobic activities, strength training, and sport-specific functional progression is permitted as tolerated.

■ Estimated Amount of Time Lost

Return to play is permitted 3 to 4 weeks after symptoms resolve.

■ Return-to-Play Criteria

The patient must delay normal activities until chest radiographs indicate that the pneumothorax has completely resolved.

Hemothorax

CLINICAL PRESENTATION

History

Blunt trauma or a penetrating chest-wall injury
Sudden, unrelieved shortness of breath
Mild to severe chest pain localized to the affected lung, which is often pleuritic

Observation

Dyspnea, especially on exertion
Dry cough
Asymmetric chest-wall expansion

Functional Status

Shock manifestations: apprehension, thirst, cold, clammy, chills, pallor, weak pulse, decreased blood pressure

Physical Evaluation Findings

Possible chest-wall tenderness
Tachypnea
Tachycardia
Diminished breath sounds

A hemothorax is the result of either blunt chest wall trauma or a penetrating chest-wall injury and often occurs in combination with a pneumothorax. The blood source can be the lung, chest wall, major or lesser vessels, diaphragm, or abdominal organs. The blood occupies the pleural space solely or in combination with air, resulting in respiratory compromise (**Figure 15-5**). With major blood loss, shock may occur. A significant hemothorax is unlikely to result from athletic competition.

Differential Diagnosis

Pneumothorax, tension pneumothorax, myocardial trauma, pulmonary embolus

Imaging Techniques

Chest radiographs are taken in the supine and lateral supine positions. If the films are not diagnostic, lateral or decubitus films can help to differentiate pleural fluid from contusion or intraparenchymal hemorrhage. Ultrasound may be beneficial in identifying pleural fluid. CT is also useful in differentiating pleural fluid from parenchymal fluid.

Definitive Diagnosis

The diagnosis is based on clinical signs and chest radiographs; CT is helpful in establishing the type of fluid present.

Pathomechanics and Functional Limitations

Loss of usable lung volume results in diminished oxygen exchange and shortness of breath. Tension pneumothorax can occur if left untreated, with resultant shock and death.

■ Immediate Management

Airway, breathing, and circulation should be monitored0 and the possible need for administration of cardiopulmonary resuscitation (CPR) anticipated. Any external bleeding must be controlled, vital signs recorded every 5 minutes, and the emergency medical system (EMS) activated when appropriate. Symptoms can vary greatly from mild to severe, including shock. The patient must be

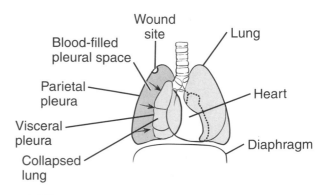

Figure 15-5 A hemothorax occurs when major blood vessels are lacerated and blood is present in the pleural space outside the lung.

continually monitored until medical evaluation is complete.

Surgical Intervention

Surgical management focuses on draining the pleural space and controlling bleeding.[5] Most bleeding responds well to chest-tube evacuation and lung re-expansion. Placement of a 32- to 36-French chest tube in the fifth or sixth intercostal space with underwater seal is required. The chest tube remains in place until no more air leaks from the lung and less than 100 to 150 mL of fluid drains in 24 hours (see ⓈⓉ 15-1). Approximately 10% of patients with traumatic hemothorax require thoracotomy to control bleeding.

Chest radiographs must be taken immediately after tube placement to confirm proper placement and reveal fluid and air evacuation. If fluid remains after chest-tube placement, a second tube may be required. If fluid persists, thoracotomy may be necessary. Daily chest radiographs are necessary until the fluid has fully resolved.

Thoracotomy indications include the immediate removal of more than 1,200 mL of blood or 200 mL/h or more of bloody output for more than 4 hours after chest-tube placement.[5]

Postinjury/Postoperative Management

Serial chest radiographs are taken to evaluate for hemothorax resolution; chest-wound healing is monitored. The patient is initially limited to bed rest due to respiratory distress. Many activities of daily living can be resumed when the chest tube is removed. With hospital discharge, the patient can slowly and progressively return to daily living habits. No long-term functional loss is expected.

Injury-Specific Treatment and Rehabilitation Concerns

Advancement through aerobic activities, strength training, and sport-specific functional progression is permitted as tolerated.

Estimated Amount of Time Lost

Return to play is allowed 3 to 4 weeks after symptoms resolve.

Return-to-Play Criteria

The patient must delay normal activities until chest radiographs demonstrate that the hemothorax has completely resolved.

Commotio Cordia (Cardiac Concussion)

CLINICAL PRESENTATION

History
Blunt trauma to the chest

Observation
Collapse and loss of consciousness

Functional Status
Unconscious

Physical Evaluation Findings
Absent pulse

Commotio cordia is a cause of sudden death due to blunt trauma to the chest wall. It can result in heart injury and sudden arrhythmia. Ventricular fibrillation is the most common arrhythmia, but complete heart block and idioventricular rhythms have also been described. The arrhythmia may be refractory to standard resuscitation measures, including defibrillation.

The blow most commonly occurs to the left precordial area and usually involves individuals 5 to 15 years of age. Trauma is related to the speed and force of impact against the chest wall and most often results from a blow due to a projectile (baseball, hockey puck, punch, or physical hit to the chest). The mortality rate of commotio cordia is high. Adolescents have a narrower anteroposterior chest diameter and greater chest-wall compliance, which are thought to contribute to greater force transmission to the heart. Usually no structural damage affects the heart or chest wall.

Chest protectors and coaching and equipment modifications may protect the heart against forces that trigger commotio cordia. Controversy remains concerning the use of low-impact balls for softball and baseball.

Differential Diagnosis
Myocardial infarction, respiratory arrest, ruptured aneurysm

Definitive Diagnosis
Because of the high mortality rate, the definitive diagnosis is often made posthumously.

Pathomechanics and Functional Limitations
The survival rate is low, approximately 10%.

Immediate Management

The patient is assessed for the presence of a pulse; if absent, a precordial thump is administered and the pulse reassessed. If the pulse is still absent, CPR and advanced cardiac life-support protocol are initiated. If an automated external defibrillator is available, the heart is defibrillated. EMS is activated immediately.

Postinjury/Postoperative Management

A cardiology workup is necessary to rule out possible underlying disease.

Injury-Specific Treatment and Rehabilitation Concerns

Autopsy studies have revealed no cardiac injury. Patients who survive the condition typically return to full activity.

Estimated Amount of Time Lost

Time loss is determined by cardiology workup.

Return-to-Play Criteria

Individuals who have recovered (spontaneously or with resuscitation) from apparent commotio cordia should undergo cardiac evaluation to determine underlying cardiac abnormalities. The patient may return to competition once recovery is complete and underlying cardiac disease has been excluded or controlled.

Costochondritis

CLINICAL PRESENTATION

History

Pain localized to the sternal border and costal angle

Observation

Swelling may be visible but is rare.

Functional Status

Deep breathing may be limited.
The Valsalva maneuver may cause pain.
Pain when exerting the thoracic musculature

Physical Evaluation Findings

Tenderness along the sternal border
Tenderness along the costal angles

Costochondritis is an inflammatory process that involves the cartilaginous junction between the ribs and sternum. The onset may be related to repetitive direct trauma or indirect trauma and is often unrelated to activity. In some individuals, chronic inflammation develops and ongoing treatment is necessary.

Differential Diagnosis

Costochondral separation, fractured rib, fractured sternum, bone tumor

Imaging Techniques

Radiographs are used to rule out rib fractures.

Definitive Diagnosis

Clinical findings, together with radiographs and occasionally bone scans for exclusion of differential diagnoses, determine the presence of costochondritis.

Pathomechanics and Functional Limitations

Pain with deep inspiration may slow the conditioning process.

Immediate Management

Ice and support such as a rib belt help reduce the pain (**Figure 15-6**).

Medications

Prescription or over-the-counter nonsteroidal anti-inflammatory drugs (NSAIDs) may be prescribed.

Postinjury Management

The inflammatory process is decreased with immediate care and the area supported with wrapping during the healing process.

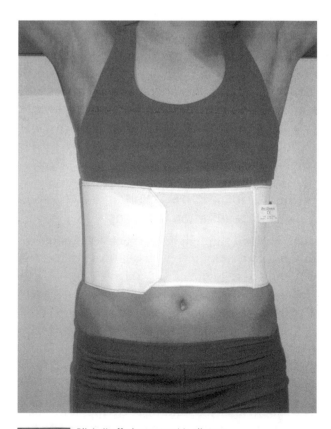

Figure 15-6   Rib belt offering support to rib cage.

■ Injury-Specific Treatment and Rehabilitation Concerns

Modalities of ice or heat (depending on the inflammatory process) and stretching exercises are instituted. Limitations are dictated by pain. Deep inspiration may be painful, and conditioning may be impaired.

■ Estimated Amount of Time Lost

This condition tends to be self-limiting, and return to full activities is possible.

■ Return-to-Play Criteria

Activity limitation is dictated by pain only, with no restrictions. A rib belt and/or chest protector (in contact sports) may reduce the patient's pain (see Figure 15-6).

Rib Stress Fractures

CLINICAL PRESENTATION

History

Insidious onset of aching, often localized at the site of injury
Sudden-onset chest pain may be described.
A sudden, sometimes audible "snap" may be described.

Observation

A guarding posture may be assumed.

Functional Status

Pain may occur during deep inspiration.

Physical Evaluation Findings

Palpable tenderness may or may not be present over the fracture site.
Pain is possible with respiration, but respiration is normal.
Other physical findings may be normal.

Rib stress fractures are an uncommon response to repetitive-motion activities, resulting in muscle-distraction forces that cause bone fatigue. Although rib stress fractures are relatively rare in athletics, the onset is often sport-specific and position-related.

Baseball pitchers may develop a stress fracture of the first rib from maximal distraction between the upward and downward muscular forces on the rib.[6] The scalenus anticus and medius muscles appear to oppose the intercostal muscles and upper serratus anterior muscle to generate sufficient force to stress the first rib.[7] This process most commonly involves the nonthrowing arm but can affect either side.

Rowers most often fracture the fourth and fifth ribs. The mechanism relates to serratus anterior muscle forces (**Figure 15-7**). Lower rib fractures have been observed in golfers and from batting in baseball players. These also appear related to repetitive muscle-contraction forces.

Differential Diagnosis

Costochondritis, muscle strain

Imaging Techniques

Chest and rib radiographs are typically normal in stress fractures. Bone scan is the test of choice when radiographs are normal and the index of suspicion is high. Bone scanning is very sensitive for fractures but not specific. Although both sensitive and specific for fractures, CT is rarely necessary.

Definitive Diagnosis

A positive bone scan confirms the diagnosis.

Pathomechanics and Functional Limitations

Deep breathing and exertion of the thoracic muscles may produce pain.

■ Immediate Management

Immediate management consists of discontinuing participation, seeking medical attention, and pursuing diagnostic testing.

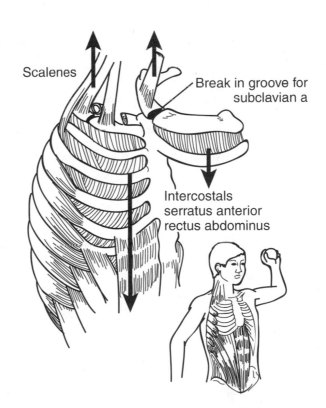

Figure 15-7 Rib stress fracture. Activities such as pitching may result in a stress fracture of the first rib. (Reproduced with permission from DeLee JC, Drez D (eds): *DeLee and Drez's Orthopedic Sports Medicine: Principles and Practices*. Philadelphia, PA, WB Saunders, 1994, p 577.)

■ Medications

Narcotics are rarely required for pain; NSAIDs are often useful for short periods. Intercostal nerve blocks are not warranted.

■ Medical Management

Rest and analgesic care are necessary until full pain relief is realized. Often rest without medication is sufficient.

■ Postinjury/Postoperative Management

Rest and NSAIDs with support during the healing process are indicated. Activities are permitted as pain allows; the condition tends to be self-limiting.

■ Injury-Specific Treatment and Rehabilitation Concerns

Aerobic activities and light-resistance upper extremity exercises are performed as pain allows. For pitchers, throwing rehabilitation should begin with a short-toss and long-toss program (see p 451). Advancement to the mound occurs with a throwing progression after a time of rest to allow fracture healing, typically 4 to 6 weeks.

■ Estimated Amount of Time Lost

Recovery takes approximately 4 to 6 weeks. The functional activities progression must be closely monitored. Any recurrent symptoms require activity modification to restore a pain-free mode. Fractures of the first rib in pitchers can be slow to respond.

■ Return-to-Play Criteria

The patient must be pain free, both to palpation and the activity stresses that caused the fracture.

Rib Fractures

Simple rib fractures are the most common injury after blunt chest trauma. Direct force to the chest wall results in nondisplaced or minimally displaced fractures at or near the point of impact. However, force transmission can result in a fracture anywhere along the rib.

The most frequent fracture sites are ribs four through nine. Fractures involving ribs one and two require considerable force and often result in injury to the underlying neurovascular structures. The flexibility of young children's rib cages makes them far less likely to fracture ribs than adults.

CLINICAL PRESENTATION

History
Blow to the chest
Chest pain
Pain increased with inspiration and forced exhalation

Observation
Respiratory muscle splinting
Possible ecchymosis
Possible swelling

Functional Status
Trunk motion reduced secondary to pain

Physical Evaluation Findings
Point tenderness over the fracture site
Pain with the rib compression test

Rib fractures to athletes occur primarily in contact and high-velocity sports. Rib fractures must always be considered as a possible indication of underlying organ injury. The number, location, and severity of the fractures must lead to a high index of suspicion; multiple fractures indicate greater force, with greater risk of underlying injury. Children require high forces to fracture ribs, increasing the potential for underlying organ damage.

Differential Diagnosis

Pneumothorax, myocardial contusion, pulmonary contusion, cardiac tamponade, costochondritis

Imaging Techniques

Chest radiographs reveal most rib fractures. Detailed rib radiographs are rarely needed but may be helpful in detecting fractures to ribs 1 and 2 and ribs 8 through 12. The possibility of a pneumothorax is increased when multiple ribs are fractured (**Figure 15-8**).

Chest radiographs repeated 2 to 3 days after injury may demonstrate the late development of intrathoracic injuries. Pneumothorax onset may be delayed for hours to days after the injury. Repeated chest radiographs are only recommended when the patient's clinical symptoms continue to suggest a rib fracture.

Definitive Diagnosis

The diagnosis is based on positive radiographic studies.

Pathomechanics and Functional Limitations

Pain limits activities. If the condition is the result of significant trauma, cardiovascular and pulmonary status must be monitored on an ongoing basis.

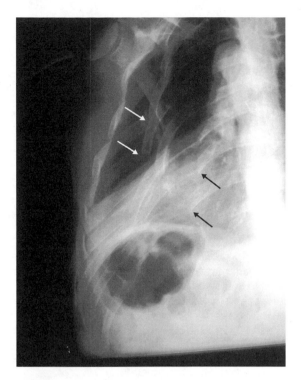

Figure 15-8   Rib fractures in a football player. Arrows indicate some of the fracture sites (not all fractures are labeled).

Immediate Management

The rate and quality of respiration are evaluated, and the pulse rate is documented. All athletic activity should be discontinued. The patient is monitored closely, with particular attention paid to the chest wall, looking for paradoxical motion that could indicate a flail chest. Physician evaluation is arranged.

Medications

Mild to moderate analgesics are usually all that is needed. Appropriate pain relief allows rest and helps normalize breathing. On occasion, intercostal nerve blocks can be administered to relieve pain.

Postinjury Management

Rest and pain relief are typically sufficient. A rib belt may be helpful in relieving pain (see Figure 15-6). However, some patients find the belt more irritating than helpful. If the patient feels the rib belt compromises breathing, its use should be discontinued.

Injury-Specific Treatment and Rehabilitation Concerns

General conditioning can resume as pain subsides. Typically aerobic activities are tolerated initially, followed by a progression of strength training, including trunk-stabilization exercises.

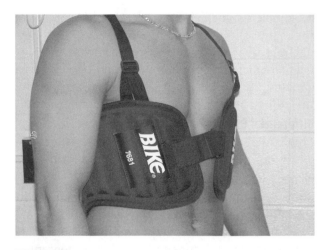

Figure 15-9   Protective rib vest. These devices can be used prophylactically to prevent rib and costochondral injuries or to prevent reinjury to these structures.

Estimated Amount of Time Lost

Pain relief is usually complete in 2 to 3 weeks. Noncontact sports may resume when pain relief is sufficient. Contact sports can normally be resumed after 3 weeks, but the patient will require rib-cage protection for 6 to 8 weeks after injury (**Figure 15-9**).

Return-to-Play Criteria

Return to activity must always be individualized according to the physical evaluation findings.

Sternal Fractures

CLINICAL PRESENTATION

History

Direct blow to the sternum
Cervical and thoracic spine hyperflexion
Complaints of sternal pain

Observation

Difficulty breathing
Swelling may develop.

Functional Status

Pain increases with respiration.
Initial shortness of breath

Physical Evaluation Findings

Anterior chest-wall tenderness
Crepitus with palpable deformity indicates displacement.

Sternal injuries can occur from direct forces, such as a football helmet or steering wheel, or indirect forces. Indirect force results from cervical and upper thoracic spine hyperflexion. The chin may strike the manubrium, driving it posteriorly.[7] Most sternal fractures involve the manubrium and midsternal body. Cervical, upper thoracic, and rib fractures and underlying soft-tissue damage may accompany this injury. Sternal fractures are extremely painful.

Differential Diagnosis

Myocardial contusion, pulmonary contusion, cardiac tamponade, rib fracture, costochondritis

Imaging Techniques

Posteroanterior and lateral chest radiographs with sternal views are usually diagnostic. Mediastinal widening on chest radiographs may indicate underlying great-vessel injury and mandate aortography.

Definitive Diagnosis

Diagnosis is based on positive radiographic findings.

Pathomechanics and Functional Limitations

This significant injury needs attentive monitoring. Activity restrictions are necessary, and functional progression is slow.

▒ Immediate Management

Participation is ceased, and the patient's pulse and respiration are monitored. Immediate medical attention is required, with diagnostic studies as needed.

▒ Medications

Analgesics may be prescribed as required for pain management; initial management may require narcotics. Later in the course of care, NSAIDs may be helpful to relieve discomfort.

▒ Medical Management

Nondisplaced sternal fractures typically respond to conservative management. Displaced fractures can be reduced using postural reduction. With the patient supine, a sandbag is placed transversely under the shoulders, slightly below the scapula.[7] The torso is hyperextended, and traction is then applied by pulling on the patient's arms (**Figure 15-10**). This reduction is used only in individuals with posterior manubrial displacement. With nondisplaced fractures and fractures that have been reduced, rest and analgesics are required. However, if underlying myocardial injury is suspected, appropriate testing should be instituted.

▒ Postinjury Management

Conservative care requires serial lateral chest radiographs approximately every 3 weeks until healing is complete. Noncontact activities are allowed as discomfort permits.

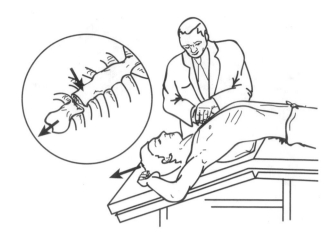

Figure 15-10 Reduction of a sternal fracture. If necessary, an assistant may apply traction by grasping the patient's arm at the axilla and pulling cephalad. Insert shows detail of the forces applied in reduction. (Reproduced with permission from DeLee JC, Drez D (eds): *DeLee and Drez's Orthopedic Sports Medicine: Principles and Practices.* Philadelphia, PA, WB Saunders, 1994, p 576.)

▒ Surgical Intervention

Surgical intervention is extremely rare and is reserved for individuals having gross displacement, with compromised respiratory function, severe pain, or nonunion. Via a midline incision over the sternum, the fracture is reduced and fixated with K-wires or a plate and screws.

▒ Postoperative Management

Surgical treatment also requires serial chest radiographs for evaluation of fracture healing and positioning. The wires or pin and plate must also be monitored.

▒ Injury-Specific Treatment and Rehabilitation Concerns

Aerobic exercise is permitted as tolerated. Initially, noncontact activities such as stationary bicycling are initiated, followed by running activities. Strength training as tolerated begins with the lower extremities, followed by trunk and upper extremity strengthening as healing allows.

▒ Estimated Amount of Time Lost

Depending on the treatment method used, 6 to 12 weeks may be required before competition can be resumed. Internal fixation, especially with K-wires, necessitates closer follow-up and no contact activities until the wires are removed.

■ Return-to-Play Criteria

Noncontact sports are allowed as tolerated. Contact sports require 6 to 12 weeks before returning, depending on pain relief and radiographic evidence of healing. Contact-sport athletes need protection similar to that described for rib fractures (eg, flak jacket, see Figure 15-9).

Flail Chest

CLINICAL PRESENTATION

History

High-velocity blunt impact to the ribs
Chest pain

Observation

Chest-wall deformity

Functional Status

Labored breathing

Physical Evaluation Findings

Chest-wall tenderness
Abnormal, segmented chest-wall motion (paradoxical breathing)
Flail-chest findings can be delayed as long as 10 days after injury.

Flail chest is the result of a severe, direct impact to the rib cage with fractures of four or more ribs in two or more places (**Figure 15-11**).[8] Because of the resulting paradoxical motion of the fractured segment of ribs, this is the most serious chest-wall injury. During inspiration and expiration, the fractured section of the ribs moves separately and in the opposite direction from the rest of the rib cage. This causes difficulty in breathing, due to diminished chest expansion with increased energy expenditure.

Because of the severe trauma, underlying lung injury is common. Pulmonary contusion occurs in about one half of patients with flail chest. Pneumothorax and hemothorax occur in more than 70% of patients.[9]

Imaging Techniques

Chest radiographs are necessary to evaluate rib fractures and lung fields. Rib radiographs may provide better detail of the fracture sites. CT is more accurate than plain films and may be necessary to further evaluate the lung parenchyma.

Definitive Diagnosis

Diagnosis is based on clinical evaluation supported by chest radiographs.

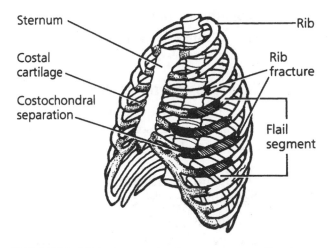

Figure 15-11 Flail chest occurs when four or more consecutive ribs are fractured in two or more places.

Pathomechanics and Functional Limitations

This injury results in loss of rib-cage integrity, compromising the ability to protect thoracic organs and maintain respiratory function. Long-term functional respiratory loss and chest deformity are common.

■ Immediate Management

Immediate management consists of maintaining airways and monitoring vital signs. A pillow placed over the flail segment may relieve pain and ease breathing.[8] The patient must be immediately transported via EMS.

■ Medications

Pain management is paramount for successful conservative management; IV narcotics and NSAIDs are most effective. Intercostal blocks, intrapleural analgesia, and patient-controlled analgesia such as procedural sedation and analgesia (PSA) pumps are all helpful.

■ Medical Management

Medical treatment requires aggressive pulmonary therapy with suctioning, incentive spirometry, early mobilization, and air humidification.[9] Effective analgesia is also important. Close observation is required to detect possible respiratory decompensation, which is an indication for endotracheal intubation and positive-pressure mechanical ventilation. Oxygen supplementation is provided to keep oxygen saturation above 90%.

15

■ Surgical Intervention

Surgical fixation with K-wires, plates, and screws to stabilize the fractures is rarely indicated.

■ Postinjury/Postoperative Management

Chest-wall protection is required for return to contact sports. A flak jacket or some other form of protection is adequate.

■ Injury-Specific Treatment and Rehabilitation Concerns

Slow progression of aerobic activity begins upon hospital discharge. The progression is in accordance with patient tolerance and fracture healing.

■ Estimated Amount of Time Lost

Splenomegaly Enlargement of the spleen.

Fracture healing requires approximately 8 weeks. Contact sports may resume approximately 3 months after injury or once complete healing is verified.

■ Return-to-Play Criteria

The patient may return to competition after clinical and radiographic evidence of complete fracture healing along with adequate sport-specific conditioning have been attained.

Spleen Injury

CLINICAL PRESENTATION

History

Mechanism of direct trauma to the abdomen or left upper quadrant
Pain in the upper left quadrant and left shoulder (Kerr sign)
A recent history of mononucleosis increases the risk of splenic trauma.

Observation

A contusion may be noted over the point of contact.
Abdominal guarding

Functional Status

Lightheadedness
Malaise
Fatigue

Physical Evaluation Findings

Point tenderness of the ribs overlying the spleen
Tenderness in the left upper abdomen
Abdominal rigidity may be noted
Hypotension
Tachycardia

Spleen injury usually results from direct abdominal force but can also occur secondary to rapid acceleration or deceleration. Most commonly, the left upper quadrant is injured by a deceleration mechanism or by displacement of left lower rib fractures, most commonly the fifth through ninth ribs; this mechanism is seen primarily in contact sports or high-speed, noncontact sports.[2]

Injury results in spleen contusion, subcapsular hematoma, rupture, or laceration. Hematoma with delayed rupture at an interval of days to weeks after injury occurs in 10% to 15% of patients. The spleen is a very vascular organ, receiving 5% of the cardiac output, primarily via the splenic artery. Accordingly, immediate and serious bleeding is common after splenic trauma.

The spleen is at particular risk when mononucleosis or another viral-related splenomegaly develops. Splenomegaly makes the spleen much more vulnerable to injury and to rupture. Therefore, patients with splenomegaly should be prohibited from contact sports until the spleen has returned to normal size.

Differential Diagnosis

Abdominal wall contusion; rib fracture; intercostal muscle strain; liver, kidney, intestines, diaphragm injuries

Medical Diagnostic Tests

Diagnostic peritoneal lavage, the test of choice in hemodynamically unstable patients, is an invasive procedure in which a catheter is placed within the peritoneal cavity. Aspiration of peritoneal blood indicates abdominal bleeding, but this finding is nonspecific.

Imaging Techniques

Improved imaging techniques have contributed vastly to the nonsurgical treatment of splenic injury. Ultrasonography is widely used in Europe and is gaining favor in the US. It can be done quickly in the emergency room, providing evidence of large amounts of abdominal fluid. Ultrasound may be helpful in determining the need for laparotomy in an unstable patient. Ultrasound can also be spleen-specific, indicating enlargement, progressive enlargement, irregular borders, and contour change, all indications of bleeding. However, the accuracy of the ultrasonic image is operator-dependent.

CT is the imaging modality of choice in hemodynamically stable patients. CT can be performed quickly with current-generation scanners, and both oral and IV contrast should be used. CT is excellent for detecting both large and small volumes of intra-abdominal blood and can be very specific for detecting splenic contusion, rupture, or laceration. CT has been instrumental in reducing the number of laparotomies in stable patients with low-grade spleen injuries, allowing the surgeon to assess and reassess the injury.

Definitive Diagnosis

The definitive diagnosis is based on positive CT scan or, in the case of a hemodynamically unstable patient with left upper abdominal trauma, bloody peritoneal lavage.

Pathomechanics and Functional Limitations

Pneumovax is recommended for spleen injuries, as well as for patients who have had their spleen removed for any reason. A heightened awareness of the immune-compromised state of these individuals is important; they may require quicker implementation of antibiotic coverage for potential bacterial illness.

■ Immediate Management

The patient's abdomen should be evaluated and checked thoroughly for signs of injury. Pulse rate, respiration rate, and blood pressure should be monitored and recorded. If an injury is suspected, the patient should be immediately transported to an emergency room. On the field, CPR protocol must be followed until EMS transport. The patient is placed in the Trendelenburg position if tachycardia or hypotension is noted (**Figure 15-12**).

■ Medications

Postoperative pain management with narcotics will likely be required. The routine use of long-term prophylactic antibiotics after splenectomy is controversial. Antibiotics (eg, amoxicillin) should be administered to any asplenic individual with the

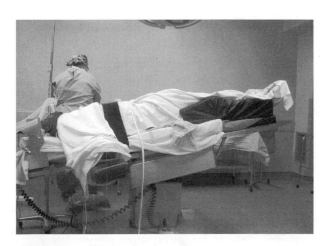

Figure 15-12 The Trendelenburg position.

first sign of infection (eg, fever, sore throat) to reduce the risk of developing postsplenectomy sepsis. Vaccinations (for pneumonia, *Haemophilus influenzae B*, and meningococcus) should also be given to a patient after splenectomy to minimize the risk of infection.

■ Medical Management

The management goal is to stop the internal bleeding and preserve the spleen.[7] Nonsurgical management is successful in 90% of children and up to 70% of adults. Although failure of conservative management most often occurs within 48 to 72 hours, late ruptures do occur and have been reported 2 weeks to several months later.

For nonsurgical management to be feasible, the patient must be hemodynamically stable without hypotension, hypovolemia, head injury, or coagulopathy. The best candidate for conservative management is a young, hemodynamically stable patient with an isolated splenic injury. Hypotension is an indication for surgical intervention.

The patient should have a large-bore IV line. Monitoring ideally occurs in the intensive care unit. Initial laboratory tests include complete blood count, urinalysis, and chemistry panel with liver enzymes. Hemoglobin and hematocrit (H/H) should be ordered every 6 hours for 24 hours. If the patient remains stable, the H/H should then be checked every 12 hours. A stable H/H and decreased abdominal pain can be expected in the first 12 hours. Strict bed rest is maintained for 2 to 3 days. The patient must refrain from oral intake until the need for surgery has been definitively eliminated and there is no sign of ileus.

Follow-up CT is recommended 3 to 5 days after injury, followed by serial evaluations. These should show signs of improvement, with hematoma resolution and normal parenchymal structure. With successful conservative management, hospitalization lasts approximately 5 to 10 days.

■ Surgical Intervention

Surgical intervention is necessary if the patient presents to the emergency room hemodynamically unstable or becomes unstable after attempts at conservative management. Other indications for surgery include decreasing hemoglobin, increasing abdominal tenderness, and persistent hypotension, tachycardia, and hypovolemia. Patients older than 55 years are more likely to require splenectomy than younger individuals.

Pneumovax A vaccination used to prevent or manage a broad range of pneumonia-causing bacteria.

Coagulopathy A disorder of the blood-clotting mechanism.

Two large-bore, peripheral IVs must be placed; prophylactic antibiotics are commonly administered perioperatively. A generous upper midline abdominal incision is typically used, with extension as needed to evaluate for other injuries. Spleen mobilization allows full spleen inspection. Laparoscopic splenectomy may be an option for the hemodynamically stable patient and allow an earlier return to athletic competition.

Surgical treatment may include suture repair (splenorrhaphy), topical and intraparenchymal application of clotting agents, and wrapping the spleen in mesh with partial resection. If the bleeding persists or the spleen is shattered, it should be removed without attempts at preservation (**Table 15-1**).

■ Postinjury/Postoperative Management

Hospitalization lasts approximately 5 to 10 days. The patient's hemodynamic status is followed closely, with repeat CT to confirm healing. After returning home, rest is recommended with slow progression of activities of daily living. No exertional activities, such as lifting, pushing, or pulling, are permitted until cleared by the surgeon.

■ Injury-Specific Treatment and Rehabilitation Concerns

With nonsurgical treatment, the primary concern is rebleeding. Close monitoring of activities is important, with the patient instructed to report symptoms and complaints promptly. Both nonsurgical and surgical care result in an extended convalescence, which causes cardiovascular and musculoskeletal detraining. Consequently, endurance training and trunk strengthening must be emphasized once the patient recovers sufficiently. Surgical treatment requires observation and management of the incision, with sutures removed at 7 to 10 days. Daily living activities are allowed with slow progression, as with conservative management.

■ Estimated Amount of Time Lost

With a mild splenic contusion, the patient is withheld from sports activity for 2 to 3 weeks. Patients with a significant injury who are treated conservatively should refrain from strenuous activity for 6 weeks, with no contact sports for up to 4 months. This time varies, however, depending on the results of follow-up CT. Laparotomy patients are not allowed strenuous activity for 4 to 6 weeks after surgery, and should not participate in contact sports for up to 2 to 3 months.

■ Return-to-Play Criteria

A CT scan 6 weeks after injury in patients treated conservatively is helpful in determining readiness for progression in conditioning and training. Surgical patients are prohibited from strenuous activity during the early postoperative period to ensure healing. Contact should be restricted for 2 to 3 months following surgery. Conditioning should be maintained once strenuous activities are allowed.

Table 15-1		

Spleen Injury Scale

Grade*		Injury Description
I	Hematoma	Subcapsular, nonexpanding, <10% surface area
	Laceration	Capsular tear, nonbleeding, <1 cm parenchymal depth
II	Hematoma	Subcapsular, nonexpanding, 10% to 50% surface area; intraparenchymal, nonexpanding, <5 cm in diameter
	Laceration	Capsular tear, active bleeding 1 to 3 cm parenchymal depth that does not involve a trabecular vessel
III	Hematoma	Subcapsular, >50% surface area or expanding; ruptured subcapsular hematoma with active bleeding; intraparenchymal hematoma >5 cm or expanding
	Laceration	>3 cm parenchymal depth or involving trabecular vessels
IV	Hematoma	Ruptured intraparenchymal hematoma with active bleeding
	Laceration	Laceration involving segmental or hilar vessels producing major devascularization (>25% of spleen)
V	Laceration	Completely shattered spleen
	Vascular	Hilar vascular injury that devascularizes spleen

* Advance one grade for multiple pnjuries up to grade III.

Reproduced with permission from Moore EE, Cogbill TH, Jurkovich GL et al: Organ injury scaling: Spleen and liver. *J Trauma* 1995;38:323.

Renal Trauma

CLINICAL PRESENTATION

History

Blunt trauma over the area of either kidney
Abdominal pain
Flank pain

Observation

Flank contusion or ecchymosis

Functional Status

Pain with trunk motion

Physical Evaluation Findings

Costovertebral angle tenderness
Abdominal mass
Urinalysis revealing gross or microscopic hematuria

Blunt force causes 80% of renal trauma, and 30% of renal injuries are sport-related. Blunt trauma is more prevalent in males, which appears to be related to their greater contact-sport participation. As in other types of abdominal trauma, injury mechanisms include a direct blow to the flank from rapid deceleration or a penetrating rib fracture.[2] The degree of renal injury depends on the amount of applied force.

Children have a higher rate of injury to the kidneys than to the spleen or liver. The explanation may be that children have less protective tissue and a large kidney size relative to trunk size. In blunt trauma, left kidney injury coexists with spleen injury roughly 30% of the time. Right kidney injury coexists with liver injury approximately 40% of the time.

Differential Diagnosis

Urinary tract infection, rib fractures, lumbar strain, muscle contusion

Medical Diagnostic Tests

Urinalysis often reveals gross or microscopic hematuria, but 25% to 40% of patients have normal urinalyses.

Imaging Techniques

Improved imaging and staging have resulted in a trend toward conservative management. Chest radiographs may reveal lower rib fractures. Lumbar spine radiographs help to evaluate possible transverse-process fractures, which are commonly associated with renal trauma. An abdominal flat-plate radiograph (also known as a KUB: kidney, ureter, bladder) may reveal a psoas shadow or loss of the renal outline.

A CT scan with IV contrast enhancement is the gold standard for evaluating renal trauma. Diagnostic accuracy is 98%, and it is excellent for identifying the extent of injury and assessing urinary extravasation.

Renal arteriograms are rarely needed. The main indication is a grade IV or V injury with planned partial nephrectomy or selective embolization. Intravenous pyelography has been replaced primarily by CT. However, pyelography can be very helpful in evaluating kidney function and gross urinary extravasation in the patient who requires emergency laparotomy for other intra-abdominal injuries.

Definitive Diagnosis

A positive CT scan provides the definitive diagnosis.

Pathomechanics and Functional Limitations

Renal trauma results in mild to severe pain; physical limitation will likewise vary. However, because of the potentially adverse prognosis, the patient must limit all activities and be monitored closely until bleeding resolves.

◼ Immediate Management

The patient's abdomen should be evaluated and checked thoroughly for signs of injury. Pulse rate, respiration rate, and blood pressure should be monitored and recorded. If an injury is suspected, the patient should be immediately transported to an emergency room. On the field, CPR protocol must be followed until EMS transport. The patient is placed in the Trendelenburg position if tachycardia or hypotension is noted (Figure 15-12).

◼ Medical Management

Approximately 80% of all patients with renal trauma can be treated conservatively. The kidney has a great capacity for spontaneous healing, and late complications are infrequent. Also, the successful use of embolization procedures, stenting, and percutaneous drainage has decreased the need for surgery. Renal lacerations, even with wide fragment separation, may exhibit spontaneous resolution.[10] However, surgical intervention is necessary in hemodynamically unstable patients with hilar or pedicle injuries.

Hematuria is the key indicator of renal trauma. Gross hematuria is a sign of significant injury, but microscopic hematuria should not be disregarded and deserves appropriate follow-up and workup. Significant vascular renal injury can occur without hematuria.

As with all abdominal injuries, adequate hemodynamic stability must be maintained through IV

Nephrectomy Surgical removal of a kidney.

Embolization Blocking an artery or vein by use of a foreign material.

Pyelography Radiographs of the kidney and ureter after the injection of a radiopaque dye.

Hematuria Microscopic or macroscopic blood in the urine.

15

Table 15-2

Renal Injury Scale

Grade*		Injury Description
I	Contusion	Microscopic or gross hematuria; urologic studies normal
	Hematoma	Subcapsular, nonexpanding without parenchymal laceration
II	Hematoma	Nonexpanding perirenal hematoma confined to the renal retroperitoneum
	Laceration	<1 cm parenchymal depth of renal cortex without urinary extravasation
III	Laceration	>1 cm parenchymal depth of renal cortex without collecting-system rupture or urinary extravasation
IV	Laceration	Parenchymal laceration extending through the renal cortex, medulla, and collecting system
	Vascular	Main renal artery or vein injury with contained hemorrhage
V	Laceration	Completely shattered kidney
	Vascular	Avulsion of renal hilum with devascularized kidney

* Advance one grade for multiple injuries to the same organ.

Reproduced with permission from Moore EE, Shackford SR, Pachter HL et al: Organ injury scaling: Spleen, liver, and kidney. *J Trauma* 1989;29:1664.

fluid replacement and maintenance. Typical routine blood tests are performed. Treatment regimens for renal injury are categorized by grade (**Table 15-2**).

Postinjury/Postoperative Management

If surgery is performed, wound care is necessary. With conservative management, bed rest is ordered until gross hematuria resolves. Limited activities are then allowed until microscopic hematuria resolves, which may take up to 4 weeks.

Injury-Specific Treatment and Rehabilitation Concerns

Return to activity should be graduated, with aerobic exercise followed by strength training and specific trunk-stabilization exercises.

Estimated Amount of Time Lost

A patient who has sustained a mild renal injury may return to activity in 2 to 4 weeks if microscopic hematuria has subsided. A severe renal injury usually resolves in 6 to 8 weeks. Return to sport activities requires complete healing with no microscopic hematuria and CT evidence of full resolution.

Return-to-Play Criteria

After surgery, 8 to 12 weeks may be needed before the patient can return to contact sports. No microscopic hematuria should be present, and a CT scan should be obtained to document full healing. Conservatively managed renal trauma can result in full resolution of microscopic hematuria, along with a normal CT scan, allowing return to sport activity in 4 to 6 weeks.

A patient who has only one functioning kidney should avoid high-impact contact sports. Most leagues disqualify individuals with only one functioning kidney from high-risk sports. Noncontact sports need not be restricted.

Abdominal Sports Hernia

CLINICAL PRESENTATION

History

Pain in lower abdominal, medial inguinal, and pubic region
Symptoms aggravated by sudden propulsive movements such as kicking

Observation

No visible abnormalities

Functional Status

Pain and tenderness with resisted sit-ups or resisted trunk rotation

Physical Evaluation Findings

Tender medial inguinal canal, lower rectus abdominus, and pubic region
Palpable gap over the external oblique and a dilated external ring
Absence of hernia bulge

Groin injuries that involve the lower abdominal and inguinal region may result in a syndrome of chronic exertional pain that has been termed abdominal sports hernia, athletic hernia, and athletic pubalgia. These injuries occur most commonly in sports associated with repetitive twisting or turning motions, such as soccer and ice hockey. Pathologic findings in

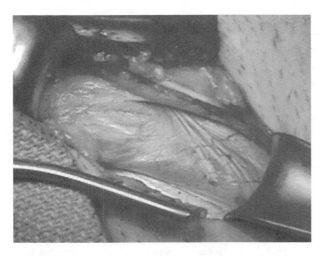

Figure 15-13 Attenuated external oblique aponeurosis in the left inguinal canal in a patient with an abdominal sports hernia.

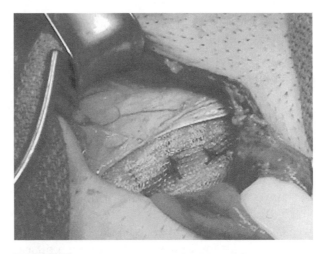

Figure 15-14 The reconstructed inguinal floor is shown, with polypropylene mesh placed deep to the external oblique layer.

the groin at surgical exploration have included a torn external oblique aponeurosis (**Figure 15-13**), torn conjoined tendon, torn conjoined tendon from the pubic tubercle, torn internal oblique muscle, disrupted posterior inguinal floor but without a direct hernia, and ilioinguinal nerve entrapment by scar tissue.

Symptom onset in athletic pubalgia may be either acute or insidious without a specific precipitating event. The pain is usually in the medial inguinal and pubic regions, occurring principally with the initial propulsive movements in running or skating. Associated adductor symptoms and adductor strain are common. Examination findings are subtle and variable but may include any or all of the features listed below. It is important to exclude an inguinal hernia on examination.

Differential Diagnosis

Muscle strain, femoral hernia, inguinal hernia, osteitis pubis, pelvic stress fracture, hip arthritis, hip adductor muscle strain

Imaging Techniques

If symptoms persist, pelvic magnetic resonance imaging (MRI) should be obtained to exclude other abnormalities. Plain pelvic radiographs may be done initially. Bone scan may be performed as an alternative to MRI to evaluate for osteitis pubis.

Definitive Diagnosis

The diagnosis is usually one of exclusion, based on history, physical examination, and imaging studies. Radiographs, MRI, and bone scan of the pelvis help to exclude other possible diagnoses.

Pathomechanics and Functional Limitations

Initially, the patient may complain of discomfort with squatting, walking stairs, and torso rotation. Most commonly, daily activities are asymptomatic.

The patient only complains with sport-specific activities (eg, agility activities, kicking, sprinting).

■ Immediate Management

Rest, NSAIDs, and avoidance of aggravating activities are recommended.

■ Medications

NSAIDs may be helpful.

■ Postinjury Management

Initial treatment is conservative—rest, NSAIDs, and ultrasound. Conservative management focuses on trunk stabilization and lower abdominal and adductor strength and flexibility. Patients whose limiting symptoms continue after 8 weeks or more of conservative management should be considered for surgical repair.

■ Surgical Intervention

Surgical options include primary pelvic-floor repair, open mesh repair, and laparoscopic posterior mesh repair (**Figure 15-14**). Other procedures carried out in some patients in conjunction with pelvic-floor repair include ilioinguinal neurolysis and adductor release.

■ Postoperative Management

In the early postoperative period, patients should be observed for wound healing and signs of infection. Active abdominal exercises and heavy lifting should be avoided for 4 to 6 weeks to allow adequate tissue healing. Rehabilitation can begin in approximately 2 weeks, when the patient is relatively pain free and wound healing is complete.

15

■ Injury-Specific Treatment and Rehabilitation Concerns

After surgical repair, rest and normal light activities are recommended for 2 weeks. Then the patient can start walking on a treadmill, progressing gradually to jogging, stationary bicycling, and pool walking. Ice should be applied to the surgical site after each workout. At 3 to 4 weeks, ultrasound and active release techniques for scar tissue at the groin site are used as needed. If necessary, NSAIDs may be continued. Progression to full activity and strength training should be as tolerated during weeks 4 through 8. Players who have had an athletic pubalgia-type injury should undergo offseason sport-specific training annually, with attention to lower abdominal and adductor strength and flexibility work to prevent recurrence or injury to the contralateral groin.

■ Estimated Amount of Time Lost

Approximately 16 weeks of activity are usually missed. A trial of conservative management should be instituted for 8 weeks, followed by 8 weeks of postoperative management if surgery is required.

■ Return-to-Play Criteria

With conservative management, return to play is allowed after symptoms have resolved. After surgery, play can resume once rehabilitation has been completed and the patient can perform normal sport activity without symptoms, usually 7 to 10 weeks after surgery.

Functional Bracing

Compression shorts may be warranted for approximately 1 year after injury (see Figure 8-3).

Inguinal Hernia

Groin hernias can occur as congenital or acquired defects. They are classified as indirect inguinal, direct inguinal, or femoral hernias (**Figure 15-15**). Most groin hernias that occur in children and young adults are indirect hernias, in which the internal inguinal ring is dilated with peritoneal protrusion into the inguinal canal. Direct hernias are the result of an acquired weakness in the transversalis fascia and floor of the inguinal canal. Femoral hernias occur almost exclusively in women and are uncommon before age 30 years; these have a high rate of **incarceration**.

Incarceration A confined or restricted hernia that is difficult to reduce.

CLINICAL PRESENTATION

History

Pain may be described as arising from the inguinal canal area, although pain may not be described by all patients.

Observation

Visible bulge around the inguinal ligament
The bulge increases with exertion and reduces with relaxation or recumbency.

Functional Status

Aching pain exacerbated by physical exertion

Physical Evaluation Findings

Tenderness and a palpable mass in the lower abdomen and/or scrotum; the mass increases with coughing and diminishes in the supine position.

A history of groin pain in combination with a noticeable bulge is present in most individuals. However, some patients may have only an asymptomatic bulge or pain without a visible bulge. Symptoms may be aggravated by strenuous physical activity. If present, the hernia bulge usually disappears when the individual is in the recumbent position. Incarceration or strangulation is a risk of any groin hernia but is not a common occurrence in young, athletically active individuals. Risk factors for hernia development, such as chronic cough or constipation, should be considered.

Differential Diagnosis

Hydrocele, lipoma, appendicitis, testicular torsion, testicular or scrotal disease

Definitive Diagnosis

The definitive diagnosis is based on the clinical findings.

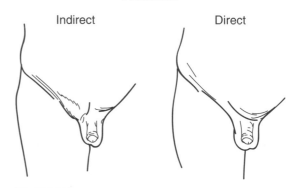

INGUINAL

Indirect   Direct

Figure 15-15 Direct and indirect hernia. Differentiation between these hernias is not always clinically possible. Understanding their features, however, improves your observation. (Reproduced with permission from Bates, B: *A Guide to Physical Examination*, ed 3. Philadelphia, PA, JB Lippincott, 1983, p 272.)

Pathomechanics and Functional Limitations

The condition results in weakness or tearing of the pelvic-wall or pelvic-floor musculature, with permanent or recurrent intestinal protrusion through the opening. Exertion increases abdominal pressure, and pain limits function.

Immediate Management

Physical examination should be performed to confirm the presence of a hernia and to determine if it is reducible. Patients with suspected groin hernias should be referred to a general surgeon for further evaluation. An acutely symptomatic patient with increased pain and an incarcerated hernia should be seen emergently by a general surgeon.

Medications

The patient requires postoperative pain management, typically the short-term use of narcotics.

Surgical Intervention

An inguinal hernia in an athlete should be surgically repaired. The repair may be carried out on an elective basis (ie, in the off-season) unless the hernia is incarcerated or symptoms limit activity. If the repair is delayed, athletic activity can continue as tolerated. An athletic truss may provide some temporary symptomatic benefit but will not prevent hernia progression or enlargement.

Surgical options include open repair under local anesthesia with sedation and laparoscopic repair under general anesthesia. Most inguinal hernia repairs in adults are performed using a tension-free, mesh-repair technique. In children and teenagers who are still growing, primary tissue repair is usually preferred.

Active abdominal exercises and heavy lifting should be avoided for 2 to 3 weeks after laparoscopic procedures and 4 to 6 weeks after open procedures to allow adequate tissue healing. Forceful Valsalva maneuvers should also be avoided during the first 7 to 14 days.

Postinjury/Postoperative Management

The patient should be monitored for wound healing, infection, hematoma, and return of bowel function the first week.

Injury-Specific Treatment and Rehabilitation Concerns

Light activities are permitted for the first 7 to 14 days after repair. Return to exercise can begin after 7 to 15 days, starting with cardiovascular conditioning and progressing to strength and functional training over 3 to 4 weeks, according to comfort level. The patient must avoid all strenuous activity, such as heavy lifting, pushing, and pulling for 2 to 3 weeks. A slow, progressive trunk-stabilization program can begin 3 weeks after surgery. The patient should apply ice after activity and use NSAIDs as needed.

Estimated Amount of Time Lost

Time lost varies but can be 4 to 7 weeks, depending on the type of repair. Laparoscopic repair may result in a more rapid return to unrestricted exercise and competitive play, as early as 3 to 4 weeks after surgery.

Return-to-Play Criteria

Return to sport is based on exercise tolerance and ability to progress with pain-free exercise.

References

1. Mullins RJ: Management of shock, in Mattox KL, Feliciano DV, Moore EE (eds): *Trauma*, ed 4. New York, NY, McGraw-Hill, 2000, pp 195-232.
2. Amaral JF: Thoracoabdominal injuries in the athlete. *Clin Sports Med* 1997;16:379-753.
3. Ferro RT, McKeag DB: Neck pain and dyspnea in a swimmer. *Physician Sportsmed* 1999;27:67-71.
4. Curtin SM, Tucker AM, Gens DR: Pneumothorax in sports. *Physician Sportsmed* 2000;28:23-32.
5. Richardson JD, Spain DA: Injury to the lung and pleura, in Mattox KL, Feliciano CV, Moore EE (eds): *Trauma*, ed 4. New York, NY, McGraw-Hill, 2000, pp 523-547.
6. Brukner P, Khan K, Sutton J: *Clinical Sports Medicine*. New York, NY, McGraw-Hill, 1993, pp 258-264.
7. Lyons FR: *Orthopaedic Sports Medicine: Principles and Practice*. Philadelphia, PA, WB Saunders, 1994, pp 572-579.
8. Martin SL, Stewart RM: Chest and thorax injuries, in Schenck RC Jr (ed): *Athletic Training and Sports Medicine*, ed 3. Rosemont, IL, American Academy of Orthopaedic Surgeons, 1999, pp 356-377.
9. Cogbill TH, Landercasper J: Injury to the chest wall, in Mattox KL, Feliciano DV, Moore EE (eds): *Trauma*, ed 4. New York, NY, McGraw-Hill, 2000, pp 483-505.
10. Peterson NE: Genitourinary trauma, in Mattox KL, Feliciano DV, Moore EE (eds): *Trauma*, ed 4. New York, NY, McGraw-Hill, 2000, pp 839-874.

15

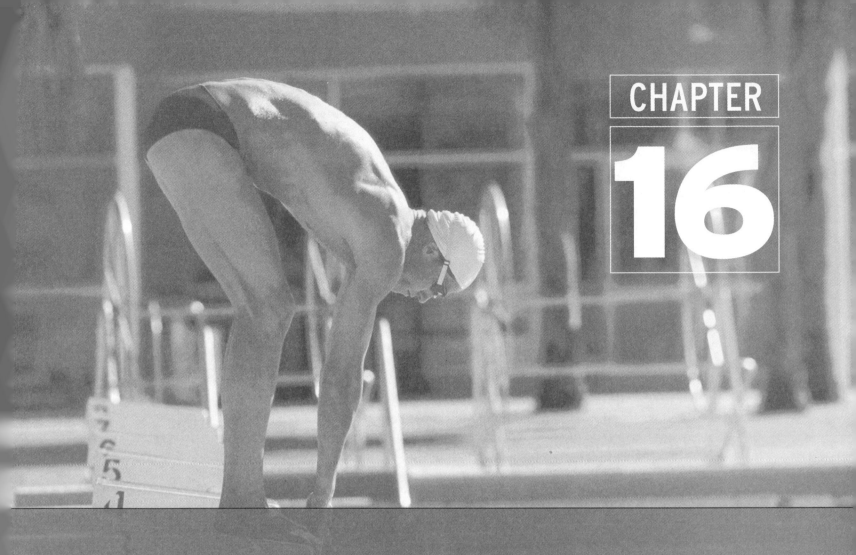

Cervical Spine Injuries

Katie Walsh, EdD, ATC
Stuart Lee, MD, FACS

Cervical Spine Fractures and Dislocations

Cervical spine fractures may or may not be associated with spinal cord injury. Unsupervised sports such as diving, surfing, and downhill skiing present the greatest risk for cervical spine fractures and dislocations. However, spinal injuries that occur during organized activities such as football, rugby, soccer, and ice hockey receive greater attention despite their relative infrequency.

The nature and treatment of cervical spine fractures depend on their location. Fractures and dislocations of the upper cervical spine (C1 and C2) are unique because of the anatomy of the craniocervical junction and the atlantoaxial junction. These fractures must be considered separately from fractures and dislocations of the lower cervical spine. Fractures of the spinous or transverse processes produce significant pain and limitations in range of motion (ROM) but do not often carry the threat of permanent disability associated with fractures or dislocations of the vertebral body.

The standard on-field and clinical evaluation techniques of palpation and ROM testing must be undertaken with caution in a patient with acute cervical spine trauma. Using too much pressure while palpating can dislodge a bony fragment and cause more severe trauma. In the presence of unstable vertebral segments or fracture, ROM testing can further traumatize the spinal cord. At the first sign of injury to a cervical vertebra or the spinal cord, the patient should be immediately immobilized and transported to an appropriate medical facility.

The general description of the immediate, on-field management of cervical spine injuries is provided on p 545 of this chapter. Also refer to p 569 of chapter 18 for information regarding the management of head injuries.

Upper Cervical Spine Fractures and Dislocations

▦ C1 Fractures

Fractures of the atlas (C1) account for 1% to 2% of all spinal fractures.[1,2] The most common C1 fracture is the Jefferson fracture, a bilateral fracture of the C1 ring caused by a blow to the top of the head producing an axial load in the cervical vertebrae (**Figure 16-1**). This can occur in diving injuries or in football, particularly when "spear tackling."

CLINICAL PRESENTATION

History

Significant neck pain associated with pain on any attempt to turn or rotate the head

Observation

The patient may posture the cervical spine and skull for comfort. No visible sign of injury may be noted.

Functional Status

Because this injury does not always present as traumatically as a lower cervical spine fracture, the patient may, in fact, attempt to return to play.

Any patient with a history of spearing and subsequent neck pain should be fully evaluated before a return-to-play decision is made.

Physical Evaluation Findings

Most fractures of C1 do not cause neurologic deficit because of the large spinal canal at the C1 level; the nature of these fractures tends to actually enlarge the spinal canal.

ROM tests should not be performed in patients with suspected cervical spine fractures or dislocations.

Differential Diagnosis

Neck strain, cervical sprain, cervical spasm

Imaging Techniques

The role of imaging in the diagnosis of C1 fractures has changed over time. Historically, the diagnosis and management of C1 fractures has been based on cervical spine radiographs, particularly the open-mouth odontoid view. If the sum of the displacement

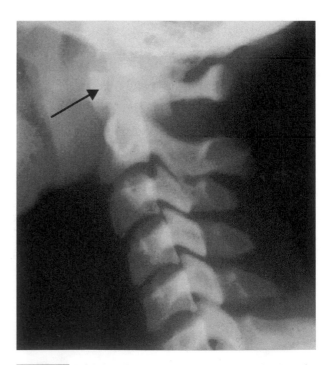

Figure 16-1 Lateral cervical spine radiograph showing a fracture of the arch of C1.

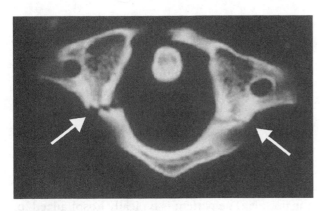

Figure 16-2 Axial CT image highlighting bilateral C1 ring fractures.

of the lateral masses of C1 over C2 is greater than 8.1 mm, taking into account magnification of the film, then the fracture is considered unstable.[2] Fractures with less lateral displacement of C1 over C2 are considered relatively stable.

The definitive evaluation of C1 fractures has been significantly aided by computed tomography (CT) and magnetic resonance imaging (MRI).[3] The ring of C1 and the fracture can be evaluated with CT scans (**Figure 16-2**). With the advent of CT technology, unilateral fractures of C1 have been shown to be more common than previously thought. The three-dimensional reconstructions available with CT allow excellent visualization of the displacement of the lateral masses of C1 over C2. MRI is useful in the diagnosis of C1 fractures

to determine if the transverse ligament of the atlas is disrupted, a determinant of fracture stability.

Definitive Diagnosis

Positive findings on radiographs, CT, or MRI (for soft-tissue and spinal cord injuries)

Pathomechanics and Functional Limitations

The loss of integrity of the C1 vertebral arch creates potential rotational instability between the C1 and C2 vertebrae. Subsequent force to the cervical spine can result in a dislocation and cause permanent spinal cord injury and/or death.

The patient experiences severe pain on cervical motion, especially rotation or flexion. Spasm of the cervical spine muscles limits motion. Trunk rotation substitutes for cervical and capital rotation.

■ Postinjury Management

The treatment of most C1 fractures is a rigid collar, such as an Aspen or Miami J collar (**Figure 16-3**), worn for 8 to 12 weeks, with follow-up radiographs every 2 to 4 weeks to evaluate fracture healing and determine if the amount of dislocation has increased.

In patients whose fractures are deemed unstable, with probable disruption of the transverse ligament (based on MRI or displacement of the lateral masses of C1 on C2), halo immobilization is recommended for 8 to 12 weeks, followed by a period of time in a rigid collar (see Surgical Intervention).

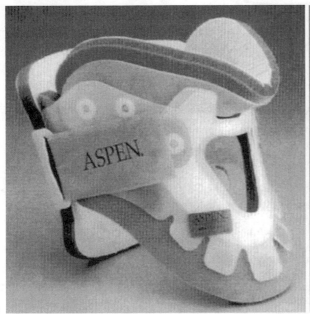
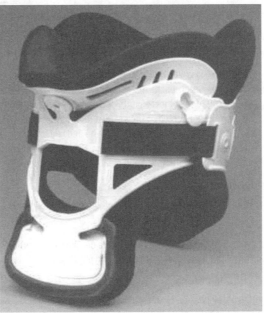

Figure 16-3 Cervical collars. **A.** Aspen collar. **B.** Miami collar.

■ Medications

Acute pain management is achieved by the use of nonsteroidal anti-inflammatory drugs (NSAIDs) and narcotic analgesics as needed. Muscle relaxants may be prescribed to treat acute muscle spasm.

■ Surgical Intervention

Surgical intervention is rarely necessary for C1 fractures. The patient may require the fitting of a halo brace to maintain constant traction on the skull, allowing C-1 to reassume proper alignment with

C2.[1] This brace is named for its resemblance to a halo as it surrounds the head. The purpose of the halo brace is to provide stability in the cervical spine above and below the injury without allowing cervical movement in any plane while the fracture or surgical site is healing (16-1).

■ Postoperative Management

Attendant postoperative care of the surgical wounds is critical because the patient cannot view several of the portals. The patient is typically hospitalized for

---

S|T Surgical Technique   16-1

Application of a Halo Brace

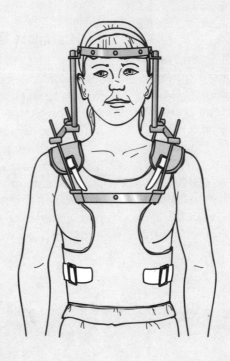

Procedure for Halo Application

1. The size of the crown (halo) and vest are determined.
2. Pin sites are determined while the ring/crown is held in place.
3. Pins are tightened at increments of 2 in-lb in a diagonal fashion until 8 in-lb of torque is achieved.
4. The crown is connected to the vest via four upright supports.
5. Tools are taped to the vest or kept at the bedside for emergency vest removal.
6. Pins are retightened to 8 in-lb 48 hours after halo application.
7. Pin sites are left uncovered and cleansed with hydrogen peroxide every other day or as needed.

Functional Limitations

Activities of daily living (ADLs) are difficult and cumbersome. The patient must sleep in a seated or semireclined position.

Implications for Rehabilitation

Muscular contractions and limited ADLs are per physician's orders while the patient is in the halo. After removal of the halo, rotation between C1 and C2 is limited or absent. The attending physician should be consulted to determine the anticipated level of function.

Potential Complications

Loosening of the pins, rings, and crowns; infection; pressure sores beneath the vest; loss of reduction secondary to poorly fitting vest or unwanted motion; bleeding at the pin sites; difficulty swallowing. (The halo will be repositioned with less extension in this situation.)[1]

2 to 3 days (if neurologically intact) after the halo is positioned for close monitoring of postoperative status. Once discharged, the patient must be aware of pressure sores that can be caused by the vest. During postoperative home care, a relative or friend should be assigned to regularly check the areas not visible to the patient. A proper hygiene routine, consisting of checking for chafing under the vest and applying absorbent powder such as cornstarch, reduces moisture and prevents pressure sores.

■ Injury-Specific Treatment and Rehabilitation Concerns

Specific Concerns
Maintain the hygiene of the halo fixation sites.
Maintain functional levels of activity as permitted by the physician.
Restrict ROM after halo removal.
Focus on ADLs.

In the rare case that the C1 fracture is a noncatastrophic event and no permanent neurologic deficits are present, the rehabilitation process is still a long one. The patient must first master ADLs within the confines of the halo. After halo removal, the patient is placed in a rigid collar for at least 3 months, followed by a soft one for an additional 2 to 3 months. Gradually, as the cervical spine regains muscular strength and endurance through rehabilitation exercises, the patient requires no additional support. Because of the underlying trauma requiring halo stabilization, these patients typically do not return to contact or collision sports.

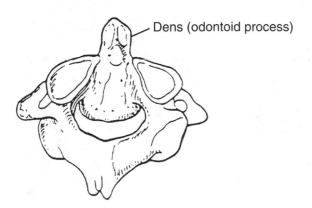

Figure 16-4 The odontoid process (dens) is a bony projection from C2 that sits posterior to C1. The articulation between the odontoid process and C1 allow for capital rotation. (Reproduced with permission from An HS, Simpson JM (eds): *Surgery of the Cervical Spine*. London, England, Martin Dunitz, 1994, p 2.)

■ Estimated Amount of Time Lost

Patients who sustain C1 fractures do not return to contact or collision sports. Ultimately, the rehabilitation goal is to return the patient to a functional lifestyle. Depending on the severity of the trauma and residual instability and in the absence of spinal cord trauma, the patient may be able to return to selected recreational activities (eg, golf or tennis) with the physician's consent.

■ C2 Fractures

C2 fractures are characterized and managed based on the unique anatomy of the C2 odontoid process, which allows for rotation of the head (**Figure 16-4**). Fractures of C2 are grouped into three categories—odontoid fractures, hangman's fractures (traumatic spondylolisthesis of the axis), and miscellaneous fractures such as vertebral body fractures.[4]

Fractures of the odontoid are classified into three types (**Figure 16-5**). Type I fractures are oblique fractures of the very tip or upper portion of the

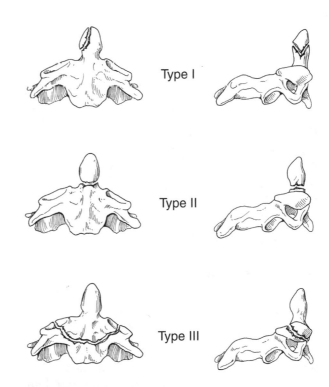

Figure 16-5 The Anderson and d'Alonzo classification system for odontoid fractures. Type I fractures are avulsion fractures of the tip of the odontoid process. Type II fractures occur at the junction of the odontoid process and the body of the axis. In the type III pattern, the fracture extends into the body of the axis through the cancellous bone. (Reproduced with permission from Chutkan NB, King AG, Harris MB: Odontoid fractures: Evaluation and Management. *J Am Acad Orthop Surg* 1997;5:199-204.)

odontoid process and are relatively uncommon. Type II fractures are the most common fracture of the odontoid process. Type III fractures extend into the vertebral body.

A hangman's fracture affects the posterior elements of C2, resulting in traumatic spondylolisthesis of the axis. The mechanism of injury is usually hyperextension of the cervical spine and commonly occurs after motor vehicle collisions; however, these fractures can also result from athletic activity when the cervical spine is forced into hyperextension.[5] This hyperextension of the neck and subsequent fracture are similar to the injury caused by judicial hangings, thus the name "hangman's fracture." Most low-velocity hangman's fractures seen clinically are not associated with spinal cord injury because they are typically low-velocity in nature, causing a bilateral fracture, which in turn opens the spinal canal. High-velocity fractures sever the spinal cord and result in almost immediate death. Patients who survive the first few minutes after fracturing the C1 have a good chance of recovery if the spinal cord is not involved, although return to contact or collision sports is often unlikely.

The classification of hangman's fractures is not well defined or accepted. One classification system describes a type I hangman's fracture as a fracture of the posterior elements of C2 without displacement of C2 on C3; a type II fracture is a fracture with subluxation of C2 on C3. Another well-accepted classification of hangman's fractures identifies a type I fracture as a posterior element fracture of C2 with 3 mm or less subluxation of C2 on C3. Type II fractures have a subluxation of C2 on C3 of 4 mm or angulation of more than 11°. Type III fractures are rare, may be associated with severe neurologic injury or death, and are confirmed with the disruption of the C2-C3 facet joints and possible locked facets.[4]

Differential Diagnosis
Cervical muscle strain, cervical sprain, spasm, other cervical fractures, degenerative osteoarthritis

Imaging Techniques
The imaging and diagnosis of C2 fractures begin with plain cervical radiographs (**Figure 16-6**). However, CT scanning—particularly with sagittal and coronal reconstructions—allows for definitive diagnosis of the fracture and better evaluation of the fracture subtype (**Figure 16-7**). MRI is rarely necessary in a neurologically intact patient with a C2 fracture.

Definitive Diagnosis
Conclusive findings on radiographs, CT scan, or MRI

Pathomechanics and Functional Limitations
Cervical rotation is limited and painful, and muscle spasm further limits motion. Trunk rotation substitutes for cervical and capital rotation. Instability of the vertebra can jeopardize the integrity of the spinal cord and/or the associated spinal nerve roots.

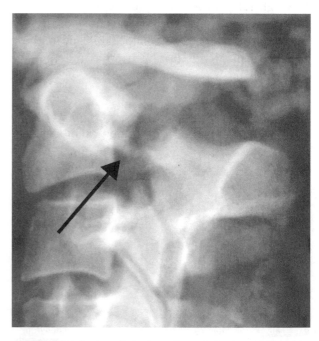

Figure 16-6 Lateral cervical spine radiograph showing a fracture of the posterior arch of C2 (hangman's fracture).

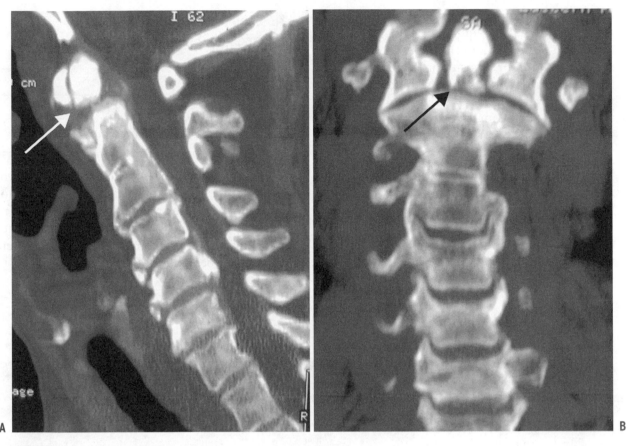

Figure 16-7 CT scans of type II odontoid fractures. **A.** Sagittal view. **B.** Coronal view.

Postinjury Management

The treatment of odontoid fractures depends on the type of fracture. Type I fractures can usually be treated with a rigid collar. Type II fractures generally require halo immobilization for 8 to 12 weeks (see ST 16-1). However, the incidence of nonunion in type II fractures increases significantly after age 40 years, and cervical fusion may be necessary. Type III fractures have been reported to heal in a rigid collar in up to 65% of cases, but some of these patients may require halo immobilization.

The management of a hangman's fracture is almost always immobilization. The fractures without dislocation can usually be managed with a rigid collar. Cervical traction and subsequent halo immobilization may be required for patients with fractures and significant dislocations at C2-C3.

Surgical Intervention

If surgery is necessary for an odontoid fracture (generally a type II fracture), posterior fusion is often performed with a C1-C2 fusion or, more recently, with transarticular stabilization at C1-C2. Anterior screw fixation of the odontoid can be performed in cer-

tain cases but is technically more demanding than posterior fusion (**Figure 16-8**).[6] Surgery is occasionally necessary for a hangman's fracture when dislocation is significant or when satisfactory alignment

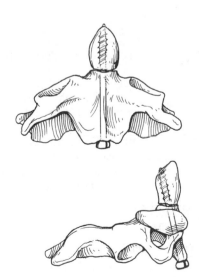

Figure 16-8 Anterior single-screw fixation of an odontoid process fracture. (Reproduced with permission from Chutkan NB, King AG, Harris MB: Odontoid fractures: Evaluation and Management. *J Am Acad Orthop Surg* 1997;5:199-204.)

cannot be maintained with a halo. The rare hangman's fractures that require surgery can be managed with either an anterior C2-C3 fusion with instrumentation or a posterior C1 to C3 fusion.[6] Miscellaneous fractures of C2 include mild fractures of the vertebral body or lateral masses of C2 that can usually be managed with rigid collar immobilization (**S T** 16-2).

Postsurgical Management

After a fusion of C1-C2, the patient may be put in a halo or, at minimum, a rigid collar for at least 3 months. Rehabilitation is limited to ADLs, and the ultimate rehabilitation goal is to return the patient to a functional lifestyle.

Injury-Specific Treatment and Rehabilitation Concerns

Specific Concerns
Prevent rotation between C1 and C2 during healing.
Limit flexion and extension activities.
Maintain cardiovascular fitness as permitted by the physician.

A soft collar replaces the hard collar and is worn for an additional 2 to 3 months before flexion-extension exercises are begun. Patients who undergo bone graft fusion and wire fixation still need 5 to 6 months of protective collar use before rehabilitation is begun.

S|T Surgical Technique 16-2

Posterior Atlantoaxial Fusion (Brooks Fusion)

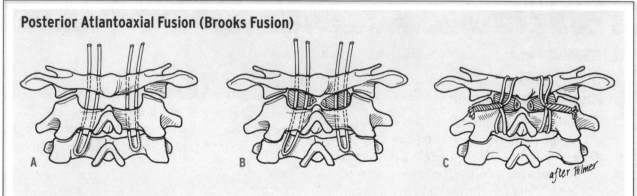

Indications

Significant dislocation of C1-C2; if satisfactory reduction cannot be achieved or maintained with a halo

Overview

Although Brooks fusion is described here, the Gallie and Sonntag procedures are similar.
1. Patient is positioned prone and a midline incision is made in the upper posterior neck from lower occiput to C4. The paraspinal muscles are dissected off the spine to expose the lower portion of the occipital bone and C1, C2, and C3.
2. Wires are passed under the C1 arch and the C2 lamina (**A**).
3. Bone may be harvested from the patient's iliac crest, or banked bone may be used.
4. Bone grafts are beveled into the space between the C1 arch and the C2 lamina (**B**).
5. The wires are tightened to fixate the graft (**C**).

Functional Limitations

Loss of rotation of C1 on C2

Implications for Rehabilitation

Rotational motions are avoided until the surgical repair has fully healed.

Comments

Patients are excluded from future contact and collision sports.

Figures reproduced with permission from An HS: Internal fixation of the cervical spine: Current indications and techniques. *J Am Acad Orthop Surg* 1995;3:194-206.

Estimated Amount of Time Lost

Time lost depends on the type of fracture, but an athlete rarely continues in contact or collision sports after such an injury. Depending on the severity of the trauma and in the absence of spinal cord trauma, the patient may be able to return to select recreational activities (eg, golf or tennis) pending the physician's consent.

Lower Cervical Spine Fractures and Dislocations

CLINICAL PRESENTATION

History
Axial loading and hyperflexion are the predominant mechanisms of history for these fractures.

Observation
The patient is typically down, and unwilling or unable to move.

Functional Status
The patient may or may not display radicular signs and symptoms.
Muscular weakness or inability to function is demonstrated.
Cardiovascular and respiratory systems may be compromised.
ROM testing should not be performed on patients suspected of suffering a cervical spine injury.

Physical Evaluation Findings
Cervical spine pain at the level of injury
Typically bilateral weakness and loss of motor function below the injury site
Usually bilateral deficit and loss of sensation below the injury site
Severe spasm and neck pain
Priapism in males

Because of the significant variety of cervical spine fractures and dislocations involving the lower cervical spine (C3 to C7), no uniform classification of these injuries is accepted. A broad way to categorize these lower cervical spine injuries is to separate the injuries with facet dislocation from those without facet dislocation (**Figure 16-9**).

Cervical spine injuries with either unilateral or bilateral facet dislocation are common.[7] Injuries with unilateral facet dislocation are usually accompanied by cervical radiculopathy (single-level root syndrome from compression of the nerve root by the dislocated facet). Injuries with bilateral facet dislocation result in approximately 50% narrowing of the spinal canal and are almost always associated with acute spinal cord injury. Facet dislocation is often accompanied by facet fracture; however,

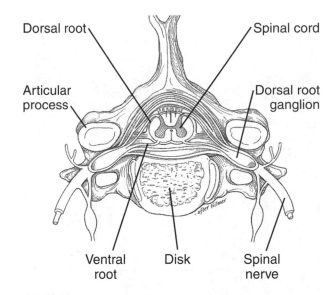

Figure 16-9 Cross-sectional view of the neural structures of the lower cervical spine. (Reproduced with permission from Levine MJ, Albert TJ, Smith MD: Cervical radiculopathy: Diagnosis and non-operative management. *J Am Acad Orthop Surg* 1996;4:305-316.)

facet dislocation can occur from severe ligamentous injury and without any obvious fracture. Lower cervical spine fractures and dislocations without facet dislocation include a number of abnormalities, such as teardrop fractures to the anterior vertebral body, significant vertebral body compression fractures or burst fractures, and ligamentous injury with subluxation of the cervical spine.

Most of these injuries are due to severe hyperflexion of the cervical spine with possible subsequent hyperextension, resulting in fractures or severe ligamentous injuries.[7,8] Axial loading is the primary mechanism of injury for cervical spine fractures with spinal cord insult.[9] Torg and associates[9] discovered that a cervical spine in a slightly flexed position converts the natural lordotic curve into a straight column, predisposing it to injury.

The clinical presentation of patients with lower cervical spine injuries with fracture and/or dislocation includes severe neck pain and neurologic deficit with either radiculopathy or evidence of acute spinal cord injury. Spinal cord syndromes are described in the section on spinal cord injury.

Differential Diagnosis
Neck strain, cervical sprain, cervical spasm

Imaging Techniques
Imaging of lower cervical spine injuries is similar to imaging of upper cervical spine injuries. Plain lateral radiographs usually demonstrate fracture and/or dislocation; however, radiographs may be normal (**Figure 16-10**). CT is optimal; scans should be taken as soon as possible because of better fracture

16

Priapism Abnormal, painful, continued erection of the penis, often the result of a spinal cord lesion.

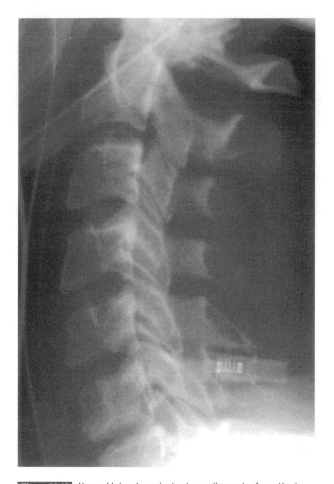

Figure 16-10 Normal lateral cervical spine radiograph of a patient subsequently found to have multiple cervical fractures.

delineation and the ability to obtain sagittal and coronal reconstructions (**Figure 16-11**). Cervical CT scanning also identifies narrowing of the spinal canal caused by **retropulsed** bone fragments or vertebral subluxation. MRI is useful to evaluate the spinal cord for hemorrhage and edema and can help iden-

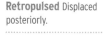

Retropulsed Displaced posteriorly.

tify ligamentous disruption and the presence of a herniated cervical disk.[7]

Definitive Diagnosis
Radiographs, CT scan, or MRI confirming the presence of a fracture

Pathomechanics and Functional Limitations
Pain with cervical movement and neck spasm can prohibit movement. Pressure on the spinal cord results in paralysis of the lower extremities and possibly the upper extremities, depending on the location of the injury.

■ Immediate Management

The immediate management of cervical fractures and dislocations must provide in-line stabilization and immobilization of the cervical spine. The patient should be transported by professionals to the nearest trauma center (see Immediate Management of On-Field Cervical Spine Injuries, p 545). The patient may also have accompanying injuries that must be managed. Therefore, respiratory and circulatory function must be closely monitored.

■ Postinjury Management

If dislocation is significant, the immediate management is to reduce the dislocation and restore normal spinal canal and foraminal anatomy. This reduction is generally performed using cervical skeletal traction with either a halo or Gardner-Wells tongs. Dislocations may be difficult to reduce with skeletal traction and may require open reduction.

Some lower cervical spine fractures that do not jeopardize the spinal cord, such as transverse or spinous process fractures, can be managed simply with a rigid collar, such as the Miami or Aspen collar (see Figure 16-3). These include

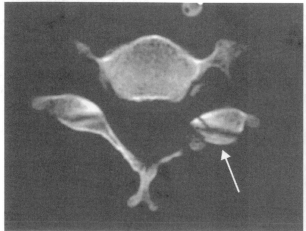
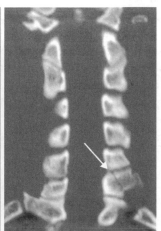

Figure 16-11 CT scan of the same patient shown in Figure 16-10. **A.** Axial view of a left C6-C7 facet fracture. **B.** Coronal view of a fracture of the C7 facet.

slight chip fractures off a vertebral body, mild compression fractures of a single vertebral body, and mild facet fractures without dislocation. The rigid collar is generally applied for 8 to 12 weeks, followed by a period in a soft collar. In the past, many severe injuries of the lower cervical spine were managed with initial reduction and long-term halo immobilization. However, morbidity is significant with 3 to 4 months of halo immobilization, and long-term immobilization is used less commonly than in the past. Nevertheless,

halo traction and even long-term halo immobilization are still used in the management of some fractures (see 16-1).

■ Surgical Intervention

Surgical stabilization, particularly with cervical instrumentation, has become more widely used. The most commonly performed procedure for stabilization of lower cervical spine fractures and dislocations is the anterior cervical diskectomy with fusion (S T 16-3). The relatively recent in-

---

S|T Surgical Technique 16-3

Anterior Cervical Diskectomy and Fusion

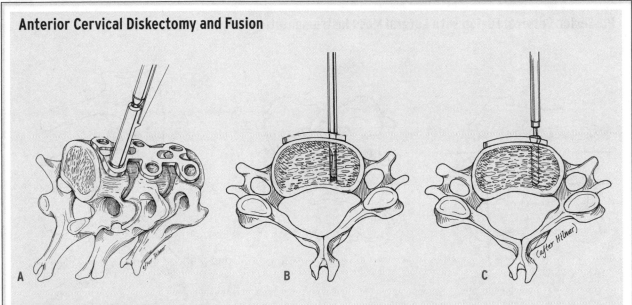

Indications

Failure to achieve satisfactory closed reduction or inability to maintain reduction with an external orthosis; significant ligamentous injury with evidence of severe facet instability; angulation of the spine of more than 15°; more than 40% compression of a vertebral body; subluxation of 20% or more of one vertebral body on another

Overview

1. The patient is placed supine with the head slightly turned to one side.
2. Cervical traction is maintained during the procedure.
3. A transverse or longitudinal incision is made in the anterior neck, and dissection is carried down through the platysma and along the anterior border of the sternocleidomastoid muscle to the spine.
4. An anterior cervical diskectomy at the affected level is performed, and the bone graft is placed in the disk space.
5. The appropriate anterior plate is selected and held in place. Holes are drilled into the vertebral bodies above and below the bone graft, and then screws are placed with a special locking system unique to the plate used (**A, B, C**).

Functional Limitations

Decreased cervical ROM. The presence of an associated spinal cord injury determines the patient's overall level of function.

Implications for Rehabilitation

The patient is placed in a rigid protective collar for 4 to 6 weeks, followed by a soft collar.

Complications

Hardware failure, bone graft displacement, injury to the trachea or esophagus with swallowing problems or hoarseness, neurologic deficit related to spinal cord manipulation

Figures reproduced with permission from An HS: Internal fixation of the cervical spine: Current indications and techniques. *J Am Acad Orthop Surg* 1995;3:194-206.

troduction of various anterior instrumentation systems has improved fusion rates and decreased the time patients must wear an external orthosis postoperatively. Anterior cervical diskectomy and fusion are performed with a bone graft placed in the disk space. Although iliac crest bone can be harvested from the patient, it is now more common to use banked bone. The use of banked bone results in decreased morbidity from pain due to an incision in the iliac crest. Once the bone graft is placed, a decision must be made about anterior instrumentation, which is generally used in the setting of acute trauma.

Posterior cervical fusion is also often used for fractures and dislocations of the cervical spine (ST 16-4). Occasionally a patient has such severe ligamentous injury that both anterior and posterior cervical fusions are necessary to maintain adequate stability and alignment of the cervical spine. These procedures can be performed on the same day or as a staged procedure, depending on the medical condition of the patient.

S|T Surgical Technique 16-4

Posterior Cervical Fusion with Lateral Mass Instrumentation

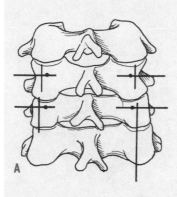
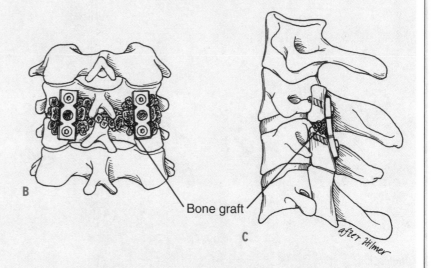

Bone graft

Indications

Fracture and/or dislocation of the cervical spine involving the posterior ligaments, irreducible facet dislocations; severe anteroposterior ligamentous injury in which a posterior fusion may be used to supplement an anterior fusion; severe anterior soft-tissue trauma, swelling, or presence of a tracheotomy

Overview

1. The patient is placed prone.
2. A midline cervical incision is made, and the cervical paraspinous muscles are dissected off the lamina and facets bilaterally.
3. Fusion is carried out one segment above and below the affected level.
4. Drill holes are made in the lateral masses of the involved segments bilaterally (**A**).
5. Screws are placed in the holes and attached to titanium rods or plates for stabilization (depending on the instrumentation used) (**B**).
6. Posterior instrumentation is supplemented with fusion of the facets, and bone can be laid along the facets and lamina bilaterally (**C**).

Functional Limitations

Mild loss of cervical flexion and extension. The total amount of ROM decrease is related to the number of segments fused; an increased number of fusions results in a greater amount of ROM deficit.

Implications for Rehabilitation

Patient is placed in a rigid protective collar for 4 to 6 weeks, followed by a soft collar. Weight lifting is limited to 10 lbs for 6 weeks.

Complications

Hardware failure, bone graft displacement, and neurologic deficit related to the manipulation of the spinal cord

Figure reproduced with permission from An HS: Internal fixation of the cervical spine: Current indications and techniques. *J Am Acad Orthop Surg* 1995;3:194-206.

Postoperative Management

The postoperative management is determined by the bony injury and associated spinal cord trauma. In the absence of neurologic deficit, protected cervical motion and generalized upper and lower extremity exercises may be initiated to prevent muscular atrophy and maintain cardiovascular and respiratory function. If spinal cord injury is significant, the patient will require extensive care and rehabilitation.

Estimated Amount of Time Lost

Time lost depends on the type and location of fracture, but it is rare for the individual to continue in contact and collision sports after such an injury. Permanent trauma to the spinal cord results in permanent disability, and all too often, the patient depends on a wheelchair. If the spinal cord is spared, the patient may be able to return to select low-risk sports, such as golf or tennis.

Injury-Specific Treatment and Rehabilitation Concerns

Specific Concerns

Restrict flexion and extension as indicated by physician.
Maintain cardiovascular levels during convalescence.
Restore strength and gain available ROM (may be restricted by the surgical technique used).

Generally, absent neurologic involvement, lower extremity cardiovascular conditioning (eg, stationary bicycling or elliptical machines) may begin right after the initial protective period. Cardiovascular equipment involving the upper extremities, such as stair steppers and cross-country ski machines, should be used more cautiously because of the potential for stressing the cervical musculature and causing pain or spasm. After the fracture heals completely, gentle ROM and strengthening exercises may begin with the physician's approval (see Rehabilitation, p 547).

Return-to-Activity Criteria

If the surgery was the result of trauma, return to competitive sport is unlikely; however, if the surgery was necessitated by degenerative arthritis or disk disease, the patient's outcome depends on the quality of the surgery and subsequent rehabilitation. Overall, the time lost due to lower cervical spine fractures without spinal cord injury generally ranges from 6 to 18 months.

Spinal Cord Injury

CLINICAL PRESENTATION

History

Axial loading and/or hyperflexion

Observation

The patient may be unable or reluctant to move unassisted. There may be no residual movement of the extremities. Decorticate or decerebrate postures may be noted.

Functional Status

Bilateral neuromuscular involvement, including muscular weakness/paralysis and radicular symptoms below the injury
Airway and cardiac function must be assessed and maintained.
ROM tests should not be performed in the presence of suspected cervical spine injury.

Physical Evaluation Findings

Pain on palpation of the cervical spine (note that palpation should not be performed on patients with known or suspected vertebral fractures)
Neuromuscular involvement ranges from weakness to paralysis.

Injury to the spinal cord with resulting neurologic deficit is perhaps the most feared of any athletic-related injury. Spinal cord trauma can cause significant temporary or permanent disability and may be accompanied by injury to the bony cervical spine; in older patients with cervical spondylosis, however, significant spinal cord injury may occur without obvious spinal fracture. Cervical spine injuries resulting in permanent paralysis have significantly declined since the antispearing rule was implemented for football in 1976.[8]

The clinical presentation of spinal cord injury varies. Complete spinal cord injury results in a total loss of spinal function below the level of the injury. Trauma to the spinal cord itself is rarely reversible, but occasionally neurologic function improves some with reduction of a severe dislocation, such as in a patient with bilateral dislocated facets.

A number of patterns of incomplete spinal cord injury are seen clinically (**Figure 16-12**). The most commonly observed incomplete spinal cord injury is the central spinal cord syndrome. This condition results in incomplete loss of motor function, with upper extremity weakness being more pronounced than lower extremity weakness. This disproportionate weakness is due to the anatomy of the spinal cord; the fibers in the corticospinal tract that supply the cervical nerve roots are more central in the spinal cord than those supplying the lower extremities.[8] Central spinal cord syndrome results in

16

hemorrhage and ischemia of the corticospinal tracts, with a disproportionate injury to the more central nerve fibers supplying the upper extremities.[8,10] The cervical central spinal cord syndrome may also be due to actual damage to anterior horn cells in the gray matter of the cervical spinal cord. Central spinal cord syndrome has historically been described in older patients with cervical spondylosis and osteophytic ridges who suffer a hyperextension injury of the cervical spine. Transient compression results in hemorrhage and ischemia in the spinal cord. However, central spinal cord syndrome is often seen in young patients with spinal trauma and incomplete spinal cord injury.

The Brown-Séquard syndrome is a **hemisection** of the spinal cord, with loss of motor function on the side of the injury and loss of pain and temperature on the side contralateral to the injury. This syndrome occurs because of the **decussation** of the spinothalamic tracts one or two segments above their entry into the spinal cord. The corticospinal tracts, which supply motor function, have already crossed in the medulla and maintain an ipsilateral course throughout the spinal cord. Classic Brown-Séquard syndrome is rarely seen in the absence of penetrating trauma, such as a bony fragment. The condition usually occurs as a "modified" Brown-Séquard syndrome, in which the patient has some motor weakness on one side of the body and decreased pain and temperature on the opposite side. The central cord syndrome may be seen with a modified Brown-Séquard syndrome in which weakness is more pronounced in the upper extremities than the lower extremities.

Name (Figure Element)	Description	Deficit Patterns
Central spinal cord syndrome (**A**)	Hemorrhage and ischemia of the corticospinal tracts	Weakness of the upper extremities more pronounced than the lower extremities
	Trauma to the cells within the anterior horn of the cervical spinal cord	
Anterior spinal cord syndrome (**B**)	Trauma to the anterior two thirds of the spinal cord	Loss of motor function and pain and temperature sensation below the level of the injury
		Touch, pressure, and proprioceptive function are usually present
Brown-Séquard syndrome (**C**)	Hemisection of the spinal cord involving the spinothalamic tracts	Loss or weakness of motor function on the side of the trauma
		Loss of pain and temperature sensation on the side opposite the trauma

Adapted with permission from Spivak JM, Vaccaro AR, Cotler JM: Thoracolumbar spine trauma: I. Evaluation and classification. *J Am Acad Orthop Surg* 1995;3:345-352.

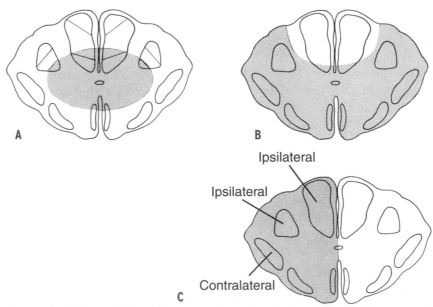

Figure 16-12 Patterns of neurologic deficit associated with incomplete lesions of the spinal cord. Injury is indicated by shaded area.

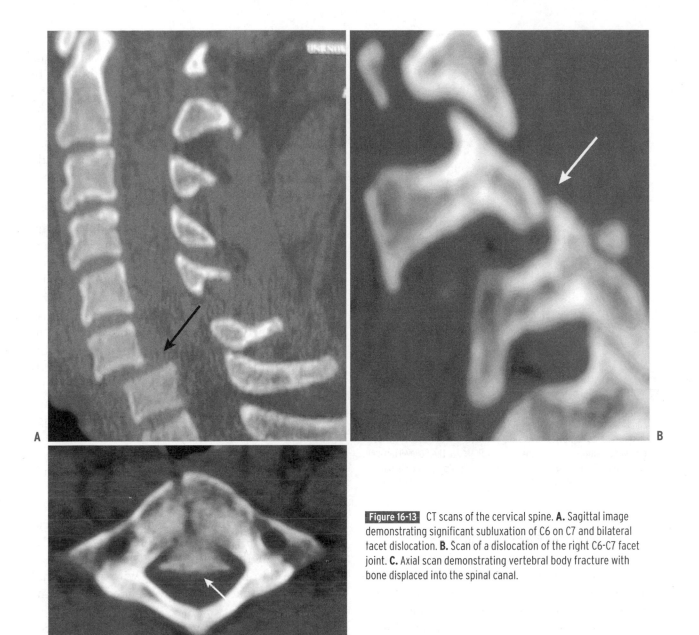

Figure 16-13 CT scans of the cervical spine. **A.** Sagittal image demonstrating significant subluxation of C6 on C7 and bilateral facet dislocation. **B.** Scan of a dislocation of the right C6-C7 facet joint. **C.** Axial scan demonstrating vertebral body fracture with bone displaced into the spinal canal.

Anterior spinal cord syndrome is an injury to the anterior two thirds of the spinal cord in the region of the anterior spinal artery. The neurologic deficit consists of loss of all motor function below the level of the injury and loss of pain and temperature sensation below the level of injury (the spinothalamic tracts). The motor deficit is usually equal in the upper and lower extremities, unlike the central spinal cord syndrome. Touch, pressure, and proprioceptive function are typically preserved due to sparing of the dorsal columns.

Differential Diagnosis
Cervical radiculopathy, cervical disk disease, cervical fracture, primary or metastatic tumor, brachial plexus injury, neurapraxia, hysterical paralysis

Imaging Techniques
A lateral cervical spine radiograph is indicated when the neurologic examination suggests a spinal cord injury. All patients with suspected spinal cord injury should undergo CT scanning to evaluate the cervical spine for fracture, dislocation, or compromise of the spinal canal (**Figure 16-13**). MRI is useful for evaluating hemorrhage or edema within the spinal cord itself and identifying a disk herniation, which may compress or sever the spinal cord (**Figure 16-14**).[3]

Definitive Diagnosis
The definitive diagnosis is based on the clinical examination, possible neurologic findings, and confirmation by MRI or CT scans.

Metastatic The spreading of a cancerous growth from one body area to another.

Hysterical paralysis The inability to move brought on by fear and/or anxiety.

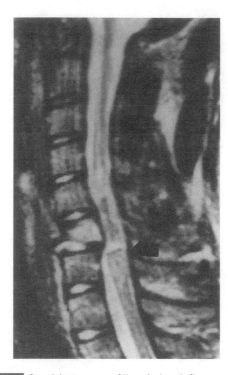

Figure 16-14 Complete severance of the spinal cord after a severe C6 fracture-subluxation. The 18-year-old male patient sustained a diving injury and immediate C6 quadriplegia. This MRI, obtained 90 minutes after the injury, depicts complete severance of the cord at the base of the C6 vertebra and hemorrhage into the cord cephalad to the C6 level (arrow). (Reproduced with permission from Delamarter RB, Coyle J: Acute management of spinal cord injury. *J Am Acad Orthop Surg* 1999;7:166-175.)

Cephalad Toward the head.

Pathomechanics and Functional Limitations

The patient may experience quadriplegia or paraplegia, depending on the level of spinal cord involvement. The degree of spinal cord trauma determines the patient's functional limitations. Complete trauma to the spinal cord results in the loss of all sensory, motor, and reflex function distal to the site of the lesion. When the lesion occurs above the C4 level, the phrenic nerve, which controls breathing, is impaired and the patient is placed on a respirator. Incomplete spinal cord trauma may result in the selective loss of motor, sensory, and/or reflex function (see Figure 16-12).

■ Medications

Drug treatment for acute spinal cord injury remains quite controversial. A number of medications, including corticosteroids, naloxone (an opioid antagonist), and GM-1 ganglioside have been tested (also see Corticosteroids for Acute Spinal Cord Trauma, chapter 4, p 55).

The medications that have undergone the most rigorous human investigation in acute spinal cord injury include corticosteroids, predominantly methylprednisolone.[8,11-14] The National Acute Spinal Cord Injury Study II (NASCIS 2), published in 1990, indicated statistically significant improvement in motor function and sensation at 6 months postinjury in patients treated with high-dose methylprednisolone within 8 hours of trauma.[12] The dose of methylprednisolone used in this study was 30 mg/kg as a loading dose and 5.4 mg/kg/h constant infusion for 23 hours.

The NASCIS 3, published in 1997, compared the efficacy of methylprednisolone administered for 24 hours and 48 hours, depending on the timing of administration of the drug. The authors concluded that patients with spinal cord injury who receive methylprednisolone within 3 hours of injury should be given a 24-hour infusion and those patients receiving methylprednisolone from 3 to 8 hours after injury should be given a 48-hour infusion.[13] For a number of years after these studies were published, the use of methylprednisolone in acute spinal cord injury was considered standard practice. However, critiques of both studies and recent reports have suggested that the available evidence does not warrant the routine use of methylprednisolone in the treatment of acute spinal cord injury. The risk of harmful side effects of such high-dose corticosteroid administration may be greater than any demonstrated clinical benefit obtained from the drug.[14] The administration of methylprednisolone is now regarded as an option in treating a patient with acute spinal cord injury that should be considered on an individual basis.[11]

The use of naloxone was evaluated in NASCIS 2 and has also been tested in other studies. At this time, no clear efficacy has been shown for the use of naloxone in the management of acute spinal cord injury. Similarly, no evidence demonstrates clinical benefit in the use of GM-1 ganglioside in the treatment of acute spinal cord injury.[11]

■ Surgical Techniques/Medical Intervention

Although surgical techniques cannot repair an injured spinal cord, the procedures described elsewhere in this chapter may be necessary to treat the bony cervical spine injuries that often accompany acute spinal cord injury. In those patients with cervical spine dislocations, immediate reduction is indicated to restore spinal canal diameter and decompress the spinal cord.[8,15] Stabilization, either with an external orthosis or surgery (for example,

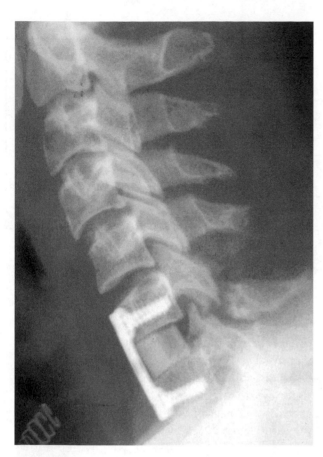

Figure 16-15 Immediate postoperative lateral cervical spine radiograph demonstrating normal alignment with fixation.

see ⓢⓣ 16-4) may be necessary to prevent secondary injury due to cervical spine instability (**Figure 16-15**). If a disk herniation is causing spinal cord compression, diskectomy is necessary.

With no definitive treatment for a spinal cord injury, the treatment is primarily supportive. Prevention of secondary injury and early initiation of mobilization and rehabilitation are the goals. Because of the poor prognosis, efforts to prevent cervical spinal cord injuries from athletic participation are of paramount importance.

Postoperative Management

Patients with acute cervical spinal cord injury (particularly of the upper cervical spinal cord) may develop respiratory failure and require intubation and ventilatory support.[8,10] Patients with cervical spinal cord injuries may also have significant hypotension due to neurogenic shock and may need vasopressors to maintain adequate circulation to the spinal cord. Maintenance of mean arterial blood pressure of 85 to 90 mm Hg for the first 7 days af-

ter acute spinal cord injury has been advocated to improve spinal cord perfusion.[16]

Available motion to the extremities should be exploited as early as possible to preserve the intact motor units, maintain sensory function, and prevent flexion contractures.

Injury-Specific Treatment and Rehabilitation Concerns

Rehabilitation for patients with spinal cord injury traditionally is directed at regaining functional ADLs. No set exercises or protocols are universal to all of these injuries, and most patients with severe and lasting neurologic deficit spend some posthospital time at a spinal cord rehabilitation center.

Spinal cord injury rehabilitation centers are available for patients with significant neurologic injury who have profound sequelae. These centers are equipped with the personnel, modalities, and exercise equipment necessary to assist in regaining activities of normal living. The centers attend to the patient's physical, mental, and emotional health, and some facilities also offer educational seminars for family members to help them adjust to the patient's limitations. More information about these centers can be obtained from the American Spinal Injury Association (www.asia-spinalinjury.org).

Estimated Amount of Time Lost

Permanent trauma to the spinal cord results in permanent disability, with the total amount of lost function related to the proportion of the spinal cord that is injured and the level at which the injury occurred. Some patients are unable to resume any level of physical activity; others may be able to participate in wheelchair sports or similar activities.

Time lost due to a spinal cord injury depends on the severity of injury, completeness of recovery, and type of activity desired after recovery. The patients who fully recuperate from such trauma do not usually return to contact or collision sports but may engage in noncontact activities and sports as soon as they regain sufficient muscular endurance, strength, ROM, and neurologic soundness.

Return-to-Play Criteria

Typically, patients with a spinal cord injury do not return to their prior level of competition. Select activities may be possible, pending the approval of the attending physician. (See chapter 24.)

16

Transient Quadriparesis (Cervical Spinal Cord Neurapraxia)

CLINICAL PRESENTATION

History

An episode of bilateral muscular weakness/paresis
Bilateral neurologic symptoms associated with areas of muscular involvement

Observation

The patient may be unable or reluctant to move unassisted.
There may be no residual movement from the extremities.
Decorticate or decerebrate postures may be noted.

Functional Status

Neurologic and muscular weakness symptoms are self-limiting.

Physical Evaluation Findings

Cervical spine is pain free and has no deformities.
Resolving bilateral neurologic and muscular weakness symptoms
No activity is allowed until the patient recovers full, bilaterally equal strength, ROM, and sensation, and is pain and symptom free

---

Table 16-1

Grading System for Neurapraxia

Grade	Duration of Symptoms
1	All neurologic symptoms resolve in less than 15 minutes
2	All neurologic symptoms resolve in more than 15 minutes but less than 24 hours
3	Neurologic symptoms persist for more than 24 hours

Reproduced with permission from Torg JS, Guille JT, Jaffe S: Injuries to the cervical spine in American football players. *J Bone Joint Surg Am* 2002;84:112-122.

Transient quadriparesis (cervical spinal cord neurapraxia) is a type of spinal cord injury that probably results from the effect of a transient compression of the spinal cord. Clinical manifestations include dysesthesia (burning pain), numbness, tingling of the extremities, and weakness or complete motor paralysis of the upper or lower extremities. An episode of transient quadriparesis generally resolves within 10 to 15 minutes, although sensory symptoms may persist for 24 to 48 hours[17,18] (**Table 16-1**). This is a spinal cord syndrome because it is bilateral and often involves all four extremities. Transient quadriparesis should not be confused with brachial plexus injury.

Spinal stenosis, or narrowing of the spinal column, has long been thought to be the culprit of several neurologic conditions in the cervical spinal canal. However, other evidence suggests stenosis of the spinal foramen is neither an indicator nor a predictor of neurologic injury.[19] On the basis of current data, cervical stenosis without instability is not thought to be a strong predictor of neurologic susceptibility; however, the findings are still controversial.

Differential Diagnosis

Cervical radiculopathy, cervical disk disease, tumor (primary or metastatic), brachial plexus injury, brachial plexus neurapraxia, hysterical paralysis (conversion disorder)

Imaging Techniques

Cervical spine radiographs in a patient with cervical spinal cord neurapraxia are negative for vertebral fracture or dislocation. Often, narrowing of the spinal canal is congenital in origin (**Figure 16-16**). The Torg ratio has been developed for determining the diameter of the spinal canal based on the anterior-to-posterior width of the spinal canal divided by the anterior-to-posterior width of the vertebral body at the same level.[19] However, this ratio was devised before the widespread use of MRI, which allows direct measurement of spinal canal diameter.

A patient with suspected cervical spinal cord neurapraxia must be assumed to have a cervical fracture or ligamentous injury until proved otherwise and should undergo CT scanning to rule out fractures. MRI should be used to evaluate the patient for cervical disk herniation and degenerative changes of the cervical spine and to assess spinal canal diameter. If these studies are negative, flexion-extension radiographs of the lateral cervical spine should be obtained to rule out any evidence of instability.

Definitive Diagnosis

Findings of the clinical examination, symptoms indicating the condition, significant imaging findings, and exclusion of other possible conditions

Pathomechanics and Functional Limitations

Initially, the patient displays the signs and symptoms of a frank spinal cord injury. These symptoms are transient, and full function gradually returns. Repeated episodes of transient quadriparesis can indicate significant spinal stenosis and increase the risk of permanent neurologic damage with each episode.

■ Immediate Management

The immediate management of a patient with cervical spinal cord neurapraxia is the same on the field as that for all suspected spinal injuries (see

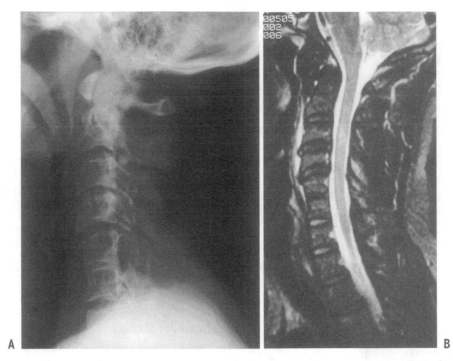

Figure 16-16   **A.** Lateral radiograph shows congenital failure of segmentation at C5-C6 (Torg type II) with no acute fractures or subluxations. **B.** Sagittal T2-weighted MRI demonstrates signal change within the cord. Subsequent flexion-extension radiographs showed a stable spine. The patient was permanently restricted from contact sports. (Reproduced with permission from Thomas BE, McCullen GM, Yuan HA: Cervical spine injuries in football players. *J Am Acad Orthop Surg* 1997;7:338-347.)

p 545). The spine should be immobilized and the patient's respiratory or circulatory function monitored. By the time the patient reaches the hospital, the symptoms have usually resolved except for mild sensory symptoms. The neurologic examination is typically normal.

Postinjury/Postoperative Management

Cervical spinal cord neurapraxia is a reversible phenomenon that generally does not require postinjury treatment. In some instances, high-dose methylprednisolone has been used to limit edema formation, but the need for this approach is questionable and somewhat controversial (see p 532).[11,14]

The patient should undergo a thorough orthopaedic and neurologic examination to identify predisposing factors to transient neurapraxia (eg, cervical stenosis, cervical disk disease, etc). Often such a finding is incidental after the injury, but its identification could serve as a predictor of further episodes.

Estimated Amount of Time Lost

The patient cannot return to play while still symptomatic. The severity and duration of the symptoms are good indicators of how quickly participation can resume. The longer and more severe the symptoms, the greater the amount of time lost. If, however, the recovery is lengthy or anatomic anomalies are present, then any possible return to play is contingent on the ultimate recovery and findings.

Injury-Specific Treatment and Rehabilitation Concerns

Specific Concerns
Provide palliative treatment for pain and muscle spasm.
Restore ROM.
Strengthen cervical muscles.

By definition, neurapraxia is a 24- to 48-hour transient quadriparesis; however, neurologic symptoms may persist much longer.[18] Rehabilitation depends on cessation of symptoms and gradual muscular reconditioning. If the episode completely resolves in hours, specific rehabilitation may not be necessary. If the episode has long-lasting symptoms, an exercise program beginning with isometric cervical exercises and progressing to isotonic training can be beneficial. Examples of these exercises and specific targeted muscles are found later in this chapter (see Brachial Plexus Injury) and in chapter 17.

Return-to-Play Criteria

Evidence suggests that a single episode of transient quadriparesis in the presence of a congenitally narrow spinal canal does not reflect a particular predisposition to permanent neurologic deficit.[17,18] Although the patient can return to contact sports, such an episode of transient and severe neurologic deficit is frightening to the patient and the patient's family. Return to competition after an episode of transient quadriparesis should be thoroughly discussed with the patient and the patient's family. The importance of returning to athletic competition (eg, for a professional athlete versus a high school athlete who will not participate in sports after high school) must be considered.

Patients who have spinal cord dysfunction and ligamentous instability, significant degenerative disease, cervical disk disease with cord compression, symptoms that last more than 36 hours, or more than one recurrence of transient quadriparesis should not be allowed to participate again in collision sports. **Table 16-2** presents guidelines for return to competition after transient neurapraxia.[17]

Cervical Disk Disease and Herniation (Cervical Degenerative Disk Disease)

CLINICAL PRESENTATION

History

Neck and/or unilateral arm pain, numbness, paresthesia, or weakness

Observation

The cervical spine may be postured to relieve radicular symptoms.
Muscle spasm in the cervical spine and possibly the associated myotomes
In prolonged cases, atrophy of the associated muscles may be noted.

Functional Status

Unilateral muscular weakness, perhaps associated with one or more myotomes
Radicular symptoms along associated dermatomes
Strength and ROM may be limited secondary to pain and muscle spasm.

Physical Evaluation Findings

Associated muscle weakness
Possible sensory impairment along the associated dermatomes
Associated reflexes may be diminished or absent.
Upper-quarter screen produces the findings described in Table 16-3.
The following special tests may be positive:
  Shoulder abduction test
  Cervical compression test
  Cervical distraction test
  Spurling test

Cervical disk herniation is less common than lumbar disk herniation.[20-22] This lower incidence is related to the fact that the cervical disks are smaller and under less stress from weight bearing than the lumbar disks.

Most cervical disk injuries are related to degenerative disease and are relatively uncommon as acute conditions.[23] A cervical disk herniation that presents after acute trauma is likely related to previous disk degeneration. The incidence of cervical disk disease increases with age and may be somewhat related to activity.[22,23] The levels most affected by cervical disk disease are C5-C6 and C6-C7.

Most cervical disk herniations occur posterolaterally, which explains the usual clinical syndrome of neck and unilateral arm pain (cervical radiculopathy). However, some disks protrude centrally and posteriorly through the posterior longitudinal ligament and cause compression of the spinal cord but do not affect the spinal nerve roots (**Figure 16-17**). These central disks can result in profound myelopathy and acute spinal cord syndromes.

The clinical symptoms most commonly associated with a herniated cervical disk are neck pain and unilateral arm pain that may be accompanied by numbness, paresthesias, and weakness (**Table 16-3**). In a patient with obvious cervical radiculopathy with weakness, numbness, and reflex changes, the

Table 16-2

Return-to-Play Guidelines for Cervical Neurapraxia

No Contraindications

Asymptomatic with a spinal canal to vertebral body ratio of less than 0.8

Relative Contraindications

One episode of neurapraxia with a spinal canal to vertebral body ratio of more than 0.8

Documented episode of cervical cord neurapraxia (CCN) associated with intervertebral disk disease and/or degenerative changes

Documented episode of CCN associated with MRI evidence of cord deformation

Absolute Contraindications

Documented episode of CCN associated with MRI evidence of cord defect or cord edema

Documented episode of CCN associated with ligamentous instability, neurologic symptoms lasting more than 36 hours, and/or multiple episodes

Reproduced with permission from Torg JS, Guille JT, Jaffe S: Injuries to the cervical spine in American football players. *J Bone Joint Surg Am* 2002;84:112-122.

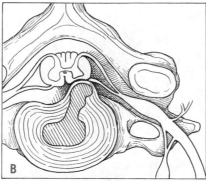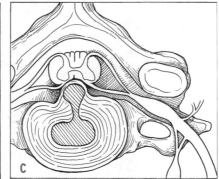

Figure 16-17 Types of disk herniations. **A.** Intraforaminal, producing symptoms along the distribution of the involved nerve root. **B.** Posterolateral radicular symptoms occur in a more diffuse pattern, but tend to remain on one side of the body. **C.** Midline herniations produce diffuse radicular symptoms on both sides of the body. (Reproduced with permission from Levine MJ, Albert TJ, Smith MD: Cervical radiculopathy: Diagnosis and nonoperative management. *J Am Acad Orthop Surg* 1996;4:305-316.)

diagnosis of cervical disk disease can be made by clinical examination alone.

Differential Diagnosis

Cervical spondylolysis, cervical strain, degenerative osteoarthritis, tumor (primary or metastatic)

Imaging Techniques

Imaging studies may be obtained for patients with signs and symptoms of cervical disk herniations that have not improved with conservative therapy. Cervical spine radiographs may demonstrate degenerative change such as disk-space narrowing or vertebral "beaking" caused by osteophytes but do not provide visualization of a herniated disk (**Figure 16-18**). MRI is the most useful test in the evaluation of a cervical herniated disk, allowing visualization of the disks and compression of the nerve roots or the spinal cord.

Despite the usefulness of MRI, cervical myelography with postmyelogram CT scanning may still be necessary (**Figure 16-19**). Myelography and CT are particularly useful in patients who have

multilevel abnormalities on MRI or have previously undergone cervical surgery.

Definitive Diagnosis

The definitive diagnosis is based on the clinical findings and a positive radiograph, MRI, or CT myelogram.

Pathomechanics and Functional Limitations

Functional status is related to pain and arm weakness but is typically self-regulated by patient tolerance. Advanced cases of disk degeneration create a neuropathy in the involved nerve roots and can paralyze the associated muscles. Secondary muscle spasm may develop in the scapular and cervical muscles.

■ Immediate Management

The initial management of a patient with a suspected cervical herniated disk is conservative. Cervical pain and muscle spasm can be treated with cold packs, and a soft collar may be applied to reduce pressure on the cervical vertebrae. The patient may experience reduced symptoms when lying or reclining.

Myelogram/ myelography A radiographic record of the spinal cord and nerves.

16

Table 16-3

Single Cervical Nerve Root Syndrome

	Cervical Disk			
	C4-C5	**C5-C6**	**C6-C7**	**C7-T1**
Compressed root	C5	C6	C7	C8
Percentage of cervical disks involved at this level	2%	19%	69%	10%
Reflex(es) diminished	Deltoid, pectoralis	Biceps, brachioradialis	Triceps	Finger jerk
Motor weakness	Deltoid	Forearm flexion	Forearm extension (wrist drop)	Hand intrinsic muscles
Paresthesia and hypesthesia	Shoulder	Upper arm, thumb, radial forearm	Fingers 2 and 3, all fingertips	Fingers 4 and 5

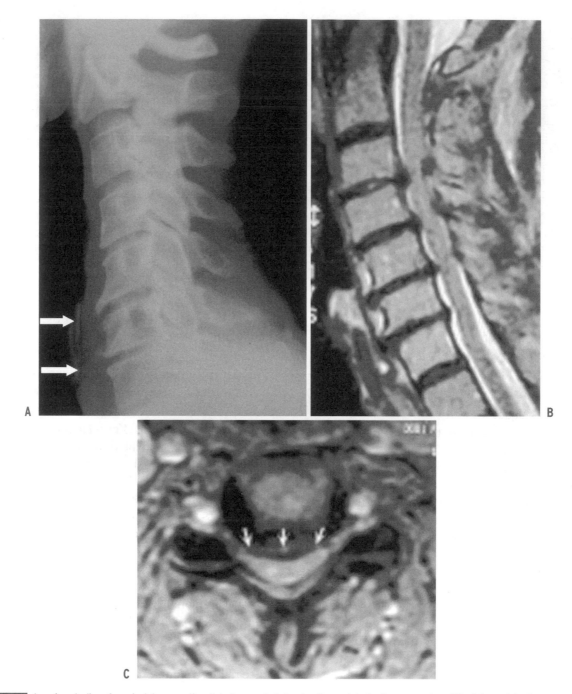

Figure 16-18 Imaging studies of cervical degenerative disk disease. **A.** Lateral radiograph indicating narrowing of the intervertebral space and osteophyte formation consistent with degenerative disk disease. Note the "beaked" formation of the vertebrae (arrows). **B.** Sagittal MRI demonstrating degenerative disk disease at multiple levels. **C.** Axial MRI showing a bulge of the cervical disk (arrows). (Parts B and C are reproduced with permission from Khanna AJ, Carbone JJ, Kebaish KM, et al: Magnetic resonance imaging of the cervical spine: Current techniques and spectrum of disease. *J Bone Joint Surg Am* 2002;84(suppl 2);70-80.)

▦ Medications

In patients with severe, acute pain, a course of an oral corticosteroid, such as methylprednisolone or dexamethasone, may be used. The course of corticosteroids is followed by NSAIDs, such as ibuprofen. In patients with acute and intense pain, narcotics may be necessary for at least the first 5 to 7 days.

▦ Postinjury Management

Approximately 60% to 70% of patients with a cervical herniated disk improve significantly or recover completely without surgical intervention.[22] The patient continues with palliative treatments and collar use and segues into more specific rehabilitation (see p 547).

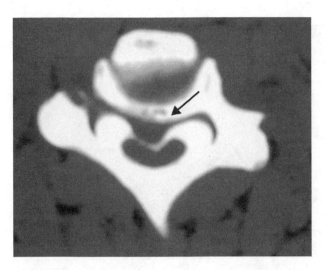

Figure 16-19 Postmyelogram axial CT image of large central disk herniation causing spinal cord compression.

Surgical Techniques

The decision about surgical technique for a herniated cervical disk (ie, an anterior or posterior approach) is based on the location of the disk herniation (central or lateral), whether the cervical spine is unstable, and whether contralateral disk disease is present (even if asymptomatic). Some surgeons operate on all herniated cervical disks using an anterior approach.

The posterior cervical laminectomy and foraminotomy can be performed at more than one level if there is adjacent symptomatic disk disease or spondylosis (ST 16-5). The posterior laminectomy and foraminotomy is less disruptive of normal anatomy and motion of the cervical spine than an anterior cervical diskectomy with or without fusion.

In the presence of cervical disk disease, some surgeons elect to perform an anterior cervical diskectomy without placing a bone graft; in most instances, the spine goes on to fuse spontaneously at the affected level (ST 16-6). Other surgeons always place a bone graft, with or without anterior cervical instrumentation. The technique of anterior cervical diskectomy for cervical disk disease is the same as that described for cervical spine stabilization after fractures and dislocations (see p 527).

In patients who have a posterior laminotomy or anterior cervical diskectomy with or without fusion, the hospital stay is usually one night. Some patients can be discharged on the same day as surgery.

Postoperative Management

Range of motion is protected and lifting is restricted for 2 to 3 weeks after surgery. The patient may wear an external orthosis such as an Aspen or Miami J collar for several weeks or several months (see Figure 16-3). If internal hardware is used, the patient may wear a soft collar for several weeks to decrease pain and prevent muscle spasm.

Injury-Specific Treatment and Rehabilitation Concerns

> **Specific Concerns**
>
> Control inflammation with modalities and/or medications.
> Provide symptomatic treatment for radicular pain and muscle spasm.
> Decrease the compressive forces on the cervical nerve roots.
> Increase facet joint motion.

A treatment protocol including heat, massage, and gentle ROM exercises may be helpful for symptomatic management. A period of soft-collar immobilization may reduce muscle spasm associated with the injury.[22] Cervical traction is often advocated. Although it can be helpful for chronic cervical spondylotic radiculopathy, it is usually not helpful with an acute herniated cervical disk and may actually aggravate the patient's pain.[23] Cervical epidural steroids may also be helpful in the management of these patients but probably should be performed only after imaging techniques confirm a cervical herniated disk.

If conservative measures fail to decrease the patient's symptoms after several weeks of treatment or the patient develops significant weakness of the arm or signs and symptoms of cervical spinal cord dysfunction (cervical myelopathy), surgical intervention should be considered.

Estimated Amount of Time Lost

After surgery 6 to 8 weeks of activity may be lost, but the type of injury and surgical technique dictate whether or not patient will return to contact and collision sports. Patients treated conservatively lose various amounts of time from activity. A patient who recovers quickly from an acute episode and does not require surgery may be allowed to return to diving, for example, but not if the episode resulted in a large herniation, surgical intervention, or fusion. Return to activity is contingent on the severity of injury and the type and extensiveness of treatment, amount of invasion, and success of rehabilitation.

16

Posterior Cervical Laminectomy and Foraminotomy

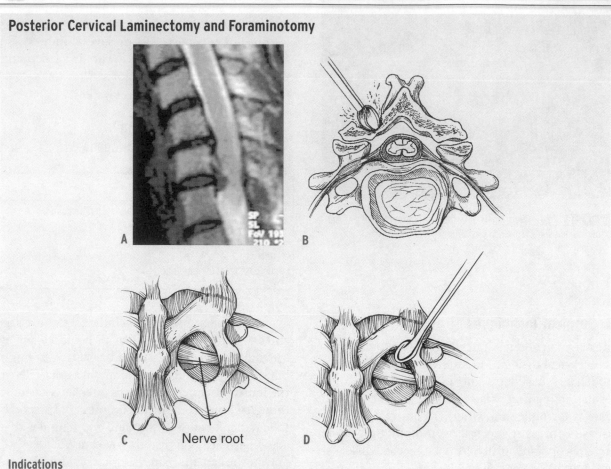

Nerve root

Indications

A documented cervical herniated disk that continues to produce significant pain after 4 to 6 weeks of conservative therapy (**A**); patients with significant weakness or spinal cord dysfunction; lateral herniated disk causing unilateral nerve root compression without evidence of spinal cord compression

Overview

1. The patient is placed prone in a fixed head holder.
2. A midline skin incision is made, and the paraspinous muscles are dissected off the laminae and facet joints on the appropriate side (**B**).
3. Laminectomy is performed, and the nerve root is identified and decompressed laterally as it enters the foramen (**C**).
4. The herniated disk fragment or fragments are generally found in the axilla of the nerve root and are removed (**D**).

Functional Limitations

ROM and strengthening exercises are necessary, especially with a preoperative neurologic deficit. Lifting is limited to less than 10 to 15 lb (4.50 to 6.75 kg) postoperatively for 2 to 3 weeks and no more than 25 lb (11.25 kg) for 6 to 8 weeks.

Implications for Rehabilitation

For patient comfort, a soft collar may be worn for a few days (if single-level laminectomy).

Comments

Normal activities may resume within 2 to 3 months of surgery.

Figures reproduced with permission from Albert TJ, Murrell SE: Surgical management of cervical radiculopathy. *J Am Acad Orthop Surg* 1999;7:368-376.

■ Return-to-Play Criteria

The presence of a symptomatic herniated disk with spinal cord or nerve root compression causing significant pain, weakness, or numbness is an absolute contraindication to athletic activity. In a patient who has had a posterolateral laminectomy and foraminotomy for a lateral herniated disk, return to contact and collision sports is possible after sufficient recovery, provided there is no residual neurologic deficit and no abnormal ROM of the cervical spine.

S|T Surgical Technique 16-6

Anterior Cervical Diskectomy

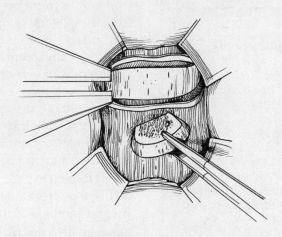

Indications

Documented cervical herniated disk that continues to produce debilitating pain after 4 to 6 weeks of conservative therapy, earlier in patients with significant weakness or spinal cord dysfunction surgery; central disk herniation with spinal cord compression; possibly patients with bilateral disk herniations, even if one side is asymptomatic

Overview

1. The patient is placed supine with the head slightly turned to one side.
2. A longitudinal incision is made in the anterior neck, and dissection is carried down through the platysma and along the anterior border of the sternocleidomastoid muscle to the spine.
3. A bone graft is harvested, often from the patient's iliac crest.
4. An anterior cervical diskectomy at the affected level is performed, and bone graft is placed in the disk space (see figure).
5. An anterior plate may be used to secure the graft (see Surgical Technique 16-3).

   This procedure is the same as for cervical spine stabilization after fracture-dislocation described for anterior cervical diskectomy and fusion; with disk disease, however, hardware is not always used. The use of hardware/fixation depends on the activity level of the patient and the preference of the surgeon. For example, athletes are more likely to have fixation than sedentary workers.

Functional Limitations

Many patients require ROM and strengthening exercises, especially with a preoperative neurologic deficit.

Implications for Rehabilitation

Lifting is limited to less than 10 to 15 lb (4.50 to 6.75 kg) postoperatively for 2 to 3 weeks and no more than 25 lb (11.25 kg) for 6 to 8 weeks.

Comments

Normal activities may resume within 2 to 3 months of surgery.

Figure reproduced with permission from Albert TJ, Murrell SE: Surgical management of cervical radiculopathy. *J Am Acad Orthop Surg* 1999;7:368-376.

16

Patients who have had anterior cervical diskectomy and fusion for symptomatic cervical disk herniation should not be allowed to return to contact or collision sports because of the possibility of altered biomechanics surrounding the fused segments. Depending on the severity of injury and surgical intervention, patients who regain full preinjury strength and functional status may return to sports. However, it is unlikely that those with hardware will return to contact and collision sports. It is also unlikely that a surgeon would allow an athlete who has sustained an axial load-type force to return to sports such as football, ice hockey, gymnastics, soccer, cheerleading, or wrestling. The level of risk, age of the patient, and specific position played (in football) all factor into the return-to-play decision.

Brachial Plexus Injury

CLINICAL PRESENTATION

History

Cervical spine forced laterally away from the shoulder
Forcible depression of the shoulder while the cervical spine remains neutral or slightly lateral to the shoulder
Rotation of the cervical spine away from the affected shoulder
Compression of the Erb point
The combination of any of these mechanisms

Observation

The patient most often carries the affected arm hanging loosely at the side, with the body leaning toward the affected shoulder.
Typically no signs of this injury are visible; the most characteristic aspects of this condition are the mechanism of injury and the symptoms described by the patient.

Functional Status

Radicular neurologic symptoms of numbness and tingling throughout the brachial plexus dermatomes immediately postinsult
Muscular weakness or transient paralysis along the myotomes

Physical Evaluation Findings

Unilateral muscular weakness and radicular symptoms along the C5 to T1 myotomes and dermatomes
Subjective neurologic assessment of dermatomes
Pain-free cervical spine on palpation and ROM
The following special tests may be positive:
  Brachial plexus traction/compression test
  Spurling test
  Shoulder abduction test

The brachial plexus is formed by the C5 to T1 nerve roots. These roots exit the cervical spine and pass through the cervicoaxillary canal under the clavicle to provide innervation to the upper extremity. Trauma to the brachial plexus occurs when the cervical spine moves away from the shoulder in a forcible fashion, often when the head or shoulder hits an unyielding object or an opponent. This mechanism primarily occurs in football players when the helmet and neck are hyperextended or moved laterally away from a depressed shoulder, such as during a tackle.[18,24]

The resulting force can either stretch the nerves on the opposite side of the motion or compress the nerves on the side toward which the cervical spine is bending. Another mechanism for brachial-plexus trauma is compression of the Erb point, the most superficial aspect of the brachial plexus, located 2 to 3 cm superior to the clavicle. The typically brief, transient motion stresses the brachial plexus, and the resulting condition includes radicular symp-

toms and muscular weakness along the path of the neurologic cords to the affected hand and fingers (Figure 16-20).

Often referred to as a "stinger" or "burner" by the lay public, a brachial plexus injury produces unilateral symptoms and must be differentiated from the bilateral symptoms associated with spinal cord injury. In athletes, brachial plexus neuropathy is typically traumatic, but symptoms have been reported from activity as simple as carrying too heavy a pack on one shoulder, which depresses it to the point of causing chronic but steady traction on the brachial plexus of the ipsilateral shoulder.

A complete rupture of the brachial plexus from a traction injury is rare and must be recognized in a timely fashion to prevent permanent disability. A delay of 6 months or longer is the most significant negative prognostic factor in recovery via a surgical graft.[25]

Differential Diagnosis

Spinal cord trauma, subluxated or dislocated humerus, abnormally shaped clavicle compressing the thoracic outlet

Imaging Techniques

It is rare for true brachial plexus injuries to require further testing or imaging, let alone surgical intervention. If the injury is not limited to a few episodes over time but instead becomes chronic, further diagnostic evaluation should be initiated. Plain radiography or CT rule out stenosis or osteophytes of the intervertebral foramen that impinge on the cervical nerve roots; MRI is used to identify injury to the spinal cord and associated nerve roots.

Definitive Diagnosis

Identification of the mechanism of injury, symptoms limited to the involved dermatomes (in most cases, symptoms are unilateral), rapid fading of symptoms, and the exclusion of the conditions identified in the Differential Diagnosis section above. Repeated episodes of brachial plexus trauma warrant radiographs and/or MRI to rule out a structural predisposition to this condition.

Chronic episodes of brachial plexus neuropathy without trauma may be caused by cervical stenosis, breast or lung carcinoma, regional hematoma, or thoracic outlet syndrome.

Pathomechanics and Functional Limitations

Neuropathy of the involved nerve roots results in paresthesia of the associated dermatomes and muscle weakness of the associated myotomes (see Figure 16-20). Associated spasm of the upper trapezius, sternocleidomastoid, levator scapulae, or scalene muscles can cause pain and restrict ROM in the cervical spine.

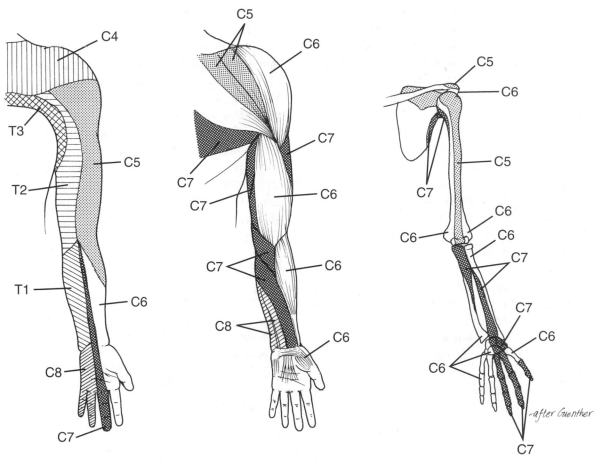

Figure 16-20 Dermatomes, myotomes, and sclerotomes of the upper extremity. The patient will have sensory and/or motor nerve symptoms within these regions corresponding with the associated spinal nerve root(s) involved. (Reproduced with permission from Levine MJ, Albert TJ, Smith MD: Cervical radiculopathy: Diagnosis and nonoperative management. *J Am Acad Orthop Surg* 1996;4:305-316.)

■ Immediate Management

If cervical spine instability or spinal cord injury is a possibility, the patient must be splinted and placed on a backboard. If the mechanism and resulting symptoms indicate brachial plexus injury, the paresthesia and muscular weakness typically resolve within a few seconds to several minutes.

■ Postinjury/Postoperative Management

The primary goal for postacute brachial plexus insult is to return to full functional and neurologic status as quickly as possible. Immediate treatment of brachial plexus neuropathy should include ice and physical agents (such as electric stimulation) that are designed to decrease muscle spasm in the upper back and shoulder area. However, these modalities are only palliative and should not be the focus of long-term treatment of this or any other cervical spine condition. Rest and a soft cervical collar may also be indicated.

■ Injury-Specific Treatment and Rehabilitation Concerns

Specific Concerns

Control pain and muscle spasm.
Strengthen cervical muscles.
Restore ROM.

The primary goals of rehabilitation after a brachial plexus injury are to strengthen and condition the musculature affiliated with the cervical spine. Determination of the patient's neurologic status largely depends on subjective information obtained during the evaluation. Muscular strength and coordination can be ascertained through exercises specific to maintaining cervical stability. The muscles that provide support and protection to the cervical spine—including the trapezius, sternocleidomastoid, levator scapulae, scalene, splenius, and longissimus groups—must be strengthened to lessen the likelihood of reinjury. Additionally, the patient must have regained full functional ROM. Manual interventions should focus on general manual traction while the patient is in a comfortable position, for example with some lateral cervical flexion, usually to the side of the injury.

Brachial plexus neuropathy occasionally returns after the initial episode and may become chronic. A treatment scheme based on the Maitland approach to treatment of acute and chronic nerve root abnormality is indicated.[26] In this approach, manual traction is initially performed at the angle in which the cervical spine is postured with little additional motion. The cervical spine is generally found laterally flexed to the side of the injury. As time elapses and symptoms permit (ie, less pain with ROM), lateral flexion and rotation to the opposite side are indicated. For example, if the injury is on the left side, then a slow progression to right lateral flexion and right rotation is appropriate. As the condition becomes chronic, palliative measures can progress to moist heat rather than ice and, as pain allows, traction should progress to the neutral position. In addition, rotation away from the side of the injury is initiated and continued until the patient has full, pain-free motion, rotation, and lateral flexion away from the affected side.

■ Estimated Amount of Time Lost

Brachial plexus neuropathy can result in only a few minutes of playing time being lost or, depending on the magnitude of the symptoms and the underlying injury, may result in several months of absence from contact or collision sport activity.

■ Return-to-Play Criteria

Two criteria must be met before the patient can return to participation. First, cervical spine abnormality must be ruled out. Any patient suspected of having a cervical spine injury should not be allowed to return to play until potentially catastrophic conditions have been ruled out. Second, both dermatomes and ROM should be evaluated: the patient may return to competition when cervical ROM is full and pain free and strength and sensation of the upper extremity are equal bilaterally. Strength of shoulder abduction (deltoids), elbow flexion (biceps), elbow extension (triceps), wrist extension, wrist flexion, and finger abduction and adduction must be ascertained.

Functional Bracing

Cervical collars alone do not provide protection from brachial plexus trauma, and collars custom-made by nonprofessionals may increase the chance of injury to the cervical spine and should be avoided. Wearing a collar does not preclude an athlete from the obligation to use proper tackling technique or maintain cervical strength and conditioning. Athletes who sustain multiple brachial plexus injuries should be evaluated for other cervical conditions, tackling technique, and a cervical conditioning program before a decision is made to recommend a cervical collar.

Cervical Strains

CLINICAL PRESENTATION

History

Sudden contraction or overstretching of the muscles
Pain over the involved muscle(s)
Muscle spasm placing pressure on nerves, producing radicular symptoms

Observation

The head is postured for comfort.
Muscle spasm causes the head and cervical spine to tilt along the muscle's line of pull.

Functional Status

Active and resisted ROM in the muscle's antagonistic pattern produces pain.
Passive ROM in the muscle's antagonistic pattern produces pain.
Strength is decreased.
Motion is limited.

Physical Evaluation Findings

Palpable tenderness over the injured site
Confirmation of the findings noted in Functional Status

A cervical strain can be determined largely by history of injury and reproducible pain with muscular contraction. It is rare, although possible, for a muscular injury to cause radicular symptoms, but muscle spasm or edema may impinge on specific nerves as they pass by the affected muscle.

The patient's functional status following a cervical strain depends on the severity of the strain. A minor strain may only be annoying, yet function is still possible; a muscular tear, on the other hand, may be prohibitive in athletics. Full cervical ROM in addition to functional strength should be ascertained before making any determination on activity.

Differential Diagnosis

Cervical sprain, brachial plexus injury, disk injury, infectious illness (eg, meningitis)

Imaging Techniques

An abnormal radiograph can confirm the presence of muscular injury. Although imaging is not typically obtained, MRI indicates muscular damage.

Definitive Diagnosis

Limited ROM and strength deficit for the affected muscle

Pathomechanics and Functional Testing

Specific muscle testing to determine the exact muscle afflicted or motion involved, as well as strength testing of that muscle to assess injury severity

Immediate Management

Any underlying injury should be ruled out and followed by application of ice and stretching to retard additional spasm and swelling. A soft collar may be warranted in the acute stages to decrease pain and spasm.

Medications

NSAIDs may be used to alleviate pain and inflammation. If spasm is severe, muscle relaxants and antianxiety medications may be helpful.

Surgical Intervention

It is unusual for a cervical strain to require surgical repair. Most muscles in the neck have reciprocal muscles that provide a similar function; consequently the loss of a specific muscle, although cosmetically damaging, may not affect overall cervical function.

Postinjury/Postoperative Management

Ice is administered while the inflammatory response is still active, followed by heat and gentle exercises specific to the injured and complementary muscles. Use of a soft collar should be discontinued as soon as practical.

Injury-Specific Treatment and Rehabilitation Concerns

> **Specific Concerns**
>
> Control muscle spasm.
> Maintain ROM.
> Strengthen cervical muscles.

Management of a cervical strain includes limiting swelling and spasm. Once these are under control, early ROM should be initiated, followed by gentle strengthening. ROM includes working on cervical flexion and extension, rotation, and lateral bending. Strengthening exercises can begin with isometric cervical exercises in all directions, increasing to free weights using the shoulder and cervical musculature. All major muscles must be strengthened, not merely the affected ones.

Estimated Amount of Time Lost

Time lost due to a cervical strain may vary from no time lost to 6 weeks or longer in the event of a complete muscle tear. The time lost depends on how quickly the patient regains ROM and functional strength.

Return-to-Play Criteria

Return to play can occur when full ROM is regained and the athlete can see and protect himself or herself in competition.

Functional Bracing

Bracing is not indicated for a cervical strain. Cervical braces are intended for postsurgical or postinjury protection, not for use during competition.

Immediate Management of On-Field Cervical Spine Injuries

A cervical spine injury should be assumed when the patient is unconscious on the playing field. If the airway is obstructed, the patient should be log-rolled into a supine position while the cervical spine is stabilized using in-line traction. If the athlete is conscious but down on the field, a complete physical examination of the cervical spine and the associated myotomes/dermatomes should be conducted before the athlete is removed from the field. The Intra-Association Task Force on the Prehospital Care of the Spine-Injured Athlete described the recommended on-field management of acute spine injuries.[27] Any unconscious athlete or one with signs or symptoms indicating trauma to the cervical spine or spinal cord should be placed on a backboard and transported immediately to a hospital[27] (**Table 16-4**).

Considerable debate has focused on when and where to remove the helmet and shoulder pads. If cardiopulmonary resuscitation (CPR) is indicated,

Table 16-4

Guidelines for Appropriate Care of the Spine-Injured Athlete

General Guidelines

Any athlete suspected of having a spinal injury should not be moved and should be managed as though a spinal injury exists.

The athlete's airway, breathing, circulation, neurologic status, and level of consciousness should be assessed.

The athlete should not be moved unless absolutely essential to maintain airway, breathing, and circulation.

An athlete who must be moved to maintain airway, breathing, and/or circulation should be placed in a supine position while maintaining spinal immobilization. When moving an athlete with a suspected spine injury, the head and trunk should be moved as a unit. One accepted technique is to manually splint the head to the trunk by placing the hands on the trapezius muscle of the injured athlete and bracing his or her head with the forearms of the rescuer.

The Emergency Medical Services (EMS) system should be activated as soon as it is ascertained that the athlete is either unconscious or has a suspected spinal injury.

Face-Mask Removal

The face mask should be removed immediately with appropriate face-mask removal instruments regardless of current respiratory status.

Those involved in the prehospital care of injured football players should have the tools for safely removing face masks readily available.

Football Helmet Removal

The athletic football helmet and chin strap should only be removed:

- if the helmet and chin strap do not hold the head securely, such that immobilization of the helmet does not also immobilize the head;
- if the design of the helmet and chin strap is such that even after removal of the face mask, the airway cannot be controlled or ventilation cannot be provided;
- if the face mask cannot be removed after a reasonable period of time; and
- if the helmet prevents immobilization for transportation in an appropriate position.

Helmet Removal

Spinal immobilization must be maintained while removing the helmet.

Helmet removal should be frequently practiced under proper supervision in a controlled environment.

Specific guidelines for helmet removal need to be developed. In most circumstances, it may be helpful to remove cheek padding and/or deflate air padding, and cut the chin straps before helmet removal.

Equipment

Appropriate spinal alignment must be maintained.

The fact that the football helmet and shoulder pads elevate an athlete's trunk when in the supine position should be recognized.

If the football helmet is to be removed, the shoulder pads must also be removed at the same time.

The front of the shoulder pads can be opened without helmet removal to allow access for CPR and defibrillation.

Note: The Task Force encourages the development of a local emergency care plan regarding the prehospital care of the athlete with a suspected spinal cord injury. This plan should include communication with the institution's administration and those directly involved with the assessment and transportation of the injured athlete.[27]

All providers of prehospital care should practice and be competent in all of the skills identified in these guidelines before they are needed in an emergency situation.

Adapted with permission from *Intra-Association Task Force for Appropriate Care of the Spine-Injured Athlete: Prehospital Care of the Spine-Injured Athlete*. Dallas, TX, National Athletic Trainers' Association, 2000.

---

the athlete's face mask must be removed, and the jersey and lacing on the anterior shoulder pad can be cut to allow administration of CPR. The football helmet assists in stabilizing the cervical spine, and shoulder pads help to maintain a slight degree of extension. The football helmet and shoulder pads should not be removed until radiographs are obtained, but the need for CPR warrants removal of the helmet and shoulder pads.

Established guidelines specific to certain sports (eg, football and ice hockey) address the efficacy of helmet removal; the common theme is to leave the helmet on because removal can cause further cervical insult.[28,29]

Rehabilitation for Noncatastrophic Cervical Spine Trauma

The premise for rehabilitation of cervical spine injuries is to continue to protect the cervical spine and regain normal strength. The achievable ROM depends on the surgical procedure performed, because some repair techniques permanently limit ROM. The onset of ROM activities may be delayed as long as 3 months in order to allow complete healing to occur. Typically, the first goals of rehabilitation are to protect the repair or injury from further harm and decrease swelling and pain. Gradually, with the physician's permission, exercises to strengthen and protect the cervical spine can be initiated. The muscles primarily involved in these functions are the trapezius, latissimus dorsi, levator scapulae, sternocleidomastoid, and scalene. In addition, the rotator cuff, scapular stabilizers, and pectoralis muscles may be stretched and strengthened to facilitate proper posture and ROM and to encourage balance among muscle groups. Finally, core-stabilization exercises are paramount to maintaining a healthy cervical spine.

Other aspects of cervical rehabilitation include teaching correct lifting techniques, proper posture (while sitting, standing, and walking), and balance. Challenges to this rehabilitation program begin at the onset of therapy, when limitations (ROM, weight restrictions, etc) are in place to protect the injury.

See chapter 17 for more spinal-stabilization techniques. Manual therapy and ROM exercises should not be performed in the presence of an unhealed fracture.

Manual Therapies

Massage

Soft-tissue massage can be used to reduce muscle spasm and break up scar tissue. Deep pétrissage and effleurage increase circulation, decrease pain, and help to resolve muscle spasm (**Figure 16-21**). Cross-friction massage and myofascial release techniques can be used to help reduce soft-tissue restrictions that limit ROM. Cross-friction massage is performed by positioning the cervical spine so that the muscle is lax. Pressure is then applied to the muscle perpendicular to the direction of its fibers.

Cervical Traction

Manual or mechanical cervical traction can be used to decrease the weight-bearing forces on the facet joints, reduce pressure on the intervertebral disks and the cervical nerve roots, and elongate the cervical musculature (**Figure 16-22**). Laterally bending the cervical spine during traction opens the facet joints and stretches the soft tissues but compresses the structures on the side toward the bend. Flexing the cervical spine stretches the posterior structures, and extending it targets the anterior structures.

16

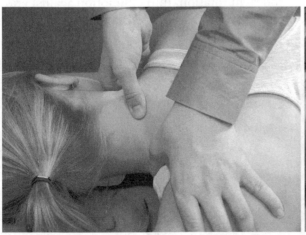 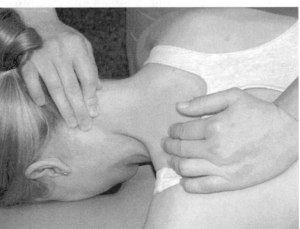

A   B

Figure 16-21 Soft-tissue mobilization techniques for the cervical spine musculature. **A.** Cross-friction massage of the upper trapezius muscle. **B.** Myofascial release.

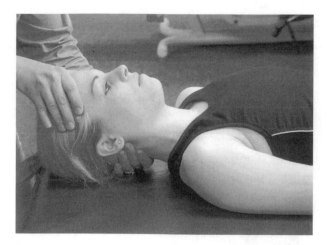

Figure 16-22 Manual traction to the cervical spine. This technique can reduce pressure on the disks, facets, and nerve roots. Changing the angle of pull allows specificity of the structures being stressed.

■ Vertebral Glides

Vertebral glides are used to restore normal joint motion to a hypomobile segment. Typically, mobilizations are graded from I to V. The mobilization grade selected for use is based on the amount of passive ROM needed at the segment (**Figure 16-23**).

The central posteroanterior (PA) glide, which is simply the spring test applied with grades of mobilization, is commonly used to treat facet hypomobility (see Figure 16-23A). To mobilize the entire segment, the thumbs are placed over the spinous process and pressure is exerted in an anterosuperior direction. To isolate individual facets, the pressure is applied directly over the target joint.

The thumbs are placed over the spinous process of the segment in question to introduce rotation. The lower mobilization grades are used for more acute dysfunctions. Transverse glides introduce a rotational force to the segment by moving the spinous process laterally (see Figure 16-23B).

Flexibility Exercises

Flexibility, including ROM exercises, is critical for cervical spine rehabilitation, particularly for those cases involving disk disease and brachial plexus trauma. Some cervical spine conditions, however, are in a rare group for which ROM exercises are contraindicated for safe recovery; these conditions include many surgical corrections, spinal cord injury, and some fractures. As with any rehabilitation program, the physician must be consulted before exercises are initiated after injury or surgery. The following exercises are for stretching specific muscles associated with the cervical spine, and performing these stretches will enhance the ROM of the particular muscle or group.

The average ROM of the cervical spine is 0° to 45° of flexion, extension, and lateral flexion and 60° of rotation. The most effective method of stretching the cervical spine is manual resistance. Only the force necessary to achieve a gentle, pain-free stretch is applied (**Figure 16-24**). An alternative is to have the patient apply his or her own resistance to the stretch. Using elastic bands or weights to assist stretching is not recommended for the cervical spine. For all of these stretches, the patient sits or lies down; force is applied in a steady fashion for 15 to 20 seconds and repeated 3 to 4 times.

Strengthening Exercises

The patient can progress through a range of isotonic strengthening exercises, including flexion, extension, left and right lateral bending, and left and right rotation. Initially, motion against gravity may provide sufficient resistance to strengthen the

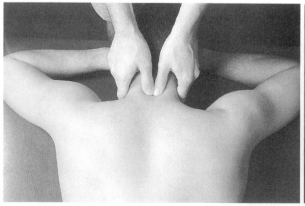

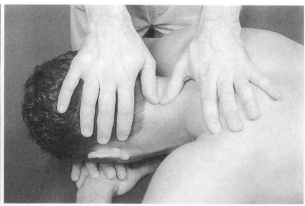

Figure 16-23 Cervical vertebral glides. **A.** Central posteroanterior glide, which applies pressure to the spinous process in an anterior direction. **B.** Transverse glide, in which the spinous process is gently mobilized left and right.

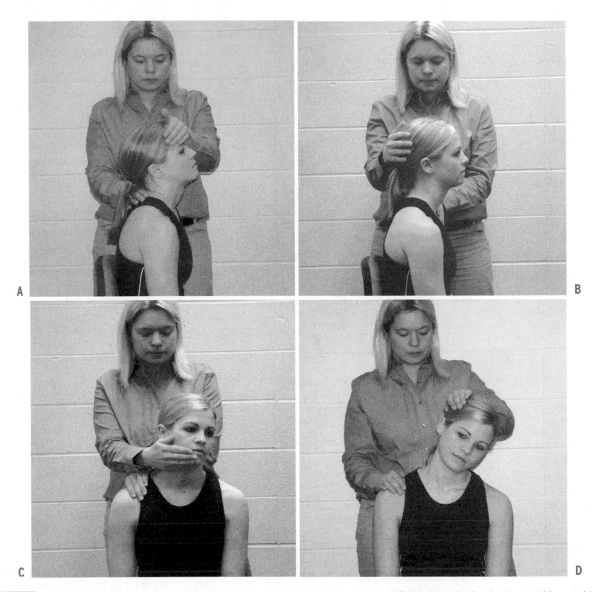

Figure 16-24 Cervical passive ROM exercises. **A.** Flexion for the upper trapezius, rotators, and multifidi. **B.** Extension for the sternocleidomastoid and multifidi. **C.** Rotation for the sternocleidomastoid on the side toward the motion, scalenes, rotators, and multifidi. Exercise is repeated in each direction. **D.** Lateral bending for the upper trapezius, sternocleidomastoid, and scalenes. Adding cervical flexion to the lateral bending targets the levator scapulae. Exercise is repeated in each direction.

16

muscle for flexion-extension and lateral bending. As the patient progresses, manual resistance can be used to strengthen the cervical muscles. The techniques used for manual resistance exercises are similar to those used for flexibility, but the patient moves against the resistance (see Figure 16-24).

Options are limited for free-weight or weight-machine training of the cervical muscles. Some commercial isotonic weight machines provide options for cervical flexion, extension, and lateral bending motions. Although free weights can be attached to a belt that fits around the patient's head, these techniques are not advocated for rehabilitation because of the risk of further traumatizing the area.

Refer to chapter 17 for a description of strengthening techniques for the extrinsic cervical spine muscles.

Core Stabilization Exercises

Exercise programs designed to strengthen stabilizing muscles are crucial to the proper treatment of hypermobile spinal segments. These programs should also be a part of spinal rehabilitation after hypomobile segments have been effectively mobilized and the patient has normal ROM. Refer to chapter 17 for a description of spinal core-stabilization exercises.

References

1. Botte MJ, Byrne TP, Abrams RA, Garfin SR: Halo skeletal fixation: Techniques of application and prevention of complications. *J Am Acad Orthop Surg* 1996;4:44-53.

2. Joint Section on Disorders of the Spine and Peripheral Nerves of the American Association of Neurological Surgeons and the Congress of Neurological Surgeons: Management of acute cervical spine and spinal cord injuries: Isolated fractures of the atlas in adults. *Neurosurgery* 2002;50(suppl 3):S120-S124.

3. Khanna AJ, Carbone JJ, Kebaish KM, et al: Magnetic resonance imaging of the cervical spine: Current techniques and spectrum of disease. *J Bone Joint Surg Am* 2002; 84(suppl 2);70-80.

4. Anderson LD, d'Alonzo RT: Fractures of the odontoid process of the axis. *J Bone Joint Surg Am* 1974;56:1663-1674.

5. Chutkan NB, King AG, Harris MB: Odontoid fractures: Evaluation and management. *J Am Acad Orthop Surg* 1997;5:199-204.

6. Joint Section on Disorders of the Spine and Peripheral Nerves of the American Association of Neurological Surgeons and the Congress of Neurological Surgeons: Management of acute cervical spine and spinal cord injuries: Isolated fractures of the axis in adults. *Neurosurgery* 2002;50(suppl 3):S125-S139.

7. Joint Section on Disorders of the Spine and Peripheral Nerves of the American Association of Neurological Surgeons and the Congress of Neurological Surgeons: Management of acute cervical spine and spinal cord injuries: Treatment of subaxial cervical spine injuries. *Neurosurgery* 2002;50(suppl 3):S156-S165.

8. Delamarter RB, Coyle J: Acute management of spinal cord injury. *J Am Acad Orthop Surg* 1999;7:166-175.

9. Torg J, Vegso JJ, O'Neill MJ, Sennett B: The epidemiologic, pathologic, biomechanical, and cinematographic analysis of football-induced cervical spine trauma. *Am J Sports Med* 1990;18:50-57.

10. Joint Section on Disorders of the Spine and Peripheral Nerves of the American Association of Neurological Surgeons and the Congress of Neurological Surgeons: Management of acute cervical spine and spinal cord injuries: Management of acute spinal cord injuries in an intensive care unit or other monitored setting. *Neurosurgery* 2002;50(suppl 3):S51-S57.

11. Joint Section on Disorders of the Spine and Peripheral Nerves of the American Association of Neurological Surgeons and the Congress of Neurological Surgeons: Pharmacologic therapy after acute cervical spinal cord injury. *Neurosurgery* 2002;50(suppl 3):S63-S72.

12. Bracken MB, Shepard MJ, Collins WF, et al: A randomized, controlled trial of methylprednisolone or naloxone in the treatment of acute spinal-cord injury: Results of the Second National Acute Spinal Cord Injury Study. *N Engl J Med* 1990;322:1405-1411.

13. Bracken MB, Shepard MJ, Holford TR, et al: Administration of methylprednisolone for 24 or 48 hours or tirilazad mesylate for 48 hours in the treatment of acute spinal cord injury: Results of the Third National Acute Spinal Cord Injury Randomized Controlled Trial. National Acute Spinal Cord Injury Study. JAMA 1997;277:1597-1604.

14. Carlson GD, Gorden CD, Oliff HS, Pillai JJ, LaManna JC: Sustained spinal cord compression: Part I. Time-dependent effect on long-term pathophysiology. *J Bone Joint Surg Am* 2003;85:86-94.

15. Carlson GD, Gorden CD, Nakazawa A, Wada E, Smith JS, LaManna JC: Sustained spinal cord compression: Part II. Effect of methyprednisolone on regional blood flow and recovery of somatosensory evoked potentials. *J Bone Joint Surg Am* 2003;85:95-101.

16. Joint Section on Disorders of the Spine and Peripheral Nerves of the American Association of Neurological Surgeons and the Congress of Neurological Surgeons: Blood pressure management after acute spinal cord injury. *Neurosurgery* 2002;50(suppl 3):S58-S62.

17. Torg JS, Guille JT, Jaffe S: Injuries to the cervical spine in American football players. *J Bone Joint Surg Am* 2002;84: 112-122.

18. Thomas BE, McCullen AGM, Yuan HA: Cervical spine injuries in football players. *J Am Acad Orthop Surg* 1999; 7:338-347.

19. Torg JS, Naranja RJ, Pavlov H, Galinat BJ, Warren R, Stine RA: The relationship of developmental narrowing of the cervical spinal canal to reversible and irreversible injury of the cervical spine cord in football players: An epidemiological study. *J Bone Joint Surg Am* 1996;78:1308-1314.

20. Mundt DJ, Kelsey JL, Golden AL, et al: An epidemiologic study of sports and weight lifting as possible risk factors for herniated lumbar and cervical discs: The Northeast Collaborative Group on Low Back Pain. *Am J Sports Med* 1993;21:854-860.

21. Rao R: Neck pain, cervical radiculopathy, and cervical myelopathy: Pathophysiology, natural history, and clinical evaluation. *J Bone Joint Surg Am* 2002;84:1872-1881.

22. Levine MJ, Albert TJ, Smith MD: Cervical radiculopathy: Diagnosis and nonoperative management. *J Am Acad Orthop Surg* 1996;4:305-316.

23. Fager CA: Cervical disc herniation, in Long DM (ed): *Current Therapy in Neurological Surgery*. Toronto, Ontario, Canada, BC Decker, 1985, pp 164-167.

24. Torg J: The cervical spine, spinal cord, and brachial plexus, in Scuderi GR, McCann PD, Burno PJ (eds): *Sports Medicine: Principles of Primary Care*. St Louis, MO, Mosby, 1997, pp 186-201.

25. Bentolila V, Nizard R, Bizot P, Sedel L: Complete traumatic brachial plexus palsy: Treatment and outcome after repair. *J Bone Joint Surg Am* 1999;81:20-28.

26. Maitland GD: *Vertebral Manipulation*, ed 4. London, England, Butterworths, 1977.

27. *Intra-Association Task Force for Appropriate Care of the Spine-Injured Athlete: Prehospital Care of the Spine-Injured Athlete*. Dallas, TX, National Athletic Trainers' Association, 2000.

28. *Inter-Association Task Force for Appropriate Care of the Spine-Injured Athlete: Prehospital Care of the Spine-Injured Athlete*. Dallas, TX, National Athletic Trainers' Association, 1999.

29. Laprade RF, Schnetzler KA, Broxterman RJ, Wentorf F, Gilbert TJ: Cervical spine alignment in the immoblized ice hockey player: A computed tomographic analysis of effects of helmet removal. *Am J Sports Med* 2000;28:800-803.

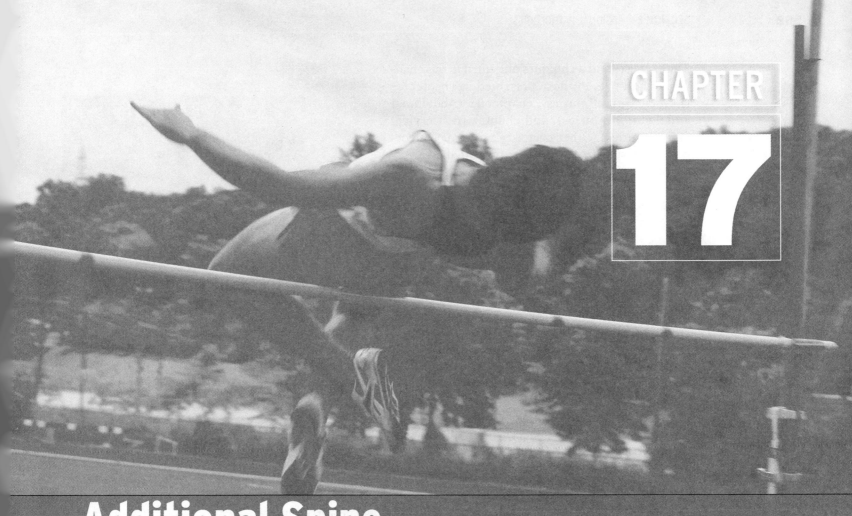

Additional Spine and Torso Therapeutic Exercises

Christopher D. Ingersoll,
PhD, ATC, FACSM
Dilaawar J. Mistry, MD,
MS, ATC

The exercises and techniques presented in this chapter are adjuncts to those presented in chapter 14 (Lumbar Spine Injuries), chapter 15 (Abdominal and Thorax Injuries), and chapter 16 (Cervical Spine Injuries). Other exercises can also be incorporated or substituted for those presented here. Additionally, most exercises can be modified based on the patient's needs, equipment on hand, or personal preference. To construct a complete rehabilitation program, cross-referencing among these chapters may be required.

Flexibility Exercises

Refer to chapters 6, 8, and 9 for lower extremity flexibility exercises and chapter 13 for upper extremity flexibility exercises.

> ### Cross-references
>
> Lumbar spine:
>   Lumbar spine joint mobilization (p 482)
>   Lumbar rotation stretch (p 482)
>   Cat-cow stretch (p 483)
>   Williams' flexion exercises (p 484)
>   McKenzie extension exercises (p 484)
> Cervical spine:
>   Cervical spine vertebral glides (p 548)
>   Cervical ROM exercises (p 549)

Core Strengthening Exercises

Core muscles are those muscles most centrally located to the core of the body. They provide stability to the spine, whereas the larger muscles on the periphery provide spine and trunk movement. The core muscles include the transverse abdominis, lower internal obliques, and multifidus, and the trunk muscles are the erector spinae, external obliques, and rectus abdominis. The core muscles cocontract to provide stiffness and stability to the lumbar spine and pelvis during static and dynamic activities. Multifidus recovery after low back injury does not occur without specific strengthening exercises, and the most important abdominal muscle providing stabilization is the transverse abdominis. For these reasons, the exercises in this section should be taught to patients with low back pain or sacroiliac instability.

Refer to chapter 14, p 484 for a description of pelvic-neutral exercises.

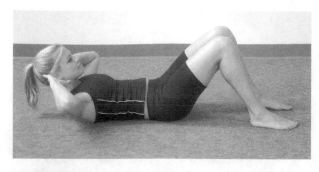

Figure 17-1 Crunches.

Transverse Abdominis Strengthening

In the supine, hook-lying position, the patient actively pulls the umbilicus to the spine as far as possible and holds it for 5 to 10 seconds. The patient should be instructed to breathe while performing this exercise.

Lumbar Multifidus Strengthening

The multifidus is recruited when the pelvic floor muscles are tensed, so the best way to facilitate strengthening is to have the patient tense the pelvic floor muscles. Instructions given to the patient include, "Tighten your muscles as if stopping urination midstream." Hold for 5 to 10 seconds.

Cocontraction

Once the patient can perform each of the above exercises correctly, the next step is to perform an isometric cocontraction of both muscles. These activities are repeated to build strength and muscle endurance. The patient progresses to performing cocontraction sitting, then standing, and then during functional activities.

Abdominal Muscle Strengthening

Crunches In the supine, hook-lying position with the feet unanchored, the patient performs a curl-up until the scapulae are off the floor (**Figure 17-1**). The patient can progress from the arms being crossed over the chest to the hands held behind the head.

Straight-leg Curls In the supine position with the legs extended but not anchored, the patient performs a sit-up in a smooth, continuous motion.

Obliques In the hook-lying position with the hips and knees rotated to one side and the shoulders flat on the floor, the patient lifts the upper trunk toward the upper hip (**Figure 17-2**). When the repetitions are completed on this side, the patient reverses the position, so the hips and knees are rotated to the opposite side, and repeats the exercise.

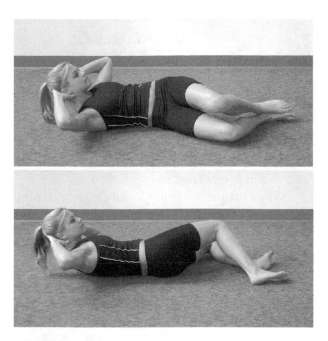

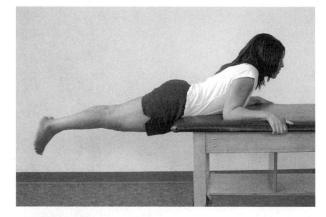

Figure 17-2 Obliques.

Figure 17-4 Prone leg lifts.

Paraspinal Muscle Strengthening

The patient can progress each of these exercises to performing them on a Swiss ball. The unstable surface makes the exercise more difficult.

Superman In the prone position, the patient maintains the pelvic-neutral position, tightens the gluteals, and raises the arms and legs upward for a count of five (**Figure 17-3**).

Prone Leg Lifts Lying on the end of a table with both feet on the floor and the hands grasping the table, the patient tightens the abdominals and gluteals and raises both legs until they are level with the trunk (**Figure 17-4**). A Roman chair can also be used for this exercise.

Prone Trunk Lifts Lying prone on the end of a table with the legs on the table and the trunk extended

over the end and inclined toward the floor, no more than about 30°, the patient contracts the gluteal and paraspinal muscles to elevate the trunk until it is level with the lower extremities (**Figure 17-5**). This exercise can also be performed on a Roman chair. The patient should not bend too far forward; this would place undue stress on the lumbar disks.

Bridging Exercises Lying supine with the knees bent and the feet flat on the surface, the patient tightens the abdomen and buttocks, pressing the small of the back into the surface. While keeping the abdomen and buttocks contracted, the back straight, and the body in a straight line from the knees to the shoulders, the patient lifts the hips off the surface. This position is held for a count of three to five and then released.

Medicine-Ball Exercises

Crunch Toss In the hook-lying position on the floor, the patient positions the arms overhead. While

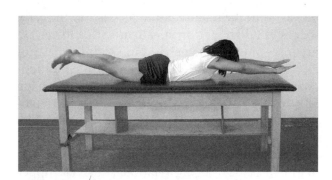

Figure 17-3 Superman.

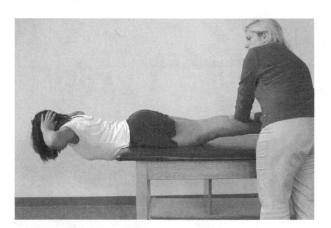

Figure 17-5 Prone trunk lifts.

17

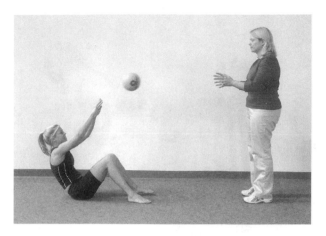

Figure 17-6   Crunch toss.

standing about 10 ft from the patient, the clinician tosses a medicine ball to the patient, so the ball is caught with the arms extended overhead as the patient performs an abdominal crunch (**Figure 17-6**). The patient returns the ball to the clinician and returns to the starting position on the floor. Pelvic-neutral position should be maintained throughout this exercise.

Standing Rotations   Standing about an arm's length apart with backs to each other, the patient and partner rotate to the side with the shoulders flexed and abducted to 90°. The medicine ball is passed back and forth, and the exercise is then repeated on the opposite side (**Figure 17-7**).

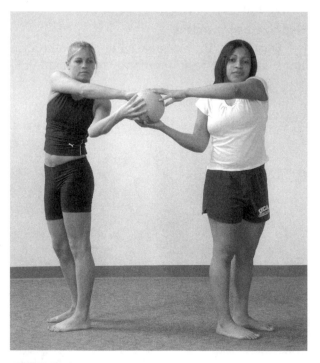

Figure 17-7   Standing rotations.

Spinal Stabilization Exercises

Exercise programs designed to strengthen stabilizing muscles are crucial to the proper treatment of hypermobile spinal segments. These programs should also be an integral part of proper follow-up care, after hypomobile segments have been effectively mobilized by the clinician and the patient is able to achieve normal range of motion.

When the patient can maintain a neutral spine, movement of the arms and legs is introduced (**Figure 17-8**). This is a difficult maneuver for the patient in the early stages of any stabilization program; however, with minimal training, the patient can generally learn to maintain a neutral spine while in motion. Once this skill is mastered, the stabilization program is relatively simple. The patient begins by superimposing easy movements over the neutral spine and progresses in sequence to more difficult maneuvers. Stabilization exercises for the cervical spine require movements of the upper extremities. In one exercise, the patient assumes a prone position on an inflated exercise ball while slowly rotating the shoulders (**Figure 17-9**).

The spinal stabilization exercises presented in chapter 14 (see p 483) can be performed on foam or inflatable rollers (**Figure 17-10**). The perturbating surface requires paraspinal and core muscle activation to maintain balance and stabilize the kinetic segment.

Cross-references

Pelvic-neutral exercises (p 484)

Cardiovascular Exercises

Cardiovascular fitness should be maintained throughout the rehabilitation process. In the early stages of rehabilitation, a patient with a lower extremity injury to the pelvis, hip, or thigh may not be able to use the injured extremity to condition. Many cardiovascular exercises also improve range of motion and strength. Therefore, methods to maintain or improve cardiovascular function must be determined. A patient's cardiovascular system can be exercised during different stages of the rehabilitation process by using a stationary bicycle, upper body exerciser, stair stepper, or rowing machine. Swimming or other water-supported exercises are also useful.

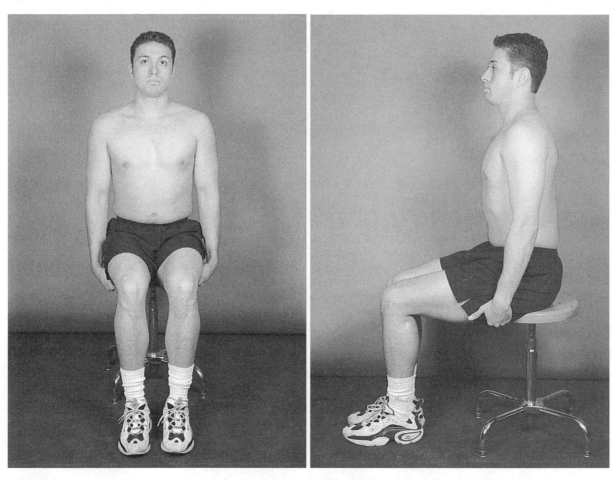

Figure 17-8 Spinal stabilization exercises. Movement of the arms and legs is introduced when the patient achieves a neutral spine.

■ Sport-Specific Activities

Sport-specific activities will depend on the patient's sport and position within the sport. For example, a basketball forward's activities may include forward sprints the distance of a court length, sprints to a lay-up, a sudden stop and jump shot, or vertical jumping. A volleyball player's activities would more likely include lateral movements to the left and right with jumps for blocking or hitting, dives, squats for setting, and diagonal sprints for the ball. Each of these activities should be performed in pelvic-neutral position. If the clinician is unfamiliar with the specific activities and demands of the patient's sport and position, a coach should be consulted to obtain assistance or instruction in useful activities for this stage of the rehabilitation program. The goal in the final stages of sport-specific activities should be normal performance without signs of hesitation in performing any activity.

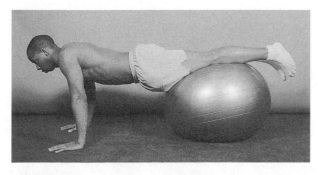

Figure 17-9 Stabilization exercise for the cervical spine.

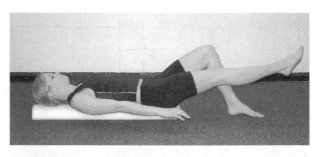

Figure 17-10 Foam or inflatable rollers.

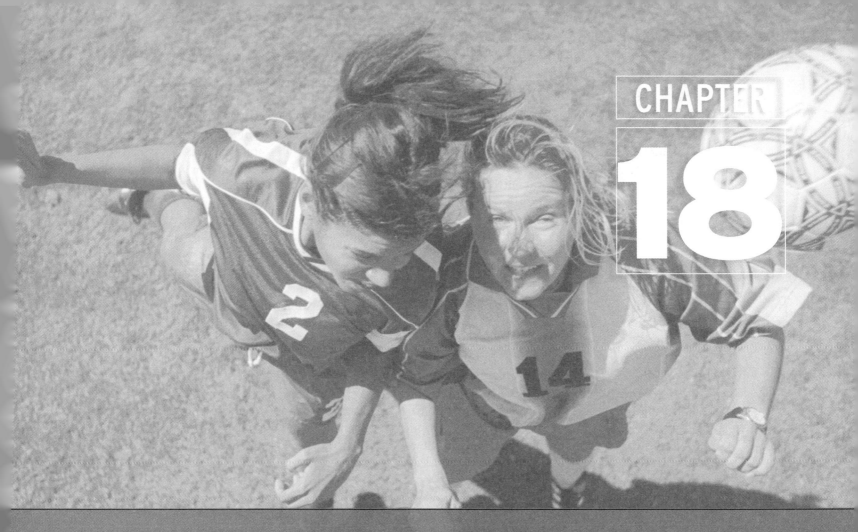

CHAPTER 18

Head Injuries

Kevin M. Guskiewicz,
PhD, ATC
Michael McCrea, PhD,
ABPP

Mechanics of Traumatic Brain Injury

Unlike most injuries sustained in sport, cerebral concussions have the potential for catastrophic outcomes if managed inappropriately. These injuries must be managed cautiously, with awareness of the potential dangers of prematurely returning an athlete to competition after injury. The evaluation process begins with the ability to identify the signs and symptoms associated with a head injury, including the ability to recognize deteriorating conditions that indicate a more serious situation. Clinical decision making should follow an assessment plan that uses a multifactorial approach, including objective measures of symptoms, cognitive function, and postural stability. Traditionally, the evidence-based literature on concussion in sport has been limited in comparison with injuries of the spine and extremities. During the past few years, however, several notable articles have been published on sport-related concussion that are beginning to shape the practice of concussion management.[1-25]

A forceful blow to a resting, moveable head usually produces maximum brain injury beneath the point of cranial impact (coup injury). A moving head hitting an unyielding object usually produces maximum brain injury opposite the site of cranial impact, as the brain shifts within the cranium (con-trecoup injury). When the head is accelerated before impact, the brain lags toward the trailing surface, squeezing away the cerebrospinal fluid (CSF) and producing maximal shearing forces at this site (**Figure 18-1**). This brain lag thickens the layer of CSF under the point of impact, explaining the absence of coup injuries when the head is moving. However, when the head is stationary before impact, neither brain lag nor disproportionate CSF distribution occurs, accounting for the absence of contrecoup injury and the presence of coup injury. Many sport-related concussions involve a combined coup-contrecoup mechanism, but this is not necessarily considered more serious than an isolated coup or contrecoup injury.[4]

Pathology

Perhaps the most challenging aspect of concussion management is recognizing the injury, especially when there are no observable signs that a concussion has actually occurred. Traumatic brain injury (TBI) can be classified into two types: focal and diffuse. *Focal*, or posttraumatic intracranial mass lesions include subdural hematomas, epidural hematomas, cerebral contusions, and intracerebral hemorrhages and hematomas. *Diffuse* brain injuries can result in widespread or global disruption of neurologic function and are not usually associated with macroscopically

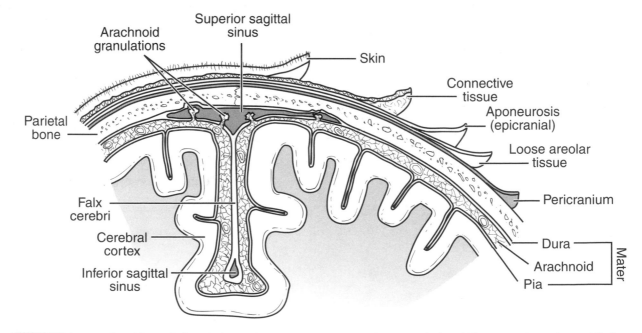

Figure 18-1 Cross-section of the skull. The outer layer is formed by the skin and its subcomponents, the middle layer by the cranium, and the inner layer by the meninges (dura mater, arachnoid mater, and pia mater). The cerebrospinal fluid is located in the subarachnoid space, between the arachnoid mater and pia mater.

visible brain lesions (although cerebral edema may be noted). Most diffuse injuries involve an acceleration-deceleration motion, either within a linear plane or rotational model. In both cases, lesions are caused by the brain being shaken within the skull. For example, with a linear acceleration-deceleration mechanism, the head experiences a violent movement (side to side or front to back) before impact.

The resulting trauma to the head is determined by how fast the head moves (acceleration and deceleration speeds), rate of deceleration, and how much force has occurred.[4,26] Rotational or rotational acceleration-deceleration injuries are believed to be the primary injury mechanism for diffuse brain injuries. Structural diffuse brain injury (diffuse axonal injury, or DAI) is the most severe type of diffuse injury because the axonal disruption can result in impairment. Such injuries can disrupt centers of the brain responsible for breathing, heart rate, consciousness, memory, and cognition. Nonstructural diffuse injuries, such as cerebral concussions, are typically less severe than structural brain lesions, because the anatomic integrity of the central nervous system is maintained. Although these injuries are less severe, they can still result in disrupted consciousness, memory, or cognition and can place the individual at higher risk for second-impact syndrome.[26]

Studies in basic neuroscience have demonstrated that mild TBI, or concussion, is followed by a complex cascade of ionic, metabolic, and physiologic events that can adversely affect cerebral function for several days to weeks.[27,28] Concussive brain injuries trigger a pathophysiologic sequence characterized earliest by an indiscriminate release of excitatory amino acids, massive ionic flux, and a brief period of hyperglycolysis, followed by persistent metabolic instability, mitochondrial dysfunction, diminished cerebral glucose metabolism, reduced cerebral blood flow, and altered neurotransmission. These events culminate in axonal injury and neuronal dysfunction.[27] Clinically, concussion results in neurologic deficits, cognitive impairment, and somatic symptoms.[29]

The immediate management of head injuries depends on the nature and severity of the injury (see Management of Sport-Related Head Injuries, p 569).

Classification of Traumatic Brain Injury

All medical personnel must understand the immediate, delayed, and associated findings and the known complications of TBI. An injury that initially appears minor may gradually worsen and reveal the signs and symptoms of a more serious injury.

Three types of stresses can injure the brain: compressive, tensile, and shearing (see Figure 3-5, p 34). *Compression* is a crushing force such that the tissue cannot absorb any additional force or load. *Tension* is the pulling or stretching of tissue. *Shearing* involves a force that moves across the parallel organization of the tissue. Uniform compressive stresses are fairly well tolerated by neural tissue, but shearing stresses are poorly tolerated.[2,30,31]

Cerebral Concussion

CLINICAL PRESENTATION

History
Direct or rotational blow to the head
Complaints of headache, dizziness, visual disturbances, concentration difficulties, etc
Distinct changes in personality may be noted (eg, sadness, impulsivity, aggressiveness).

Observation
Light and noise sensitivity
Poor balance and coordination
Dizziness
Nausea and vomiting
Memory loss or disorientation

Functional Status
Altered level of consciousness (loss of consciousness is not a prerequisite finding)
Vision disturbances
Concentration difficulties
Inability to maintain balance

Physical Evaluation Findings
Positive findings on neuropsychological tests
The following special tests may be positive:
- Balance Error Scoring System (BESS)
- Romberg test
- Tandem walk

These findings vary with the severity of the injury.

Fortunately the most common sport-related injury to the brain is the least severe. *Cerebral concussion* is an injury that results from a blow to the head, which causes altered mental status and one or more of the following symptoms: headache, nausea, vomiting, dizziness, balance problems, fatigue, trouble sleeping, drowsiness, sensitivity to light or noise, blurred vision, difficulty remembering, and difficulty concentrating.[32] It is important to realize that loss of consciousness (LOC) does not have to occur

Table 18-1

Cantu Evidence-Based Grading System for Concussion

Grade 1 (mild)	No LOC,[†] PTA < 30 min, PCSS < 24 h
Grade 2 (moderate)	LOC < 30 min **or** PTA ≥ 30 min **or** PCSS ≥ 24 h < 7 d
Grade 3 (severe)	LOC ≥ 1 min **or** PTA ≥ 24 h **or** PCSS ≥ 7 d

[†]LOC indicates loss of consciousness; PTA, posttraumatic amnesia (anterograde/retrograde); and PCSS, postconcussion signs and symptoms other than amnesia. Reprinted with permission from Cantu RC: Posttraumatic retrograde and anterograde amnesia: Pathophysiology and implications in grading and safe return to play. *J Athl Train* 2001;36:244-248.

for the patient to be diagnosed with a concussion. The definition of concussion is often expanded to include mild (grade 1), moderate (grade 2), and severe (grade 3) (**Table 18-1**). Although these distinctions are important for treatment and prognosis, they are less significant than previously thought.

Retrograde amnesia
Memory loss of events occurring prior to injury.

■ Mild Concussion

For the most part, experts concur on the definition of mild concussion, but disagreement persists regarding the definitions of "moderate" and "severe" concussions. Mild concussions are the most difficult to recognize and diagnose[30] but are the most frequently occurring (approximately 85%) and often are not reported until after the practice or game.[33,34] The force of impact causes a transient irregularity in the electrophysiology of the brain substance, altering mental status. Although mild concussion involves no LOC, the patient may experience impaired cognitive function, especially in remembering recent events (posttraumatic amnesia) and in assimilating and interpreting new information.[6,17,30,31] Dizziness and tinnitus may also occur, but rarely can a gross loss of coordination be detected with a Romberg test. The presence of a headache, which tends to occur with nearly all concussions, should not be underestimated.[33] The intensity and duration of the headache can indicate if the injury is improving or worsening with time.

Serial observation
Repeated assessment of the same injury.

■ Moderate Concussion

Moderate concussions are associated with transient mental confusion, tinnitus, moderate dizziness, unsteadiness, and prolonged posttraumatic amnesia (longer than 30 minutes). A momentary LOC often occurs, lasting from several seconds to 1 minute. Blurred vision and nausea may also be present. Moderate concussions demand careful clinical observation and skillful judgment, especially regarding return-to-play decisions at a later date.

■ Severe Concussion

It is not difficult to recognize a severe concussion, which presents with signs and symptoms lasting significantly longer than those for mild and moderate concussions. The patient experiences more signs and symptoms than described in the previous two levels, and tinnitus, blurred vision, and nausea are more likely to be present. Most experts agree that any concussion resulting in prolonged LOC should be classified as a severe concussion. Some authors[35,36] classify brief LOC (including momentary blackout) as a severe concussion instead of the more widely accepted moderate concussion. Severe concussions may also involve posttraumatic amnesia lasting longer than 24 hours as well as some **retrograde amnesia**. Prominent disorientation may be observed in more severe grades of concussion. In addition, neuromuscular coordination is markedly compromised, with severe mental confusion, tinnitus, and dizziness. Despite the emphasis often placed on LOC and amnesia, it is important to consider the duration of all signs and symptoms when classifying the injury. **Serial observations** for signs and symptoms should be conducted to identify progressive underlying brain damage.

Differential Diagnosis
Subdural hematoma, epidural hematoma, intracerebral hemorrhage, second-impact syndrome, skull fracture

Medical Diagnostic Tests
Systematic assessment may reveal significant postconcussive symptoms. Neuropsychological tests can identify subtle changes in the patient's cognitive status, reaction time, attention span, and concentration (see p 571). Postural-stability tests may reveal motor deficits or sensory-integration problems that indicate a concussion has been sustained.

Imaging Techniques
Radiographic imaging, computed tomography (CT), or magnetic resonance imaging (MRI) may be obtained to rule out the presence of a cerebral hematoma, hemorrhagic lesion, or other traumatic injury that would indicate a medical emergency (see Figure 18-3) but are not diagnostic for a concussion.

Definitive Diagnosis
Several grading scales have been proposed for classifying and managing sport-related cerebral concussion.[6,35-42] None have been universally accepted or followed with any consistency by the sports medicine community. Some scales are more conservative than others; however, most are useful in

managing concussion. Sports medicine staffs should work together to choose one scale and ensure it is consistently used.

Although most scales are based primarily on level of consciousness and amnesia, other signs and symptoms associated with concussion must be considered because most concussions do not involve LOC or observable amnesia. Approximately 8.9% involve LOC, and only 27.7% involve amnesia.[33] Regardless of the grade of injury, the diagnostic focus should be on the duration of the symptoms associated with the injury. See **Table 18-2** for a list of signs and symptoms associated with cerebral concussion, which can be checked off or graded for severity on an hourly or daily basis after an injury.

The graded symptom checklist is best used in conjunction with the Cantu Evidence-Based Grad-ing System for Concussion[6] (see Table 18-1), which very appropriately emphasizes signs and symptoms in addition to LOC and amnesia in the grading of the injury. It is also important to grade the concussion only after the symptoms have resolved, as the duration of symptoms is believed to be a good indicator of overall outcome.[6,34,43]

■ Immediate Management

Management of the three types of concussive injuries is not substantially different, as the standard of care is removal from participation and serial evaluations. In the event of prolonged LOC (severe concussion), the patient should be evaluated by a physician, with consideration given to neuroimaging of the brain. No athlete should be returned to participation while still experiencing symptoms.

Table 18-2

Graded Symptom Checklist for Concussion*

Symptom	Time of Injury	2-3 h After Injury	24 h After Injury	48 h After Injury	72 h After Injury
Blurred vision					
Dizziness					
Drowsiness					
Easily distracted					
Excess sleep					
Fatigue					
Feel "in a fog"					
Feel "slowed down"					
Headache					
Irritability					
Loss of consciousness					
Loss of orientation					
Memory problems					
Nausea					
Nervousness					
Personality change					
Poor balance/coordination					
Poor concentration					
Ringing in ears					
Sadness					
Seeing stars					
Sensitivity to light					
Sensitivity to noise					
Sleep disturbance					
Vacant stare/glassy eyed					
Vomiting					

*A graded symptom checklist is used not only for the initial evaluation but for subsequent follow-up assessments and is periodically repeated until all postconcussion signs and symptoms have returned to baseline or cleared at rest and during physical exertion. The items can be either checked as "present" or scored on a scale of 0-6, with 0 representing "not present" to 6 representing "severe."

18

More specific assessment guidelines are presented in the management section of this chapter (p 569).

Medications

Most physicians advise against the use of pain medications immediately after a cerebral concussion, as their use may mask symptoms. Once it is evident that a more serious head injury has not occurred, acetaminophen may be considered to treat headache symptoms associated with the concussion. Medications containing aspirin or nonsteroidal anti-inflammatory drugs (NSAIDs) that decrease platelet function and may increase intracranial bleeding should be avoided, as they can accelerate hematoma formation.

Cerebral Hematoma

The skull fits the brain like a custom-made helmet, leaving little room for space-occupying hematomas. Two primary types of hematomas can occur after head trauma: epidural and subdural, depending on whether they are outside or inside the dura mater (**Figure 18-2**). Each can increase intracranial pressure and shift the cerebral hemispheres away from the hematoma. As the hematoma develops, intracranial pressure increases, and neurologic signs deteriorate.

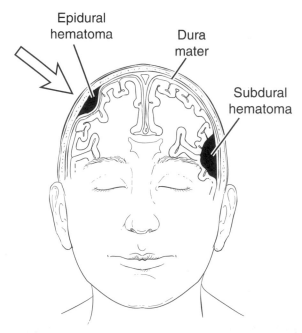

Figure 18-2 Types of cerebral hematoma. Epidural hematomas form between the dura mater and the skull. Subdural hematomas form between the dura mater and the brain.

Epidural Hematoma

An epidural hematoma is an accumulation of blood between the dura mater and the inner surface of the skull as a result of arterial bleeding, most often from the middle meningeal artery. The accumulation of blood typically leads to a rapid degradation in the patient's neurologic status. The patient may lose consciousness from the concussive force, then have a period of altered consciousness, and subsequently appear asymptomatic with normal neurologic examination results.[2]

The problem arises when the injury leads to a slow accumulation of blood in the epidural space, causing the patient to initially appear asymptomatic until the hematoma reaches a critically large size and begins to compress the underlying brain.[44] Immediate surgery may be required to decompress the hematoma and control the hemorrhage. The clinical manifestations of an epidural hematoma depend on the type and amount of energy transferred, the time course of the hematoma formation, and the presence of simultaneous brain injuries. Often the size of the hematoma determines the clinical effects.[45,46]

Subdural Hematoma

The mechanism of a subdural hematoma is more complex than that of an epidural hematoma. The force of a blow to the skull thrusts the brain against the point of impact. The subdural vessels stretch and tear, leading to a hematoma developing within the subdural space. Subdural hematomas are classified as acute, with symptoms presenting 48 to 72 hours after injury, and chronic, with more variable clinical manifestations occurring in a later time frame.[2] Low pressure causes the clot to form slowly, delaying the onset of symptoms for hours or days (acute) or even weeks or months (chronic) after the actual trauma, when the clot may absorb fluid and expand. The clinical presentation of an acute subdural hematoma varies. The individual may be awake and alert with no focal neurologic deficits, but typically persons with any sizable acute subdural hematoma have significant neurologic deficits, including altered states of consciousness.[2]

Intracerebral Hemorrhage

A cerebral contusion is a heterogeneous zone of brain damage that consists of hemorrhage, cerebral infarction, necrosis, and edema. Cerebral contusion is a frequent sequela of head injury and is often considered the most common traumatic lesion of the brain visualized on radiographic evaluation.[2,47]

This injury is usually the result of an inward deformation of the skull at the impact site. Contusions can vary from small, localized areas of injury to large, extensive areas of involvement. An intracerebral hematoma is similar in pathophysiology and radiographic appearance to a cerebral contusion. The intracerebral hematoma, a localized collection of blood within the brain tissue itself, is usually caused by a torn artery from a depressed skull fracture, penetrating wound, or acceleration-deceleration mechanism. These injuries are not typically associated with a lucid interval and are often rapidly progressive; however, the formation of a traumatic intracerebral hematoma can be delayed. Intracerebral hematomas and subdural hematomas are the most common causes of lethal sport-related brain injuries.[2]

The brain substance may suffer a cerebral contusion (bruising) when an object hits the skull or vice versa. The impact causes injured vessels to bleed internally, and consciousness is lost. A cerebral contusion may be associated with partial paralysis or hemiplegia, one-sided pupil dilation, or altered vital signs and may last for a prolonged period. Progressive swelling can further compromise brain tissue not injured in the original trauma. Even with a severe contusion, however, eventual recovery without intracranial surgery can occur. The prognosis is often determined by the supportive care delivered from the moment of injury, including adequate ventilation and cardiopulmonary resuscitation, proper transport techniques (if necessary), and prompt expert evaluation.

Differential Diagnosis

Concussion, second-impact syndrome, skull fracture

Medical Diagnostic Tests

Thorough neurologic examination involving special tests for cognitive function and postural stability, cranial nerve assessment, and neuroimaging (CT or MRI)

Hemiplegia Paralysis of one side of the body.

CLINICAL PRESENTATION

Epidural Hematoma	Subdural Hematoma	Intracerebral Hemorrhage/ Cerebral Contusion
History		
Coup or contrecoup mechanism (acceleration-deceleration) resulting in inward deformity	Coup or contrecoup mechanism	Direct blow to an immoveable head or coup or contrecoup mechanism (acceleration-deceleration) and inward deformation of the skull at the site of impact
Pathology (Injury or Mechanism)		
Dural detachment from inner table of skull; middle meningeal artery is usually ruptured	Subdural venous bleeding resulting from stretching or tearing of subdural veins; if acute, presents within 48-72 hours after trauma; if chronic, presents at 3 weeks after trauma	Cerebral contusions of underlying brain tissue at the site of impact; multiple small areas of contusions may coalesce into large area resembling a lesion
Observation		
Size of hematoma determines the clinical presentation; can demonstrate lucid intervals or persistent unconsciousness	Acute presentation can vary and include those who are awake and alert with no focal neurologic deficits to altered consciousness and often a state of coma with major focal neurologic deficits; chronic presentation typically involves symptoms suggestive of increased intracranial pressure	Normal function or any type of neurologic deterioration, including coma
Functional Status		
Neurologic status deteriorates within 10 minutes to 2 hours	Neurologic status deteriorates within hours to days (acute) or weeks to months (chronic)	Rapid deterioration of neurologic status
Physical Evaluation Findings		
Skull fracture may be noted on radiographs	Skull fracture less common; usually involves slower bleeding causing altered consciousness	Possible depressed skull fracture

18

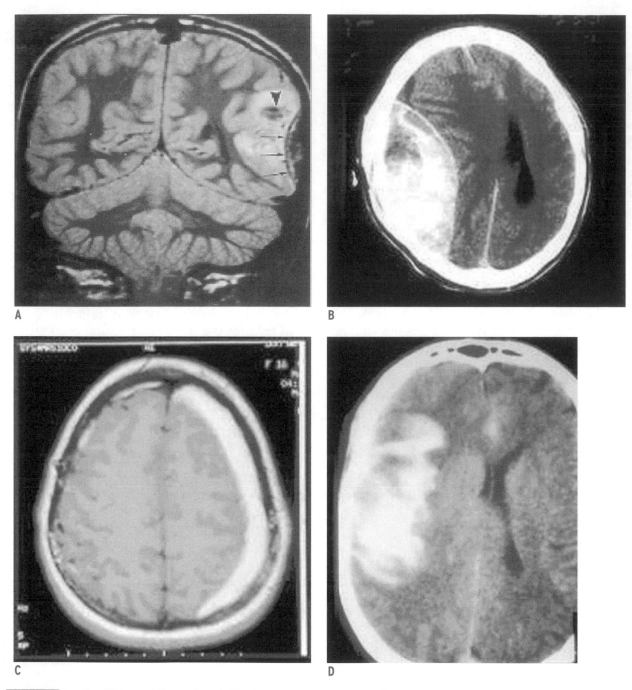

Figure 18-3 Imaging of intracranial hemorrhage. **A.** MRI of epidural hematoma compressing the underlying brain tissue (arrows). **B.** CT scan of a large epidural hematoma. **C.** MRI of a subdural hematoma. **D.** CT scan of an intracranial hematoma.

Imaging Techniques

An epidural hematoma results in the classic appearance of a biconvex or lenticular shape of the hematoma on CT scans (**Figure 18-3**).[2] A subdural hematoma is confirmed by MRI demonstrating extra-axial, low-density fluid collection in the subdural space. An intracerebral hemorrhage results from inward deformation of the skull, leading to

transient compression of the brain against the skull and hemorrhagic contusions present on CT scan.

Definitive Diagnosis

The definitive diagnosis is based on the findings of the neurologic examination and cognitive and postural-stability testing. Although CT and MRI scans can help to rule out a more serious injury such as a hemorrhage, these tests do not indicate the severity of a cerebral concussion. A variety of cognitive and motor tests must be employed to obtain an accurate diagnosis, because deficits may be present in one area but not another.

Immediate Management

When symptoms present acutely, the patient must be provided with adequate ventilation, including intubation and/or CPR if necessary. Cranial nerve inhibition is a sign of increased intracranial pressure (**Figure 18-4**). The patient must be transported to the nearest appropriate hospital in the event that surgical decompression of the brain is necessary.

Because of the latent symptoms associated with a subdural hematoma, a patient demonstrating early neurologic symptoms should be monitored closely. If the cause or magnitude of the injury is in doubt, immediately refer the patient to a physician. Even with delayed onset, any signs of rapid deterioration in neurologic status should be addressed emergently.

More specific assessment guidelines are presented in the management section of this chapter (p 569).

Medications

Aspirin and NSAIDs should not be administered while a person is experiencing postconcussion symptoms. These medications and other cyclooxygenase-1 inhibitors prevent blood coagulation and can lead to increased intracranial hemorrhage. Dexamethasone or another corticosteroid may be administered to minimize cerebral edema. Emergency antiseizure and anticonvulsive medication may be prescribed based on the patient's symptoms. These medications can affect the patient's apparent neurologic status, causing slurred speech, lethargy, and poor psychomotor control.

Surgical Intervention

If pharmacologic attempts to control intracranial hemorrhage are not successful or if the rate of hematoma formation is too rapid, surgical decompression of the skull may be required. The mechanical release of pressure is often sufficient to save the patient's life, but permanent neurologic deficit may still result.

Postinjury/Postoperative Management

The treatment for any athlete who has suffered loss of consciousness or altered mental status should include prolonged observation and monitoring for several days, because slow bleeding can cause subsequent deterioration of mental status. In such a case, surgical intervention may be necessary to evacuate (drain) the hematoma and decompress the brain.

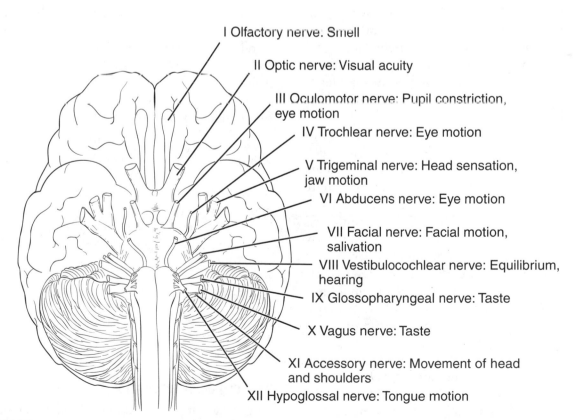

I Olfactory nerve. Smell

II Optic nerve: Visual acuity

III Oculomotor nerve: Pupil constriction, eye motion

IV Trochlear nerve: Eye motion

V Trigeminal nerve: Head sensation, jaw motion

VI Abducens nerve: Eye motion

VII Facial nerve: Facial motion, salivation

VIII Vestibulocochlear nerve: Equilibrium, hearing

IX Glossopharyngeal nerve: Taste

X Vagus nerve: Taste

XI Accessory nerve: Movement of head and shoulders

XII Hypoglossal nerve: Tongue motion

Figure 18-4 The cranial nerves comprise 12 pairs of nerves that have specific sensory and motor function.

Second-Impact Syndrome

CLINICAL PRESENTATION

History

A second blow to the head, typically within a short period of time (up to 10 days) after a concussion

Symptoms from the original concussion were unresolved at the time of the second impact.

LOC may or may not occur.

Observation

The patient typically collapses within seconds to 1 minute of impact.

Rapid onset of pupil dilation and loss of eye movement

Evidence of respiratory failure

Functional Status

Control of eye motion is lost.

Respiratory failure occurs.

Coma occurs rapidly.

Physical Evaluation Findings

Inhibited cranial nerve function

Impaired cognition progressing to eventual LOC

Loss of motor function

Rapid deterioration in vital signs

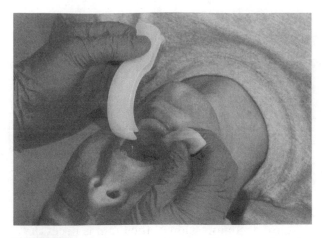

Figure 18-5 To maintain an open airway, qualified personnel may be required to intubate an athlete with a head injury. This technique can be performed with the helmet on and the face mask pulled back.

Second-impact syndrome (SIS) occurs when a patient who has sustained an initial head trauma, most often a concussion, experiences a second injury before symptoms associated with the first have totally resolved. During the past two decades, athletic-related SIS has been the topic of much discussion and debate.[30,31,35,40,42,48-51]

Often, the first injury was unreported or unrecognized. The SIS usually occurs within 1 week of the initial injury and results in cerebral edema caused by the brain's inability to autoregulate its blood supply. Brain stem failure develops in 2 to 5 minutes, eventually leading to coma and respiratory failure. Unfortunately, the mortality rate of SIS is 50%, and the morbidity rate is 100%. Although the number of reported cases is relatively low, the potential for SIS in an athlete with a mild head injury should be a major consideration when making a return-to-play decision.[37]

The structures involved in these head injuries vary depending on the impact acceleration-deceleration and the mechanism. However, the presentation of signs and symptoms and recommended care are standard.

Differential Diagnosis

Subdural hematoma, epidural hematoma, intracerebral hemorrhage, concussion, skull fracture

Imaging Techniques

MRI is more sensitive in identifying cranial edema than CT (see Figure 18-3).

Definitive Diagnosis

The definitive diagnosis is based on the history of two substantial concussive forces within a 1-week period or sustaining a second concussion while the symptoms of a prior concussion are still present. Cerebral imaging, intracranial pressure tests, and neurologic status also contribute to the final diagnosis.

■ Immediate Management

On-field management of SIS includes the removal of any helmet or pads to allow for rapid intubation of the patient (**Figure 18-5**). Suspicion of SIS warrants immediate transport to an emergency department.

More specific assessment guidelines are presented in the management section of this chapter (p 569).

■ Medications

If the condition worsens, the patient may be managed pharmacologically as described for cerebral hematoma.

■ Surgical Intervention

Surgical decompression and/or cranial clot removal may be necessary.

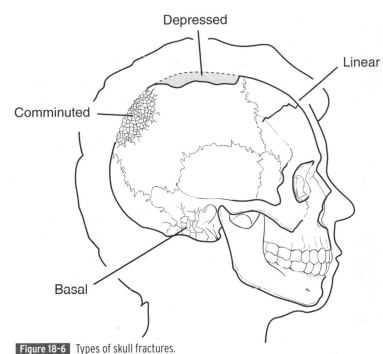

Type	Description
Depressed	Portion of the skull is indented toward the brain
Nondepressed	Minimal indentation of skull toward the brain
Linear	Fracture line runs circumferentially with no indentation of the skull
Comminuted	Multiple fracture fragments
Basal/basilar	Involves base of skull

Figure 18-6   Types of skull fractures.

Skull Fractures

CLINICAL PRESENTATION

History

Blunt trauma or high-velocity blow to the skull
LOC may have occurred after the injury.

Observation

Bleeding may be present.
Deformity of the skull may be noted.
Posterior auricular ecchymosis (Battle's sign) may be evident.
Periorbital ecchymosis ("raccoon eyes") may indicate a fracture of the anterior portion of the skull.
Otorrhea may be present with basilar skull fractures.
Possible **rhinorrhea**

Functional Status

The signs and symptoms of a TBI may also be noted.
Skull fractures may affect the inner or middle ear and result in hearing loss.
Anterior skull fractures may affect cranial nerves V, VI, VII, and VIII.

Physical Evaluation Findings (Do not palpate open wounds)

Point tenderness over the site of injury
Possible crepitus over the fracture line
The "halo test" confirms CSF leakage from the nose or ears.

With a skull fracture, coup and contrecoup mechanisms of brain injury frequently do not occur because the bone itself, either transiently (linear skull fracture) or permanently (depressed skull fracture)

displaced at the moment of impact, absorbs much of the trauma energy or directly injures the brain tissue (**Figure 18-6**). The bones of the skull are relatively thick, but thin areas of bone in the parietal and temporal regions and the inherently thin bones of the sphenoid sinus, foramen magnum, and sphenoid wings forming the base of the skull increase the risk of fracture at these sites. Focal lesions are most common at the anterior tips and the inferior surfaces of the frontal and temporal lobes because the associated cranial bones have irregular surfaces.[2,31]

Linear skull fractures and basilar skull fractures tend to result when a wide area of the skull receives a low-energy force during a fall to the turf or court or from contact with another stationary object. These injuries carry the risk of a concurrent epidural hematoma, thrombosis of the venous sinus, or dysunion of the cranial sutures. Basilar fractures may also cause damage to the dura mater.

Skull fractures may be difficult to diagnose clinically. A depressed skull fracture may be confused clinically with a deep scalp hematoma. Therefore, radiographic evaluation is needed for the prompt detection and proper management of skull fractures. An associated brain injury must always be considered when evaluating skull fractures.

High-energy trauma to a limited area of the skull, such as being struck by a moving bat, causes a depressed fracture. The rounded nature of the skull results in the comminution of depressed skull fractures. Open depressed or comminuted fractures

Otorrhea Cerebral spinal fluid draining from the ear canal.
Rhinorrhea Cerebral spinal fluid draining from the nose.

18

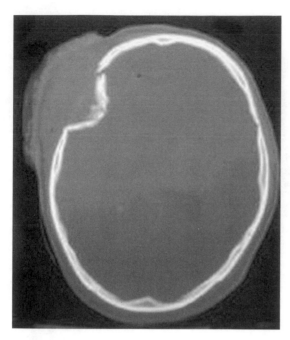

Figure 18-7 CT scan of a depressed skull fracture.

may expose the underlying meninges and allow the introduction of foreign matter into the cranial vault.

Differential Diagnosis

Subdural hematoma, epidural hematoma, intracerebral hemorrhage, concussion, SIS

Imaging Techniques

The imaging technique of choice for identifying most types of skull fractures is CT; plain-film radiographs are not sensitive enough to identify most linear fractures. The preferred imaging views on CT are sagittal and helical (**Figure 18-7**).

Definitive Diagnosis

The definitive diagnosis of the type of skull fracture is based on imaging findings, preferably a CT scan.

Pathomechanics and Functional Limitations

Closed skull fractures (eg, linear) create weakened areas that result in the decreased ability of the skull to absorb and dissipate force, thereby increasing the risk of expanding the fracture line and losing the ability to protect the brain from concussive forces. However, as long as the patient is not subjected to concussive forces while the skull is healing, ADLs are not normally inhibited.

Depressed skull fractures decrease the volume of the cranial vault. Any loss of volume reduces the space available for the brain. As the volume of the vault decreases, the forces placed on the brain increase, potentially fatally inhibiting its function. Bony segments of the fracture can also lacerate the underlying brain, vascular, and meningeal tissue. Open fractures can result in profuse blood loss and expose the underlying tissue to contaminants.

Immediate Management

Patients with suspected or known skull fractures should be transported in a reclining position. Open fractures and associated skin wounds should be covered with a sterile gauze bandage. (Note: A suspected cervical fracture must take precedence in the management options.)

More specific assessment guidelines are presented in the management section of this chapter (p 569).

Medications

Pharmacologic options are based on the suspicion of underlying brain trauma. In the absence of brain injury, narcotic analgesics, aspirin, ibuprofen, or acetaminophen may be prescribed for pain. A patient with an open fracture is prescribed a course of prophylactic antibiotics.

Surgical Intervention

Surgery is required if the bony segments of a depressed fracture are displaced more than 5 mm, if a cerebral hematoma has formed, or if the dura mater or venous sinus is torn. With a depressed fracture, the surgeon cleans and manually realigns the displaced fragments of bone. Large pieces of bones may be wired together. The bony fixation may be improved through the use of a titanium mesh or bone cement.

Postinjury/Postoperative Management

Signs of underlying brain trauma must be evaluated. Many skull fractures are treated conservatively, including linear fractures and simple depressed skull fractures. With time, most fragments of depressed skull fractures realign, and the normal contour of the skull returns. The physician may elect to treat occipital and basilar condyle fractures with a hard cervical collar.

The patient is restricted to bed rest for a few days after injury and then restricted to modified activity until healing occurs.

Estimated Amount of Time Lost

Simple linear fractures usually heal in 4 to 6 weeks, but the patient should remain out of sport participation for a lengthier recovery period once the fracture is stable. The amount of time lost increases as the complexity of the fracture increases.

Return-to-Play Criteria

The fracture must be stable and completely healed on radiographic evaluation. Any underlying injury such as brain trauma or inner ear disruption must also be resolved.

Protective Headgear

Patients should be encouraged to wear appropriate helmets when returning to competition, especially in sports not mandating headwear, such as roller blading, bicycling, and skiing.

Management of Sport-Related Head Injuries

Recognition of a concussion is straightforward if the athlete has LOC. However, 90% to 95% of all cerebral concussions involve no LOC, only a transient loss of alertness or the presence of mental confusion. The patient appears dazed, dizzy, or disoriented. These injuries are more difficult to recognize and even more challenging to classify, given the numerous grading scales available and the inability to quantify most signs and symptoms.

The primary objectives for managing head injuries are:

- Recognize the injury and its severity.
- Determine if the athlete requires additional attention or assessment.
- Decide when the athlete may return to sport activity.

This section focuses on the important findings of the initial evaluation after head injury.

Initial On-Site Assessment

The approach to the initial assessment differs, depending on whether the athlete is "down" or ambulatory. *Athlete down* conditions are signified by the response of the athletic trainer or team physician (or both) to the athlete on the field or court. *Ambulatory* conditions involve the patient being seen by the clinician at some point after the injury. Head trauma in an athletic situation requires immediate assessment for appropriate emergency action, and if at all possible, the initial evaluation should be performed with the patient at the site where the injury occurred.

Primary Survey

The primary survey takes only 10 to 15 seconds, as respiratory and cardiac status are assessed to rule out a life-threatening condition. A patient who is unconscious or is regaining consciousness but is still disoriented and confused should be managed as if a cervical spine injury is present (see chapter 16). An unconscious patient should be transported from the field or court on a backboard with his or her head and neck immobilized.

Vital signs should be monitored at regular intervals (1 to 2 minutes) while talking to the patient in an attempt to help bring about full consciousness. If LOC is brief, lasting less than 1 minute, and the remainder of the examination is normal, the patient may be observed on the sideline and referred to a physician at a later time. Prolonged unconsciousness, lasting 1 minute or longer, requires immobilization and transfer to an emergency facility so the patient can undergo a thorough neurologic examination.

Secondary Survey

A thorough history is the most important part of the evaluation because it can quickly narrow down the assessment. The presence of LOC, mental confusion, and amnesia are evaluated. Confusion can be determined rather quickly by noting facial expression (dazed, stunned, "glassy eyed") and any inappropriate behavior, such as running the wrong play or returning to the wrong huddle (**Table 18-3**).

Table 18-3

Neural Watch Chart

Unit		Time
1. Vital signs	Blood pressure	_____
	Pulse	_____
	Respiration	_____
	Temperature	_____
2. Conscious and . . .	Oriented	_____
	Disoriented	_____
	Restless	_____
	Combative	_____
3. Speech	Clear	_____
	Rambling	_____
	Garbled	_____
	None	_____
4. Will awaken to . . .	Name	_____
	Shaking	_____
	Light pain	_____
	Strong pain	_____
5. Nonverbal reaction	Appropriate	_____
	Inappropriate	_____
	"Decerebrate"	_____
	None	_____
6. Pupils	Size on right	_____
	Size on left	_____
	Reacts on right	_____
	Reacts on left	_____
7. Ability to move	Right arm	_____
	Left arm	_____
	Right leg	_____
	Left leg	_____

18

Amnesia testing is conducted by first asking simple questions directed toward recent memory and progressing to more involved questions. Asking the patient what the first thing he or she remembered after the injury tests for length of posttraumatic amnesia. Asking what the play was before the injury or who the opponent was last week tests for retrograde amnesia, which is generally associated with a more serious head injury. Questions of orientation (name, date, time, and place) may be asked; however, research suggests that they are not good discriminators between injured and uninjured athletes.[52] Facing the patient away from the field and asking the name of the opposing team may be helpful. Questions should be posed to determine if tinnitus, blurred vision, or nausea are being experienced. A concussion symptom checklist similar to that found in Table 18-3 may be used to facilitate the follow-up assessment of signs and symptoms.

Portions of the observation and palpation plan should take place during the initial on-site evaluation. While the history is obtained, any deformities or abnormal facial expressions (cranial nerve VII), speech patterns, respirations, or extremity movements should be noted. Additionally, gentle palpation of the skull and cervical spine should be performed to rule out an associated fracture. The athlete who is conscious or who was momentarily unconscious should be transported to the sideline or locker room for further evaluation after the initial on-site evaluation. **Table 18-4** highlights the primary and secondary survey.

■ Sideline Assessment

A more detailed examination can be conducted on the sideline or in the athletic training clinic once the helmet has been removed. A quick cranial nerve assessment should first be performed. Visual acuity (cranial nerve II: optic) can be checked by asking the patient to read or identify selected objects (at near range and far range). Eye movement (cranial nerves III and IV: oculomotor and trochlear) should be checked for coordination and a purposeful appearance by asking the patient to track a moving object. The pupils should be equal in size and reaction to light; the pupils should constrict when light is shined into eyes. Observation of the pupils also assesses the oculomotor nerve. Abnormal movement of the eyes or changes in pupil size or reaction to light often indicate increased intracranial pressure. The possibility of a skull fracture should also be ruled out, especially if the patient was not wearing a helmet at the time of injury.

If the patient's outward condition appears to worsen, the pulse rate and blood pressure should be assessed. An unusually slow heart rate or increased pulse pressure (increased systolic and decreased diastolic pressures) after the individual has calmed down may be signs of increasing intracranial pressure. Most individuals with cerebral concussions do not have abnormal findings; however, vital signs are important considerations for detecting a more serious injury such as an epidural or subdural hematoma. Significant deviations in the patient's vital signs require referral for more extensive evaluation and possible life support.

Special Tests for the Assessment of Coordination

The use of a quantifiable clinical balance test, such as the Balance Error Scoring System (BESS), is recommended over the standard Romberg test, which for years has been used as a subjective tool to assess balance. The BESS provides a quick, cost-effective method of objectively assessing postural stability in athletes on the sideline or in the athletic training clinic after a concussion and has been found to be a reliable and valid assessment tool for managing sport-related concussion.[12,53,54] Balance test

---

Table 18-4

On-site Assessment

Primary Survey	Secondary Survey	
Rule out life-threatening condition	History	Mental confusion
Check respirations (breathing)		Loss of consciousness
Check cardiac status		Amnesia
	Observation	Monitor eyes
		Graded symptom checklist
		Deformities, abnormal facial expressions, speech patterns, respirations, extremity movement
	Palpation	Skull and cervical spine abnormalities
		Pulse and blood pressure (if condition is deteriorating)

results during injury recovery are most reliable when they are compared with baseline measurements. Clinicians who work with athletes or patients on a regular basis should attempt to obtain baseline measurements before competition.

More sophisticated balance assessment using computerized forceplate systems and sensory organization testing (SOT) has identified deficits up to 3 days after a mild concussion.[12,55,56] These tests are recommended for making return-to-play decisions, especially when preseason baseline measurements are available for comparison.

Special Tests for Assessment of Cognition

A brief mental status examination should be conducted to evaluate any deficits in orientation, memory, concentration, and general coherence after injury. Recently, attention has focused on developing more systematic methods to evaluate mental status on the sideline, beyond the traditional questions of "where are we" and "how many fingers." The Standardized Assessment of Concussion (SAC) is a brief screening instrument designed for the neurocognitive assessment of concussion by a medical professional with no prior expertise in neuropsychological testing.[57,58] Several prospective studies have demonstrated the psychometric properties and clinical sensitivity of the SAC in assessing concussion and tracking postinjury recovery.[19-21,59] The SAC requires approximately 5 minutes to administer and assess four domains of cognition: orientation, immediate memory, concentration, and delayed recall. A composite total score (of 30 possible points) is summed to provide an overall index of cognitive impairment and injury severity. The SAC also contains a brief neurologic screen and documentation of injury-related factors (eg, LOC, posttraumatic amnesia, retrograde amnesia) (**Table 18-5**). Equivalent alternate forms of the SAC are available and should be used to minimize practice effects from serial testing after an injury. In lieu of the SAC, a series of questions to properly evaluate concentration (**Table 18-6**) and recent memory (**Table 18-7**) can be asked.

Other neuropsychological (cognitive) tests have been used to identify and manage TBI in athletes.[12,13,56,60,61] Although most of these tests are difficult to administer as part of a sideline examination, they are useful for subsequent follow-up assessments. On most paper-and-pencil neuropsychological tests, young, healthy, well-motivated athletes who experience mild cerebral concussion can demonstrate significant cognitive decline immediately after injury.[12,56,60,61] **Table 18-8** lists several paper-and-pencil tests that have been used by neuropsychologists in cooperative efforts with athletic trainers and team physicians to evaluate recovery of neurocognitive function in symptomatic players.

Computerized Neuropsychological Testing

As neuropsychological testing has become more popular in the sports medicine setting, experts have attempted to find more practical assessment tools. Several factors have greatly limited the widespread application of formal neuropsychological testing at the secondary school and collegiate levels. The time and financial costs typically required for conventional neuropsychological testing are often unfeasible in a sports setting. Additionally, many institutions lack the necessary personnel to implement the recommended model of individual preseason baseline neuropsychological testing of all athletes for comparison with postinjury test results.

Neuropsychologists have made recent advancements in the development of computerized applications for the assessment of concussion and TBI. Certain computerized test modules have been designed specifically to assess concussion in athletes. Computerized testing may offer several scientific and practical advantages over conventional paper and pencil batteries. Most computerized batteries require 20 to 30 minutes per athlete. To save time, computerized testing can be conducted in large group settings, with several athletes being tested simultaneously on separate computers. Computerized neuropsychological testing thereby greatly reduces the time, cost, and personnel demands associated with baseline testing of one athlete at a time with traditional tests.

Computerized testing allows a more precise measurement of subtle deficits associated with concussion, including reaction time, cognitive processing speed, and response latency. For example, computerized neuropsychological tests permit highly accurate measurement of simple and complex reaction time, with near-millisecond timing accuracy.[62,63] This level of timing resolution has become increasingly important to neuropsychological research, especially in the areas of concussion and TBI. Finally, these newer methods allow the individual's data to be stored and easily accessed for clinical management after a concussion and large data sets to be archived for research purposes.

The following three computerized neuropsychological test batteries are currently available to athletic trainers and other sports medicine personnel.

The National Rehabilitation Hospital Mild Brain Dysfunction Automated Neuropsychological Assessment Metrics (ANAM) was designed to assess cerebral concussion and other conditions characterized by

Table 18-5

Standardized Assessment of Concussion (SAC)

1) Orientation:

Month:	_____	0 1
Date:	_____	0 1
Day of week:	_____	0 1
Year:	_____	0 1
Time (within 1 h):	_____	0 1
Orientation Total Score	_____	/5

2) Immediate Memory: (All 3 trials are completed regardless of score on trial 1 and 2; total score equals sum across all 3 trials.)

List	Trial 1	Trial 2	Trial 3
Word 1	0 1	0 1	0 1
Word 2	0 1	0 1	0 1
Word 3	0 1	0 1	0 1
Word 4	0 1	0 1	0 1
Word 5	0 1	0 1	0 1
Total			

Immediate Memory Total Score _____ /15

(Note: Subject is not informed of Delayed Recall testing of memory)

Neurological Screening:

Loss of Consciousness: (occurrence, duration)

Pretraumatic and Posttraumatic Amnesia: (recollection of events before and after injury)

Strength:

Sensation:

Coordination:

3) Concentration:

Digits Backward (If correct, go to next string length. If incorrect, read trial 2. Stop after incorrect on both trials)

4-9-3	6-2-9	_____	0 1
3-8-1-4	3-2-7-9	_____	0 1
6-2-9-7-1	1-5-2-8-6	_____	0 1
7-1-8-4-6-2	5-3-9-1-4-8	_____	0 1

Months in reverse order: (entire sequence correct for 1 point)

Dec-Nov-Oct-Sep-Aug-Jul

Jun-May-Apr-Mar-Feb-Jan	_____	0 1

Concentration Total Score _____ /5

EXERTIONAL MANUEVERS
(when appropriate)

5 jumping jacks	5 push-ups
5 sit-ups	5 knee-bends

4) Delayed Recall

Word 1	0 1
Word 2	0 1
Word 3	0 1
Word 4	0 1
Word 5	0 1
Delayed Recall Total Score _____	/5

Summary of Total Scores:

Orientation	_____	/5
Immediate Memory	_____	/15
Concentration	_____	/5
Delayed Recall	_____	/5
TOTAL SCORE	_____	/30

Reprinted with permission from McCrea M, Randolph C, Kelly JP: *The Standardized Assessment of Concussion (SAC): Manual for Administration, Scoring and Interpretation*, ed 2. Waukesha, WI, CNS, 2000.

Table 18-6

Tests of Concentration

Questions	Correct Response?
Recite the days of the week backward beginning with today.	
Recite the months of the year backward beginning with this month.	
Serial 3s: count backward from 100 by 3 until you get to single digits.	
Serial 7s: count backward from 100 by 7 until you get to single digits.	

Table 18-7

Tests of Recent Memory

Questions	Correct Response?
Where are we playing (name of field or site)?	
Which quarter (period, inning, etc) is it?	
Who scored last?	
Who did we play last week?	
Who won last week?	
Repeat the words used to determine anterograde amnesia.	

Table 18-8

Selected Neuropsychological Tests and Abilities Evaluated

Tests	Ability Evaluated
Hopkins Verbal Learning Test (HVLT)	Verbal memory
Trail Making Test: A and B	Visual scanning, mental flexibility, attention
Brief Visuospatial Memory Test (BVMT)	Visual memory
Stroop Color-Word Test	Mental flexibility, attention
Wechsler Digit Span Test	Attention span
Symbol Digit Modalities Test	Visual scanning, attention
Grooved Pegboard Test	Motor speed, coordination
Paced Auditory Serial Addition Test	Attention, concentration, immediate memory recall, rapid mental processing

mild or subtle brain dysfunction. The ANAM measures factors similar to those assessed by traditional neuropsychological tests frequently used in concussion research, including the Paced Auditory Serial Addition Test, Stroop Color-Word Test, Trail Making Test Part B, Consonant Trigrams Test, California Verbal Learning Test, and Hopkins Verbal Learning Test.[64] The current ANAM sports battery includes more than 1,000 test versions and takes approximately 18 minutes to complete. The battery includes a test of Simple Reaction Time, which is repeated at the end of the battery; Matching to Sample assesses visual memory; Continuous Performance Test assesses attention and concentration; Math Processing assesses mental processing speed and mental efficiency; and Sternberg Memory assesses working memory.[65]

The HeadMinder Concussion Resolution Index (CRI) is a relatively new (1999) web-based neuropsychological test that was developed specifically to compare an athlete's postconcussion performance with his or her own preinjury baseline performance. The CRI can be administered from any computer with an Internet connection. The baseline assessment takes less than 25 minutes, and the postconcussion assessment takes approximately 20 minutes. Alternate forms are available, so that multiple follow-up assessments can be administered to track resolution of cognitive symptoms. The CRI measures memory, reaction time, speed of decision making, and speed of information processing through a variety of cognitive tests. Reaction Time and Cued Reaction Time assess simple reaction time. The Visual Recognition Test allows for assessment of the athlete's speed of decision making or complex reaction time. Animal Decoding and Symbol Scanning assess processing speed.[8,65]

The University of Pittsburgh Medical Center's Immediate Postconcussion Assessment and Cognitive Testing (ImPact) was developed approximately 10 years ago and is probably the most widely used computerized cognitive testing battery in the sports medicine community. Like the CRI, ImPact was designed to provide sensitive information in the form of cognitive data and symptom reporting. Administration is relatively self-explanatory. Baseline testing takes approximately 22 minutes, and postconcussion testing takes about 18 minutes. The ImPact software package consists of a Self-Report Symptom Questionnaire (21 symptoms commonly associated with concussion), a Concussion-History Form that precedes the neuropsychological measures, and tests of cognitive function: attention span, working memory, sustained attention, selective attention, nonverbal problem solving, reaction time, visual and verbal memory, and response variability.[16,18]

Computerized testing undoubtedly offers several practical and methodologic advantages, especially related to baseline testing of large numbers of athletes. Further research is required, however, to provide clinical validity data on these measures and to determine how these measures compare with one another. Issues related to user qualifications for administration and interpretation of computerized neuropsychological testing also require further consideration.

Other Tests

If the patient successfully completes the special tests and return to participation on the same day is anticipated, sensory (dermatome) testing and range-of-motion testing should be performed, followed by strength testing. These tests are conducted to ensure that the patient has normal sensory and motor function, which could have been compromised by an associated brachial plexus injury. These tests can be performed in a systematic order, as described for upper and lower quarter screenings.

If the patient has been asymptomatic for at least 15 minutes and has cleared all tests to this point, functional tests should be performed to assess readiness to return to participation. Functional testing should include exertional tests on the sideline, such as sit-ups, push-ups, short sprints, and sport-specific tasks. The objective of these tests is to seek evidence of early postconcussive symptoms. Often these exercises increase intracranial pressure in the head-injured athlete and cause symptoms to increase. The patient should be withheld from competition if the symptoms return during exertion.

The initial and follow-up findings of head-injury evaluations must be documented.

18

Rehabilitation

Rehabilitation After Cerebral Concussion

The literature on medical treatment and rehabilitative therapies for sport-related concussion is sparse. During the emergence of sport-concussion research, most researchers have focused on measuring acute effects and recovery, with little emphasis on treatment interventions. The current standard of care involves a period of rest during the acute postinjury period, followed by a gradual return to noncontact exercise without risk for reinjury and eventual return to full participation once the athlete has been symptom free under exertional conditions for several days. An emphasis on wellness is also critical during the acute recovery period, especially with regard to a regulated sleep cycle, limited physical exertion, and avoidance of alcohol, recreational drugs, and medications that have not been approved by the attending physician. The need is clear for prospective studies examining the potential benefit from pharmacologic agents and rehabilitation techniques on the rate and completeness of recovery after concussion. In the general brain injury literature, the efficacy of cognitive rehabilitation remains a topic of great debate. Similar to recent studies on methods of assessing sport concussion, this type of research in a sports medicine setting may inform us about effective treatments for head injury in a general trauma setting. With the use of the computerized neuropsychological testing devices, treatment and rehabilitation techniques may be quantified and more efficient research will be conducted.

Return to Competition After Sport-Related Concussion

During the past two decades, a number of grading scales for severity of concussion and return to play have been proposed.[6,26,35-42] The lack of consensus among experts is because few of the scales or guidelines are derived from conclusive scientific data but rather were developed from anecdotal literature and clinical experience. The Cantu Evidence-Based Grading Scale (see Table 18-1) is currently recommended because it emphasizes all signs and symptoms without placing too much weight on LOC and amnesia. This scale should be used only after the patient is declared symptom free, as duration of symptoms is important in grading the injury. Regardless of injury grade, no athlete should return to participation while still symptomatic.

The question of return to competition after a head injury is handled on an individual basis, although conservatism seems the wisest course in all cases. The athlete whose confusion resolves promptly (within 20 minutes) and has no associated symptoms at rest or during or after functional testing may be a candidate to return to play. *Any LOC eliminates a player from participation that day.* **Table 18-9** offers a guide to making restricted and unrestricted return-to-play decisions after concussion. The following factors should also be considered when making decisions regarding an athlete's readiness to return after head injury:

- History of concussion, including the frequency and severity of each episode
- The sport of participation (contact versus noncontact)
- Availability of experienced personnel to observe and monitor the athlete during recovery
- Early follow-up to determine when a disqualified athlete can return to participation
- Repeated assessment should be the rule to establish the athlete's recovery course. The athletic trainer and team physician must be assured that the athlete is asymptomatic before a return to participation is permitted. This can be done through a comprehensive assessment battery that involves a neurologic examination and neuropsychological, functional, exertional, and postural stability testing.
- Any athlete who has experienced LOC should not return to play on that day.
- Any athlete whose symptoms deteriorate should be sent for neurologic evaluation and possible hospital admission.

Athletes who have been unconscious for a period of time or those who have headaches or other persistent symptoms require evaluation and monitoring by a physician. Although most people with head trauma recover without any permanent neurologic deficit or need for surgery, head trauma can

Table 18-9

Guidelines for Return to Play After Concussion*

Mild Remove from contest. Examine immediately and at 5-min intervals for development of abnormal concussive symptoms at rest and with exertion. May return to contest if examination is normal and no symptoms develop for at least 20 min.

If any symptoms develop within the initial 20 min, return on that day should not be permitted.

If the athlete is removed from participation as a result of developing symptoms, follow-up evaluations should be conducted daily. May return to restricted participation when the athletic trainer and team physician are assured the athlete has been asymptomatic at rest and with exertion for at least 2 d, followed by return to unrestricted participation if asymptomatic for 1 additional day. Neuropsychological assessment and balance and coordination testing are valuable criteria, especially if preseason baseline measures are available.

Moderate Remove from contest and prohibit return on that day. Examine immediately and at 5-min intervals for signs of evolving intracranial injury. Reexamine daily. May return to **restricted** participation when the athletic trainer and team physician are assured the athlete has been asymptomatic at rest and with exertion for at least 4 d, followed by return to **unrestricted** participation if asymptomatic for an additional 2 d. The performance during restricted participation should be used as a guide for making the decision for unrestricted participation. Neuropsychological assessment and balance and coordination testing are valuable criteria, especially if preseason baseline measures are available.

Severe Treat on field or court as if there has been a cervical spine injury. Examine immediately and at 5-min intervals for signs of evolving intracranial injury. Reexamine daily. Return to play is based on how quickly the athlete's initial symptoms resolve:

1. If symptoms totally resolve within the first week, athlete may return to **restricted** participation when the athletic trainer and team physician are assured the athlete has been asymptomatic at rest and with exertion for at least 10 days, followed by return to **unrestricted** participation if asymptomatic for an additional 3 days.

2. If symptoms fail to totally resolve within the first week, athlete may return to **restricted** participation when the athletic trainer and team physician are assured the athlete has been asymptomatic at rest and with exertion for at least 17 days, followed by return to **unrestricted** participation if asymptomatic for an additional 3 days.

Performance during restricted participation should be used as a guide for making the decision for unrestricted participation. Neuropsychological assessment and balance and coordination testing are valuable criteria, especially if preseason baseline measures are available.

*Asymptomatic means the athlete's scores have returned to baseline on the graded symptom checklist.

Any second concussion sustained within a 3-month period of the first concussion requires that the athlete rest for twice the maximum number of days recommended for the respective severity level.

be very serious and perhaps life threatening. Several guidelines have been proposed for return to play after multiple head injuries in the same season.[35-37] Most experts agree that athletes should be held from competition for extended periods of time (1 to 3 additional weeks) after a second concussion to ensure that all postconcussive symptoms have resolved and that participation in contact sports should be terminated for the season after three concussions.

References

1. Aubry M, Cantu RC, Dvorak J, et al: Summary and agreement statement of the 1st International Symposium on Concussion in Sport, Vienna 2001. *Clin J Sport Med* 2002;12:6-11.

2. Bailes JE, Hudson V: Classification of sport-related head trauma: A spectrum of mild to severe injury. *J Athl Train* 2001;36:236-243.

3. Barr WB: Methodologic issues in neuropsychological testing. *J Athl Train* 2001;36:297-302.

4. Barr WB, McCrea M: Sensitivity and specificity of standardized neurocognitive testing immediately following sports concussion. *J Int Neuropsychol Soc* 2001;7:693-702.

5. Bleiberg J, Halpern EL, Reeves D, Daniel JC: Future directions for neuropsychological assessment of sports concussion. *J Head Trauma Rehabil* 1998;13:36-44.

6. Cantu RC: Posttraumatic retrograde and anterograde amnesia: Pathophysiology and implications in grading and safe return to play. *J Athl Train* 2001;36:244-248.

7. Collins MW, Lovell MR, Iverson GL, Cantu RC, Maroon JC, Field M: Cumulative effects of concussion in high school athletes. *Neurosurgery* 2002;51:1175-1181.

8. Erlanger D, Saliba E, Barth JT, Almquist J, Webright W, Freeman J: Monitoring resolution of postconcussion symptoms in athletes: Preliminary results of a Web-based neuropsychological test protocol. *J Athl Train* 2001;36:280-287.

9. Ferrara MS, McCrea M, Peterson CL, Guskiewicz KM: A survey of practice patterns in concussion assessment and management. *J Athl Train* 2001;36:145-149.

10. Giza CC, Hovda DA: The neurometabolic cascade of concussion. *J Athl Train* 2001;36:228-235.

11. Grindel SH, Lovell MR, Collins MW: The assessment of sport-related concussion: The evidence behind neuropsychological testing and management. *Clin J Sport Med* 2001;11:134-143.

12. Guskiewicz KM, Ross SE, Marshall SW: Postural stability and neuropsychological deficits after concussion in collegiate athletes. *J Athl Train* 2001;36:263-273.

13. Macciocchi SN, Barth JT, Littlefield LM, Cantu RC: Multiple concussions and neuropsychological functioning in collegiate football players. *J Athl Train* 2001;36:303-306.

14. Halstead DP: Performance testing updates in head, face, and eye protection. *J Athl Train* 2001;36:322-327.

15. Kelly JP: Loss of consciousness: Pathophysiology and implications in grading and safe return to play. *J Athl Train* 2001;36:249-252.

16. Lovell MR, Collins MW, Iverson GL, et al: Recovery from mild concussion in high school athletes. *J Neurosurg* 2003;98:296-301.

17. Lovell MR, Iverson GL, Collins MW, McKeag D, Maroon JC: Does loss of consciousness predict neuropsychological decrements of concussion? *Clin J Sport Med* 1999;9:193-198.

18. Maroon JC, Lovell MR, Norwig J, Podell K, Powell JW, Hartl R: Cerebral concussion in athletes: Evaluation and neuropsychological testing. *Neurosurgery* 2000;47:659-669.

19. McCrea M: Standardized mental status assessment of sports concussion. *Clin J Sport Med* 2001;11:176-181.

20. McCrea M: Standardized mental status testing on the sideline after sport-related concussion. *J Athl Train* 2001;36:274-279.

21. McCrea M, Kelly JP, Randolph C, Cisler R, Berger L: Immediate neurocognitive effects of concussion. *Neurosurgery* 2002;50:1032-1042.

22. Oliaro S, Anderson S, Hooker D: Management of cerebral concussion in sports: The athletic trainer's perspective. *J Athl Train* 2001;36:257-262.

23. Osborne B: Principles of liability for athletic trainers: Managing sport-related concussion. *J Athl Train* 2001;36:316-321.

24. Powell JW: Cerebral concussion: Causes, effects, and risks in sports. *J Athl Train* 2001;36:307-311.

25. Randolph C: Implementation of neuropsychological testing models for the high school, collegiate, and professional sport settings. *J Athl Train* 2001;36:288-296.

26. Ommaya A: Biomechanical aspects of head injuries in sports, in Jordan B, Tsairis P, Warren R (eds): *Sports Neurology.* Rockville, MD, Aspen Publishers, Inc, 1990, pp 75-83.

27. Hovda DA, Prins M, Becker DP, et al: Neurobiology of concussion, in Bailes JE, Lovell MR, Maroon JC (eds): *Sports-Related Concussion.* St Louis, MO, Quality Medical Publishing, Inc, 1999, pp 12-51.

28. Giza CC, Hovda DA: The neurometabolic cascade of concussion. *J Athl Train* 2001;36:228-235.

29. Alexander MP: Mild traumatic brain injury: Pathophysiology, natural history, and clinical management. *Neurology* 1995;45:1253-1260.

30. Cantu RC: Athletic head injuries. *Clin Sports Med* 1997;16:531-542.

31. Cantu RC: Reflections on head injuries in sport and the concussion controversy. *Clin J Sports Med* 1997;7:83-84.

32. Committee on Head Injury Nomenclature of the Congress of Neurological Surgeons: Glossary of head injury including some definitions of injury to the cervical spine. *Clin Neurosurg* 1966;12:386-394.

33. Guskiewicz KM, Weaver NL, Padua DA, Garrett WE Jr: Epidemiology of concussion in collegiate and high school football players. *Am J Sports Med* 2000;28:643-650.

34. Guskiewicz KM, McCrea M, Marshall SW, et al: Cumulative effects of recurrent concussion in collegiate football players: The NCAA Concussion Study. *JAMA* 2003;290:2549-2555.

35. Practice parameter: The management of concussion in sports (summary statement). Report of the Quality Standards Subcommittee of the American Association of Neurology. *Neurology* 1997;48:581-585.

36. Report of the Sports Medicine Committee: Guidelines for the Management of Concussion in Sports. Denver, CO, Colorado Medical Society, 1990 (revised 1991).

37. Cantu RC: Guidelines for return to contact sports after a cerebral concussion. *Physician Sportsmed* 1986;14:75-83.

38. Jordan B: Head injuries in sports, in Jordan B, Tsairis P, Warren R (eds): *Sports Neurology.* Rockville, MD, Aspen Publishers, Inc, 1989, pp 84-97.

39. Nelson W, Jane J, Gieck J: Minor head injuries in sports: A new system of classification and management. *Physician Sportsmed* 1984;12:103-107.

40. Roberts W: Who plays? Who sits? Managing concussion on the sidelines. *Physician Sportsmed* 1992;20:66-72.

41. Torg J (ed): *Athletic Injuries to the Head, Neck & Face.* St Louis, MO, Mosby-Year Book, 1991.

42. Wilberger JJ, Maroon J: Head injuries in athletes. *Clin Sports Med* 1989;8:1-9.

43. McCrea M, Guskiewicz KM, Barr W, et al: Acute effects and recovery time following concussion in collegiate football players: The NCAA Concussion Study. *JAMA* 2003;290:2556-2563.

44. Jamieson KG, Yelland JDN: Extradural hematoma: Report of 167 cases. *J Neurosurg* 1968;29:13-23.

45. Bricolo AP, Pasut LM: Extradural hematoma: Toward zero mortality, a prospective study. *Neurosurgery* 1984;14:8-12.

46. Servadei F: Prognostic factors in severely head injured adult patients with epidural haematomas. *Acta Neurochir (Wien)* 1997;139:273-278.

47. Schonauer M, Schisano G, Cimino R, Viola L: Space occupying contusions of cerebral lobes after closed brain injury: Considerations about 51 cases. *J Neurosurg Sci* 1979;23:279-288.

48. Mueller FO: Catastrophic head injuries in high school and collegiate sports. *J Athl Train* 2001; 36:312-315.

49. Kelly JP, Nichols JS, Filley CM, Lillehei KO, Rubinstein D, Kleinschmidt-DeMasters BK: Concussion in sports: Guidelines for the prevention of catastrophic outcome. *JAMA* 1991;226:2867-2869.

50. Saunders RL, Harbaugh RE: The second impact in catastrophic contact-sports head injuries. *JAMA* 1984;252:538-539.

51. Hugenholtz H, Richard MT: Return to athletic competition following concussion. *Can Med Assoc J* 1982;127:827-829.

52. Maddocks D, Saling M: Neuropsychological sequelae following concussion in Australian rules footballers. *J Clin Exp Neuropsychol* 1991;13:439-442.

53. Riemann BL, Guskiewicz KM, Shields EW: Relationship between clinical and forceplate measures of postural stability. *J Sport Rehabil* 1998;8:71-82.

54. Riemann BL, Guskiewicz KM: Objective assessment of mild head injury using a clinical battery of postural stability tests. *J Athl Train* 2000;35:19-25.

55. Guskiewicz KM, Perrin DH, Gansneder BM: Effect of mild head injury on postural sway. *J Athl Train* 1996;31:300-306.

56. Guskiewicz KM, Riemann BL, Perrin DH, Nashner LM: Alternative approaches to the assessment of mild head in-

juries in athletes. *Med Sci Sports Exerc* 1997;29(7 suppl):S213-S221.

57. McCrea M, Kelly JP, Randolph C, et al: Standardized Assessment of Concussion (SAC): On-site mental status evaluation of the athlete. *J Head Trauma Rehabil* 1998;13:27-35.

58. McCrea M, Randolph C, Kelly JP: *Standardized Assessment of Concussion (SAC): Manual for Administration, Scoring and Interpretation*. Waukesha, WI, CNS Inc, 1997.

59. McCrea M, Kelly JP, Kluge J, Ackley B, Randolph C: Standardized assessment of concussion in football players. *Neurology* 1997;48:586-588.

60. Barth JT, Alves WM, Ryan TV, et al: Mild head injury in sports: Neuropsychological sequelae and recovery of function, in Levin HS, Eisenberg HA, Benton AL (eds): *Mild Head Injury in Sport*. New York, NY, Oxford University Press, 1989, pp 257-275.

61. Collins MW, Grindel SH, Lovell MR, et al: Relationship between concussion and neuropsychological performance in college football players. *JAMA* 1999;282:964-970.

62. Kane RL, Kay GG: Computerized assessment in neuropsychology: A review of tests and test batteries. *Neuropsychol Rev* 1992;3:1-117.

63. Kane RL, Reeves DL: Computerized test batteries, in Horton A (ed): *The Neuropsychology Handbook*. New York, NY, Springer, 1997, vol 2, pp 426-467.

64. Bleiberg J, Garmoe WS, Halpern EL, Reeves DL, Nadler JD: Consistency of within day and across day performance after mild brain injury. *Neuropsychiatry Neuropsychol Behav Neurol* 1997;10:247-253.

65. Erlanger DM, Feldman DJ, Kaplan D, Theodoracopolus A, Kutner KC: Development and validation of a Web-based protocol for management of sports-related concussion [abstract]. *Arch Clin Neuropsychol* 2000; 15:675.

18

Face and Related Structures Pathologies

Christine Heilman,
MS, ATC
Michael Ellerbusch, MD

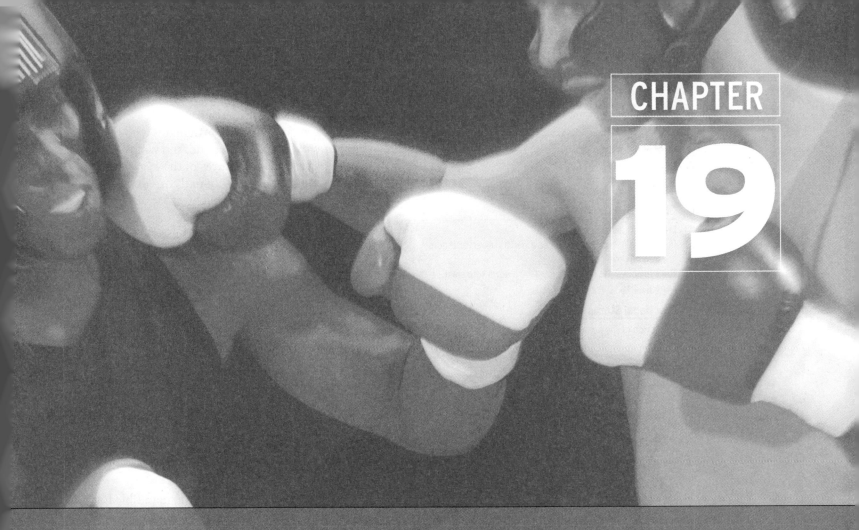

Zygomatic Fractures

CLINICAL PRESENTATION

History

Direct blow to the face, especially the zygoma

Observation

Bruising at the site of impact

Depression of the zygomatic bone may be observed before swelling develops.

The eye above the fracture may have a downward slant.

Enophthalmos may be observed.

Functional Status

Disruption of the bony contour of the eye may restrict eye motility.

Physical Evaluation Findings

A step-off deformity may be palpated at the fracture site.

Extraoral or intraoral palpation may reveal crepitus at the fracture site.

If numbness is present, it follows the distribution of the infraorbital nerve.

Enophthalmos
A protruding globe.

The facial skeleton is formed by a series of bony horizontal and vertical buttresses that serve as shock absorbers for the craniofacial complex. These relatively dense, bony pillars are surrounded by more delicate areas of bone that form the bony sinuses in the face. The facial buttresses absorb and dissipate the force of an impact, preventing injury to the underlying structures such as the brain, eyes, and other neurovascular structures. Fractures of the facial bones have unique risks and complications, such as blood from a hemorrhage collecting in the pharynx and obstructing the airway.[1]

The zygomatic bone articulates with the frontal bone, maxilla, temporal bone, and wing of the sphenoid (**Figure 19-1**). Fractures of the zygomaticomaxillary complex (ZMC) usually involve several of these articulations and account for approximately 10% of sport-related facial fractures.[2]

Zygomatic fractures occur when significant force is applied to the prominent cheekbone. The bony complex is forced posteriorly and rotates laterally and inferiorly. The medial and lateral canthal tendons that support the eye attach to the medial and lateral orbital rims, respectively. Thus, any malalignment of the rim bones changes the axis of the intercanthal line, giving the eye a downward-sloping appearance (**Figure 19-2**).

The Manson system can be used to classify ZMC fractures based on the findings of computed tomography (CT) scans (**Table 19-1**). Most sport-related zygomatic fractures are low- or medium-velocity injuries, such as being "elbowed" in the ZMC.

Differential Diagnosis

Orbital fracture, malar fracture, mandible fracture, facial contusion

Imaging Techniques

CT is the most accurate imaging technique for identifying ZMC fractures (**Figure 19-3**).[3] Subtle fractures are frequently not visible on standard radiographs. The type of zygomatic fracture can be classified using the Manson system (see Table 19-1).

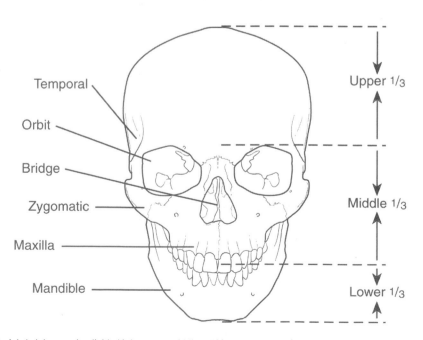

Temporal
Orbit
Bridge
Zygomatic
Maxilla
Mandible

Upper ⅓
Middle ⅓
Lower ⅓

Figure 19-1 The craniofacial skeleton can be divided into upper, middle, and lower components.

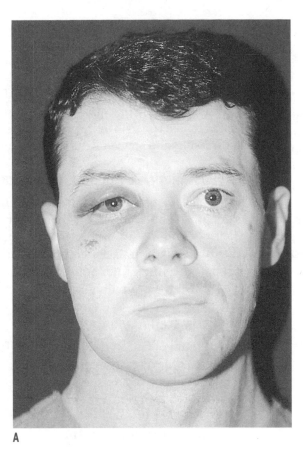
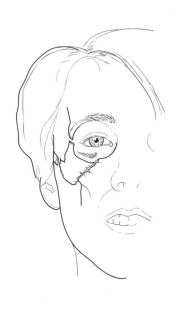

A   B

Figure 19-2   Clinical findings associated with a ZMC fracture include periorbital ecchymosis, downward slant of the lateral canthus, and a depressed cheekbone (**A**). Compare this with the underlying bony injury (**B**).

Table 19-1

Manson Classification System for Zygomatic Fractures

Classification	Description
Low energy	No displacement
	No instability of the fragment
Middle energy	Complete fracture
	Moderate displacement
	Comminution
High energy	Fracture line extends through the glenoid fossa of the temporomandibular joint

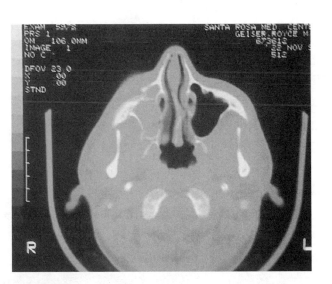

Figure 19-3   CT scan demonstrating a fracture of the left zygomatic bone. Note the absence of the sinus, which appears as a large, dark area on the right side of the image.

Definitive Diagnosis

The definitive diagnosis and subsequent management approach are based on the findings of radiographs or CT scans (or both).

Pathomechanics and Functional Limitations

Derangement of the periorbital architecture can disrupt the normal alignment of the eyes, causing diplopia and other vision deficits. Surgical repair is required to correct the vision disturbance. However, rigid internal fixation is not as strong as the patient's own intact facial skeleton. If a similar blow occurs to the repaired fracture site before bone healing is complete, the patient is at risk for a more severe fracture pattern than the initial injury. The second injury is likely to damage the underlying vital structures.

Immediate Management

Because facial trauma may disrupt the airway, the patient's airway, breathing, and circulation (ABCs) must be evaluated and continually monitored. If the ABCs have been compromised, their management takes precedence. If the ABCs are normal and a fracture is suspected, remove the athlete from competition and evaluate for trauma to the brain and cervical spine. Treat the injured area with ice to control the formation of edema and refer the patient to a specialist.

Medications

Acetaminophen or narcotic analgesics can be started for pain relief after a closed head injury has been ruled out. Nonsteroidal anti-inflammatory drugs (NSAIDs) are a treatment option, but they may increase bleeding in acute injuries and have been implicated in delaying bone healing time.

Surgical Intervention

If indicated, surgical repair should be performed within 7 to 10 days to prevent early fracture consolidation. Rigid fixation of these fractures is usually obtained with titanium miniplates and screws specifically designed for facial bones. The surgical approach helps to minimize facial scars by internally fixating the plates and screws under the eyelid (**Figure 19-4**). The use of rigid fixation has decreased the need for extended intermaxillary fixation (wiring the jaws together) and resulted in more predictable, stable, long-term results and fewer nutrition-related difficulties.[4]

Postinjury/Postoperative Management

The goals for managing all facial fractures are the same: make an accurate diagnosis; obtain precise anatomic reduction of the fracture; stabilize the fracture to achieve facial contour, symmetry, and primary healing of the bones; and, if applicable, reestablish the pretraumatic dental occlusion.

Estimated Amount of Time Lost

A minimum of 6 to 8 weeks is required for fracture healing. Athletes who are prohibited from wearing facial protection (eg, boxers) may be withheld from competition for up to 3 months.

Return-to-Play Criteria

The patient can return to competition when the fracture site is stable and no residual vision deficit exists.

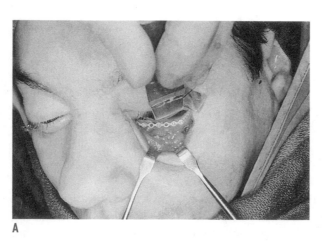
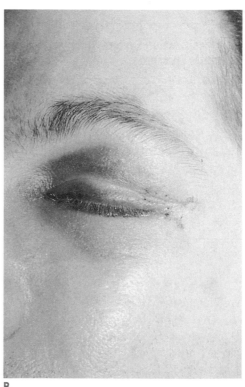

Figure 19-4 Surgical treatment of a ZMC fracture. **A.** Rigid fixation is obtained using titanium miniplates and screws. **B.** Early postsurgical results of the fracture reduction and fixation.

Functional Bracing

Properly constructed protective facial devices may allow the patient to return to competition earlier.

Nasal Fractures

CLINICAL PRESENTATION

History

Direct blow to the nose

Observation

Epistaxis
Possible deformity
With time, suborbital ecchymosis ("raccoon eyes") may develop.

Functional Status

The patient is often unable to breathe through the nose, especially during inspiration.

Physical Evaluation Findings

Pain and possible crepitus during palpation of the nasal bone
Intranasal inspection may identify the presence of a septal hematoma, deviated septum, or fracture that occludes the airway.

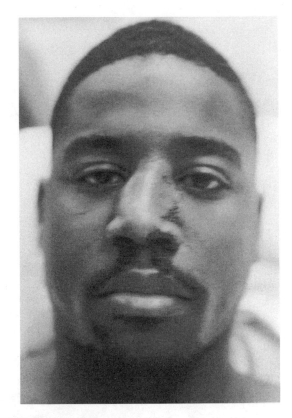

Figure 19-5 Swelling and gross deviation of the nasal dorsum indicate a possible nasal fracture.

Nasal fractures account for approximately half of all sport-related facial fractures, with 15% being recurrent fractures.[5] Because these fractures are so frequent, their severity may be underestimated, and, therefore, they may be undertreated.[5] The late effects of poorly managed nasal fractures can include functional breathing difficulties and an unacceptable cosmetic appearance; the latter can ultimately have a negative psychological effect on the patient (**Figure 19-5**).

Although the cosmetic effects of nasal injury are the most outwardly notable, the risk of secondary complications is significant. The external nose and nasal passages are intricately associated with the sebaceous glands, eustachian tubes, and nasal sinuses. Deviation of the septum, nasal bones, or lateral cartilages can have a profound effect on nasal airflow.

The nasal bones can be fractured from an anterior (frontal) or lateral force. A frontal blow causes the nasal bones to splay apart, much like the pages of an open book, giving the nose a wide, flat appearance. More commonly, a nasal fracture occurs when the impact comes from a lateral direction, causing the nose to deviate to the side away from the direction of the blow. The nasal bone on the side of the impact is forced inward, and if the blow is severe enough, the opposite nasal bone is pushed outward

(**Figure 19-6**). Because of the intimate relationship between the septum and the nasal bones, if the nasal bones fracture, the septum may deviate and fracture.

Epistaxis

Several blood vessels that supply the nose join at the anterior septum in a confluence known as the Little area or Kiesselbach plexus. This confluence of blood vessels is readily subject to environmental insults such as excessive heat and dryness and trauma; 90% of all nosebleeds occur in the anterior portion of the septum.[6]

Differential Diagnosis

Epistaxis, nasal cartilage separation

Imaging Techniques

A CT scan defines the bony anatomy and the fracture configurations. Radiographs have a 60% false-negative rate of interpretation, and suture lines are sometimes incorrectly interpreted as fractures (**Figure 19-7**).[5]

Definitive Diagnosis

The diagnosis of a nasal fracture is frequently based entirely on the clinical findings, especially intranasal observation, palpation of asymmetric nasal bones, and visible deviation of the nasal septum. Nasal injuries produce rapid swelling that can mask the

19

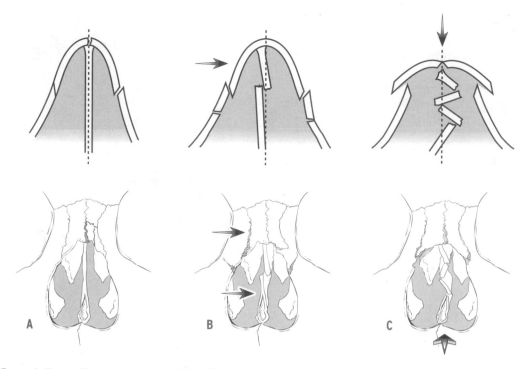

Figure 19-6 Trauma to the nasal bones can take on a variety of forms. **A.** Isolated nasal bone fracture with no septal displacement. **B.** Lateral forces that result in a fracture of nasal bones and septal deformation. **C.** Frontal blow that results in splayed fractures of the nasal bones and septum.

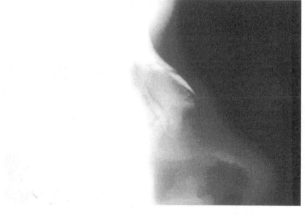

Figure 19-7 Lateral radiograph depicting a nasal fracture.

Mucoperichondrium
The structure overlying the nasal cartilage that provides it with blood supply and nutrients.

underlying tissues. This factor and the relative unreliability of radiographic findings increase the importance of performing a thorough examination of the nose as soon as possible after the injury. Prompt diagnosis is also required to obtain a closed reduction. Delaying the diagnosis may necessitate an open reduction.

The intranasal examination should be conducted with proper lighting, a nasal speculum, and, if necessary, suction. The intranasal structures are sprayed with a vasoconstrictor such as phenylephrine to control epistaxis. The septum is inspected for deviation or fractures severe enough to occlude or obstruct the airway and to identify intranasal lacerations. Small amounts of blood in the saliva are common with

nasal fractures.[7] A slow, steady unilateral drip is considered traumatic rather than spontaneous epistaxis.

Particular emphasis should be placed on diagnosing a septal hematoma. Trauma to the nose can cause blood to accumulate between the septal cartilage and the overlying mucoperichondrium, similar to what occurs with a hematoma of the ear. The septum bulges and may appear darker than the surrounding nasal mucosa as a result of the accumulated blood. A suspected septal hematoma demands immediate attention.

Pathomechanics and Functional Limitations

An untreated fracture or deviated septum can decrease nasal airflow, causing the patient to rely on breathing through the mouth. Permanent deformity may result. If a septal hematoma is not diagnosed, the cartilage can become ischemic and necrotic, leading to collapse of the nasal dorsum with a resultant "saddlenose" deformity. Edema within the nasal passage can block one or both eustachian tubes, thereby affecting hearing or balance, or both.

■ Immediate Management

The nose should be evaluated for asymmetry or other deformity as soon as possible after the injury occurs and before edema forms. Associated injury to the head, mouth, and the eye's bony orbit should be ruled out at this time. The nose should be treated with ice to limit swelling and control epistaxis. An open wound that exposes cartilage or bone is treated as an open fracture. The wound should be thoroughly irrigated and the patient placed on appropriate antibiotics.

Epistaxis as a result of nasal trauma is usually of a limited nature and can almost always be controlled with digital pressure on the anterior nose and placing the patient in a seated position with the head upright. Nasal packing is only required when severe bleeding cannot be controlled with digital pressure.

The anterior nasal chamber can be packed using commercially available nose packs, a sectioned tampon, or less preferably, sterile gauze. A physician may elect to soak the pack in thrombin to further control the bleeding. The pack should not be forced deep into the nasal cavity, and care must be used to prevent overpacking. The posterior nasal chamber should only be packed in an emergency department.

Nasal packs should not be left in place for more than 72 hours. Keeping the nose packed for a longer period of time increases the risk of infection, including meningitis.

■ Medications

NSAIDs or narcotic analgesics can be started for pain relief after a closed head injury has been ruled out (see the pharmacology precautions listed on p 53). If closed reduction is required, a local or mild general anesthetic or sedative may be administered.

■ Surgical Intervention

In managing a septal hematoma, the physician incises the affected mucosa and evacuates the hematoma. The nasal passage is then packed with gauze impregnated with petrolatum or a vasoconstrictor (such as Lacrilube).

Repair can be limited to a simple closed reduction of the nasal bones using topical and local anesthesia in the physician's office setting or be a more involved open reduction of a fractured or severely dislocated septum in the operating room. The realigned nasal bones or septum are then splinted externally and internally (**Figure 19-8**). The splints are usually removed in 7 to 10 days.

■ Postinjury/Postoperative Management

The indications for treatment of nasal injuries by a physician are nasal airway obstruction or obvious external nasal deformity. Acute fractures or displacements should be managed as soon as possible after injury. Swelling that occurs over time obscures the deformity and makes proper repair difficult. If swelling has occurred, it is usually prudent to wait at least 4 to 7 days in adults and 4 days in children for the swelling to subside. The patient can then be reexamined and definitive repair performed if needed.

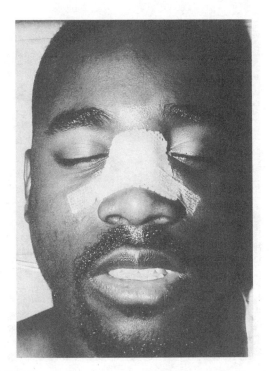

Figure 19-8 The displaced nasal bones and septum are realigned and splinted to maintain proper alignment during the healing process.

A septal hematoma must be identified and drained early to prevent a saddlenose deformity. Drainage can be performed under local anesthesia, such as lidocaine without epinephrine, with subsequent drainage using an 18-gauge needle and packing of the passage, or the area may require anesthesia for incision, drain insertion, and packing of the area to ensure the hematoma does not return.

Recurrent epistaxis can be decreased with use of a humidifier or vaporizer at night while sleeping. Petrolatum gel is applied twice daily to control bleeding until the injury is completely healed.

■ Estimated Amount of Time Lost

Depending on the amount of protection that can be provided to the nose, the patient may lose no time from activity. A surgically repaired nasal fracture may keep the patient from competition for 7 to 10 days.

■ Return-to-Play Criteria

The decision to return the athlete to competition and the need for nasal protection should be carefully weighed. The nasal bones generally heal sufficiently within 4 to 8 weeks, allowing the athlete to return to competition in contact sports.

Functional Bracing

A protective facial device of sufficient strength to prevent further injury should be used if the athlete resumes competition soon after repair (**Figure 19-9**).

19

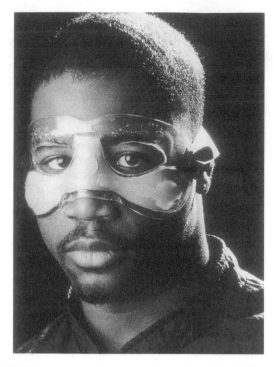

Figure 19-9   A custom-designed protective facial mask can protect the nose and allow the athlete to resume competition. This device can also protect the nasal structures from repetitive injury.

Because repeated nasal injuries are possible, prophylactic use of a protective facial device should be considered after a nasal fracture.

Mandible Fractures

CLINICAL PRESENTATION

History
Direct blow to the mandible.

Observation
Swelling forms over the fracture site.
Malocclusion of the teeth may be noted.
Possible intraoral bleeding
Ecchymosis forms on the floor of the mouth.
A step deformity (malalignment of the teeth) may be noted between the teeth on each side of the fracture site.

Functional Status
Difficulty opening the mouth
Pain with biting down or inability to bite down
Possible maltracking of the mandible during motion

Physical Evaluation Findings
Intraoral examination may reveal a step deformity.
Intraoral or extraoral palpation may reveal pain and crepitus along the fracture site.
Pain is produced when stressing the mandible.
The tongue-blade test may be positive.
Anterior distraction of the mandible produces pain.

Malocclusion
Improper alignment of the teeth when the mouth is closed.

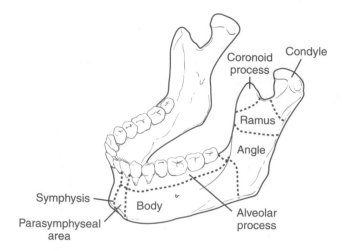

Figure 19-10   The bony mandible and its associated dental structures.

The horseshoe-shaped mandible articulates with the base of the skull at the temporomandibular joints (TMJs). It is a strong cortical bone but is relatively weak at its angles, the neck of the condyles, and the distal body, where the long root of the canine tooth and the mental foramen are located (**Figure 19-10**). Because of the mandible's arched shape and several weak, thin areas, it is common for the lower jaw to fracture in two places.

The subcondylar regions are the most commonly fractured areas of the lower jaw. These areas are thinner than the rest of the mandible; therefore, forces generated at impact are transmitted to these areas. A subcondylar fracture can have devastating, long-term functional and cosmetic sequelae.

The condylar region of the mandible is a growth center, and suspected fractures to this region in young patients require extraordinary attention. Trauma to an immature epiphysis may result in shortened mandible height and lead to occlusion problems. Injuries to this region can also result in hemorrhage into the TMJ, potentially leading to fibrosis and ankylosis.

Differential Diagnosis
TMJ sprain or dislocation, tooth fracture

Imaging Techniques
Simple anteroposterior radiographs, such as the modified Towne view, Walter view, or an orthopantograph, usually reveal condylar head, mandibular arch, and subcondylar fractures (**Figure 19-11**). A CT scan can reveal more subtle fractures and provide valuable information about displacement of the fractured segments and possible intracranial injuries (**Figure 19-12**).

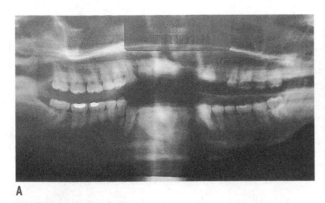
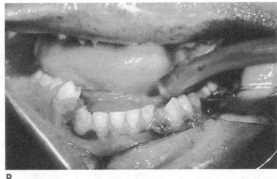

A   **B**

Figure 19-11 Methods used to evaluate step-off deformities. **A.** Panorex-type radiograph demonstrating a right mandibular body fracture with a step-off deformity of the teeth. **B.** Clinical view reveals intraoral bleeding from a mucosal tear and the step-off deformity of the teeth.

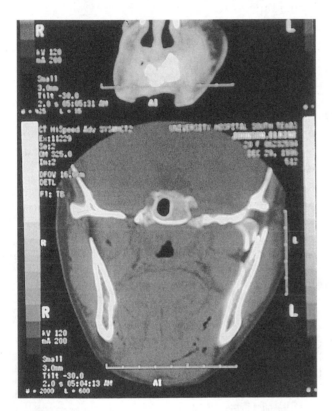

Figure 19-12 A CT scan demonstrating a left subcondylar fracture.

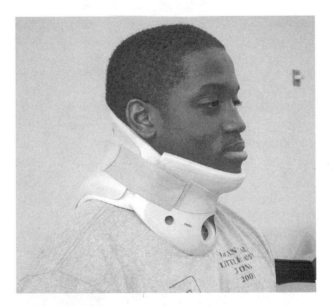

Figure 19-13 A hard cervical collar used for immobilizing the cervical spine can also be used to immobilize the mandible.

Definitive Diagnosis
Positive physical and radiographic findings for fracture

Pathomechanics and Functional Limitations
The patient has difficulty opening and closing the mouth, and chewing is painful. Functional limitations are created by the malocclusions and instability of the fracture. Over time, asymmetry of the mandible can create unequal pressures within the TMJ, resulting in degenerative changes and dysfunction.

Immediate Management
Fractures that occur on both sides of the jaw can become unstable. At the time of injury, the anterior segment can shift backward, causing the tongue to block the airway. Pulling the tongue or the anterior jaw forward can open the airway. The tongue or jaw should be stabilized in this position and the patient transported to the emergency department, with proper cervical spine immobilization if necessary. Refer to the immediate management of zygomatic fractures regarding airway compromise.

A secondary survey should be conducted to rule out trauma to the brain, cervical spine, face, teeth, and eyes. A hard cervical collar or Barton bandage should be applied to limit jaw motion while the patient is referred for further medical attention (**Figure 19-13**).

19

Medications

NSAIDs or narcotic analgesics can be begun for pain relief once a closed head injury has been ruled out.

Surgical Intervention

Displaced fractures must be reduced, either by placing the patient in maxillomandibular fixation with the jaws wired together for 4 to 6 weeks or by rigidly fixing the segments with plates and screws using an open technique. Rigid fixation has the advantage of allowing the patient to open and close the jaws, thereby preventing long-term injury to the TMJs through early motion and improved nutritional status (**Figure 19-14**).

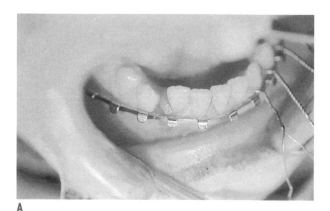

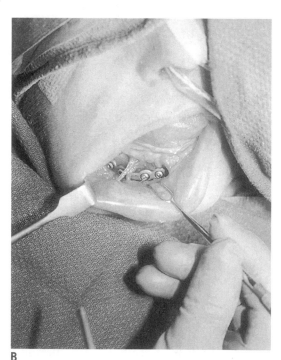

Figure 19-14 The management of a displaced fracture includes maxillomandibular fixation. **A.** Arch bars and wires placed on the upper and lower teeth can be used to fixate the jaws into proper occlusion and allow for healing of minimally displaced or nondisplaced fractures over a 4- to 8-week period. **B.** Rigid fixation of the fracture with titanium plates and screws allows for immediate postsurgical jaw motion.

Postinjury/Postoperative Management

Nondisplaced fractures with easily reproducible occlusion can be managed with close observation and a diet of soft foods. If the patient's jaw has been fixated, the diet should be modified to include sufficient caloric intake with proper nutritional balance. Several commercially available supplements can be used to achieve these goals.

Estimated Amount of Time Lost

An athlete with a jaw fracture should not be allowed to return to play until healing has occurred, which generally takes 6 to 8 weeks, but protective devices can permit an earlier return (see Functional Bracing).

Return-to-Play Criteria

Return-to-play criteria may depend on the sport and fixation techniques. Generally, the more rigid the internal fixation technique, the quicker the return to play. Wiring of the jaw can compromise nutritional status and make it difficult and time consuming to take in adequate oxygen to satisfy the demand created by high-intensity activity.

Functional Bracing

A protective cage or helmet with a jaw extension can allow athletes in selected sports to return to competition earlier.

Temporomandibular Joint Dislocations

CLINICAL PRESENTATION

History

Most TMJ dislocations occur traumatically, secondary to a lateral blow to the mandible.
Pain occurs when attempting to open and close the mouth.

Observation

In a frank dislocation, the patient is unable to close the mouth.
Malocclusion of the teeth

Functional Status

The patient may be unable to voluntarily open and close the mouth.
The mandible may track laterally when the mouth is opened and closed.

Physical Evaluation Findings

If the TMJ is still dislocated, spasm of the masseter and temporal muscles can be felt during palpation.
The tongue-blade test may be positive. A popping or clicking noise is heard when a stethoscope is placed on the TMJ.

The TMJ is the only synovial joint in the skull and is surrounded by a loose capsule. The articular surfaces are covered with a fibrous cartilage rather than the hyaline cartilage found in other joints. A cartilaginous disk divides the joints into upper and lower compartments. The superior temporal articulation is formed by the articular tubercle, articular eminence, glenoid fossa, and posterior glenoid spine.

The TMJ subluxates during normal opening and closing of the mouth. Traumatic dislocations tend to occur when the TMJ muscles are relaxed and a lateral blow is sustained by the mandible. However, dislocations can occur during sneezing, eating, or other times when the mouth is opened widely. Progressive joint degeneration can lead to a chronically dislocating TMJ.

Simple dislocations are marked by the mandible displacing anteriorly relative to the joint and most frequently occur unilaterally. Complex dislocations are characterized by an upward displacement, commonly involving a fracture of the skull, or posterior displacement, fracturing the auditory canal.

Differential Diagnosis
Mandibular fracture

Imaging Techniques
CT and magnetic resonance imaging are the imaging techniques of choice.

Definitive Diagnosis
The definitive diagnosis is based on the clinical symptom of the TMJ locking or catching and is confirmed through radiographic studies.

Pathomechanics and Functional Limitations
The TMJ subluxates anteriorly each time the mouth is opened and closed. Chronic TMJ disorders can interfere with the patient's ability to chew, speak, yawn, and sneeze. Embarrassing moments can occur when the TMJ locks in social situations.

Patients who have sustained a traumatic posterior TMJ dislocation may experience hearing deficits. The auditory canal can be fractured when the condyle displaces posteriorly; narrowing of the canal and the subsequent inflammatory response can reduce hearing temporarily or permanently.

■ Immediate Management
A Barton bandage should be applied to limit jaw motion while the patient is referred for further medical attention (see Figure 19-13). A physician should attempt to reduce a frank dislocation as soon as possible after the injury (see Postinjury Management).

■ Medications
Mild sedatives or anesthetics may be required to reduce the dislocation. NSAIDs or narcotic analgesics can be started for pain relief after a closed head injury has been ruled out.

■ Surgical Intervention
Reducing an anterior TMJ dislocation is relatively easy if the patient is relaxed. Relaxation is made easier if mild sedatives or anesthetics are administered. The physician grasps the lower molars with the thumbs and the symphysis of the mandible with the index fingers. The thumbs on the molars then apply downward pressure while the fingers rotate the anterior portion of the mandible upwardly.

■ Postinjury/Postoperative Management
After reduction, the patient must be restricted from widely opening the mouth for up to 2 months. Ideally, the patient makes a conscious effort to prevent yawning or chewing large, hard foods and so voluntarily abides by this restriction. With a severe or recurrent dislocation or if the patient is unwilling or unable to restrict mandibular motion, the jaw may need to be wired shut.

As with mandibular fractures, patients sustaining a TMJ dislocation eat a modified diet emphasizing soft, nutritional foods. If the patient's jaw has been fixated, the diet should be modified to include sufficient caloric intake while maintaining proper nutritional balance.

■ Estimated Amount of Time Lost
An athlete with a TMJ dislocation treated conservatively normally does not lose time from competition, although a first-time dislocation may require 4 to 14 days of healing before returning to competition. Surgical repair extends the amount of time lost.

■ Return-to-Play Criteria
The TMJ should be properly located, and the patient should be able to open the mouth to the point necessary to breathe and speak without recurrent locking.

Functional Bracing
Facial protection similar to that used for mandibular fractures can help to prevent recurrent traumatic dislocations. Custom-designed mouthpieces may also be effective in reducing the frequency of dislocations in a chronically dislocating TMJ.

Tooth Fractures

CLINICAL PRESENTATION

History

A blow to the teeth
Biting on a hard object
Depending on the nature of the injury, discomfort may vary from minimal pain to constant pain (see Table 19-2).

Observation

Fractures to the crown may produce obvious defects, although type I fractures may be less visible.
The tooth may be luxated (see p 591).
Bleeding may be noted with type III fractures.

Functional Status

Depending on the type of fracture, the patient may be unable to eat or drink without pain.

Physical Evaluation Findings

Palpation of the teeth may reveal deformity.

Tooth fractures can involve the crown or the root. A fracture of the crown usually does not require urgent attention unless it involves the neurovascular tissue or the pulp of the tooth (**Figure 19-15**). Fractures that expose the tooth's nerves can be extremely painful (**Table 19-2**).

Root fractures are more difficult to diagnose. Any mobility of a tooth, pain on palpation, or movement suggests a root fracture. These fractures are described by their location: cervical third, middle third, or apical third.

A dentoalveolar fracture is a fracture of the alveolar bone and the associated teeth. The involved teeth may or may not have associated fractures of the crown or root, or they may be subluxated or avulsed. Dentoalveolar fractures should be treated as open fractures. Eighty percent of dental injuries involve the four anterior teeth.[8]

Differential Diagnosis

Tooth luxation, tooth avulsion, mandible fracture, maxillary fracture, TMJ dislocation or sprain

Imaging Techniques

Radiographs are used to identify fracture lines, especially of the root, and the depth of the fracture. They also serve as a reference for future procedures.

Definitive Diagnosis

The definitive diagnosis is based on gross observation or dental radiographic findings.

Pathomechanics and Functional Limitations

The fracture type and the associated pain limit the patient's ability to eat and drink. A type I crown fracture may simply cause irritation as the tongue passes over the fracture site. Other fractures of the crown or root must be evaluated by a dentist as soon as possible to prevent infection and decrease the risk of losing the tooth.

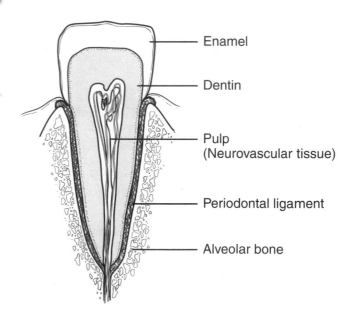

Figure 19-15 The dentoalveolar process includes the tooth, alveolar bone, and the periodontal ligament.

Table 19-2

Fractures of the Crown

Type	Portion Involved	Symptoms
I	Only the enamel is fractured.	Pain is minimal, but the patient may report irritation of the tongue as it rubs across the fracture site.
II	The dentin is fractured, but the pulp is not exposed.	The tooth is sensitive to cold.
III	The fracture has exposed the pulp.	Pain is constant.

Immediate Management

Inspect the mouth for lost pieces of the tooth, some of which may be embedded within the lips, cheek, or gum. Recovered segments of a tooth fracture should be managed like a tooth avulsion. To reduce the risk of aspiration, the mouth should be thoroughly inspected for residual tooth fragments. If the tooth is fragmented, transport the segment using a commercially available kit or place it in milk or a saline solution. To prevent infection of a fractured crown or root, have the patient gargle with saline solution.

Medications

NSAIDs or narcotic analgesics may be started for pain relief after a closed head injury has been ruled out. The dentist will also determine the need for tetanus prophylaxis and antibiotic medications.

Postinjury Management

Type I fractures most often present cosmetic concerns, especially when the front teeth are involved.

Treatment of tooth fractures includes covering the exposed pulp and dentin with calcium hydroxide paste supported by an acid-etched composite resin, alleviating discomfort and allowing healing to begin.[9] If the crown is superficially fractured and has a resultant sharp edge that bothers the patient, the edge can be gently filed down with an emery board.

Estimated Amount of Time Lost

Athletes sustaining type I and II fractures of the crown may be immediately returned to competition but should be evaluated by a dentist immediately after the game. Type III fractures must be evaluated by a dentist before the patient is cleared to play.

Return-to-Play Criteria

The tooth should be stable, with no risk of dislodging and becoming trapped in the airway during competition.

Functional Bracing

The incidence of injury or reinjury of the teeth when athletes are wearing intraoral mouthguards is low.

Tooth Luxations and Tooth Avulsions

CLINICAL PRESENTATION

History

A direct blow to the mouth or teeth
Complaints of pain, discomfort, or an abnormal sensation when biting

Observation

The tooth may be visibly malaligned; with an avulsion, the tooth is completely dislodged from the gum.
Bleeding may be present.

Functional Status

The patient is unable to bite down.

Physical Evaluation Findings

A luxated tooth is mobile during palpation.

Tooth Luxation

Luxation or dislocation of a tooth has occurred when the tooth is malpositioned in its bone socket. Malposition generally indicates some damage to the periodontal ligaments and neurovascular structures. The tooth should be gently manipulated into position, the surrounding alveolar bone palpated for fractures, and the patient referred to a dentist. An intruded tooth is characterized by the displacement of the root into the bone, resulting in a fracture of the mandible or maxilla and the possible rupture of the periodontal ligament. An extruded tooth involves the displacement of the tooth out of its socket, jeopardizing the neurovascular supply and tearing the periodontal ligaments. The prognosis for long-term damage depends on the amount of displacement from the tooth's normal position.[8]

Tooth Avulsion

An avulsion injury is described as a partial or total separation of the tooth from the alveolus, creating damage similar to that of an extruded tooth, and is an urgent situation. The prognosis for viability of the tooth and successful replantation is inversely proportional to the length of time the tooth is out of its socket. Generally, the tooth should be replanted within 20 minutes to 2 hours.

Differential Diagnosis

Tooth fracture, mandible fracture, maxillary fracture, TMJ dislocation or sprain

19

Imaging Techniques

Radiographs are used to identify concomitant injury to the root or socket. They also serve as a reference for future procedures.

Definitive Diagnosis

The diagnosis of a tooth luxation or avulsion can be made based on the patient's signs and symptoms. However, radiographs are required to identify possible fracture of the root or bony socket.

Pathomechanics and Functional Limitations

If the periodontal ligament fibers undergo desiccation or are removed as a result of rough handling, the tooth may undergo resorption or ankylosis to the surrounding bone and ultimately be lost.

Desiccation The process of tissue dehydration or drying out.

■ Immediate Management

The keys to successful replantation are maintaining the nourishment and preserving the tooth's periodontal ligament. As such, prompt attention by a dentist is imperative to save the tooth.

Tooth Luxation

The patient can be asked to gently bite down on a piece of folded sterile gauze to stabilize the tooth during transport.

Tooth Avulsion

The root of the tooth, where the ligaments are attached, should be handled carefully. Do not scrub or brush the root of the avulsed tooth. Instead, gently handle the tooth by the crown and irrigate it with normal saline. If the tooth cannot be immediately replanted into its socket, it should be cleansed with care and simply placed in the buccal vestibule of the mouth (between the cheek and gum), and the patient should be transported immediately to a dentist. If the patient is unable to hold the tooth in the cheek, it should be placed in fresh cold milk, sterile saline, the patient's saliva, or cool tap water. Milk is an ideal storage medium; activity in periodontal cells has been maintained for up to 6 hours when a tooth is stored in milk. Commercially available transport systems for avulsed teeth may also be used.

Dystopia Change in the position of the pupil relative to the unaffected side.

■ Medications

NSAIDs and narcotic analgesics can be started for pain relief after a closed head injury has been ruled out.

■ Surgical Intervention

For a tooth luxation, the dentist will replant the tooth into its socket, splint the tooth, prescribe analgesics and antibiotics and a diet of soft foods, and follow the athlete closely. Often the tooth re-

quires endodontic therapy (root canal treatment) for ultimate salvage.

■ Postinjury/Postoperative Management

Treatment of a tooth luxation may involve splinting the affected tooth with bonded acrylic and monofilament nylon or wiring by a dentist.[9] A diet consisting of soft food may be necessary during the healing process for both surgical and nonsurgical management.

■ Estimated Amount of Time Lost

The amount of time lost will vary from the immediate return to competition to 2 to 3 days missed if oral surgery is required.

■ Return-to-Play Criteria

A player should not return to competition if the tooth is displaced 3 mm or more.

Functional Bracing

The incidence of injury or reinjury of the teeth is quite low when athletes wear intraoral mouthguards.

Orbital Fractures ("Blowout" Fractures)

CLINICAL PRESENTATION

History

A blow to the orbital rim or periorbital region
Pain when opening the mouth

Observation

Infraorbital ecchymosis
Enophthalmos
Vertical dystopia

Functional Status

Entrapment of the inferior rectus muscle can limit upward gaze of the affected eye.
If the fracture involves the sinus, air may escape from the lower portion of the globe when the patient attempts to blow the nose.

Physical Evaluation Findings

Numbness in the cheek can result from inhibition of the infraorbital nerve.

The bony orbit of the eye is formed by portions of the frontal, maxillary, and zygomatic bones and the wings of the sphenoid, lacrimal, and ethmoid bones (**Figure 19-16**). The orbit serves to support the globe. A strong orbital rim is created by thick-

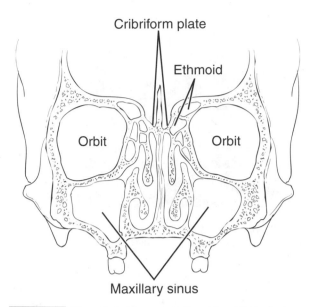

Figure 19-16 The orbital walls separate the orbit and its contents from the various sinuses of the face.

ened portions of the frontal, maxillary, and zygomatic bones, protecting the eye from large, solid objects.

Orbital fractures can occur independently or in combination with interior wall fractures; interior wall fractures can also occur alone. A direct blow to the orbital rim may be insufficient to fracture the bony rim; however, it can increase intraorbital pressure sufficiently to fracture the thin interior bones. The interior bones most commonly fractured are those of the inferior medial portion, or the floor of the orbit, a "blowout" fracture (**Figure 19-17**).

A circumferential bony framework protects the vital structures of the orbital complex. The aperture of the bony rim does not allow objects with diameters greater than 10 cm to penetrate to the globe.[10] The circumferential bony rim should be palpated during the examination. Fractures of the orbital rim can occur at any point; however, frac-

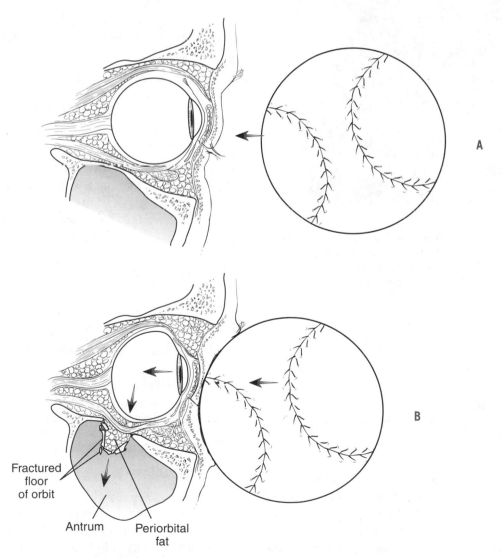

Figure 19-17 Orbital rim fracture. **A.** The opening of the periorbital rim does not allow objects with a diameter greater than 10 cm to penetrate. **B.** The force generated at impact causes a blowout fracture of the thin, bony walls of the orbital floor.

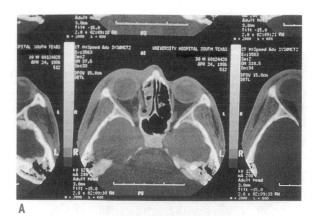

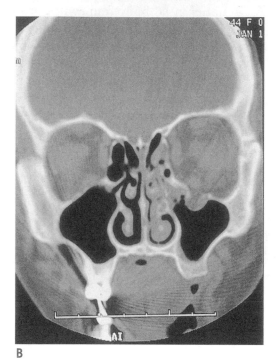

Figure 19-18   **A.** A CT scan demonstrates a fracture of the medial wall of the orbit, showing its contents communicating with the ethmoid sinus. **B.** A CT scan showing an orbital floor fracture with displacement of the orbital soft tissues into the maxillary sinus.

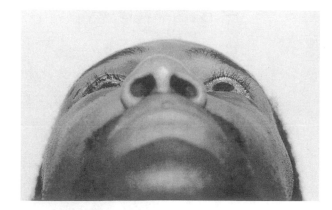

Figure 19-19   A worm's eye view demonstrating enophthalmos of the patient's right eye after a fracture of the orbital floor.

tures of the inferior rim are the most common type.

Differential Diagnosis
Zygomatic fracture, neuropathy of the ocular motor nerves

Medical Diagnostic Tests
A forced duction test is used to determine if limited ocular movements are caused by entrapped soft tissues, edema, or a contused motor nerve or muscle. First, the affected eye is anesthetized with a topical anesthetic. Next, the sclera is grasped with a fine-toothed forceps at the level of the inferior rectus muscle insertion. Last, the eye is gently moved

in the superior and inferior directions. If the globe moves easily, entrapment of the ocular contents can be ruled out.

Imaging Techniques
A CT scan from the coronal view (bird's eye) is ideal for evaluating the interior walls of the orbit and can accurately reveal a blowout fracture (**Figure 19-18**).

Definitive Diagnosis
The diagnosis of an orbital fracture can be made based on the patient's signs and symptoms, especially enophthalmos or exophthalmos, and is confirmed through radiographs or CT scan, or both (**Figure 19-19**).

Pathomechanics and Functional Limitations
Diplopia on upward gaze can be due to restricted movement of the eye from direct entrapment of the inferior rectus muscle or swelling or contusion of the muscle.

■ Immediate Management
Shield the affected eye, and transport the patient for appropriate medical care. Because of the possibility of surgery, withhold food and fluids until an ophthalmologist evaluates the patient.

■ Medications
NSAIDs and narcotic analgesics can be started for pain relief once a closed head injury has been ruled out.

■ Surgical Intervention
Because soft-tissue swelling, hemorrhage, or damage to the oculomotor nerves can mimic the signs and symptoms of an orbital floor fracture, the surgical correction of a blowout fracture is controversial.[2] Often, the combination of CT scan findings, clinical examination including limited upward gaze,

and significant enophthalmos leads to the decision to surgically repair the orbital floor defect. Orbital rim fractures are repaired with open reduction techniques through aesthetic incisions and stabilized with miniplates and screws.

Postinjury/Postoperative Management

Patients should be restricted from forcibly blowing the nose until the fracture site is healed. The associated pressure can cause motion in the fractured bone separating the orbit and the facial sinuses and delay the healing process. If eye motion causes pain, the patient may be instructed to use a forward gaze and rely on head motion to obtain the needed field of view.

Estimated Amount of Time Lost

Protective facial devices sufficient to prevent reinjury should be used if the player returns to competition before 4 to 8 weeks have passed.

Return-to-Play Criteria

Radiographic evidence of healing of the involved bones is usually required before returning to competition. The patient's vision must be adequate to safely participate in sport.

Functional Bracing

Protective eyewear can prevent both acute injuries and reinjuries.

References

1. Crow RW: Diagnosis and management of sports-related injuries to the face. *Dent Clin North Am* 1991;35:719-732.
2. Torg JS (ed): *Athletic Injuries to the Head, Neck and Face*, ed 2. Philadelphia, PA, Lea & Febiger, 1991, pp 611-649.
3. Manson PN, Markowitz B, Mirvis S, Dunham M, Yaremchuk M: Toward CT-based facial fracture treatment. *Plast Reconstr Surg* 1990;85:202-214.
4. Garza JR, Baratta RV, Odinet K, et al: Impact intolerances of the rigidly fixated maxillofacial skeleton. *Ann Plast Surg* 1993;30:212-216.
5. Schendel SA: Sport-related nasal injuries. *Physician Sportsmed* 1990;18:59-74.
6. Friedrich C: Therapy of recurring epistaxis of the anterior nasal septum. *Arch Otorhinolaryngol* 1982;236:131-134.
7. Linn LW, Vrijhoef MM, de Wijn JR, Coops RP, Cliteur BF, Meerloo R: Facial injuries sustained during sports and games. *J Maxillofac Surg* 1986;14:83-88.
8. Padilla RR, Felsenfeld AL: Treatment and prevention of alveolar fractures and related injuries. *J Craniomaxillofac Trauma* 1997;3:22-27.
9. Camp JH: Diagnosis and management of sports-related injuries to the teeth. *Dent Clin North Am* 1991;35:733-756.
10. Guyette RF: Facial injuries in basketball players. *Clin Sports Med* 1993;12:247-264.

19

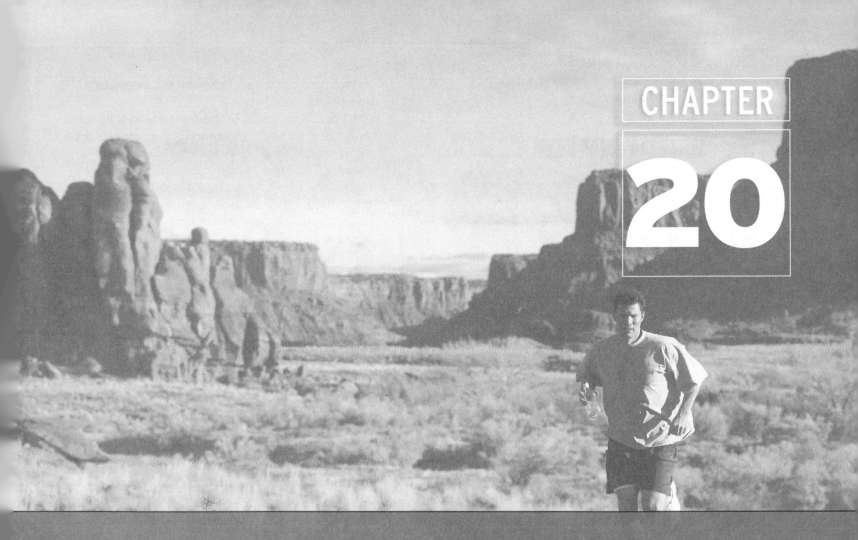

Exertional Heat Illnesses

Douglas J. Casa, PhD,
ATC, FACSM
Randy Eichner, MD,
FACSM

Heat Cramps

CLINICAL PRESENTATION

History

Recent history of intense exercise in a hot environment
Lack of heat acclimatization
Insufficient sodium intake during meals and practices
Irregular access to meals and fluids
Previous history of cramping
Chronic dehydration

Observation

Profuse sweating
Obvious muscle cramping

Functional Status

Increased fatigue
Cramping inhibits routine muscle activity and function.

Physical Evaluation Findings

Dehydration
  - Mucous membranes
  - Skin **turgor**
  - Decreased body weight
Thirst
Sweat that is high in salt content

Turgor The skin's resistance to being deformed. Tested by lifting a small nap of skin on the hand and noting how quickly it returns to normal. In dehydrated individuals, the skin will slowly return to normal.

Recent evidence suggests that heat cramps are related to an electrolyte deficit.[1] A sodium deficiency, whether caused by inadequate intake of sodium or excessive amounts of sodium lost in sweat or, most likely, a combination of the two, increases the risk of heat cramps.[1] Individuals who experience heat cramps should have their rehydration and dietary protocols analyzed to determine if their sodium intake is insufficient.[2] Increasing the amount of sodium in the diet and rehydration beverages during practices and games seems to decrease the incidence of heat cramping. Extra sodium intake early in practice may ward off heat cramps later in the session—for example, adding 0.5 to 1.0 g of sodium to the first 30 to 40 oz (0.9 to 1.18 L) of the sports drink consumed during a practice, with a regular sports drink consumed for the remainder of the practice. These considerations are even more relevant during periods of two practices a day in the heat, when sweat sodium losses are exacerbated.[1] Consumption of additional sodium without proper dilution in a rehydration beverage is not recommended.[3]

Rehydrating with a sports drink becomes even more critical when faced with sodium replacement issues. The flavor of the sports drink, compared with water, makes the added sodium more palatable.[3] Sports drinks also provide additional sodium to complement the sodium obtained from meals and snacks.

The cause of muscle cramps is not well understood and may be mulifactorial. Heat cramps are often present in athletes who perform strenuous exercise in the heat, who become dehydrated or fatigued, and who have decreased blood sodium concentrations.[1,3-6] Conversely, cramps can also occur in the absence of warm or hot conditions (eg, ice hockey players).[3]

Whether cramps are heat related or not, they tend to occur later in an activity in conjunction with muscle fatigue and after fluid and electrolyte imbalances have reached critical levels. Dehydration, a diet containing insufficient electrolytes, and large losses of sodium and other electrolytes in sweat appear to increase the risk of severe, often wholebody, muscle cramps.[7] Muscle cramps can often be avoided with adequate conditioning, acclimatization, rehydration, and electrolyte replacement and appropriate dietary practices.[5,8-12]

The current hydration and electrolyte status of athletes who experience heat cramps should be identified to develop conditioning and acclimatization strategies. If problems persist, the athlete should be referred to the team physician, registered dietitian, or both.

Differential Diagnosis

Muscle strain

Definitive Diagnosis

The most critical criteria are intense pain (not associated with acute muscle strain) and persistent muscle contractions in working muscles during and after prolonged exercise and most often associated with exercise in heat.[3,7]

Pathomechanics and Functional Limitations

The presence of muscle spasm interferes with the athlete's ability to ambulate or compete.

Immediate Management

The following procedures are recommended if heat cramps are suspected:[3,7,8]

- Reestablish normal hydration status and replace some sodium losses with an electrolyte sports drink.

- Some additional sodium may be needed (especially in athletes with a history of heat cramps) earlier in the activity (before cramps begin) and is best administered by dilution in a sports drink. For example, 0.5 to 1 g of sodium dissolved in 1 L of a sports drink early in the exercise session provides ample fluids and sodium and is palatable.

- Light stretching, relaxation, and massage of the involved muscle may help the acute pain of a muscle cramp.
- Ice can help relieve cramping pain.
- Refer to the supervising physician if the condition does not improve with the recommended course of action.

Medications

Intravenous (IV) normal saline may be given by the medical staff (**Figure 20-1**). The IV amount and sodium concentration are dictated by the supervising physician, with the aims of ameliorating the fluid deficit and replacing electrolyte losses.[3,7]

Postinjury Management

Modify the athlete's electrolyte intake to avoid future episodes. Weight charts and urine specific gravity may be used to monitor hydration and rehydration (see Identifying the Level of Hydration or Dehydration, p 608).[3,7]

Estimated Amount of Time Lost

The amount of time lost is dictated by the severity of the condition and the length of time it took to initiate treatment. Generally, athletes can return to play within a few hours or by the next day.[3,7]

Return-to-Play Criteria

Athletes should be assessed to determine if they can perform at the level needed for safe and successful participation. After an acute episode, diet,

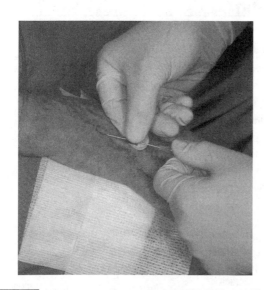

Figure 20-1 Intravenous sodium may be administered by qualified personnel to rehydrate the patient and replace electrolytes.

rehydration practices, electrolyte consumption, fitness status, level of acclimatization, and use of dietary supplements should be reviewed and possibly modified to decrease the risk of recurring heat cramps.[3,7] Rehydration status can be assessed with weight charts and physical examination.

Heat Exhaustion

CLINICAL PRESENTATION

History

Intense exercise in a hot environment
Dehydration and/or electrolyte depletion

Observation

Physical fatigue and dizziness
Profuse sweating
Pallor
The patient may experience nausea, vomiting, or diarrhea.
Central nervous system (CNS) inhibition (confusion, slurred speech, ataxia, etc) may be apparent.

Functional Status

Unable to continue exercise or difficulty exercising in a hot environment
Persistent muscle cramps

Physical Evaluation Findings

Ataxia and coordination problems
Syncope

Ameliorating Improving a condition.

Heat exhaustion is a moderate illness characterized by the inability to sustain adequate cardiac output as a result of strenuous physical exercise and environmental heat stress. Inherent needs to maintain blood pressure and essential organ function, combined with a loss of fluid due to acute dehydration, create a challenge the body cannot sustain.[3,13] Intense exercise in the heat challenges the cardiovascular system to deliver enough blood to the working muscles so that exercise intensity can be maintained. Additionally, the body is working hard to keep itself cool, primarily by shunting heat via warm blood to the skin, where it is cooled by the atmosphere. Ultimately, a safe body temperature is maintained by evaporating sweat or by losing heat through a thermal gradient via convection and radiation. If the air temperature is extremely hot, the only means of losing heat may be through the evaporation of sweat. In some cases when the intensity of exercise and environmental conditions are extreme, the cardiovascular system cannot meet the demands of blood supply to the muscles and skin while also maintaining blood pressure.[14]

This situation can be exacerbated by dehydration and sodium loss from profuse sweating.[14] The consequence may be cardiovascular insufficiency and slowing or cessation of activity.[14]

Differential Diagnosis

Exertional heat stroke, exertional hyponatremia, heat syncope, postural hypotension, exercise-associated collapse[7,8]

Definitive Diagnosis

The most critical criteria are obvious difficulty continuing intense exercise in the heat, lack of severe hyperthermia (usually <104°F [40°C]), although mild hyperthermia is common (100° to 103°F [37.7° to 39.4°C]), and lack of severe CNS dysfunction. If any CNS dysfunctions (see those described for exertional heat stroke) are present, they are mild and subside quickly with treatment and rest.[3,7,8]

■ Immediate Management

The following procedures are recommended if heat exhaustion is suspected[3,7,8,15,16]:

- Remove the athlete from play and immediately move to a shaded or air-conditioned area.
- Remove excess clothing and equipment.
- Cool the athlete until rectal temperature is approximately 101°F (38.3°C).
- Have the athlete lie comfortably with the legs propped above heart level.
- If the athlete is not nauseated, vomiting, or experiencing CNS dysfunction, rehydrate orally with chilled water or a sports drink. If the athlete is unable to take oral fluids, start a normal saline IV.
- Monitor heart rate, blood pressure, respiratory rate, core temperature, and CNS status.
- Transport to an emergency facility if rapid improvement is not noted with the prescribed treatment.

■ Medications

An IV may be recommended if consciousness is altered or if the patient is nauseated or vomiting and dehydrated. Note that this is not necessarily the case for exertional hyponatremia; some of these patients require only sodium without rehydration.[8]

■ Postinjury Management

The athlete should work with the medical staff to optimize hydration, acclimatization, fitness level, and other possible contributing factors to reduce the likelihood of another episode.[7,8,17-21]

■ Injury-Specific Treatment and Rehabilitation Concerns

Specific Concerns

Maintain cardiovascular status.
Ensure adequate hydration.
Resolution of all symptoms

If the underlying cause of heat exhaustion was a lack of acclimatization or a poor fitness level (or both), correct the problem before the athlete returns to full-intensity training in heat (especially in sports with equipment).[3,7,8]

■ Estimated Amount of Time Lost

Avoid intense practice in heat until at least the next day to ensure recovery from fatigue and dehydration. In severe cases, intense practice in heat should be delayed for more than 1 day.[3]

■ Return-to-Play Criteria

Physician clearance or, at minimum, a discussion with the supervising physician is recommended before the athlete returns to intense exercise. Any underlying conditions that might predispose the patient to continued problems such as improper nutrition or a disease state must be ruled out.[3,7]

Exertional Heat Stroke

CLINICAL PRESENTATION

History

Recent history of intense exercise in a hot environment

Observation

The patient may be experiencing nausea, vomiting, or diarrhea (each further dehydrating the body).
The skin is hot and may be either wet or dry.

Functional Status

The patient is unable to function normally.
Cognitive impairments may hinder normal communication with the patient.

Physical Evaluation Findings

Rectal temperature greater than 104°F (40°C)
CNS dysfunction
Increased heart rate
Decreased blood pressure
Increased respiratory rate
Dehydration
Combativeness

During exercise (usually intense) in warm and hot environments (especially when humidity is high), body temperature increases can exceed the physiologic capacity to dissipate heat. If this increase is sustained, hyperthermia may result, and exertional heat stroke (EHS) can be the consequence. As thermoregulatory capacity is exceeded, body temperature rises, and extreme circulatory and metabolic stresses can produce tissue damage and severe physiologic dysfunction, leading to EHS and possible death. Exertional heat stroke is a leading killer of high school and collegiate athletes in the United States.[22-25]

Prevention and early identification of EHS are key to avoiding fatalities.[26] Incipient EHS can resemble less serious conditions, such as heat exhaustion or exercise-related collapse.[8,26] As such, the immediate medical evaluation must differentiate among these. Many cases of fatal EHS can be attributed to delayed recognition and treatment. The first hour (often termed the "golden hour") appears to be the critical period in which aggressive treatment can be lifesaving.[26]

Prompt assessment of the core body temperature and CNS function is critical to the appropriate evaluation of EHS. Axillary, oral, temporal artery, and tympanic (aural canal) temperatures are not valid measurements of core temperature for this purpose. The medical staff should be trained and equipped to assess core temperature via rectal thermometer or an ingestible thermistor (**Figure 20-2**).[3,26-30] If the measuring device can be kept in place while whole-body cooling is conducted (ie, a rectal thermistor),

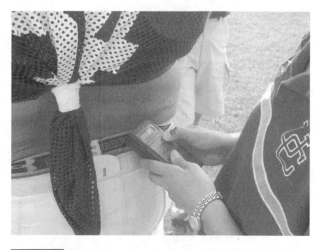

Figure 20-2 Core temperature using an ingestible thermistor. Before competition, the athlete swallows a capsule-sized thermistor. As the thermistor passes through the digestive tract, core temperature is transmitted via radio waves to a handheld unit that displays and records the information. The thermistor passes naturally through the digestive tract and is not reusable.

the point at which body cooling can be halted can be objectively determined. An additional benefit is that the continuous monitoring of core temperature allows for cooling to continue unimpeded (ie, the patient need not be removed from the bath to check body temperature).[26] If rectal temperature cannot be measured accurately, the medical staff should rely on CNS alterations to discriminate between heat exhaustion and EHS and not on potentially inaccurate oral, axillary, or tympanic measurements. Relying on an inaccurate temperature measurement may cause death if treatment is delayed as a result.[8,26]

If hyperthermia is untreated, physiologic changes will likely occur within vital organ systems (eg, muscle, heart, brain) and result in fatal consequences. Aggressive and immediate whole-body cooling is the key to optimizing treatment.[26]

Differential Diagnosis

Heat exhaustion, seizure, syncope, exercise-associated collapse, hyponatremia, postural hypotension[26]

Definitive Diagnosis

The most critical criteria for the definitive diagnosis of EHS are hyperthermia, usually defined as a rectal temperature greater than 104°F (40°C) immediately postincident, and CNS dysfunction, such as altered consciousness, coma, convulsions, disorientation, irrational behavior, decreased mental acuity, irritability, emotional instability, confusion, hysteria, or apathy.[3,4,7,8,26,31-34]

■ Immediate Management

If rapid on-site cooling is possible (ie, appropriate medical staff such as a certified and/or licensed athletic trainer [ATC] or physician is on-site and airway, breathing, and circulation [ABC] are stable), the patient should be cooled first and transported later. Immediate whole-body cooling (ice water immersion) is considered the best treatment for EHS and should be initiated within minutes after an incident (**Figure 20-3**). Increasing the rate of cooling minimizes the mortality rate because the likelihood of organ failure is directly correlated with the length and degree of hyperthermia. Anecdotal and textbook reports of full-body cold immersion therapy not being recommended for EHS due to the risk of inducing cardiovascular shock, peripheral vasoconstriction, or hypothermic overshoot are unfounded. Medical organizations that oversee the education of ATCs, emergency medical technicians, and physicians should ensure that curriculums teach ice water immersion for EHS and rectal temperature as-

20

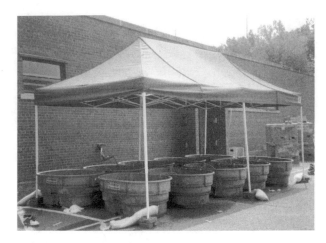

Figure 20-3 Full-body cooling station. These ice-filled and water-filled tubs, maintained in a shaded area, are used to immerse the athlete's body and rapidly lower the core temperature.

Heat capacity The quantity of heat required to raise the temperature of a unit of mass by a specific unit change in temperature. Thermal capacity.

sessment to provide the public they serve with optimal care.[3,26,35-43]

Immersion therapy produces the best cooling rates due to thermal conductivity and the volume-specific heat capacity of the water. The lower the temperature, the faster the cooling occurs.[41] If conditions allow, an immersion of 35°F (1.7°C) is recommended for the acute treatment of EHS. This may not be feasible to attain or maintain in hot conditions, in which case the immersion bath should simply be kept as cold as possible.

Cooling can be successfully verified by measuring rectal temperature. If on-site cooling is not an option, the patient must be immediately transported to the nearest medical facility.

The following procedures are recommended for the immediate treatment of a patient with EHS (assuming ABCs have been assessed and appropriate medical staff is on-site):

- Remove clothing and equipment.
- Immediately immerse the athlete in a tub of cold water in the range of 35° to 58°F (1.7° to 14.5°C).
- Constant monitoring of core temperature by rectal thermistor or thermometer is necessary during immersion therapy.

If immersion is not possible, alternative cooling strategies must be implemented. Immediately move the patient to a shaded area or air-conditioned facility. Cooling techniques such as cold water spraying, fans, ice bags, or ice over as much of the body as possible and cold towels (replaced frequently) must be used.

As the patient is being cooled, continue to monitor ABCs, core temperature, and CNS function (eg, cognition, convulsions, orientation, and conscious-

ness). Once the patient's core temperature reaches 101°F (38.3°C), cooling can be stopped, but the patient's vital signs, including core temperature, must continue to be monitored. Transport the patient to a medical facility for further evaluation.

■ Medications

Normal saline via IV may be given if medical staff is available.[8,26]

■ Postinjury Management

Physiologic changes can occur after an episode of EHS. For example, the athlete's heat tolerance may be temporarily or permanently compromised. A careful return-to-play strategy should be provided by the athlete's physician and implemented with the assistance of the ATC or other qualified health care professional.[3,7,8,26,44-47]

■ Injury-Specific Treatment and Rehabilitation Concerns

Specific Concerns

Rule out secondary injury to the body's organ systems.
Ensure adequate hydration.
Reacclimatize the athlete.

Physician clearance is required before returning to exercise. The athlete should avoid all exercise until completely asymptomatic and laboratory test results are normal. The athlete should cautiously begin a gradual return to physical activity to regain peak fitness and acclimatization under the supervision of the ATC and team physician. The type and length of exercise should be determined by the athlete's physician. The following is a suggested exercise pattern leading to the return to full activity:[3,26]

1. Easy to moderate exercise in a climate-controlled environment, followed by strenuous exercise in a climate-controlled environment.
2. Easy to moderate exercise in heat, followed by strenuous exercise in heat.
3. (If applicable) Easy to moderate exercise in heat with equipment, followed by strenuous exercise in heat with equipment. Ideally, core temperature should be monitored.

■ Estimated Amount of Time Lost

The severity of the incident dictates the length of recovery time. The patient should avoid exercise for at least 1 week after release from medical care.

A much longer time may be required in severe cases or in athletes with residual heat intolerance. See the rehabilitation concerns discussed previously.[3,26]

■ Return-to-Play Criteria

Physician clearance is required before the patient returns to activity. The patient should have no residual effects from the heat stroke, restoration of the body's thermoregulatory system, and adequate rehydration and nutrition.[3,26] The athlete must be reacclimatized to the environmental conditions. See the rehabilitation concerns discussed previously.

Exertional Hyponatremia

CLINICAL PRESENTATION

History

Overconsumption of fluids
Salty sweat
Inadequate sodium intake in the diet or during prolonged
    activity

Observation

Nausea, vomiting (often repeated)
Swelling of extremities (hands and feet)
CNS dysfunction
Respiratory distress

Functional Status

Lethargy
Increasing headache
Extreme fatigue
Apathy
Agitation

Physical Evaluation Findings

Urine has low specific gravity.
CNS dysfunction develops as the condition progresses.

When an athlete consumes more fluids (especially water) than necessary, sodium in the bloodstream can become diluted and result in exertional hyponatremia; ultimately, if the decrease in blood sodium is severe enough, complications such as cerebral and pulmonary edema can arise and prove fatal.[8] Exertional hyponatremia tends to occur during activities that extend for 4 hours or more in warm or hot weather.[48] Exertional hyponatremia becomes potentially serious when plasma sodium levels decrease to less than 130 mmol/L. The more pronounced the drop, the greater the risk of medical consequences.[3,8,48] Sodium lost through sweat and urine, coupled with inadequate sodium intake during lengthy events, can increase the rate at which hyponatremia develops.[3] Although excessive fluid intake is likely the most common cause of exertional hyponatremia, especially in marathon runners and athletes participating in shorter events, it can also occur in the absence of overhydration in athletes who do not adequately replace sodium (**Table 20-1**).[3,7,8,48-50] In fact, in long, hot races such as the Hawaii Ironman Triathlon, exertional hyponatremia can occur even in athletes who are also volume depleted (dehydrated). Athletes need adequate sodium in the diet before an event or long practice session. Also, ingesting fluids and foods that contain sodium during long-duration activities helps to replace lost sodium.[3] In certain circumstances, individuals who lose a great deal of sodium in sweat may need to specifically supplement sodium during the event by using Gatorlytes diluted in a sports drink or Pedialyte.

The possibility of developing hyponatremia is significantly reduced when fluid consumption during activity does not exceed fluid losses.[8] Because progressive dehydration can also compromise thermoregulatory function, athletes must be aware of their individual fluid needs to protect against both dehydration and overhydration.[3,5,8]

Table 20-1

Factors Leading to Exertional Hyponatremia

Factor*	Cause
Excessive fluid intake	More fluid is ingested than is lost through sweat and urine over a given period of time, resulting in hyperhydration and decreased blood sodium levels.
Sodium intake/output imbalance (eg, high sweat sodium levels, low sodium levels in fluids and foods)	Sodium lost in sweat during lengthy exercise sessions, especially in athletes with salty sweat
	Low sodium levels in diet leading up to event, low sodium levels in fluids and foods during event

*Note: The combination of these two conditions exacerbates the patient's condition.

Fluid needs can be determined by establishing an athlete's sweat rate (L/h) during a given intensity of activity, while wearing a given amount of clothing and equipment, for a given set of environmental conditions.[5] Variations can exist in sweat rates, so individual assessments can be helpful.[5] When fluid needs are being established, it is best to mimic the conditions of the athletic event to establish an accurate sweat rate[5] (see Developing an Individualized Hydration Protocol, p 606).

Although significant attention has been devoted to the need to rehydrate athletes, caution must also be taken to prevent overhydrating athletes. Several deaths have occurred from exertional hyponatremia.[22]

Differential Diagnosis

Heat stroke, heat exhaustion, postural hypotension, heat syncope, exercise-associated collapse[8,48]

Definitive Diagnosis

Urine with low specific gravity is produced during the event and tends to appear after activity—for example, in the medical tent. In fact, high levels of antidiuretic hormone with minimal urine production seem to be a contributing factor in some cases. If the condition progresses, CNS changes (eg, altered consciousness, confusion, coma, convulsions, altered cognitive functioning) and respiratory changes result from cerebral and pulmonary edema, respectively.

Exertional hyponatremia is more likely to occur during physical activity that lasts for longer than 4 hours, providing enough time for the athlete to consume fluids and lose large amounts of fluids through sweating. This condition may also be more likely to develop during lower-intensity endurance exercises when the athlete has extra opportunity to consume a large volume of fluid.[3,7,8,48,49]

The most critical criteria for determination of exertional hyponatremia include the following:[3,8]

- The absence of severe hyperthermia (temperature most commonly <104°F [40°C])
- Low blood sodium levels (<130 mmol/L); the severity of the condition increases as sodium levels decrease.
- The likelihood of excessive fluid consumption before, during, and after exercise (weight gain during activity)
- Low sodium intake
- Indications of sodium deficits before, during, and after exercise
- Progressively worsening headache

Immediate Management

The possibility of hyperthermia (heat stroke or heat exhaustion) must be ruled out. If either condition is present, treat the patient appropriately.[3,7,8,48]

Symptoms that complicate the diagnosis are feeling dizzy or weak and collapsing. When this occurs after the athlete has stopped competition, rather than during competition, the likely cause is postural hypotension, a pooling of blood in the legs and inadequate blood supply to the upper body.[13] This can be avoided by walking or flexing the legs when standing in place. When an athlete collapses from postural hypotension, the legs should be raised above the head and held there for 3 to 4 minutes to relieve symptoms.[8]

The following procedures are recommended if exertional hyponatremia is suspected:

- If blood sodium levels cannot be determined on-site, delay rehydrating the patient (which may worsen the condition) and transport immediately to a medical facility.
- The administration of sodium, certain diuretics, or IV solutions may be necessary. Administration is monitored by the physician on-site or in the emergency department to ensure no complications develop.

Medications

An IV of a hypertonic sodium replacement, diuretic (if hyperhydrated), and/or anticonvulsive drug (if the patient has seizures) may be administered by a physician on-site or in the hospital.[8]

Postinjury

Physician clearance is strongly recommended for all patients and required for patients who were hospitalized.[3,7,8]

Estimated Amount of Time Lost

In minor cases, activity can resume a few days after the athlete completes an educational session on establishing an individual hydration protocol (see p 607). This will ensure that the proper amounts and types of beverages and meals are consumed before, during, and after physical activity.[3,7]

Return-to-Play Criteria

In minor cases, participation can resume in a few days, assuming actions have been taken to modify fluid intake and sodium ingestion. In extreme cases in which system damage occurred, the physician must dictate an appropriate and gradual return to participation when the recovery is complete.[3,7]

Hydration Needs for Athletes

Proper hydration influences the quality of athletic performance. The evaporation of sweat from the skin's surface is a powerful cooling mechanism that releases the heat being produced by the working muscles. Replenishing the body's fluids is an important consideration in any type of physical exertion. Athletes have sometimes been told to consume "as much fluid as possible" to ward off the dangers of dehydration. More recently, athletes and medical staff have been told to limit hydration due to the potential dangers associated with overhydrating.

Not drinking enough during activity and thus inducing dehydration can impair performance and health. Yet overdrinking (beyond what is lost) can cause exertional hyponatremia (see p 603).

How does the competitive athlete balance the risks of dehydration and hyponatremia? The answer lies in individualizing fluid needs and tailoring a hydration plan. This is a simple process that can maximize performance and minimize risks. The following is an overview of dehydration, with guidelines to determine an individual's fluid needs.

Dehydration

Dehydration is the acute change in fluid stores from a steady-state condition of normal body water to something less than normal body water.[14] Dehydration is caused by two distinct factors that may occur during exercise (**Table 20-2**): (1) the loss of fluids by sweating, urinating, and respiration, and (2) fluid intake that is less than fluid losses.[1-6,9,11,48,51-61]

If the body remains in a state of decreased body water stores for an extended period of time, the individual is said to be hypohydrated, a steady-state condition of decreased body water.[14] Because the human body is approximately 65% water, a signif-

Table 20-2

Factors Leading to Dehydration [1-6,9,11,48,51-61]

Condition	Effect
During moderate and intense activity	Sweat rate increases proportionally to the intensity of the activity.
	At high-intensity levels (eg, >75% $\dot{V}_{O_{2max}}$), the rate at which fluid can be processed by the stomach and intestines and emptied into the bloodstream is decreased.
	Increasing intensity likely decreases the amount of time the individual can focus on rehydration.
During activity in warm and hot conditions	As the temperature increases, the sweat rate increases.
Individuals with high sweat rates	The need to consistently replenish fluids.
Inadequately hydrated at the start of exertion	Dangerous levels of dehydration can be reached more rapidly.
Multiple practices the same day	As the number of daily exercise sessions increases, the amount of fluid needed during the course of the day increases.
Improper eating	Most fluid consumption occurs during meal times, so a disturbance in normal meals may alter the ability to maintain proper hydration.
Inadequate access to fluids	Significantly increased risk of dehydration.
Poor vigilance	Athletes do not follow, or are unaware of, directions for proper hydration before, during, and after exercise.
Somatotype	A person's size influences the sweat rate: larger individuals generally have a higher sweat rate than smaller individuals.
Characteristics of the rehydration fluid	If the temperature of the rehydration fluid is too hot or cold, if it is made of nonideal compounds, or if the person dislikes the flavor, the degree of voluntary rehydration may be altered.
Individual fluid tolerance	Some individuals cannot comfortably handle the amounts of fluid needed to approximate fluid losses during activity; one solution may be to gradually drink small amounts of fluids over time rather than larger amounts of fluid in a shorter timeframe.
	Athletes may be able to alter the amount when the hydration protocol is practiced during training sessions.

20

icant decrease in body water stores alters normal physiologic function. For example, cardiovascular function (heart rate), thermoregulatory capacity (sweating), and muscle function (endurance capacity) can be impaired if dehydration reaches critical thresholds, altering the physiologic function of these processes.[14]

When fluid consumption is less than fluid losses, dehydration occurs. Fluid can be lost in sweat, urine, and feces and during respiration. During exercise, most fluid loss is in the form of sweat. Fluid losses can be replaced by fluids consumed orally or by IV and those produced during metabolism (a small amount of water is formed by the metabolic pathways that allow muscles to contract). Most fluid intake occurs from the oral consumption of fluids or fluids in food products. Generally speaking, during exercise, when sweat losses exceed fluid intake via oral consumption, dehydration occurs. Mild dehydration, about 1% to 2% of total body weight, is likely to occur and is not a great concern, but losses beyond this point should be avoided if possible.[5]

Recognizing Dehydration

Although dehydration is an important factor that contributes to hyperthermia associated with exercise, other factors also contribute. For example, intensity of activity, environmental conditions (humidity, temperature, shade or cloud cover), level of fitness, degree of heat acclimatization, amount of clothing and equipment worn, and illness all contribute to the rate of rise in body temperature. Athletes should consider these factors when trying to decrease the risk associated with exercise in warm and hot conditions.[3,5,7,8]

Athletes, coaches, and the medical staff must be adept at recognizing and treating hyperthermia. If it is mild, the runner needs to slow down or stop, depending on the symptoms. If the symptoms are more severe, an immediate effort must be made to reduce core body temperature. Athletes should be able to recognize the basic signs and symptoms of heat illness, for which dehydration may be a cause—irritability and general discomfort, headache, weakness, dizziness, cramps, chills, vomiting, nausea, head or neck heat sensations, disorientation, and decreased performance.

Treating Dehydration

A dehydrated athlete should be moved to a cooler environment (indoor air conditioning, shaded area, etc), if possible, and appropriately rehydrated. A conscious, cognizant, dehydrated athlete with-

out gastrointestinal distress can aggressively rehydrate orally. Patients who are experiencing mental deterioration from dehydration or gastrointestinal distress should be transported to a medical facility for IV rehydration. If an exertional heat illness beyond dehydration is suspected, medical treatment is necessary. Additionally, dehydration itself, if severe, may require medical assistance.[5]

An athlete with CNS dysfunction or who is nauseated or vomiting may have EHS or hyponatremia and should be treated or transported for immediate medical attention and laboratory evaluation. If an athlete's weight loss is greater than 2% within a given day or on consecutive days, the athlete should return to normal hydration status before being allowed to practice.[3,5]

If the degree of dehydration is minor and the athlete is symptom free, continued participation is acceptable. The athlete must maintain adequate hydration status and should receive periodic checks from on-site medical personnel.[3,5]

▓ Developing an Individualized Hydration Protocol

Optimum hydration is based on the premise that fluid intake should approximately match fluid losses. When these processes are synchronized, the hazards of underhydrating or overhydrating are reduced, and the likelihood of a safe and productive exercise session is enhanced.[5]

Determining Sweat Rates

Hydration strategies must take into account the sweat rate, sport dynamics (eg, rest breaks, fluid access), environmental factors, acclimatization state, exercise duration, exercise intensity, and individual preferences. To assess an individual's rehydration needs, the individual's sweat rate must be determined using the following calculation[5]:

Sweat rate = body weight prepractice − body weight postpractice + fluid intake − urine volume/exercise time (h)

The most valuable measurements are those obtained during a representative range of environmental conditions, practices, and competitions.[5] **Table 20-3** presents a sample worksheet for calculating sweat rates.

Sweat rate calculation is the most fundamental consideration when establishing a hydration protocol. Average sweat rates from the scientific literature or other athletes can vary from 0.5 L/h to more than 2.5 L/h (1.1 lb/h to 5.5 lb/h) and are insuffi-

Table 20-3

Sample Sweat Rate Calculations

A	B	C	D	E	F	G	H	I	J
		Body Weight							
		Before Exercise	**After Exercise**				**Sweat Loss**	**Exercise Time**	**Sweat Rate (H/I)**
Name	**Date**			**ΔBW (C−D)**	**Drink Volume**	**Urine Volume†**	**(E + F − G)**		
		kg (lb/2.2)	kg (lb/2.2)	g (kg × 1000)	g (oz × 30)	mL (oz × 30)	mL (oz × 30)	min h	mL/min mL/h
		kg (lb/2.2)	kg (lb/2.2)	g (kg × 1000)	g (oz × 30)	mL (oz × 30)	mL (oz × 30)	min h	mL/min mL/h
		kg (lb/2.2)	kg (lb/2.2)	g (kg × 1000)	g (oz × 30)	mL (oz × 30)	mL (oz × 30)	min h	mL/min mL/h
		kg (lb/2.2)	kg (lb/2.2)	g (kg × 1000)	g (oz × 30)	mL (oz × 30)	mL (oz × 30)	min h	mL/min mL/h
Kelly K.†	9/15	61.7 kg (lb/2.2)	60.3 kg (lb/2.2)	1400 g (kg × 1000)	420 mL (oz × 30)	90 mL (oz × 30)	1730 mL (oz × 30)	90 min 1.5 h	19 mL/min 1153 mL/h

Reprinted with permission from Murray R: Determining sweat rate. *Sports Sci Exch.* 1996;9(Suppl 63).

†Weight of urine should be subtracted *if urine was excreted prior to postexercise body weight.*

‡In the example, Kelly K. should drink about 1 L (32 oz) of fluid during each hour of activity to remain well hydrated.

ciently accurate to create individual hydration plans.[5]

When calculating an individual's sweat rate for application during competition, have the athlete practice at a similar intensity in a 1-hour training session in climatic conditions that are similar to the expected conditions.[5] The following procedure is recommended to determine the sweat rate[5]:

- Perform a warm up until perspiration is generated.
- Urinate if necessary.
- Disrobe and weigh on an accurate scale.
- Conduct practice for 1 hour at an intensity similar to that of the targeted competition.
- Drink a measured amount of a beverage of choice during the practice.
- Do not urinate during the practice (unless the amount of urine is measured).
- Disrobe and weigh again on the same scale after the practice.
- Enter the data into Table 20-3.

Metabolism of carbohydrates, fats, and protein during exercise accounts for a small amount of the weight lost during activity, so weight changes after an activity can largely be attributed to sweat losses, and, thus, the previously described calculation of fluid needs is a viable option.

When sweat rate is not known or measurement is not feasible, the easiest way to monitor and enhance behavior is to weigh athletes before and af-ter practice. Athletes who lose weight during the practice should be encouraged to drink more during the next practice. Conversely, if they gain weight during the practice, encourage them to drink less during the next practice.[3,62]

Heat acclimatization produces dramatic physiologic changes that enhance an athlete's ability to tolerate exercise in the heat, but it may alter individual fluid-replacement considerations (**Table 20-4**).[4] Sweat rate generally increases after 10 to 14 days of heat exposure, requiring a greater fluid intake for a similar bout of exercise. An athlete's sweat rate should be reassessed after acclimatization.[5] Also, moving from a cool environment to a warmer one increases the overall sweat rate during exercise (independent of the sweat changes associated with heat acclimatization). Athletes must closely monitor their hydration status for the first week of exercise in a warm environment. Increased sodium intake is recommended during the first 3 to 5 days of heat exposure, because the increased thermal strain and sweat rate increase the sodium lost in sweat. Adequate sodium intake optimizes fluid palatability and absorption during the first few days and may decrease exercise-associated muscle cramping. After 5 to 10 days, sweat sodium concentration decreases, but the overall sweat rate is higher, so the athlete should still be conscientious about sodium ingestion.[5]

Fluid replacement beverages should be easily accessible in individual fluid containers and fla-

20

Table 20-4

Strategies for a Successful Heat Acclimatization Program

1. Attain adequate fitness in cool environments before attempting to heat acclimatize.

2. Exercise at intensities (>50% $\dot{V}_{O_{2max}}$) and gradually increase the duration (up to 90 min/d) and intensity of the exercise sessions during the first 2 weeks.

3. Initially, perform the highest intensity workouts during the cooler morning or evening hours and other training during the hottest time of the day. After about 10 to 14 days of exercise in the heat, most of the benefits of acclimatization have occurred, and some of the intense exercise should now take place during the hotter times of the day.

4. Monitor body weight to ensure that proper hydration is maintained as sweat rate increases.

5. When necessary, monitor rectal temperature so that body temperature stays within safe limits.

6. Athletes who live in a cool environment but will travel to a hot environment for competition can induce partial acclimatization by wearing insulated clothing, although they should leave some skin surface uncovered and monitor rectal temperature to avoid hyperthermia. Additionally, if the athlete can arrive 3 to 5 days before competition in a hot environment, many of the benefits of acclimatization can be attained.

7. Be sure to have ample sodium in the diet and rehydration beverages in the initial week of practices in a hot environment because sweat sodium losses are greater than before training commenced or while training in a cooler environment. Extra sodium also ensures optimal expansion of plasma volume, a cardinal component of acclimatization.

Adapted with permission from Casa DJ: Exercise in the heat: II. Critical concepts in rehydration, exertional heat illness, and maximizing athletic performance. *J Athl Train* 1999;34:253-262.

vored to the athlete's preference. Individual containers permit easier monitoring of fluid intake.[5] Clear water bottles marked in 100-mL (3.4-oz) increments provide visual reminders to help athletes gauge proper amounts.[5] Carrying water bottles or other hydration systems during activity when ac-

cess to fluid is limited encourages greater fluid volume ingestion.[5]

Athletes should begin exercise sessions well hydrated. Hydration status can be monitored by athletes in several ways. Assuming proper hydration, preexercise body weight should be relatively consistent across exercise sessions. However, body weight is dynamic. Frequent exercise sessions can induce non–fluid-related weight loss influenced by timing of meals and defecation, time of day, and calories expended in exercise.[3,5]

■ Identifying the Level of Hydration or Dehydration

The simplest way to assess hydration status is by comparing urine color (from a sample in a container) to a urine color chart. A urine color of 1 to 3 indicates sufficient hydration, whereas 6 to 8 indicates some degree of dehydration.[3,5,63-65] Urine volume is another general indicator of hydration status. An athlete should need to urinate frequently during the course of the day. Remember that body weight changes during exercise give the best indication of hydration needs.[5] A more objective way to assess hydration status than urine color is with urine-specific gravity. **Table 20-5** indicates how urine-specific gravity correlates with hydration status. If the athlete's hydration status is unclear at the time of the baseline body weight before a practice (especially in at-risk individuals), it would be wise to also assess urine-specific gravity at that time to ensure this weight reflects a hydrated condition. If not, the athlete should be hydrated before practice and a new baseline body weight obtained, or at the least, the athlete should be monitored (if minimally dehydrated) more closely.[3,5]

To ensure proper preexercise hydration, the athlete should consume approximately 500 to 600 mL (17 to 20 oz) of water or a sports drink 2 to 3 hours before exercise and 200 to 300 mL (7 to 10 oz) of water or a sports drink 10 to 20 minutes

Table 20-5

Indices of Hydration Status

	% of Body Weight Change*	Urine Color	Urine-Specific Gravity
Well hydrated	+1 – −1	1, 2, or 3	<1.020
Minimal dehydration	−1 – −3	4 or 5	1.020–1.024
Significant dehydration	−3 – −5	5 or 6	1.025–1.029
Serious dehydration	>5	6, 7, or 8	>1.030

*% Body weight change = $\dfrac{\text{Preexercise body weight} - \text{postexercise body weight} \times 100}{\text{Preexercise body weight}}$

Note that a seriously dehydrated athlete may not be able to provide a urine sample.

Also, these entities are physiologically independent, and the numbers provided are only general guidelines.

Adapted with permission from Casa DJ, Armstrong LE, Hillman SK, et al: National Athletic Trainers' Association position statement: Fluid replacement for athletes. *J Athl Train* 2000;35:212-224.

before exercise.[5] These preexercise amounts should be less if the individual has a small frame and low body mass (ie, a female marathon runner). Fluid temperature influences the amount consumed. Although individual preferences exist, a cool beverage at 10° to 15°C (50° to 59°F) is recommended.[5]

Postexercise hydration should aim to correct any fluid loss occurring during the practice or event and encourage the rapid restoration of physiologic function. Ideally, the rehydration process should be completed within 2 hours if another exercise session is planned for the day. If not, the athlete can freely rehydrate through the course of the day. Rehydration should contain water to improve the hydration status, carbohydrates to replenish glycogen stores, and electrolytes to speed rehydration. Additionally, a small amount of protein post exercise in the rehydration beverage can enhance muscle recovery.[66] When rehydration must be rapid, the athlete should compensate for obligatory urine losses incurred during the rehydration process and drink about 25% to 50% more than sweat losses to ensure optimal hydration 4 to 6 hours after the event (see Table 20-5).[3,5] When the rehydration must occur during a brief period between two exercise sessions (ie, between events, halftime), it is critical to educate athletes that full rehydration may not be possible given the time constraints and gastrointestinal intolerance for large quantities of fluids. In these circumstances, partial rehydration is absolutely necessary. Rehydrating only 50% of the fluid deficit during a 20-minute period provides a number of performance and physiologic advantages during the next exercise session.[67] The goal, therefore, to begin the next exercise session properly hydrated may not be feasible, but drinking the maximal tolerable amount (never to exceed fluid losses) in a process of partial rehydration can still be an effective hydration strategy.

Sports Drinks

In many situations, athletes benefit from including carbohydrates (CHOs) and electrolytes (ie, sodium and potassium) in their rehydration drinks. Rehydration fluids should contain CHOs if the exercise session lasts more than 45 to 50 minutes or is intense. An ingestion rate of approximately 1 g/min (0.04 oz/min) maintains optimal carbohydrate metabolism (eg, 1 L of a 6% carbohydrate drink per hour of exercise, less for those who have sweat rates less than 1 L per hour).[5] Carbohydrate concentrations greater than 8% increase the rate of CHO delivery to the body but compromise the rate of fluid emptying from the stomach and absorption from the intestine. Fruit juices, CHO gels, sodas, and some sports drinks have CHO con-

centrations greater than the 8% threshold and are not recommended as the sole source of fluids during an exercise session.[5] Athletes should consume CHOs at least 30 minutes before the normal onset of fatigue and earlier if the environmental conditions are unusually extreme, although this may not apply for very intense, short-term exercise, which may require earlier intake of CHOs.[5] Most CHO forms (ie, glucose, sucrose, maltodextrins) are suitable, and the absorption rate is maximized when multiple forms are consumed simultaneously. Substances to be limited include fructose (which may cause gastrointestinal distress), and substances to be avoided include alcohol, very high amounts of caffeine (which may increase urine output and reduce fluid retention), and carbonated beverages (which may decrease voluntary fluid intake due to stomach fullness).[5]

A modest amount of sodium (0.5 to 0.7 g/L) is an acceptable addition to all hydration beverages because salt stimulates thirst, increases voluntary fluid intake, may decrease the risk of hyponatremia, and causes no harm.[5] Additional sodium should be added to the athlete's fluid intake when there is a history of poor nutrition (meals not eaten) or heat cramps, the duration of physical activity exceeds 4 hours, and the activity occurs in notably hot weather. Under these conditions, adding modest amounts of sodium (0.5 to 0.7 g/L) can offset sodium lost in sweat and minimize the physiologic events associated with electrolyte imbalances (eg, muscle cramps, hyponatremia).[5]

Strategies for Preventing Exertional Heat Illnesses

Each athletic organization should establish an emergency plan related to exertional heat illnesses. A thorough plan includes steps to reduce the risk of heat illness, identify the signs and symptoms of the early stages of exertional heat illnesses, and describe the immediate care protocol should these conditions arise.

Some factors leading to the onset of heat illness, such as fitness level, can be optimized to reduce the individual's predisposition to these conditions. Other factors, however, such as intrinsic metabolic disorders, cannot (**Table 20-6**).[1,3,4,7,8,13,26,52,63,68-86] The medical staff must educate coaches, athletes, and parents regarding the basic signs and symptoms of the exertional heat illnesses, so problems can be identified and referred to the team's ATC as soon as possible.[3,5,7]

Medical personnel can predict when complications will arise while athletes exercise in hot environments. The rate of core temperature in-

Table 20-6

Intrinsic and Extrinsic Factors Predisposing Heat Illness

Intrinsic Factors	Extrinsic Factors
History of exertional heat illnesses	Intense or prolonged exercise (several hours) with minimal breaks
Inadequate heat acclimatization	Limited access to fluids before and during practice and rest breaks
Lower level of fitness status	High ambient temperature, humidity, and/or sun exposure
High percentage of body fat	Recent exposure to heat and humidity
Dehydration	High wet bulb globe temperature
Overhydration	Inappropriate clothing and/or equipment for climatic conditions (ie, amount of football gear can be minimized during initial days when practices occur twice a day)
Fever	
Gastrointestinal illness	
Salt deficiency	Inappropriate work/rest ratios based on exercise intensity
Inadequate meals or insufficient calorie intake	No shaded areas to escape environmental conditions
Skin condition (eg, sunburn, rash)	Lack of education and awareness of heat illnesses among coaches, athletes, and medical staff
Certain medications (eg, antihistamines, diuretics)	
Dietary supplements (eg, ephedra)	No emergency plan to identify and treat exertional heat illnesses
Motivation to push oneself: "warrior mentality"	A delay in recognition of early warning signs
Reluctance to report problems, issues, or illness	
Prepubescence	

Table 20-7

Critical Factors Influencing Core Temperature Increase (Key Factors to Consider when Attempting to Reduce Risk of Exertional Heat Illness)

Factor	Modification in Hot/Humid Environment
Intensity of exercise	Decrease intensity of exercise
	Decrease work/rest ratio
Heat acclimatization status and fitness level (see Table 20-5)	Institute a fitness/acclimatization program before the start of formal practices
	Exclude from participating in 2-a-day practices those who have not attained an adequate level of fitness and/or acclimatization
Hydration status	Monitor hydration status before, during, and after activity
Amount of equipment and clothing	Wear less equipment or clothing, especially during initial days of exercise in the heat
Wet bulb globe temperature (especially level of humidity)	Exercise during times of day when wet bulb globe temperature is lower or at least have shade during rest breaks

crease is influenced by several factors (**Table 20-7**).[1,3,5,7,8,13,26,58,63,66,68,73,79,80,81,83,87-92] Prevention is best augmented by the early identification of heat-related problems. Headaches, dizziness, and nausea, for example, are not normal responses to exercise in the heat and may provide early warnings of a problem. Athletes should be encouraged to report any abnormal symptoms early to coaches and the medical staff.

Individual athletes may have predispositions to heat illness. Awareness allows closer monitoring of the athlete's status. For example, athletes who are overweight, not acclimatized, ill, lacking sleep or rest, or "overmotivated" and those with extremely high sweat rates may be at increased risk and require more attention on the part of the medical staff (**Table 20-8**).[3,7,8,48]

Table 20-8

Preventing Heat-Related Illness and Exertional Hyponatremia

Provide education and implement rehydration strategies that ensure athletes drink based on fluid losses and do not exceed the fluids lost in sweat and urine.

Encourage athletes to be well acclimatized to the heat, because this is an effective way to decrease sweat sodium losses.

Encourage athletes to maintain normal meal patterns and do not restrict dietary sodium intake, so sodium levels are normal before the event starts.

Encourage athletes to consume a little extra sodium with meals and snacks during continuous days of exercise in hot weather to help maintain blood sodium levels.

The wet bulb globe temperature is a good measure of the environmental risks during exercise (**Figure 20-4**). **Table 20-9** shows a conservative approach that may be appropriate for athletes who are not accustomed to extreme heat (ie, those who live in the northern climates of the United States).[93] **Table 20-10** shows a slightly more liberal approach, which may be more appropriate for athletes who are accustomed to living and exercising in hot environments.[94]

If the medical staff does not have access to a wet bulb globe thermometer, another option for determining practice schedules is the use of heat and humidity measures, which can be ascertained with a simple sling psychrometer (**Figure 20-5**). EHS risk rises with increasing heat and relative humidity.

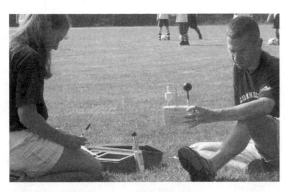

Figure 20-4 Recording the wet bulb globe temperature (WBGT). The WBGT produces an index based on the air temperature, relative humidity, and radiant heat. WBGT measurements should be recorded before practice or competition and repeated at regular intervals during the activity.

Table 20-9

Wet Bulb Globe Temperature (WGBT) Risk Chart

WBGT	Flag Color	Level of Risk	Comments
<18°C (<65°F)	Green	Low	Risk is low but still exists
18°C–23°C (65°F–73°F)	Yellow	Moderate	Risk level increases as event progresses through the day
23°C–28°C (73°F–82°F)	Red	High	Everyone should be aware of injury potential; individuals at risk should not compete
>28°C (>82°F)	Black	Extreme or hazardous	Consider rescheduling or delaying the event until conditions are safer; if the event must take place, be on high alert. Take steps to reduce risk factors (eg, more and longer rest breaks, reduced practice time, reduced exercise intensity, access to shade, minimal clothing and equipment, and cold tubs at practice site).

Adapted with permission from Roberts WO: Medical management and administration manual for long distance road racing, in Brown CH, Gudjonsson B (eds): *IAAF Medical Manual for Athletics and Road Racing Competitions: A Practice Guide*. Monaco, International Amateur Athletic Federation Publications, 1998, pp 39-75.

Table 20-10

Activity Restrictions for Outdoor Physical Conditioning in Hot Weather

WBGT* (°F)	Flag Color	Guidance for nonacclimatized personnel in boldface *Guidance for fully acclimatized personnel in italics*
<78.0°F	No flag	**Extreme exertion may precipitate heat illness** *Normal activity*
78.1°F-82.0°F	Green	**Use discretion in planning intense exercise** *Normal activity* Pay special attention to at-risk individuals in both cases.
82.1°F-86.0°F	Yellow	**Limit intense exercise to 1 hour, limit total outdoor exercise to 2.5 hours** *Use discretion in planning intense physical activity* Pay special attention to at-risk individuals in both cases. Be on high alert: watch for early signs and symptoms in both cases.
86.1°F-89.9°F	Red	**Stop outdoor practice sessions and outdoor physical conditioning** *Limit intense exercise to 1 hour, limit total outdoor exercise to 4 hours (Be on high alert: watch for early signs and symptoms throughout)*
≥90°F	Black	**Cancel all outdoor exercise requiring physical exertion** *Cancel all outdoor exercise involving physical exertion*

WGBT indicates wet bulb globe temperature.
*Calculation of WBGT: 0.7 Twb + 0.2 Tbg + 0.1 Tdb, where Twb indicates wet bulb temperature; Tbg, black globe temperature; and Tdb, dry bulb temperature.
Guidelines assume that personnel are wearing summer-weight clothing; all activities require constant supervision (ie, via athletic trainer) to ensure early detection of problems. When equipment must be worn, as in football, please use guidelines for one flag color level below. Example: If WBGT is 86° F (yellow), use the guidelines for red.
Adapted from Nunnelly SA, Reardon MJ: Prevention of Heat Illness, in Pandolf KB, Burr RE (eds): *Medical Aspects of Harsh Environments, vol 1*. Washington DC, Borden Institute, Office of The Surgeon General, US Army 2002, p 223.

20

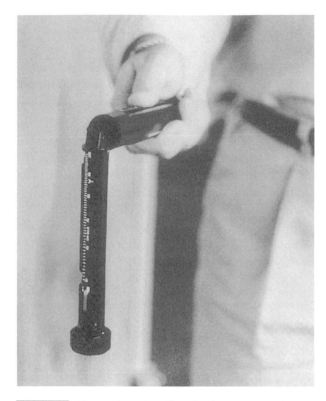

Figure 20-5 Sling psychrometer. Although not as comprehensive as a wet bulb globe temperature, a sling psychrometer can be used to measure the ambient conditions.

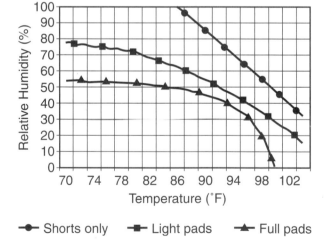

Figure 20-6 Heat stress risk temperature and humidity graph.[95] Conditions that plot between squares and circles: use work/rest ratio with 15 to 20 minutes of activity followed by 5- to 10-minute rest and fluid breaks; practice should be in shorts only (with all protective equipment removed, if used for activity).

Conditions that plot between triangles and squares: use work/rest ratio with 20 to 25 minutes of activity followed by 5- to 10-minute rest and fluid breaks; practice should be in shorts (with helmets and shoulder pads only, not full equipment if used for activity).

Conditions that plot beneath triangles: use work/rest ratio with 25 to 30 minutes of activity followed by 5- to 10-minute rest and fluid breaks.

Fluid breaks should be scheduled for all practices and more frequently as the heat stress rises. With reference to **Figure 20-6**, add 5° to the temperature between 10 AM and 4 PM from mid May to mid September on bright, sunny days. Practices should be modified to reflect heat stress conditions. Regular practices with full practice gear can be conducted for conditions that plot to the left of the triangles. Cancel all practices when the temperature and relative humidity plot to the right of the circles; practices can be moved into air-conditioned spaces or held as walk-through sessions with no conditioning activities.

■ References

1. Bergeron MF: Exertional heat cramps, in Armstrong LE (ed): *Exertional Heat Illnesses*. Champaign, IL, Human Kinetics, 2003, pp 91-102, 230-234.

2. Bergeron MF: Heat cramps during tennis: A case report. *Int J Sport Nutr* 1996;6:62-68.

3. Casa DJ, Almquist J, Anderson S, et al: Inter-association task force on exertional heat illnesses consensus statement. *NATA NEWS* June 2003;24-29.

4. Casa DJ: Exercise in the heat: II. Critical concepts in rehydration, exertional heat illnesses, and maximizing athletic performance. *J Athl Train* 1999;34:253-262.

5. Casa DJ, Armstrong LE, Hillman SK, et al: National Athletic Trainers' Association position statement: Fluid replacement for athletes. *J Athl Train* 2000;35:212-224.

6. Convertino VA, Armstrong LE, Coyle EF, et al: American College of Sports Medicine position stand: Exercise and fluid replacement. *Med Sci Sports Exerc* 1996;28:i-vii.

7. Binkley HM, Beckett J, Casa DJ, Kleiner DM, Plummer PE: National Athletic Trainers' Association position statement: Exertional heat illnesses. *J Athl Train* 2002;37:329-343.

8. Casa DJ, Roberts WO: Considerations for the medical staff: Preventing, identifying and treating exertional heat illnesses, in Armstrong LE (ed): *Exertional Heat Illnesses*. Champaign, IL, Human Kinetics, 2003, pp 169-196, 255-259.

9. Armstrong LE, Epstein Y: Fluid-electrolyte balance during labor and exercise: Concepts and misconceptions. *Int J Sport Nutr* 1999;9:1-12.

10. Gisolfi CV: Fluid balance for optimal performance. *Nutr Rev* 1996;54(4 Pt 2):S159-S168.

11. Maughan RJ: Optimizing hydration for competitive sport, in Lamb DR, Murray R (eds): *Optimizing Sport Performance*. Carmel, IN, Cooper Publishing, 1997, pp 139-183.

12. Murray R: Fluid needs in hot and cold environments. *Int J Sports Nutr* 1995;5(suppl):S62-S73.

13. Armstrong LE, Anderson JM: Heat exhaustion, exercise-associated collapse, and heat syncope, in Armstrong LE (ed): *Exertional Heat Illnesses*. Champaign, IL, Human Kinetics, 2003, pp 57-90, 234-241.

14. Casa DJ: Exercise in the heat: I. Fundamentals of thermal physiology, performance implications, and dehydration. *J Athl Train* 1999;34:246-252.

15. Armstrong LE, Epstein Y, Greenleaf JE, et al: American College of Sports Medicine position stand: Heat and cold illnesses during distance running. *Med Sci Sports Exerc* 1996;28:i-x.

16. Armstrong LE, Hubbard RW, Kraemer WJ, DeLuca JP, Christensen EL: Signs and symptoms of heat exhaustion during strenuous exercise. *Ann Sports Med* 1987; 3:182-189.

17. Armstrong LE, Maresh CM: The induction and decay of heat acclimatisation in trained athletes. *Sports Med* 1991;12:302-312.

18. Gisolfi C, Robinson S: Relations between physical training, acclimatization, and heat tolerance. *J Appl Physiol* 1969;26:530-534.

19. Kenney WL: Physiological correlates of heat intolerance. *Sports Med* 1985;2:279-286.

20. Mitchell D, Senay LC, Wyndham CH, van Rensburg AJ, Rogers GG, Strydom NB: Acclimatization in a hot, humid environment: Energy exchange, body temperature, and sweating. *J Appl Physiol* 1976;40:768-778.

21. Piwonka RW, Robinson S, Gay VL, Manalis RS: Preacclimatization of men to heat by training. *J Appl Physiol* 1965;20:379-384.

22. Armstrong LE: Classification, nomenclature, and incidence of the exertional heat illnesses, in Armstrong LE (ed): *Exertional Heat Illnesses*. Champaign, IL, Human Kinetics, 2003, pp 17-28, 227-230.

23. Bijur PE, Trumble A, Harel Y, Overpeck MD, Jones D, Scheidt PC: Sports and recreation injuries in US children and adolescents. *Arch Pediatr Adolesc Med* 1995;149:1009-1016.

24. Hawley DA, Slentz K, Clark MA, Pless JE, Waller BF: Athletic fatalities. *Am J Forensic Med Pathol* 1990;11:124-129.

25. Mueller FO, Schindler RD: Annual survey of football injury research, 1931-1984. *Athl Train J Natl Athl Train Assoc* 1985;20:213-218.

26. Casa DJ, Armstrong LE: Heatstroke: A medical emergency, in Armstrong LE (ed): *Exertional Heat Illnesses*. Champaign, IL, Human Kinetics, 2003, pp 26-56, 230-234.

27. Armstrong LE, Maresh CM, Crago AE, Adams R, Roberts RO: Interpretation of aural temperatures during exercise, hyperthermia, and cooling therapy. *Med Exerc Nutr Health* 1994;3:9-16.

28. Deschamps A, Levy RD, Coslo MG, Marliss EB, Magder S: Tympanic temperature should not be used to assess exercise-induced hyperthermia. *Clin J Sport Med* 1992;2:27-32.

29. Knight JC, Casa DJ, McClung JM, et al: Assessing if two tympanic temperature instruments are valid predictors of core temperature in hyperthermic runners and does drying the ear canal help [abstract]. *J Athl Train* 2000;35:S21.

30. Roberts WO: Assessing core temperature in collapsed athletes: What's the best method? *Physician Sportsmed* 1994;22(8):49-55.

31. Epstein Y: Exertional heatstroke: Lessons we tend to forget. *Am J Med Sports* 2000;2:143-152.

32. Knochel JP: Environmental heat illness: An eclectic review. *Arch Intern Med* 1974;133:841-864.

33. Roberts WO: Exercise-associated collapse in endurance events: A classification system. *Physician Sportsmed* 1989;17(5):49-55.

34. Shapiro Y, Seidman DS: Field and clinical observations of exertional heat stroke patients. *Med Sci Sports Exerc* 1990;22:6-14.

35. Armstrong LE, Crago AE, Adams R, Roberts WO, Maresh CM: Whole-body cooling of hyperthermic runners: Comparison to two field therapies. *Am J Emerg Med* 1996;14:355-358.

36. Brodeur VB, Dennett SR, Griffin LS: Exertional hyperthermia, ice baths, and emergency care at the Falmouth Road Race. *J Emerg Nurs* 1989;15:304-312.

37. Clements JM, Casa DJ, Knight JC, et al: Ice-water immersion and cold-water immersion provide similar cooling rates in runners with exercise-induced hyperthermia. *J Athl Train* 2002;37:146-150.

38. Golden F, Tipton M: *Essentials of Sea Survival*. Champaign, IL, Human Kinetics, 2002.

39. Hayward JS, Collis M, Eckerson JD: Thermographic evaluation of relative heat loss areas of man during cold water immersion. *Aerosp Med* 1973;44:708-711.

40. Marino F, Booth J: Whole body cooling by immersion in water at moderate temperature. *J Sci Med Sport* 1998;1:73-82.

41. Proulx CI, Ducharme MB, Kenny GP: Effect of water temperature on cooling efficiency during hyperthermia in humans. *J Appl Physiol* 2003;94:1317-1323.

42. Sandor RP: Heat illness: On-site diagnosis and cooling. *Physician Sportsmed* 1997;25(6):35-40.

43. Wyndham C, Strydom N, Cooks H, et al: Methods of cooling subjects with hyperpyrexia. *J Appl Physiol* 1959;14:771-776.

44. Armstrong LE, De Luca JP, Hubbard RW: Time course of recovery and heat acclimation ability of prior exertional heatstroke patients. *Med Sci Sports Exerc* 1990;22:36-48.

45. Epstein Y: Heat intolerance: Predisposing factor or residual injury? *Med Sci Sports Exerc* 1990;22:29-35.

46. Mehta AC, Baker RN: Persistent neurological deficits in heat stroke. *Neurology* 1970;20:336-340.

47. Royburt M, Epstein Y, Solomon Z, Shemer J: Long-term psychological and physiological effects of heat stroke. *Physiol Behav* 1993;54:265-267.

48. Armstrong LE: Exertional hyponatremia, in Armstrong LE (ed): *Exertional Heat Illnesses*. Champaign, IL, Human Kinetics, 2003, pp 103-136, 244-249.

49. Speedy DB, Noakes TD, Schneider C: Exercise-associated hyponatremia: A review. *Emerg Med* 2001;13:17-27.

50. Armstrong LE, Casa DJ, Watson G: Exertional hyponatremia: Unanswered questions and etiological perspectives. *J Athl Train*. In press.

51. Sawka MN, Young AJ, Francesconi RP, Muza SR, Pandolf KB: Thermoregulatory and blood responses during exercise at graded hypohydration levels. *J Appl Physiol* 1985;59:1394-1401.

52. Armstrong LE: *Keeping Your Cool in Barcelona: The Effects of Heat Humidity and Dehydration on Athletic Performance Strength and Endurance*. Colorado Springs, CO, United States Olympic Committee Sports Sciences Division, 1992, pp 1-29.

53. Armstrong LE, Hubbard RW, Szlyk PC, Matthew WT, Sils IV: Voluntary dehydration and electrolyte losses during prolonged exercise in the heat. *Aviat Space Environ Med* 1985;56:765-770.

20

54. Bijlani R, Sharma KN: Effect of dehydration and a few regimes of rehydration on human performance. *Indian J Physiol Pharmacol* 1980;24:255-266.

55. Cheung SS, McLellan TM: Heat acclimation, aerobic fitness, and hydration effects on tolerance during uncompensable heat stress. *J Appl Physiol* 1998;84:1731-1739.

56. Morimoto T, Miki K, Nose H, Yamada S, Hirakawa K, Matsubara D: Changes in body fluid and its composition during heavy sweating and effect of fluid and electrolyte replacement. *Jpn J Biometeorol* 1981;18:31-39.

57. Murray R: Dehydration, hyperthermia, and athletes: Science and practice. *J Athl Train* 1996;31:248-252.

58. Nadel ER, Fortney SM, Wenger CB: Effect of hydration state on circulatory and thermal regulations. *J Appl Physiol* 1980;49:715-721.

59. Pichan G, Gauttam RK, Tomar OS, Bajaj AC: Effects of primary hypohydration on physical work capacity. *Int J Biometerorol* 1988;32:176-180.

60. Sawka MN, Coyle EF: Influence of body water and blood volume on thermoregulation and exercise performance in the heat. *Exerc Sport Sci Rev* 1999;27:167-218.

61. Walsh RM, Noakes TD, Hawley JA, Dennis SC: Impaired high-intensity cycling performance time at low levels of dehydration. *Int J Sports Med* 1994;15:392-398.

62. Murray R: Determining sweat rate. *Sports Sci Exch* 1996;9(suppl)63.

63. Armstrong LE: *Performing in Extreme Environments.* Champaign, IL, Human Kinetics, 2000.

64. Armstrong LE, Maresh CM, Castellani JW, et al: Urinary indices of hydration status. *Int J Sport Nutr* 1994;4:265-279.

65. Armstrong LE, Soto JA, Hacker FT Jr, Casa DJ, Kavouras SA, Maresh CM: Urinary indices during dehydration, exercise, and rehydration. *Int J Sport Nutr* 1997;8:345-355.

66. Ivy JL, Goforth HW, Damon BM, McCauley TR, Parsons EC, Price TB: Early postexercise muscle glycogen recovery is enhanced with a carbohydrate-protein supplement. *J Appl Physiol* 2002;93:1337-2002.

67. Casa DJ, Maresh CM, Armstrong LE, et al: Intravenous versus oral rehydration during a brief period: Responses to subsequent exercise in the heat. *Med Sci Sports Exerc* 2000;32:124-133.

68. Armstrong LE, Casa DJ: Predisposing factors for exertional heat illnesses, in Armstrong LE (ed): *Exertional Heat Illnesses.* Champaign, IL, Human Kinetics, 2003, pp 151-168, 250-255.

69. Armstrong LE, Hubbard RW, Askew EW, et al: Responses to moderate and low sodium diets during exercise-heat acclimation. *Int J Sport Nutr* 1993;3:207-221.

70. Armstrong LE, Maresh CM: Exercise-heat tolerance of children and adolescents. *Pediatr Exerc Sci* 1995;7:239-252.

71. Armstrong LE, Szlyk PC, DeLuca JP, Sils IV, Hubbard RW: Fluid-electrolyte losses in uniforms during prolonged exercise at 30 degrees C. *Aviat Space Environ Med* 1992;63:351-355.

72. Bar-Or O: Thermoregulation in females from a life span perspective, in Bar-Or O, Lamb DR, Clarkson PM (eds): *Exercise and the Female: A Life Span Approach.* Carmel, IN, Cooper Publishing, 1996, pp 249-284.

73. Cadarette BS, Sawka MN, Toner MM, Pandolf KB: Aerobic fitness and the hypohydration response to exercise-heat stress. *Aviat Space Environ Med* 1984;55:507-512.

74. Chung NK, Pin CH: Obesity and the occurrence of heat disorders. *Mil Med* 1996;161:739-742.

75. Dawson B: Exercise training in sweat clothing in cool conditions to improve heat tolerance. *Sports Med* 1994;17:233-244.

76. Fortney SM, Vroman NB: Exercise, performance and temperature control: Temperature regulation during exercise and implications for sports performance and training. *Sports Med* 1985;2:8-20.

77. Gardner JW, Kark JA, Karnei K, et al: Risk factors predicting exertional heat illness in male Marine Corps recruits. *Med Sci Sports Exerc* 1996;28:939-944.

78. Hayward JS, Eckerson JD, Dawson BT: Effect of mesomorphy on hyperthermia during exercise in a warm, humid environment. *Am J Phys Anthropol* 1986;70:11-17.

79. Kark JA, Burr PQ, Wenger CB, Gastaldo E, Gardner JW: Exertional heat illness in Marine Corps recruit training. *Aviat Space Environ Med* 1996;67:354-360.

80. Montain SJ, Sawka MN, Cadarette BS, Quigley MD, McKay JM: Physiological tolerance to uncompensable heat stress: Effects of exercise intensity, protective clothing, and climate. *J Appl Physiol* 1994;77:216-222.

81. Nadel ER, Pandolf KB, Roberts MF, Stolwijk JA: Mechanisms of thermal acclimation to exercise and heat. *J Appl Physiol* 1974;37:515-520.

82. Nielsen B: Solar heat load: Heat balance during exercise in clothed subjects. *Eur J Appl Physiol Occup Physiol* 1990;60:452-456.

83. Pandolf KB, Burse RL, Goldman RF: Role of physical fitness in heat acclimatisation, decay and reinduction. *Ergonomics* 1977;20:399-408.

84. Pascoe DD, Shanley LA, Smith EW: Clothing and exercise: I. Biophysics of heat transfer between the individual clothing and environment. *Sports Med* 1994;18:38-54.

85. Shapiro Y, Pandolf KB, Goldman RF: Predicting sweat loss response to exercise, environment and clothing. *Eur J Appl Physiol Occup Physiol* 1982;48:83-96.

86. Shvartz E, Saar E, Benor D: Physique and heat tolerance in hot dry and hot humid environments. *J Appl Physiol* 1973;34:799-803.

87. Elias SR, Roberts WO, Thorson DC: Team sports in hot weather: Guidelines for modifying youth soccer. *Physician Sportsmed* 1991;19(5):67, 68, 72-74, 77, 80.

88. Francis K, Feinstein R, Brasher J: Optimal practice times for the reduction of the risk of heat illness during fall football practice in the southeastern United States. *Athl Train J Natl Athl Train Assoc* 1991;26:76-78, 80.

89. Pandolf KB, Cadarette BS, Sawka MN, Young AJ, Francesconi RP, Gonzalez RR: Thermoregulatory responses of middle-aged and young men during dry-heat acclimation. *J Appl Physiol* 1998;65:65-71.

90. Buskirk ER, Iampietro PF, Bass DE: Work performance after dehydration: Effects of physical conditioning and heat acclimatization. *J Appl Physiol* 1958;12:789-794.

91. Maughan RJ, Shirreffs SM: Preparing athletes for competition in the heat: Developing an effective acclimatization strategy. *Sports Sci Exch* 1997;10:1-4.

92. Tilley RI, Standerwick JM, Long GJ: Ability of the wet bulb globe temperature index to predict heat stress in men wearing NBC protective clothing. *Mil Med* 1987;152:554-556.

93. Roberts WO: Medical management and administration manual for long distance road racing, in Brown CH, Gudjonsson B (eds): *IAAF Medical Manual for Athletics and Road Racing Competitions: A Practical Guide.* Monaco, International Amateur Athletic Federation Publications, 1998, pp 39-75.

94. Nunnelly SA, Reardon MJ: Prevention of heat illness, in Pandolf KB, Burr RE (eds): *Medical Aspects of Harsh En-vironments.* Washington, DC: TMM Publications, 2002, pp 209-230.

95. Kulka J, Kenney WL: Heat balance limits in football uniforms: How different uniform ensembles alter the equation. *Physician Sportsmed* 2002;30(7):29-39.

20

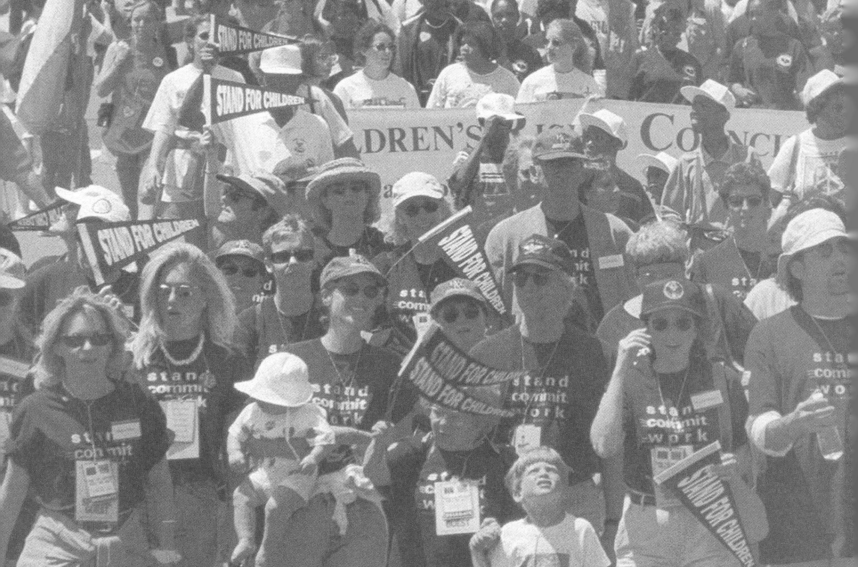

SECTION
3

Specific Populations

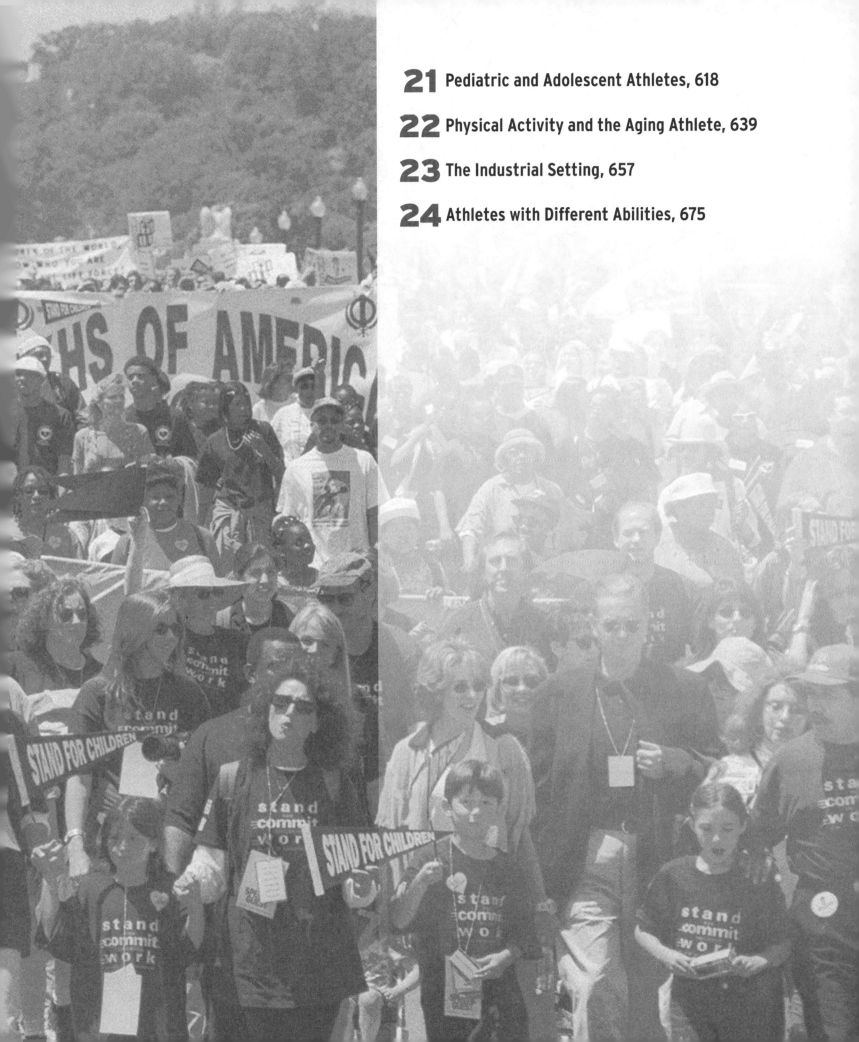

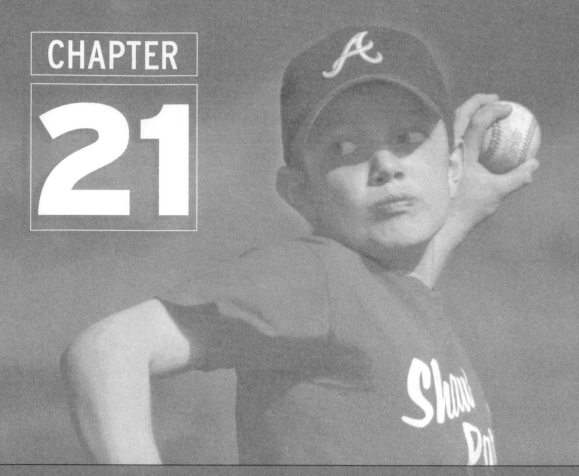

Pediatric and Adolescent Athletes

Ronald P. Pfeiffer, EdD,
LAT, ATC
Kevin Shea, MD
Peter J. Apel, BA

Description of the Population

Participation by children and adolescents in youth sports and recreational activities continues to flourish in the United States. Approximately 30 million preadolescents and adolescents are involved in organized sports.[1] This participation is beneficial to the overall health of these children but is not without risk. Large-scale epidemiologic studies of sports injuries in children are rare, but two recent studies are noteworthy. In a survey of 11,840 children and adolescents aged 5 to 17 years, the estimated annual number of injuries resulting from sports and recreational activities participation was 4,379,000, with 1,363,000 classified as serious (resulting in hospitalization, surgical treatment, missed school, or a half day or more in bed).[2,3] On the basis of these data, sports injuries were estimated to account for 36% of all injuries reported for this age group. These data, however, also included non–sport-related injuries, such as those sustained on playground equipment or skateboards. A study of children and adolescents aged 7 to 13 years involved in community organized baseball, softball, soccer, and football was conducted over two playing seasons.[4] Injury rates, in injuries per 100 **athlete exposures**, were 1.7 for baseball, 1.0 for softball, 2.1 for soccer, and 1.5 for football. Football produced the highest frequency of injuries per team per season at 14, compared with 3 and 2 for baseball and softball, respectively. Contusions were the most common injury and, except for softball, the odds of being injured were higher during games than practices.

Influence of Gender

In sports that involve running and cutting, jumping, and landing, females sustain higher rates of knee injuries than males,[5-11] but most authors have surveyed adult populations. No differences in injury rates between genders were noted during a study of youth soccer participants, but the specific incidences of knee injuries were not reported.[4] In contrast to similar studies,[4] the American Academy of Pediatrics (AAP) reported a male-to-female overall injury rate ratio of 1:2 in youth soccer, assuming similar risk exposure. In contrast, another study of injuries in youth soccer demonstrated a male-to-female overall injury rate ratio of 1:2, assuming similar risk exposures, yet no significant differences between males and females were noted in some injury categories, such as fractures.[12] This finding agrees with the work of previous researchers who also examined gender differences in injury rates in youth soccer.[13,14] In a survey of approximately 6 million injury claims from a single company providing coverage for youth soccer leagues, anterior cruciate ligament (ACL) injuries in female youth soccer players aged 12 through 15 years were more common than ACL injuries in males of the same age.[15]

Changes in Participation Levels

To determine if injury rates are increasing or decreasing over time, injuries sustained in 17 different sporting activities by children aged 16 years and younger during two time periods (September through December 1983 and 1998) and evaluated at the same hospital in Wales were investigated.[16] The total number of injuries increased from 561 in 1983 to 953 in 1998. In 1998, the risk of injury for boys aged 10 to 15 years was 1 in 22 and for girls of the same age, 1 in 55. These rates were 3.52 and 2.12 times, respectively, the rates seen in boys and girls aged 10 to 15 years in 1983. The increases in injury rates were concluded to be the result of increased participation by both boys and girls within the geographic region, as the population had remained relatively constant over the 15-year study period.[16]

General Conclusions

Because of differences in methods and injury definitions, direct comparisons of available studies are not possible; however, some general conclusions can be made. First, it seems probable that the overall number of pediatric and adolescent athletes being injured while participating in sports will continue to increase. In addition, evidence suggests that with respect to general injury categories, such as fractures, sprains, or strains, no significant gender differences in injury rates exist. Yet it is also likely that, with regard to specific body areas (for example, the knee), females may have a higher risk of injury. Thus, injury-prevention programs similar to those advocated for older athletes in recent years should be targeted to help reduce this injury risk.[17-20] Because these studies included children as young as 5 years, medical personnel charged with providing care to these young athletes must be familiar with the unique, age-related anatomy and injuries specific to this population.

Athlete exposure
A single practice session or athletic event.

21

Unique Anatomy and Implications for Injury

The phrase "pediatric and adolescent athletes are not simply little adults" is most certainly cliché within the sports medicine community. It is an important and valid concept, however. Sports medicine practitioners must have a good understanding of the process of puberty when treating athletic pediatric and adolescent patients. Aside from the obvious body-mass differences between children and adults, anatomic differences are also present within the musculoskeletal system (**Table 21-1**). American children begin their growth spurt (take-off) at age 11 years for boys and 9 years for girls, with peak height velocity occurring at 13.5 years for boys and 11.5 years for girls.[21] Puberty involves profound changes within the child, both physically and psychologically, and brings significant increases in both long-bone growth and muscle mass. For example, growth during puberty accounts for 17% to 18% of the final height for boys and 17% for girls. In addition, boys on average double their total muscle mass between the ages of 10 and 17 years.[22] The major anatomic changes associated with puberty in both boys and girls are shown in Table 21-1.

The Physis

The physis (growth plate) is specialized cartilaginous tissue interposed between the metaphysis and the epiphysis in the long bones of children.[23] The physis is a multilayered structure that physiologi-

cally transcends zones of cartilaginous matrix to complete ossification, resulting in increased length of the bone. Both sides of the physis are active in the process of bone formation: proximally (intramembranous), resulting in both cylinderization and funnelization, and distally, directly beneath the articular cartilage layer (endochondral formation) and resulting in hemispherization[24] (**Figure 21-1**). The physis is said to be open until the child reaches skeletal maturity, after which the physis is no longer active, or is closed. The open physes are easily seen on magnetic resonance imaging, as shown in the sagittal view of the knee (**Figure 21-2**). The region of greatest risk for injury is the area between the hypertrophic cells and the region of calcification[25] (**Figure 21-3**).

Injuries to the Physis

Physeal fractures occur from an array of mechanisms, both acute and chronic in nature. The Salter-Harris classification system for physeal fractures describes five distinct types of fractures (see p 41). If not properly diagnosed and treated, physeal fractures can be serious because of their potential to cause growth disturbances, with partial or complete physeal arrest, subsequent limb-length inequality, and angular deformities. Examples of Salter-Harris fractures are discussed throughout this chapter.

Table 21-1

Anatomic Changes Associated with Puberty (Mean Age)

Boys	Girls
Testicular enlargement (11.5 years)	Breast development (10 years)
Pubic-hair development (12.5 years)	Pubic hair development (11 years)
Peak height velocity (13 years)	Peak height velocity (11 years) Menarche (12 years)
Adult pubic hair configuration (15 years)	Adult pubic hair configuration (14 years)
Skeletal maturity (16 years)	Skeletal maturity (14 years)

Reproduced with permission from Koester MC: Adolescent and youth sports medicine: A "growing" concern. *Athl Ther Today* 2002;7:6-12. Copyright 2002, Human Kinetics (Champaign, IL).

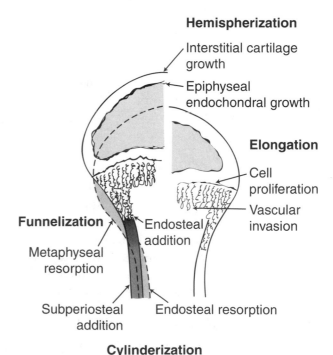

Figure 21-1 The growing-remodeling process of a typical long bone. Selective bone resorption coupled with new bone deposition in the epiphyseal, metaphyseal, and diaphyseal regions results in growth and shape changes. Reproduced with permission from Morrissy RT, Weinstein SL (eds): *Pediatric Orthopaedics*, ed 4. Philadelphia, PA, Lippincott-Raven, 1996, Fig. 1-25.

The Apophysis

The apophysis is anatomically similar to the epiphysis and represents the attachment site for tendons. The apophyses are under constant tension during puberty. As bone growth accelerates, tension can

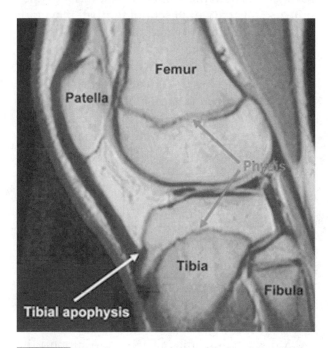

Figure 21-2 Magnetic resonance imaging of the knee in a skeletally immature patient.

further increase as the musculotendinous system falls behind the skeletal system in rate of growth.[22] The mechanisms of apophyseal injuries are similar to those causing muscle strains in adults. Apophysitis can also result from overuse and may worsen during periods of rapid growth associated with puberty. Areas commonly involved include the tibial tubercle, calcaneus, medial distal humerus (epicondyle), base of the fifth metatarsal, iliac crest, ischial tuberosity, distal patella, and tarsal navicular.[22]

Other Injuries Common to this Population

Two additional areas of concern regarding potential injury are the growth cartilage located on the articular surfaces of joints and the ligaments supporting articulations. Before puberty, ligaments may be weaker relative to adjacent skeletal tissues, including the physis.[22] Major ligament injuries should be suspected when the injury mechanism appeared to be of adequate magnitude to result in a sprain. Prepubertal children generally exhibit more joint laxity than their older, postpubescent counterparts, so it is critical that any physical examination of such injuries include assessment of the contralateral joint to avoid a false-positive test. Children tend to demonstrate more laxity in their

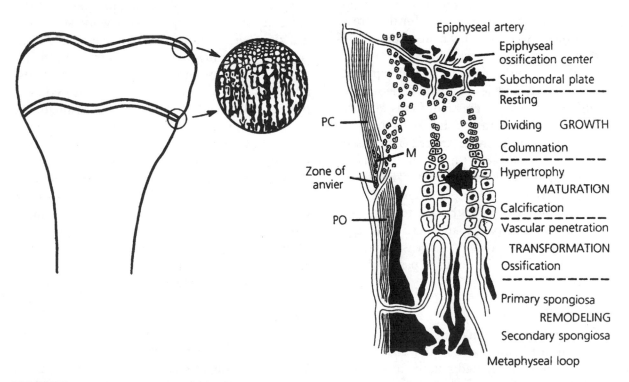

Figure 21-3 Zones of the growth plate contain different cellular architecture and intracellular matrix arrangements. PC, perichondrium; PO, periosteum; M, matrix.

joints from higher ratio of type III to type I collagen. Type III is more elastic; however, aging results in a gradual shift to type I, which is less elastic. The implication for major joints (eg, glenohumeral joint) is that dislocations sustained early in life result in a higher risk of recurrent dislocations.[26]

The major forms of articular cartilage conditions are osteochondroses, including osteochondritis dissecans. In children, the regions most vulnerable to this type of injury are the elbow, knee, and ankle.[27] The precise cause remains unknown but is most likely multifactorial, involving trauma, ischemia, genetics, and other factors.[28-30]

Resistance Training for Injury Prevention

Resistance training, also known as strength training, is a well-accepted practice for both performance enhancement and injury prevention in the adult athletic population. Although resistance training is typically associated with weight lifting (eg, barbells, dumbbells), other forms of resistance are also used, including hydraulic systems, isokinetic machines, plyometrics (eg, bounding and jumping exercises), elastic bands, and body weight.

Strength Gains

Historically, the medical profession discouraged children from strength training for fear their musculoskeletal systems were not ready for the stress imposed by lifting weights.[31] It was also commonly believed that prepubescent children were unable to increase their strength beyond what was expected from normal growth and development because they lacked sufficient hormone concentrations.[32] However, studies conducted in the late 1970s into the 1980s showed that properly structured, supervised strength training could result in strength gains in very young children without injury.[33-37] The mechanism of strength gain in the prepubescent age group is thought to be neurologic in that the training improves muscle-activation capabilities.[38-40] Under appropriate training conditions, increases in muscle mass can be expected as children pass through adolescence.

Injury Prevention

Substantial evidence demonstrates a relationship between weight training and injury reduction. Two of the earliest published studies to address this question yielded intriguing results, but both involved subjects of high school age and not prepubescents.[41,42] In an 8-year study, a preseason, total-body conditioning program that included weight training was associated with a significant reduction in both the number and severity of knee injuries in varsity high school football players.[41] Other authors investigated the effects of "diversified variable resistance isokinetic and isotonic exercises" on the incidence of injury in a cohort of high school male and female athletes involved in basketball, gymnastics, volleyball, wrestling, and football.[42] A time-loss injury resulted in removal from a practice or game or a subsequent missed practice or competitive event. One group completed the weight-training program only during the preseason and competitive season, whereas a second group completed a year-round conditioning program, and a third (control) group did not use weight training during the off-season and was limited to once per week or less during the competitive season. The combined weight-training groups had an overall injury rate of 26.2%, and the control group had an injury rate of 72.4%.

More recent studies also seem to support the premise that resistance training may lower both overall injury rates and the rate of injury to specific joints such as the knee. Forty-two of 300 female soccer players aged 14 to 18 years participated in a 7-week preseason conditioning program (cardiovascular conditioning, plyometric work, sport-cord drills, strength training, flexibility exercises, and acceleration training).[43] Over the next year, the injuries severe enough to cause the athlete to miss either a game or practice were monitored. The trained group had a significantly lower incidence of overall injury (14.3%) than the control group (33.7%). All injuries involved the lower extremities, with most being at the knee and ankle. ACL injury rates were not significantly different between the groups, but a trend toward fewer injuries in the treatment group was noted. The treatment group sustained one ACL injury, representing 2.4% of the total injuries; the control group sustained eight ACL injuries, representing 3.1%. The lack of a significant difference may have resulted from the small sample size rather than the lack of a training effect.

The effectiveness of a preseason conditioning program in reducing knee injuries was tested in a large-scale study of high school–aged female soccer, basketball, or volleyball athletes.[19] The female teams were divided into training and control groups; a male athlete control group was also included for comparison purposes. The intervention program included strength training with weights and plyometric training. Over one playing season, the incidence of knee injuries was 0.12 in the training group and 0.43 in the untrained group. Stated another way, the incidence of knee injuries in the untrained group was 3.6 times higher than the incidence in their trained counterparts. The rate in the male athletes was 0.09; thus, the incidence in untrained females was 4.8 times higher than the incidence in males.

Strength-Training Guidelines

The decision to include some form of strength training in the overall activity program of pediatric and adolescent athletes should be based on the availability of proper equipment, instruction in lifting techniques, and supervision. Personnel should be well versed in currently accepted practices with respect to both the design and implementation of age-appropriate resistance-training programs. Preventing training-related injuries is of the utmost importance and is best accomplished by incorporating the principles of periodization: the volume and intensity of training are varied throughout the year in an effort to maximize benefits while avoiding overtraining.[44] Whenever possible, personnel providing instruction and supervision in resistance training should have received specialized, formal instruction by organizations such as the National Strength and Conditioning Association (NSCA) or the National Athletic Trainers' Association (NATA). Credentials indicating expertise in exercise prescription include Certified Strength and Conditioning Specialist (CSCS), granted by the NSCA, and Certified Athletic Trainer (ATC), granted by the NATA Board of Certification, Inc. In the absence of these credentials, personnel should at least have a bachelor's or advanced university degree in a field such as physical education, exercise or movement science, or kinesiology.

Position and Policy Statements

Two major professional organizations, the AAP and the NSCA, have published position or policy statements on resistance training for pediatric and adolescent age groups.[45,46] Although a com-

---

Table 21-2

Recommendations for Pediatric and Adolescent Weight Training

1. Follow proper resistance-training techniques and safety precautions.

2. Avoid power lifting, body building, and maximum lifts until physically and skeletally mature to handle the forces.

3. A pediatrician and/or sports medicine physician should perform a medical evaluation prior to participation in a weight training program. Any injuries occurred during weight training should be properly evaluated before returning to activity.

4. Specific weight-training programs should include a warm-up and cool-down period and aerobic conditioning.

5. All major muscle groups should be initially included in the weight training program.

6. Exercises should be performed with no resistance to teach the technique. Once the technique has been mastered loads (weight) can be added.

7. Weight can be increased when the individual can complete 8 to 15 repetitions and maintain proper lifting technique.

Adapted from Faigenbaum A, Kraemer W, Cahill B, et al: Youth resistance training: Position statement paper and literature. *Strength Condition* 1996;18:62-75.

---

plete listing of the details of these statements is beyond the scope of this chapter, the reader is encouraged to obtain and review these documents. The AAP recommendations are presented in **Table 21-2**.

Acute Injuries to the Upper Extremity

Acute injuries to the upper extremity most often occur when a pediatric athlete falls onto an outstretched hand, although other mechanisms of injury are possible. Fractures of the upper extremity in children and adolescents usually heal well, but they may require surgical treatment. Thus, if the mechanism of injury and physical assessment suggest a fracture or dislocation, referral for radiographic evaluation and surgical consultation is recommended. If distal pulses are weak or absent or a neurologic deficit is present at the time of injury, immediate emergency care is needed.

21

Shoulder Injuries

Shoulder injuries in the pediatric athlete are often due to instability, especially in sports with overhead movements, such as swimming and baseball. Repeated overhead motions can stretch the joint capsule and allow excessive motion of the humeral head. Acute shoulder dislocation may result in stretching of the joint capsule or other glenohumeral joint problems.

Individuals 11 to 20 years old demonstrated approximately the same incidence of glenohumeral joint dislocation as their counterparts 51 to 60 years old.[47] However, athletes with a history of a pediatric dislocation had more than an 80% chance of reinjury.[47] The reason is thought to be related to the high ratio of type III to type I collagen in children and adolescents (see p 14). Pediatric dislocations are believed to stretch the capsule more than adult dislocations and diminish the capsule's ability to provide the support needed for proper articulation. Surgical treatment for instability is generally successful[48,49] and is often recommended.[50,51] Pediatric athletes with an acute shoulder dislocation should receive similar care as an adult but should also be referred to a shoulder surgeon for consultation concerning long-term treatment options.

Elbow Injuries

Historically, the focus of the sports medicine community relative to pediatric elbow injuries has been on throwing-related problems. Perhaps the best known of these is "Little League elbow," which received great attention from the research community in the mid 1970s.[52,53] These injuries are discussed later in this chapter. Most acute injuries to the elbow involve fractures that result from falling on an outstretched arm.

Supracondylar Fractures

Although rare in adults, fractures of the distal humerus are relatively common injuries in pediatric and adolescent athletes. Supracondylar fractures of the humerus are the most common fractures in pediatric patients younger than 7 years and account for 60% of elbow fractures in children [54,55] (**Figure 21-4**). Up to 70% of these injuries result from a fall on an outstretched hand.[56] Girls are more likely to experience supracondylar elbow fractures, usually to the nondominant hand. An athlete with an acute supracondylar fracture has localized pain and point tenderness over the distal humerus, with possible ecchymosis or deformity. Radiographic assessment is necessary to gauge injury severity and plan treatment. The potential for numerous complications exists with these fractures, including compartment syndrome, neurovascular injury, and malunion, especially with fractures that are more severely displaced. Such injuries require prompt orthopaedic evaluation. A nondisplaced fracture is treated with casting; a displaced fracture requires surgical reduction in most cases. In children, these fractures heal rapidly, usually without long-term complications.[57,58]

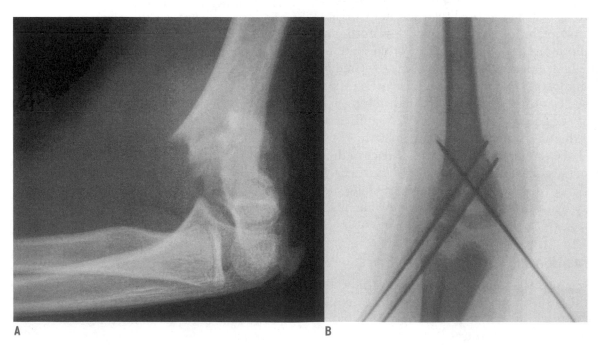

A   B

Figure 21-4 Supracondylar elbow fracture on radiograph (**A**) and the typical treatment of reduction and pinning for fracture stabilization on fluoroscopic imaging (**B**).

Lateral Condylar Fractures

Lateral condylar fractures account for about 12% of elbow fractures seen in children.[54] Although they are less common than supracondylar fractures, they are considered more severe because of the potential for growth plate involvement. These injuries are frequently seen when a child falls on an outstretched hand. Lateral condylar fractures may disrupt the articular surface of the distal humerus or damage the physis (**Figure 21-5**). As previously discussed, physeal damage can lead to physeal arrest and abnormal growth and deformities.[59] Displaced fractures usually require surgery.[59] Nondisplaced fractures can be treated with casting, although they can become displaced within the cast because of the anatomic origin of the forearm extensors on the bony fragment. Thus, close radiographic and functional follow-up is necessary.[60]

Elbow Dislocations and Medial Epicondylar Fractures

Elbow dislocations can constitute an orthopaedic emergency if distal pulses are not present or if neurologic compromise exists. Unreduced elbow dislocations typically appear deformed, and the child has little functional ability. Medial epicondyle and medial condylar fractures are commonly seen with posterior elbow dislocations, and the radiographic presence of such a fracture should always increase the suspicion of an elbow dislocation that may have spontaneously reduced (**Figure 21-6**).

Fractures of the medial epicondyle are more common than dislocations and account for about 10% of elbow fractures in children.[61] Because of the physeal anatomy of the skeletally immature elbow, the ulnar collateral ligament and flexor muscles frequently avulse a fragment from the medial epicondyle. Elbow dislocations and fractures of the medial epicondyle are usually the result of falling with the forearm supinated and the elbow in full or partial extension. Nearly 50% of medial epicondyle fractures are associated with dislocation of the elbow, and often the displaced fragment becomes trapped in the joint,[62,63] preventing closed reduction of the dislocated elbow.

An elbow dislocation may appear deformed, and if the medial epicondyle is fractured, the medial aspect of the elbow is typically point tender.[64-66] With neurologic compromise or absent distal pulses, an elbow dislocation constitutes an orthopaedic emergency. Treatment of medial epicondyle fractures is controversial, especially for minimally displaced fractures. Nondisplaced fractures are typically treated with casting, but displaced fractures may require surgery.[67]

■ Forearm Injuries

Fractures of the forearm are common in young athletes, with the distal radius being the most common site of fracture in children[55] (**Figure 21-7**). As with most upper extremity injuries, fractures of the distal radius often involve a fall onto an outstretched

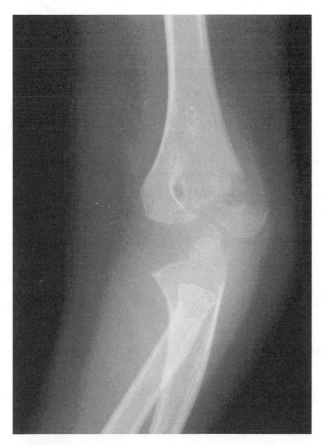

Figure 21-5 Radiograph of a lateral condylar fracture in a skeletally immature patient.

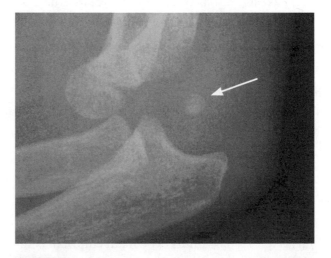

Figure 21-6 Radiograph of a posterior elbow dislocation. The medial epicondyle (arrow) is displaced and incarcerated in the joint.

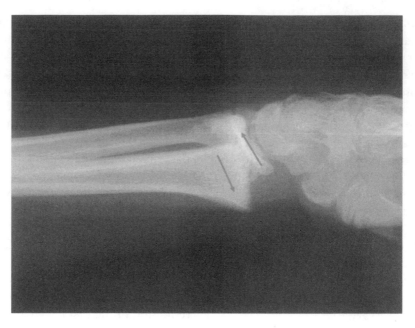

Figure 21-7   Radiograph of a displaced Salter-Harris II growth-plate fracture of the distal radius.

hand. With skeletal maturation, the fracture site tends to move from proximal to distal.[68] In younger patients, fractures usually involve the distal metaphysis of the radius and ulna, but as patients approach skeletal maturity, fractures through the distal radial physis become more common.

If displacement is present, the forearm may be deformed; however, not all forearm fractures are displaced. Skeletal point tenderness also indicates a fracture. A fracture through the growth plate usually requires surgical reduction and fixation, especially if displacement is significant.[69] Midshaft fractures of the forearm in younger patients frequently require only closed reduction and casting, but as patients mature, internal fixation is often necessary. With growth-plate involvement, abnormal shortening of the radius or ulna is possible. Still, injuries of the forearm tend to heal well, and serious long-term complications are rare.[70]

Acute Injuries to the Lower Extremity

The mechanisms of athletic injuries in children and adolescents are typically similar to those seen in adults, but the immature skeletal anatomy of the pediatric and adolescent athlete produces unique injuries not seen in adults. The main culprit in pediatric athletic injuries is the cartilaginous growth plate (physis) at the ends of long bones, separating the metaphysis from the epiphysis. In children and adolescents, ligaments are typically stronger than bone, and bone is stronger than cartilage. Thus, mechanisms that would be expected to cause ligamentous injuries in adults may cause fractures of the bone (eg, tibial eminence avulsion) **(Figure 21-8)** or cartilaginous fractures (eg, Salter-Harris type II) in children.

Fractures

Apophyseal Avulsions of the Pelvis

Among the acute injuries of the pelvic region, apophyseal avulsions are the most common.[71] An apophysis is the point on the bone at which a muscle attaches, and occasionally a fragment of bone is wholly or partially dislodged by the muscle (see Figure 8-10, p 235). Apophyseal avulsions are usually caused by a sudden or violent muscle contraction.[72] Common sites for apophyseal avulsions in pediatric and adolescent athletes include the ischial tuberosity (hamstrings), pubis (adductors), lesser trochanter (iliopsoas), anterior superior iliac spine (tensor fascia lata), anterior inferior iliac spine (rectus femoris), and iliac crest (gluteus medius). Sudden or violent muscle activity is typically seen in sports such as gymnastics, tackle football, sprinting, field events in track and field, and soccer and any activity involving quick or powerful muscle contractions.

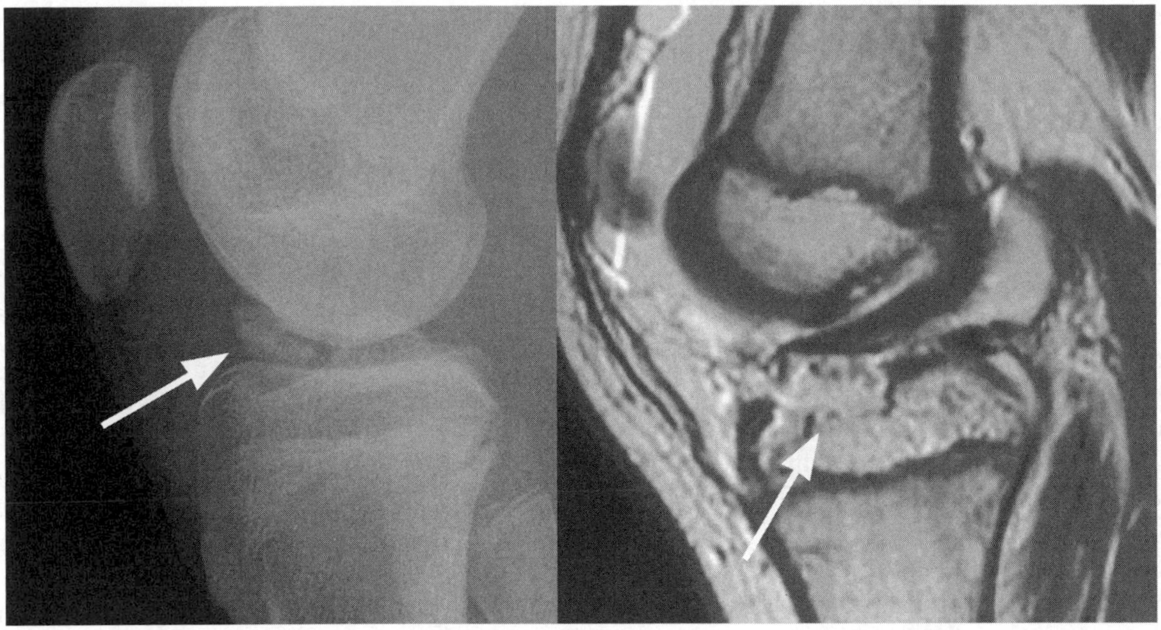

Figure 21-8 Radiograph (**A**) and magnetic resonance imaging scan (**B**) of a displaced tibial spine fracture. The ACL fibers of the tibial insertion are displaced proximally (arrows).

The athlete typically reports having felt a sudden "pop" or "letting go" near the site of injury, followed immediately by considerable pain and loss of function. In many respects, these injuries mimic muscle strains and are often initially misdiagnosed as such. Careful physical examination differentiates muscle strains from apophyseal avulsions. The initial evaluation should include a history of the activity immediately preceding the injury and palpation of the painful area. Functional testing should include manual muscle testing of the suspected muscle group, with attention to increases in pain or significant weakness. Point tenderness is demonstrated, and pain may also be referred to another region of the hip.[71] Walking with a limp indicates a more severe injury.[73]

Initial treatment for apophyseal avulsions includes rest, ice, compression, and elevation (RICE). The athlete should be fitted with crutches to limit weight bearing and then referred to a physician for a more complete medical evaluation. Radiographic evaluation confirms the diagnosis; however, this injury can be difficult to visualize due to its size and location.[74] Definitive treatment is usually conservative and includes rest, ice, and pain management, followed by a gradual return to activity concomitant with a general strength and flexibility program. Surgical intervention is rarely required,

because most injuries involve minimal displacement of the avulsed fragment.[72]

■ Physeal (Salter-Harris) Fractures

The strength of the ligament relative to the physis predisposes the growth plate to injuries in pediatric and adolescent athletes. The cartilaginous physes are approximately one third as strong as their associated ligaments, and this difference becomes more disparate during growth spurts.[75] Fractures involving the physis are categorized according to the Salter-Harris system[76] (see p 41).

Physeal Fractures of the Knee

Physeal fractures of the knee are commonly associated with tackle football and involve either the distal femoral or proximal tibial physeal plate. The injury usually results from a valgus stress, similar to the mechanisms commonly associated with tears of the ACL and medial collateral ligament in adults.[71] A major concern with physeal trauma is the long-term prognosis for an arrested growth plate, which, as mentioned earlier, can lead to limb-length inequality, angular deformity, or both.

Fractures of the distal femoral physis occur 10 times more frequently than proximal tibial physeal fractures and are most common in boys age 10 to 14 years.[75] The signs and symptoms of femoral physeal injury include pain at the site of the proximal attachment of the medial or lateral collateral ligament and local swelling (**Figure 21-9**). A physeal fracture of the knee may also present with associated ligament laxity.[77] When this injury is suspected, excessive force must not be applied when performing a valgus or varus stress test. Restrict the test to a gradually applied force to test for relative laxity compared with the uninjured knee.

Although less likely, injuries of the proximal tibial physis do occur. The mechanism is typically direct trauma, such as a blow to the anterior knee.[75] With proximal tibial physeal fractures, symptoms include pain upon weight bearing and point tenderness in the region of the joint line and just distal to it, directly over the region of the proximal tibial physis.

Any pediatric or adolescent athlete with the appropriate history for one of these injuries and with the signs described above should be treated with RICE and referred to an orthopaedist with expertise in the management of Salter-Harris fractures. Radiographic evaluation is necessary to confirm a diagnosis of physeal fracture; however, the diagnosis may be elusive because some of these injuries spontaneously reduce, and specialized imaging techniques such as stress or oblique radiographs may be required.[71] Treatment for physeal injuries ranges from closed reduction with casting to open reduction and internal fixation.

Physeal Fractures of the Ankle

When evaluating a pediatric or adolescent athlete with an apparent ankle sprain, an injury to the physis or other fracture should always be suspected. Careful examination of the injured area, palpation, functional testing, and, when appropriate, imaging studies are needed to rule out a growth-plate injury. Pain and swelling localized to the site of the commonly sprained ligaments (ie, anterior talofibular and calcaneofibular) usually represent a "simple" ankle sprain. Such injuries are treated with RICE, external support (such as taping), and appropriate rehabilitation exercises. If, however, the pain appears to be more closely associated with the physeal anatomy of the ankle and foot, a physeal fracture should be suspected.

A common physeal injury of the ankle in the pediatric and adolescent populations is the triplane (Salter-Harris type IV) fracture (**Figure 21-10**), which is more prevalent in patients approaching skeletal maturity. The fracture is typically associated with an external-rotation mechanism and can be described radiologically as three separate fractures: (1) within the coronal plane, through the posterior aspect of the medial malleolus; (2) in the axial plane, through the physis; and (3) in the sagittal plane, through the epiphysis of the tibia.[71]

An inversion ankle injury that may be mistaken for an ankle sprain is a type I injury of the distal

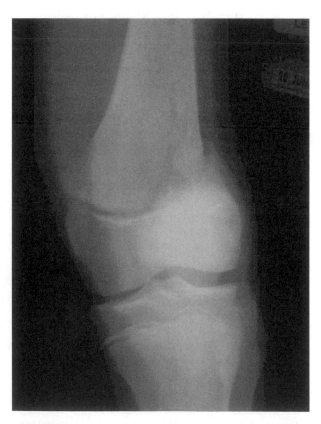

Figure 21-9 Radiograph of a displaced Salter-Harris II growth-plate fracture of the distal femur. Clinically, this injury may present as a medial collateral ligament sprain.

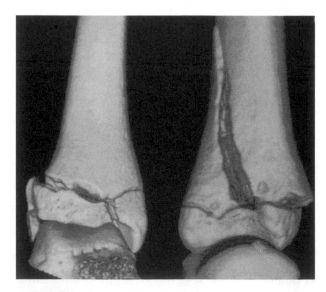

Figure 21-10 Computed tomography scan of a distal tibial triplane fracture involving the growth plate.

fibula. Localizing pain can be helpful in differentiating this injury from a simple sprain. In a Salter-Harris type I fracture of the distal fibula, swelling and tenderness are directly over the distal fibular growth plate, proximal to the lateral malleolus. Radiographic evaluation of a type I injury is usually negative,[78] unlike that of other ankle fractures discussed here. Salter-Harris type II fractures of the ankle and triplane fractures are both seen radiographically.

Physeal fractures of the ankle require various degrees of treatment, ranging from simple immobilization with casting to open reduction with internal fixation. The initial treatment is RICE, followed by referral to an orthopaedist with experience in treating these types of injuries in children. The risk of growth-plate arrest can be relatively high with some of these fractures.

Other Acute Fractures of the Foot and Ankle

Two acute injuries of the foot and ankle specific to pediatric and adolescent athletes are noteworthy. The first is an avulsion fracture involving the peroneus brevis tendon and its insertion on the proximal aspect of the fifth metatarsal. This apophyseal fracture is often caused by a severe inversion mechanism. Signs and symptoms include pain and point tenderness over the proximal fifth metatarsal with pain in resisted eversion. Radiographic evaluation may reveal a displaced fragment proximal to the fifth metatarsal. Treatment is usually conservative, with most injuries responding well to temporary immobilization via crutches and elastic bandaging.[79]

Another foot injury is the Lisfranc sprain, an injury to the tarsometatarsal joints. Radiographic evaluation is necessary to look for evidence of displacement or fracture. Treatment depends on the patient's ability to bear weight and the presence of radiographic abnormalities. If weight bearing is possible with correct anatomic positioning, treatment consists of casting for 4 to 6 weeks (non-weight bearing), followed by protected walking.[80] In more severe cases involving major ligamentous disruption, surgery is necessary.

▪ Ligamentous Injuries

A frequent ligamentous athletic injury in adults, an ACL tear is less common in children. Because of the relative strengths of the ligament, bone, and physis, tibial eminence avulsion injuries are more commonly seen in children and adolescents.[71,79] Yet recent research suggests that ACL tears are becoming more common in pediatric and adolescent patients.[15] The ACL pulls a fragment of bone from its tibial insertion, the tibial eminence (also referred to as the intercondylar eminence). Although tibial eminence avulsions are more frequent, evidence suggests that ACL tears without tibial eminence involvement seem to be increasingly common.[81] Interestingly, females, especially those of high school age, are at higher risk for ACL injury relative to males.[81,82]

Anterior Cruciate Ligament Injury

Although epidemiologic data on injury types and rates are scarce in pediatric and adolescent athletes, the incidence of knee ligament injury has increased with the growth in participation of youth sports.[81,83] In the case of the ACL, the relative incidence of intrasubstance ligament rupture compared with avulsion of the tibial eminence is unknown. As the athlete approaches skeletal maturity, an intrasubstance tear of the ACL becomes more likely than an avulsion injury (**Figure 21-11**). However, sport-related intrasubstance ACL injuries have been documented in skeletally immature males and females.[15,84]

Research in both adult and adolescent patients has shown females have a higher risk of knee and ACL injuries.[5,82] In a study of high school-aged athletes, Powell and Barber-Foss[82] found that in basketball, females had rates of knee injury, knee surgery, and surgery for ACL injury that were four times as high as rates for the male basketball players. In soccer, females had rates of knee injury, knee surgery, and ACL injury 3.41 times higher than the rates for males.[82] Numerous factors have been identified as possible causes of the difference in ACL injury rate between males and females, including athletic technique, muscular strength, shoe-surface interface, skill level, joint laxity, limb alignment, notch dimensions, hormonal and menstrual factors, and ligament size.[7,85-92] Presently, the contribution of each of these factors is unknown.

The mechanisms of injury that cause ACL tears in the pediatric and adolescent athlete population are probably similar to those of adults. Two general categories of mechanisms exist: contact and noncontact. Noncontact injuries typically involve landing from a jump with a hyperextended knee or with the knee out of position relative to the body's center of mass, producing a valgus stress on the knee combined with axial rotation. Noncontact ACL injuries can also be caused by rapid deceleration or directional changes when running (see p 136). Despite extensive research, a consensus group concluded that the precise mechanism of injury for noncontact ACL injuries is still to be determined.[7]

A thorough examination is critical in the pediatric and adolescent athlete, as the child's ability to

21

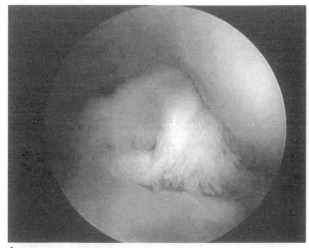

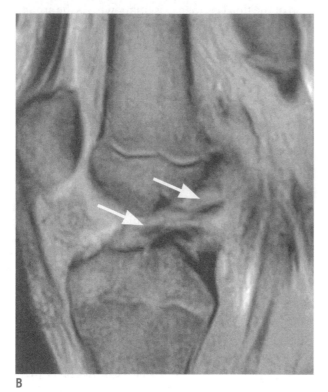

Figure 21-11 Anterior cruciate ligament tears. **A.** Arthroscopic appearance of a torn anterior cruciate ligament. **B.** Sagittal magnetic resonance imaging scan of a torn anterior cruciate ligament in a skeletally immature athlete. Note the anterior subluxation of the tibia.

recall the history of the injury is often unreliable. As is the case with an adult athlete, a child reporting a pop or snap within the joint at the time of injury raises the level of suspicion for a major ligament injury. Often a parent or other adult observer can be of great help when attempting to determine the precise mechanism of injury. It is also important to remember that increased laxity of the major ligaments is normal in females of this age group.[83] As

such, it is critical to compare all examinations with the uninjured, contralateral knee. The knee should be evaluated for all the major ligamentous restraints using the standard functional tests. Additionally, the integrity of the medial and lateral menisci should be evaluated, especially in the presence of a positive test for an ACL or collateral ligament injury.

The integrity of the ACL can be effectively assessed within minutes of the injury using the Lachman test.[79] The on-field evaluation can be key to diagnosis, as the patient's ability to relax for this examination decreases soon after the injury occurs. If the injured knee demonstrates increased laxity or a soft endpoint on the Lachman examination, the possibility of an ACL injury or tibial spine avulsion should be considered. Unilateral laxity of more than 3 to 5 mm should be considered positive evidence for either an ACL rupture or an avulsion fracture. When significant laxity is found, imaging studies are necessary to determine the specific nature of the injury (ie, true ligament rupture versus avulsion of the tibial eminence, as tibial eminence fractures are readily identified on radiographs). Magnetic resonance imaging may be helpful for evaluating knee injuries because of its unique ability to visualize soft tissues such as the ACL and menisci. Meniscal injury and entrapment has also been described.[93]

Treatment of tibial spine fractures depends on the degree of displacement. Nondisplaced fractures can be treated with casting. Fractures with significant displacement may require surgery. Numerous recent authors have demonstrated excellent outcomes with arthroscopically repaired fractures. Arthroscopic repair also allows for evaluation of meniscal injury, such as entrapment or tear.[93]

The decision regarding conservative treatment versus surgical repair of this injury in a child is complex, as both surgical and nonsurgical treatments have potential complications. Chronic absence of the ACL subsequent to injury can result in meniscal damage, osteoarthritis, and poor outcomes.[94-98] Limited published studies support surgical (intra-articular) reconstruction of the ACL in pediatric and adolescent athletes who intend to return to their preinjury activity level.[95,96,98-100] Most concerns related to surgical reconstruction focus on avoiding intrusion into the distal femoral or proximal tibial physes, which can lead to physeal arrest and result in leg-length discrepancies or angular deformities.[98] In spite of these concerns, it appears that reconstructions can be successful[84,94,97,101] when the placement of hardware and transphyseal tunnels is taken into account. Nonetheless, ACL reconstruction remains a controversial topic among pediatric orthopaedists, and growth-plate complications from this procedure are still reported.[93,102,103]

Tibial Eminence Avulsion

Tibial eminence avulsions, usually seen only in children, are the result of mechanisms that would lead to an ACL tear in an adult. Tibial eminence avulsion fractures are classified based on relative radiographic displacement. Type I fractures are nondisplaced and are treated conservatively with immobilization in a long-leg cast for 4 to 6 weeks. Type II fractures are minimally displaced, and type III fractures are completely displaced. Type II and type III tibial eminence avulsions may be secured with internal fixation placed either arthroscopically or with open reduction.[104] Reports of meniscal entrapment with more displaced fractures are concerning, and these patients may be best treated with arthroscopic evaluation.[93] Treatment of tibial spine fractures depends on the degree of displacement. Nondisplaced fractures can be treated with casting. Fractures with significant displacement may require surgery. Numerous recent investigators have demonstrated excellent outcomes with arthroscopic repair of these fractures. Arthroscopic repair also allows for evaluation of meniscal injury, such as entrapment or tear.[93]

Overuse Injuries

As sports participation in this age group has increased significantly in recent years, so have the frequency, intensity, and volume of exercise associated with this participation. As a result, just as in adult athletes, overuse injuries are occurring in pediatric and adolescent athletes. Approximately half of the sports injuries in children are of the overuse variety, with no apparent gender-related difference in injury frequency.[3,105]

Skeletal Growth and the Apophyses

The cause of overuse injuries in children is the same as that in the adult population. In short, overuse occurs when activity levels exceed the body's ability to recover. Contributing to the problem is the fact that adolescent athletes undergo periods of accelerated long-bone growth, typically between the ages of 6 and 14 years, resulting in length increases by a factor of 1.4.[106] The associated soft tissues (muscles, tendons, and apophyses) cannot immediately adapt to these sudden changes in limb length. There-

Table 21-3

Common Sites for Apophysitis

Anatomic Site	Condition
Base of fifth metatarsal	Iselin disease
Calcaneus	Sever disease
Medial distal humerus	Little League elbow
Tibial tubercle	Osgood-Schlatter disease
Iliac crest	
Ischial tuberosity	

Adapted with permission from Koester MC, Amundson CL: The adolescent athlete: Special medical concerns, in Pfeiffer RP, Mangus BC (eds), *Concepts of Athletic Training.* Sudbury, MA, Jones & Bartlett, 2002, p 276.

fore, children undergoing rapid growth may experience increased tension within these associated soft tissues. Common sites for apophysitis are shown in **Table 21-3**. Apophysitis tends to be self-limiting and resolves with maturation of the apophyses.

Osgood-Schlatter Disease

Osgood-Schlatter disease is characterized by pain, tenderness, and swelling of the tibial tubercle.[107,108] The diagnosis is made based on the clinical examination, with radiographs recommended to confirm the absence of other, potentially more serious conditions.[108] Treatment of Osgood-Schlatter disease includes reduced activity, application of ice after activity, and stretching of the quadriceps muscles. Also, nonsteroidal anti-inflammatory drugs (NSAIDs) may be prescribed for intermittent use. Commercial knee straps may be helpful, presumably by decreasing the traction forces acting on the tibial tubercle.[108]

Sever Disease

Sever disease is characterized by pain in the area of the calcaneal apophysis. Associated with running and jumping sports, Sever disease occurs frequently before or during peak growth in both genders.[109] The diagnosis can be based on the physical findings, including a positive squeeze test in association with a tight Achilles tendon[109] as well as pain over the calcaneal apophysis. Treatment includes rest and Achilles stretching exercises. Passive stretching is highly effective and should be done at least once daily. A heel lift should be placed in the sports shoes to reduce the tension on the plantar flexors.

Little League Elbow

Little League elbow can involve either the medial or lateral epicondyle, depending on the specific pathogenesis. Pain over the medial elbow is related to valgus overload and concomitant stress on the

21

medial joint capsule and associated ligaments. The mechanisms of injury are the early and late cocking phases of the overhand throw[110] (see Figure 10-13). Pain over the lateral elbow region in throwers is associated with compressive forces related to the late cocking and early acceleration phases of the overhand throw.[110] Specific damage may involve osteochondritis of the radial head or capitellum or both. Conservative treatment includes rest and strengthening and stretching exercises.

Limiting both the number of innings per game and pitches thrown per week is the best method of preventing elbow injuries in young pitchers. The number of innings should be limited to three or four per game, and the player's pitch count should be held to fewer than 200 pitches per week.[108] Consideration should also be given to the athlete's age and the type of pitch being thrown. Certain pitches place greater stress on the anatomic components of the arm: for example, USA Baseball recommends that children younger than 14 years not be taught to throw a curve ball[111] (**Table 21-4**).

Iselin Disease

Iselin disease involves the insertion of the peroneus brevis tendon at the proximal tuberosity of the fifth metatarsal. The apophysis becomes inflamed by undue stress from foot inversion associated with sporting activities that involve running and cutting, resulting in a traction apophysis.[112,113] Symptoms include pain at the tubercle, which can be reproduced by resisting eversion.[113] Treatment is application of ice and pain management (NSAIDs) in conjunction with ankle resistance exercises to improve peroneal strength.[107,113] A short period of casting may be necessary in some instances.

Pelvic Apophysitis

Apophysitis of the pelvis, specifically involving either the iliac crest or the ischial tuberosity, occurs between the ages of 8 and 15 years in the active adolescent population.[114] With iliac apophysitis, pain occurs bilaterally on trunk rotation in the absence of any history of crest contusion. Osteomyelitis, Perthes disease, slipped capital femoral epiphysis, and other hip and pelvis disorders should be ruled out in these patients.[107] With ischial apophysitis, the pain is periarticular in the region of the tuberosity, again in the absence of any reported acute injury trauma. If the athlete reports a popping or tearing sensation in the region of the tuberosity, an avulsion must be considered. Treatment for pelvic apophysitis is conservative: rest, ice, and NSAIDs, and flexibility and strengthening exercises.[107,114,115]

Prevention of Overuse Injuries

Injury prevention must be a priority for everyone involved in sporting activities. This is particularly true for overuse injuries, because as many as 50% may be preventable.[116] **Table 21-5** presents steps that

---

Table 21-4

Age (In Years) Recommended for Learning Various Pitches (Mean ± SD)

Fastball	8 ± 2
Change-up	10 ± 3
Curveball	14 ± 2
Screwball	17 ± 2
Slider	16 ± 2
Forkball	16 ± 2
Knuckleball	15 ± 3

Reproduced with permission from Andrews JR, Fleisig G: Medical and safety advisory committee: Special report. How many pitches should I allow my child to throw? *USA Baseball News* April 1996.

Table 21-5

Prevention of Overuse Injuries in Pediatric and Adolescent Athletes

Preparticipation examinations

Screening by a physician can identify risk factors for injury and provide an opportunity to develop specific recommendations for addressing them.

Proper adult supervision and coaching

Leagues and parents should ensure that coaches have the resources to become educated about recognizing and preventing overuse injuries common in their sports and to ensure that athletes are properly supervised.

Training programs that emphasize general fitness and avoid excessive training volumes

Although individual situations vary, the 10% rule—limiting increases in training frequency, intensity, and duration to no more than 10% per week—serves as a general guide.[3,116] Periodization of training, which systematically varies training volume and incorporates scheduled rest periods, should also be considered.

Delaying sport specialization

Allow children to experiment with different activities to develop a variety of skills and interests.

Careful monitoring of training for children undergoing growth spurts

It might be appropriate to modify training during this time period because of the growth-related factors that can lead to injury.

Adapted with permission from DiFiori JP: Overuse injuries in young athletes: An overview. *Athl Ther Today* 2002;7:25-29. Copyright 2002, Human Kinetics (Champaign, IL).

should be considered to help prevent overuse injuries in pediatric and adolescent athletes.

Female Athlete Triad

Three interrelated conditions often seen in female athletes are **disordered eating**, menstrual dysfunction, and osteoporosis or osteopenia (**Figure 21-12**). Together, these constitute the female athlete triad.[117] Disordered eating can lead to amenorrhea, and both disordered eating and **amenorrhea** can lead to a loss of bone density and osteoporosis. The precise physiologic mechanism for this condition is complex and not yet fully understood. In the female athlete triad, disordered eating is often the most responsible factor, either by intent or oversight. Treatment can be as simple as helping the athlete to understand her caloric needs or may require multidisciplinary intervention, counseling, and possibly hormone or calcium supplementation. Early identification of disordered eating and amenorrhea can assist in preventing long-term harm to the athlete. Any adolescent female with a stress fracture needs to have a thorough nutritional assessment and possibly an endocrinology consultation. Be aware of the possibility of associated eating disorders or other causes of osteopenia.

Disordered Eating

Disordered eating describes a number of conditions, some of which are easily treated, whereas others require more complex intervention. Physically active athletes have higher caloric needs than those who are not active and may be in negative energy balance if their caloric output exceeds calories consumed. This imbalance may be inadvertent if the athlete lacks knowledge concerning her caloric needs, or it may be intentional, by fasting, purposeful undereating, purging, or the use of laxatives, diet pills, or diuretics. In addition, abnormal compulsive exercise beyond that of the normal training regimen is also a form of disordered eating. Often, disordered eating arises from an unrealistic body image or actual or perceived pressure to be thin.[118] The degree of disordered eating ranges from mild to severe, and the condition is more frequent in sports in which body image is important (ballet, figure skating) or perceived to be important (long-distance running) and in sports with weight classifications or limits (rowing, martial arts).[119] The incidence of disordered eating in athletes is unknown.

Menstrual Dysfunction

Neither amenorrhea nor **oligomenorrhea** is a normal consequence of exercise, and the presence of either in the athlete should be viewed as abnormal.[120] An athlete with primary amenorrhea, or no menses by age 16 years, requires an extensive medical workup to determine the cause and should be referred to a gynecologist or endocrinologist. Secondary amenorrhea, or an absence of three to six consecutive periods in the first few years after menarche, or oligomenorrhea, more than 35 days between menstrual periods, may be due to a number of factors, all of which must be ruled out in order to confirm a diagnosis of exercise-induced amenorrhea.[121]

The incidence of menstrual dysfunction in athletes is unknown, although estimates range from 1% to 67%, depending on the sport and measure of dysfunction.[117,122] Of 97 college-aged runners, 36% had menstrual dysfunction.[123] Of the runners with menstrual dysfunction, 6% had osteoporosis, and 48% had osteopenia. These bone-density changes can be serious because of the body's inability to recover lost minerals, even after resumption of normal menses. In addition, female athletes who menstruate irregularly are more likely to experience musculoskeletal injuries.[124]

Osteoporosis

Prolonged amenorrhea can lead to an irreversible loss of bone mineral density, and even after normal menses resume, osteoporosis can persist.[125-128] A delay in menarche and prolonged intervals of amenorrhea predispose ballet dancers to both scoliosis and stress fractures.[129] In addition to amenorrhea, decreased caloric intake correlates with lower bone densities, even when menses are normal.[123,130] Thus, preventing osteoporosis and future musculoskeletal injuries is the primary goal in treating the female athlete triad. First, nutritional deficiencies are addressed, and then other treatment options are explored, including oral contraceptives for normalization of menses and calcium supplements.

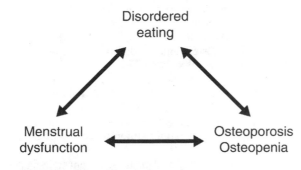

Figure 21-12 The female athlete triad involves disordered eating, menstrual dysfunction, and osteoporosis or osteopenia.

■ Treatment

Women who are oligomenorrheic or amenorrheic may have significantly lower bone mineral density than women who menstruate normally. Thus, the aim of treatment in these patients is to restore normal menses.[120,131] In addition, women with eating disorders but normal menstrual periods may also be at risk for osteoporosis.[123] For these patients, the goal of treatment is to restore appropriate caloric balance. In patients with both an eating disorder and dysfunctional menstruation, treating the eating disorder may solve both problems.

Athletes who are simply unaware of their caloric needs may only need nutritional counseling. Athletes who are suspected of having anorexia nervosa or bulimia may need professional intervention. Regardless of the cause of the triad, a multidisciplinary approach involving parents, coaches, physicians, ATCs, and behavioral counselors is needed to diagnose and treat this syndrome.[132]

■ References

1. National Athletic Trainers' Association Research & Education Foundation: Requests for proposals: Epidemiology study pediatric sports health care, 2001. Available at http://www.natafoundation.org/rfpepidemiological.html. Accessed May 4, 2004.

2. Bijur PE, Trumble A, Harel Y, Overpeck MD, Jones D, Scheidt PC: Sports and recreation injuries in US children and adolescents. *Arch Pediatr Adolesc Med* 1995;149:1009-1016.

3. Dalton SE: Overuse injuries in adolescent athletes. *Sports Med* 1992;13:58-70.

4. Radelet MA, Lephart SM, Rubinstein EN, Myers JB: Survey of the injury rate for children in community sports. *Pediatrics* 2002;110:e28.

5. Arendt E, Dick R: Knee injury patterns among men and women in collegiate basketball and soccer: NCAA data and review of literature. *Am J Sports Med* 1995;23:694-701.

6. Biondino CR: Anterior cruciate ligament injuries in female athletes. *Conn Med* 1999;63:657-660.

7. Griffin LY, Agel J, Albohm MJ, et al: Noncontact anterior cruciate ligament injuries: Risk factors and prevention strategies. *J Am Acad Orthop Surg* 2000;8:141-150.

8. Gray J, Taunton JE, McKenzie DC, Clement DB, McConkey JP, Davidson RG: A survey of injuries to the anterior cruciate ligament of the knee in female basketball players. *Int J Sports Med* 1985;6:314-316.

9. Harmon KG, Ireland ML: Gender differences in noncontact anterior cruciate ligament injuries. *Clin Sports Med* 2000;19:287-302.

10. Kirkendall DT, Garrett WE Jr: The anterior cruciate ligament enigma: Injury mechanisms and prevention. *Clin Orthop* 2000;372:64-68.

11. Zelisko JA, Noble HB, Porter M: A comparison of men's and women's professional basketball injuries. *Am J Sports Med* 1982;10:297-299.

12. American Academy of Pediatrics Committee on Sports Medicine and Fitness: Injuries in youth soccer: A subject review. *Pediatrics* 2000;105(3 Pt 1):659-661.

13. Schmidt-Olsen S, Jorgensen U, Kaalund S, Sorensen J: Injuries among young soccer players. *Am J Sports Med* 1991;19:273-275.

14. Maehlum S, Dahl E, Dalijord O: Frequency of injuries in a youth soccer tournament. *Physician Sportsmed* 1986;14(7):73-79.

15. Shea K, Pfeiffer RP, Wang JH, Curtin M, Apel PJ: Anterior cruciate ligament injury in pediatric and adolescent soccer players: An analysis of insurance data. *J Pediatr Orthop*. In press.

16. Jones SJ, Lyons RA, Sibert J, Evans R, Palmer SR: Changes in sports injuries to children between 1983 and 1998: Comparison of case series. *J Public Health Med* 2001;23:268-271.

17. Soderman K, Werner S, Pietila T, Engstrom B, Alfredson H: Balance board training: Prevention of traumatic injuries of the lower extremities in female soccer players? A prospective randomized intervention study. *Knee Surg Sports Traumatol Arthrosc* 2000;8:356-363.

18. Caraffa A, Cerulli G, Projetti M, Aisa G, Rizzo A: Prevention of anterior cruciate ligament injuries in soccer: A prospective controlled study of proprioceptive training. *Knee Surg Sports Traumatol Arthrosc* 1996;4:19-21.

19. Hewett TE, Lindenfeld TN, Riccobene JV, Noyes FR: The effect of neuromuscular training on the incidence of knee injury in female athletes: A prospective study. *Am J Sports Med* 1999;27:699-706.

20. Junge A, Rosch D, Peterson L, Graf-Baumann T, Dvorak J: Prevention of soccer injuries: A prospective intervention study in youth amateur players. *Am J Sports Med* 2002;30:652-659.

21. Abbassi V: Growth and normal puberty. *Pediatrics* 1998;102(2 Pt 3):507-511.

22. Koester MC: Adolescent and youth sports medicine: A "growing" concern. *Athl Ther Today* 2002;7:6-12.

23. Greene WB (ed): *Essentials of Musculoskeletal Care*, ed 2. Rosemont, IL, American Academy of Orthopaedic Surgeons, American Academy of Pediatrics, 2001.

24. Gamble J: Development and maturation of the neuromusculoskeletal system, in Morrissy RT, Weinstein SL (eds): *Lovell and Winter's Pediatric Orthopaedics*. Philadelphia, PA, Lippincott-Raven, 1996, p 23.

25. Guy J, Micheli LJ: Pediatric and adolescent athletes, in Schenck RC (ed): *Athletic Training and Sports Medicine*, ed 3. Rosemont, IL, American Academy of Orthopaedic Surgeons, 1999, pp 799-816.

26. Walton J, Paxinos A, Tzannes A, Callanan M, Hayes K, Murrell GA: The unstable shoulder in the adolescent athlete. *Am J Sports Med* 2002;30:758-767.

27. DiFiori JP: Overuse injuries in children and adolescents. *Physician Sportsmed* 1999;27(1):75-89.

28. Federico DJ, Lynch JK, Jokl P: Osteochondritis dissecans of the knee: A historical review of etiology and treatment. *Arthroscopy* 1990;6:190-197.

29. Ralston BM, Williams JS, Bach BR, Bush-Joseph CA, Knopp WD: Osteochondritis dissecans of the knee. *Physician Sportsmed* 1996;24(6):73-84.

30. Pappas AM: Osteochondroses: Diseases of the growth centers. *Physician Sportsmed* 1989;17(6):51-62.

31. U.S. Consumer Product Safety Commission. National electronic injury surveillance system. Directorate for Epidemiology. National Injury Information Clearinghouse. Washington, DC, 1979.

32. American Academy of Pediatrics: Weight training and weight lifting: Information for the pediatrician. *Physician Sportsmed* 1983;11(3):157-161.

33. Weltman A, Janney C, Rians CB, et al: The effects of hydraulic resistance strength training in pre-pubertal males. *Med Sci Sports Exerc* 1986;18:629-638.

34. Servedio F, Bartels R, Hamlin R, Teske D, Shaffer T, Servedio A: The effects of weight training, using Olympic style lifts, on various physiological variables in prepubescent boys [abstract]. *Med Sci Sports Exerc* 1985;17:288.

35. Sewall L, Micheli L: Strength training for children. *J Pediatr Orthop.* 1986;6:143-146.

36. Pfeiffer R, Francis R: Effects of strength training on muscle development in prepubescent, pubescent, and post-pubescent males. *Physician Sportsmed* 1986;14(9):134-143.

37. Vrijens F: Muscle strength development in the pre- and post-pubescent age. *Med Sport* 1978;11:152-158.

38. Ramsay JA, Blimkie CJ, Smith K, Garner S, MacDougall JD, Sale DG: Strength training effects in prepubescent boys. *Med Sci Sports Exerc* 1990;22:605-614.

39. Kraemer W, Fry A, Frykman P, Conroy B, Hoffman J: Resistance training and youth. *Pediatr Exerc Sci* 1989;1:336-350.

40. Ozmun JC, Mikesky AE, Surburg PR: Neuromuscular adaptations following prepubescent strength training. *Med Sci Sports Exerc* 1994;26:510-514.

41. Cahill BR, Griffith EH: Effect of preseason conditioning on the incidence and severity of high school football knee injuries. *Am J Sports Med* 1978;6:180-184.

42. Hejna W, Rosenberg A, Buturusis D, Krieger A: The prevention of sports injuries in high school students through strength training. *Natl Strength Condition Assoc J* 1982;4:28-31.

43. Heidt RS Jr, Sweeterman LM, Carlonas RL, Traub JA, Tekulve FX: Avoidance of soccer injuries with preseason conditioning. *Am J Sports Med* 2000;28:659-662.

44. Stone M, O'Bryant H, Garhammer J: A hypothetical model for strength training. *J Sports Med Phys Fitness* 1981;21:342-351.

45. Bernhardt DT, Gomez J, Johnson MD, et al: Strength training by children and adolescents. *Pediatrics* 2001;107:1470-1472.

46. Faigenbaum A, Kraemer W, Cahill B, et al: Youth resistance training: Position statement paper and literature. *Strength Condition* 1996;18:62-75.

47. Rowe CR: Prognosis in dislocations of the shoulder. *J Bone Joint Surg Am* 1956;38:957-977.

48. Paxinos A, Walton J, Tzannes A, Callanan M, Hayes K, Murrell GA: Advances in the management of traumatic anterior and atraumatic multidirectional shoulder instability. *Sports Med* 2001;31:819-828.

49. Pollock RG, Owens JM, Flatow EL, Bigliani LU: Operative results of the inferior capsular shift procedure for multidirectional instability of the shoulder. *J Bone Joint Surg Am* 2000;82:919-928.

50. Kirkley A, Griffin S, Richards C, Miniaci A, Mohtadi N: Prospective randomized clinical trial comparing the effectiveness of immediate arthroscopic stabilization versus immobilization and rehabilitation in first traumatic anterior dislocations of the shoulder. *Arthroscopy* 1999;15:507-514.

51. Burkhead WZ Jr, Rockwood CA Jr: Treatment of instability of the shoulder with an exercise program. *J Bone Joint Surg Am* 1992;74:890-896.

52. Gugenheim JJ Jr, Stanley RF, Woods GW, Tullos HS: Little League survey: The Houston study. *Am J Sports Med* 1976;4:189-200.

53. Larson RL, Singer KM, Bergstrom R, Thomas S: Little League survey: The Eugene study. *Am J Sports Med* 1976;4:201-209.

54. Landin LA, Danielsson LG: Elbow fractures in children: An epidemiological analysis of 589 cases. *Acta Orthop Scand* 1986;57:309-312.

55. Cheng JC, Ng BK, Ying SY, Lam PK: A 10-year study of the changes in the pattern and treatment of 6,493 fractures. *J Pediatr Orthop* 1999;19:344-350.

56. Farnsworth CL, Silva PD, Mubarak SJ: Etiology of supracondylar humerus fractures. *J Pediatr Orthop* 1998;18:38-42.

57. Arino VL, Lluch EE, Ramirez AM, Ferrer J, Rodriguez L, Baixauli F: Percutaneous fixation of supracondylar fractures of the humerus in children. *J Bone Joint Surg Am* 1977;59:914-916.

58. Nacht JL, Ecker ML, Chung SM, Lotke PA, Das M: Supracondylar fractures of the humerus in children treated by closed reduction and percutaneous pinning. *Clin Orthop* 1983;177:203-209.

59. Badelon O, Bensahel H, Mazda K, Vie P: Lateral humeral condylar fractures in children: A report of 47 cases. *J Pediatr Orthop* 1988;8:31-34.

60. Foster DE, Sullivan JA, Gross RH: Lateral humeral condylar fractures in children. *J Pediatr Orthop* 1985;5:16-22.

61. Wilkins K: Fractures and dislocations of the elbow region, in Wilkins K (ed): *Fractures in Children*. Philadelphia, PA, JB Lippincott, 1991, pp 509-828.

62. Kilfoyle RM: Fractures of the medial condyle and epicondyle of the elbow in children. *Clin Orthop* 1965;41:43-50.

63. Tachdjian MO: Fractures of the medial epicondyle of the humerus, in Tachdjian MO (ed): *Pediatric Orthopaedics*, ed 2. Philadelphia, PA, WB Saunders, 1990, pp 3121-3123.

64. Wilson NI, Ingram R, Rymaszewski L, Miller JH: Treatment of fractures of the medial epicondyle of the humerus. *Injury* 1988;19:342-344.

65. Farsetti P, Potenza V, Caterini R, Ippolito E: Long-term results of treatment of fractures of the medial humeral epicondyle in children. *J Bone Joint Surg Am* 2001;83:1299-1305.

66. Hines RF, Herndon WA, Evans JP: Operative treatment of medial epicondyle fractures in children. *Clin Orthop* 1987;223:170-174.

67. Case SL, Hennrikus W: Surgical treatment of displaced medial epicondyle fractures in adolescent athletes. *Am J Sports Med* 1997;25:682-686.

68. Tredwell SJ, Van Peteghem K, Clough M: Pattern of forearm fractures in children. *J Pediatr Orthop* 1984;4:604-608.

69. Gibbons CL, Woods DA, Pailthorpe C, Carr AJ, Worlock P: The management of isolated distal radius fractures in children. *J Pediatr Orthop* 1994;14:207-210.

70. Cannata G, De Maio F, Mancini F, Ippolito E: Physeal fractures of the distal radius and ulna: Long-term prognosis. *J Orthop Trauma* 2003;17:172-179.

71. Auringer ST, Anthony EY: Common pediatric sports injuries. *Semin Musculoskel Radiol* 1999;3:247-256.

72. Micheli LJ: *Pediatric and Adolescent Sports Medicine*. Boston, MA, Little Brown, 1984.

73. Combs J: Hip and pelvis avulsion fractures in adolescents: Proper diagnosis improves compliance. *Physician Sportsmed* 1994;22(7):41-49.

74. Dalzell D, Auringer ST: Problem children: Common fractures commonly missed. *Postgrad Radiol* 1998;18:170-183.

21

75. Stanitski CL, Sherman C: How I manage physeal fractures about the knee. *Physician Sportsmed* 1997;25(4):108-121.

76. Salter RB, Harris WR: Injuries involving the epiphyseal plate. *J Bone Joint Surg Am* 1963;45:587-622.

77. Bertin KC, Goble EM: Ligament injuries associated with physeal fractures about the knee. *Clin Orthop* 1983;177:188-195.

78. Marsh JS, Daigneault JP: Ankle injuries in the pediatric population. *Curr Opin Pediatr* 2000;12:52-60.

79. Sullivan JA, Anderson SJ (eds): *Care of the Young Athlete,* Rosemont, IL, American Academy of Orthopaedic Surgeons, American Academy of Pediatrics, 2000.

80. Funk D, Clanton, TO, Bonci CM: Leg, ankle, and foot injuries, in Schenck RC (ed): *Athletic Training and Sports Medicine,* ed 3. Rosemont, IL, American Academy of Orthopaedic Surgeons, 1999, pp 489-523.

81. Micheli LJ, Metzl JD, Di Canzio J, Zurakowski D: Anterior cruciate ligament reconstructive surgery in adolescent soccer and basketball players. *Clin J Sport Med* 1999;9:138-141.

82. Powell JW, Barber-Foss KD: Sex-related injury patterns among selected high school sports. *Am J Sports Med* 2000;28:385-391.

83. Iobst CA, Stanitski CL: Acute knee injuries. *Clin Sports Med* 2000;19:621-635,vi.

84. Matava MJ, Siegel MG: Arthroscopic reconstruction of the ACL with semitendinosus-gracilis autograft in skeletally immature adolescent patients. *Am J Knee Surg* 1997;10:60-69.

85. Hewett TE: Neuromuscular and hormonal factors associated with knee injuries in female athletes: Strategies for intervention. *Sports Med* 2000;29:313-327.

86. Harmon KG, Dick R: The relationship of skill level to anterior cruciate ligament injury. *Clin J Sport Med* 1998;8:260-265.

87. Rozzi SL, Lephart SM, Gear WS, Fu FH: Knee joint laxity and neuromuscular characteristics of male and female soccer and basketball players. *Am J Sports Med* 1999;27:312-319.

88. Teitz CC, Lind BK, Sacks BM: Symmetry of the femoral notch width index. *Am J Sports Med* 1997;25:687-690.

89. Barrett GR, Rose JM, Ried EM: Relationship of anterior cruciate ligament injury to notch width index (a roentgenographic study). *J Miss State Med Assoc* 1992;33:279-283.

90. Good L, Odensten M, Gillquist J: Intercondylar notch measurements with special reference to anterior cruciate ligament surgery. *Clin Orthop* 1991;263:185-189.

91. Wolman RL: Association between the menstrual cycle and anterior cruciate ligament in female athletes [letter]. *Am J Sports Med* 1999;27:270-271.

92. Wojtys EM, Huston LJ, Boynton MD, Spindler KP, Lindenfeld TN: The effect of the menstrual cycle on anterior cruciate ligament injuries in women as determined by hormone levels. *Am J Sports Med* 2002;30:182-188.

93. Kocher MS, Micheli LJ, Gerbino P, Hresko MT: Tibial eminence fractures in children: Prevalence of meniscal entrapment. *Am J Sports Med* 2003;31:404-407.

94. Aichroth PM, Patel DV, Zorrilla P: The natural history and treatment of rupture of the anterior cruciate ligament in children and adolescents: A prospective review. *J Bone Joint Surg Br* 2002;84:38-41.

95. Angel KR, Hall DJ: Anterior cruciate ligament injury in children and adolescents. *Arthroscopy* 1989;5:197-200.

96. Janarv PM, Nystrom A, Werner S, Hirsch G: Anterior cruciate ligament injuries in skeletally immature patients. *J Pediatr Orthop* 1996;16:673-677.

97. McCarroll JR, Rettig AC, Shelbourne KD: Anterior cruciate ligament injuries in the young athlete with open physes. *Am J Sports Med* 1988;16:44-47.

98. Pressman AE, Letts RM, Jarvis JG: Anterior cruciate ligament tears in children: An analysis of operative versus nonoperative treatment. *J Pediatr Orthop* 1997;17:505-511.

99. Werner A, Wild A, Ilg A, Krauspe R: Secondary intra-articular dislocation of a broken bioabsorbable interference screw after anterior cruciate ligament reconstruction. *Knee Surg Sports Traumatol Arthrosc* 2002;10:30-32.

100. Nystrom M, Samimi S, Ha'Eri GB: Two cases of irreducible knee dislocation occurring simultaneously in two patients and a review of the literature. *Clin Orthop* 1992;277:197-200.

101. McCarroll JR, Shelbourne KD, Porter DA, Rettig AC, Murray S: Patellar tendon graft reconstruction for midsubstance anterior cruciate ligament rupture in junior high school athletes: An algorithm for management. *Am J Sports Med* 1994;22:478-484.

102. Barber FA: Anterior cruciate ligament reconstruction in the skeletally immature high-performance athlete: What to do and when to do it? *Arthroscopy* 2000;16:391-392.

103. Koman JD, Sanders JO: Valgus deformity after reconstruction of the anterior cruciate ligament in a skeletally immature patient: A case report. *J Bone Joint Surg Am* 1999;81:711-715.

104. Lastihenos M, Nicholas SJ: Managing ACL injuries in children: Are kids' injuries different? *Physician Sportsmed* 1996;24(4):59-70.

105. Watkins J, Peabody P: Sports injuries in children and adolescents treated at a sports injury clinic. *J Sports Med Phys Fitness* 1996;36:43-48.

106. Hawkins D, Metheny J: Overuse injuries in youth sports: Biomechanical considerations. *Med Sci Sports Exerc* 2001;33:1701-1707.

107. Busch M: Sports medicine, in Morrissy RT, Weinstein SL (eds): *Lovell and Winter's Pediatric Orthopaedics,* ed 4. Philadelphia, PA, Lippincott-Raven, 1996, vol 2, pp 1063-1064.

108. Adirim TA, Cheng TL: Overview of injuries in the young athlete. *Sports Med* 2003;33:75-81.

109. Madden CC, Mellion MB: Sever's disease and other causes of heel pain in adolescents. *Am Fam Physician* 1996;54:1995-2000.

110. Klingele KE, Kocher MS: Little League elbow: Valgus overload injury in the paediatric athlete. *Sports Med* 2002;32:1005-1015.

111. McFarland EG, Ireland ML: Rehabilitation programs and prevention strategies in adolescent throwing athletes. *Instr Course Lect* 2003;52:37-42.

112. Canale ST, Williams KD: Iselin's disease. *J Pediatr Orthop* 1992;12:90-93.

113. Omey ML, Micheli LJ: Foot and ankle problems in the young athlete. *Med Sci Sports Exerc* 1999;31:S470-S486.

114. Peck DM: Apophyseal injuries in the young athlete. *Am Fam Physician* 1995;51:1891-1895,1897-1898.

115. Kujala UM, Orava S, Karpakka J, Leppavuori J, Mattila K: Ischial tuberosity apophysitis and avulsion among athletes. *Int J Sports Med* 1997;18:149-155.

116. The prevention of sport injuries of children and adolescents. *Med Sci Sports Exerc* 1993;25(8 suppl):1-7.

117. Nattiv A, Agostini R, Drinkwater B, Yeager KK: The female athlete triad: The inter-relatedness of disordered eating, amenorrhea, and osteoporosis. *Clin Sports Med* 1994;13:405-418.

118. Manore MM: Nutritional needs of the female athlete. *Clin Sports Med* 1999;18:549-563.

119. Johnson MD: Disordered eating in active and athletic women. *Clin Sports Med* 1994;13:355-369.

120. American Academy of Pediatrics Committee on Sports Medicine and Fitness: Medical concerns in the female athlete. *Pediatrics* 2000;106:610-613.

121. Shangold M, Rebar RW, Wentz AC, Schiff I: Evaluation and management of menstrual dysfunction in athletes. *JAMA* 1990;263:1665-1669.

122. Loucks AB: Effects of exercise training on the menstrual cycle: Existence and mechanisms. *Med Sci Sports Exerc* 1990;22:275-280.

123. Cobb KL, Bachrach LK, Greendale G, et al: Disordered eating, menstrual irregularity, and bone mineral density in female runners. *Med Sci Sports Exerc* 2003;35:711-719.

124. Lloyd T, Triantafyllou SJ, Baker ER, et al: Women athletes with menstrual irregularity have increased musculoskeletal injuries. *Med Sci Sports Exerc* 1986;18:374-379.

125. Cann CE, Martin MC, Genant HK, Jaffe RB: Decreased spinal mineral content in amenorrheic women. *JAMA* 1984;251:626-629.

126. Cann CE, Genant HK, Ettinger B, Gordan GS: Spinal mineral loss in oophorectomized women: Determination by quantitative computed tomography. *JAMA* 1980;244:2056-2059.

127. Drinkwater BL, Nilson K, Chesnut CH III, Bremner WJ, Shainholtz S, Southworth MB: Bone mineral content of amenorrheic and eumenorrheic athletes. *N Engl J Med* 1984;311:277-281.

128. Drinkwater BL, Nilson K, Ott S, Chesnut CH III: Bone mineral density after resumption of menses in amenorrheic athletes. *JAMA* 1986;256:380-382.

129. Warren MP, Brooks-Gunn J, Hamilton LH, Warren LF, Hamilton WG: Scoliosis and fractures in young ballet dancers: Relation to delayed menarche and secondary amenorrhea. *N Engl J Med* 1986;314:1348-1353.

130. Miller KK: Mechanisms by which nutritional disorders cause reduced bone mass in adults. *J Womens Health (Larchmt)* 2003;12:145-150.

131. Kazis K, Iglesias E: The female athlete triad. *Adolesc Med* 2003;14:87-95.

132. Sanborn CF, Horea M, Siemers BJ, Dieringer KI: Disordered eating and the female athlete triad. *Clin Sports Med* 2000;19:199-213.

21

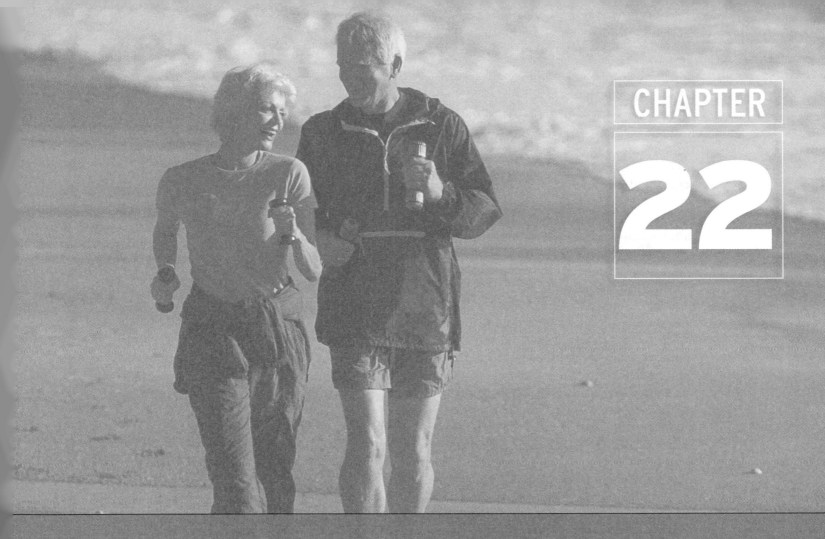

Physical Activity and the Aging Athlete

Paula Sammarone
Turocy, EdD, ATC
Mitchell D. Seemann, MD

Introduction

By 2030, an estimated 70 million individuals in the United States will be aged 65 years and older; persons 85 years and older will be the fastest growing segment of the population.[1] Aging, and its associated structural and functional losses, is a natural process of life. However, aging is an individual process that is influenced by genetic, lifestyle, disease, and other factors.[2] With no control over the genetic factors and very little control over past disease, the only factor influencing aging that can be modified is lifestyle.

The lifestyle goal of many aging individuals is to remain physically active and to participate in sport and fitness activities until late into their lives. This group is referred to by several names, the most common being masters athletes, senior athletes, and older athletes. The age range is 18 years to more than 100 years,[3] with most athletes being older than 35 years.[4] Masters swimming, an organized program of swimming for adults, includes more than 40,000 members who are age 18 years and older.[3] The National Senior Games Association boasts of serving 250,000 constituents, from age 50 years to more than 100 years, in 50 member organizations across the United States.[4] The ever-growing variety of senior athletic events reflects the increased involvement of the aging population in physical activity and athletic participation (**Figure 22-1**).

This group of athletes will be more prominently represented in the population of physically active adults and will require more attention to their needs for injury prevention and enhanced performance. Most athletic health care providers will come in contact with these athletes at organized events, races, local community centers, recreation facilities, and sports medicine facilities and through involvement with senior sport leagues.

Aging accounts for only half of the functional decline that occurs between the ages of 30 and 70 years; deconditioning and disuse account for the other half.[5] Some of the physiologic and structural changes associated with aging include decreases in strength, muscle fibers (affecting type II fibers more than type I), aerobic capacity, stroke volume, cardiac output, and maximum heart rate and reduced amounts of mucopolysaccharides in cartilage, leading to irreversible changes. The rate and magnitude of many of these changes can be reduced through regular participation in exercise. Moderate to vigorous physical activity produces physiologic im-

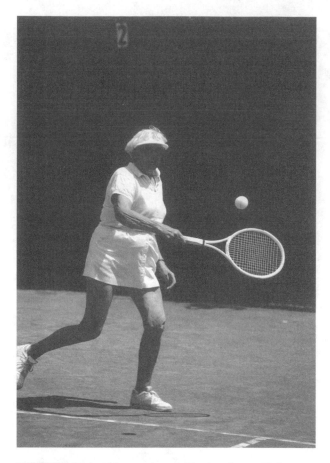

Figure 22-1   The growing number of older Americans adds to the increasing number of persons who remain physically active. (Image © Photodisc.)

provements, regardless of the age of the athlete. Performance improvements in senior athletes require the same commitment to training demanded of younger athletes, with appropriate modifications and safety considerations for changes associated with aging.

Preparticipation and Safety Considerations

Current health status, inherent changes in physiology, and comorbid conditions should be carefully examined and considered when working with aging athletes. All athletes, regardless of age, should receive a complete physical examination before beginning an exercise program. The examination should include a comprehensive medical history, physical examination, and laboratory tests. Laboratory tests include serum chemistry analysis, a complete blood count, a comprehensive lipoprotein profile, and pulmonary function.[6] Other components may include body composition assessment, comprehensive orthopaedic examination, and electrocardiogram and stress tests.[7]

When examining a patient who desires to begin an exercise regimen, the physician should consider the patient's underlying health conditions and medications before determining activity status. As compared with younger athletes, senior athletes are more likely to have other and often multiple health concerns that require special monitoring, medications, and considerations during exercise. Common comorbidities that may affect a senior athlete's activity status include cardiovascular and pulmonary diseases, metabolic diseases, and immunologic and hematologic disorders such as cancer[8] (**Table 22-1**). These conditions often require multiple and possibly interacting medications that could affect exercise.

Other tools used to determine an individual's health and preparedness to begin a physical fitness or sport activity are the Physical Activity Readiness

Comorbidities (Comorbidity)
Pathologic or disease processes that coexist but are unrelated (eg, diabetes and muscle strain)

Table 22-1

Common Comorbid Conditions in Senior Athletes

Category of Disease	Specific Condition	Considerations for Exercise Programming
Cardiovascular	Hypertension	Monitor for signs of cardiorespiratory distress during exercise.
		Cardiorespiratory endurance training should not begin until drug therapy is initiated; training is then performed within 40% to 70% $\dot{V}_{0_{2max}}$.
		Strength or resistive training is not recommended as the only form of exercise, because it places too much stress on the cardiovascular system.
		Resistance training with high resistance and a low number of repetitions may elevate blood pressure; recommend beginning the program with low resistance and a high number of repetitions.
		MEDICATION CONSIDERATIONS[10]:
		Beta blockers reduce heart rate response to submaximal and maximal exercise; therefore, heart rate should not be used to monitor exercise. Perceived exertion scales should be used to gauge intensity of work.
		Beta blockers may contribute to early fatigue in endurance activities.
		Antihypertensive drugs lower exercise blood pressure and increase systolic pressure, while diastolic pressure remains unchanged or decreases slightly.
	Peripheral artery disease	Exercise is not permitted when the athlete has other comorbid conditions that may limit exercise tolerance.
		Monitor for signs of cardiorespiratory distress during exercise.
		Exercise is permitted; however, peripheral pain should be used to gauge exercise intensity. Pain scale: 1 = pain onset, 2 = moderate pain, 3 = intense pain, 4 = maximal pain.
		Initial workouts should include 20 minutes of interval walking or stair climbing 3 times a week at 40% of heart rate reserve. Exercise should stop when pain is assessed at 3/4 and may begin again only when the athlete is recovered fully (pain = 0/4). Over a 6-month period, gradually increase the program to 40 minutes at 70% of **heart rate reserve**.
		Full recovery (no pain) should be achieved between exercise bouts.
		Warm up and cooldown activities should be required before non-weight-bearing tasks to assist circulation.
		MEDICATION CONSIDERATIONS[9]:
		Intermittent **claudication** medications (pentoxifylline, dipyridamole, aspirin, and warfarin) may improve time to claudication but may also cause additional bleeding in the case of injury.
		Beta blockers may decrease time to claudication but may also reduce the ability to use heart rate to monitor intensity; use perceived exertion to evaluate intensity.

Heart rate reserve
Method of determining a safe exercise heart rate (target heart rate) that takes into consideration both age and resting heart rate.

22

Claudication
Ischemia in muscles that results in lameness (limp) and pain.

Table 22-1

Common Comorbid Conditions in Senior Athletes—continued

Category of Disease	Specific Condition	Considerations for Exercise Programming
Metabolic	**Diabetes**	No exercise permitted if • active retinal hemorrhage or recent therapy for retinopathy, or • active illness or infection, or • blood glucose level >250-300 mg/dL and ketones present, or • blood glucose level of 80-100 mg/dL (increased risk of hypoglycemia); ingest carbohydrates to maintain glucose levels Athlete should be monitored for signs of hypoglycemia throughout exercise program. Food intake with exercise is important to maintain blood glucose levels; an additional 15 g of carbohydrates needed either before or after exercise. If exercise is vigorous or of longer duration, an additional 15-30 g of carbohydrate is required every hour to decrease the risk of hypoglycemia. MEDICATION CONSIDERATIONS[10]: **Insulin and hypoglycemic agents** come in many different forms with various onsets, peaks, and hours of effective duration; these medications may cause hypoglycemia in exercising athletes.
Hyperlipidemia	**Hyperlipidemia**	Monitor for signs of cardiorespiratory distress during exercise. Need to control weight and blood lipid levels through low-fat diet and aerobic exercise. Begin moderate exercise 40% to 70% $\dot{V}O_{2max}$ program 5 days a week, once a day for 15 minutes MEDICATION CONSIDERATIONS[9]: No conclusive evidence exists that **antilipemic agents** alone affect the ability to exercise; however, when used in conjunction with 3-hydroxy-3-methylglutaryl coenzyme A reductase inhibitors, they may lead to myopathy.
Immunologic/ Hematologic	**Cancer**	Regular communication with the athlete and physician is essential when working with cancer patients. Recovered patients require monitoring of the exercise program and consultation with physician when appropriate. Postsurgical patients may have resulting pain, loss of flexibility, and motor and sensory damage. Caution should be taken when initiating new activities, assessing injury pain, and using therapeutic modalities. Patients who have received radiation treatments may experience a loss of flexibility in irradiated joints and cardiac or lung scarring that may limit cardiorespiratory capacity. Aerobic exercise may be contraindicated in these patients. MEDICATION CONSIDERATIONS[10]: **Chemotherapy** may cause peripheral nerve damage, cardiomyopathy, pulmonary fibrosis, myopathy, and/or anemia.

Heart rate reserve is calculated by the Karvonen method[6]:
Maximal heart rate (HR_{max}) = 220 − age (±10-12 beats/min)
Resting heart rate (HR_{rest}) = pulse (beats/min) for 1 minute
Target heart rate = ([HR_{max} − HR_{rest}] × 0.55 + HR_{rest}

Adapted with permission from American College of Sports Medicine: *ACSM's Exercise Management for Persons with Chronic Diseases and Disabilities.* Champaign, IL, Human Kinetics, 1997.

Questionnaire (PAR-Q), developed by the Canadian Society for Exercise Physiology, Inc; the American College of Sports Medicine (ACSM) Risk Stratification system[6]; and preexercise field and baseline testing within the seven aspects of fitness: aerobic capacity, anaerobic capacity, cardiorespiratory endurance, strength, flexibility, neuromuscular function, and functional performance.[9]

The PAR-Q was designed to identify adults, aged 15 to 69 years, who should not become involved in exercise programs or who should seek further medical advice before participating and is

Table 22-2

Risk Factors and Associated Signs and Symptoms of Coronary Artery and Pulmonary Disease

Risk Factors for Coronary Artery Disease	Signs and Symptoms of Possible Cardiovascular and Pulmonary Disease
Family history	Pain, discomfort, angina in chest, neck, jaw, arms, or other areas
Cigarette smoking	Shortness of breath at rest or with mild exertion
Hypertension	Dizziness or syncope
Hypercholesterolemia/ hyperlipidemia	Orthopnea or paroxysmal nocturnal dyspnea
Impaired fasting glucose	Ankle edema
Obesity	Palpitations or tachycardia
Sedentary lifestyle	Intermittent claudication
	Known heart murmur
	Unusual fatigue or shortness of breath with activity

Adapted with permission from American College of Sports Medicine: *Exercise Prescription: Exercise Testing and Prescription for Others*, ed 6. Baltimore, MD, Lippincott Williams & Wilkins, 2000, pp 226-229.

Table 22-3

Warm Up and Cooldown Activities

Warm Up Activities	Cooldown Activities
5 to 10 minutes of low-intensity calisthenics and stretching exercises • At least 1 exercise for each major muscle group/joint • Slow, controlled movement (static stretching) • Duration of each stretch: 10 to 30 seconds • Repetitions: 4 (minimum) • Rest interval: 10 to 15 seconds between stretches 5 to 10 minutes of progressive aerobic activity (eg, bicycle riding, brisk walking, or jogging)	Exercises of decreasing intensities (performed until heart rate returns to approximately 40% of heart rate reserve) Stretching exercises as described under Warm Up Activities

Adapted with permission from American College of Sports Medicine: *Exercise Prescription: Exercise Testing and Prescription for Others*, ed 6. Baltimore, MD, Lippincott Williams & Wilkins, 2000, pp 226-229.

considered a minimal standard for entry into moderate-intensity exercise programs.[6] In conjunction with the PAR-Q evaluation, senior athletes also should be evaluated for selected risk factors associated with the development of coronary artery disease (CAD) and for signs or symptoms that may indicate cardiovascular, pulmonary, or metabolic disease (**Table 22-2**). Athletes must also be monitored for signs and symptoms of cardiovascular and pulmonary distress during activity, because these conditions may develop after the initial evaluation.

Individuals of the same age do not necessarily have the same physiology. The degenerative changes associated with age and disuse vary on a continuum; therefore, an athlete's activity status also should be considered on a continuum, and exercise programs should be developed based on individual needs. Although research on elderly individuals has increased and is readily available, research specific to this population of athletes is very limited. Most of the findings described in this chapter, therefore, are based on studies of both the general elderly population and senior athletes.

■ Preparing for Physical Activity— Warm Up and Cooldown

As with younger athletes, exercise in senior athletes should be preceded by a warm-up activity and followed by a cooldown activity (**Table 22-3**). Warm-up activities prepare the body for exercise by improving muscular flexibility and joint range of motion (ROM) and enhancing metabolism and circulation. A warm-up should progress from a 5- to 10-minute session of low-intensity calisthenics and stretch to a 5- to 10-minute session of progressive aerobic activity that allows the body to reach the lower limits of the target heart rate (55% of maximal heart rate) for endurance training.[6] The target heart rate is calculated using the formula in Table 22-1.

Cooldown activities allow the body to return to its resting state by lowering heart rate and blood pressure to resting levels, enhancing venous return, reducing the potential for postexercise hypotension or dizziness, decreasing body heat, and removing lactic acid. Cooldown activities include exercises of diminishing intensities and stretching. Omitting a cooldown immediately after exercise has been associated with an increased incidence of cardiovascular complications.[6] A cooldown should always be incorporated into a senior athlete's exercise program and is especially important in athletes with comorbid conditions that predispose them to cardiovascular distress.

The stretching phase of these activities should involve all major muscle groups. The exercises should incorporate slow, controlled movements such as static stretching, in which the stretch is held for 10 to 30 seconds at the end of the ROM, the point at which the stretch causes minor discomfort but not pain.[11] The athlete should not attempt to push past the point of discomfort, because this is the body's natural protection mechanism. Each stretching exercise should be performed for at least four repetitions per muscle group, with a few seconds of rest between repetitions.[11]

Types of Training

Recommended training routines for older adults include cardiorespiratory endurance (endurance) and muscular training (strength).[6] Although many more facets of physical fitness and training can be incorporated, these two types of exercise are recommended for all older adults. Older, healthy individuals respond similarly to strength and endurance overload as do younger athletes, but overload training for older athletes should be introduced more gradually in the early stages of training.[5] Appropriate exercise can alter, slow, or even partially reverse some of the age-related physiologic changes seen in older athletes, including sarcopenia and decreases in lean muscle mass and force production, and it can create an overall improved mental and physical well-being.[5,12]

An overall training plan for senior athletes should follow **periodization** similar to that in training plans appropriate for younger athletes. Senior athletes can increase the intensity of this generalized exercise program with gradual and correct progression of training. These progressions should be individualized, activity specific, and designed specifically to meet the senior athlete's goals and current health status. Periodization may result in higher levels of strength, muscular power, and muscular endurance, increased speed, and reduced reaction times. The appropriateness and extent of physical adaptation, however, depend on the intensity, frequency, duration, and mode of exercise used by the athlete.

Social support, facility access, availability of appropriate activities, and neighborhood safety influence the amount and type of exercise performed by the senior athlete. Successful senior athletes often seek out other seniors to assist them in maintaining their interest and motivation to participate in sport and recreational activities in their sixth and seventh decades of life.[13]

Cardiorespiratory endurance training is directed at improving the duration of strenuous and aerobic activity ($\dot{V}O_{2max}$) a senior athlete can maintain.[5] Thirty to 50 minutes of aerobic exercise per day, performed 3 to 5 days per week, and one set of re-

Sarcopenia
Progressive decrease in muscle mass and muscle fiber size that is often associated with aging.

Periodization
Organized year-round exercise plan that delineates exercise goals and programming to ensure maximal fitness gains and adequate rest and recovery.

Table 22-4

Health Benefits of Exercise in Seniors

1. Reduces premature mortality from stroke, coronary artery disease, hypertension, diabetes, and some cancers
2. Slows age-associated decline in metabolism
3. Enhances aerobic capacity, improving the ability to manage obesity
4. Correlates with longevity and improved physical and mental well-being
5. Reduces age-related bone loss
6. Increases muscle mass
7. Improves muscular strength and neuromuscular coordination
8. Assists in limiting bone resorption
9. Improves function
10. Reduces the risk of falls

Adapted with permission from Galloway MT, Jokl P: Aging successfully: The importance of physical activity in maintaining health and function. *J Am Acad Orthop Surg* 2000;8:37-44.

---

sistance exercises targeting major muscle groups, performed twice a week, produce significant health benefits in seniors[12] (**Table 22-4**). Senior athletes also experience reduced heart rate and lactate production, as well as decreased perceived exertion at defined $\dot{V}O_{2max}$.[14] Older athletes engaged in vigorous running or other aerobic activities also have lower mortality rates and slower development of disability than their peers who do not exercise.[15]

The increased number of older athletes means that health care providers must understand the aging process and the needs of older individuals who wish to become and remain more active. It also will be incumbent upon health care providers to discover new methods to assist these senior athletes in participating safely while still achieving their personal and activity-related goals.

Structural Changes Associated with Aging

Impairments or injuries to one structural component may influence the health and function of other components. In the senior athlete, however, the effects may be longer lasting, cause more secondary changes elsewhere in the body, or require greater modifications in exercise programs than typically needed in younger athletes. Therefore, when working with senior athletes, an increased emphasis is placed on recognizing conditions and situations that may place the individual at risk while still max-

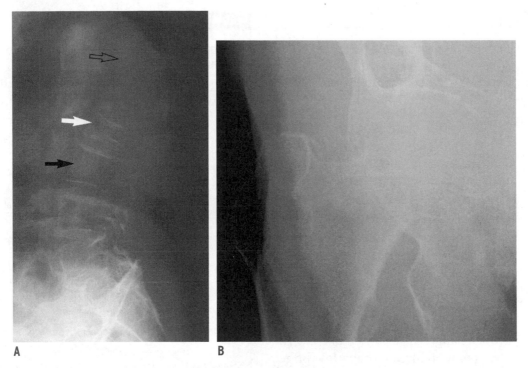

Figure 22-2 Osteoporosis and osteopenia. **A.** Three characteristics of osteoporosis as seen in an 83-year-old woman: "Empty-box" appearance of the vertebra (black arrow) caused by the relative increase in the density of the vertebral endplates; biconcave "codfish" vertebra (white arrow) caused by an expansion of the nucleus pulposus into the weakened endplates; and a wedge-shaped fracture of the vertebra (open arrow). **B.** Antero-posterior radiograph of a 76-year-old woman who demonstrates poor bony detail as the result of osteopenia. (Reproduced with permission from Johnson TR, Steinback LS (eds): *Essentials of Musculoskeletal Imaging.* Rosemont, IL, American Academy of Orthopaedic Surgeons, 2004, pp 14, 81.)

imizing the athlete's performance, minimizing the risks associated with age and inactivity, and delaying the effects of aging.

Bone

By age 18 years, 97% of adult bone mass is achieved; bone density continues to increase until age 30.[16] The amount of bone density achieved by age 18 years and enhanced through moderate exercise in the 20s is the key to maintaining adequate bone density later in life.[16] Bone formation and resorption is a perpetual cycle in younger athletes. Old bone is constantly resorbed through osteoclastic activity, and new bone is deposited in its place. With aging, this process of resorption and redeposition of bone slows, resulting in weakened bone.[17] In women, a decrease in bone mineral density of 0.75% to 1.0% per year begins in the early 30s. This rate may triple after menopause, resulting in a loss of 30% of bone mass before 70 years of age.[11] Men also experience bone mineral loss, decreasing 0.4% per year beginning at age 50 years. However, major injury associated with bone loss is usually not evident until 80 years of age.[12] The risk of osteoporosis-related fractures increases exponentially with age and affects both men and women of all races. In women after menopause to age 85 years, the incidence of vertebral body fractures increases sixfold.[5]

Bone strength is determined by both bone density and bone quality. Bone density is determined by peak bone mass and the amount of bone loss. Bone quality is the structure, turnover, damage (eg, microfractures), and mineralization of bone. The risk of fracture increases when bone mineral density and quality become compromised by osteoporosis and osteopenia, respectively.[18]

Osteoporosis and Osteopenia

Osteopenia, a decrease in the bone mineral density of 1.0 to 2.5 standard deviations below the young adult mean in the hip and lumbar spine, indicates mild to moderate bone deficiency and is often the precursor to osteoporosis[5]; 37% to 50% of women and 28% to 47% of men are diagnosed with osteopenia.[16] Osteoporosis, a bone mass of more than 2.5 standard deviations below the ideal peak bone mass, is characterized by marked bone deficiency and increased risk of fracture[5] (**Figure 22-2**). Of women 50 years or older, 13% to 18% have osteoporosis, as do 3% to 6% of men of the same age, increasing this population's risk of fracture to approximately 1.5 million fractures per year.[16] Several risk factors and behaviors increase the potential to develop osteoporosis (**Table 22-5**).

Bone density Bone mineral content that is determined by a combination of peak bone mass and the amount of bone loss; determining factor for osteoporosis/osteopenia.

Osteoporosis Deterioration of bone tissue resulting in an increased risk of fracture as the result of a low-calcium diet.

Bone strength Strength of bone determined by bone density and bone quality.

Bone quality Structure, turnover, damage/injury, and mineralization of bone.

Osteopenia Decrease in bone mineral density, indicating mild to moderate bone deficiency; often a precursor to osteoporosis.

22

Table 22-5

Risks and Behaviors Associated with Osteoporosis

Risks Associated With Osteoporosis	Behaviors Associated With Osteoporosis
Gender (females > males)	Diet low in calcium and vitamin D
Advanced age	Use of medications (steroids, anticonvulsants, thyroid hormone)
Family history	
Premature menopause	
Hormonal changes (estradiol, testosterone, progesterone, cortisol, parathyroid, thyroxine, growth hormone, insulin)	Sedentary lifestyle
	Cigarette smoking
	Excessive alcohol intake
	High caffeine intake
	High-protein and high-phosphorus diets

Adapted with permission from Lane JM, Nydick M: Osteoporosis: Current modes of prevention and treatment. *J Am Acad Orthop Surg* 1999;7:31.

Table 22-6

Weight-bearing Activities to Preserve or Increase Skeletal Mass

Type of Activity	Examples of Appropriate Activities
Impact	• Jogging, walking, climbing stairs
	• Trampoline bouncing, dance, aerobics
	• Racquet sports: tennis, squash, racquetball
	• Field sports: soccer, lacrosse, field hockey
	• Court sports: basketball, volleyball
Strength development	• Multijoint exercises[15]
	50% of 1 RM* or 70% of 3 RM
	2-3 sets of 8 repetitions
	2 days a week for 20-40 minutes
	• Axial and core exercises (caution: trunk flexion)
Balance	• Proprioceptive exercises, tai chi, yoga, dance

*RM indicates repetition maximum.
Adapted with permission from Williams GN, Higgins MJ, Lewek MD: Aging skeletal muscle: Physiologic changes and the effects of training. *Phys Ther* 2002;82:26-28.

Osteoporotic changes are a particular concern for senior athletes who already have low bone mass or who begin their physical activities after age 50 years. For seniors who were physically active throughout their lives, osteoporosis is much less of a concern, because physical activity counteracts the demineralization of bone.[2] Seniors with low bone mass but without additional risk factors also have a reduced chance of developing an osteoporotic (low-energy) fracture; however, athletes demonstrating only modest bone loss (osteopenia) may be at greater risk of developing a fracture.[5] Risk factors include low body weight (less than 85% of ideal), recent loss of body weight (10 lb), history of low-energy fractures, history of low-energy familial fractures in siblings or parent, and a history of smoking or use of certain medications, including corticosteroids and chemotherapy.[5]

Exercise and Bone

Preventing osteoporosis is important for senior athletes because the two most critical factors of osteoporotic fracture, attainment of peak bone mass and the prevention of postmenopausal resorption, are influenced by the person's behaviors.[13] Peak bone mass is achieved during the late 20s.[5,14] Personal behaviors and conditions, such as lack of weight-bearing exercise, inadequate caloric intake, abnormal menstrual status, and inadequate calcium intake (<1,000 mg/d) and vitamin D intake (<400 U/d) that may occur during childhood, adolescence, and into the college years, influence the athlete's ability to achieve peak mass and should be corrected as soon as recognized.[5] If bone loss persists, individualized therapy and intervention may include the use of antiresorptive agents (eg, hormone replacement

therapy, calcium, vitamin D), bone-stimulating agents, and weight-bearing exercise.

Exercises requiring weight bearing are most effective in preserving and increasing skeletal mass.[5] The most effective weight-bearing exercises require impact loading, strength development, and balance (**Table 22-6**). Impact-loading exercises directly stimulate osteoblastic formation and deter resorption, whereas strengthening exercises affect the bones underlying the exercised muscles. Balance exercises assist in maintaining correct body mechanics and decrease the incidence of falls.[5] Results of partial weight-bearing activities such as swimming, water aerobics, and kayaking in preserving strength and increasing skeletal mass are mixed. However, these activities do assist with strength development and should not be discounted. These alternative exercises also can be used in place of impact-loading exercises for athletes who have arthritic joint changes. Caution is necessary for strengthening exercises that require trunk flexion, because these activities increase the loads across the vertebral bodies and may result in stresses that exceed the capacity of the bone.[5]

■ Joints

Stiffness, loss of flexibility, decreased ROM, and degenerative joint changes occur in the aging population.[12] These functional changes are associated with changes in the structure and function of collagen. Collagen is present in all joint components: articular cartilage of bone, tendons, and ligaments. Decreased collagen solubility, tendon flexibility, and strength result from age-dependent biochemical and biomechanical changes in the structure of collagen.[16] The subsequent structural stiffness and weakness predispose the athlete to sprains, strains, and tendinitis. A history of sprains or strains also adds to the senior athlete's risk of joint injury. Previous joint injuries result in permanent disturbances to the normal stress-strain characteristics of collagen fibers, causing irreversible changes and increased joint stiffness and susceptibility to stretching injuries.[2]

In addition to collagen changes in ligaments and tendons, the senior athlete also experiences changes in the collagen matrix of articular cartilage. Normal articular cartilage has a unique load-support mechanism that protects the bone by shielding the collagen matrix from excessive stresses and reducing friction at the articular surfaces by decreasing shear and compressive forces.[19] In the aging athlete, the amount of mucopolysaccharides decreases, leading to reduced water content in the matrix.[12] These changes result in fibrillation, thinning, and ultimately loss of articular cartilage, which reduce function and further stress the already stressed joint.[2,18] These changes in joint structure and mechanics make senior athletes more susceptible to osteoarthrosis, osteoarthritis, and degenerative joint disease.[2,12]

Osteoarthritis (Degenerative Joint Disease)

Arthritis is a general term encompassing more than 100 different rheumatologic diseases that affect the joints and, sometimes, muscle and other tissues. The two most common types of arthritis are osteoarthritis (degenerative joint disease) and rheumatoid arthritis[9] (**Figure 22-3**). Symptoms of arthritis include stiffness, pain, and swelling in joints, making routine daily tasks difficult.

Osteoarthritis is the most common form of arthritis, with most individuals displaying some pathologic changes in weight-bearing joints by age 40 years. Twenty-five percent of that population has some pain or disability related to osteoarthritis.[20] The common signs and symptoms of osteoarthritis include complaints of morning stiffness (usually <30 minutes in duration), crepitus, joint effusion, increased tissue temperature, bone tenderness, decreased ROM, and hypertrophic bony changes.[21] Weight-bearing activities worsen these symptoms, and rest improves them.

Opinions conflict as to the cause of osteoarthritis. Factors that increase the risk for development of osteoarthritis include genetic predisposition and secondary causes of chronic joint instability, prior surgical procedures to remove tissue, obesity, injury, infection, lack of activity, crystalline disease, malalignment, and other anatomic derangements.[20,22] Normal joints have low coefficients of friction and do not wear out with typical use and trauma. Senior athletes with internal joint derangements or other secondary risk factors, however, must be advised to be more careful of their joints, limiting themselves to moderate- to low-impact activities.[19] Both athletes and nonathletes involved in long-term, vigorous weight-bearing exercise, have similar risks for the development of osteoarthritis.[9]

In the early stages of osteoarthritis, bone begins to replace the cartilaginous surface, changing the physical properties of the cartilage. The bone becomes stiffer and less yielding, resulting in conditions ranging from less serious inflammatory synovitis and bony osteophytosis to more serious subchondral pressure, bone angina, subchondral microfractures, and periostitis.[21] As the condition worsens, the resulting fibroblastic and osteoblastic cellular reactions cause further roughening, pitting, and irregularities in the cartilaginous surface. This

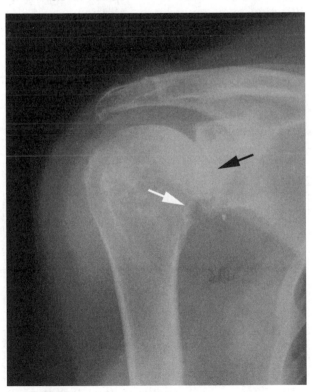

Figure 22-3 Rheumatoid arthritis of the glenohumeral joint. The characteristic findings of rheumatoid arthritis include the loss of joint space (black arrow), erosive changes in the medial humeral neck (white arrow), and the absence of osteophytes. (Reproduced with permission from Johnson TR, Steinbach LS (eds): *Essentials of Musculoskeletal Imaging*. Rosemont, IL, American Academy of Orthopaedic Surgeons, 2004, p 224.)

22

increased wear on the cartilaginous surface lessens the ability of the cartilage to dissipate the force across the whole surface, increasing stress on the rim of the cartilage and the edges of the pitted areas. As the wear continues, the gaps in the cartilage get bigger, exposing more bone; complete loss of cartilage can result, leaving only eburnated bony surfaces.[23] Soft-tissue structures in and around the arthritic joint also are affected. The synovium may become inflamed, the joint becomes stiffer, and the associated musculature becomes weakened.[19] The articular cartilage has no innervation, so the pain associated with this condition is a result of irritation of the exposed nerves in the periosteum.

Eburnated A change in bone density causing it to become hard; resembling ivory.

Management of Osteoarthritis

Degenerative joint disease is managed either surgically or nonsurgically. The nonsurgical approach is the most common and is based on the athlete's pain level and function. The standard approach follows the traditional four-stage rehabilitation plan (**Table 22-7**).

The goal of stage 1 is to control inflammation, improve ROM, and reeducate muscles.[21] The use of nonsteroidal anti-inflammatory drugs (NSAIDs) and, to a lesser degree, intra-articular corticosteroid injections may control pain. Effusion should also be controlled via cryotherapy, elevation, and compression.[21] In stage 2, open kinetic chain and non–weight-bearing exercises are introduced. These exercises are designed to retrain the musculature to protect the joint and prepare it for weight bearing. Isometric exercises are progressed to isotonic exercise within comfortable ROMs (**Figure 22-4**).

Overall cardiovascular conditioning that does not irritate the affected joint (eg, swimming, cycling, kayaking) also is emphasized in this phase. In stage 3, the athlete progresses to closed kinetic chain exercises with increased ROM. Nonirritating, sport-specific exercises and movements can be introduced in this phase. In stage 4, rehabilitation is geared toward return to sport or function. Activities are increased as tolerated; however, progression must not be too quick during this phase. Recovery time for a senior athlete is slower than that for an adolescent or younger athlete. Emphasis also should be placed on correct technique and eliminating the predisposing causes or conditions that contribute to injury.[21] Athletes should be counseled to avoid hard surfaces and high-impact activities and encouraged to use shock-absorbing insoles.[16]

Vigorous exercise is contraindicated in joints with acute inflammation or uncontrolled systemic disease. Heating arthritic joints and initiating proper warm-up activities before exercise, as well as performing cooldown activities and using cold therapy after exercise, may help to keep arthritic joints asymp-

Table 22-7

Rehabilitation Plan for Athletes with Osteoarthritis

Stage of Rehabilitation	Goal of Stage
Stage 1 (acutely symptomatic)	Reduce swelling, control inflammation, manage pain, improve range of motion, reeducate muscles
Stage 2	Retrain muscles to protect joint and prepare for weight bearing; improve cardiovascular fitness as tolerated
Stage 3	Progress strength development and introduce more sport-specific activities
Stage 4	Return to sport and function

Reproduced with permission from Felson DT, Lawrence RC, Dieppe PA, et al: Osteoarthritis: New insights. Part I: The disease and its risk factors. *Ann Intern Med* 2000;133:635-646.

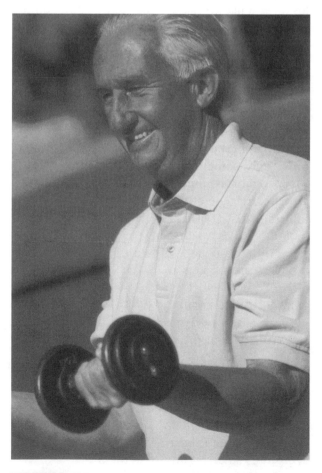

Figure 22-4 Light isotonic (free-weight) exercises are used as a transition between stage 1 and stage 3 rehabilitation exercises. (Image © Photodisc.)

tomatic.[22] Health and safety recommendations that must be considered when working with senior athletes with arthritis are shown in **Table 22-8**.

Rehabilitation programs are often accompanied by regimented pharmaceutical intervention plans. Aging athletes with osteoarthritis may be treated using five different types of medications—acetaminophen, NSAIDs, chondroprotective oral supplements, corticosteroid injections, and viscosupplementation—designed to decrease inflammation and associated pain and to encourage matrix and synovial fluid normalization within a joint (see chapter 4 for further discussion of these medications).[23]

Acetaminophen is an analgesic agent that relieves pain with few side effects. NSAIDs have both anti-inflammatory and analgesic properties that are prescribed to manage swollen, painful joints. Their role is to block the production of proinflammatory agents; however, associated side effects include decreasing the protective effects of prostaglandins on the gastric mucosal lining, renal blood flow, and sodium balance. A temporary platelet effect lengthens bleeding times, but this effect is reversed 24 hours after the medication is discontinued.[25]

The chondroprotective oral supplements, glucosamine and chondroitin, have become increasingly more popular; glucosamine is thought to stimulate chondrocyte and synoviocyte metabolism, whereas chondroitin inhibits degradative enzymes and prevents the formation of fibrin thrombi in periarticular tissues.[25] Intra-articular corticosteroid injections also are helpful for patients whose conditions fail to improve with anti-inflammatory therapy or who have contraindications to the use of acetaminophen or NSAIDs. When injected, corticosteroids are potent anti-inflammatory agents that have very low risk for systemic side effects or complications; however, this treatment is contraindicated in patients with recent fractures, microtrauma, or suspected septic joints.[25] Finally, viscosupplementation is an injectable treatment that is designed to add to the concentrations of hyaluronate available in osteoarthritic joints in hopes of improving elastoviscosity, making the synovial fluid more effective in absorbing joint loads and lubricating articular surfaces.[25] When a senior athlete is taking these medications, the potential side effects must be recognized and proper referral made back to the athlete's physician as needed.

Arthritic athletes need to be observed for signs and symptoms that the exercise program is too vigorous or beyond their level of tolerance. These signs and symptoms include unusual or persistent fatigue, increased weakness, decreased ROM, increased joint swelling, and pain lasting longer than 1 hour after exercise.[24] Athletes with these signs or symptoms should be restricted from activities and an appropriate rehabilitation program initiated. The workout program and other activities in which the athlete is involved should be reviewed and modified to better suit the athlete's joint health and abilities.[9]

Joint Replacement (Arthroplasty)

As more older individuals decide to remain active, it is logical to assume that more senior athletes will attempt to return to sport after joint replacement. Currently in the United States, more than 500,000 individuals have knee and hip joint replacements,[26] and the numbers of ankle procedures increase as the quality of ankle arthroplasties improves.[27]

Joint replacement involves removing diseased joint cartilage and a small amount of underlying bone and replacing those surfaces with metal and plastic[16] (**Figure 22-5**). A metal portion of the arthrosis is affixed to bone, and a plastic component recreates the load-bearing surfaces of the joint.[26] Although the load-bearing surfaces of the ankle are smaller than those of the hip or knee, weight bearing in the ankle is estimated at 1.5 to 7 times the athlete's normal body weight, depending on the activity.[27]

Artificial joints do not have the same ability to adapt to the stresses of sport movement as do normal joints. Even the simplest movements of walking cause microscopic wearing of the plastic components of the replacement joint, thereby shortening the lifespan of the joint replacement.[26] The

---

Table 22-8

Recommendations for Exercise Programming

1. Select low-impact activities and avoid stair climbing, jogging, and running activities if arthritis of the hip or knee is present.

2. Include flexibility and joint range-of-motion exercises, but avoid overstretching and causing hypermobility in joints.

3. Reduce loads on joints when possible (aquatic exercise, biking, rowing).

4. Use activities of low intensity and duration during the initial training phases.

5. If necessary, have the athlete perform several shorter exercise sessions throughout the day instead of a single, long session.

6. Interval training may be more comfortable for the athlete than continuous training.

7. Set time goals, rather than distance goals, to control the pace of activity.

Adapted with permission from American College of Sports Medicine: *ACSM's Exercise Management for Persons with Chronic Diseases and Disabilities.* Champaign, IL, Human Kinetics, 1997.

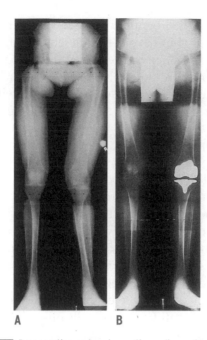

A   B

Figure 22-5 Preoperative and postoperative radiographs of a total knee arthroplasty (TKA). **A.** Preoperative radiograph demonstrating a valgus deformity of the left knee. **B.** Postoperative radiograph after TKA showing proper alignment of the knee. (Reproduced with permission from Favorito PJ, Mihalko WM, Krackow KA: Total knee arthroplasty in the valgus knee. *J Am Acad Orthop Surg* 2002;10:16-24.)

Table 22-9

Exercise Guidelines Following Arthroplasty

Activities Permitted After Joint Replacement Surgery	Prior Experience Needed to Participate After Arthroplasty?
Stationary bicycling, dancing, golf, swimming, walking, doubles tennis	No
Low-impact aerobics, road bicycling, bowling, hiking, horseback riding, cross-country skiing	Yes

Adapted with permission from Sherbondy PS: Stay active after joint replacement: Fit society page. *Exerc Older Adult* Summer 2003;6,11.

lifespan can be further shortened by continued sport or recreational activities. Age, activity level, and the complexity of the surgery affect the success and lifespan of a replacement joint.[28] Several other complications are associated with joint replacements. The interface between the bone and the implant may break down, resulting in implant loosening. The implant can break or dislocate, and the bone can fracture above or below the implant.[26]

The patient should fully understand all the ramifications of the procedure before the surgery. Before surgery, the orthopaedic surgeon must discuss the desired outcomes and the potential complications of postsurgical activity. The patient should identify the level of activity desired after surgery, and the orthopaedic surgeon must inform the athlete if the goals and expectations are realistic and possible.[26]

When making decisions about a patient's sport participation after arthroplasty, the physician must consider the patient's prior experience with the desired activity.[26] After joint replacement surgery, it is more realistic for a patient to continue with existing exercises or sports than to begin a new activity. Many physicians do not encourage beginning a new sport activity after joint replacement surgery.[26] Guidelines for return to function for athletes with joint replacements are shown in **Table 22-9**; how-

ever, the condition of each patient should be evaluated and recommendations determined on a case-by-case basis. Regardless of past athletic experience, athletes are advised not to return to high-impact sports, including racquetball, singles tennis, football, basketball, and softball or heavy lifting, carrying, or intensive manual labor activities after arthroplasty. Opinions vary on return to weight training and downhill skiing.[26]

Exercise and Joints

Aging increases crystallinity of collagen fibers, resulting in increased collagen-fiber diameter that reduces the fiber's extensibility.[1] Exercise improves joint mobility, decreases joint stiffness, and allows muscles to assist with joint mobility. Stronger muscles allow for normal joint mechanics, thereby decreasing the mechanical stressors that may facilitate injury.[2] Flexibility is the key to maintaining acceptable musculoskeletal function, balance, and agility in older adults; the level of function plays an important role in decreasing muscle and tendinous injury, as well as improving overall activity-specific abilities.[23] Flexibility programs are effective in improving joint ROM in older adults who participate in regular exercise.[1] Flexibility exercises should be performed at least 2 to 3 days per week as part of the warm-up and cooldown activities described earlier in this chapter.

The health and function of articular cartilage depend on compression and release of weight.[23] All seniors should remain as active as possible to provide for better nutrition of the cartilage and to slow the decline associated with the lack of movement in the weight-bearing joints. It also is important to strengthen the muscles that support a joint and to stretch the soft tissues that may limit or alter the ROM of a joint. Modifications in the athlete's activities also may be indicated, including more opportunities for cross-training activities, replacing high-impact activities with low-impact or no-impact activities such as swimming or bicycling, and eliminating activities that cause pain (eg, performing squats).[29]

Muscles

Sport and recreational activities require high levels of muscle performance, regardless of age.[30] The changes in skeletal muscle associated with aging demand special consideration in senior athletes. Muscle mass decreases 15% to 30% by age 80 years, with most of that loss occurring in the type II (fast-twitch) muscle fibers.[5,17,19, 31-37] This decrease in muscle mass is characterized by a 40% decrease in total muscle area and a 39% decrease in total muscle fiber.[31] Lost tendon flexibility and increased muscle stiffness accompany the aging process. This increased muscle stiffness can occur as a result of changes in muscle tone (actin-myosin cross-linking) or alterations in the extracellular matrix (collagen), or both. Age-related matrix changes result from both biochemical and biomechanical changes that decrease tendon flexibility and strength.[12]

Sarcopenia is the phenomenon of muscle-mass loss that occurs as a result of reduced sizes and numbers of muscle fibers.[5,12] The underlying causes for this reduction in muscle are still unclear.[32] Regardless of the cause, all seniors are affected by this loss, as the size of a muscle and its ability to create force are highly correlated.[17] A loss of muscle mass can decrease mechanical function (generating force, power, or braking movements), reduce the muscle's role as a dynamic metabolic store that affects an athlete's maximum aerobic capacity, and limit the protection muscle mass provides for the skeleton.[5,32]

Age-related muscular changes present the senior athlete with many more challenges not typically experienced by younger athletes. Although senior athletes are no more prone to injuries than younger athletes who train a comparable amount,[12,19] aging skeletal muscle is damaged more easily with loading than is skeletal muscle in younger athletes. Therefore, senior athletes often are more susceptible to muscular injuries and soreness after exercise.[5]

Tendinitis and muscle strains are the most common diagnoses in athletes of all ages.[12] Most overuse injuries result from training errors. Training errors are more prevalent in senior athletes beginning new activities and are related to the total volume of activity and the adaptive abilities of the aging muscle and tendon.[12] More than 80% of all injuries resolve uneventfully, and less than 5% of all senior athletic injuries require surgical intervention.[12]

Recovery from injury is an important consideration for any athlete. However, little research exists on how senior athletes recover. Symptoms and athletic disability last longer than in younger athletes, and senior athletes appear to require more time to recover.[12] Yet healing time does not differ for overuse and acute injuries in senior athletes, unlike these injuries in younger athletes.[12]

Age is not the only factor to affect the healing process. Degenerative joint changes in response to injuries incurred in youth or as a result of current training practices also may adversely affect recovery.[2] To prevent additional debilitating injuries in senior athletes, all injuries should be treated promptly. Injuries that would normally have little impact on sedentary, aging individuals can cause considerable debilitation in a senior athlete.[2] Unfortunately, aging athletes tend not to consult physicians immediately after they are injured. They wait to see if the symptoms resolve themselves, allowing injuries to become chronic before treatment is begun.[33] Like their younger counterparts, senior athletes are reluctant to discontinue their exercise regimens or participation in competition.[2] Essential to the athlete's ability to return to activity are a correct diagnosis, an active and progressive rehabilitation program, modification and correction of technique, allowing sufficient time for full recovery (including alternative training methods) to prevent the senior athlete from becoming immobile, taping or bandaging to assist with proprioception and stability, and the use of anti-inflammatory medications.[2,33] In the senior athlete, surgery should always be the last resort.

Common injuries to the senior athlete are consistent with the types and locations of those found in younger athletes who train with comparable methods. Again, with few published, comprehensive epidemiologic studies of injuries to senior athletes, little evidence exists beyond the anecdotal to support an increased incidence of one type of injury over another. The only general statement that can be made is that a history of injury and decreases in muscular strength and proprioception change the normal mechanics of all joints and increase the risk of joint and muscular injury.

Exercise and Muscles

Resistance training is as important for older athletes as it is for younger athletes in preventing injury and improving performance. Senior athletes can increase overall strength with training, resulting in hypertrophy and an associated increase in the volume of type I and type II fibers. The hypertrophy can be as extensive as in younger athletes, but the strength developed is in proportion to the number and relative sizes of the muscle fibers activated. Exercise training increases the proficiency of muscle-fiber recruitment, with evidence of increased dendrite arborization. Early changes in strength occur as a result of an overall increase in the neural factors responsible for strength; however, a regular regimen of strength training not only enhances the neurologic functions of muscle, it also assists in preserving the functional reaction time of muscle.[5]

Maximal strain and tendon-aponeurosis stiffness increase with age. Viscosity decreases, but low-load resistance training improves the elasticity of the tendon-aponeurosis structures.[34] The ability to train muscle is unaffected by age, even in the oldest athletes. The senior athlete can improve muscle mass up to 15% with correct training.[14] This increase in muscle mass results from an improved rate of resting protein turnover that occurs with strength training.[35]

One caution for strength training in this population is that eccentric exercise causes more pronounced skeletal muscle damage in senior athletes than in younger athletes. This damage results in greater rates of myofibrillar protein breakdown.[36] Vitamin E supplementation may improve the rate of muscle repair after muscle damage from exercise,[36] but senior athletes should limit the amount of eccentric muscle work included in both training and rehabilitation programs.

Resistance-training programs for senior athletes must be individualized and consider the patient's current health, fitness status, and fitness goals.[6] Programs should incorporate all the same safety considerations as weight programs used by younger athletes with regard to ROM, slow and rhythmic movements, and proper breathing techniques.[6,12] Senior athletes should incorporate more multijoint than single-joint exercises and consider using machines over free weights to ensure correct and safe technique.[6] Arthritic athletes should not participate in strength training during periods of active pain or inflammation.[6]

The maximum strength (1-repetition maximum, or 1 RM) must be established before beginning a strength program. To ensure safety, submaximal predictors should be used to determine weight as opposed to direct measurement methods.[6] Senior athletes may require a longer adaptation phase when initiating a periodized weight-training program to allow muscle and connective tissue to adjust.[6] When returning from a period away from exercise, the senior athlete should begin at a level of 50% or less of previous training, gradually increasing to prior levels. When overloads are introduced, increases in the

Table 22-10
American College of Sports Medicine Guidelines for Initiating Resistance Training in the Senior Athlete
8-10 exercises
Program should not exceed 60 minutes; average program length should be 20-30 minutes
Exercises should incorporate major muscle groups: gluteals, hamstrings, pectorals, latissimus dorsi, deltoids, and abdominals
1 set of 10-15 repetitions at an exertion level perceived as "somewhat hard"
Workouts should occur at a minimum of twice a week with a minimum 48-hour rest interval between workouts
Adapted with permission from American College of Sports Medicine: *Exercise Prescription: Exercise Testing and Prescription for Others*, ed 6. Baltimore, MD, Lippincott Williams & Wilkins, 2000, pp 226-229.

number of exercise repetitions should occur before the resistance lifted is increased.[6]

The American College of Sports Medicine has developed recommendations for senior athletes beginning weight-training programs[6] (**Table 22-10**). After weight training is introduced, a plan for periodization should be developed and adapted for the specific needs of the athlete; however, caution should be taken to ensure that the athlete avoids performing too many sets or loads that are near the 1 RM.

■ Proprioception

The function and adaptability of the somatosensory system in the senior athlete are specifically related to muscular function. The somatosensory system is the peripheral afferent motor mechanism related to postural control.[37] It provides information to the body on the orientation of body segments to one another and to the support surface. Input to the somatosensory system is classified as either tactile or proprioceptive and comes from the peripheral sensory receptors located in the skin, muscles, and joints.[37] Improved proprioception in athletes is a growing area of research that has a direct impact on athletic performance. Proprioception is defined as a specialized variation of touch that encompasses the sensation of joint movement (kinesthesia) and joint position (static joint position sense).[37]

Senior athletes have demonstrable alterations in proprioception and vestibular function that occur as a result of changes in the central nervous system, the peripheral nervous system, and the senses of sight, hearing, and taste. These changes include cortical atrophy, associated with a 20% decline in neurotransmitter levels and cerebral blood flow,

Table 22-11

Methods to Improve Proprioception

Level of Central Nervous System Motor Activation	Activities to Enhance Performance
Spinal cord	Adjustments to sudden changes in joint position
Brainstem	Balance exercises
Neuromuscular	Plyometric exercises

Adapted with permission from Griffin LY: Neuromuscular training and injury prevention in sports. *Clin Orthop* 2003;409:53-60.

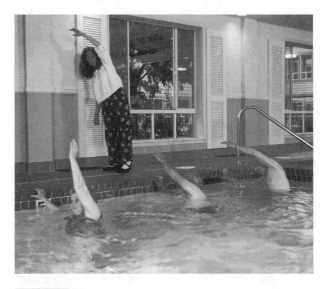

Figure 22-6 Aquatic exercises can provide resistance without overloading the joint's articular surfaces. (Image © Photodisc.)

and a 10% to 15% decrease in nerve conduction velocity.[14,31] Decreased nerve-conduction velocities impair coordinated complex motor activities and maintenance of balance and slow reaction time up to 20% over younger athletes.[2,26,38] Proprioception deteriorates with age, and at least one group concluded that changes in proprioception may be a sensitive method for detecting subclinical osteoarthritis.[38] A theory currently being evaluated is that changes in proprioception result in changes in joint function that may lead to degenerative joint disease. These changes correlate with changes in muscle fiber types[31] and directly affect the performance of both the activities of daily living and sports.

Exercise and Proprioception

To enhance proprioceptive-mediated neuromuscular controls, rehabilitation and conditioning programs should be structured to address all three levels of central nervous system motor activation: the spinal cord, brainstem, and neuromuscular levels (**Table 22-11**).[37] Spinal cord reflexes can be improved by emphasizing activities that necessitate reflex, neuromuscular-controlled responses to sudden alterations in joint positioning. Postural (balance) exercises should be incorporated to enhance motor function at the brainstem level, and repeating motor patterns (plyometrics) should be added to assist in converting conscious to unconscious motor patterns. Plyometric work improves neuromuscular control and feed-forward processing.[37]

Special precautions should be incorporated for senior athletes when neuromuscular control work involves plyometrics. Because of the effects of impact and the potential harm that could result to aging bones and joints, alternative environments and surfaces, such as pools or unweighting devices, and lower-impact activities should be incorporated (**Figure 22-6**). Plyometric activities should be avoided in senior athletes who have arthritis or joint re-

placement or who may experience adverse effects from the workouts.

Cardiopulmonary Function

A final consideration for the senior athlete is cardiopulmonary function. Many significant changes in cardiopulmonary structure and function associated with aging play a role in the performance and health of the senior athlete. Decreased aerobic performance, total lung and vital capacities, inspiratory air flow and maximum blood flow, and expiratory air flow and increased residual volumes and ventilation perfusion result.[2] The structural changes associated with these physiologic and performance changes include increased vascular stiffness, endothelial cell degeneration, increased left ventricular thickness, increased circumference of cardiac valves, and a thicker aorta and arterial tree. These alterations result in lengthened contraction duration and an increased refractory period, decreased vascular tone, and decreased dilation of arterioles in response to the stimulus of physical activity.[14] The physiologic responses to these changes include reduced responsiveness of the cardiovascular system, which results in lower heart rates at submaximal and maximal work loads, as well as decreased arterial vasodilation. Resting heart rate remains the same, but maximal attainable heart rate declines.[13] The result is a drop in $\dot{V}O_{2max}$ and limits in cardiac output and maximum aerobic capacity; $\dot{V}O_{2max}$ and heart rate are directly correlated.[2]

These structural and functional changes place the senior athlete at increased risk of developing coronary artery disease or manifesting congenital

22

or acquired heart disease (eg, hypertrophic cardiomyopathy, aortic stenosis) and arrhythmias and conduction abnormalities (eg, atrial fibrillation and flutter, atrioventricular block).[7] Senior athletes, particularly males, are at four times greater risk of experiencing these changes than are college-aged athletes, although the absolute risk of a major event during physical activity is small in asymptomatic patients who do not have known heart disease.[7] Nevertheless, masters athletes with moderate- to high-risk profiles for coronary artery disease and who desire to enter vigorous competitive situations should undergo preparticipation exercise testing.

Preparticipation cardiovascular testing should be a part of every senior athlete's preparticipation physical examination. The examination should include methods to identify occult cardiovascular diseases that can cause sudden cardiac death, nonfatal myocardial infarction, stroke, angina, acute coronary syndromes, and heart failure brought on by intense athletic activity or abrupt burst exertion[7] (**Table 22-12**). The American Heart Association Consensus Panel recommended that all examinations include a review of family history, with special attention to premature sudden death and heart disease in surviving relatives. Athletes who have a personal history of heart murmur, systemic hypertension, fatigability, syncope, exertional dyspnea, or exertional chest pain should undergo a physical examination that checks for heart murmurs (taken both sitting and standing), femoral pulses, stigmata of Marfan syndrome, and blood pressure.[7]

Exercise and Cardiopulmonary Function

Endurance training improves the oxidative capacity of aging skeletal muscle and has demonstrated benefits for senior athletes.[5] Regular aerobic exercise offers many health benefits, may reduce the risk of fatal and nonfatal myocardial infarctions and other coronary events, and is involved in preventing primary and secondary cardiovascular disease.[7]

Aerobic activities involve continuous, rhythmic movements performed for a minimum of 15 minutes that are designed to stimulate aerobic metabolism and improve cardiorespiratory function. These activities may involve upper, lower, and combined

Ischemia Insufficient blood supply to an area as a result of a mechanical obstruction (blood vessel narrowing) of the blood supply

Table 22-12

Participation Considerations for Specific Cardiac Conditions

Condition	Participation Consideration
Documented ischemic heart disease	Restrict high-intensity competitive sports
	May participate in low-intensity competitive sports (eg, golf, bowling)
Impaired left ventricular systolic function under resting conditions	Restrict high-intensity competitive sports
Evidence of exercise-induced myocardial **ischemia**, including angina, abnormal electrocardiogram, or abnormal imaging findings with exercise testing	Restrict high-intensity competitive sports
Evidence of exercise-induced frequent or complex supraventricular or ventricular arrhythmias, including nonsustained ventricular tachycardia	Restrict high-intensity competitive sports
Exercise-induced systolic hypotension	Restrict high-intensity competitive sports
Moderate to severe systemic hypertension (stage 2 or 3)	Avoid high-intensity static competitive sports (eg, weight lifting, gymnastics)
Congenital and valvular heart disease conditions	Avoid high-intensity sports and confine competition to low-intensity sports
Cardiomyopathy or arrhythmogenic right ventricular cardiomyopathy	No competitive sports
Myocarditis (with and without dilated cardiomyopathy)	May return to competition when there is no longer evidence of active infection (usually 6 months)
Chagas' disease	Unrestricted sports competition if no objective signs or symptoms of cardiac involvement are evident (and resting and exercise electrocardiograms are normal)
Athletes using cardioactive drugs	Discuss competitive sports interests and needs with physician; however, drugs may impair performance during intense competitive sports
Mild atherosclerosis, normal left ventricular function, and no inducible ischemia or arrhythmias	May be able to participate in more vigorous competitive sports but should be decided on individual basis

Adapted with permission from Maron BJ, Araujo GS, Thompson PD, et al: Recommendations for preparticipation screening and the assessment of cardiovascular disease in masters athletes. *Circulation* 2001;103:327-334.

upper and lower body activities that are performed at a designated intensity. Factors to consider before determining the type and level of exercise intensity are the individual's level of fitness, medications that may influence heart rate (eg, beta blockers), risks of cardiovascular and orthopaedic injury associated with higher intensity exercise programs, individual preferences for exercise, and individual program goals and objectives.[6] The athlete must not exercise at intensity levels exceeding the maximum heart rate ($HR_{max} = 220 - $ age) as described earlier in this chapter. Athletes who exceed this level place unsafe and potentially harmful stresses on the cardiorespiratory system; activities that cause the athlete to exceed the HR_{max} should be stopped immediately and modified to ensure safe participation.

To ensure a safe aerobic exercise plan, the athlete must be aware of his or her heart rate throughout the exercise program. To minimize medical problems and promote long-term compliance, cardiopulmonary exercise intensity should progress to tolerance and preference; the intensity guidelines used for the general population for aerobic exercise training generally apply to the elderly, using close measures of heart rate, perceived exertion, and percentage of heart rate reserve.[6] The following guidelines should be used for senior athletes:[6]

- Exercise at 70% to 80% of maximum heart rate or 60% to 80% of heart rate reserve for 20 to 30 minutes, excluding warm up and cooldown. For persons beginning aerobic exercise training who have not previously been physically active, time and intensity should be lessened. The recommended initial stage begins with three exercise sessions (15 to 20 minutes) per week at an intensity level of 40% to 50% of heart rate reserve. The intensity level should be maintained throughout the exercise program.

- To avoid injury and ensure safety, older individuals should initially increase duration rather than intensity of exercise. The maximum heart rate should never be exceeded at any point during an exercise program, and perceived exertion should be considered in addition to heart rate in athletes who are taking medications that may affect heart rate (eg, beta blockers).

- Endurance exercise sessions should occur three to five times per week; the additional benefits of more frequent training appear to be minimal, but the incidence of lower extremity injuries increases abruptly.

- It is important to consider the rate of progression. Additional endurance exercise should be based on functional capacity, medical and health status, age, individual activity preferences and goals, and the individual's tolerance to the current level of training.

- Aerobic exercise programs may use upper body, lower body, or combined upper and lower body activities. However, upper extremity activities increase the stress on the cardiorespiratory system to a greater degree than either lower extremity or combined activities, and lower extremity activities increase blood pressure to a greater extent than do combination activities.[39]

Regular aerobic exercise increases pulmonary gas exchange and decreases breathlessness, probably via strengthened respiratory musculature and reduced ventilatory demand.[2] Expected patterns of cardiac alterations normally seen in response to age are modified in the older athlete, suggesting that exercise training is an effective stimulus in shaping left ventricular structure and function in the older heart.[40]

References

1. Mazzeo RS, Cavanaugh P, Evans WJ, et al: Exercise and physical activity for older adults. *Med Sci Sports Exerc* 1998;30:992-1008.
2. Menard D, Stanish WD: The aging athlete. *Am J Sports Med* 1989;17:187-196.
3. United States Masters Swimming. USMS frequently asked questions. Available at: http://www.usmms.org/faq.htm. Accessed April 26, 2003.
4. Senior Games/Olympics. Senior Olympics and Games. Available at: http://www.seniorsomething.com/srolym.html. Accessed April 26, 2003.
5. Williams GN, Higgins MJ, Lewek MD: Aging skeletal muscle: Physiologic changes and the effects of training. *Phys Ther* 2002;82:26-28.
6. American College of Sports Medicine: *Exercise Prescription: Exercise Testing and Prescription for Others*, ed 6. Baltimore, MD, Lippincott Williams & Wilkins, 2000, pp 226-229.
7. Maron BJ, Araujo GS, Thompson PD, et al: Recommendations for preparticipation screening and the assessment of cardiovascular disease in masters athletes: An advisory for healthcare professionals from the working groups of the World Heart Federation, the International Federation of Sports Medicine, and the American Heart Association Committee on Exercise, Cardiac Rehabilitation, and Prevention. *Circulation* 2001;103:327-334.
8. Dirckx JH (ed): *Stedman's Concise Medical Dictionary for the Health Professions,* ed 4. Baltimore, MD, Lippincott Williams & Wilkins, 2001.
9. American College of Sports Medicine: *ACSM's Exercise Management for Persons with Chronic Diseases and Disabilities.* Champaign, IL, Human Kinetics, 1997.

22

10. Reents S: *Sport and Exercise Pharmacology*. Champaign, IL, Human Kinetics, 2000.

11. Lonner JH: A 57-year-old man with osteoarthritis of the knee. *JAMA* 2003;289:1016-1025.

12. Galloway MT, Jokl P: Aging successfully: The importance of physical activity in maintaining health and function. *J Am Acad Orthop Surg* 2000;8:37-44.

13. Booth ML, Owen N, Bauman A, Clavisi O, Leslie E: Social-cognitive and perceived environment influences associated with physical activity in older Australians. *Prev Med* 2000;31:15-22.

14. Daley MJ, Spinks WL: Exercise, mobility, and aging. *Sports Med* 2000;29:1-12.

15. Fries JF, Singh G, Morfeld D, Hubert HB, Lane NE, Brown BW Jr: Running and the development of disability with age. *Ann Intern Med* 1994;121:502-509.

16. Lane JM, Nydick M: Osteoporosis: Current modes of prevention and treatment. *J Am Acad Orthop Surg* 1999; 7:19-31.

17. Wilmore JH: The aging of bone and muscle in sports medicine in the older athlete. *Clin Sports Med* 1991;10:231-244.

18. Lane JM, Riley EH, Wirganowicz PZ: Osteoporosis: Diagnosis and treatment. *J Bone Joint Surg Am* 1996;78:618-632.

19. Maharam LG, Bauman PA, Kalman D, Skolnik H, Perle SM: Masters athletes: Factors affecting performance. *Sports Med* 1999;28:273-285.

20. American College of Sports Medicine: Position stand: Osteoporosis and exercise. *Med Sci Sports Exerc* 1995; 27:i-vii.

21. Felson DT, Lawrence RC, Dieppe PA, et al: Osteoarthritis: New Insights. Part 1: The disease and its risk factors. *Ann Intern Med* 2000;133:635-646.

22. American Medical Association: Arthritis overview. Available at: http://www.medem.com/search/article_display.cfm?path=\\TANQUERAY\M_ContentItem&mstr=M_ContentItem/ZZZEV1FZQBC.html&soc=AMA&rsrch_typ=NAV_SERCH. Accessed November 17, 2003.

23. Goldstein TS: *Geriatric Orthopaedics: Rehabilitative Management of Common Problems*, ed 2. Gaithersburg, MD, Aspen Publishers, 1999, p 2.

24. Arthritis Foundation: Arthritis and exercise. Available at: http://www.medem.com/search/article_display.cfm?path=\\TANQUERAY\M_ContentItem/ZZZ9QAS8MDC.html&soc=NIH&srch_typ=NAV_SERCH. Accessed November 17, 2003.

25. Cole BJ, Harner CD: Degenerative arthritis of the knee in active patients: Evaluation and management. *J Am Acad Orthop Surg* 1999;7:389-402.

26. Sherbondy PS: Stay active after joint replacement: Fit society page. *Exerc Older Adult* Summer 2003;6, 11.

27. Easley ME, Vertullo CJ, Urban WC, Nunley JA: Total ankle arthroplasty. *J Am Acad Orthop Surg* 2002;10:157-167.

28. Sanchez-Sotelo J, Berry DJ, Trousdale RT, Cabanela ME: Surgical treatment of developmental dysplasia of the hip in adults: II. Arthroplasty options. *J Am Acad Orthop Surg* 2002;10:334-344.

29. Spector TD, Harris PA, Hart DJ, et al: Risk of osteoarthritis associated with long-term weight-bearing sports: A radiologic survey of hips and knees in female ex-athletes and population controls. *Arthritis Rheum* 1996;39:988-995.

30. Gauchard GC, Tessier A, Jeandel C, Perrin PP: Improved muscle strength and power in elderly exercising regularly. *Int J Sports Med* 2003;24:71-74.

31. Bostrom PG, Buckwalter A: The physiology of aging, in Koval KJ (ed): *Orthopaedic Knowledge Update 7*. Rosemont, IL, American Academy of Orthopaedic Surgeons, 2002, pp 85-93.

32. Hameed M, Harridge SDR, Goldspink G: Sarcopenia and hypertrophy: A role for insulin-like growth factor-1 in aged muscle? *Exerc Sport Sci Rev* 2002;30:15-19.

33. Kallinen M, Markku A: Aging, physical activity and sports injuries: An overview of common sports injuries in the elderly. *Sports Med* 1995;20:41-52.

34. Kubo K, Kanehisa H, Miyatani M, Tachi M, Fukunaga T: Effect of low-load resistance training on the tendon properties in middle-aged and elderly women. *Acta Physiol Scand* 2003;178:25-32.

35. Phillips SM, Parise G, Roy BD, Tipton KD, Wolfe RR, Tarnopolsky MA: Resistance-training–induced adaptations in skeletal muscle protein turnover in the fed state. *Can J Physiol Pharmacol* 2002;80:1045-1053.

36. Evans WJ: Exercise, nutrition and aging. *J Nutr* 1992;122(3 suppl):796-801.

37. Griffin LY: Neuromuscular training and injury prevention in sports. *Clin Orthop* 2003;409:53-60.

38. Skinner HB, Barrack RL, Cook SD: Age-related decline in proprioception. *Clin Orthop* 1984;184:208-211.

39. Katch WD, Katch FI, McArdle VL: *Exercise Physiology: Energy, Nutrition, & Human Performance*, ed 5. Baltimore, MD, Lippincott Williams & Wilkins, 2001.

40. Douglas PS, O'Toole M: Aging and physical activity determine cardiac structure and function in the older athlete. *J Appl Physiol* 1992;72:1969-1973.

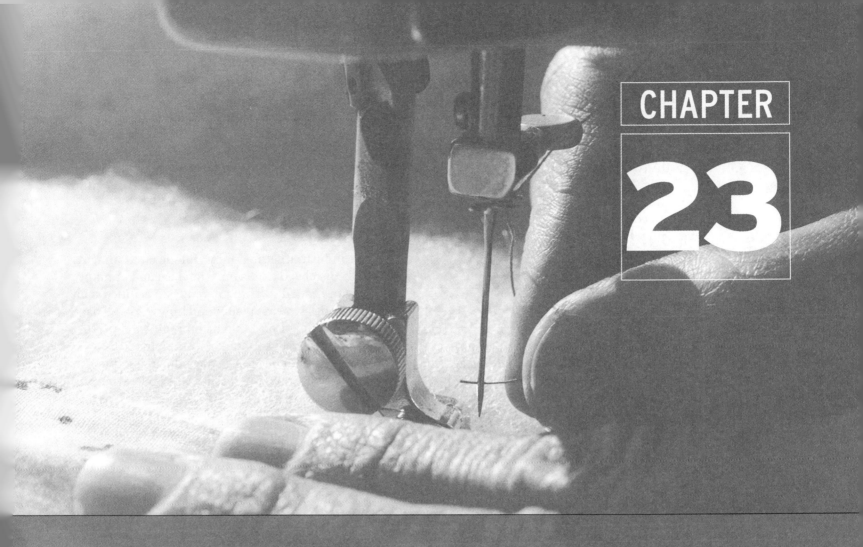

The Industrial Setting

Samuel Bradbury, MAOM,
ATC, CEA

Health care providers employed in the industrial setting face unique challenges. The patient population, work hazards, union rules, and reimbursement issues all influence the provision of health care. The health care worker's contractual arrangement also affects the type of services provided (**Table 23-1**).

Musculoskeletal injuries are the primary form of trauma in the industrial setting.[1] These injuries result in costs to the employer, with the employee averaging 9 days away from work, although this varies by occupation (**Table 23-2**).[1]

Union Employers

An important union function is to ensure that the components of a collective bargaining agreement are maintained, improved, or altered in the best interest of the employee, yet keeping the employer in mind. Collective bargaining agreements are made with employers. What health care professionals say and do as representatives of the employer can affect the employer's relationship with the union members. The local shop steward or management representative can assist in ensuring that communications are professional, effectively documented, and consistent with the collective bargaining agreement.

This local representation relationship and the union hierarchy affect the return-to-work process. The union's role is to support the worker in all areas of collective bargaining. Inappropriate actions or communications by those representing the employer can result in a grievance being filed against management under the collective bargaining agreement (**Table 23-3**).

Environmental Concerns

Industrial settings vary, influenced by the type of plant, weather conditions, and products involved. Environmental temperature, moving machinery, heavy labor, and noise create potentially volatile and hazardous working conditions.

Heat

The industrial setting offers unique environments for heat-related exposure. High heat and humidity are not limited to outdoor venues. Facilities such as foundries, steam plants, and iron works all have components of heat and/or humidity, the precursors to heat-related illness (see chapter 20).

Metabolic concerns in the industrial setting become more prevalent because workers are usually older and may have systemic diseases such as diabetes, hypertension, and obesity. Poor physical fitness can be complicated by increased metabolic demands. When these factors are combined with heat, humidity, physical exertion, minimal water consumption, and alcohol or drug use, the potential for heat-related illness is magnified. Monitor-

Table 23-1

Health Care Provider Roles

Role	Service Provided
Onsite	Contracted to provide onsite prevention, treatment, and rehabilitation services. May also function as a fitness or wellness director.
Outpatient	Clinic-based prevention and acute treatment or specialty rehabilitation, such as work-hardening and work-conditioning programs
Consultant	Individual is paid, usually under contract, to provide ergonomic or advanced injury care and injury management programs.

Table 23-2

Work-Related Musculoskeletal Disorders Involving Lost Work Days, 2002

	Number (in 1,000s)	Median Days Away from Work
Total musculoskeletal disorders	487.9	9
Nursing aides, orderlies, and attendants	44.4	6
Truck drivers	36.8	12
Laborers, nonconstruction	24.9	8
Janitors and cleaners	15.2	7
Assemblers	15.2	14
Construction laborers	11.1	10
Registered nurses	10.8	6
Supervisors and proprietors, sales occupations	9.9	7
Cashiers	9.3	8
Stock handlers and baggers	8.8	5
Sales workers, other commodities	7.8	7

Adapted with permission from United States Department of Labor, Bureau of Labor Statistics: News: Lost-worktime injuries and illness. Characteristics and resulting days away from work, 2002. (3/25/04 News Release USDL 04-460)

ing workers' heart rates and hydration status (see p 605) and ensuring adequate ventilation in indoor facilities containing heat-producing equipment decreases the workers' risk of heat illness.

Dehydration onset can be an insidious but potentially hazardous process. Physiologic performance begins to decrease when 3% of the body's weight is lost through dehydration, and hallucinations begin at 7%.[2] Forced ventilation, adequate water supplies, monitoring at-risk individuals, and education programs can reduce the occurrence of dehydration and heat illness.

Cold

Occupations such as meat packing, food distribution, oil production, delivery, mining, and open-cab heavy-equipment operation all involve cold and cold exposure. Cold exposure should be monitored per industry standards and the advice of medical professionals. Cold exposure, in conjunction with tobacco use and exposure to upper extremity vibration, predisposes the individual to hand-arm vibration syndrome (HAVS) (see p 665).

Table 23-3

Grievances Related to Workers' Compensation Issues

Violation of the negotiated agreement

Improper working conditions

Unequal or unfair treatment

Improper disciplinary action

Disagreement over interpretation of agency policies

Violations of health and safety standards

Table 23-4

OSHA Standards for Hearing Protection

Duration (h/d)	dB(A)
8	90
6	92
4	95
3	97
2	100
1.5	102
0.5	110
0.25 or less	115

Hearing damage begins at 90 dB(A).

Noise

Audiometry, the study and monitoring of the hearing system, is used to identify hazardous sound levels, track the hearing of at-risk workers over time, and protect the employer against fraudulent hearing-loss claims. The Occupational Safety and Health Administration (OSHA) has set the threshold for required hearing protection at 85 dB(A) over an 8-hour day.[3] These standards are based on the length of exposure and intensity of the sound (**Table 23-4**).

Noise collection samples are obtained with noise **dosimeters** or sound-level meters (**Figure 23-1**). Data are collected over time to determine peak sound thresholds and identify safe and unsafe areas (**Figure 23-2**). "Hearing protection required" areas can then be determined.[4]

> **Dosimeter** A device that monitors the total accumulated exposure (dose) to an environmental condition.

Ergonomic Evaluation of Work Skills

The purpose of ergonomic evaluation is to ensure a safe, efficient, and effective work environment by maximizing the biomechanical efficiency of workers' tasks and reducing unwanted or repetitive stresses on the body. Ergonomics incorporates theories from engineering design, biomechanics, psychology, information technology, industrial hygiene, industrial safety, epidemiology, work physiology, and occupational medicine.

Error reduction is a primary function of the ergonomist, who approaches the problem by designing a system in which the human makes the fewest number of errors. Engineers are statistically and empirically driven. They understand systems design, redundancy patterns, and anthropometric usage and focus on the fact that the hu-

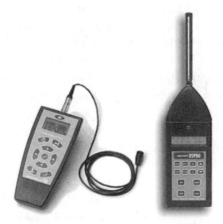

Figure 23-1 Examples of noise-monitoring devices (dosimeters). (Printed with permission from Larson Davis, Provo, UT. www.lardav.com.)

23

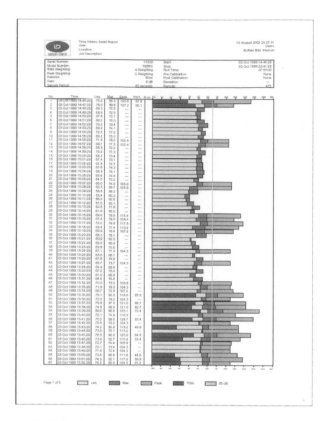

Figure 23-2 Sample industrial noise report. (Printed with permission from Larson Davis, Provo, UT. www.lardav.com.)

man's major role in a system is to make decisions. This error reduction is achieved by incorporating an understanding of psychology and organizational behavior patterns, human tendencies, and population biases.

Risk Assessment

Risk assessment is a specific evaluation that uses established ergonomic tools and injury data to identify and quantify the ergonomic risks associated with a task or job. Commercial tools such as the Rapid Upper Limb Assessment, National Institute of Occupational Safety and Health Lifting Equation, Rapid Entire Body Assessment, and cycle-time video analysis of jobs assist in identifying the potential injury risk. These tools are also used to determine work/rest ratios to help companies assess risk factors associated with production rates. This information is useful to the medical, production, and management staffs to develop plans to decrease risk patterns.

Risk assessments with standardized ergonomic tools may require some additional knowledge to analyze the resultant data and make appropriate recommendations about workplace improvement or redesign. Experienced professionals

such as certified professional ergonomists or certified ergonomics associates are often needed to make sound, cost-effective suggestions to company management.

Physical Demand Assessment

Physical demand assessment involves collection of weight, distance, load, and frequency measurements of a task in real time as a worker performs the normal job functions. The purpose of the physical demand assessment is to define each job task's physical demands or functions, using tools such as a stopwatch, scale, strain gauge, and measuring tape and/or video observation.

A physical demand assessment identifies physical requirements under specific conditions and with the specific tools needed to complete the task. Physical demand assessment is similar to a sport-skills analysis of an athlete. Current physical job requirements are reviewed, such as lifting amounts and frequencies, pushing and pulling, postures (eg, reaching or standing), and dynamic movements (eg, crawling and climbing). If a worker is injured, data can be collected from the workers who are currently performing that job.

Postoffer Assessment

By identifying the tasks required to successfully complete a job and be a productive employee, the evaluation process identifies skills the worker is lacking in order to safely return to the job after injury, or it can be used for preemployment screening. In industry, preemployment screening is known as a postoffer assessment. Consisting of both physical and cognitive components, the assessment determines if an employee who has been hired on a pending basis can perform the minimum job functions as determined by the employer. According to the **Americans with Disabilities Act** (ADA), postoffer assessments must be job-specific and directly related to the company's productivity.[5]

The ADA requires an employer to focus on the essential job functions to determine whether a person with a disability is qualified. This is an important nondiscrimination requirement. Many people with disabilities who can perform essential job functions are denied employment because they cannot do tasks that are only marginal.

If an individual meets all other job prerequisites, employment cannot be denied because of a disability that prevents the individual from performing all but the most essential job functions

Americans with Disabilities Act Federal legislation that prohibits discrimination against individuals with disabilities, requires organizations to remove physical barriers that prevent access to areas, and requires employers to make reasonable accommodations to compensate for an individual's disability.

with the benefit of reasonable accommodations. Selection criteria related to marginal functions that exclude an individual because of his or her disability are not consistent with business necessity.

Postoffer assessment should be directly related to those job tasks considered **essential functions**. A function may be essential for several reasons, including the following:

- Performance of the function can be distributed among a limited number of available employees

- The position exists so that an employee will perform the function

- The function is highly specialized

- The function cannot be removed from the job requirements without fundamentally altering the position.

Postoffer assessments should not include marginal functions, those tasks that can be easily transferred to another employee without hurting the employer's business. Thus an employer may choose to restructure a job as a form of reasonable accommodation. Job restructuring may include modifications, such as reallocating or redistributing marginal job functions an employee is unable to perform because of a disability and altering when and/or how a function—essential or marginal—is performed. Although an employer may wish to reallocate essential functions as a reasonable accommodation, the employer is never required to do so.

■ Functional Capacity Evaluation

A functional capacity evaluation (FCE) objectively measures the individual's function level within the context of employment and job-specific skills (**Table 23-5**). The employee's functional measures are compared with the job's functional demands or normative data to make return-to-work or disability determinations or as the basis for a rehabilitation plan. The FCE data also can be used to predict the employee's ability to sustain these tasks over a predetermined time frame.

Typically in the FCE process, objective and subjective information is collected about how a worker performs a specific procedure. These standardized assessments usually include basic postures such as standing, sitting, bending, and reaching, as well as dynamic movements such as squatting, climbing, and walking. The process typically includes a specific protocol for deter-

Table 23-5
Uses of a Functional Capacity Evaluation
Determine return-to-work capabilities.
Compare current worker capabilities with the demands.
Evaluate the progress of an injured worker within the rehabilitation program in comparison to return-to-work physical demands.
Determine final levels of function if an employee with a work injury does not improve or the employee is unlikely to return to the previous job.
Determine current levels of functions compared with standard *Dictionary of Occupational Titles* or ONET for placement and vocational assessment purposes.*
Determine levels of participation and motivation in the return-to-work process.
Aid in determining conscious behavior or manipulation of test data in an effort to gain from an injury.
Provide evidence in legal cases.
*_Dictionary of Occupational Titles_, ed 4. Washington, DC, Department of Labor, 1991. ONET (Occupational Information Network) is available online to find occupations at http://online.onetcenter.org/gen_search_page. Accessed July 14, 2004.

Essential functions
Tasks an individual must be able to complete in order to hold a specific position, with or without accommodation. The tasks are inherent in the position, and specialized skills are required to perform them.

mining the worker's lifting limits. For some workers, these limits are determined by comparing static lifting (pulling on a dynamometer) with normative data or by using kinesiophysical determinants while the individual lifts progressively weighted objects. The subjective data consist of the worker's reported pain, task difficulty, and replies to standardized self-administered questionnaires; an interview; and the evaluator's observations of behaviors and responses to the tasks placed before the worker.

A number of standardized FCE testing tools are commercially available to evaluate human body physical functions, although differences exist in how the systems collect and analyze data, the equipment required, and the statistical analysis used. These tools are also used to identify workers who may benefit from other psychosocial services. Testing specificity is significant in determining the tool to be used. Some tools are better designed for identifying behavior patterns, whereas others use criterion-based statistics or work physiology data to determine report outcomes.

State practice regulations and the methods used can restrict those who perform or provide an FCE report. Most tools have been developed by physical therapists or occupational therapists, thereby restricting their availability to these health care professionals. Some suppliers provide training for other users.

Injury Prevention

The patient base in the industrial setting is heterogeneous, with a wide range of ages and various body builds, levels of physical fitness, and motivations. Some patients may have underlying diseases such as diabetes, cancer, or cardiorespiratory conditions. All these conditions can predispose the individual to injury and may influence the rehabilitation process.

Information obtained from the workplace and ergonomic evaluation of job tasks forms the foundation of injury prevention programs. Although injury prevention programs focus on individual workers, many techniques (eg, job rotation and job sequencing) alternate workers' roles and tasks to decrease the cumulative stress placed on the body. Limiting worker exposure to environmental hazards such as heat, cold, sound, and vibration must also be addressed. Employers can modify the work environment and job demands to help prevent work-related injury and decrease time lost through effective evaluation, treatment, and rehabilitation programs.

Job Rotation

Job rotation is a preventive procedure in which groups of employees who are exposed to ergonomic risk factors alternate through different job duties on a time-based schedule. A physical demand analysis or job-cycle outline that includes muscle actions and patterns is needed to develop an effective job rotation cycle. Alternating roles helps to prevent repetitive stress injuries by changing the primary muscle groups being stressed and the motion being performed. Job rotation is an inexpensive, effective strategy for injury reduction. However, many employers fail to evaluate job rotations for biomechanical patterns, planes of movement, and muscle group involvement.

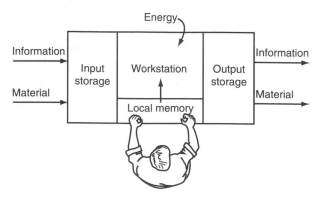

Figure 23-3 Processes involved with job sequencing. (Reproduced from Konz, S: *Work Design Occupational Ergonomics,* ed 6. Copyright © 2004 by Holcomb Hathaway Publishers Inc., Scottsdale, Arizona, p 179. Used with permission.)

Job Sequencing

The job sequencing process involves the effective flow of both product and mental information (**Figure 23-3**). Each job task has a mental component that must be sequenced fluidly for proficient completion. The packaging process provides a good example. A job sequencing analysis determines if the patterns and movements used to pick up the parts, place them in the box, close the box, and dispatch the box are the most efficient and are biomechanically sound.

Because they have mastered job-cycle biomechanics and sequencing, experienced workers are more efficient than new line workers. Mentoring programs and training in specified techniques should be encouraged as part of the hiring and placement process to prevent injuries when new employees start working rather than after an injury has occurred.

Hierarchy of Controls

The best way to protect workers is to eliminate workplace hazards and risks, which can be done in a variety of ways. Control of hazards and risks is best performed in the following sequence, listed from most effective to least effective and known as the "hierarchy of controls."

- *Substitution:* Using safer chemicals or other products to keep chemical hazards from entering the workplace from the start; finding effective alternatives to eliminate risks and hazards before they begin
- *Engineering controls:* A reliable means of eliminating or designing out hazards in the workplace, eg, having machines instead of humans complete jobs
- *Ergonomics:* Changing the job to fit the needs of the worker, instead of making the worker fit the job
- *Administrative controls:* Changing how workers perform their jobs through policies and training, in an effort to reduce their exposure to hazards
- *Personal protective equipment (PPE):* Personal protective equipment is the least desirable way to protect workers because if the PPE fails, the workers are exposed to the hazard. PPE includes respirators, hard-hats, face and eye protection, hearing protection, gloves, and protective clothing and footwear.

Ergonomists prefer engineering controls, because selection of control technologies should be based on their reliability and efficacy in eliminating or reducing workplace hazards or risks. Engineering controls are preferred because they are reliable, consistent, effective, measurable, and not dependent on human behavior (that of managers, supervisors, or workers) for their effectiveness. Also, they do not introduce new hazards into the process.

The hierarchy of controls should be kept in mind when considering job tasks, because substituting or engineering out the hazard may be more effective than ergonomic or other intervention strategies to make the job safer.

Manual Handling Issues

Manual handling is the worker's ability to manipulate an object in a job-specific manner by lifting, pulling, and/or pushing the object. The frequency, load, distance, duration, and the posture used during manual handling determine the worker's injury risk. Manual handling creates potential workplace injury issues when the worker is not strong or fit enough to handle the specific load. Some manual handling tasks may require the use of specific equipment, such as pallet jacks or hand trucks. Repetitive performance of the same task over time can lead to overuse injuries. Physiologically, the worker is only capable of manually handling limited loads or can only tolerate so many repetitions of that load before breakdown occurs.

Historically, the most common preventive tools have been "back schools"[6,7] and the "back-belt"[8] devices designed to support the back when moving objects (**Figure 23-4**). However, much of the research on these approaches has failed to demonstrate a decrease in the number of injuries.[8]

Decreasing manual handling weight and repetition is an effective method of reducing injuries. Physical strength and the maximum weight that can be lifted are not closely correlated. The National Institute of Occupational Safety and Health lifting standards begin at a maximum of 51 lb for males and are reduced by a specific percentage if certain factors are present.[9]

Vibration Issues

Many industrial workers use a large number of tools or drive equipment as part of their job. At certain frequencies and in specific body positions, vibration can cause reflex sphincter muscle closure or blood vessel vasoconstriction, resulting in severely reduced blood circulation to the affected extremities. This de-creased blood supply starves the working tissues of oxygen and nutrients, increasing muscular fatigue.

Mechanical vibration of a machine is caused by its moving components; each component has a certain frequency associated with its movement. The individual moving components transmit a range of vibration frequencies to the body. This is an important consideration when the effects of vibration on humans are measured, because the body is not equally sensitive to all vibration frequencies.

The effects of vibration-related responses can be experienced in the extremities or systemically. The body's response to vibration is directly related to the frequency (Hz) and acceleration. When a person is seated, vibration has the following effects at given frequencies:[10]

- Less than 2 Hz at accelerations of 3 to 4 g: interference with breathing
- From 4 to 14 Hz at accelerations of 1.2 to 3.2 g: increases in chest, abdominal, and back pain. The threshold for pain will vary from person to person.
- Greater than 14 Hz at accelerations of 5 to 9 g: muscular tension, headaches, eye-strain, and speech disturbances

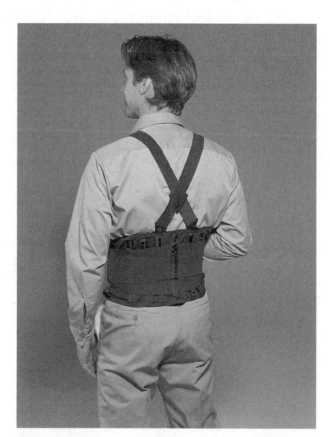

Figure 23-4 Example of a back support worn to reduce low back injuries. (Printed with permission from Safco Products, a division of Liberty Diversified Industries (LDI), New Hope, MN. www.safcoproducts.com.)

23

To understand why humans are more sensitive to some frequencies, it is useful to consider the human body as a mechanical system. Each body part has specific sensitivities to different frequency ranges, in part because the body is not symmetric, thus the vibratory forces are not evenly distributed. Vibration's effect on the body is measured in three distinct ranges—low (0 to 2 Hz) as from ships and cranes, middle (>2 to 20 Hz) as from vehicles and aircraft, and high (greater than 20 Hz) as from tools.

With segmental vibration, the frequency range of primary interest is from approximately 8 to 1,000 Hz. Most handheld tools generate random vibrations over a frequency range from 2 to 2,000 Hz. Long-term exposure to these frequencies can lead to serious health issues, including degenerative spinal changes; HAVS (see p 665); arthritis; tendinous changes; atrophy leading to calcium loss and stress fractures; and "dead finger" or "white finger" syndrome, in which the fingers become bluish or white, cold, and numb.

Injuries Common to the Industrial Setting

Most musculoskeletal injuries that occur in the industrial setting are similar to those seen in other settings. Common injuries include carpal tunnel syndrome (p 433), lumbar and cervical disk injuries (p 536), lumbar strains (chapter 14), shoulder injuries (chapter 10), and hand injuries (chapter 12). The wide range of employee ages and fitness levels and the repetitive nature of work-related movement patterns can lead to overuse injuries. Heavy lifting and accidental contact with moving parts increase the risk of acute trauma.

Acute Trauma

Attention to injury prevention programs (see p 662) has resulted in decreased rates of acute and overuse injuries and reduced the total number of work days missed as the result of workplace-related trauma.[1] However, machinery and moving equipment can result in severe acute injuries. Onsite care is often limited to immediate management and late-stage rehabilitation.

Crush Injuries

Crush injuries involve limb entrapment in equipment, resulting in tissue compression, shear, and avulsion (**Figure 23-5**). Additional trauma can occur as the limb is extracted from the machine. The fingertips are the most frequently crushed appendage

in the workplace. Also, because most machinery is not sterile, the tissues may be infiltrated with foreign bodies, requiring multiple surgeries and debridement procedures.

Management of crush injuries involves controlling bleeding by applying sterile gauze over the site. If bleeding is severe, several layers may be required. New layers of gauze should be applied over the existing layers, rather than removing the original layers. Sterile gauze can be secured with roller bandages. Although contamination is possible, the embedded material should not be removed from the wound. Removal can increase bleeding, further embed the material in the tissue, or remove viable tissue. If foreign matter is present, the bandages can be saturated with sterile saline solution to keep the wound moist. Unless prior physician approval has been granted, the wound should not be treated with any type of topical antiseptic.

During the healing process, tendons may adhere to the surrounding tissue, slowing the restoration of range of motion (ROM). Because of extensive damage to the skin, subcutaneous tissue, tendons, nerves, blood vessels, joints, and bones, crush injuries are difficult to manage and rehabilitate. Complications include tissue necrosis, edema, decreased ROM, and loss of use of the extremity.

Impalement by Small Objects

Impaled objects can include such items as nails, screws, heavy wires, needles, plastic, glass, or wood that have been forcefully embedded in a worker's skin, typically in an extremity (**Figure 23-6**). Sometimes the embedded objects are attached to other, larger objects such as a board, large piece of cabling, or a syringe.

The embedded object should not be removed. If attached to a larger object, the embedded item

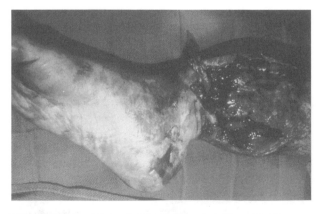

Figure 23-5 Crush injury to the leg. (Reproduced from American Academy of Orthopaedic Surgeons: *Emergency Care and Transportation of the Sick and Injured*, ed 8. Sudbury, MA, Jones and Bartlett Publishers, 2002, p 570.)

should be cut away from the larger object with wire cutters, pin cutters, or a similar tool to avoid leverage at the wound. The embedded object should be secured by applying a bulky dressing around the limb and object, and the patient then transported to a medical facility.

Once the worker is under a physician's care, radiographs may be taken of the limb to rule out other possible underlying trauma and to identify hazards associated with extracting the impalement. The object is commonly removed under local anesthesia, although complicated extrications may require general anesthesia. After removal, the wound is irrigated and debrided. If needed, tetanus prophylaxis and antibiotics are administered.[11]

Degloving Injuries

A degloving injury occurs when an extremity is caught in, dragged by, or pulled from a piece of equipment or has fallen with some velocity, resulting in stripping away of the skin and subcutaneous tissues. The most common injuries are to the hand and arm, when a worker is dragged into a large machine such as a mixer or conveyor system. The worker instinctively pulls while the machine maintains hold onto the extremity, causing the skin to be stripped off the limb. This injury can also occur when a worker's jewelry gets caught in equipment or snagged on a protruding object such as a nail.

Initial injury management is to control bleeding, treat for shock, and transport the patient to the hospital for emergency care. Bleeding is controlled using direct pressure, as described for crush injuries, and pressure points. Postsurgical management of degloving injuries depends on the severity, location, and surgeon's discretion. Once the patient has completed hand therapy and reached maximum expected ROM for all associated joints, neurologic function, and functional movements, job-specific rehabilitation of the involved extremity can begin.

Amputations and Avulsions

Avulsions result in separation of soft-tissue layers and either total removal of the tissue from the body or hanging of the tissue as a flap. Complete avulsions, especially of the extremities, are frequently referred to as amputations (**Figure 23-7**). Traumatic amputations can occur from saws, cutting instruments, and other types of machinery.

Although the primary immediate management goal is to control bleeding and save the patient's life, every effort should be made to preserve the avulsed or amputated tissue. In many cases, the tissue can be surgically reattached, but proper prehospital tissue care is vital to a successful outcome. Avulsed tissues should be stabilized to the body using bulky compression dressings and a splint to prevent further injury. Amputated tissue should be wrapped in a sterile dressing and placed in a plastic bag covered with ice for transportation. Physicians' opinions about keeping the tissue wet or dry during transportation vary. The preferred protocol should be identified in the employer's standard operating procedures.[12]

■ Hand-Arm Vibration Syndrome

HAVS is caused by repeated and prolonged exposure to vibrating equipment and is most prevalent in cold environments (see Vibration Issues p 663).

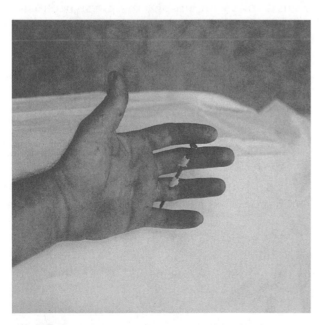

Figure 23-6 Impalement of finger by a nail. (Reproduced from American Academy of Orthopaedic Surgeons: *Emergency Care and Transportation of the Sick and Injured*, ed 8. Sudbury, MA, Jones and Bartlett Publishers, 2002, p 569.)

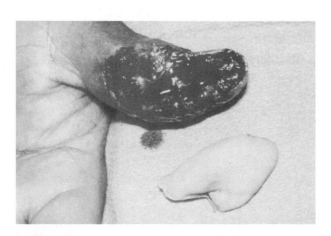

Figure 23-7 Thumb amputation. (Reproduced from American Academy of Orthopaedic Surgeons: *Emergency Care and Transportation of the Sick and Injured*, ed 8. Sudbury, MA, Jones and Bartlett Publishers, 2002, p 574.)

23

The signs and symptoms of HAVS include vascular and neurologic components; however, the pathophysiology and cause and effect between the two types of symptoms are not clearly understood.

Initial HAVS symptoms are similar to those of carpal tunnel syndrome (see p 433). With continued exposure to vibration, the fingertips blanch (similar to frostbite), the sign that an irreversible process has begun. In the early stages, the blanching attacks persist for 5 to 15 minutes, with long intervals between attacks. As the syndrome progresses, the attacks increase in frequency, duration, and intensity (**Table 23-6**). In the late stages, blanching attacks occur in all seasons and whenever the fingers come into contact with cold. Nicotine's vasoconstrictive effects may increase HAVS severity. Medical treatment is generally palliative and includes calcium channel blocker antihypertensive medications.[13]

Rehabilitation Services

Treatment, rehabilitation, and specialty work-hardening and work-conditioning programs may be provided onsite. Traditional rehabilitation is followed by incorporation of ergonomic tasks to assess the risk factors and physical demands of the job or provide FCE testing to determine readiness to return to work.

Onsite programs designed to improve care through prompt, physician-defined treatment or standard protocols are effective, cost-saving rehabilitation and preventive strategies and are becoming more popular with employers.[14] Work-conditioning and work-hardening programs are specific rehabilitation approaches that focus on returning the employee to work (**Table 23-7**).[15]

Case Management and Case Containment

Case management is a primary function of health care providers in the industrial setting. It begins once an injury occurs and includes the immediate treatment, reassurance, and directing of appropriate care. Proper case management can make a significant difference in the outcome of a work injury case. Communicating with supervisors and safety, human resources, and insurance personnel to keep them informed of the worker's current status is much like working with coaches, keeping them informed of who is on the injury list and which drills can be performed. When managed correctly, the injured worker can return to the job in a meaningful progression; however, education, communication, and sometimes mediation are required to effectively address all the associated issues.

Work Conditioning

Work conditioning involves intensive, work-related, goal-oriented rehabilitation programs designed to restore normal body function and enable an employee to return to work.[16] Most work-conditioning programs are short (2 to 4 weeks) and target specific physical deficits. A typical program involves 4 hours of activity designed to develop cardiovascular endurance, improve manual handling skills, enhance strength, increase flexibility, provide nutritional education, and instill injury prevention techniques. The worker also must begin to mentally prepare for return to work. Objective testing demonstrates that the worker can perform safely in the return to work.

Work Hardening

Work hardening is a more specific type of rehabilitation program than work conditioning. This program uses vocational methods to address the medical, physical, behavioral, and psychological aspects of employability and return to work and is characterized by daily work assignments and weekly functional testing. Many work-hardening programs are multidisciplinary, focusing on real or simulated work activities, and designed for clients who have stringent physical requirements for return to work, chronic pain issues, pending workers' compensation legal issues, and motivational issues about re-

---

Table 23-6

Disorders and Categories Associated with HAVS

Stage	Description
I	Occasional blanching of one or more fingers without loss of work capacity
II	Repeated blanching of one or more fingers (especially in the winter) with slight loss of work capacity and daily activities
III	Extensive blanching involving all fingers in summer and winter and interference with social, work, and personal activities
IV	Same as stage III, but the worker is unable to continue in the same line of work

Reproduced from Taylor W, Pelmear PL, eds: *Vibration White Finger in Industry*. New York, NY: Academic Press, 1975.

turn. Most clients have been out of work longer than 4 months and may be in poor physical condition. Most programs are 2 to 8 weeks in duration but have become more focused and goal-driven than earlier programs, which were as long as 18 weeks.

Work-hardening programs are progressive, starting at 2 to 4 hours/day, 5 days/week, and progressing to 8 hours/day. At about 6 hours/day, however, many workers prefer to return to work rather than continue to simulate working tasks.

■ Transitional Work Programs

Transitional work programs are designed to reduce time lost from the job, either by keeping the employee at a defined job or by returning the injured worker to the job with restrictions. Employees who cannot return to work as part of their own work team are shared with another team until they can transition back into their original job responsibilities. They also may work in floating positions, allowing them to function within their capabilities and according to their knowledge for a number of teams.

The patient's work status is regularly evaluated and modified by the work transition team. To determine the employee's appropriate role in a transitional work program, the transition team must have a firm understanding of the job tasks and the associated physical demands and work cooperatively with the employer.

In some cases, such as a unionized workplace, work transition programs must be closely monitored to avoid potential problems with collective bargaining issues, such as placing an injured worker into a job that requires a more experienced worker. Many

unionized workplaces address job transition issues in the collective bargaining agreement and, with the union's support, effectively return workers to the job.

■ Return-to-Work Issues

Although in most cases a simple algorithm (**Figure 23-8**) is useful in determining the return-to-work process, unique challenges still arise. The health care provider must accurately explain the condition being treated and its implication for return to work. For example, with a disk herniation, the worker needs to know that pain and disability are often self-limiting and that many other individuals with the same condition maintain normal lifestyles.

Information provided by the physician can be reinforced or contradicted by other caregivers. Contradictory information is a major cause of worker distress and can lead to physician shopping and prolonged recovery time. Workers exceeding the expected recovery time should be reevaluated by the physician. If appropriate, a multidisciplinary program is then initiated to address psychosocial issues (**Table 23-8**).

Differences Between Job Tasks and Physical Demands

The inability to return an employee to work may be related to the restrictions placed by the employer's defined job demands. In some cases, the employer may have considered only the heaviest, most difficult, or most awkward job to establish the demands. In reality, the worker may be required to perform at these levels only rarely.

A physical demand assessment can aid in definitively describing the job and job tasks, rates and frequencies, heights, weights, tools used, and metabolic

Algorithm A step-by-step procedure for solving a problem or accomplishing some end.

Table 23-7

Comparison of Work-Conditioning and Work-Hardening Programs

	Work Conditioning	Work Hardening
Definition	Program addresses physical and functional needs and may be provided by a single discipline.	Program addresses physical, functional, psychosocial, and pain issues and is likely provided by a multidisciplinary team.
Intake Process	Intake examination typically includes a general fitness assessment and general job duties review for determining deficits. Program goals are built based on this comparative review.	Intake examination typically includes participation in a standardized FCE before entry. It may also include a psychological review or testing, as well as vocational testing. Goals are specific and established weekly.
Program Structure	The program is structured around general physical conditioning and functional activities related to work. Manual handling education may also be a part of the program.	The program is structured around gradual but intense physical strength and endurance progression programs, specific and increasing work simulations, and a significant education and/or pain-coping process.
Session Duration and Frequency	Starting at 2 to 3 hours/day, 3 days/week, for 2 to 4 weeks	Progressing up to 8 hours/day, 5 days/week, for 2 to 8 weeks

Adapted with permission from APTA Board of Directors. *Occupational Health Guidelines: Work Conditioning and Work-Hardening Programs (BOD 03-01-17-58)*. Alexandria, VA. American Physical Therapy Association; 2001.

23

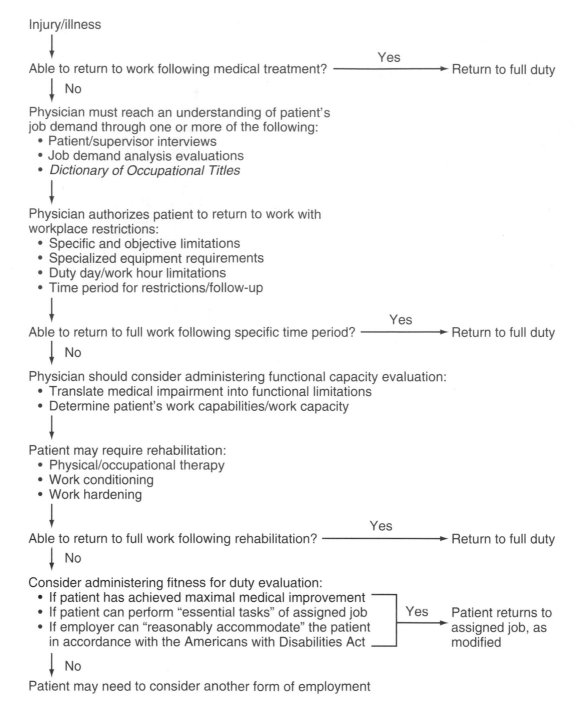

Injury/illness

Able to return to work following medical treatment? ——— Yes ——→ Return to full duty

↓ No

Physician must reach an understanding of patient's job demand through one or more of the following:
- Patient/supervisor interviews
- Job demand analysis evaluations
- *Dictionary of Occupational Titles*

↓

Physician authorizes patient to return to work with workplace restrictions:
- Specific and objective limitations
- Specialized equipment requirements
- Duty day/work hour limitations
- Time period for restrictions/follow-up

↓

Able to return to full work following specific time period? ——— Yes ——→ Return to full duty

↓ No

Physician should consider administering functional capacity evaluation:
- Translate medical impairment into functional limitations
- Determine patient's work capabilities/work capacity

↓

Patient may require rehabilitation:
- Physical/occupational therapy
- Work conditioning
- Work hardening

↓

Able to return to full work following rehabilitation? ——— Yes ——→ Return to full duty

↓ No

Consider administering fitness for duty evaluation:
- If patient has achieved maximal medical improvement
- If patient can perform "essential tasks" of assigned job
- If employer can "reasonably accommodate" the patient in accordance with the Americans with Disabilities Act

——— Yes ——→ Patient returns to assigned job, as modified

↓ No

Patient may need to consider another form of employment

Figure 23-8 Algorithm for the return-to-work process. (Reproduced with permission from Wyman DO: Evaluating patients for return to work. *Am Fam Physician* 1999;59:844-848.)

demands. A job trial or FCE can then be performed to determine the worker's capabilities. By comparing the two assessments, an objective determination about a safe return to work can be established.

Psychosocial and Cultural Considerations

Many injured employees have psychosocial issues that must be addressed, such as alcohol abuse, depression, or other psychiatric disorders.[17] Conflict may exist between the worker and the employer. The injured worker may place the blame for the injury on the workplace or employer and feel that the em-

ployer is more focused on the injury's financial aspects than on the employee. The employer may blame the employee and perceive that the employee is manipulating the system to gain undeserved benefits.

Lack of understanding by the worker and a hands-off approach by the employer create poor communication and a "me versus them" environment. In many cases, the employee makes serious attempts to return to work, only to be challenged by suspicious employers or attorneys who discourage returning to work for short-term gains. The worker may fall into the disabled role as a means

Table 23-8

Biopsychosocial Model of Injury Care

Onset of Pain

Explain the biopsychosocial model

Address concerns about pain, including the course, diagnosis, and prognosis

Emphasize the patient's role in recovery

Make appropriate referral if indicated

2 Weeks after Onset

Address concerns again, old and new

Address social factors, including attitudes about work, as well as the responses of family and friends

Reinforce patient's role in recovery

Make appropriate referral if indicated

4 Weeks after Onset

Address concerns again, old and new

Address social factors again

Reinforce patient's role in recovery again

Refer for multidisciplinary evaluation and possible treatment

Adapted with permission from Weiser S: Psychosocial aspects of occupational musculoskeletal disorders, in Nordin M, Pope MH, Andersson G (eds): *Musculoskeletal Disorders in the Workplace*. St Louis, MO, Mosby, 1997, p 58.

of adapting and surviving in this social system and as one way of being validated.

Worker's Response to Injury

Musculoskeletal complaints can be influenced by personality type, anxiety, depression, and psychological distress. Family dynamics may also create a "disabled support system" when the worker has a family member who is also disabled and who negatively influences the injured worker. Other factors may also influence the employee's self-determination to recover from an injury, prolonging rehabilitation.

Underlying conditions such as chronic pain syndrome or complex regional pain syndrome may also complicate the rehabilitation process.

Chronic Pain Syndrome

Chronic pain manifests in a client who complains of persistent pain but has disproportionate clinical evidence of physical impairment and has failed to respond to traditional pain-control techniques. Chronic pain involves multiple factors, including psychological components, and may begin as physical pain that has failed to resolve or has worsened. Pain networks may become a "learned pattern" and can lead to unhealthy lifestyles, creating problems in daily functioning. Existing problems may be exacerbated when poor biomechanical patterns replace proper movement, leading to overuse, exaggerated movements, and increased atrophy at the injury site and causing pain in associated areas along the nerve distribution. Other problems linked with chronic pain syndrome include sleep and appetite disturbances; overuse, abuse, or dependence on pain medications; alcohol abuse; social withdrawal; depression; and hypochondria.

Poor biomechanics are sometimes used to reduce discomfort caused by other trauma. Psychological blocks may prevent the patient from engaging in activities that may produce pain and subsequently produce anxiety-related symptoms. Part of the recovery process may involve interrupting the cycle through a gradual return to activity.[18]

Persons suffering from chronic pain syndrome can become excessive users of health care resources, seeking multiple medical examinations and unnecessary surgeries. The presence of an attorney in a workers' compensation case may be associated with the failure to return to work after pain treatment. Potential litigation can change the injured worker's focus from adjusting to the present situation with pain to one of ego and pride because he or she has been wronged by the employer.[19]

Complex Regional Pain Syndrome

Complex regional pain syndrome (CRPS), formerly known as reflex sympathetic dystrophy syndrome, is a broad-scope term categorizing a wide range of diagnoses.[20,21] CRPS occurs when the normal healing process of tissues becomes aberrant. An extremity's normal physiologic response to injury involves hormonal and neural signals that cause increased blood flow, edema, decreased joint movement, and pain. These signs and symptoms are usually proportional to injury severity and resolve with healing of the traumatized tissue. In some cases, however, the prolonged healing response results in chronic, painful symptoms arising from the injury site and may involve the entire extremity. If left unchecked, this process may lead to persistent swelling, increased pain, decreased range of motion, and ultimately a functionless limb (**Table 23-9**).

The pathophysiology of CRPS is unknown but may involve a pathologic sympathetic reflex, catecholamine hypersensitivity, abnormal autoregulation in response to local inflammatory factors, and abnormal neuronal connections created by an injured peripheral nerve. No definitive tests exist for CRPS. The diagnosis is based primarily on exclusion of other causes of pain on physical examination and on the clinical and radiographic features listed in Table 23-9. Response to sympathetic blockades, osteopenia on radiographs, and abnormal bone scan and thermography may support the CRPS diagnosis.

23

Stages of Complex Regional Pain Syndrome

Stage	Usual Time Course (mo)	Clinical Features	Radiographic Findings
Acute	0 to 3	Warm, red, edematous extremity; burning pain; intolerance to cold; altered sweat pattern; joint stiffness without any significant effusion; hyperesthetic skin; no fixed joint contractures	Normal plain radiographs; may have abnormal uptake of imaging agent on bone scan
Dystrophic	3 to 6	Cool, cyanotic, edematous extremity; shiny, hyperesthetic skin; fixed contractures; fibrotic changes occur in synovium	Subchondral osteopenia; patellar and medial femoral condyle osteopenia on sunrise view; may have abnormal uptake of imaging agent on bone scan
Atrophic	6 to 12	Loss of hair, nails, skin folds; fixed contractures; muscle wasting	Bone demineralization

Reproduced with permission from Hogan CJ, Hurwitz SR: Treatment of complex regional pain syndrome of the lower extremity. *J Am Acad Orthop Surg* 2002;10:281-289.

Medical Record Documentation

Paperwork associated with the industrial setting includes documentation of work-related injuries and illnesses, treatment, rehabilitation, attendance at educational programs, rehabilitation treatments, and outcomes measures when discharging the patient. Documentation should be objective. Quotation marks are used for items reported by the worker, and remarks are cited verbatim to avoid any discrepancy if records are subpoenaed.

Documentation becomes the principal defense in malpractice cases, which are more likely when dealing with individuals who may be unmotivated to return to work. Medical records should not be kept with human resource records. Medical records are confidential, and both paper and electronic records must be stored in a manner that restricts access to designated officials.[5]

In certain instances, medical information may be disclosed to employers, supervisors, and managers—when reasonable ADA accommodations must be made to meet an employee's work restrictions, during first-aid or emergency treatment, to individuals investigating ADA (or similar regulatory agency) compliance issues, and for workers' compensation legal issues.[5]

Medication Use and Abuse

In the industrial setting, additional knowledge and understanding of prescription and over-the-counter medications, recreational drug and alcohol use, and drug-testing procedures are required. The regulations governing these processes and knowledge and awareness of the recreational, habitual, or inappropriate use of illegal and prescription medications are critical to creating a safe work environment. With motor carriers, legal ramifications are significant because of an additional layer of federal regulations.

Medications and OSHA Recordability

Under the OSHA 300 injury/illness recording process, an injury must be recorded if medical treatment is provided to the injured or ill worker. Injury recordability is based on a number of factors, but work-related injuries and illnesses are considered recordable if they result in death, loss of consciousness, days away from work, restricted work activity or job transfer, or medical treatment beyond first aid.

OSHA states that the employer must record any significant work-related injury or illness diagnosed by a physician or other licensed health care professional. Thus if a physician writes a prescription for medication, the injury meets the recordability criteria. Employers may attempt to prevent recordability by limiting or working to prevent the writing of a prescription for medication. This is an attempt to meet the definition of first-aid treatment—if the injury or illness is treated with nonprescription medications and is treated with nonprescription dosages, then the treatment is considered first aid and not a recordable injury or illness.

Medication Use Around Moving Equipment

Many pain medications cause drowsiness or, when mixed with other substances, can significantly impair judgment, reflex time, and psychomotor control. Workers who use heavy machinery, drive vehicles, or operate worksite machinery while impaired place themselves, their coworkers, and the public at risk.

Substance Use in Motor Carriers

The trucking and motor transportation industries have stringent regulations and testing procedures that require adherence. Drug and alcohol testing in the motor carrier industry may be a contributing factor to the decline in alcohol-related fatalities. Accidents involving blood alcohol concentrations of 0.01 g/dL or more have substantially decreased since the Federal Motor Carrier Safety Administration began its monitoring and enforcement program in 1982.[22]

Medication Use in the Industrial Setting

Analgesics, muscle relaxants, and anti-inflammatory medications are often used to treat acute and chronic musculoskeletal injuries. Narcotics listed in the Drug Enforcement Administration's (DEA) Scheduled Medications II and III[23] should be prescribed with caution because of the risk of dependency. The use of narcotics or any of the medications on the DEA Schedules is prohibited by anyone operating commercial or industrial motor vehicles.

Chronic pain is often associated with depressed mood or clinical depression, in which case a selective serotonin-reuptake inhibitor may be added to the treatment regimen to improve the patient's mood, thereby decreasing perceived pain intensity.

Drug Interactions

The patient's medication usage must be closely monitored to prevent unwanted drug interactions. Information regarding the employee's prescribed medications and medication allergies must be communicated to the attending physician. The *Physician's Desk Reference* (www.pdr.net) is a standard tool to review drug interactions.[24]

■ Drug Abuse

The term "abuse" implies that a substance or medication is used in a manner other than that intended by the prescribing physician. This includes recreational use and use in greater than the prescribed amounts, at increased frequencies, or for different indications or by different routes of intake than intended, usually resulting in adverse consequences. Self-medicating with drugs prescribed to family members or friends is a common example of drug abuse.

Drug Addiction

Drug addiction is the progression of drug abuse in which loss of control increases and an obsessive-compulsive pattern begins. In many cases, the obsessive-compulsive behavior becomes the primary illness. Physiologic changes lead to tolerance, withdrawal, and sensitization. Cognitive changes are also common.

Drug Dependence

Dependence is the physiologic process associated with substance abuse and a predictable event when opioids, benzodiazepines, barbiturates, and stimulants are prescribed. Dependence on these medications is related to dose, time, and potency and may result in tolerance while they are taken and withdrawal symptoms when they are decreased or stopped. Physiologic dependence is not necessarily an addiction. For example, cancer patients depend on medication for pain relief, but unlike addicts, they medicate at prescribed times and at prescribed dosages.

Addictive Behavior Patterns

"Drug-seeking behavior" is a poorly defined term that refers to a behavior pattern that includes manipulative means or demanding actions to obtain medications. The individual may imply that the medication is the only possible solution to a medical problem. Patients go to extreme measures to obtain the desired medication, including presenting false or exaggerated symptoms, claiming that other medications do not work, and rejecting less potent medications because of fictitious allergies.

In addition to manipulative behavior, such as pitting physicians' opinions against each other, some addictive behavior patterns involve criminal activity. If desperate enough, addicted individuals may forge a physician's prescription, commit burglary or robbery to obtain the medication, or offer bribes, including sexual favors.

> **Scheduled medications** Federal regulations grouping prescription medications into 5 groups based on their potential for abuse and/or addiction: Group I medications have high abuse potential and are not prescribed in the US. Group V medications offer the least potential for abuse.

Regulations

State, federal, and union regulations influence industry-based health care. Each state has specific regulations governing the rights and reimbursement of injured workers and the health care providers who treat them. Third-party reimbursement adds another regulatory thread that influences industrial health care.

Workers' compensation laws, frequently based on state workers' compensation statutes, are designed to reduce the need for litigation after an employee's injury by ensuring financial compensation for job-related injury, illness, or fatality. Employers and coworkers also receive protection under workers' compensation acts by limiting the financial amount an employee can receive after injury and eliminating the liability of coworkers in most instances.[25] Federal statutes are restricted to individuals employed in some aspect of interstate commerce (**Table 23-10**).

23

Table 23-10

Examples of Federal Workers' Compensation Programs

Act	Group Protected
Federal Employees' Compensation Act[26]	Includes all nonmilitary federal employees; provides financial awards for accidental job-related disability or death; disabled workers may be required to undergo job retraining
Federal Employment Liability Act[27]	Protects railroad workers against negligent acts of their employers
Merchant Marine Act (the Jones Act)[28]	Protects seamen against negligent acts of their employers
Longshore and Harbor Workers' Compensation Act[29]	Provides workers' compensation to specific employees of private maritime employers
Black Lung Benefits Act[30]	Compensation for coal miners who suffer from "black lung" disease; awards may be paid directly by the mine operator or, in the case of insidious onset, by the Department of Labor

Table 23-11

Selected Federal Regulatory Agencies

Agency	Function
Department of Labor	Promotes the welfare of employees and job seekers by protecting retirement benefits and health care coverage, supporting employment opportunities, and facilitating union/employer relations; also protects employees' health and safety, works to prevent discriminatory practices, and provides unemployment insurance
Mine Safety and Health Administration[32]	Enforces the provisions of the Federal Mine Safety and Health Act to promote safe and healthy working environments for miners
Department of Transportation	Regulates transportation industries and companies that build or maintain the US transportation infrastructure; injured employees are covered under the Federal Employees Compensation Act[33]
National Institute for Occupational Safety and Health (NIOSH)	Part of the Centers for Disease Control and Prevention, NIOSH is responsible for research and making recommendations to prevent work-related disease and injury. NIOSH also investigates potentially hazardous work conditions.
Federal Aviation Administration (FAA)	Oversees flight training, air traffic control, and flight operations, including airport planning and safety standards in the US
Occupational Safety and Health Administration (OSHA)	Oversees the provisions of the Occupational Safety and Health Act of 1970;[34] primary responsibility is to protect the health and physical welfare of workers by cooperating with state governments to establish protective standards, enforce those standards, and reach out to employers and employees through technical assistance and consultation programs; OSHA standards vary from state to state

Not all workers are covered under state workers' compensation programs, and some states operate under a number of compensation acts and federal regulatory agencies (**Table 23-11**). Similarly, both federal and state workers' compensation acts vary among states and are subject to legislative changes. Workers' compensation acts establish the rate (dollar amount) for reimbursement services and restrict reimbursable rehabilitation services to specific professions.[31]

■ References

1. United States Department of Labor, Bureau of Labor Statistics: News: Lost-worktime injuries and illness. Characteristics and resulting days away from work, 2002. (3/25/04 News Release USDL 04-460) Available at: http://www.bls.gov/news.release/pdf/osh2.pdf. Accessed July 14, 2004.

2. Konz S: *Work Design: Industrial Ergonomics*, ed 5. Scottsdale, AZ, Halcomb Hathaway Publishers, 2000.

3. Occupational Safety and Health Administration: Guidelines for noise enforcement, appendix A, CPL 2-2.35A-29 CFR 1910.95(b)(1). Washington DC, US Department of Labor, Occupational Safety and Health Administration, December 19, 1983, OSHA Directive No. CPL 2-2.35A.

4. Brandt Instruments: Spark noise dosimeters, sound level meters and human vibration analysis systems from Larson-Davis. Available at: http://www.brandtinst.com/LarsonDavis/SoundLevelMeters/index.html. Accessed July 14, 2004.

5. Americans with Disabilities Act of 1990, 42 USC §41705 (1990).

6. Hsieh CY, Adams AH, Tobis J, et al: Effectiveness of four conservative treatments for subacute low back pain. *Spine* 2002;27:1142-1148.

7. Keijsers J, Steenbakkers M, Meertens RM, Bouter LM, Kok G: The efficacy of the back school: A randomized trial. *Arthritis Care Res* 1990;3:204-209.

8. National Institute of Occupational Safety and Health: Back belts: Do they prevent injury? Available at: http://www.cdc.gov/niosh/backbelt.html. Accessed July 14, 2004.

9. National Institute of Occupational Safety and Health: Application manual for the revised NIOSH lifting equation. Available at: http://www.cdc.gov/niosh/94-110.html. Accessed July 14, 2004.

10. Kroemer K, Grandjean E: *Fitting the Task to the Human: A Textbook of Occupational Ergonomics*, ed 5. Philadelphia, PA, Taylor and Francis, 1997.

11. Buttaravoli and Stair: Common simple emergencies, 10.16 minor impalement injuries. Available at: http://www.ncemi.org/cse/cse1016.htm. Accessed July 14, 2004.

12. Langdorf M, Kazzi D: Replantation. Available at: http://author.emedicine.com/emerg/topic502.htm. Accessed July 14, 2004.

13. Wasserman DE: *Occupational Vibration: A Brief Overview*. Knoxville, TN, The Institute for the Study of Human Vibration, University of Tennessee College of Engineering, 1999. Available at: http://www.engr.utk.edu/ishv/newpaper.html. Accessed July, 14 2004.

14. Hochanadel CD, Conrad DE: Evolution of an on-site industrial physical therapy program. *J Occup Med* 1993; 35:1011-1016.

15. Commission for Accreditation of Rehabilitation Facilities: *Medical Rehabilitation Standards Manual with Survey Preparation Questions*. Tucson, AZ, Commission for Accreditation of Rehabilitation Facilities, 2003, p 26.

16. Occupational Health Physical Therapy Guidelines: Work Conditioning and Word Hardening Programs 03-01-17-58 (Program 32) [Retitled: Occupational Health Guidelines: Work Conditioning and Work Hardening Programs, Amended BOD 03-00-25-62; BOD 03-99-16-49; BOD 11-94-33-109; Initial BOD 11-92-29-134].

17. Dersh J, Gatchel R, Polatin T, Mayer P: Prevalence of psychiatric disorders in patients with chronic work-related musculoskeletal pain disability. *J Occup Environ Med* 2002;4:459-468.

18. Weitz S, Witt PH, Greenfield DP: Treatment of chronic pain syndrome. Available at: http://njspine.com/patientinfo/chronic-pain.html. Accessed July 14, 2004.

19. Brain Injury Association, The Head Injury Center of Pennsylvania: Chronic pain syndrome. Available at: http://www.uphs.upenn.edu/tbilab/rehab/chronic_pain_mgnt.shtml. Accessed July 14, 2004.

20. Galer BS, Bruehl S, Harden RN: IASP diagnostic criteria for complex regional pain syndrome: A preliminary empirical validation study. *Clin J Pain* 1998;14:48-54.

21. Pain Research Institute, Department of Neurological Science, The University of Liverpool: Chronic regional pain syndrome (reflex sympathetic dystrophy). Available at: http://www.liv.ac.uk/pri/html/pain_rsd.html. Accessed July 14, 2004.

22. Federal Motor Carrier Safety Administration. Results from 2001 drug testing survey. Available at: http://www.fmcsa.dot.gov/factsfigs/dashome.htm. Accessed July 14, 2004.

23. Drug Enforcement Administration: Title 21, Food and Drugs, chapter 13, Drug abuse prevention and control, Subchapter I, Control and enforcement, Part B, Authority to control standards and schedules, Section 812c, Schedules II and III. Available at: http://www.usdoj.gov/dea/pubs/csa/812.htm#c. Accessed July 14, 2004.

24. *2004 Physician's Desk Reference*. Montvale, NJ, Thomson Healthcare, 2003.

25. Legal Information Institute, Cornell Law School: Workers compensation: An overview. Available at: http://www.law.cornell.edu/topics/workers_compensation.html. Accessed July 14, 2004.

26. Federal Employees' Compensation Act. §8101-8193 (1993).

27. Federal Employment Liability Act, 45 USC §51-60 (1908).

28. Merchant Marine Act, 15 USC §688 (1920).

29. Longshore and Harbor Workers' Compensation Act, 33 USC §901-950 (1927).

30. Black Lung Benefits Act, 30 USC §901-945 (1972).

31. Physical medicine and rehabilitation ground rules. *Schedule of Medical Fees, September 1997*. Topeka, KS, Kansas Department of Human Resources, Division of Workers' Compensation, 1997, pp 226-229.

32. Federal Mine Safety and Health Act of 1977, Public Law 91-173 (1977).

33. US Department of Labor, Department of Employment Standards, Division of Federal Employees Compensation, Federal Employees Compensation Act (FECA). Available at: http://dothr.ost.dot.gov/Toolkit/WorkComp/Injured_at_work/injured_at_work.html. Accessed July 14, 2004.

34. Occupational Safety and Health Act of 1970, 84 Stat. 1597, Title 29, USC 656.

23

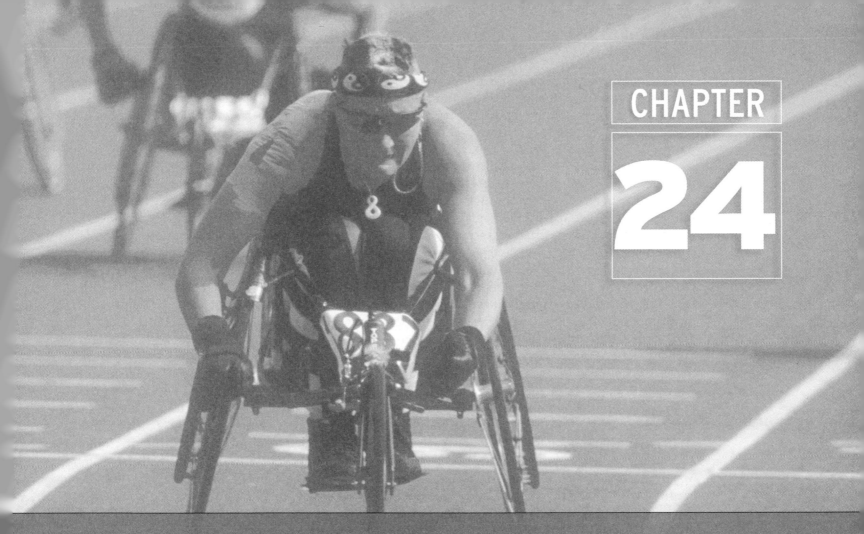

Athletes with Different Abilities

Michael S. Ferrara, PhD, ATC

Sport opportunities for people with disabilities have increased exponentially with recent advances in wheelchair and prosthetic designs that improve mobility. Developments in the treatment and rehabilitation of people with disabilities have provided vast opportunities for therapeutic recreation. Opportunities are also increasing for participation in sport and recreation offered through local community centers (eg, YMCAs), organized community sports, and sport organizations specific to people with disabilities. Athletes with disabilities have been integrated into sports for those without disabilities. Within the United States Olympic Committee, many national governing bodies such as those for swimming and cycling have vertically integrated athletes with disabilities into their Olympic Development Model. One example of this integration is Marla Runyan, an athlete with a visual impairment who was a member of the 2000 United States Olympic Track and Field Team and has participated in the New York City Marathon, demonstrating her athletic ability and not her disability.

Sir Ludwig Guttmann, Director of the Stoke Mandeville Hospital in Aylesbury, England, has been credited with developing sports for people with disabilities as part of the hospital's rehabilitation program after World War II. His model promoted active lifestyles for individual with disabilities. Since the initial efforts of Guttmann, competitive sports have grown tremendously. The Paralympics provide international competitive sporting opportunities for athletes with physical (amputation, spinal injured, spina bifida, cerebral palsy, polio) and sensory (visual impairment) disabilities.[1] The Special Olympics provide competition for athletes with cognitive impairments.

The Paralympics are held in the same city and venue after the summer and winter Olympic Games. At the 2004 Paralympics Games in Athens, Greece, more than 4,000 Paralympians from 130 countries participated in 19 sports. Fourteen of these sports have Olympic equivalents, such as swimming, athletics, volleyball, and cycling, with minimal modifications in the rules (**Figure 24-1**). Four sports are unique to the Paralympics: goalball (for those with visual impairment), bocce (for those with cerebral palsy), and power lifting and wheelchair rugby (for those with various disabilities).

International sports opportunities are offered for athletes with cognitive impairment, such as the 11th International Special Olympic Games, most recently held in 2003 in and around Dublin, Ireland, at which more than 7,000 athletes participated in 21 different sports. At the 2005 Melbourne, Australia Deaflympics, athletes with hearing impairments were expected to represent 80 countries.

All these elite international events require medical supervision and event coverage. Further, medical staffs are appointed to provide medical care to country teams. Team USA, for example, includes a staff of physicians, athletic trainers, and physical therapists. Typically, the US staffs are organized and structured following the United States Olympic Committee medical model for providing health care.

In addition to traditional elite and competitive sports activities, many individuals with disabilities also participate in extreme sports such as rock climbing, mountaineering, surfing, and skiing and a host of other athletic endeavors. These sports activities challenge the physical and mental abilities of the individual to maximize the fulfillment of life goals. Many people with disabilities also participate in more traditional activities, such as golf, tennis, walking, and cycling. Just as for people without disabilities, sport and physical activity provide health benefits, including reduction of the health risks associated with inactivity and an improved psychosocial outlook.

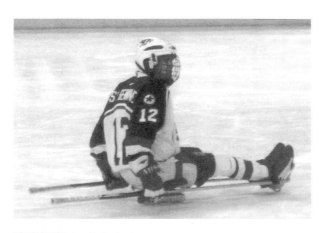

Figure 24-1   Ice sledge hockey.

The Preparticipation Physical Examination

People acquire a wide range of disabilities through disease, injury, and congenital deficits. Before embarking on competitive activities, the individual should undergo a comprehensive preparticipation physical examination (PPE). The PPE criteria developed for able-bodied athletes are frequently not applicable to athletes with unique needs. PPEs for special-needs athletes have been developed, many of them by specific athletic organizations.

The PPE for an athlete should entail a comprehensive screening program that is tailored to the individual's disability and/or condition; rather than focus on excluding the individual from participation, the program should direct the athlete toward the most appropriate activities.[2] The examination should identify predisposing conditions and co-morbidities and provide a complete needs assessment. To accurately determine the athlete's physical ability and limitations, the following factors must be assessed during the PPE:

- range of motion and flexibility of the extremities and trunk
- strength
- balance and equilibrium skills
- postural discrepancies
- associated reactions produced by increased activity (particularly important in athletes with central nervous system involvement)
- sensory discrimination and circulation problems
- rhythmic and coordination skills
- leg-length and other discrepancies of bone growth or size
- visual or auditory accuracy
- orthopaedic or other special appliances worn by the athlete
- level of cognitive function (if applicable)

From the PPE findings, the individual's functional level and class can be determined (**Table 24-1**). Once abilities and limitations have been identified through an accurate assessment of these factors, realistic goals and sport participation levels can be established (**Table 24-2**). In addition, the assessment helps to determine guidelines for exercise prescription and sport adaptation.

Types of Disabilities

This section focuses on the most prevalent disabilities found in athletes and provides a basic description of each. A number of available resources provide further information on each disability. The International Paralympic Committee also offers detailed descriptions of the disabilities its athletes possess (www.paralympic.org).

Amputations

An estimated 3 million amputees live in the United States.[3] Major lower extremity amputations are hip disarticulations and above-knee (AK), below-knee (BK), below-ankle (Syme), and midfoot amputations. Upper extremity amputations are forequarter disarticulations and above-elbow (AE), below-elbow (BE), hand, and finger amputations. A wide variety of prosthetics made from the lightest materials to provide maximum function are available for the upper and lower extremities. Also, a number of prosthetics have been developed specifically for sports, particularly track and field athletes.

Blindness or Visual Impairment

Each year, 50,000 Americans become blind. Blindness most often occurs with advancing age; half of all blind people are older than 65 years. A significant number of blind people, however, are children or young adults. Common causes of blindness include cataracts, diabetic retinopathy, glaucoma, macular degeneration, retinitis pigmentosa, and trauma. Athletes who are blind or visually impaired have various degrees of visual acuity. In general, the limits of legal blindness range from not being able to see well enough to drive a car to total light and dark insensitivity.

Cerebral Palsy

Cerebral palsy (CP) is a disorder of movement and posture caused by an irreparable central nervous system lesion and is graded on a scale of 1 (most severe) to 8 (least severe).[2] Individuals with CP may have musculoskeletal and other abnormalities, speech and hearing difficulties, visual problems, and seizures. Musculoskeletal abnormalities include scoliosis, kyphosis, and lordosis or a combination of these. Hip and shoulder subluxations and dislocations are common. Muscle spasticity may predispose this population to an unusually high number of muscle strains. Individuals with CP can undergo a variety of surgical tenotomies to release spastic contractures and facilitate improved function by balancing muscle forces and providing for more normal range of motion. These procedures can include combinations of Achilles tendon lengthening and adductor and hamstring releases (**Figure 24-2**).

Multiple musculoskeletal abnormalities may be present; therefore, all physical examinations should address the individual's ability to sit, stand (with or without assistance), and walk (with or without assistance or equipment). The effects of CP vary from individual to individual. At its mildest, CP may result in a slight awkwardness of movement in either an upper or lower extremity. At its most severe, CP results in the loss of muscle

24

Table 24-1

Functional Classification System Categories and Classes for Athletes with Disabilities

Visually Impaired: Athletics

T10	No light perception; unable to recognize shapes
T11, F11	2/60 and/or visual field of less than 5°*
T12, F12	2/60-6/60 and visual field of more than 5° and less than 20°*

Amputee

T42	Single above-the-knee; combined lower and upper limb amputations; minimum disability
T43	Double below-the-knee; combined lower and upper limb amputations; normal function in throwing arm
T44	Single below-the-knee; combined lower and upper limb amputations; moderate reduced function in one or both limbs
T45	Double above-the-elbow; double below-the-knee
T46	Single above-the-elbow; single below-the-elbow; upper limb function in throwing arm
F40	Double above-the-knee; combined lower and upper limb amputations; severe problems when walking
F41	Standing athletes with no more than 70 points in the lower limbs†
F42	Single above-the-knee; combined lower and upper limb amputations; normal function in throwing arm
F43	Double below-the-knee; combined lower and upper limb amputations; normal function in throwing arm
F44	Single below-the-knee; combined lower and upper limb amputations; normal function in throwing arm
F45	Double above-the-elbow; double below-the-elbow
F46	Single above-the-elbow; single below-the-elbow; upper limb function in throwing arm

Cerebral Palsy

T30	Severe to moderate involvement; uses one or two arms to push wheelchair; control is poor; affects both arms and legs
T31	Severe to moderate involvement; foot-propelled wheelchair push; affects both arms and legs
T32	Limited control of movements; some throwing motion
T32, F32	Full upper strength in upper extremity; propels wheelchair independently; affects both arms and legs, or same-side arm and leg
T33, F33	Good functional strength with minimal limitation or control problems in upper limbs and trunk; affects lower legs
T34, F34	May use assistive devices; slight loss of balance; affects lower legs or both legs and one arm
T35, F35	Walks or runs without assistive devices; balance and fine motor control problems
T36, F36	Good functional ability in dominant side of body; affects arm and leg on same side of body
T37, F37	Minimal involvement; could be present in lower legs, arm and leg on same side of body, or one leg, or demonstrate problems with balance

Wheelchair

T50	Uses palms to push wheelchair; may have shoulder weakness
T51	Pushing power comes from elbow extension
T52	Normal upper limb function; no active trunk
T53	Backwards movement of trunk; uses trunk to steer; double above-the-knee amputations
F50	No grip with nonthrowing arm; may have shoulder weakness
F51	Difficulty gripping with nonthrowing arm
F52	Nearly normal grip with nonthrowing arm
F53	No sitting balance
F54	Fair to good sitting balance
F55	Good balance and movements backward and forward; good trunk rotation
F56	Good movements backward and forward; usually to one side (side-to-side movements)
F57	Standard muscle chart of all limbs must not exceed 70 points†

Functional: Swimming

S1	Unable to catch water; restricted range of motion; no trunk control; leg drag; assisted water start
S2	Unable to catch water; restricted range of motion; no trunk control; slight leg propulsion; unassisted water start
S3	Wrist control limited; limited arm propulsion; minimal trunk control; hips below water; water start
S4	Wrist control; arms not full fluent; minimal trunk control; hips below water; better body position
S5	Full propulsion in catch phase; limited arm movement; trunk function; leg propulsion; sit or stand starts
S6	Catch phase present; arm movement efficient; trunk control; leg propulsion; push start, sit or stand
S7	Good hands; good arms; good trunk; hips level; stand or sit dive start
S8	Hand propulsion; arm cycle good; trunk good; hips and legs level; use of start blocks
S9	Full hand propulsion; full arm propulsion; full trunk control; propulsive kick; dive start from blocks
S10	Full hand and arm propulsion; full trunk control; strong leg kick; dive start and propulsion in turns

Visually Impaired: Cycling, Goalball, Judo, and Swimming

B1	No light perception, unable to recognize hand shapes
B2	Visual acuity of 2/60 with less than 5° field of vision
B3	Visual acuity of 2/60-6/60 and field of vision from 5°-20°

* Normal field of vision is approximately 120°-180°.

† The extent of the disability is represented by an evaluation that tests function and strength of the muscle groups. Function and muscle strength are represented by point values for each class (ie, less than 70 points equals an F41 or F57 athlete).

From the *Xth Paralympic Games Official Commemorative Program*. Oakville, Ontario, Canada: Disability Tolay Publicity Group, 1996:79.

Adapted with permission from Booth DW, Grogono BJ: Athletes with a disability, in Harris M, Williams C, Stanish WD, Micheli LJ (eds): *Oxford Textbook of Sports Medicine*. Oxford, England, Oxford University Press, 1998, pp 815-831.

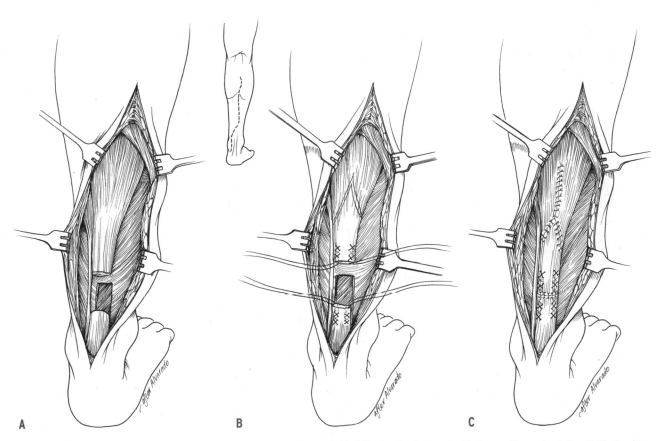

Figure 24-2 Technique for V-Y lengthening of the triceps surae. **A.** A medial incision is extended proximally in a gently curving S (inset). The tendon ends are debrided, and the repair site is prepared by windowing the deep posterior fascia. **B.** A V cut is made in the triceps surae aponeurosis. **C.** After approximation of the tendon ends, the aponeurosis is closed. (Reproduced with permission from Saltzman CL, Tearse DS: Achilles tendon injuries. *J Am Acad Orthop Surg* 1998;6:316-325.)

control and profoundly affects movement and speech. Depending on which areas of the brain have been damaged, one or more of the following may occur:

- muscle tightness or spasm
- involuntary movement
- difficulty with gross motor skills, such as walking and running
- difficulty with fine motor skills, such as writing and speaking
- abnormal perception and sensation
- decreased cognitive skills in the most extremely affected **pentaplegics**.

Short Stature

Dwarfism describes an unusually short stature that can arise from a variety of genetic and other conditions. Dwarfism occurs in about 1 in 10,000 births; most children with dwarfism are born of average-stature parents. The Little People of America, one of the largest and most active support groups for people with dwarfism, considers dwarfism to be an adult height of 4 feet 10 inches, or less. Dwarfism may be the result of skeletal **dysplasias**, conditions

marked by abnormal bone metabolism and growth, and is divided into two types—short-trunk and short-limb dysplasias.

One of the hallmark physical examination findings in this population is restricted range of motion of the major joints and spine. The vertebral segments may also contain short pedicles, which decrease the diameter of the spinal canal and thus predispose the athlete to congenital spinal stenosis.

Spinal Cord Injuries

Spinal cord injury (SCI) occurs when trauma damages cells within the spinal cord (see chapter 16); the cause is usually trauma, such as a car accident or athletic injury, but may be incomplete spinal-cord formation, as in spina bifida. The level of the SCI determines the level of function. Quadriplegia involves both lower extremities, with various degrees of upper extremity involvement. Paraplegia involves the lower extremities, with minimal or no upper extremity impairment. Symptoms such as pain or sensitivity to stimuli, muscle spasms, and sexual dysfunction may develop from the disability. Many athletes with SCI also have

Pentaplegia Paralysis of the extremities, trunk, and diaphragm.

24

Dysplasia The abnormal growth and development of cells or tissues.

Table 24-2

Participation Possibility Chart

Conditions	Archery	Bicycling	Tricycling	Bowling	Canoeing/Kayaking	Diving	Fencing	Field Events*	Fishing	Golf	Horseback Riding	Rifle Shooting	Sailing	Scuba Diving	Skating: Roller & Ice	Skiing: Downhill	Skiing: Cross-country	Swimming	Table Tennis
Amputations																			
Upper extremity	RA	R	R	R	RA	R	R	R	R	RA	R	RA	R	R	R	R	R	R	R
Lower extremity																			
Above-knee	R	R	R	R	R	R	I	R	R	R	R	R	R	R	I	RA	RA	R	R
Below-knee	R	R	R	R	R	R	R	R	R	R	R	R	R	R	R	R	R	R	R
Cerebral palsy																			
Ambulatory	R	R	R	R	R	R	I	R	R	R	R	R	I	R	R	RA	RA	R	R
Wheelchair	R	I	I	R	R	I	I	I	R	I	I	R	R	–	–	–	–	I	R
Spinal cord disruption																			
Cervical	RA	–	RA	RA	IA	–	–	I	R	–	X	RA	R	–	–	IA	IA	R	RA
High thoracic: T1-T5	R	–	R	R	R	–	RA	R	R	RA	I	R	R	R	–	IA	IA	R	R
Low thoracolumbar: T6-L3	R	–	R	R	R	–	RA	R	R	RA	R	R	R	R	–	RA	RA	R	R
Lumbosacral: L4-sacral	R	R	R	R	R	R	R	R	R	R	R	R	R	R	I	R	R	R	R
Neuromuscular disorders																			
Muscular dystrophy	RA	I	R	R	I	I	–	R	R	R	I	RA	R	I	I	I	I	R	R
Spinal muscular atrophy	RA	I	R	R	I	I	–	R	R	R	I	RA	R	I	I	I	I	R	R
Charcot-Marie-Tooth syndrome	R	R	R	R	R	R	R	R	R	R	R	R	R	R	R	R	R	R	R
Ataxias	R	I	I	R	I	I	–	R	R	I	I	R	R	I	I	I	I	R	R
Others																			
Osteogenesis imperfecta	R	I	R	R	R	I	R	R	R	R	I	I	R	R	I	I	I	R	R
Arthrogryposis	R	I	I	R	R	I	I	R	R	I	R	R	R	I	I	I	I	R	R
Juvenile rheumatoid arthritis	RA	I	I	RA	R	I	I	I	R	I	I	R	R	I	I	I	I	R	R
Hemophilia	RA	R	R	R	R	R	R	R	R	R	R	R	R	R	I	I	R	R	R
Skeletal dysplasias	R	R	R	R	R	R	R	R	R	R	R	R	R	R	R	RA	R	R	R

R = recommended, X = not recommended, A = adapted, I = individualized, – = no information or not applicable.

* Clubthrow, discus, javelin, shot put.

Adapted with permission from Chang FM: The disabled athlete, in Stanitski CL, DeLee JC, Drez D: *Pediatric and Adolescent Sports Medicine*. Philadelphia, PA, WB Saunders, 1994, vol 3, pp 48-76.

spinal deformities because of trunk-muscle paralysis and may require supports to aid in balance while sitting.

Patients with SCI are prone to develop secondary medical problems, such as bladder infections, lung infections, and pressure sores. Also, depending on the level of the injury, bowel and bladder function may be affected. Recent advances in functional electric stimulation have allowed certain individuals with SCI to ambulate and others with high-level injuries to breathe without a respirator.

Injuries to Athletes with Disabilities

Injury rates and types in athletes with disabilities are similar to those in athletes without disabilities.[4-6] As would be expected, individuals who use wheelchairs tend to have more upper extremity injuries, specifically rotator cuff tendinitis, ulnar nerve injury, and carpal tunnel syndrome. Those with visual impairment or CP tend to have more knee and ankle injuries.[7-10] Injuries by sport tend to follow patterns similar to those of athletes without disabilities.[9] For

Conditions	Individual Sports						Team Sports											
	Tennis	Tennis: Wheelchair	Track	Track: Wheelchair	Weight Lifting	Wheelchair Poling	Baseball	Softball	Basketball	Basketball: Wheelchair	Football: Tackle	Football: Touch	Football: Wheelchair	Ice Hockey	Sledge Hockey	Soccer	Soccer: Wheelchair	Volleyball
Amputations																		
Upper extremity	R	–	R	–	R	–	R	R	R	–	R	R	–	R	–	R	–	R
Lower extremity																		
Above-knee	I	R	–	R	R	R	RA	RA	–	R	I	I	R	–	R	I	R	R
Below-knee	R	I	R	I	R	I	R	R	R	I	R	R	I	I	I	R	I	R
Cerebral palsy																		
Ambulatory	R	–	R	–	R	–	R	R	I	–	I	I	–	I	–	R	–	R
Wheelchair	–	R	–	R	R	R	I	I	–	R	–	–	R	–	I	–	R	I
Spinal cord disruption																		
Cervical	–	IA	–	R	–	I	–	–	–	I	–	I	–	I	–	–	–	IA
High thoracic: T1-T5	–	R	–	R	R	R	RA	RA	–	R	–	–	R	–	R	–	R	RA
Low thoracolumbar: I6-L3	–	R	–	R	R	R	RA	RA	–	R	–	–	R	–	R	–	R	RA
Lumbosacral: L4-Sacral	R	–	R	–	R	–	R	R	R	I	I	R	I	I	–	R	–	R
Neuromuscular disorders																		
Muscular dystrophy	I	I	I	I	–	R	I	I	I	I	–	–	I	I	I	I	I	I
Spinal muscular atrophy	I	I	I	I	–	R	I	I	I	I	–	–	I	I	I	I	I	I
Charcot-Marie-Tooth																		
syndrome	R	–	R	–	R	–	R	R	R	–	R	R	–	I	–	R	–	R
Ataxias	R	R	I	R	I	R	I	I	I	R	–	I	I	I	I	I	R	I
Others																		
Osteogenesis imperfecta	R	R	R	R	I	R	I	I	I	R	X	I	I	X	X	X	R	I
Arthrogryposis	R	–	R	X	I	X	R	R	R	–	X	R	I	I	–	I	–	R
Juvenile rheumatoid arthritis	I	I	I	I	I	I	I	I	I	I	I	I	I	I	I	I	I	I
Hemophilia	I	–	R	–	I	–	I	R	R	–	X	I	–	X	–	I	–	R
Skeletal dysplasias	R	–	R	–	I	–	R	R	R	–	I	R	–	R	–	R	–	R

example, swimmers and cyclists tend to incur similar injuries to the shoulder. However, wheelchair basketball athletes have more shoulder, wrist, and hand injuries, while basketball athletes without a disability tend to sustain lower extremity injuries to the knee and ankle.[7,8,11]

■ Disability and Injury Patterns

Although certain disabilities and sports are associated with certain types of injuries, most injuries occur from the traditional injury mechanisms and predisposing factors previously outlined in this text.

Knowledge of the disability and resulting impairment is important, but assessing the injury requires a traditional evaluation: a thorough medical history, a comprehensive medical examination, and appropriate special tests such as radiographs and magnetic resonance imaging to determine the nature and extent of the injury.

Athletes with Amputations

Athletes with amputations participate in many sport activities, including volleyball, track and field, and cycling, with no changes in the rules. The injury

24

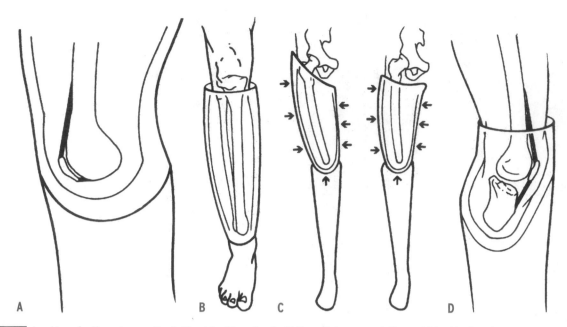

Figure 24-3 Load transfer through a prosthesis. Direct load transfer via (**A**) through-knee amputation and (**B**) ankle disarticulation. **C.** Indirect load transfer in an above-knee amputation with either a standard quadrilateral socket (left) or an adducted narrow medial-lateral socket (right). **D.** Indirect load transfer in a below-knee amputation. (Reproduced with permission from Greene WB (ed): *Essentials of Musculoskeletal Care*, ed 2. Rosemont, IL, American Academy of Orthopaedic Surgeons, 2000, p 13.)

Ground reaction force The reaction to the force that the body exerts on the surface and is subsequently transmitted up the extremity.

patterns for these athletes are similar to those of able-bodied athletes in the same sport.

Lower extremity prosthetics transfer body weight and ground reaction forces up the extremity via direct or indirect load transfers (**Figure 24-3**). Direct transmission is used when the amputation occurs directly at the level of the knee or ankle joint. In the case of through-bone amputations, the distal end of the stump cannot withstand the forces; they are transferred over the remainder of the limb.

Athletes with an amputation require additional attention for the care of their residual limb (stump). Knowledgeable athletes usually know when skin irritation is occurring from the prosthesis. A proper-fitting prosthesis prevents problems caused by a fit that is too loose or too tight. Advances in prosthetic design have reduced the number of residual limb-related problems, and protective padding and skin-protection devices reduce friction and aid in the healing process after an irritation. However, frequent prosthetic adjustments are needed to accommodate exercise-related hypertrophy and normal growth and development patterns.

Proper residual limb care is important for the athlete's comfort and prevention of blisters and pressure-related ulcerations. If the athlete is diabetic or has decreased sensation in the residual limb, visual inspection is necessary to identify pressure points.

Overgrowth is an excess of bone production at the site of transection and is a common occurrence in children with acquired amputations. The overgrowth can produce bony spikes at the bone–soft tissue interface and lead to blisters and other forms of skin breakdown (**Figure 24-4**).[2,12]

The residual limb must be regularly inspected for blisters, pressure sores, edema, dermatitis, and other skin conditions. Sweat collects between the limb and the prosthesis, increasing the need to regularly clean the residual limb itself, the sock, and the prosthetic socket to prevent bacterial infection. Proper hygiene consists of normal washing with fragrance-free soap and water and then thoroughly rinsing the area. The soap should not contain substances that will dehydrate the skin or make it slippery. If the skin is dry, a light moisturizing cream may be applied at night, but moisturizer should not be used before the prosthesis is worn. The sock must be changed regularly and washed using a light detergent or soap and water. When the sock becomes worn or frayed, uneven pressure distribution can occur, and the sock should be discarded. The skin covering the residual limb was not intended to assume weight-bearing forces, which combine with skin friction to predispose the area to blisters and pressure sores. Blisters that form in the area should be cleaned and dressed using standard protocol. Sweat accumulation in a

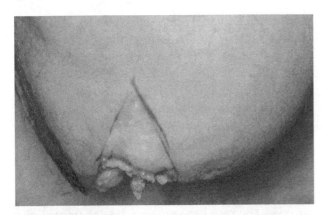

Figure 24-4 A sharp spike of bone overgrowth eroded through the skin, necessitating revision of the remaining limb. (Reproduced with permission from Krajbich JI: Lower-limb deficiencies and amputations in children. *J Am Acad Orthop Surg* 1998;6:358-367.)

Table 24-3

Increased Metabolic Demands of Athletes Using Limb Prostheses

Amputation Level	% Energy Increase Beyond Baseline
Long below-knee	10
Medium below-knee	25
Short below-knee	40
Bilateral, medium below-knee	41
Average above-knee	65

Note that the energy expenditure for a bilateral below-knee amputation is less than that of a unilateral above-knee amputation.

Reprinted from Miller MD: *Review of Orthopaedics*, ed 4. Saunders, 2004. Chapter 9: Rehabilitation: Gait, amputations, prosthetics, and orthotics. With permission from Elsevier Inc.

dark, damp environment can lead to bacterial infection. In the event of signs of ulcerations, the patient must immediately be referred to a physician for evaluation. The prosthesis should not be worn if large blisters or pressure sores are present.

Phantom pain is common after an amputation and is experienced by most individuals with amputations at one time or another. Some have very little pain. Others experience severe pain on a daily basis. The term phantom sensation is not just the feeling of having a limb when no limb is present (which usually goes away), but describes any sensation or pain originating from a residual limb; it can range from tingling sensations to severe, sharp, stabbing pain that can only be controlled by advanced pain-management techniques.

The sound limb is commonly injured and should be evaluated in the normal fashion. For example, if a volleyball player with an above-knee amputation injures the remaining ankle in competition, the resulting condition and impairment are the same as in any other volleyball player. Thus, standard treatment and rehabilitation protocols are used to restore function and activity as quickly and safely as possible.

Athletes who compete using prostheses have increased metabolic demands for participation; the metabolic demands are inversely proportional to the length of the remaining limb and the number of remaining functioning joints, even during slower speed movements such as walking (**Table 24-3**).[2] The shorter the remaining limb, the greater the metabolic demand. Many lower extremity prostheses are designed to store potential energy and convert it into kinetic energy during athletic activities. Extra attention is required to prevent heat-related illness and promote electrolyte restoration.[2]

Athletes with Blindness or Visual Impairment

The lack of visual cues in relation to road surface and conditions—as well as barriers such as walls, curbs, and other athletes—can lead to an increased rate of lower extremity injuries, most commonly of the foot and ankle (26%), with only 10% affecting the knee. Because the impairment is limited to the optic system and does not involve the musculoskeletal system, the resulting condition and injury evaluation are similar to those of able-bodied athletes, but the lack of visual cues can decrease proprioceptive function. Athletes in sports such as track and distance running employ guide runners for assistance. The guide and runner are typically matched based on running speed and fitness level, so the athlete can perform maximally. Disability-specific medical problems are few and usually related to medications. However, some visual impairments are associated with albinism, or a lack of skin pigment. For these athletes, protection from sunburn is critical.

Athletes with Cerebral Palsy

Lower extremity injuries to athletes with CP are most frequent at the knee and ankle. The number of such injuries may be related to muscle spasticity and biomechanical changes in the running gait. Therefore, lower extremity strength and flexibility should be carefully analyzed. People with CP have tight lower extremity musculature, particularly of the hamstrings and gastrocnemius. Shoulder, wrist, and hand conditions are common in those who use wheelchairs (see Athletes Who Use Wheelchairs section for more information). A variety of flexibility techniques should be used to achieve maximum flexibility of the major joints and muscle groups, including the hips, low back, and shoulders.

24

Active and passive range of motion of the individual with CP should be evaluated. An athlete with spasticity may have an exaggerated stretch reflex, such that the muscle contracts with great force, displaying an apparent lack of motion. Some athletes have athetoid CP, which is associated with continuous, slow, arrhythmic motions.

Because an athlete with CP may have speech difficulties, medical professionals must take the time to listen carefully. An athlete with CP who has a speech impairment may use a speech synthesizer or word board to communicate.

Athletes with Down Syndrome

In 1983, Special Olympics International issued a directive to all medical personnel, coaches, parents, and athletes restricting the participation of athletes with Down syndrome until they underwent medical examinations for atlantoaxial instability (**Figure 24-5**).[2] Researchers had demonstrated that individuals with Down syndrome had collagen and ligament laxity that could lead to cervical instability. The incidence rate has been estimated at 10% to 20% of the Down syndrome population. Atlantoaxial instability is detected radiographically in conjunction with the physical examination. The radiographic examination should include anteroposterior, lateral, flexion-extension, and odontoid views of the spine.

Longitudinal radiographic examination should also be performed to detect changes in spinal stability over time. Those with positive findings must eliminate or restrict certain activities that result in possible axial loading, hyperflexion, or hyperextension mechanisms. Spinal fusion may be indicated to stabilize the joint with symptomatic dislocations.

Other orthopaedic conditions associated with Down syndrome include hip dysplasia, genu valgum with associated knee laxity, patella alta, patellar instability, scoliosis, malaligned or malpositioned fingers and toes, and increased rates of femoral neck stress fractures. General medical conditions common in this population include hearing loss, cardiovascular and respiratory disorders, obesity, and immunologic deficiency.[2]

Athletes Who Use Wheelchairs

A number of advances in wheelchair design have allowed for maximum shoulder range of motion in order to provide effective and efficient propulsion strokes. The rapid growth in wheelchair athletics has furthered improvements in the design of competition chairs. In accordance with Wheelchair Sports USA, these chairs cannot have gears, levers, or chains that affect speed. Improvements have also been made in maneuverability.

The mechanics of wheelchair propulsion techniques predispose the shoulder and wrist to overuse injuries—tendinitis or bursitis of the shoulders and, not surprisingly, carpal tunnel syndrome. Blisters and lacerations of the hands and arms are also problems. Wheelchair racers should protect their hands with specially designed gloves.[8,13]

In the shoulder, rotator cuff injuries occur, with associated pectoral muscle tightness. A comprehensive shoulder examination identifies the structures involved in the injury so that an appropriate treatment and rehabilitation program can be implemented. Carpal tunnel syndrome occurs from the constant impact of the heel of the hand on the racing wheel with the wrist in slight hyperflexion.[7,11]

The loss of protective skin sensation below the level of injury requires extraordinary care to prevent and treat pressure sores. Pressure sores usually occur over bony prominences, such as the greater trochanters, ischial spines, and medial and lateral

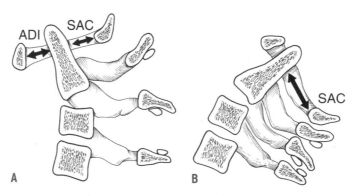

Figure 24-5 Sagittal cross-section through the base of the upper cervical spine and skull. **A.** In atlantoaxial instability, the atlanto-dens interval (ADI) increases in flexion (arrow), and the space available for the spinal cord (SAC) decreases (arrow). **B.** With neck extension, C1 and C2 are realigned in their normal relationship, and the SAC increases (arrow). (Adapted with permission from Chang FM: The disabled athlete, in Stanitski CL, DeLee JC, Drez D (eds): *Pediatric and Adolescent Sports Medicine.* Philadelphia, PA, WB Saunders, 1994, vol 3, pp 48-76.)

malleoli or wherever clothing or equipment applies prolonged pressure to the skin. Proper padding in the wheelchair is usually effective in preventing this problem, as is periodic removal from the wheelchair during times of rest.[10,11]

Another potentially serious problem for the athlete with SCI is thermoregulatory control. Because the internal thermostat operates less efficiently in an individual with SCI, the athlete cannot tolerate temperature extremes, particularly excessive heat. Thus evaporative skin cooling with mist bottles and the like may be necessary. Protection from direct sunlight must be provided for athletes at competition sites.

SCI above the level of T8 results in the loss of sympathetic control to the lower body. The most serious health concern for this athlete may be **autonomic dysreflexia**. Symptoms of autonomic dysreflexia include dizziness, sweating, headache, and potentially severe hypertension. An obstructed urethral catheter is the most common trigger for autonomic dysreflexia; simply draining the bladder may prevent autonomic dysreflexia. Other causes of autonomic dysreflexia are fecal impaction, renal calculi or infection, pressure sores, and other noxious stimuli.

General Medical Conditions

▪ Pharmacologic Concerns

Athletes with disabilities often use prescription medications for a variety of medical conditions. Physicians and health care personnel should be aware of the indications, contraindications, and synergistic effects of using multiple medications. Although many of these medicines are needed to allow the athlete to participate, some medications may cause significant cognitive effects or have other consequences that could reduce the athlete's performance. The International Paralympic Committee has an active doping control program and adheres to the banned drug list of the World Anti-Doping Agency (www.wada-ama.org). The athlete and the physician must be aware of medications that are on the banned drug list. If the medication is banned, the physician should determine if there is a suitable substitute.

▪ Seizures

Medications taken by athletes who have seizures may reduce their awareness and reflex responses and can have significant cognitive effects. The usual medications prescribed for seizures include phenobarbital, phenytoin, and carbamazepine. Carbamazepine is the preferred medication because it has the fewest side effects and should not adversely affect the athlete's performance.

An athlete who is having a seizure must be protected from harm. After the seizure, the athlete should rest before attempting to resume activity and should not be allowed to participate in sport or recreational activities without first obtaining medical clearance from a physician. The medical team should be aware of the athlete's compliance with the medication regimen and other factors that could induce a seizure, such as stress and changes in sleep pattern and diet. To address any potential changes in medications, the athlete should discuss plans for participation in sport activities with the primary physician.

▪ Heat Illness and Prevention

Athletes with SCI have increased risk for heat injury secondary to decreased sensory awareness, sympathetic nervous system dysfunction, and inability of the body to warm and cool itself. Those with quadriplegia or a lesion above T8 typically lack an effective sweating response; when combined with decreased vasodilatation below the level of the injury, the normal cooling response to environmental conditions is reduced.

Because of the increased metabolic demands, amputee athletes are at an increased risk for heat-related illness.[2] Also, precaution is advised when albino athletes as well as those with high blood pressure, diabetes, and sweat-gland dysfunction are exposed to the sun.

The standards of care for practice and participation in the heat should be followed.[14] In addition, a heat and hydration plan should be developed to protect the health of the athletes (see chapter 20). Athletes should be encouraged to drink plenty of fluids during practice and competition and educated about proper hydration. Athletes with swallowing disorders or drooling caused by an upper motor neuron lesion may have difficulty drinking. These athletes need to be counseled on drinking frequently, using swallowing strategies, and monitoring the volume and color of urine. Shade, tents, and appropriate clothing should also be incorporated into the heat-illness prevention plan. Exposure time should be limited for those susceptible to sunburn due to decreased sensation or lack of skin pigmentation.

Autonomic dysreflexia Occurs in spinal cord injuries above level T8 and results in dizziness, sweating, headaches, and potentially severe hypertension; may be caused by a plugged urethral catheter, fecal impaction, renal calculi, infections, or pressure sores.

24

Injury Prevention Techniques

Injury prevention is as important for athletes with disabilities as it is for all other athletes. Those who establish injury prevention programs must be familiar with specific physical problems and special precautionary measures that diminish the risk of injury for these participants. Part of the injury prevention program is the physical assessment to determine any contraindications to specific types of activities or exercises. For the body part with limited range of motion, activities should be performed within the functional range.

A comprehensive injury prevention program focuses on the traditional areas of flexibility, strength training, and cardiovascular conditioning. General body fitness and sport-specific activities are emphasized. For example, a swimmer who is visually impaired needs a specialized, sport-specific conditioning program emphasizing the shoulder, upper back, and neck regions to improve strength and flexibility and reduce or minimize injury to this area. Cuff weights and tubing can be used in a rotator cuff injury prevention program. To complement the conditioning program, core stability training can provide benefits in both sport and activities of daily living.

In addition to traditional conditioning programs, a biomechanical analysis of movement may be helpful to determine joint actions or forces that may predispose the athlete to injury. For example, in a runner, gait analysis can demonstrate any foot, ankle, knee, or hip abnormalities. Based on this analysis, corrective procedures can be implemented to prevent injury, such as orthotics or a specific program to increase flexibility or strength and target specific muscle groups. Further, the results of the biomechanical analysis can be shared with the coach, who works with the athlete to improve motor-pattern efficiency and thus improve sport performance.[14]

The greatest challenge for athletes with disabilities may be in access to coaches, facilities, and equipment. The medical professional can serve as a liaison to coaches and strength and conditioning personnel to assist in the design, development, and monitoring of an injury prevention program. Access to facilities and equipment has improved tremendously with the implementation of the Americans with Disabilities Act. Most health and fitness facilities are now accessible to wheelchair users. Equipment manufacturers have designed weight training equipment that is completely accessible to the wheelchair user and eliminates unnecessary transfers (**Figure 24-6**).[14]

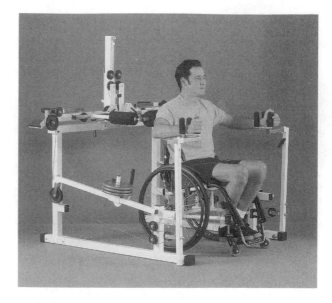

Figure 24-6 A weight machine adapted for use with wheelchair-bound individuals. (Printed with permission from GPK, Inc.)

■ References

1. Reynolds J, Stirk A, Thomas A, Geary F: Paralympics: Barcelona 1992. *Br J Sports Med* 1994;28:14-17.
2. Wind WM, Schwend RM, Larson J: Sports for the physically challenged child. *J Am Acad Orthop Surg* 2004; 12:126-137.
3. Kegel B, Malchow D: Incidence of injury in amputees playing soccer. *Palaestra* 1994;10:50-54.
4. Ferrara MS, Palutsis GR, Snouse S, Davis RW: A longitudinal study of injuries to athletes with disabilities. *Int J Sports Med* 2000;21:221-224.
5. Ferrara MS, Peterson CL: Injuries to athletes with disabilities: Identifying injury patterns. *Sports Med* 2000; 30:137-143.
6. Ferrara MS, Buckley WE: Athletes with disabilities injury registry. *Adapt Phys Act Q* 1996;13:50-60.
7. Burnham RS, May L, Nelson E, Steadward R, Reid DC: Shoulder pain in wheelchair athletes: The role of muscle imbalance. *Am J Sports Med* 1993;21:238-242.
8. Curtis KA, Black K: Shoulder pain in female wheelchair basketball players. *J Orthop Sports Phys Ther* 1999; 29:225-231.
9. Curtis KA, Dillon DA: Survey of wheelchair athletic injuries: Common patterns and prevention. *Paraplegia* 1985;23:170-175.
10. Ferrara MS, Davis RW: Injuries to elite wheelchair athletes. *Paraplegia* 1990;28:335-341.
11. Burnham RS, Higgins J, Steadward RD: Wheelchair basketball injuries. *Palaestra* 1994;10:43-49.
12. Krajbich JI: Lower-limb deficiencies and amputations in children. *J Am Acad Orthop Surg* 1998;6:358-367.
13. Wilson PE, Washington RL: Pediatric wheelchair athletics: Sports injuries and prevention. *Paraplegia* 1993; 31:330-337.
14. Ferrara MS, Buckley WE, McCann BC, Limbird TJ, Powell JP, Robl R: The injury experience of the athlete with a disability: Prevention implications. *Med Sci Sports Exerc* 1992;24:184-188.

APPENDIX

Following is manufacturer information for products referenced in this book.

Aspen collar (Aspen Medical Products, Inc., Long Beach, CA)

Betadine (Purdue Frederick, Norwalk, CT)

Bodyblade (Hymanson Inc., Playa Del Ray, CA)

Celebrex (Pfizer, New York, NY)

Drytex (DonJoy Orthopedics, Inc., Vista, CA)

Gatorlytes (Gatorade, Chicago, IL)

Histoacryl blue (Dermabond, Ethicon, Inc., Somerville, NJ)

Hypaque (Sterling Winthrop Inc., New York, NY)

Kenalog (Bristol-Myers Squibb, Lakewood, NJ)

Kinesio Taping (Kinesio Taping Association, Albuquerque, NM)

Lacri-Lube (Allergan, Irvine, CA)

Marcaine (Hospira, Inc., Lake Forest, IL)

Miami J collar (Jerome Medical, Moorestown, NJ)

National Institute of Occupational Safety and Health Lifting Equation (available at http://www.cdc.gov/niosh/94-110.html and http://www.lni.wa.gov/Safety/Topics/HazardInfo/Ergonomics/ServicesResources/Tools/default.asp)

Orthoplast (Johnson & Johnson Corp., New Brunswick, NJ)

Pedialyte (Abbott Laboratories, Abbott Park, IL)

Plyoball (JUMPUSA.com, Sunnyvale, CA)

Pneumovax (Merck & Co, Inc., Whitehouse Station, NJ)

Protonics (Empi, St. Paul, MN)

Rapid Entire Body Assessment (NexGen Ergonomics, Inc.; also available at http://hsc.usf.edu/~tbenard/hollowhills/REBA_M11.pdf)

Rapid Upper Limb Assessment (NexGen Ergonomics, Inc., Point Claire, Quebec, Canada; also available at http://www.ergonomics.co.uk/Rula/Ergo)

TheraBand (Hygenic Corp., Akron, OH)

TheraPutty (Spri Medical & Rehab Products, Northbrook, IL)

Toradol (Syntex LLC, Palo Alto, CA)

Xylocaine (AstraZeneca LP, Wilmington, DE)

INDEX/GLOSSARY

Boldface page numbers refer to illustrations.